Encyclopedia of
Sleep and Dreaming

Encyclopedia of
Sleep and Dreaming

Mary A. Carskadon
Editor in Chief

Macmillan Publishing Company
NEW YORK

Maxwell Macmillan Canada
TORONTO

Maxwell Macmillan International
NEW YORK OXFORD SINGAPORE SYDNEY

Macmillan Publishing Company
866 Third Avenue, New York, NY 10022

Maxwell Macmillan Canada, Inc.
1200 Eglinton Avenue East, Suite 200, Don Mills, Ontario M3C 3N1

Macmillan, Inc., is part of the Maxwell Communication Group of Companies.

Library of Congress Catalog Card Number: 92-38048

Printed in the United States of America

printing number
1 2 3 4 5 6 7 8 9 10

Library of Congress Cataloging-in-Publication Data

Encyclopedia of sleep and dreaming / Mary A. Carskadon, editor in
   chief.
      p.   cm.
   Includes bibliographical references and index.
   ISBN 0-02-897085-3 (hardcover) : $95.00
   1. Dreams—Encyclopedias.   2. Sleep—Encyclopedias.   3. Sleep
disorders—Encyclopedias.   I. Carskadon, Mary A.
   BF1078.E63   1993
   154.6′03—dc20   92-38048
                                                                         CIP

The paper used in this publication meets the minimum requirements of
American National Standard for Information Sciences—Permanence of Paper for
Printed Library Materials. ANSI Z39.48–1984.

CONTENTS

Editorial and Production Staff

Philip Friedman
Publisher

Elly Dickason
Editor in Chief, Macmillan Reference

David Eckroth
Executive Editor

Jonathan Wiener
Project Editor

Karin K. Vanderveer
Assistant Editor

Josephine Della Peruta   Stephen Van Leeuwen
Copy-editors

Donald Spanel
Proofreader

Cynthia Crippen
Indexer

Rose Capozzelli
Production Manager

PREFACE

The "modern" era of sleep and dreaming research was launched in 1953 by the description of rapid eye movement bursts during sleep and their association with dreaming by Eugene Aserinsky and Nathaniel Kleitman. This discovery inspired physiologists, psychologists, and psychiatrists to begin a red-eyed voyage of scientific discovery. Forty years later, a new era of research has taken wing, borne aloft by advances in sleep disorders medicine, molecular biology, the neurosciences, and biological rhythms. The *Encyclopedia of Sleep and Dreaming* represents a bridge from past to future, covering the field across a broad front that includes biological, medical, and psychological approaches. Because of its scientific focus, a reader looking for the meaning of a specific dream image, for example, will not find this *Encyclopedia* useful. On the other hand, the reader with a curiosity about how and when dreaming occurs, what sleep disorders are, how aging affects sleep, what circadian rhythms have to do with sleep and wakefulness, which brain centers modulate sleep, and so forth, is looking in the right place. As we compiled the *Encyclopedia*, our target audience was the inquisitive student interested in learning about the current scientific knowledge base of sleep and dreaming, how the phenomena are studied, and what future opportunities await young people who aspire to engage in the scientific study of this endlessly intriguing, yet curiously obscure field. Others who will find the volume useful are their teachers and parents, for whom the entries having to do with maturation (see DEVELOPMENT), ADOLESCENCE AND SLEEP, and daytime SLEEPINESS may be particularly salient. Sleep professionals will find the field's minutiae in the *Encyclopedia*, and perhaps some key morsels of information may activate new directions in their thinking.

Sleep and dreaming are occult in the sense of hidden, shrouded by the cover of darkness. Sleep is commonly considered a time of minimal physical, physiological, and psychological activity; thus, sleep and dreaming have rarely attracted the attention of the scientific community at large.

Nevertheless, the field is growing at an increasingly rapid pace, and the opportunities for new scientific input are numerous. Therefore, young people reading this book should be encouraged, not discouraged, if they cannot find answers to their every question—as a young and growing field, sleep and dreaming research contains far more unanswered than answered questions.

Because the *Encyclopedia* is organized alphabetically, rather than thematically, the reader may initially have difficulty acquiring an overview of broad topics. Nevertheless, a number of opportunities within the volume may make such an overview possible, if the reader chooses entries judiciously in a sequential fashion. For example, an overview of sleep processes in general might begin with the entry on NORMAL SLEEP and progress from this initial entry to several others cross-referenced within it. Thus, one might next go to the entry on STAGES OF SLEEP for a description of how sleep is assessed in normal humans; the entry on CYCLES OF SLEEP ACROSS THE NIGHT offers another view of normal sleep. A second approach to broadly based information in the *Encyclopedia* can come through "guidepost" entries. Guideposts—printed in italic type—have been prepared by the editorial board to provide informational nodes pointing to relevant articles on a given topic. Thus, for example, the guidepost on DEVELOPMENT designates a variety of entries that discuss how sleep changes across the maturational span, from fetal life to old age. Allan Rechtschaffen's inclusive guidepost on DREAMS AND DREAMING leads the interested reader toward entries that introduce topics ranging from the brain mechanisms underlying dreaming to the psychoanalytic interpretations of dreams, with many stops in between. The effects of drugs on sleep are described in a number of entries, and the guidepost on PHARMACOLOGY written by Tom Roth indicates relevant entries that might be missed by simply looking for a specific drug. In addition, the composite article on the CHEMISTRY OF SLEEP begins with a description of how synapses transmit chemical messages and then describes many of the chemical interactions that affect sleep and dreaming. Jerome Siegel wrote, among others, a guidepost on BRAIN MECHANISMS, which includes references to entries detailing the involvement of many brain areas in the control of sleep and dreaming. Other examples of crucial guideposts are BIOLOGICAL RHYTHMS and CIRCADIAN RHYTHM DISORDERS, prepared by Gary Richardson and referring to a coherent set of related entries.

Many readers will have a single topic they wish to pursue, and there are several options for such an approach to the book. The first is to choose a few key words about the topic and then look them up in the Index. As the entries are read, take note of cross-references indicated in parentheses, such as "(See EXERCISE)," or listed directly in the text in small capital letters, such as CONTENT OF DREAMS. When searching the list of article titles for key words, keep in mind that we made a conscious effort to avoid using the words sleep or dream in entry titles. These words are used only when they were integral to the title, usually because of common colloquial or scientific usage.

My vision of this *Encyclopedia* is that it will become a fundamental resource found in every high school and college library. This vision guided the preparation of the book and led us to include sufficient information to answer as many questions as we could anticipate and also to provide information in a way that we hope will fuel a student's interest in the topic. My hope is that students will not stop their quest with the *Encyclopedia*, but that they will look beyond this volume, aided by citations to primary and secondary references in journals and books. I have also insisted that the *Encyclopedia* contain a bit of whimsy through material that is both edifying and fun, such as entries on the sandman, pajamas, pillows, myths and legends, teddy bears, nudity, music, movies, literature, and art. Thus, I hope that the *Encyclopedia* engages the reader and conveys a sense of the many ways in which sleep and dreaming influence our lives.

I would like to take this opportunity to thank many people without whose assistance the *Encyclopedia* could not have been completed. First, of course, the brilliant crew of associate editors, Al Rechtschaffen, Jerry Siegel, Tom Roth, and Gary Richardson—all of whom are colleagues, scientists, and experts in the field of sleep research, all generous in their offers of support and assistance, and all very special friends. Over 200 individual authors contributed their insights and expertise to the over 400 individual topics in the *Encyclopedia*; the overwhelmingly positive and energetic input from these authors was especially gratifying. Virtually every pioneering icon in sleep and dreaming research and sleep disorders medicine contributed to the *Encyclopedia*, among them Nathaniel Kleitman, William Dement, Michel Jouvet, Al Rechtschaffen, Bernie Webb, Gerry Vogel, Rosalind Cartwright, Mircea Steriade, Irwin Feinberg, Roger Broughton, Robert Van de Castle, Ernest Hartmann, David Foulkes, Montague Ullman, Peter Hauri, Howard Roffwarg, Christian Guilleminault, and Elio Lugaresi. Particularly special to me are the contributors by my present and former students (Semi, Pam, Steve, Jenny, Kate, Joan, Jodi, Mark, Avi, Lakshyan, Katie, John, Max, Russ, Cecilia, Tom, David, Jennie, and James); by the experts in related fields who generously agreed to integrate their work for the *Encyclopedia*, such as Zach Boukydis, Greg Fritz, Kenn Kaufman, Freddi Kronenberg, John Lauber, and Sig Pueschel; by astronaut Jim Bagian; and most especially by the many women scientists whose support and inspiration I treasure. In addition to Philip Friedman, several members of the Macmillan Publishing Company were instrumental in preparing the *Encyclopedia*. They include David Eckroth, whose energetic enthusiasm got the ball rolling; Jonathan Wiener, whose editorial expertise carried it along; and Elly Dickason, whose most emphatic encouragement pushed the work over the top.

Finally, I must acknowledge the help of Kate Herman, a very special and enormously talented young woman. Kate's keen eye for typos is legendary around our lab; moreover, her facility with written English is exceptional and helped to salvage more than a few awkward entries. Kate's unflagging charm, wit, and good spirits served us all well in her role as liaison among the editorial board members, authors, and Macmillan. Kate provided me with steadfast support through the difficult times, meeting my bad humors with good, keeping us organized, and providing gentle reminders of tasks that lay ahead. I knew from the start that I could not do this task without Kate . . . how perfectly right I was!

MARY A. CARSKADON

LIST OF ARTICLES

LIST OF CONTRIBUTORS

Acebo, Christine
Brown University

Ontogeny
Premature Infants
Smoking and Sleep

Ackerman, Sigurd H.
St. Luke's/Roosevelt Hospital Center, New York

Eating Disorders
Nutrition and Sleep

Aldrich, Michael
University Hospital, Ann Arbor, MI

Cataplexy
Electroencephalogram
Epilepsy
Hypnagogic Hallucinations
K-Complex
Sawtooth Waves
Sleep Paralysis
Vertex Sharp Waves

Ancoli-Israel, Sonia
V.A. Medical Center, San Diego, CA

Epidemiology of Sleep Complaints and Disorders

Anderson, Janis
Brigham and Women's Hospital, Boston

Light Therapy
Seasonal Affective Disorder

Antrobus, John
City College of New York

Characteristics of Dreams
Recall of Dreams

Ariagno, Ronald L.
Stanford University

Sudden Infant Death Syndrome

Aytur, Semra
Bradley Hospital, East Providence, RI

Chocolate
Sandman

Badia, Pietro
Bowling Green University

Amnesia
Learning
Smell During Sleep

Baghdoyan, Helen A.
Pennsylvania State University

Anesthesia
Chemistry of Sleep: Acetylcholine

Bagian, James P.
NASA, Houston, TX

Space Shuttle Sleeping Arrangements

Benca, Ruth M.
University of Chicago

Genetics of Sleep
Immune Function

Bergmann, Bernard
University of Chicago

Deprivation, Total: Physiological Effects

Biber, Michael P.
Harvard Medical School

Kleine-Levin Syndrome

Bigler, Pamela J.
Bradley Hospital, East Providence, RI

Early Birds and Night Owls
Lullaby

Bliwise, Donald L.
Stanford University Medical Center

Aging and Sleep
Alzheimer's Disease
Dementia

Bonnet
V.A. Medical Center, Dayton, OH

Deprivation, Partial
Deprivation, Total: Behavioral Effects
Depth of Sleep
Fragmentation

Bootzin, Richard R.
University of Arizona

Cognition
Stimulus Control for Insomnia

Boukydis, C. F. Zachariah
Bradley Hospital, East Providence, RI

Colic

Broughton, Roger J.
Ottawa General Hospital, Ottawa, Ontario

Passing Out
Sentinel Hypothesis

Brown, Lawrence W.
Sleep Disorders Center, Philadelphia

Mental Retardation

Buchsbaum, Monte S.
V.A. Medical Center, San Diego, CA

Cerebral Metabolism

Bulkley, Kelly
University of Chicago

Jung's Dream Theory

Buysse, Daniel J.
Western Psychiatric Institute, Pittsburgh, PA

Affective Disorders Other Than Major
   Depression
Antidepressants
Depression

Campbell, Scott S.
*New York Hospital/Cornell Medical Center,
   White Plains, NY*

Seasonal Effects on Sleep
Slow-wave Sleep

Carskadon, Mary A.
Brown University

Echidna
Instantaneous Dreaming

Microsleep
Multiple Sleep Latency Test
Normal Sleep
Oversleeping
Polysomnography
Stages of Sleep

Cartwright, Rosalind D.
*Rush-Presbyterian-St. Luke's Medical
   Center, Chicago*

Functions of Dreams
Interpretation of Dreams

Chase, Michael H.
University of California at Los Angeles

Motor Control

Coble, Patricia A.
Western Psychiatric Institute, Pittsburgh, PA

Childhood, Sleep During

Cohn, Martin A.
*Sleep Disorders Center of Southwest
   Florida, Naples*

Sleep Therapy

Czeisler, Charles A.
Brigham and Women's Hospital, Boston

Light

Davis, Stephen S.
Bradley Hospital, East Providence, RI

Ondine's Curse

Dawson, William Andrew
*Queen Elizabeth Hospital, Adelaide,
   Australia*

Aboriginal Dreaming

Dement, William C.
Stanford University

Canine Narcolepsy
REM Sleep, Discovery of
Sleepiness

Dinges, David F.
University of Pennsylvania

Napping
Sleep Inertia

Dorsey, Cynthia M.
McLean Hospital, Belmont, MA
Monoamine Oxidase Inhibitors

Duffy, Jeanne F.
Brigham and Women's Hospital, Boston
Constant Routine

Dumont, Marie
Hôpital Sacré-Coeur, Montreal, Quebec
Advanced Sleep Phase Syndrome

Engelhardt, Christin L.
Deaconess Hospital, St. Louis, MO
Antihistamines
Myths About Dreaming
Myths About Sleep

Engle-Friedman, Mindy
Baruch College
Female Sexual Response

Eveloff, Scott E.
Rhode Island Hospital, Providence
Sudden Death in Asian Populations

Feinberg, Irwin
University of California at Davis
Cycles of Sleep Across the Night

Ferber, Richard
Children's Hospital, Boston
Rhythmic Movement Disorder

Foulkes, David
Georgia Mental Health Institute, Atlanta
Adler's Dream Theory
Children's Dreams
Cognitive Dream Theory

Franzblau, John
World Federation of Sleep Research Societies, Beverly Hills, CA
Movies, Dreams in

Franzblau, Susan
World Federation of Sleep Research Societies, Beverly Hills, CA
Movies, Dreams in

Fritz, Gregory K.
Rhode Island Hospital, Providence
Bedwetting

Fujita, Shiro
Oakland Otology and Apnea Clinic, Troy, MI
Uvulopalatolaryngoplasty

George, Charles F. P.
Victoria Hospital, London, Ontario
Human Leukocyte Antigen
L-Tryptophan

Gillin, J. Christian
V.A. Medical Center, San Diego, CA
Cerebral Metabolism

Glotzbach, Steven F.
Stanford University
Sudden Infant Death Syndrome

Glovinsky, Paul B.
City College of New York
Sleep Hygiene
Sleep Restriction, Therapeutic

Graeber, R. Curtis
Boeing Commercial Airplane Group, Seattle, WA
Microgravity and Space Flight

Greene, Robert W.
V.A. Medical Center, Brockton, MA
Midbrain
REM Sleep, Physiology of

Guilleminault, Christian
Stanford University
Hypersomnia
Hypnic Jerks
Maxillofacial Surgery
Mononucleosis

Hall, Janet E.
Massachusetts General Hospital, Boston
Menstrual Cycle

Harper, Ronald M.
University of California at Los Angeles
Autonomic Nervous System
Heart Regulation During Sleep

Hartmann, Ernest
Shattuck Hospital, Boston

Nightmares
Personality and Dream Recall
Sexual Symbolism

Hartse, Kristyna M.
St. Louis University

Reptiles, Sleep in

Hauri, Peter
Mayo Clinic, Rochester, MN

Alpha-Delta Sleep
Aspirin
Panic Disorder

Hayes, Boyd
Brigham and Women's Hospital, Boston

Allergies
Ambulatory Monitoring
Daylight Saving Time

Heller, H. Craig
Stanford University

Hibernation

Hendricks, Joan C.
University of Pennsylvania

English Bulldogs as an Animal Model of
Sleep Apnea

Hennager, Krista
Luther College

Flying in Dreams
Pictorial Representation
Senoi Dream Theory
Symbolism in Dreams

Henriksen, Steven J.
Scripps Clinic, La Jolla, CA

Chemistry of Sleep: Peptides

Herman, Ivan
Greenwich, CT

Teddy Bears

Herman, John H.
*University of Texas Southwest Medical
Center, Dallas*

Color in Dreams
Eye Movements and Dreaming

Herman, Kate B.
Bradley Hospital, East Providence, RI

Alarm Clocks
Echidna
Oversleeping
Stages of Sleep

Herman, Phyllis
Cos Cob, CT

Folk and Other Natural Remedies for
Sleeplessness

Hicks, Robert A.
San Jose State University

Personality and Sleep

Hirshkowitz, Max
V.A. Medical Center, Houston, TX

Erectile Dysfunction
Erections
Nocturnal Penile Tumescence
Sex and Sleep
Sexual Activation

Hoddes, Eric
*Presbyterian–St. Luke's Hospital, Aurora,
CO*

Stanford Sleepiness Scale

Hoppenbrouwers, Toke
Woman's Hospital, Los Angeles

Fetal Sleep–Wake Patterns

Horne, J. A.
*Loughborough University, Leicestershire,
England*

Exercise

Hoyt, Grant
Stanford University

Drockle

Hua, Jenny
Brown University

Bedtime Stories

Jaffe, Linda S.
Brigham and Women's Hospital, Boston

Gonadotropic Hormones

Jofe, Stephanie
Massachusetts General Hospital, Boston
Premenstrual Syndrome

Johnson, T. Scott
Brigham and Women's Hospital, Boston
Altitude
Cheyne-Stokes Respiration

Jones, Barbara E.
McGill University, Montreal, Quebec
Chemistry of Sleep: Amines and Other
 Transmitters
Sleeping Sickness

Jouvet, Michel
Université Claude Bernard, Lyons, France
Metabolic Control of REM Sleep

Kapen, Sheldon
V.A. Medical Center, Allen Park, MI
Stroke

Kaufman, Kenn
American Birds, Tucson, AZ
Birds

Keenan, Sharon A.
School of Sleep Medicine, Stanford, CA
Alpha Rhythm
Electroencephalography
Electromyography
Electrooculography
Polysomnography
Stages of Sleep

Kerr, Nancy H.
Oglethorpe University
Blindness: Dreams of the Blind

Kihlstrom, John F.
University of Arizona
Cognition

Kilduff, Thomas S.
Stanford University
Estivation
Torpor

Kim, Eleanore S.
Brigham and Women's Hospital, Boston
Zeitgebers

Kleitman, Nathaniel
University of Chicago
Basic Rest–Activity Cycle

Klerman, Elizabeth
Brigham and Women's Hospital, Boston
Deprivation, Selective: NREM Sleep

Kracke, Waud H.
Chicago
Cultural Aspects of Dreaming

Kribbs, Nancy Barone
*Unit for Experimental Psychiatry,
 Philadelphia*
All-Nighters
Siesta

Kripke, Daniel F.
University of California, San Diego
Longevity

Krippner, Stanley
Saybrook Institute, San Francisco
Telepathy and Dreaming

Kronenberg, Fredi
Columbia University
Menopause

Krueger, James M.
University of Tennessee
Chemistry of Sleep: Sleep Factors

Kryger, M.
*St. Boniface General Hospital, Winnipeg,
 Manitoba*
Snoring

Kupfer, David J.
Western Psychiatric Institute, Pittsburgh, PA
Affective Disorders Other Than Major
 Depression
Antidepressants
Depression

LaBerge, Stephen
Stanford University

Lucid Dreaming

Landis, Carol A.
University of Washington

Pain

Lauber, John K.
*National Transportation Safety Board,
Washington, DC*

Public Safety in Transportation

Lavie, Peretz
Sleep Disorders Center, Haifa, Israel

Posttraumatic Nightmares
Religion and Dreaming

Lee, Kathryn
University of California, San Francisco

Pregnancy, Sleep in

Lee, Richard
Brigham and Women's Hospital, Boston

Sleep Positions
Time Zones

Lucas, Edgar
All Saints Episcopal Hospital, Fort Worth, TX

Dogs
Twitches

Luebke, Jennifer I.
V.A. Medical Center, Brockton, MA

REM Sleep, Physiology of

Lugaresi, Elio
Clinica Neurologica, Bologna, Italy

Fatal Familial Insomnia

Lydic, Ralph
Reciprocal Interaction Theory

Mahowald, Maren L.
V.A. Medical Center, Minneapolis

Arthritis and Other Musculoskeletal Disorders

Mahowald, Mark W.
*Hennepin County Medical Center,
Minneapolis*

Headaches, Nocturnal
Incubus Attacks
Sleep Terrors
Sleeptalking
Sleepwalking
Violence

Mamelak, Adam N.
University of California, San Francisco

Coma

Manber, Rachel
University of Arizona

Adolescence and Sleep

Mancuso, Joan
Yale University

Art, Sleep and Dreams in Western

Marks, Gerald A.
*University of Texas Southwestern Medical
Center, Dallas*

Lateral Geniculate Nucleus
PGO Waves
Thalamus

Martens, Heinz
Brigham and Women's Hospital, Boston

Blindness: Effects on Sleep Patterns and
Circadian Rhythm

McCarley, Robert W.
V.A. Medical Center, Brockton, MA

Visual System

McGinty, Dennis
V.A. Medical Center, Sepulveda, CA

Amphibians
Basal Forebrain
Energy Conservation
Thermoregulation

McKenna, James J.
Pomona College

Co-Sleeping

Mendelson, Wallace B.
State University of New York, Stony Brook

Barbiturates
Benzodiazepines

Growth Hormone
Sleeping Pills

Meyer, Thomas J.
Rhode Island Hospital, Providence

Pressurization

Mignot, E.
Stanford University

Canine Narcolepsy

Miller, James C.
Miller Ergonomics, Lakeside, CA

Truckers

Millman, Richard P.
Rhode Island Hospital, Providence

Sudden Death Syndrome in Asian Populations
Tonsillitis

Mindell, Jodi A.
St. Joseph's University

Infancy, Normal Sleep Patterns in
Infancy, Sleep Disorders in

Mitler, Merrill M.
Scripps Clinic, La Jolla, CA

Amphetamines
Death
Fatigue-Recovery Model
Public Safety in the Workplace
Stimulants
Truckers

Moldofsky, Harvey
Toronto Western Hospital, Ontario

Chronic Fatigue Syndrome
Nonrestorative Sleep

Moline, Margaret L.
New York Hospital/Cornell Medical Center, White Plains, NY

Cortisol
Jet Lag

Monk, Timothy H.
Western Psychiatric Institute, Pittsburgh, PA

Morningness/Eveningness
Shiftwork

Moorcroft, William H.
Luther College

Condensation
Pregnancy and Dreaming
Problem Solving and Dreaming
Psychic Dreams
Unconscious

Morairty, Stephen
V.A. Medical Center, Sepulveda, CA

Parasympathetic Nervous System
Sympathetic Nervous System

Morales, Francisco
University of California at Los Angeles

Motor Control

Morrison, Adrian
University of Pennsylvania

Animals' Dreams
Animals in Sleep Research

Nitz, Douglas
V.A. Medical Center, Sepulveda, CA

Early Sleep Theories

Nofzinger, Eric A.
Western Psychiatric Institute, Pittsburgh, PA

Antidepressants

Norman, Suzan E.
Mount Sinai Medical Center, Miami, FL

Night Sweats

O'Connor, Kevin A.
Hennepin County Medical Center, Minneapolis

Internal Desynchronization

Ogilvie, Robert D.
Brock University, St. Catherine's, Ontario

Perception During Sleep
Sleep Onset

Orem, John
Texas Technical University

Respiration Control in Sleep

Orr, William C.
Baptist Medical Center Foundation, Oklahoma City

Heartburn
Tracheostomy

Parsons, L. Claire
University of Arizona
Head Injury

Petro, Ellen
Brigham and Women's Hospital, Boston
Endocrinology

Phillips, Nathan H.
University of California, Santa Cruz
Metabolism

Pivik, R. T.
Ottawa General Hospital, Ontario
Attention Deficit Hyperactivity Disorder
Marijuana

Poe, Gina Rochelle
V.A. Medical Center, Sepulveda, CA
Paradoxical Sleep

Pollak, Charles P.
New York Hospital/Cornell Medical Center, White Plains, NY
Chronotherapy
Delayed Sleep Phase Syndrome
Noise

Pressman, Mark R.
Lankenau Hospital, Wynnewood, PA
Brain Mapping
Electrodermal Activity
Evoked Potentials
Galvanic Skin Response
Periodic Leg Movements
Pupillometry

Prospero-Garcia, Oscar
Scripps Clinic, La Jolla, CA
Chemistry of Sleep: Peptides

Provine, Robert R.
University of Maryland
Yawning

Pueschel, Siegfried M.
Rhode Island Hospital, Providence
Down Syndrome

Radulovacki, Miodrag
University of Illinois
Chemistry of Sleep: Adenosine

Rechtschaffen, Allan
University of Chicago
Phasic Integrated Potentials

Redline, Susan
University Hospital, Cleveland, OH
Heritability of Sleep and Sleep Disorders

Reynolds, Charles F., III
Western Psychiatric Institute, Pittsburgh, PA
Affective Disorders Other Than Major
  Depression
Antidepressants
Depression

Richardson, Gary S.
Brigham and Women's Hospital, Boston
Circadian Rhythms
Neuroendocrine Hormones
Thyroid Disease and Sleep

Roehrs, Timothy A.
Sleep Disorders Center, Detroit, MI
Alcohol
Caffeine
Drugs of Abuse
Memory

Roffwarg, Howard P.
University of Texas Southwestern Medical Center, Dallas
Middle Ear Muscle Activity
Sleep Disorders Centers

Rosekind, Mark R.
NASA Ames Research Center, Moffett Field, CA
Behavioral Modification
Biofeedback
Pilots
Relaxation Therapy

Rosenberg, Richard S.
Evanston Hospital, Evanston, IL
Aging and Circadian Rhythms

Rosenthal, Leon D.
Henry Ford Hospital, Detroit, MI

Electrocardiogram
Narcolepsy
Over-the-Counter Sleeping Pills
Over-the-Counter Stimulants
Sleep Attacks

Ross, Richard J.
V.A. Medical Center, Philadelphia

Recurring Dreams

Roth, Thomas
Henry Ford Hospital, Detroit, MI

Drugs for Medical Disorders
Early Morning Awakening
Hallucinations
Hypersomnia
Sleep Extension

Rothenberg, Saul
*Rush-Presbyterian-St. Luke's Medical
    Center, Chicago*

AIDS and Sleep

Sadeh, Avi
Tel Aviv University, Israel

Activity-Based Measures of Sleep
Milk Allergy and Infant Sleep
Night Waking in Infancy
Thumbsucking
Transitional Objects

Salin-Pascual, Rafael J.
Henry Ford Hospital, Detroit, MI

Narcotics

Satinoff, Evelyn
University of Illinois

Temperature Effects on Sleep

Satlin, Andrew
McLean Hospital, Belmont, MA

Sundown Syndrome

Schanzer, Lakshyan
*Massachusetts School of Professional
    Psychology*

Meditation and Sleep

Schenck, Carlos H.
*Hennepin County Medical Center,
    Minneapolis*

REM Sleep Behavior Disorder

Schulz, Hartmut
Free University, Berlin, Germany

Ultradian Rhythms

Schwartz, William
University of Massachusetts

Suprachiasmatic Nucleus of the Hypothalamus

Shanahan, Theresa L.
Brigham and Women's Hospital, Boston

Melatonin
Pineal Gland

Sharkey, Katherine M.
Bradley Hospital, East Providence, RI

Coffee
Nightcaps
Pajamas and Nightwear
Short Sleepers in History and Legend
Tea

Shiromani, Priyattam J.
V.A. Medical Center, Brockton, MA

Nicotine

Siegel, Diane J.
V.A. Medical Center, Sepulveda, CA

Pillows

Siegel, Jerome
V.A. Medical Center, Sepulveda, CA

Medulla
Pons
REM Sleep, Function of
REM Sleep, Mechanisms and Neuroanatomy

Spencer, John P.
Bradley Hospital, East Providence, RI

Popular Music, Sleep and Dreams in

Spielman, Arthur J.
City College of New York

Sleep Hygiene
Sleep Restriction, Therapeutic

Spinweber, Cheryl L.
*University of Southern California at San
    Diego*

Gardner, Randy
Rest

Stepanski, Edward J.
Sleep Disorders Center, Detroit, MI

Insomnia
Minnesota Multiphasic Personality Inventory
Toothgrinding

Steriade, M.
University of Laval, Quebec

Arousal
Sleep Spindles

Stevens, Janice R.
St. Elizabeth's Hospital, Washington, DC

Blinking

Stone, Max
Bradley Hospital, East Providence, RI

Creativity in Dreams
Phase-Response Curve

Stoyva, Johann
University of Colorado

Deafness and Dreaming
Hypnosis and Dreaming

Suessle, Amy E.
Brigham and Women's Hospital, Boston

Light–Dark Cycles

Sullivan, Jason
Brigham and Women's Hospital, Boston

Beds
Waking Up

Szymusiak, Ronald
V.A. Medical Center, Sepulveda, CA

Hypothalamus
NREM Sleep Mechanisms

Tobler, Irene
University of Zurich, Switzerland

Fish
Insects, Sleeplike States in

Toth, Linda A.
University of Tennessee

Infection

Trosman, Harry
University of Chicago

Freud's Dream Theory

Uchida, Sunao
University of California at Davis

Cycles of Sleep Across the Night

Ullman, Montague
Albert Einstein College of Medicine

Experiential Dream Groups

Van de Castle, Robert L.
Blue Ridge Hospital, Charlottesville, VA

Content of Dreams

Van Gelder, Russell N.
Stanford University

Entrainment
Free Running
Temporal Isolation

Verdone, Paul
California State University, Sacramento

Psychophysiology of Dreaming

Vieira, Cecilia M.
Bradley Hospital, East Providence, RI

Nudity in Dreams

Vogel, Gerald W.
Georgia Mental Health Institute, Atlanta

Activation–Synthesis Hypothesis
Deprivation, Selective: REM Sleep
Hypnagogic Reverie
Incorporation into Dreams

Wagner, Daniel R.
*New York Hospital/Cornell Medical Center,
    White Plains, NY*

De Mairan, Jean Jacques d'Ortous
Flower Clock
Hypernychthemeral Syndrome
Irregular Sleep–Wake Cycle
Wagner, Robert

Wagner, Robert
Sealy, Inc., Middlebury Heights, OH

Mattress

Waldstreicher, Joanne
Massachusetts General Hospital, Boston

Prolactin

Walhof, Laura
Brigham and Women's Hospital, Boston

Gradual Sleep Reduction
Thyroid-Stimulating Hormone

Walsh, James K.
Deaconess Hospital, St. Louis, MO

Antihistamines
Myths About Dreaming
Myths About Sleep

Ware, J. Catesby
Sentara Norfolk General Hospital, Norfolk, VA

Tranquilizers

Webb, Wilse B.
University of Florida, Gainesville

Cultural Aspects of Sleep
Dream Theories of the Ancient World
Functions of Sleep
Individual Differences
Instinct

Welsh, David K.
Harvard Medical School

Hippocampal Theta
Timing of Sleep and Wakefulness

Wen, Patrick
Brigham and Women's Hospital, Boston

Brain Tumors

Westbrook, Carol C.
National Sleep Foundation, Los Angeles

Appendix: Organizations Concerned with
Sleep

Westbrook, Philip R.
Cedars-Sinai Medical Center, Los Angeles

Apnea

Wheatland, Thomas
Bradley Hospital, East Providence, RI

Literature, Sleep and Dreams in

Wicks, Jenifer
Bradley Hospital, East Providence, RI

Cocaine
Cola
Counting Sheep
Long Sleepers in History and Legend

Winkelman, John
McLean Hospital, Belmont, MA

Parkinson's Disease

Wittig, Robert M.
Sleep Disorders Center, Detroit, MI

Continuous Positive Airway Pressure
Sports and Sleep

Wooten, Virgil
St. Vincent Infirmary Medical Center, Little Rock, AR

Medical Illness and Sleep

Wu, Joseph C.
V.A. Medical Center, San Diego, CA

Cerebral Metabolism

Wu, M. F.
V.A. Medical Center, Sepulveda, CA

Sensory Processing and Sensation During Sleep

Wyatt, James K.
University of Arizona

Encephalitis

Zammit, Gary K.
St. Luke's/Roosevelt Hospital Center, New York

Eating Disorders
Nutrition and Sleep

Zarcone, Vincent P., Jr.
V.A. Medical Center, Palo Alto, CA

Alcoholism
Delirium Tremens
Psychopathology, Nondepression

Zepelin, Harold
Oakland University

Evolution of Sleep
Internal Alarm Clock
Mammals

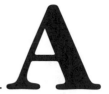

ABORIGINAL DREAMING

In traditional Australian aboriginal culture, *the Dreaming* refers to everything known and understood in the past, the present, and the future. The Dreaming is the focal point of traditional aboriginal existence and simultaneously determines their way of life, their culture, and their relationship to the physical and spiritual environment. For the traditional aborigines, the Dreaming is a collection of creation stories that demonstrate and define their history, culture, and law, determining in minute detail every aspect of their relationship to the land and other aboriginal people.

The words *dreaming* and *dreamtime* are terms used by traditional aboriginals because links and insights into the spiritual world are frequently established during dreams. For the traditional aboriginal, dreams are a parallel reality that form an important link with the spiritual world. The distinction between dreams and reality, common in Western belief systems, carries little meaning to traditional aboriginal culture. For the tribal aboriginal, the dream is a spiritual connection into the collective unconscious, and the Dreaming is one pathway to this spiritual consciousness.

The Dreaming beliefs are passed from one generation to the next by way of storytelling. A complex set of dream stories is used to educate the young aboriginal child. These stories make up a powerful influence on the aboriginal child because they combine myths, legends, art, music, and ceremony in an integrated spiritual and social matrix. Through the Dreaming, aboriginal people are connected to the land, and the custodial role of aboriginal culture is clearly defined.

Through the journeys and deeds of the creator spirits who inhabit every part of the natural environment, the Dreaming stories acculturate the young aboriginal child. Trees, rocks, and mountains, plants, animals, and insects all contain their own spirit. Each spirit has a lesson for the young child. Through these stories, the Dreaming defines the roles and relationships between the natural world and traditional aboriginal culture.

This spiritual component that animates the land changes how the traditional aborigines perceive their world. Their physical world carries an additional metaphysical dimension. In simple terms, the land is living and it is considered the body of ancestral creator spirits. Every aspect of the physical world is a reflection of this metaphysical animistic concept. For example, a river might be considered as the body of a great snake who traveled the land many years ago. A line of hills might be thought of as a giant sleeping lizard. This view of the land, shaped over 40,000 years, is similar to the emerging Western notion of the "Gaia principle."

For the traditional aborigines, the Dreaming confers specific individual and community responsibility. For each family or tribal group, the land is a collection of sacred sites to be tended carefully. Responsibility for each site is determined by reference to the Dreaming, and this automatically confers specific individual and community responsibility. Thus, in traditional aboriginal culture, the Dreaming and custodial responsibility, rather than ownership, is the basis for deciding what territory belongs to a specific tribal group.

In addition to its communal functions, this custodial relationship to the natural world carries important responsibilities and obligations for individual aboriginals. These obligations take the form of conservation practices, observance of community laws, and continued practice of sacred and or secret rituals. In addition to its spiritual content, the Dreaming covers many aspects of daily living through codes of practice related to hunting, food-gathering, storytelling, and social behavior. It is only by observing the natural order explained within the Dreaming that the aboriginal culture ensures it survival.

Unlike Western religions, which emphasize an external spiritual reality that is shared by the community, the Dreaming is also an intense personal experience. Although there are specific aspects of the Dreaming that are communal, every individual's experience of it is unique. Thus, each traditional aboriginal has a personal Dreaming through which he or she connects to a universal collective unconscious.

This connection typically occurs through the spirit that inhabits each individual. This inhabiting spirit (or *totem*) determines the fundamental spiritual identity of each aboriginal. On the basis of this spiritual identity, the Dreaming will define many of the individual's social roles and responsibilities within normal daily life. The acquisition of spiritual identity plays a fundamental role in defining the individual both within the social or family group and with respect to custodial responsibilities to the ancestral creator spirits.

The importance of this spiritual identity is demonstrated by the manner in which it is acquired. Importantly, the spiritual identity is acquired before the individual is born, emphasizing the fact that one's spiritual identity precedes one's individual social identity. The spiritual identity is acquired through the mother, and in most aboriginal groups this occurs at the time and place where the mother first becomes aware of the pregnancy. At this time, the fetus is adopted by the "spirit baby" who inhabits this particular part of the physical environment.

Because each part of the environment is clearly defined by the Dreaming, each individual has a clear spiritual identity and his or her role as custodian of that spirit and place is subsequently defined. The spirit enters the fetus through physical proximity, thereby making the mother aware of the impending birth. Through this association, each individual's personal Dreaming is clearly defined and this belief reinforces the spiritual ties between the aboriginal, his or her totem, and custodial responsibilities to the living land.

William Andrew Dawson

ACCIDENTS

See Head Injury; Public Safety in Transportation; Public Safety in the Workplace

ACETYLCHOLINE

See Chemistry of Sleep: Acetylcholine

ACTIVATION–SYNTHESIS HYPOTHESIS

The activation–synthesis hypothesis is a theory about dreams. The hypothesis proposes that physiological events during REM sleep explain the occurrence and unique characteristics of dreams (Hobson and McCarley, 1977). The hypothesis is intended to replace Freud's psychoanalytic hypothesis that psychological events explain the occurrence and characteristics of dreams (Freud, 1953). Briefly, the psychoanalytic hypothesis is that dreams are instigated by the rise of meaningful though unconscious, unacceptable wishes during sleep. The wishes are made less objectionable by distortion that disguises their true nature. The dream narrative continues the disguise to fulfill the unacceptable wish in a hallucinated way. Thus, according to Freud, dreams are disguised wish fulfillments; they function to protect sleep by decreasing the growing tension created by the strong unfulfilled wishes, much the same way that daydreaming relieves waking tension. Thus, according to psychoanalytic theory, dreams are instigated by meaningful psychological events, namely, wishes; the dream narrative has psychological meaning, namely, the fulfillment of a wish; and the dream has the function of protecting sleep from the arousal created by an unfulfilled wish. (See also FREUD'S DREAM THEORY.)

The activation–synthesis hypothesis rejects all these psychological explanations of dreams. It explains dreams as the result of physiological events during REM sleep, a state from which dreams are usually reported. Physiologically, REM sleep is generated by the electrical activity of neurons in a part of the brain called the PONS (Hobson and McCarley, 1977). The pons is located in the hindbrain, which in evolutionary terms is a primitive brain region. By itself the hindbrain does not support higher mental activity such as consciousness, thought, psychologically meaningful wishes, perception, and intentional movement. Hence, the pontine generation of REM sleep implies that physicochemical events in the pons, rather than meaningful wishes, initiate dreaming. The pontine neurons that generate REM sleep send electrical signals to many brain areas. The targets include the forebrain, which involves brain regions responsible for conscious thought, voluntary movement, conscious sensations (such as sight, touch, and hearing), and conscious feelings (such as love, hate, and fear). The pontine electrical signals activate the targeted forebrain areas responsible for these conscious mental activities.

According to the activation–synthesis hypothesis, the activation of the forebrain areas generates the conscious dream experience. For example, pontine activation of brain areas responsible for walking will produce the dream image of walking. Pontine activation of brain areas responsible for seeing a beach scene will produce the visual dream image of a beach scene. Pontine activation of brain areas responsible for fear will produce the dream experience of fear.

The forebrain also has the higher mental function of synthesizing or integrating different experiences into a coherent whole. For instance, the forebrain might synthesize the preceding examples into a dream that portrays a frightened dreamer walking on a beach, though the reason for the fear is unknown. Thus, according to the activation–synthesis hypothesis, the dream narrative is a forebrain synthesis of a hindbrain activation pattern—hence the term *activation-synthesis hypothesis*. The narrative is determined by physiological events, not by meaningful psychological events such as the disguised fulfillment of unconscious wishes.

In the activation–synthesis hypothesis, dream distortion also occurs for physiological reasons, not for the psychological purpose of disguise (Hobson and McCarley, 1977). The pattern of neural electrical signals originating in the pontine hindbrain during REM sleep is random rather than orderly or psychologically meaningful. The

targeted forebrain attempts to make sense of its random activation. It does so by comparing and interpreting its random activation pattern with the presumably ordered activation patterns of stored memories. The forebrain then does the best it can to synthesize its random patterns into a meaningful whole. Dream distortion results from the forebrain's incapacity to successfully synthesize random patterns of activation. Thus, rather than serving the psychological purpose of disguise, dream distortion represents only "the best of a poor job" by the forebrain.

The activation–synthesis hypothesis is consistent with some laboratory evidence and not consistent with other evidence. On the supportive side, the hypothesis predicts the frequency of visual, auditory, and other sensations in dreams; the frequency of limb movements in dreams; and the occurrence of dream distortion and of dream bizarreness, such as dreams of paralysis (McCarley and Hoffman, 1981; Hobson et al., 1987). Most significantly, the hypothesis makes REM dream properties consistent with physiological events during REM sleep. On the nonsupportive side (Vogel, 1978), the activation–synthesis hypothesis cannot easily explain laboratory findings that, contrary to popular views, dreams are usually coherent narratives and not bizarre. Random forebrain activation requires an almost kaleidoscopic sequence of meaningless images. Also, the activation–synthesis hypothesis, which explains dreams as outcomes of REM sleep physiology, cannot easily explain the frequent dreaming that occurs during sleep onset and NREM sleep in the absence of REM sleep. On balance, then, the activation–synthesis hypothesis is a current, reasonable, but unproven physiological theory about the occurrence and properties of dreams.

REFERENCES

Freud S. 1953. The interpretation of dreams (1900). In Strachey J, ed./transl. *Complete psychological works,* stand. ed., vols 4 and 5. London: Hogarth Press.

Hobson JA, Hoffman SA, Helfand R, Kostner D. 1987. Dream bizarreness and the activation–synthesis hypothesis. *Hum Neurobiol* 6:157–164.

Hobson JA, McCarley RW. 1977. The brain as a dream state generator: An activation–synthesis hypothesis of the dream process. *Am J Psychiatry* 134: 1335–1348.

McCarley RW, Hoffman E. 1981. REM sleep dreams and the activation–synthesis hypothesis. *Am J Psychiatry* 138:904–912.

Vogel GW. 1978. An alternative view of the neurobiology of dreaming. *Am J Psychiatry* 135:1531–1535.

Gerald W. Vogel

ACTIVITY

[*In the context of sleep research, the term* activity *generally refers to coordinated and purposeful behaviors, such as feeding and ambulation. Although complex motor activity can occur during sleep (as in* SLEEPWALKING*), the term generally refers to waking behavior. When electroencephalographic definitions of sleep–wake states are not available, observed periods of activity and* REST *are used synonymously with wakefulness and sleep.*

Much of the research on CIRCADIAN RHYTHMS *in animals is performed by measuring regular daily periods of activity. In studies of rodents, motor activity is typically quantified by counting the number of revolutions of a running wheel or the number of times the animal changes position in its cage. The active portion of the animal's circadian activity–rest cycle is designated* alpha, *while the quiet portion is called* rho. *If alpha and rho are assumed to reflect wake and sleep, this measure overestimates sleep duration, because it cannot discriminate periods of quiet wakefulness from sleep. Such behavioral measures nevertheless provide a consistent and easily quantified index of circadian timing processes.*

Variations in relative amounts of physical activity may occur very frequently within the 24-hour day. In humans, for example, a pattern of approximately 90-minute variations in activity level may constitute a BASIC REST-ACTIVITY CYCLE, *which may, in turn, be a daytime manifestation of the REM–NREM* CYCLES OF SLEEP ACROSS THE NIGHT.

In spite of the significant overlap of wakefulness and activity, the distinction between them is important. For example, the amount of physical activity within a period of wakefulness appears to be related to subsequent sleep. Additional discussion of this phenomenon can be found in the entries on EXERCISE *and the* FATIGUE-RECOVERY MODEL *of sleep.*]

ACTIVITY-BASED MEASURES OF SLEEP

Sleep–wake cycles are highly correlated with rest–activity cycles. In addition, levels of motility (movement) vary with sleep states and the related changes in muscle tone. These facts provide the rationale for activity-based sleep–wake assessment. This type of sleep measurement started as early as 1922 with the use of a special bed equipped to record body movements (Szymansky, 1922).

Since then, several different technologies have been devised to record body movements during sleep. Basically, these techniques involve transformation of the physical attributes of a body movement into an analog signal that can be directly recorded or further transformed to a digital count and stored in electronic memory for prolonged periods. Certain methods are similar in principle to the playing of audio recordings on a phonograph; instead of a stylus moving along the tracks of the phonograph record, there is an accelerator responding to body movements, and the audio signal is replaced by a numeric representation (see Tyron, 1991, for a detailed review of the physical and psychometric properties of different methods for activity measurements in psychology and medicine). Techniques for measuring body movements in sleep include photographic monitoring, polysomnographic recording, use of body and bed transducers, and direct visual observation.

One instrument commonly used in sleep research is the pressure-sensitive mattress (Thoman and Glazier, 1987). Motility signals, generated by changes in pressure on the mattress, are recorded by a small device placed near the bed. Special filters and algorithms may be applied to the signal to provide information regarding respiration as well as larger body movements during sleep. Since the use of the mattress does not involve any electrodes or sensors directly attached to the subject, this method of measurement has been particularly useful in sleep studies with young children.

An increasingly popular means of assessing sleep–wake cycles through activity levels is actigraphy (or actometry) (Kripke et al., 1978). The actigraph is a small monitor that may be worn continuously on the wrist for prolonged periods, providing activity data that can be translated to sleep–wake measures. The primary advantage of the actigraph is that it makes possible a cost-effective, naturalistic study of sleep–wake patterns while subjects continue their normal daytime routines and sleep in their usual environment. A number of studies have shown the usefulness of actigraphic sleep–wake measurement in adults, children, and infants, as well as its capacity to identify sleep disturbances and to distinguish between sleep-disturbed individuals and normal control subjects. For instance, Sadeh and colleagues (1989) reported 91 percent agreement between actigraphic and polysomnographic sleep–wake scoring in normal subjects, and 85.7 percent and 78 percent scoring agreement in sleep APNEA patients and insomniacs, respectively (see POLYSOMNOGRAPHY).

Because of its cost-effectiveness and flexibility, actigraphy has often been used in clinical drug trials and other intervention studies. One study that illustrates this method's unique potential examined the disruptive effects of JET LAG on sleep–wake cycles, and the use of drugs to alleviate these effects: Normal subjects wore actigraphs for several weeks while flying across time zones westward and eastward under various drug and placebo conditions (Lavie, 1990).

Actigraphy and other activity-based measures have a number of limitations. The methods are generally informative, more flexible, and less intrusive than laboratory polysomnography; when sleep disturbances are detected by actigraphy,

however, the reason or underlying mechanisms remain obscure unless a full laboratory study is then conducted. In addition, since the methods are based solely on activity, serious misclassification may occur: for example, if a subject is in bed, motionless and trying to fall asleep but unsuccessful for a prolonged period—as often occurs in insomnia. In such an instance, the actigraph may automatically record the time as sleep although the subject is actually awake.

Figure 1 is a plot of actigraphic data from a patient experiencing schedule difficulties. Each row represents a 24-hour period, with midnight represented by zero. The black bars indicate the activity level in a given sampling epoch. White areas represent sleep periods, and black areas represent periods of wakefulness. As can be seen, this subject's sleep periods varied dramatically during the week of the study.

(See also AMBULATORY MONITORING; ELECTROEN-CEPHALOGRAPHY; ELECTROMYOGRAPHY.)

REFERENCES

Kripke DF, Mullaney DJ, Messin S, Wyborney VG. 1978. Wrist actigraph measures of sleep and rhythms. *Electroencephalogr Clin Neurophysiol* 44:674–678.

Lavie P. 1990. The effects of 7.5 mg midazolam vs placebo on sleep disturbances associated with west-

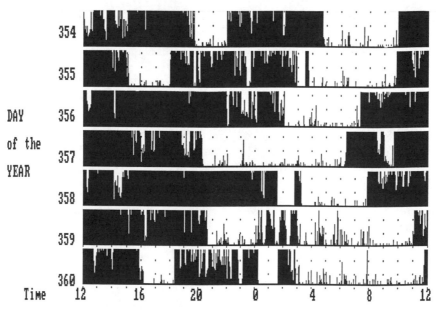

Figure 1.   A record of a patient's activity level as measured with an actigraph.

ward and eastward flights. *Psychopharmacology* 101:250–254.

Sadeh A, Alster J, Urbach D, Lavie P. 1989. Actigraphically based automatic bedtime sleep–wake scoring: Validity and clinical applications. *Ambulatory Monitoring* 2(3):209–216.

Szymansky JS. 1922. Aktivitaet und Ruhe bei den Menschen. *Zeitschrift für Angewandte Psychologie* 20:192–222.

Thoman EB, Glazier RC. 1987. Computer scoring of motility patterns for states of sleep and wakefulness: Human infants. *Sleep* 10:122–129.

Tyron WW. 1991. *Activity measurement in psychology and medicine.* New York: Plenum.

Avi Sadeh

ADENOSINE

See Caffeine; Chemistry of Sleep: Adenosine

ADLER'S DREAM THEORY

Alfred Adler (1870–1937), an Austrian psychiatrist at one time closely associated with Sigmund Freud, separated from him to develop an alternative to psychoanalysis known as individual psychology (Ansbacher and Ansbacher, 1956). Adler did not devote the same degree of attention as did Freud to dream phenomena, and his ideas are neither extensive nor consistent enough to constitute a genuine theory. Nevertheless, his writings (Adler, 1931/1958; Adler, 1927/1963) anticipated many later neo-Freudian dream theories and even some of the more recent changes in psychoanalytic theory itself.

One of the basic principles of Adler's general theory is the pervasive influence of a striving toward mastery that originates during a period of infantile helplessness. Thus, mind develops as the means by which infantile inadequacy is overcome and world mastery is achieved. As a mental act, dreaming also is imagined to be harnessed to the goal of mastery. Specifically, for Adler, dreaming is an anticipation of or preparation for future situations. It attempts to solve interpersonal problems rather than, as for Freud, to discharge intrapsychic tensions.

Problem-solving theories of dream function face a number of problems: dreams do not seem to contain many obvious problem solutions; many people do not take their dreams seriously enough to act on any suggestions about waking life that might be found there; and the particular content of most dreams is too quickly forgotten to be useful later. Adler developed one ingenious way around such difficulties. He admits that the *ideational* and *perceptual* content of the dream has little adaptive value. Instead, he focuses on the *mood* or *feeling state* created by the dream. Adler notes the common experience of carrying a dream-instigated mood well into the following day, even though the events that created the mood are quite fictitious and readily forgotten. But Adler vacillates on how adaptive these dream-created moods actually are. He allows that dreams and dream-instigated moods may provide only unrealistic or deceptive solutions to problems in waking life.

Adler does not entirely neglect the ideational and perceptual content of dreams. Here, too, however, he vacillates on its unrealistic versus adaptive nature. For example, he links a fantastic or unrealistic (bizarre) quality of some dream imagery to the diminished reality contact of sleep, a state in which the dreamer is not stimulated to deal honestly with real-life situations. And yet, Adler also holds that dream imagery is largely expressive in nature; that is, particular dream portrayals emerge for their ability, not to disguise the dreamer's underlying thoughts, but to express them.

Adler's theory, though not always internally consistent, nevertheless offers significant alternatives to Freud's: that the dream itself is concerned with present and future experience rather than with the infantile period alone; that waking and dreaming are related aspects of mental life and more continuous than discontinuous; that the process of dreaming is driven by realistic adaptive needs rather than by childish wishes; and that dream imagery is a unified expression of the dreamer's character rather than a piecemeal construction designed to conceal its origins. In the hands of later psychologists (for example, Hall, 1966; French, 1954), many of these ideas found more consistent expression and greater acceptance.

(See also CONTENT OF DREAMS; FREUD'S DREAM THEORY.)

REFERENCES

Adler A. 1931/1958. *What life should mean to you.* New York: Capricorn.

Adler A. 1927/1963. *Understanding human nature.* New York: Premier.

Ansbacher HL, Ansbacher R, eds. 1956. *The individual psychology of Alfred Adler.* New York: Basic.

French TM. 1954. *The integrative process in dreams.* Chicago: University of Chicago Press.

Hall CS. 1966. *The meaning of dreams,* rev. ed. New York: McGraw-Hill.

David Foulkes

ADOLESCENCE AND SLEEP

The second decade of life is a period of profound physiological and psychological changes that accompany the transition from childhood to adulthood. These include changes in endocrine secretions related to the pubertal process as well as increases in psychological stress due to increasing maturational demands. These changes affect many aspects of an adolescent's life, and sleep is no exception. Several aspects of sleep are affected, including sleep behaviors, the ELECTRO-ENCEPHALOGRAM (EEG) of sleep, and the development of sleep disorders.

Sleep-Wake Behavior

Perhaps the most pronounced changes in sleep-wake behavior during this period of life are a decrease in the total amount of sleep and the development of irregular sleep-wake schedules. These changes are commonly associated with an increase in daytime sleepiness that affects daytime functioning. Sleep-wake schedules change in several ways. There is a steady delay in bedtime from about 9:00–10:00 P.M. at age 10 to about 1:30–2:30 A.M. during early college years (at age 18). Moreover, adolescents often state that they enjoy staying up late and that they tend to go to bed much later on weekend nights than on school nights. On the other hand, because of school schedules, wakeup time on school days becomes earlier with the transition from middle school to high school. The result is a reduction in the total hours of sleep during the week and an attempt to catch up for lost sleep by delaying wakeup time until the later morning hours on weekends. The average sleep time declines from about 10 hours before puberty through 8.5 hours in midadolescence to 7 hours in the late teen years (Carskadon and Dement, 1987). The decrease in total sleep time is accompanied by an increase in the discrepancy between sleep behavior on school nights and weekend nights.

Many factors may work together to bring about these changes in the duration of sleep and in the irregularity of the sleep-wake patterns during the second decade of life. Research in the 1980s suggests that the reduction in total sleep time is unlikely to be due to an actual decrease in the *need* for sleep. In fact, sleep need during the pubertal process is at least as high as it is before the onset of puberty (Carskadon et al., 1980). The reduction in total sleep time and the development of an irregular sleep-wake schedule are more likely due to increased demands on an adolescent's time. These increased demands stem from several sources: an increase in school work and extracurricular activities, an increase in interest and involvement in social life, and, in many cases, an increase in the total number of hours an adolescent may spend working for wages. Many adolescents find it hard to manage their time efficiently under these demanding conditions and tend to postpone their bedtime and to shorten their sleep. Consequently, adolescents who spend more hours on these activities are more likely to report that they sleep fewer hours per night and with less regular timing.

Daytime Sleepiness

Large surveys of adolescents indicate that more than half wish to have more sleep (Strauch and Meier, 1988) and many report that they are sleepy at some point during the day. The severity of the problem in this population is confirmed by objective laboratory measures. When adolescents are deprived of one or two nights of sleep, they show marked reductions in alertness and in performance levels on tasks that require attention, memory, cognitive skills, and motor skills. These reductions in performance are due to a very high level of sleepiness as evidenced by the presence of short sleep episodes during the performance of these tasks. These studies suggest that the high prevalence rate of daytime sleepiness in this age group may have marked effects on school performance and could be linked to the increased automobile accident rate of adolescents. Moreover, daytime sleepiness could affect mood and may contribute to the increased use and abuse of drugs and alcohol.

Several factors contribute to the increased daytime sleepiness in adolescence. First, as mentioned above, contrary to popular belief, sleep needs are not reduced during adolescence. A series of studies of sleep and daytime sleepiness in which participants in summer sleep camps were allowed to sleep for 10 hours show that, regardless of the time spent asleep, the occurrence of daytime sleepiness increased with age, peaked at midpuberty, and remained at the higher level through the rest of the second decade of life (Carskadon et al., 1980). Although poor sleep at night is a common cause of daytime sleepiness, the prevalence of poor sleep is very low compared with the prevalence of daytime sleepiness, implying that other factors may contribute to daytime sleepiness. Chief among them is the chronic sleep deprivation resulting from the decrease in total sleep time. Another predisposing factor for daytime sleepiness is the irregularity of the sleep-wake schedule, as it may weaken the underlying biological rhythm. Studies show that young adults with irregular sleep-wake schedules tend to experience more daytime sleep episodes and to be more sleepy than individuals with regular sleep-wake schedules (e.g., Billiard and Alperovitch, 1988). Although susceptibility to sleepiness following sleep deprivation varies greatly from person to person, there is evidence that teenagers who work more than 20 hours per week are at a high risk of daytime sleepiness (Carskadon, 1990).

Morning sleepiness and difficulties in starting the day are more common than problems with sleepiness during other parts of the day. Whereas preadolescents tend to wake up spontaneously in the morning and to feel ready to start the day, adolescents and young college students need several reminders to wake up and may take a longer time to feel wide awake. This is likely due to the effects of sleep deprivation resulting from delayed bedtime and to the possibility of a mild delayed sleep phase (a circadian rhythm disorder discussed below). Ferber (1990) has hypothesized that the difficulty in getting out of bed in the morning in this age group is a manifestation of oppositional behavior and a form of asserting control on the environment.

Sleep Electroencephalogram

The most marked changed in the EEG of sleep in the second decade of life is a reduction in slow-wave (stages 3 and 4) sleep. By the end of the second decade of life, time spent in slow-wave sleep is only 70 percent of what it was at the beginning of the decade. In addition, the ratio between stage 4 and stage 3 of slow-wave sleep decreases. On the other hand, there is an increase in stage 1 and 2 NREM sleep. Far less marked changes occur in REM sleep. There seems to be a slight reduction in total REM sleep time because of the general reduction in sleep duration, but no marked changes in the percentage of REM sleep (Carskadon and Dement, 1983). As adolescents progress through the pubertal process, the time elapsed from sleep onset until the first REM sleep period becomes shorter (however, girls tend to have an increased latency to REM sleep after midpuberty). The role that the pubertal process plays in the changes occurring in sleep architecture during the second decade of life is seen in a study of children who experienced precocious (early) puberty. These are typically children in the first decade of life who, for some reason, started puberty very early in their life. The sleep of these young children was reported to fall in the range of values appropriate for adolescents and did not change back to age-appropriate norms following hormonal treatment that stopped the pubertal process (Rothenberg et al., 1989).

Sleep Disorders

During the second decade of life, the prevalence rates of different sleep disorders change. Insomnia and daytime sleepiness become significantly more prevalent, parasomnias become less prevalent, and several adult sleep disorders, such as NARCOLEPSY and restless legs syndrome, show initial symptoms.

Insomnia

Many adults who seek help for their poor sleep report onset of the problem in their teen years. It is hard to tell how prevalent insomnia is during the teen years. About 12 percent to 14 percent of adolescents report frequent insomnia symptoms, but many more report less frequent and very short-term symptoms. The most prevalent insomnia symptom during this developmental stage is the difficulty in falling asleep, which is commonly assumed to be caused by rising levels of stress associated with the maturation process. When adolescents experience poor sleep, they most commonly attribute it to depression, anxiety, and "being worried." Treatment of insomnia in adolescence is similar to treatment of adult insomnia (see INSOMNIA). One aspect of the treatment that is particularly important for adolescents is regulation of the sleep-wake schedule, as a regular sleep-wake rhythm is a basic precondition for good sleep. Unfortunately, because of social, academic, and work pressures, it is extremely difficult to convince adolescents and young college students to adopt a regular sleep-wake pattern.

Delayed Sleep Phase

The tendencies to push bedtime to later hours and to maintain irregular sleep schedules predispose adolescents and young college students to biological rhythm disorders. Many physiological functions such as body temperature, hormone secretion, and sleep-wake cycle follow a circadian (daily) rhythm. A disturbance of the sleep-wake circadian rhythm occurs when the "biological clock" does not correspond to the individual's usual bedtime hours. The most likely rhythm disturbance in adolescence is delayed sleep phase. Individuals in this category report they have a hard time falling asleep at a desired time, but have normal sleep in the absence of an imposed schedule. The disorder is associated with daytime sleepiness, particularly in the morning. There are case study reports on the disorder in adolescents and young adults. Moreover, adults who suffer from delayed sleep phase syndrome often report childhood onset of the symptoms. In mild cases, the regulation of sleep-wake patterns coupled with exposure to light early in the day may suffice to correct the problem. In more severe cases, however, chronotherapy may be required. Chronotherapy is a process by which bedtime is progressively delayed by 3 hours each day until the desired bedtime is reached (see CHRONOTHERAPY).

Excessive Daytime Sleepiness

Although adolescents as a group tend to complain of daytime sleepiness, these complaints usually do not reach clinical levels. When symptoms of excessive daytime sleepiness occur, it is important to rule out disorders of excessive daytime sleepiness, such as narcolepsy and sleep apnea. Narcolepsy is a rare but rather disabling disorder of excessive daytime sleepiness that is accompanied by sleep attacks along with other alarming symptoms such as sleep paralysis (see NARCOLEPSY). Its prevalence rate is 0.02 percent to 0.09 percent and it typically begins its clinical course between the ages of 15 and 25 (Bootzin and Chambers, 1990). Sleep APNEA is a disorder of abnormal breathing during the night that results in brief awakening and fragmented sleep. Although the disorder typically starts much later in life, about 3 percent of adolescents experience brief awakenings because of difficulties in breathing during the night that could be related to sleep apnea. Another adult sleep disorder that results in fragmented sleep and daytime sleepiness is the restless legs syndrome. The disorder is associated with irresistible movement of the leg during sleep. It is typically diagnosed during the fourth decade of life but its symptoms may appear in a subclinical intensity during the second decade of life.

Disorders of Partial Arousals

Disorders of partial arousals constitute a subclass of the parasomnias that occur during partial arousal from SLOW-WAVE SLEEP. Included are SLEEPWALKING, nocturnal enuresis (BEDWETTING), and night terrors. These disorders are developmental in nature. Their prevalence rates are higher in childhood and decline markedly during adolescence. Although prevalence rates during the second decade of life vary according to severity and frequency of the problem, they are estimated as less than 1 percent for night terrors and as about 3 percent for nocturnal enuresis. Sleepwalking peaks around age 12 but declines sharply by late adolescence. The presence of these three disorders in late adolescence and adulthood is commonly associated with psychological or other medical conditions, such as nocturnal seizures and sleep apnea.

REFERENCES

Billiard MC, Alperovitch A. 1988. Epidemiology of excessive somnolence in draftees. In Koella WP, Obal F, Schulz H, Visser P, eds. Sleep '86, pp 194–195. New York: Gustav Fischer Verlag.

Bootzin RR, Chambers MJ. 1990. Childhood sleep disorders. In Gross AM, Drabman RS, eds. *Handbook of clinical behavioral pediatrics*, pp 205–227. New York: Plenum.

Carskadon MA. 1990. Adolescent sleepiness: Increased risk in a high-risk population. *Alcohol Drugs Driving* 6 (1):317–328.

Carskadon MA, Dement WC. 1983. Evolution of sleep and daytime sleepiness in adolescents. In Guilleminault C, Lagaresi E, eds. *Sleep/wake disorders: natural history, epidemiology, and long term evaluation,* pp 201–216. New York: Raven.

Carskadon MA, Dement WC. 1987. Sleepiness in the normal adolescent. In: Guilleminault C, ed. *Sleep and its disorders in children,* pp 53–66. New York: Raven.

Carskadon MA, et al. 1980. Pubertal changes in daytime sleepiness. *Sleep* 2:453–460.

Cashman MA, McCann BS. 1988. Behavioral approaches to sleep/wake disorders in children and adolescents. In Hersen M, Eisler RM, Miller PM, eds. *Progress in behavior modification*, pp 215–283. Newbury Park, Calif.: Sage.

Ferber R. 1990. Sleep schedule-dependent causes of insomnia and sleepiness in middle childhood and adolescence. *Pediatrician* 17:13–20.

Rothenberg SA, Sklar CA, Regginardo D, Blumberg D, David R. 1989. Sleep structure before and after sex-steroid suppression in children with central precocious puberty. *Sleep Res* 18:97.

Strauch I, Meier B. 1988. Sleep need in adolescents: A longitudinal approach. *Sleep* 11:378–386.

Rachel Manber

ADVANCED SLEEP PHASE SYNDROME

Advanced sleep phase syndrome (ASPS) is a sleep disorder in which the problem is not the quality of sleep but rather the timing of the sleep episode. Those with this disorder experience an overwhelming sleepiness too early in the evening and awakening that occurs too early in the morning. The sleep episode is thus advanced in relation to the desired sleep time. Typically, sleep onset occurs between 6 P.M. and 9 P.M. and the patient wakes up before 5 A.M., sometimes as early as 1 A.M., feeling alert and refreshed, but frustrated. A person with ASPS may thus complain simultaneously of HYPERSOMNIA and INSOMNIA: hypersomnia because of excessive sleepiness and inability to stay awake in the evening, and insomnia because of inability to sleep through the night.

When patients with ASPS follow their spontaneous rhythm, they get a normal quantity and quality of sleep. However, most patients with ASPS suffer from the negative social consequences of the syndrome, which keep them from sharing in normal evening activities. When the patients force themselves to stay awake in the evening, they cannot wake up later in the morning. Consequently, after repeated efforts to go to sleep later, patients may suffer from chronic sleep DEPRIVATION and from excessive daytime SLEEPINESS.

Relationship with Aging

Advanced sleep phase syndrome is very uncommon and seems most likely to occur in elderly individuals. In normal aging, awakening tends to occur earlier (see AGING AND SLEEP), and it has been suggested that ASPS could be an excessive expression of normal age-related changes in circadian physiology (see AGING AND CIRCADIAN RHYTHMS). Research suggests that the circadian oscillator has an earlier phase and a shorter period in older people than in young adults (Czeisler et al., 1986; Weitzman et al., 1982). A very early phase of the circadian oscillator could cause the sleep episode to happen too early in the daytime and result in awakening at an unacceptably early hour.

Treatment

Sleep medication is usually ineffective in the treatment of ASPS. Two nonpharmacological treatments have had some success. One, CHRONOTHERAPY, takes advantage of the less impaired patient's ability to go to sleep at an earlier rather than a later time. Chronotherapy lasts about 2 weeks, during which the patient's bedtime is set 3 hours earlier every 2 days, going backward around the clock until the desired bedtime is achieved. The other treatment, LIGHT THERAPY, makes use of the fact that bright LIGHT enhances the phase-shifting capability of the circadian oscillator. The patient is exposed to 5 hours of bright light in the evening for 3 consecutive days. Phototherapy moves the phase of the oscillator to a later time, thus facilitating a later bedtime and wake time. These treatments are still experimental, and more studies are needed to confirm their efficiency and determine their long-term effects.

REFERENCES

Advanced sleep phase syndrome. 1990. In Diagnostic Classification Steering Committee, Thorpy MJ, chairman, *International classification of sleep disorders; Diagnostic and coding manual,* pp 133–137. Rochester, Minn.: American Sleep Disorders Association.

Czeisler CA, Kronauer RE, Johnson MP, Allan JS, Johnson TS, Dumont M. 1989. Action of light on the human circadian pacemaker: Treatment of patients with circadian rhythm sleep disorders. In Horne J, ed. *Sleep '88—proceedings of the Ninth European Congress on Sleep Research,* pp 42–47. Stuttgart: Gustav Fischer.

Czeisler CA, Rios DC, Sanchez R, Brown EN, Richardson GS, Ronda JM, Rogacz S. 1986. Phase advance and reduction in amplitude of the endogenous circadian oscillator correspond with systematic changes in sleep-wake habits and daytime functioning in the elderly. *Sleep Res* 15:268.

Moldovsky H, Musini S, Phillipson EA. 1986. Treatment of a case of advanced sleep phase syndrome by phase advance chronotherapy. *Sleep* 9:61–65.

Weitzman ED, Moline ML, Czeisler CA, Zimmerman JC. 1982. Chronobiology of aging: Temperature, sleep-wake rhythms and entrainment. *Neurobiol Aging* 3:399–309.

Marie Dumont

AFFECTIVE DISORDERS OTHER THAN MAJOR DEPRESSION

Many studies have examined the electroencephalographic sleep characteristics of patients with serious depression, usually referred to as major depressive disorder (see DEPRESSION). Far fewer studies have focused on patients with other forms of affective (mood) disorders. These other mood disorders include atypical depression, mania, dysthymia, and bereavement-related depression.

Patients with atypical depression are characterized by sensitivity to interpersonal rejection, anxiety and phobic symptoms, and an extreme loss of energy ("leaden paralysis") when depressed. These patients have electroencephalographic sleep characteristics similar to those of other depressed patients, including short REM sleep latency, but they have long sleep durations (HYPERSOMNIA) rather than INSOMNIA.

Patients with bipolar mood disorder, also known as manic depression, have repeated and sustained mood swings. During depressed phases, which last weeks to months, they have clinical symptoms virtually identical to those of other patients with depression. Episodes of mania are characterized by abnormally elevated or irritable mood, grandiose thoughts, and socially destructive behavior (for instance, substance abuse, promiscuity, excessive spending, and other types of impulsive behavior). When depressed, patients with bipolar mood disorder have electroencephalographic sleep findings very similar to those of other depressed patients. Bipolar depressives who have extreme loss of energy may not have the typical shortening of REM latency or loss of slow-wave sleep and may also have hypersomnia. Surprisingly, bipolar patients in manic episodes have shorter REM sleep latencies than healthy subjects, similar to the classic finding in depression. The short REM sleep latency during mania is evident despite shortened sleep time.

Dysthymia is a milder, more chronic form of depression. Electroencephalographic sleep findings in patients with dysthymia are similar to those of major depression, but less severe.

Recent studies have examined electroencephalographic sleep characteristics of older adults who are grieving the death of a spouse. Some of these patients are clinically depressed and others are not. Still others fall into a middle ground of "subsyndromal" depression. Electroencephalographic sleep findings in bereaved patients with depression resemble those in other elderly depressed patients, in terms of poor sleep continuity, enhanced measures of REM sleep, decreased slow-wave sleep, and short REM sleep latency. Nondepressed bereaved subjects have electroencephalographic sleep characteristics indistinguishable from those of healthy elderly subjects. Those with milder, subsyndromal depression during bereavement report subjectively disturbed sleep, but their electroencephalographic sleep profiles are similar to those of healthy subjects, with the exception of minor changes in slow-wave sleep.

Like older adults with bereavement-related depression, middle-aged adults who develop a reactive depression in the course of divorce are characterized by abnormal REM sleep findings, including short REM latency. Dream reports of such subjects, when collected in the sleep laboratory upon awakening from REM sleep, tend to be short, sparse in content, and dominated by themes of helplessness or victimization. In general, sleep after a mood-disturbing event, such as loss of a spouse through death or divorce, tends to be more disturbed among subjects with symptoms of depression (or a negative shift in "affect balance") and less disturbed among patients who do not experience depression.

Daniel J. Buysse
Charles F. Reynolds
David J. Kupfer

AGE

See Adolescence and Sleep; Aging and Circadian Rhythms; Aging and Sleep; Childhood, Sleep During; Children's Dreams; Development; Fetal Sleep-Wake Patterns; Infancy, Normal Sleep Patterns in; Infancy, Sleep Disorders in; Ontogeny; Premature Infants; Puberty

AGING AND CIRCADIAN RHYTHMS

The regular alternation of sleep and wakefulness is one of the most evident examples of circadian rhythmicity. With rare exceptions, we observe rhythms in a state of entrainment to the 24-hour variations of a variety of environmental factors, such as light, temperature, and social interactions, and this limits our ability to observe the function of the body's internal clock. Despite these constraints, a number of studies have consistently documented age-related changes in sleep rhythms (see also AGING AND SLEEP). These changes include (1) a decrease in the amplitude of entrained human sleep rhythms (more awakenings during the night and more naps during the day), (2) advanced phase of the sleep–wake rhythm (earlier bedtime and early-morning awakening; see ADVANCED SLEEP PHASE SYNDROME), and

(3) diminished entrainment (poor tolerance of jet lag and shift work). These changes in circadian sleep patterns may have important consequences; for example, nocturnal awakenings are frequently cited as a critical factor in the decision to institutionalize the elderly.

Observed changes in sleep pattern may reflect age-related changes in a variety of aspects of the circadian system. With age, changes may occur in the extent of exposure to ZEITGEBERS, or in the ability to perceive and respond to the zeitgebers. For example, the lifestyle and health of older persons might lessen or prevent exposure to outdoor sunlight. Alternatively, eye disease in an older person might diminish the entraining effects of light.

Several researchers have suggested that a fundamental alteration of the circadian clock itself may occur with age. A few heroic efforts have explored the function of the circadian clock in elderly human subjects, using "unmasking" protocols; however, much of our understanding of age-related changes of the circadian clock comes from animal studies.

Animal Models

Animal studies of age-related changes in circadian rhythms have been useful because a stringent degree of environmental control can be exerted for an extended time, allowing exploration of underlying circadian mechanisms. In most studies of the circadian clock, environmental conditions are held constant with the exception of a single variable, most often exposure to light. Differences between experimental groups are limited to the age of the subjects; similar housing, lighting, and feeding conditions are used for young and old animals. In rats, age-related changes in sleep rhythms have been measured that are similar in many respects to those reported to occur in humans. Several studies have documented decreases in the amplitude of entrained circadian rhythms of sleep (e.g., Rosenberg, Zepelin, and Rechtschaffen, 1979), with older animals sleeping relatively more during the active portion of the day and relatively less during the inactive portion. Decreases in the length of sleep episodes with age have also been reported.

Older animals also show a shift of the timing of

activity rhythms analogous to the shift to earlier bedtimes in humans. Young hamsters typically wait about 30 minutes after lights out to begin running-wheel activity and continue through the dark period. In contrast, old animals begin running-wheel activity prior to the time lights go out and end activity considerably before the lights come on.

Age-related changes in ability to reentrain following an abrupt phase shift of the light cycle have also been reported. Old rats require more time to adjust their sleep pattern to a 12-hour inversion of the light cycle than do young rats. In recent studies, old hamsters required significantly more time to adjust wheel-running rhythms to a delay of the light cycle (requiring them to "stay up late"), whereas an advance shift (requiring them to "go to bed early") was accomplished more quickly by the old hamsters than the young hamsters.

Changes in Zeitgebers

For many years, humans were thought to be insensitive to LIGHT as a zeitgeber; recent studies have demonstrated an important role for bright light in the entrainment of human sleep rhythms. Exposure to sunlight, however, may be minimal in the elderly, and 24-hour variation in light exposure in the elderly may be quite small as well. In humans, strong social time cues are removed with retirement, an event concurrent with reported increases of complaints of insomnia. Institutionalization frequently results in a further diminution of environmental stimulation of all types. Some results seem to indicate that age-related differences in temperature rhythms are minimal when variable exposure to environmental influences is controlled, suggesting that behavioral differences are an important component of the altered circadian profile (Monk, 1989). To date there has not been a systematic evaluation of the effects of changes in environmental stimuli on the aging circadian clock.

Recent studies have addressed the complex interactions between sleep, activity, and temperature rhythms that complicate interpretation of age-related changes in rhythms. Vigorous activity appears to increase the amplitude of entrained rhythms (Welsh, Richardson, and Dement, 1986), whereas restriction of activity (e.g., by forced bed rest) clearly reduces the amplitude of some rhythms. In general, older animals are less active than the young, and this chronic change in activity level may be responsible for some of the observed age-related decreases in sleep rhythm amplitude. In addition, stimuli that appear to affect the circadian clock via acute changes in activity level, such as benzodiazepines, are reported to be less effective in elderly animals. Sleep is fragmented when it occurs with elevated body temperature, and the amplitude of the entrained temperature rhythm is reduced and the phase advanced in the elderly. Therefore, early-morning arousals in the elderly may be a reflection of the earlier rise of body temperature caused by the phase advance.

Changes in the Response to Zeitgebers

In general, the elderly are not less sensitive to zeitgebers. In fact, some stimuli may be more effective in the elderly than in the young. The propensity for sound to cause arousal during sleep has been shown to be increased in elderly human subjects as compared with young adults. In a study of age group differences in the phase response curve, old animals retained the ability to respond to pulses of light with appropriate direction and magnitude shifts in the phase of their activity rhythms. Moreover, light pulses at certain circadian times, particularly those at the transition point of the PHASE RESPONSE CURVE between pulses causing advances and pulses causing delays, produced much larger phase shifts in old hamsters as compared with young hamsters. This increase in shift magnitude was interpreted as an age-related "instability" of the circadian system.

Age-Related Changes in the Circadian Clock

Perhaps the most compelling evidence of an age-related change in the circadian clock itself comes from observation of "free running" rhythms in the absence of zeitgebers. These studies are frequently complicated by the life history of the animals and "aftereffects" of lighting conditions that may persist for many months. Nevertheless, several authors using longitudinal as well as cross-sectional studies have reported that the period of the free-running locomotor activity rhythm, which is about 24.25 hours in young hamsters, grows shorter with advancing age, reaching a minimum of about 24.0 hours in animals over a year old (Pittendrigh and Daan, 1974; Morin, 1988). The period of the free-running sleep rhythm is also reported to be shortened with age in rats (van Gool, Witting, and Mirmiran, 1987). Data from studies of humans living in constant environmental regimes (see TEMPORAL ISOLATION) suggest that the period of the human circadian clock may also decrease with age.

Lesion, stimulation, and transplantation studies have localized the regulation of circadian rhythms to the SUPRACHIASMATIC NUCLEUS OF THE HYPOTHALAMUS. The overall population of neurons in this nucleus remains stable throughout the life span, but significant decreases in vasopressin-containing neurons may represent a histological correlate of observed changes in circadian rhythms. Additional studies are essential to provide an anatomical basis for observed circadian rhythm changes with age.

Implications for Human Sleep

To some extent, the age-related increase in complaints of insomnia may result from changes in the environment or in the ability to respond to time cues rather than from change in the clock itself. Efforts to increase the difference between night and day, such as a quieter sleeping environment, brighter lights during the day, and increased activity level, may reduce sleep fragmentation and daytime napping and restore more "youthful" circadian rhythms in older patients. Many elderly spend much of the day in bed and shut out potential entraining stimuli; sleep restriction therapy in the elderly may be successful in part by increasing the amount of environmental stimulation.

Some authors have minimized the effects of age-related changes in the circadian clock. Pittendrigh and Daan (1974) have observed that "there is no obvious functional meaning to the systematic increase of circadian frequency with age." The age-related decrease in period may drive the advance of sleep phase in the elderly, but in itself early-morning awakening is rarely sufficient to lead to a clinical complaint. Some authors argue that modification of the circadian

clock itself may be neither possible nor desirable, and that age-related changes of the clock compensate for age-related changes in other physiological systems, such as energy metabolism. Perhaps, as Webb (1978) has suggested, we should recognize, accept, and incorporate into our daily lives these age-related changes in sleep rhythms. On the basis of the available evidence, as we get older we should expect to go to bed earlier, awaken earlier, and require more time to adjust to jet travel.

(See also CIRCADIAN RHYTHMS.)

REFERENCES

Monk TH. 1989. Circadian rhythm. *Clin Geriatr Med* 5:331–346.

Morin LP. 1988. Age-related changes in hamster circadian period, entrainment, and rhythm splitting. *J Biol Rhythms* 3:237–248.

Pittendrigh CS, Daan S. 1974. Circadian oscillations in rodents: A systematic increase of their frequency with age. *Science* 186:548–550.

Rosenberg RS, Zepelin H, Rechtschaffen A. 1979. Sleep in young and old rats. *J Gerontol* 34:525–532.

van Gool WA, Witting W, Mirmiran M. 1987. Age-related changes in circadian sleep wakefulness rhythms in male rats isolated from time cues. *Brain Res* 413:384–387.

Webb WB. 1978. Sleep, biological rhythms and aging. In Samis HV, Capobianco S, eds. *Aging and biological rhythms*, pp 309–325. New York: Plenum.

Welsh DK, Richardson, GS, Dement WC. 1986. Effect of age on the circadian pattern of sleep and wakefulness in the mouse. *J Gerontol* 41:579–586.

Richard S. Rosenberg

AGING AND SLEEP

In both humans and animals, aging is accompanied by predictable changes in sleep. These changes have been well described, and they are equally important both in describing the aging process and in characterizing sleep. For example, many researchers have suggested that the aging process itself is characterized by a breakdown in the timing and coordination of various physiological processes within an organism. Many of the changes in sleep described below can be thought of as part of such an age-related temporal disorganization.

The question "When does aging begin?" is frequently asked. When discussing sleep, the answer depends very much on what aspect of sleep is at issue. For instance, decreases in stage 3 and 4 sleep probably are detectable in the twenties but lowered sleep efficiencies may not be detectable until the sixties.

Sleep Quality and Sleep Depth

The easiest way to study human age-related changes in sleep quality and depth is by questionnaire. Many such surveys have occurred over the last 30 years. The results are generally similar. As humans grow older, they experience frequent, disruptive nighttime awakenings. Often they have difficulty going to sleep as well. These changes show a steady increase from about age 40 on. Curiously, there is less agreement among studies concerning whether older persons also have increased difficulty falling asleep at the beginning of the night.

There are many reasons for the poorer-quality and lighter sleep accompanying aging. It is helpful to catergorize these as (1) external factors, (2) internal factors secondary to physical and psychological aspects of aging, and (3) internal factors unique to sleep. External factors include increased sensitivity of the older person's sleep to noise and disturbance from commonly used medications like antihypertensive drugs. Internal factors include not only physical illnesses such as arthritis and diabetes that are common in elderly persons and disrupt sleep, but also normal age-related events such as MENOPAUSE and frequent nocturnal urination (nocturia). Psychological factors including worries, anxieties, and feelings of sadness when a loved one has died, as so often happens in old age, may also play a role (see AFFECTIVE DISORDERS OTHER THAN MAJOR DEPRESSION). Finally, internal factors relating to the sleep process itself may lead to awakening during the night. The biological clock (see AGING AND CIRCADIAN RHYTHMS) may be set differently in older people so that they become sleepy early in the evening and wake up earlier in the morning than younger persons (Figure 1; see EARLY MORNING AWAKENING).

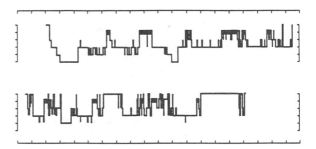

Figure 1. The progression of sleep stages. The progression of sleep stages across a single night in a representative young adult (top) and an elderly person (bottom). The lower recording illustrates the reduction of delta sleep, frequent spontaneous awakenings, and early morning awakenings that are characteristic features of sleep in the aged, even in the absence of specific medical or psychiatric disorders. Vertical axis from top to bottom: awake, REM, Stage 1, 2, 3, 4 NREM. (Reproduced, with permission, from Czeisler CA, Richardson GS, Martin JB. 1991. Disorders of sleep and circadian rhythms. In *Harrison's principles of internal medicine,* 12th ed, pp 209–217. New York: McGraw-Hill.)

This may be particularly true in older women. In addition, changes in the architecture of sleep, involving primarily alterations in the STAGES OF SLEEP, have been widely researched.

The primary changes in sleep architecture seen in aging are an increase in stage 1 sleep, a decrease in stage 3 and 4 sleep, a decrease in sleep efficiency, and an increase in brief arousals (Figure 1). Interestingly, REM sleep does not change appreciably across the adult life span, though some studies have suggested changes in REM sleep in dementia (see DEMENTIA). Stage 1 sleep is a transitional stage of sleep. Typically, it is scored when sleep lightens, and beginning at about ages 35 to 45, individuals can be observed to have relatively more of this stage of sleep. The decline in stage 3 and 4 sleep seen by the twenties may actually be one of the earliest biomarkers of aging within the brain. Specialized computerized measurements of the slow (delta) waves that make up stage 3 and 4 sleep have indicated that it is the size (i.e., amplitude) of the waves that decreases with age; for reasons that are not well understood, elderly women may have more stage 3 and 4 sleep than elderly men. Sleep efficiency is simply a percentage, it is the proportion of time in bed that the person actually spends asleep. In young adults without sleep problems, over 95 percent of the time spent in bed may be spent asleep. By the age of 65, a sleep efficiency of 80 percent or even lower is quite common. Brief arousals are very transient (typically 5 to 15 seconds): alterations in the electroencephalographic patterns occurring during sleep that typically disrupt the sleep of the older person and may occur after episodes of APNEA or PERIODIC LEG MOVEMENTS, or sometimes without any clear cause. All of these age-related changes in sleep architecture tend to result in a reduction of the quality and depth of sleep in older persons. Many of these age-related changes have been reported for other species as well, including mice, rats, hamsters, and cats.

Sleep Need

It is tempting to infer that if both sleep quality and DEPTH OF SLEEP deteriorate with aging the need for sleep must also decrease in elderly persons. This is a complicated issue, however, because there are many different ways to evaluate a "need" for sleep. One way involves the study of how much sleep adult humans typically obtain, that is, the so-called sleep quota. Another complementary approach is to study sleep after it has been restricted, that is, to study rebound effects.

Both questionnaire studies and polysomnographic studies indicate that older subjects sleep less at night than younger persons. Because sleep must be viewed as a function of both homeostatic and circadian processes (see FUNCTIONS OF SLEEP), however, the total amount of sleep over the entire 24-hour day should be taken into account when age-related changes in sleep quotas are discussed. In those few surveys that ask subjects about how much they sleep during the day and at night and compute a sum, the age-related decline in sleep amount is much less pronounced. Such surveys about NAPPING and daytime sleep may still be inaccurate, however, because in many cultures individuals may be unwilling to admit to napping, SLEEPINESS, or tiredness. Additionally, in many elderly persons (who are typically retired), napping may reflect excess leisure time rather than a biological need for sleep during the day. In fact, physiological evidence that the need for sleep may not decline with aging has been shown in several studies that have examined daytime alertness in the elderly with physiological measures. For example, some studies with the MULTIPLE SLEEP LATENCY TEST have shown elderly persons to be more physiologically sleepy than younger persons during daytime hours. Other evidence for this increased biological sleepiness in old age is provided by studies of pupillometry showing that elderly persons have a sluggish response to bright light in their pupils. Finally, many studies show decreases in reaction time in old age. For example, elderly persons take more time in responding to sound, light, or touch than younger persons. All of these studies indicate that during the daytime, elderly persons are simply less alert than younger persons. These results also imply that the need for sleep is just as strong in old age but that there is a redistribution of sleep more evenly across the 24-hour day.

Studies of aged animals offer some corroboration for these patterns. Obviously, in animals sleep quotas are unaffected by the social and cultural factors influencing humans. In both rats and mice, aged animals show this redistribution of sleep around the 24-hour day without a net change in sleep amount. These results again suggest no decline of sleep need. They also confirm the importance of animal research in general in helping to understand what happens to sleep in humans as we age. (See ANIMALS IN SLEEP RESEARCH.)

Another way of looking at the need for sleep is to examine what happens when sleep is lost (i.e., when sleep DEPRIVATION occurs). Presumably, one might infer that the same need for sleep exists in young and old persons if they both react the same way to being deprived of sleep. Several studies have examined these effects. Older persons tend to sleep somewhat longer and deeper (increased stages 3 and 4) after losing sleep than before sleep deprivation. These changes appear similar to what happens in younger adults; however, younger persons continue to sleep more deeply on the second and third nights after sleep deprivation. Older people show this pattern only on the initial night. Furthermore, when the effects of sleep deprivation on waking performance are considered, the results suggest that elderly persons may be less affected by loss of sleep than are younger persons. Thus, the sleep deprivation studies afford evidence that the need or drive to sleep is still present, though modified somewhat, in old age.

Sleep Pathologies: Sleep Apnea and Nocturnal Myoclonus

Over the last 10 years, researchers have learned that both sleep APNEA and nocturnal myoclonus (see PERIODIC MOVEMENTS IN SLEEP) are very common in old age. It is important to point out that, although these conditions may necessitate an evaluation by an expert in sleep disorders medicine, many elderly persons show mild levels of both sleep apnea and nocturnal myoclonus that probably are not harmful. In addition, in the case of sleep apnea, there is some evidence that different mechanisms may be involved in older persons. The discrimination of a mild, age-related change from a severe, clinically important disease must be made by a specialist. Suffice it to say that this differentiation of normality versus disease has been the subject of often intense debate among specialists in the field and is the focus of many research studies.

REFERENCES

Bliwise DL. 1989. Normal aging. In Kryger MH, Roth T, Dement WC, eds. *Principles and practice of sleep medicine,* pp 24–29. Philadelphia: Saunders.

Kuna ST, Remmers JE, Suratt PM, eds. 1991. *Sleep and respiration in aging adults.* New York: Elsevier.

Morgan K. 1987. *Sleep and aging: A research based guide to sleep in later life.* Baltimore: Johns Hopkins University Press.

Prinz PN, Vitiello MV, Raskind MA, Thorpy MJ. 1990. Geriatrics: Sleep disorders and aging. *N Engl J Med* 323:520–526.

Richardson GS. 1990. Circadian rhythms and aging. In Schneider EL, Rowe JW, eds. *Handbook of the biology of aging,* 3rd ed, pp 275–305. San Diego: Academic.

Samis HV, Capobianco S. 1978. *Aging and biological rhythms.* New York: Plenum.

The treatment of sleep disorders of older people. 1990. NIH Consensus Development Conference, March 26–28, 1990, Vol 8, No 3. U.S. Dept of Health and Human Services, Office of Medical Applications of Research. Building 1, Room 260, Bethesda, MD 20892. Videotape.

Donald L. Bliwise

AIDS AND SLEEP

Acquired immunodeficiency syndrome (AIDS) is caused by the human immunodeficiency virus (HIV). When a person has been infected with HIV, a blood test will be positive for antibodies to the virus well before any symptoms of disease appear. A person with a positive blood test is said to be HIV-seropositive (HIV+). AIDS occurs when the virus has compromised the immune system of an HIV+ person to the point that a variety of microorganisms, which the immune system normally prevents from causing disease, instigate serious and often fatal illnesses.

Because sleep is a function of the CENTRAL NERVOUS SYSTEM (CNS), it is especially important to understand that the CNS is an early target of this virus. On interaction of HIV with the CNS, neurological symptoms are often the first symptoms of AIDS to appear; however, changes in sleep may precede even the first neurological symptoms of AIDS. As the disease progresses, sleep continues to deteriorate. Changes in sleep are particularly interesting and important because they provide a window through which we may see early and subtle responses of the CNS and immune system to HIV infection. Analyzing the quality of sleep can help to evaluate the effectiveness of treatments for people who are HIV+ or have AIDS. In addition, understanding the effect of HIV infection on sleep can provide insights about how the immune system responds to viruses and infections and how that response is related to sleep (see IMMUNE FUNCTION).

Human Immunodeficiency Virus Infection

Sleep Structure

Systematic studies seeking to understand the effect of HIV infection and AIDS on sleep began appearing in the late 1980s. Norman and her colleagues (1990) were the first to describe a group of HIV+ people with no symptoms of AIDS who had changes in their sleep structure. They found an increase in SLOW-WAVE SLEEP (SWS) (stage 3 and 4 sleep) later in the night than is usual. This increase in SWS is exactly opposite what would be expected from the mood changes likely to follow a positive HIV test (see ANXIETY; DEPRESSION). Other sleep abnormalities Norman et al.

found included increased fragmentation of sleep and the appearance of increased alpha frequencies (8 to 12 Hz) in NREM sleep (see ALPHA–DELTA SLEEP). Both of these abnormalities reduce the quality of a night's sleep. Increased sleep FRAGMENTATION has been associated with a decrease in SWS, so the presence of fragmentation in combination with increased SWS in HIV+ people is an unusual and important finding. Figure 1 shows the difference in the amount and distribution of stages 3 and 4 between an HIV-negative subject and an HIV-infected subject. One proposed explanation is related to the immune system factor interleukin, which is released when the immune system is activated. Krueger and colleagues (1984) have shown that giving interleukin-1 to animals results in an increase in their slow-wave sleep. Norman and colleagues (1990) reasoned that a similar increase in interleukin in HIV+ people might account for their extra slow-wave sleep. This hypothesis remains to be tested.

Sleep Complaints and Sleep Habits

Nine of ten subjects in the Norman study reported a subjective problem with sleep. In a larger survey, Rothenberg and colleagues (1990) found that about one third of 68 HIV+ men and women who had no symptoms of AIDS had a current sleep problem. This proportion of sleep problems is comparable to the frequency of sleep disturbances in the general population. Thus it appears that being infected with HIV may be associated with a complaint about sleep, but the frequency of those complaints may not be any higher than for the population as a whole. In the Rothenberg sample, sleep habits, including the time of going to bed, the time of waking up, and the estimated total time slept per night, were also comparable to those in the general population of the same age.

Rothenberg and colleagues also looked at the relationship between immune system integrity in HIV+ people and their sleep complaints. A primary immune measure for severity of HIV infection is the concentration of helper T lymphocytes (CD4+ cells) in the blood. As HIV infection progresses to AIDS, the number of CD4+ cells decreases. When CD4+ cells were measured in twenty HIV+ people who had a current sleep complaint, it was found that the lower their immune cell (CD4+) levels, the more sleep problems they had. This finding supports the conclusion that deterioration of the immune system is associated with progressive decreases in the quality of sleep.

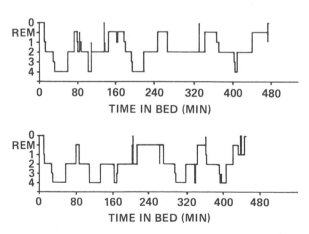

Figure 1. Comparison of normal sleep hypnogram from an HIV-negative subject (top) with the hypnogram from an HIV-infected but otherwise healthy subject (bottom). Note the increase in slow-wave sleep and its placement later in the night in the HIV-infected subject. *Reprinted with permission from Norman S, Chediak A, Kiel M, Cohn M. 1990. Sleep disturbances in HIV-infected homosexual men.* AIDS 4:775–781.

AIDS

Unfortunately, when AIDS progresses, CNS pathology is not restricted to any particular region. Neuron destruction, tumors, and infections have been found in widespread CNS locations. It is not surprising, therefore, that sleep is severely disrupted when HIV infection progresses to the point of AIDS. Kubicki and colleagues (1988) reported several sleep structure abnormalities in people with AIDS, including reduced stage 3, stage 4, and REM sleep, increased time in stage 1 sleep, increased number of arousals, increased time awake, and reduced numbers of SLEEP SPINDLES and K-COMPLEXES. Kubicki and colleagues attributed many of these changes in sleep and waking to brain infection, HIV encephalitis (see ENCEPHALITIS), and destruction related to the patients' other opportunistic diseases. Because the CNS damage was so widespread in these subjects, Kubicki et al. (1989) could not attribute specific changes in sleep structure to specific, damaged areas of the brain.

Conclusions

These studies suggest that the body's early response to HIV infection includes a change in sleep structure that precedes subjective sleep complaints as well as symptoms of AIDS. As the immune system becomes increasingly compromised and AIDS develops, the original response to the infection can no longer be mounted by the immune system and the CNS. HIV infection and opportunistic diseases in people with AIDS lead to severely distorted sleep structure, reversing the earlier increase in slow-wave sleep and causing large increases in wakefulness during the night.

REFERENCES

Krueger J, Walter J, Dinarello C, Wolff S, Chedid L. 1984. Sleep-promoting effects of endogenous pyrogen (interleukin-1). *Am J Physiol* 246:R994–R999.

Kubicki S, Henkes H, Alm D, Scheuler W, Pohle H, Ruf B, Konneke J. 1989. [Polygraphic sleep data in AIDS patients]. *Electroencephalogr Electromyogr* 20: 288–94. Largest sleep study of AIDS patients. In German with English abstract.

Kubicki S, Henkes H, Terstegge K, Ruf B. 1988. AIDS related sleep disturbances—A preliminary report. In Kubicki S et al, eds. *HIV and the nervous system,* pp 97–105. Stuttgart/New York: Fischer-Verlag.

Norman S, Chediak A, Kiel M, Cohn M. 1990. Sleep disturbances in HIV-infected homosexual men. *AIDS* 4:775–781.

Rothenberg S, Zozula R, Funesti J, McAuliffe V. 1990. Sleep habits in asymptomatic HIV-seropositive individuals. *Sleep Res* 19:342.

Saul Rothenberg

ALARM CLOCKS

Time consciousness has dogged humanity since ancient bone calendars tracked agricultural and game-hunting seasons 10,000 years ago and is perhaps best represented in Western industrialized society by that small tyrant and icon of popular culture, the alarm clock. Time tracking is now a particularly urban concern; to many of today's societies, a clock without an alarm may seem only partly functional. In much of the United States, the alarm clock is ubiquitous.

Standardized timekeeping crept slowly into the fabric of early society. Evidence of crude sundials in the Middle East dates back more than 4,000 years ago; a 24-hour day was adopted in Egypt by about 100 B.C. Successive developments, including nocturnal timekeeping measures, were stimulated by the demands of the cultural context and expanding knowledge of the world. When the sun went down, the Egyptians counted time intervals by burning measured ropes, the Chinese by burning segmented pipes of gunpowder; King Alfred the Great popularized banded candles for the same purpose in late ninth-century Wessex. Greek and Arabian astrolabes enabled early astronomers to track the regular movements of celestial bodies; sandglasses emerged from the ancient Middle East as hourglasses in fourteenth-century Europe. In 1400 B.C., the Egyptians used water-dripping clocks; the Greco-Roman water clock, or clepsydra, is thought to have included alarm-striking mechanisms.

Early measurement techniques were often motivated by the need to alert people at required times for various religious duties—in particular, the monks and priests of medieval Europe. Rural abbeys of the Benedictine order scheduled several prayer periods per day, including nocturns at night and matins before dawn, and they relied upon a water clock to trigger an alarm for the sacristan, or designated waker, who then rang bells to rouse everyone else in the monastery. Such time consciousness and discipline were considered crucial to salvation and the survival of the Christian Church (Landes, 1985).

Mechanical clocks originated in the Far East as early as the second century A.D.; subsequent Chinese horological history shows that timekeeping was monopolized by the imperial court. The greatest of royal Chinese clocks was a water-clock tower constructed by Su Sung in A.D. 1090, which featured striking gong alarms to signal hours, quarters, and night watchmen's shifts. Chinese timekeeping technology regressed, however, after invasions and war subsequent to the eleventh century, enabling seafaring Europeans of the late 1700s to bribe the Celestial Court for trading privileges with a gift of chiming alarm clocks (Landes, 1985).

The first personal alarm clock may have been

no more than a simple mirror angled to direct the rays of the rising sun at the eyes of the sleeper. Although chamber clocks probably developed around the same time as larger-scale turret clocks in the late medieval period, a clockmaker of seventeenth-century Concord, New Hampshire, is credited with one of the earliest documented alarm clocks. Inspired by his work ethic to rise at 4:00 A.M., resist laziness, and avoid oversleeping, Levi Hutchins rigged a bell inside one of his clocks to ring at a specific hour. He never patented his invention, so his only profit was being awakened on time for the next 68 years (Garrison, 1977). United States patent records show that subsequent inventors better realized the potential commercial appeal of their products. In 1882, Samuel Applegate's alarm bed dropped sixty corks on a sleeper's head; in 1900, Ludwig Ederer's device tilted the bed upright until the sleeper fell out (Grout, 1991). Of all stylish, fanciful, or imaginative timepieces, however, the best combination of form and function with humor may be the baseball-shaped alarm clock that doesn't shut off until thrown against the wall (Morris, 1989). It is questionable whether a market exists for the "ultimate" alarm clock patented in 1991, which reportedly estimates how much time one has left to live (Andrews, 1991)!

Consumers Union, a national product-rating organization, has evaluated the alarm clock radio as an able contender in the morning race against time. Cost is not correlated with reliability of noise output at the chosen arousal point, only with better radio sound and a greater number of convenient alarm-related controls and features. Advantages include display legibility, ease of alarm setting, choice of radio or buzzer with adjustable volume, a "drowse" or "snooze" option for brief sleep extension, and double-alarm setting for bedmates with different rise times ("Clock radios," 1990). Particularly high marks are given if the alarm volume automatically starts low and then increases, presumably lessening the shock of waking abruptly to a loud noise.

Researchers have demonstrated that human auditory AROUSAL thresholds vary with such factors as sleep stage, age, and sex (Zepelin, McDonald, and Zammit, 1984). Alarm clock inventors through the ages have been forced to consider the fact that perception in all sensory domains is markedly reduced in sleep (see PER-CEPTION DURING SLEEP; SENSORY PROCESSING AND SENSATION DURING SLEEP). Devices designed for the deaf or hard-of-hearing shake the bed, vibrate the pillow, or flash lights; those for the blind use Braille numbers, hands accessible to touch, or a speech synthesizer to announce the time. Alarm clocks invented in Japan are purported to work by releasing an invigorating scent for about 10 minutes until the sense of smell is stimulated enough to arouse the sleeper (Gordon, 1992). Scientific evidence, however, indicates that olfactory sensitivity is low during REM sleep, is lower still in stage 4 of NREM sleep, and results in very few arousals even from stage 2 of NREM sleep (Carskadon et al., 1990). Decreased responsivity to smell in the middle and later hours of night does not suggest much promise for the olfactory alarm clock (Badia, Boecker, and Lammers, 1991; see also SMELL DURING SLEEP).

Several inventions have recast early methods of timekeeping in newer technology, resulting in greater accuracy and utility, and the alarm clock is no exception to this trend. The rooster, a reliable rouser for centuries, was transformed by craftsmen of the Black Forest around 1775 into the ever-popular cuckoo clock, which featured carved wooden gears and decorations. A more sophisticated alarm, the microelectronic Prayer Times Clock, charts astronomical movements, enabling accurate Muslim observance of five daily prayers anywhere in the world; when programmed with a traveler's latitude and longitude, this invention sounds an alarm 5 minutes before and at the appropriate time, also indicating the specific prayer and the direction of Mecca ("Technology," 1987).

Has the alarm clock finally come of age? In later childhood and adolescence, puberty contributes to increased sleep need, and parents are often forced to assume the role of alarm clock by dragging their sleepy teenagers out of bed (Carskadon, 1990). Taking responsibility for waking oneself, or at least for setting the alarm, may be seen as one of the hallmarks of adulthood (see ADOLESCENCE AND SLEEP). With the renewed popularity of the wake-up call, the effort to "rise and shine" has again become an interpersonal event. Once a convenience previously known primarily to travelers in hotels and motels, wake-up calls have been offered to clinicians by their answering services in California, to students at Stanford University in the 1980s, and to sleepyheads across the nation by wake-up call agencies advertising a toll-free telephone number on television.

At Brown University, longitudinal surveys of sleep habits from high school through college indicate that waking up *without* an alarm clock becomes even less likely when teenagers leave home. Self-reported alarm clock dependency on weekdays increased from 71 percent of students surveyed in their final semester of high school to 81 percent of those responding in their first semester of college, and increased again to 84 percent of respondents in their second semester of college (Carskadon et al., unpublished data)—not too surprising, since these surveys indicate that a phase delay of approximately 2 hours occurred in a majority of students across the transition from high school to college (Carskadon and Davis, 1989). Predictably, self-reported dependence on alarm clocks for rising on weekends was significantly lower (15 percent, 17 percent, and 31 percent of respondents, respectively).

The real value of a clock or watch once had as much to do with the jewels inside as out, but many timepieces nowadays are inexpensive, even disposable—precious time itself is the commodity. Academic or work requirements drive activity in the early hours of the day, while desires for family time or entertainment promote a night life, and sleep is squeezed to a minimum, with the alarm clock serving as primary coordinator and whip-cracker. Stress is perhaps the most commonly cited complaint in modern society; researchers have associated anxiety with more frequent sleep complaints, including insomnia and excessive daytime sleepiness (Hirshkowitz et al., 1990) (see INSOMNIA; SLEEPINESS; ANXIETY; PSYCHOPATHOLOGY, NONDEPRESSION). Demands on one's time and energy set up a cycle of late hours, insufficient sleep, and serious sleep–wake disruption, including the sleep-disturbing side effects of self-medication with ALCOHOL, CAFFEINE, NICOTINE, or SLEEPING PILLS. As periods of work and activity move around the clock, the alarm clock's domain expands from the wee hours of morning to the entire 24-hour cycle to combat the forces of sleepiness, impaired sleep efficiency, rotating schedules, and NAPPING attendant on SHIFTWORK. The snooze button has become a universal joke as dependence on the alarm clock has become a fact of life.

(See also INTERNAL ALARM CLOCK.)

REFERENCES

Andrews S. 1991. Clock with a difference. *New York Times,* 13 July, pp 18 ff.

Badia P, Boecker M, Lammers W. 1991. Some effects of different olfactory stimuli on sleep. *Sleep Res* 19:145.

Carskadon MA. 1990. Patterns of sleep and sleepiness in adolescents. *Pediatrician* 17:5–12.

Carskadon MA, Bigler PJ, Carr J, Gelin J, Etgen G, Davis SS, Herman KB. 1990. Olfactory arousal thresholds during sleep. *Sleep Res* 19:147.

Carskadon MA, Davis SS. 1989. Sleep-wake patterns in the high-school-to-college transition: Preliminary data. *Sleep Res* 18:113.

Clock radios. 1990. *Consumer Reports* 55(12): 325–327.

Garrison W. 1977. *Why didn't I think of that?* Englewood Cliffs, N.J.: Prentice-Hall.

Gordon J. 1992. Beauty word of mouth: An alternative to your clock radio. *Glamour,* March, p 79.

Grout P. 1991. Made in America: Patently eccentric. *Amtrak Express* 11(7):30.

Hirshkowitz M, Hamilton CR III, Rando KC, Bellamy M, Williams RL, Karacan I. 1990. State-trait anxiety scores in adults with sleep complaints. *Sleep Res* 19:163.

Landes DS. 1985. *Revolution in time: Clocks and the making of the modern world.* Cambridge, Mass.: Harvard University Press.

Morris S. 1989. Clock facelifts. *Omni,* July, pp 90–92.

Technology: Beeping the faith. 1987. *Sci Am,* March, p 74.

Zepelin H, McDonald CS, Zammit GK. 1984. Effects of age on auditory awakening thresholds. *J Gerontol* 39:294–300.

Kate B. Herman

ALCOHOL

Ethyl alcohol (ethanol) is a small fat- and water-soluble molecule that is rapidly and completely absorbed from the whole gastrointestinal tract and is evenly distributed throughout all body fluids and tissues, including the brain (Ritchie, 1975). The rate of absorption is modified by the concentration of the ethanol beverage (beer at 3 percent to 6 percent ethanol is slower than whiskey at 40 percent to 45 percent), stomach contents (an empty stomach facilitates absorption), and rate of consumption. Because ethanol is distributed by the water content of tissue, a more muscular person will have lower levels of ethanol in blood than a fat person given the same dose of ethanol based on body weight. Ethanol is metabolized by the liver into carbon dioxide and water at a constant rate of about 10 to 15 milligram percent per hour (1 ounce of 80-proof whiskey, 12 ounces of beer, or 4 ounces of wine is metabolized in an hour).

As with other psychoactive substances, ethanol has profound effects on sleep and wakefulness. It is considered a sedative, but its effects on waking and sleep are complex and somewhat paradoxical. The acute bedtime administration of ethanol to normal nonalcoholic volunteers shortens the latency to sleep onset and, depending on dose, may initially increase the amount of deep slow-wave sleep (Williams and Salamy, 1972). Additionally, ethanol reduces the amount of REM sleep. An ethanol concentration in blood of 50 milligram percent (100 milligram percent is legal intoxication in most states) or greater is necessary to observe these sleep effects. Typically, the sleep effects of ethanol are observed only during the first half of an 8-hour sleep period. Ethanol is metabolized at a constant rate as noted above; consequently, the usual dose of ethanol (50 to 90 milligram percent) given in these studies is almost completely eliminated from the body after 4 or 5 hours.

After elimination of ethanol, an apparent compensatory effect on sleep occurs. During the latter half of the sleep period, an increased amount of REM sleep and increased wakefulness or light sleep are found (Williams and Salamy, 1972). Within three to four nights of repeated administration of the same dose, the initial effects on sleep are lost (technically referred to as tolerance), whereas the secondary disruption of sleep during the latter half of the night remains. REM sleep time and sleep latency return to their basal levels and effects on slow-wave sleep, if initially present, do not persist. When nightly administration of ethanol is discontinued, increased amounts of REM sleep (termed a *REM rebound*) are found, lasting for several nights. But the finding of a REM rebound after repeated nightly ethanol administration in healthy, nonalcoholic normals has not been a particularly consistent result (Vogel et al., 1990). It has been argued that the presence of a REM rebound is a characteristic of drugs with a high addictive potential. For other drugs, including morphine, BARBITURATES, and

AMPHETAMINES, the data regarding a REM rebound after repeated use are stronger.

When administered to awake nonalcoholic volunteers, ethanol has also been shown to be sedating (Roehrs, Zwyghuizen-Doorenbos, and Roth, 1990). The sedating effect has been clearly demonstrated after blood ethanol concentration (BEC) has reached a peak of 40 milligram percent or greater. On repeated tests of the latency of falling asleep during the day (see MULTIPLE SLEEP LATENCY TEST), a systematic dose-related reduction in latency to sleep onset is found. Performance tasks sensitive to sedation also are disrupted by ethanol (Mello and Mendelson, 1978). At lower ethanol concentrations and immediately after ethanol consumption when ethanol is still being absorbed, sedative effects are not as clearly evident. Subjectively, some individuals report increased arousal and euphoria, although the electroencephalographic studies have found electroencephalogram patterns suggestive of a sedative effect. The effects of ethanol typically have been characterized as biphasic (Pohorecky, 1977). At low doses and during absorption, ethanol appears to be arousing, and at high doses and during elimination, it is sedating. Some data suggest these subjective arousing effects to ethanol may be individually specific effects associated with genetic or personality-based factors.

Given the sedative effects of ethanol and its potential to disrupt performance, it is not surprising that epidemiological data indicate ethanol is associated with increased risk of industrial and traffic accidents. The National Highway Traffic Safety Administration estimated that 49 percent of all traffic fatalities in 1989 were alcohol related (i.e., a police report indicated that one or more drivers had ethanol concentrations of 10 milligram percent or more), which is a slight decline from the percentages of previous years (U.S. Department of Transportation, 1990). Assessment of the timing of the alcohol-related accidents across the 24-hour day showed alcohol-related accidents were more prevalent during the nighttime (between midnight and 6 A.M.) than the daytime. The age group showing the highest rate of alcohol-related accidents while legally intoxicated was 20-to 25-year-olds. In both cases, during the nighttime and in young adults laboratory evidence shows increased levels of sleepiness and reduced alertness (Roth et al., 1989). Thus, the epidemiological data regarding the temporal distribution and the age group distribution of alcohol-related accidents suggest that ethanol and sleepiness interact to increase the risk of alcohol-related accidents.

Recent laboratory studies provide clear evidence of a sleepiness–ethanol interaction (Roth, Roehrs, and Merlotti, 1990). Reducing bed time increases sleepiness throughout the following day. The sedative and performance disruptive effects of ethanol are enhanced when sleepiness is increased in such a way. Three drinks become the functional equivalent of six drinks after 5 hours in bed for five nights. Conversely, an extension of bed time enhances alertness (reduces sleepiness) and reduces the sedative and performance disruptive effects of ethanol. After six nights of 10 hours in bed, a moderate dose of ethanol (about four drinks producing a BEC of 50 milligram percent), which disrupted performance and increased sleep latency after a usual 8-hour bed time, no longer does so. Additionally, the same moderate ethanol dose given over the midday, when sleepiness is enhanced in most individuals, is performance disruptive, whereas that same dose in the early evening, when alertness is at a peak, has no measurable effect. Finally, after the same 8 hours of bed time, sleepy individuals perform more poorly and have greater sleepiness when given ethanol than do their alert counterparts.

The specific mechanism by which ethanol produces sedative effects is not yet known. Ethanol is known to affect the brain in two major ways (Hoffman and Tabakoff, 1988). It has long been known that ethanol (being fat soluble) alters the structure of the neuronal membrane and thereby can have broad effects on the function of the neuron, altering ion flow across the membrane and also potentially disturbing neurotransmitter receptor functions. Ethanol also has been shown to alter the function of nearly all neurotransmitter systems in various other ways.

Two transmitter systems, gamma-aminobutyric acid (GABA) and glutamate, have received much recent attention because the ethanol effects on these systems are observed at very low ethanol doses. Importantly, these two systems are implicated in control of sleep and wakefulness. GABA is a major inhibitory system in the brain, and ethanol has been shown to facilitate GABA function. Glutamate is a major excitatory system, and ethanol has been shown to inhibit activation of this system. Thus ethanol sedation may result from enhancement of GABA inhibition and antagonism of glutamate excitation (See also CHEMISTRY OF SLEEP.)

REFERENCES

Hoffman PL, Tabakoff B. 1988. Ethanol's action on brain biochemistry. In Tarter RE, Van Thiel DH, eds. *Alcohol and the brain,* pp 19–68. New York: Plenum Medical.

Mello NK, Mendelson JH. 1978. Alcohol and human behavior. In Iversen LL, Iversen SD, Snyder SH, eds. *Handbook of pharmacology drugs of abuse,* vol 12, pp 235–317. New York: Plenum Press.

Pohorecky LA. 1977. Biphasic action of ethanol. *Biobehav Rev* 1:231–240.

Ritchie JM. 1975. The aliphatic alcohols. In Goodman LG, Gilman A, eds. *The pharmacological basis of therapeutics,* pp 137–151. New York: Macmillan.

Roehrs T, Zwyghuizen-Doorenbos A, Roth T. 1990. Residual sedating effects of ethanol. In Perrine MW, ed. *Alcohol, drugs & traffic safety,* pp 157–163. Chicago: National Safety Council.

Roth T, Roehrs T, Carskadon MA, Dement WC. 1989. Daytime sleepiness and alertness. In Kryger MH, Roth T, Dement WC, eds. *Principles and practice of sleep medicine,* pp 14–23. Philadelphia: Saunders.

Roth T, Roehrs T, Merlotti L. 1990. Ethanol and daytime sleepiness. *Alcohol Drugs Driving* 6: 357–362.

U.S. Department of Transportation. 1990. *National Highway Traffic Safety Administration General Estimates System 1989 report.* Washington, DC: U.S. Govt. Printing Office. DOT HS 807 665.

Vogel GW, Buffenstein A, Minter K, Hennessey A. 1990. Drug effects on REM sleep and on endogenous depression. *Neurosci Biobehav Rev* 14: 49–63.

Williams H, Salamy A. 1972. Alcohol and sleep. In Kissin B, Begleiter H, eds. *The biology of alcoholism,* vol 2, pp 435–483. New York: Plenum.

Timothy A. Roebrs

ALCOHOLISM

Alcoholism is a psychiatric disorder characterized by a compulsive use of ALCOHOL that dominates the patient's life. Normal role functions are lost; cognitive and neurological impairment may result; there is frequent alienation from families, friends and employers; there is a marked tendency to relapse. The disease is progressive and is not secondary to an abnormal childhood environment or abnormal development of the personality. Many risk factors contribute to the prevalence of alcoholism, such as availability of alcoholic beverages, cultural acceptance of intoxicated behavior, and strength of the patient's family and occupational identity.

Sleep may or may not be disturbed in the course of alcoholism. Alcoholics in the early and middle stages (that is, before the loss of significant occupational and social identity has occurred) frequently report that alcohol allows them to sleep fairly normally. As alcoholism progresses, sleep disturbance is characterized by profoundly increasing fragmentation of REM sleep, and eventually REM sleep suppression becomes marked. In early abstinence after heavy drinking periods, the alcoholic person will usually experience a REM sleep REBOUND. Low REM sleep time during abstinence may be associated with cognitive impairment secondary to the direct toxic effects of alcohol on the brain. SLOW-WAVE SLEEP may or may not recover during abstinence periods. Alcoholics observed for as long as 2 years show continuing reduction or absence of slow-wave sleep. Alcoholism can result in prolonged fragmentation of REM sleep by intervals of stage 1 sleep (see STAGES OF SLEEP) and waking. The electromyogram (EMG) can remain active in REM sleep—rather than suppressed as is normal—during recovery periods. Alcohol has a now well-known effect on ventilation during sleep, and alcoholic patients are particularly prone to the development of sleep APNEA syndromes; the breathing of alcoholics during sleep can remain abnormal even with prolonged abstinence. The BODY TEMPERATURE cycle (see also THERMOREGULATION) is affected by alcohol; characteristically, alcohol causes a lower body temperature during the initial part of the night followed by higher-than-normal body temperature in the second half of the night. This phenomenon has not been adequately explored in the sleep of alcoholic patients. During recovery, alcoholics frequently show short REM LATENCY, which may or may not be associated with symptoms of DEPRESSION.

Alcoholism probably results in a dysregulation of serotonin and of serotonin's function in REM sleep regulation (see CHEMISTRY OF SLEEP: AMINES AND OTHER TRANSMITTERS). Alcoholic patients without slow-wave sleep in recovery periods frequently show low levels of serotonin metabolites in their cerebrospinal fluid. Furthermore, acute alcohol administration to alcoholics causes decrements in serotonin metabolite and its second messenger (i.e., the active substance produced within the neuron in response to serotonin), cyclic AMP.

Alcoholics in recovery have a high prevalence of sleep disorders, including hypersomnolence (see HYPERSOMNIA). The sleep apnea syndromes and PERIODIC LEG MOVEMENTS must be evaluated if the patient's sleep continues disturbed after the first month of recovery.

It is yet to be determined whether the sleep abnormalities that persist in prolonged abstinence periods in alcoholic patients are associated with relapse. Recent evidence indicates that the REM sleep disturbances may be associated with relapse. Failure to recover slow-wave sleep may be associated with cognitive impairment and thereby indirectly with relapse.

REFERENCES

Thompson WL. 1978. Management of alcohol withdrawal syndromes. *Arch Intern Med* 138:278–283.
Zarcone VP Jr. 1983. Sleep in alcoholism. In Chase MH, Weitzman ED, eds. *Advances in sleep research*. vol 8: *Sleep disorders: Basic and clinical research*. Flushing, N.Y.: SP Medical and Scientific Books.

Vincent P. Zarcone, Jr.

ALERTNESS

[*Although alertness is often considered as the opposite end on a continuum from* SLEEPINESS, *alertness may be a unique psychological dimension with important functional consequences. For example, the most common measure of physiological sleepiness, the* MULTIPLE SLEEP LATENCY TEST *(MSLT), does not necessarily always indicate an individual's level of alertness. Alertness in this context may be more directly assessed using a measure called the Maintenance of Wakefulness Test (MWT), in which the person is required to remain sit-*

ting quietly, but to stay awake, for 40 minutes at several 2-hour intervals across a day. In general, results of these two measures are well correlated; in certain individuals, however, the MSLT can show a very high level of sleepiness while the MWT simultaneously indicates a high degree of alertness. Thus, the distinction between alertness and sleepiness is not always clear-cut.

Nevertheless, most of the disorders of excessive sleepiness, or HYPERSOMNIA—*such as* NARCOLEPSY *and sleep* APNEA *syndrome—are associated with impaired alertness along with excessive sleepiness. Other conditions associated with severe sleepiness are also inevitably associated with impaired alertness, such as certain* CIRCADIAN RHYTHM DISORDERS, *sleep* DEPRIVATION, *and* JET LAG.

The brain mechanisms controlling alertness may be neurochemical (see CHEMISTRY OF SLEEP*), and many chemical compounds certainly affect alertness.* STIMULANTS, *including* OVER-THE-COUNTER STIMULANTS, AMPHETAMINES, NICOTINE, CAFFEINE *and so forth, are noted for their ability to increase alertness. Other compounds, such as* ALCOHOL, SLEEPING PILLS, ANTIHISTAMINES, *and* TRANQUILIZERS, *tend to decrease alertness and also to increase sleepiness.*]

ALLERGIES

Acquired hypersensitivities to contact with ordinarily harmless substances are known as *allergies*. The substances, called allergens, are usually common ones such as pollen or dust, and contact is usually with the skin, gastrointestinal tract, or respiratory system. The hypersensitivity reaction can vary from a mild rash or a sneeze to the complete life-threatening collapse of anaphylactic shock.

Allergies are the product of an overzealous immune system. Upon initial contact with an allergy-causing substance (a new pillow containing goose feathers, for example), specialized immune system cells, or lymphocytes, in the bloodstream create molecules called antibodies that are capable of recognizing and locking onto the goose feather molecules just as they would attach to a truly harmful substance such as a virus. These antibody molecules are stationed like sen-

tries on the surface of *mast cells,* which are located throughout the body but are especially common in skin and mucus membranes. Days, weeks, or even years later, new exposure to goose feathers will cause the sensitized mast cells to emit histamine, a substance responsible for the symptoms of swelling and redness associated with inflammation, as well as for narrowing of the air passages in the lungs and increased secretion of acid in the stomach.

The common mechanisms are the basis for the similarity of the symptoms of allergies to those of infectious diseases. Perhaps the most common manifestation of allergy is allergic rhinitis, or hay fever, consisting of sniffling, sneezing, nasal congestion, and feelings of tiredness that mimic a cold or the flu. Increased daytime sleepiness may accompany allergies, although perhaps by indirect mechanisms. Because many people are chronically sleep deprived, the symptoms of allergies may simply allow underlying SLEEPINESS to become unmasked by making bedrest or relative inactivity more permissible. Alternatively, nocturnal sleep may be disturbed by allergic symptoms, resulting in increased daytime sleepiness. In addition, ANTIHISTAMINES, the medications commonly used to treat hay fever, are frequently sedating—especially those available without a prescription. In fact, antihistamines are the principal ingredient in many OVER-THE-COUNTER SLEEPING PILLS.

Perhaps the most serious impact of allergies on sleep occurs when allergies precipitate nocturnal asthma attacks or when allergic rhinitis causes nasal obstruction leading to sleep APNEA. Why, when we can easily breathe through our mouth, should a stuffed-up nose prevent us from breathing? The precise cause is unclear, but when normal individuals have their nostrils sealed during the night they have significantly poorer sleep and more obstructive apneas and hypopneas than when allowed to breathe normally. In some cases, simply obstructing the nose results in sleep apnea of clinically significant severity. Studies of hay fever sufferers suggest that they have more apneas and more disturbed sleep during the seasons when they are affected by their allergies.

In addition to treating their allergies with medications, allergy sufferers may benefit from reducing their exposure to allergens by ridding their bedrooms of substances likely to cause allergic reactions and installing special air filtration systems.

REFERENCES

McNicholas WT, Tarlo S, Cole P, Zamel N, Rutherford R, Griffin D, Phillipson EA. 1982. Obstructive apneas during sleep in patients with seasonal allergic rhinitis. *Am Rev Respir Dis* 126(4):625–628.

Olsen KD, Kern EB, Westbrook PR. 1981. Sleep and breathing disturbance secondary to nasal obstruction. *Otolaryngol Head Neck Surg* 89(5): 804–810.

Boyd Hayes

ALL-NIGHTERS

Students commonly stay up all or most of the night in what is called *pulling an all-nighter* to prepare for an exam or to write a term paper. This practice, especially common among college students, of "burning the midnight oil" is made necessary by academic demands and often a good deal of procrastination.

Performance on the day following an all-nighter is affected both by the inefficient hour of study *and* by accumulated loss of sleep (see DEPRIVATION, TOTAL: BEHAVIORAL EFFECTS). Physiological and circadian rhythms reach their low point during the night (see CIRCADIAN RHYTHMS), and learning ability is not at peak. Disruptive sleep patterns can also result in decreased efficiency. For example, athletes complain of a decrease in their winning edge when undergoing JET LAG as a result of flying around the world for competitions (Wellborn, 1987).

Research has shown that studying all night results in fairly good immediate memory, but the material memorized is forgotten over time, much more so than if the studying is done during the day (Monk and Folkard, 1978; see also LEARNING; MEMORY). Logically, then, staying up all night to study immediately prior to a testing situation may be a reasonable strategy if necessary, but it is not practical in preparation for future exams.

Sleep loss affects "divergent" thinking, or the ability to think creatively, flexibly, and spontaneously (Horne, 1988). Therefore, it is possible to stay up all night doing rote memorization of exam material, but extremely difficult to accomplish a creative task. Repetitive, "busy work" kinds of tasks, and physical work are more easily accomplished during an all-nighter than are tasks

for which new and different ways of thinking are required. It follows that performance on a test taken on the day following an all-nighter will be better if the answers require strict memorization of facts, rather than combination of learned material in new and imaginative ways to answer complex essay questions.

In Japan, students study diligently for the national college entrance exam, many going to cram schools known as *juku* after their regular school hours. Students then go home and study until late into the night. The slogan heard in many Japanese high schools is "Pass with four, fail with five!" (Fallows, 1987). These numbers refer to how many hours of sleep students permit themselves while they are studying. Obviously this is not the healthiest approach to good SLEEP HYGIENE. It is not conducive to long-term retention of knowledge, nor to creative thinking. Apparently the goal in the Japanese system is to show colleges and future employers that one is tough enough to take the pressure and pass.

It may be possible to prepare in advance if you know an upcoming all-nighter is inevitable. By sleeping longer for a few nights prior to the all-nighter, you can increase your alertness during the study period. Even a nap on the afternoon before a late night will increase your alertness (see NAPPING).

Falling asleep during class and an inability to concentrate may be only the least results of an all-nighter. Students should never attempt to drive an automobile, operate any heavy machinery, or drink ALCOHOL following an all-night study session, as everyday activities become life-threatening when combined with sleep loss.

REFERENCES

Fallows J. 1987. Gradgrind's heirs: Despite what the U.S. Department of Education says, you would not want your kids to go to a Japanese secondary school. *Atlantic* 259:16–21.

Horne JA. 1988. Sleep loss and "divergent" thinking ability. *Sleep* 11:528–536.

Monk TH, Folkard S. 1978. Concealed inefficiency of late-night study. *Nature* 273:296–297.

Wellborn SN. 1987. For too many, life is just a snore: The body's sleep rhythms. *U.S. News World Rep* 102:56–57.

Nancy Barone Kribbs

ALPHA–DELTA SLEEP

Typically, alpha waves (8 to 13 cycles per second) are electroencephalographic waves indicating a state of relaxed wakefulness with eyes closed. Delta waves are slower (0.5 to 2 cycles per second) and have much higher amplitude. They indicate very deep sleep. In rare cases, however, these two electroencephalographic waveforms are mixed together (see Figure 1). This state is called *alpha–delta sleep.*

When alpha–delta sleep was first described in 1973, it was thought that alpha waves only intruded into delta sleep: hence its name. This was later found to be wrong. Alpha waves can mix with any sleep stage, including REM sleep. Therefore, the correct name would be "alpha wave intrusion into sleep." However, this name is too long, and the name alpha–delta sleep has stuck. The main daytime consequences of alpha–delta sleep are a feeling of malaise, pain, and achiness throughout the body, and a lack of energy (see NONRESTORATIVE SLEEP), although some patients show alpha–delta sleep without any daytime consequences.

Efforts to quantify the amount of alpha wave intrusion into sleep have not developed very far to date. A type of computerized analysis called fast Fourier transform is the most accurate measure of the extent to which alpha waves have intruded into a sleep record, but this procedure is cumbersome and expensive. The most commonly used procedure today is simply rating a record by the percentage of alpha waves: 1 for 0 percent to 25 percent, 2 for 25 percent to 50 percent, 3 for 50 percent to 75 percent, 4 for over 75 percent. The sample in Figure 1 would be rated 4. Ratings of 1 and 2 are considered normal; ratings of 3 and 4 indicate alpha–delta sleep.

Alpha–delta sleep occurs in many conditions. Most often it is seen in patients who suffer from various forms of pain, especially arthritis. They are also seen in patients who have taken high and chronic doses of STIMULANTS such as AMPHETAMINES. Patients with various thyroid conditions may show alpha–delta sleep. Finally, alpha waves can be introduced into the sleep of normal subjects by sounding tones that are loud enough to disturb the sleeper, but not loud enough to awaken him or her. When this is done, sleepers report vague feelings of unease, malaise, and morning stiffness, similar to patients who suffer

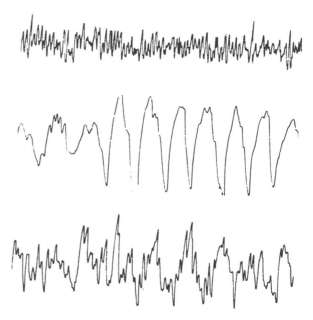

Figure 1.   The top graph shows alpha waves, typical for relaxed wakefulness (eyes closed). The middle graph shows delta waves, typical for deep NREM sleep (stage 4). The bottom graph shows alpha–delta sleep (alpha waves riding on top of the delta waves).

from fibrositis (see ARTHRITIS AND OTHER MUSCULO-SKELETAL DISORDERS).

REFERENCE

Hauri P, Hawkins DR. 1973. Alpha-delta sleep. *Electroencephalogr Clin Neurophysiol* 34:233–237.

Peter Hauri

ALPHA RHYTHM

Alpha rhythm is an electroencephalographic waveform produced by the human brain when an individual is in a relaxed awake condition with eyes closed. The frequency of alpha rhythm is 8 to 13 cycles per second (see Figure 1). Alpha rhythm predominates in electroencephalographic recordings taken from the posterior part of the cerebral cortex known as the occipital lobe. When the eyes are opened, alpha rhythm changes to a low-voltage (low-amplitude) mixture of various frequencies.

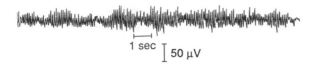

1 sec ⊺ 50 μV

Figure 1. Alpha rhythm.

An interesting phenomenon has been observed in individuals participating in sleep deprivation studies. Often, after being kept awake for one or two consecutive days and nights, individuals will have an electroencephalogram that shows a clearer alpha rhythm when the eyes are open; however, when the eyes are closed, the alpha rhythm disappears. This apparent deviation from normal occurs because the sleep-deprived individual falls asleep instantly upon closing his or her eyes.

Sharon A. Keenan

ALTERED STATES OF CONSCIOUSNESS

[Altered states of consciousness are those states of being that are not a normal or natural part of everyday life. Thus, sleep and dreaming occurring in a normal fashion would not be considered altered *states of consciousness. Many conditions that do constitute such altered states may appear similar to sleep and dreams, but in fact they differ significantly from the natural state.*

COMA, *for example, is a state in which the individual may appear to be asleep—that is, recumbent with eyes closed and high arousal threshold. Nevertheless, coma is very distinct from sleep: Fundamental differences include the inability to arouse with a strong stimulus, as well as marked changes in brain activity as measured by the* ELECTROENCEPHALOGRAM, *or* EEG. ANESTHESIA, *another altered state, is unconsciousness induced through the administration of drugs that alter the brain's* AROUSAL *mechanisms. Certainly many facets of the anesthetic state appear similar to sleep, yet the entire spectrum of brain function markedly differentiates the two states. The phenomenon of* PASSING OUT, *whether through* HEAD INJURY, ALCOHOL *intoxication, or other conditions that*

abruptly and acutely impair brain arousal, is also distinct from normal SLEEP ONSET.

HALLUCINATIONS, HYPNAGOGIC REVERIE, *and hallucinogenic drugs are all associated with perceptions that bear some similarity to dreaming.* HYPNOSIS, *while it may also incorporate features of dreaming, is clearly a different state that is induced volitionally—either externally (by another person) or through self-hypnosis. The meditative state has several external commonalities with sleep, as well as certain EEG similarities; nevertheless, sleep and* MEDITATION *are also considered two distinct entities.*

REM SLEEP BEHAVIOR DISORDER *(RBD) shares the mental content of dreaming but differs greatly from the usual dreaming experience, since the person with RBD is able to move around as if acting out his dreams. In this sense, RBD can be seen as an altered state: a normal state of consciousness (dreaming during sleep) within an abnormal physical state (absence of the normal REM sleep* ATONIA*).* NIGHTMARES, SLEEP-TALKING, *and* SLEEPWALKING, *on the other hand, are* not *necessarily altered states of consciousness, but are examples of extremes of normal behavior.*

Many MAMMALS *and* BIRDS *undergo seasonal changes in level of arousal and metabolic functioning as a means of conserving energy and regulating body temperature.* HIBERNATION, ESTIVATION, *and* TORPOR *resemble sleep and have several physiological links to the sleeping state. While these states are natural and adaptive, they differ in fundamental respects from the typical circadian cycle of sleep and wakefulness (see* CYCLES OF SLEEP ACROSS THE NIGHT*).]*

ALTITUDE

One might expect that sleep when one is sojourning in the mountains would be excellent. Cool night temperatures following a hike during the day would seem the perfect prescription for a good night's sleep. Yet it has long been recognized by mountaineers following abrupt exposure to altitude that they often awaken unrefreshed after several hours of sleep and recall the night as a disturbed and fitful one. The sleep disturbance observed at altitude is best considered a form of INSOMNIA.

The major factor that underlies this sleep disturbance is the relative lack of oxygen at terrestrial altitude compared with sea level. Other factors typical of the altitude environment may also play a role in sleep disruption, such as cold and discomfort, dehydration, ultraviolet irradiation, and the occurrence of acute mountain sickness (see below), although the contribution of these adverse influences to sleep is unknown.

Researchers have examined the characteristics of electroencephalographically recorded sleep during the first several days of altitude exposure. Such studies have established that an alteration in sleep staging (see STAGES OF SLEEP) and architecture occurs during the early period of altitude exposure. Stages 3 and 4 decline, arousals from sleep increase, and wake time is also increased. Investigators have been struck, however, by the discrepancy between subjective sleep quality, which is reported as very poor, and the modest changes observed electroencephalographically. This discrepancy highlights the limitations of the ELECTROENCEPHALOGRAM (EEG) as a means of describing sleep.

During the initial days of exposure to altitude, rather marked changes take place in the respiratory, circulatory, and endocrine systems. The quantity of oxygen in the blood is reduced, thus stimulating altitude sojourners to breathe at higher rates and depths. The quantity of carbon dioxide in the blood (and the body in general) declines as a consequence of this hyperventilation. These changes in the content of gases in the body set the stage for instability in the control of breathing and, especially during sleep, lead to periodic breathing (also known as CHEYNE-STOKES RESPIRATION). During sleep the altitude sojourner, just like the lowlander, exhibits some small decline in overall breathing. The oxygen content of the blood is low because of the altitude; consequently, the decline in ventilation promptly leads to a marked fall in the oxygen present in the lungs and body. The response of the respiratory system is then to increase ventilation rapidly to correct this deficiency. An "overshoot" develops, so that breathing momentarily ceases to correct for the hyperventilation. This alternation between rapid breathing and no breathing can occur as frequently as every 20 to 30 seconds and is responsible in part for the disturbance in sleep continuity. In particular, during the rapid breathing phase there may be an arousal or a microarousal from sleep.

Increased quantities of the hormones adrenaline and noradrenaline are produced during altitude exposure as part of the overall stress response. These substances are known for their "alerting" effects and may also contribute to poor sleep quality. (See CHEMISTRY OF SLEEP.)

Hypoxia (lack of oxygen) may adversely influence sleep directly in addition to the indirect effect on respiration described above. Animals made hypoxic show a decline in REM sleep and a reduction in the amplitudes of slow waves toward those seen in wakefulness. These studies raise the possibility that hypoxia may interfere at a cellular or subcellular level with the neurochemical processes that control sleep.

Acute mountain sickness (AMS) is the term applied to a constellation of symptoms seen in many individuals who ascend to altitudes over 8000 feet. These symptoms include headache, nausea, vomiting, fatigue, and insomnia. The acute exposure to the hypoxic environment is again central to the cause of this condition. During sleep, sojourners who are more susceptible to AMS show more severe declines in oxygen than do subjects who are more resistant to AMS.

Over a few days to a few weeks, most individuals are capable of adjusting to moderate altitudes by a process called acclimatization. The symptoms of AMS and of insomnia gradually abate. The alterations in EEG-defined sleep, however, do not always fully disappear and stages 3 and 4 may remain low. Some individuals continue to exhibit irregular breathing rhythms (not necessarily periodic breathing) and severe hypoxia during sleep. This maladaptation to altitude is referred to as *chronic mountain sickness*. Additional evidence for the adverse effect of altitude on sleep is the change in sleep seen with return to sea level: Sleep latencies decline and sleep efficiency rises. These changes are consistent with an altitude-induced state of sleep deprivation.

Generally, no treatment is indicated for altitude-related sleep disturbance, as it is often self-limited; however, the inhalation of oxygen promptly eliminates the periodic breathing at altitude in most individuals and leads to sound restful sleep. Acetazolamide, a medication that stimulates breathing, has also been shown effective both for the control of periodic breathing during sleep at altitude and for the symptoms of AMS.

REFERENCES

Pappenheimer JR. 1984. Hypoxic insomnia: Effects of carbon monoxide and acclimatization. *J Appl Physiol* 57:1696–1703.

Reite M, Jackson D, Cahoon RL, Weil JV. 1975. Sleep physiology at high altitude. *Electroencephalogr Clin Neurophysiol* 38:463–471.

Sutton JR, Houston CS, Mansell AL, McFadden MD, Hackett PM, Rigg JR, Powles AC. 1979. Effect of acetazolamide on hypoxemia during sleep at high altitude. *N Engl J Med* 301:1329–1331.

Weil JV. 1985. Sleep at high altitude. *Clin Chest Med* 6:615–621.

T. Scott Johnson

ALZHEIMER'S DISEASE

Alzheimer's disease (AD) is a progressive deterioration of the intellect occurring in some individuals as they grow old. AD is not an inevitable consequence of aging. It occurs in about 5 percent to 10 percent of the population between the ages of 65 and 84 and as many as 45 percent of the population above age 85, though a few cases have been reported as early as age 50. AD is a progressive, insidious, and inevitably fatal condition. Its course may be 10 years or longer, and it is the fourth leading cause of death in the geriatric population, following heart disease, cancer, and stroke. The disease typically begins with mild cognitive confusion, perhaps difficulty with memory, for example. As the condition progresses, there are more serious mental losses, including difficulty with understanding language; loss of recognition of friends, family, and spouse; and complete disorientation for time and location. The definitive diagnosis of AD can be made only at the time of autopsy, where certain distinctive changes (neurofibrillary tangles, plaques with amyloid deposition) can be detected by microscopic examination of brain tissue. Before death, AD is diagnosed by exclusion. This means that only when other conditions that could lead to the cognitive deterioration (certain vitamin deficiencies, metabolic abnormalities, infectious diseases, brain tumors, strokes) have been ruled out can the diagnosis of AD be made. Frequently, when a physician orders "tests for Alzheimer's disease" these are the types of diseases that need to be investigated.

The causes of AD are unknown. Abnormalities of several kinds of neurotransmitters, including acetylcholine and somatostatin, have been found in the brains of AD patients. Over the years, environmental causes (aluminum, organic solvents, mercury), viruses, and abnormal genetics have been implicated, though the evidence for all of these factors is mixed. Familial forms of AD are well documented; however, the mode of inheritance is probably complex and may depend on the age at which the disease is first seen. In 1987 some researchers reported that a region of chromosome 21 may be abnormal in patients with AD, and this area was thought to be important in the development of the enzymes leading to amyloid protein. More recently, however, other studies have placed the defect on other chromosomes, and some researchers speculate that, as in many diseases, genetic susceptibility only predisposes an individual to develop AD. The disease may then occur only if particular environmental conditions also exist.

Sleep patterns in AD patients are characterized by low sleep efficiency, low or virtually absent stage 3 and 4 sleep, and, in some studies, a reduction in REM sleep. These changes are characteristic of dementia in general (see DEMENTIA), as is the condition labeled SUNDOWNING, which refers to episodes of nocturnal confusion and agitation. Approximately 30 percent of AD patients sundown. Some studies have shown that AD patients have more sleep APNEA than age-matched controls, but there is disagreement on this issue. Because severe AD patients often show a near-total breakdown of their sleep–wake cycle (dozing during the day, awake at night), deterioration of the brain centers controlling CIRCADIAN RHYTHMS may occur. In general, although sleep disturbance may be profound in AD, it is best to view these sleep changes as secondary to the brain deterioration occurring in AD, rather than as a cause of the disorder.

At present, there are no known cures for AD. Several medications that alter levels of acetycholine in the brain may very slightly reduce the rate of decline, but they do not alter the fatal course of the disease. In recent years, developments in molecular biology have led to the discovery of genes that encode the amyloid protein found in the brains of persons with AD. These results hold promise for future treatments that might correct or block the action of the protein. Other directions for future treatments may involve substances such as nerve growth factor. More research is needed to establish more clearly the causes of and treatments for this devastating and tragic disease.

REFERENCES

Hooper C. 1991. An exciting "if" in Alzheimer's. *J NIH Res* 3:65–70.

Katzman R. 1986. Alzheimer's disease. *N Engl J Med* 314:964–972.

Oliver R, Bock FA. 1987. *Coping with Alzheimer's: A caregiver's emotional survival guide.* Los Angeles: Wilshire Book Co.

Reisberg B. 1983. *Alzheimer's disease.* New York: Free Press.

Wurtman RJ, Corkin S, Growdon JH, Ritter-Walker E. 1990. Alzheimer's disease. In *Advances in neurology,* vol 51, New York: Raven.

Donald L. Bliwise

AMBULATORY MONITORING

To ambulate is to walk around; when a person is said to be ambulatory, he or she is capable of walking around. When we speak of ambulatory monitors, in the strictest sense, we mean devices that collect physiological or behavioral data and can easily be worn while walking around. In the fields of sleep research and sleep disorders medicine, however, some of the most interesting events occur precisely when people stop walking around. As a result, the term has come to include practically any portable device that allows for the collection of data outside a laboratory, whether or not it is actually worn or carried around while in use.

Ambulatory monitors range from wristwatch-sized activity recorders, or actigraphs, used in circadian studies (see ACTIVITY-BASED MEASURES OF SLEEP) to more elaborate machines that gather information about several bodily functions at once and are nearly capable of replacing polygraphs and sleep labs for certain uses. In fact, because of their use in a naturalistic home or work setting, these portable machines may reveal information that could never be discovered by laboratory studies.

Among the first ambulatory monitors were Holter monitors, ambulatory electrocardiographic (ECG) monitors for detecting heart abnormalities. These machines, about the size of a personal cassette player and attached to the patient by wires and electrodes taped to the chest, are in use today in every major hospital. Patients typically wear them for 24 to 48 hours while the data are being collected and stored on magnetic tape or, in some cases, in solid-state computer memory inside the recorder. The tapes or computer files are then examined, often with the help of computers to reduce the large amount of information, and a diagnosis is made. Other machines commonly used in medicine can similarly measure blood pressure, stomach acidity, or seizure activity. An important component of the productive use of these monitors is the simultaneous listing in a diary of a patient's daily activities and the occurrence of symptoms. Some systems go beyond the simple recording of information and either transmit it to a remote monitoring site, such as a hospital, or present some feedback to the wearer.

Ambulatory monitors are especially well-suited to studies of CIRCADIAN RHYTHMS, in which the variables of interest need to be measured over days, weeks, or even months. Special devices that measure activity, heart rate, core body temperature, and sunlight exposure over long periods have been developed. In evaluating CIRCADIAN RHYTHM DISORDERS as well as some types of cyclical depression (for example, SEASONAL AFFECTIVE DISORDER [SAD], or bipolar illness), the use of activity and temperature monitoring has become standard even in clinical practice. Rather than a short-term symptom, it is the daily alternation of rest and activity over a period of several days or weeks that is most interesting. Ambulatory monitoring, then, provides the only objective data available (outside of a costly long-term stay in a time-isolation facility) for the diagnosis and treatment of these patients.

Sleep researchers and clinicians are often interested in more complicated physiological variables, as well as the interaction between several different physiological processes, especially those that vary with sleep state. Multichannel monitors that measure electroencephalographic activity, muscle tone, and eye movements are necessary to determine definitively whether a person is awake or asleep; however, because these sensors are often difficult to apply and keep attached over long periods, other indirect methods that do not use electroencephalography are being used, and if not overinterpreted, provide unique and useful data. Devices that measure electroencephalograms (EEGs) are useful for studying a person's nocturnal sleep in a home setting, but are probably more frequently used as a means of studying workers like airline PILOTS or railroad engineers, in whom PERFORMANCE lapses can be catastrophic. While the majority of patients recorded in sleep labs have sleep-related breathing disorders, far more people experience other forms of disrupted sleep. The advent of devices that allow home monitoring of sleep itself promises better diagnosis and treatment of these disorders than has been possible with laboratory-based studies.

Home monitoring has also come to have a role in the evaluation of ERECTILE DYSFUNCTION in men, although many studies of NOCTURNAL PENILE TUMESCENCE must still be performed in a laboratory with interventional awakenings and evaluation by specially trained personnel.

Sleep APNEA, while still most commonly studied in the laboratory, may also be monitored in the home, and devices for screening patients before lab studies and for following up with them afterwards have been developed. They may or may not include EEG-based sleep measurements, but always feature some method of determining whether pauses in breathing are occurring, and if so, what effect they are having on blood oxygen levels. Other measurements like snoring sounds, heart rate, and body position aid in the interpretation of this information. Home sleep studies, if kept simple enough, are reliable, and their easy repeatability makes them actually more sensitive than the typical single-night laboratory study in patients whose disorders are variable from night to night.

Whereas laboratory studies may allow for more kinds of esoteric procedures, more channels of information, and more control over testing conditions, ambulatory monitoring offers longer-term, more frequent, more naturalistic, and less-expensive investigations. While ambulatory monitoring cannot supply and is not meant to replace the bounty of data that laboratory studies provide, it is beginning to give researchers and clinicians an alternative to the famine of information when this feast is not available.

REFERENCES

Akerstedt T, Torsvall L, Gillberg M. 1985. In Koella WP, Ruther E, Schulz E, eds. *Sleep 1984*, pp 88–89. Stuttgart: Fischer-Verlag.
Miles LE, Broughton RJ, eds. 1990. *Medical monitoring in the home and work environment*. New York: Raven.

Boyd Hayes

AMINES

See Chemistry of Sleep: Amines and Other Transmitters

AMNESIA

The topic of amnesia for events occurring during sleep is closely related to the topic of learning during sleep. Both topics relate directly to the issue of forming memories during sleep. Can events that we experience during sleep be stored in our memories (consolidated) for later recall? The answer to this question is important as it relates directly to learning in sleep. For learning to occur during sleep, memories of events experienced in sleep must be stored and consolidated, and then remembered (retrieved) during waking. If events experienced during sleep are not remembered during waking, we then say that we are amnesic for those events.

There are both anecdotal and systematic accounts of amnesia (failure to remember) for events occurring during sleep. For example, of the four or five dreams that occur across each night, only a fragment of the very last dream— the one out of which we usually awaken—is remembered. The others are lost. Another example of amnesia involves somnambulism (SLEEPWALKING). Sleepwalkers walk and talk and respond to environmental events in the deepest sleep stage (stage 4) but when awakened do not remember any of their experiences. In addition to these anecdotal accounts, many systematic experiments have been conducted testing whether sentences or words presented to sleeping subjects were later recalled during waking. These experiments reveal subjects to be amnesic, that is, they show no evidence of retention, whether they are awakened and tested soon after the words are presented at night or the following morning (Badia, 1990). The only time that evidence for retention occurs is if the brain waves (electroencephalogram) show a waking pattern of activity for 15 seconds or more at the time information is presented (subject is essentially awake when presented with the material). The suggestion is that for memories to be formed, wakefulness is required (Emmons and Simon, 1956; Koukkou and Lehmann, 1968).

The following research illustrates that during sleep stimulus events can be detected, established memories can be accessed, and responses can be emitted and yet the individual remains amnesic to all of these events on awakening.

Subjects are instructed in the waking state that tones will be presented while they are sleeping (they store this information in memory while awake). They are also instructed that whenever a tone is perceived in sleep they are to take a deep breath (or close a small switch taped to their finger). There is considerable evidence that subjects can make both of the latter responses without awakening from sleep (Harsh and Badia, 1990). A few practice trials are given in waking to make sure that subjects understand the task and can follow instructions. They are then allowed to sleep. Then, periodically during the night (every 4 minutes), while sleeping, tones are presented to them. Subjects respond to such tones with a very high frequency, nearly 100 percent of the time in some cases, and on most trials they do so without awakening. The main point is that instructions given while awake (i.e., learning has occurred in waking) can be retrieved and acted on while sleeping. The fact that the subjects detect the stimulus (in this case the tone), recall the instructions (instructions to respond), and select the proper response (press switch or breathe deeply) while asleep indicates that information can be processed in sleep (memories formed earlier in waking can be retrieved in sleep and acted on). But when awakened, do individuals remember that tones were presented to them and that they responded to them? In a word, "no." When subjects are asked the following morning the number of tones presented to them during the night and the number to which they responded, they report

virtually no memory for hearing the tones or for having responded to them, even though they may have detected and responded to the tones over a hundred times during the night. Furthermore, it does not matter whether they are questioned in the morning or awakened after they make the response (breathing or switch closure) at night. Subjects are able to process, in sleep, information acquired in waking, but cannot remember doing so. In short, they are amnesic to events that occur in sleep (see LEARNING).

REFERENCES

Badia P. 1990. Memories in sleep: Old and new. In Bootzin BR, Kihlstrom JF, Schacter DL, eds. *Sleep and cognition,* pp 67–77. Washington, DC: American Psychological Association. The book by Bootzin et al. is an excellent review of the cognition-during-sleep literature.

Emmons WH, Simon CW. 1956. The non-recall of material presented during sleep. *Am J Psychol* 6:76–81.

Harsh J, Badia P. 1990. Stimulus control and sleep. In Bootzin BR, Kilhstrom JF, Schacter DL, eds. *Sleep and cognition,* pp 58–66. Washington, DC: American Psychological Association.

Koukkou M, Lehmann D. 1968. EEG and memory storage in sleep experiments with humans. *EEG Clin Neurophysiol* 25:455–462.

Pietro Badia

AMPHETAMINES

Amphetamines are drugs derived from phenylisopropylamine. Amphetamines are also called central nervous system sympathomimetics because they affect the sympathetic nervous system by mimicking the effect of norepinephrine, the primary neurotransmitter of the sympathetic nervous system. Structurally similar to cocaine, amphetamines are powerful stimulants that affect the peripheral nervous system and the central nervous system. Amphetamines produce intensely pleasurable sensations in humans. Animals given amphetamine injections will aggressively seek more amphetamine. It is these effects that lead to drug abuse and drug dependency and make amphetamines some of the most abused drugs in the world.

The intensity of the pleasurable response to amphetamine is related to the rate with which the drug reaches the brain. Amphetamines that are highly lipophilic and prepared in a form that can be injected or inhaled by sniffing or smoking are the most favored by amphetamine abusers. Amphetamine is generally known as "speed" or "crank." Amphetamine in the form of *d*-methamphetamine is very lipophilic and can readily be prepared in a smokable (hydrochloride) form known as "ice," "crystal," or "crystal-meth." When an amphetamine drug is taken in low doses, fatigue and sleepiness are reduced, movement is increased, and a sense of effectiveness and strength is produced. In very high doses, complex movements are replaced by stereotyped, simple movements and a sense of anxiety and danger is engendered.

The stimulating effects of amphetamines on blood pressure and respiration were first described in the 1930s. The alerting effects of these drugs were being used to treat narcolepsy and to control fatigue by 1935. Amphetamines potentiate dopamine, norepinephrine, and serotonin in the brain, leading to increased locomotor activity, prolonged wakefulness, and distortions in perception. Amphetamines have important medical uses and are most commonly prescribed to control appetite in obese patients and to increase attention in children with ATTENTION DEFICIT HYPERACTIVITY DISORDER. (See DRUGS OF ABUSE; STIMULANTS.)

REFERENCES

Gilman AG, Goodman LS, Gilman A. 1980. *Goodman and Gilman's The pharmacological basis of therapeutics.* New York: Macmillan.

Lyon M, Robbins TW. 1975. The action of central nervous system stimulant drugs: A general theory concerning amphetamine effects. In Essman WB, Valzelli L, eds. *Current developments in psychopharmacology,* vol 2, pp 79–163. New York: Spectrum.

Merrill M. Mitler

AMPHIBIANS

Amphibians (salamanders, toads, frogs) are representatives of the most primitive terrestrial animals, recapitulating in each life cycle the metamorphosis from water-bound, gill-breathing existence characteristic of fish to lung breathing like more modern vertebrates. This great evolutionary step requires a number of adaptations in addition to lungs, for example, the development of limbs for locomotion, increased skeletal rigidity to overcome effects of gravity, and a means to conserve moisture (Colbert, 1961). The nature of sleeplike behavior in such animals could provide information about the adaptive role of sleep. The fossil record indicates that some contemporary amphibians are similar to those that lived nearly 200 million years ago, so these animals do indeed represent ancient history.

When sleep is measured in submammalian species, it is important to examine both the conventional electrophysiological criteria used in mammals, such as electroencephalographic patterns, and behavioral criteria, such as sustained motor quiescence, reduced sensory responsiveness, and rhythms of rest and activity. The results of such studies indicate that there are important species differences among amphibians. The bullfrog, *Rana catesbiani,* does not exhibit changes in responsiveness to sensory stimulation over time and does not show behavioral rest–activity cycles (Hobson, 1967). Awake postures (reclining, but eyes open, reactive) can be maintained for extended periods, interrupted only by infrequent walking, jumping, or swimming. In contrast, tree frogs (genus *Hyla*) are found to be active at night and behaviorally quiescent during the day (Hobson, Goin, and Goin, 1968). Somewhat anecdotal observations suggest these frogs are less responsive to sensory stimulation during periods of inactivity.

Electroencephalograms (EEGs) from bullfrogs and tree frogs are similar but are unlike those seen in mammals. Inactive periods are characterized by low-amplitude arrhythmic patterns, like waking patterns in mammals. Behavioral activity is associated with increased electroencephalographic amplitude and occurrence of synchronous bursts—changes very unlike those of mammals. Synchronous bursts are closely associated with respirations; Hobson (1968) showed that such bursts could be evoked by blowing air through the animals' nares. These and other experiments show that synchronous bursts in the EEG result from stimulation of olfactory receptors by airflow during respirations. Increased synchrony in the EEG during behavioral activation reflects the fact that breathing is more frequent during these periods.

Behavioral and electroencephalographic patterns were also studied in the tiger salamander (*Ambystoma tigrinum*), a species with many similarities to specimens identified in ancient fossils. In this species, a 4-hour rest–activity cycle is observed during both day and night (McGinty, 1972). As in frogs, electroencephalographic patterns resemble the activated pattern of mammals at all times, with bursts of higher amplitude synchronous waves occurring only following breaths. Computerized power spectral analysis of the EEG in adults confirms the visual observations: behavioral activation is associated with increased EEG power in low and moderate frequency bands (i.e., relatively slower electroencephalographic waves), a change opposite to that of mammals. Recordings from larval (aquatic stage) specimens show lower amplitudes in the EEG than those in adults, and no episodes with slow waves. Visual analysis of the EEG in a nocturnally active toad confirms these findings (Huntley, Donelley, and Cohen, 1987). The toad is described as less responsive to stimuli during the inactive phase. Both salamanders and toads lower their heads during the quiescent phase, assuming a more relaxed "sleeplike" posture.

Thus, some amphibian species exhibit behavioral patterns analogous to the sleep–wake cycle in mammals, including circadian (about 24-hour) or ultradian (shorter than 24-hour) rest-activity cycles and reductions in sensory responsiveness. However, because even these changes are not seen in bullfrogs, it seems that sleep is not a general characteristic of all amphibians. The sleeplike state in amphibians may serve adaptation to the environmental contingencies specific to each species, such as minimizing vulnerability to predators and maximizing food gathering, without being essential for physiological stability. However, too little work has been done to be sure about these conclusions. Nevertheless, there is agreement in all studies that electroencephalographic patterns are not related to the sleep–wake cycles as in mammals. This suggests that the forebrain may have a less important function in sleep for amphibians.

REFERENCES

Colbert EH. 1961. *Evolution of the vertebrates*. New York: Science Editions.

Hobson JA. 1967. Electrographic correlates of behaviour in the frog with special reference to sleep. *Electroencephalogr Clin Neurophysiol* 22:113–121.

———. 1968. Respiration and EEG synchronisation in the frog. *Nature* 213:988–989.

Hobson JA, Goin OB, Goin CJ. 1968. Electrographic correlates of behaviour in tree frogs. *Nature* 220:386–387.

Huntley AC, Donelley M, Cohen HB. 1978. Sleep in the western toad, Bufo boreas. *Sleep Res* 7:141.

McGinty D. 1972. Sleep in amphibians. In Chase MH, ed. *The sleeping brain,* pp 7–10. Los Angeles: Brain Information Service.

Dennis McGinty

ANALYSIS

See Freud's Dream Theory; Interpretation of Dreams

ANESTHESIA

CONSCIOUSNESS can be defined as an awareness of one's feelings and surroundings. There are different levels or states of consciousness, which vary along a continuum. Examples of naturally occurring states of consciousness include wakefulness, RAPID EYE MOVEMENT (REM) sleep, and HIBERNATION. Because states of consciousness are generated by the brain, they can be pharmacologically manipulated. People manipulate their own states daily with drugs such as NICOTINE, CAFFEINE, and ALCOHOL. States of consciousness can also be manipulated for medical purposes, and anesthesiologists pharmacologically manipulate the brain to produce states of anesthesia. *Anesthesia* is defined as a reversible drug-induced absence of perception of all sensation. The five features that characterize general anesthesia are unconsciousness, analgesia (imperception of pain), amnesia, skeletal muscle relaxation, and reduced autonomic responses.

The routine use of anesthesia for surgical procedures is a very recent addition to the practice of medicine. Before the 1840s, surgery was considered a last resort and death during surgery was frequent. The development of modern anesthesia began in 1776 with Joseph Priestley's synthesis of nitrous oxide (N_2O) and his notation that it might be used for surgical procedures. In 1818, Michael Faraday proposed that diethyl ether could be useful for surgical procedures. Nevertheless, ether continued to be used only for amusement and for inducing altered states of consciousness at social gatherings called ether frolics. It was William Morton, a medical student in Boston, who successfully demonstrated to the medical community the use of ether for the surgical removal of a tumor on October 16, 1846 at the Massachusetts General Hospital. At the end of the operation, the surgeon, Dr. Warren, turned to the crowd and said, "Gentlemen, this is no humbug." Henry Bigelow, a prominent surgeon, published an account of this demonstration in the *Boston Medical and Surgical Journal,* and the term *anesthesia* was introduced by Oliver Wendell Holmes.

Natural sleep and anesthetically induced unconsciousness are similar in some ways and quite distinct in others. At the behavioral level, an anesthetized person may at first glance resemble a sleeping person, and both states are characterized by reduced muscle tone. However, an anesthetized person will not make any spontaneous movements, whereas a sleeping person will make many large posture shifts throughout the night. The electroencephalogram (EEG) of a sleeping person will predictably and spontaneously change patterns throughout the night, and the changes in the electroencephalographic pattern of a sleeping person are endogenously generated by the brain. The electroencephalographic pattern of an anesthetized person, however, depends upon which anesthetic agents and which dosages are used. Barbiturates produce spindles in the EEG that resemble the spindles occurring during natural sleep, but other anesthetic procedures reduce the amplitude of the EEG to barely perceptible levels. Physiological measurements made during natural sleep reveal that heart rate, blood pressure, respiration, and a host of other varia-

bles become slow and regular during NREM sleep and rapid and irregular during REM sleep. As with sleep-dependent changes in the EEG, these physiological changes are spontaneously and endogenously generated by the brain. These same physiological variables are profoundly affected by anesthetics and may become rapid and irregular upon emergence from anesthesia. Many anesthetic drugs that eliminate pain also severely depress heart rate and respiration. One of the challenges faced by modern anesthesiologists is to administer the correct combination of drugs to produce insensibility to pain while controlling autonomic variables.

Anesthetic agents can be divided into two major types based on their routes of administration. General anesthetics are administered by means of the lungs and are thus called inhalation anesthetics. These agents are very useful because they produce unconsciousness, analgesia, amnesia, and muscle relaxation, which are four of the five desired features of anesthesia. Examples of widely used inhalation anesthetics include halothane, enflurane, and isoflurane.

Intravenous agents constitute the second major type of anesthetic. The four major classes of intravenously administered drugs used in the practice of anesthesia include BARBITURATES, BENZODIAZEPINES, opiates, and dissociative agents. Barbiturates are used mainly to induce anesthesia because they enter the brain rapidly and produce unconsciousness within 10 to 20 seconds after injection. Thiopental (Pentathol) is the barbiturate most widely used today. A second class of intravenous agents is the benzodiazepines. These drugs are widely used as preanesthetic medication because they reduce anxiety, produce amnesia, and provide some skeletal muscle relaxation. (Benzodiazepines are also frequently prescribed for use as sleeping pills in the nonoperative setting.) Benzodiazepines commonly used in the operating room include diazepam, lorazepam, and midazolam.

Opiates are a third class of intravenous anesthetics. They are excellent analgesics, but they depress respiration and do not produce skeletal muscle relaxation. A fourth class of anesthetic intravenous agents is referred to as dissociative anesthetics, the most common of which is ketamine hydrochloride. The term dissociative anesthesia derives from the feeling of dissociation from one's surroundings that patients report after receiving ketamine. A patient who has received ketamine does not appear to be asleep, as do patients treated with any of the agents listed previously.

Despite the fact that anesthetics are widely, routinely, and expertly used, it is fascinating to note that the mechanisms of anesthetic action remain unknown. There are several reasons why the mechanisms by which anesthetics alter consciousness and physiology are poorly understood. First, anesthetic agents have widely varying chemical structures, so it is difficult to elucidate structure–activity relationships. Second, there are no specific antagonists of anesthetic agents, which suggests that these agents do not act at any single class of cellular receptor. Third, the molecular sites at which anesthetics act on a cell are unknown. Fourth, brain mechanisms that generate natural states of consciousness are incompletely understood.

It should be clear that anesthetically induced states and naturally occurring sleep states are distinctly different. At the same time, both REM sleep and anesthesia are characterized by decreases in muscle tone (ATONIA) and an impaired ability to regulate body temperature (see REM SLEEP, PHYSIOLOGY OF; THERMOREGULATION). To date, there has been little discourse between neuroscientists studying sleep and neuroscientists interested in mechanisms of anesthetic action. It is highly probable that brain mechanisms regulating naturally occurring states of sleep and wakefulness are preferentially involved in generating anesthetically induced states. The study of brain mechanisms underlying the generation of states of consciousness promises to be an exciting area for future neuroscientific research.

REFERENCES

Kennedy SK, Longnecker DE. 1990. History and principles of anesthesiology. In Gilman AG, Rall TW, Nies AS, Taylor P, eds. *The pharmacological basis of therapeutics,* 8th ed., pp 269–284. New York: Pergamon.

Miller RD, ed. 1990. *Anesthesia,* 3rd ed. New York: Churchill and Livingston.

Roth SH, Miller KW, eds. 1986. *Molecular and cellular mechanisms of anesthetics.* New York: Plenum.

Helen A. Baghdoyan

ANIMALS' DREAMS

Anyone who has carefully watched dogs or cats sleep has observed that they periodically twitch their toes, ears, and whiskers. Dogs will whine and yelp like hounds at these times no matter what breed they are; cats are generally quite silent, even big cats like tigers. The very careful observer will see that the pattern of breathing is very irregular—sometimes deep, other times shallow. This behavior occurs during REM sleep. The various movements briefly break through the otherwise complete paralysis (ATONIA) of the body muscles (see REM SLEEP MECHANISMS AND NEUROANATOMY).

Long before REM sleep was clearly recognized as a distinct, physiologically unique phase of sleep, dog owners in particular believed that such behavior signified their dogs were dreaming, perhaps hunting in their sleep. Ironically, they had predicted what was later found to be true for humans: that REM sleep is a period of intense, complicated mental activity.

Do animals dream, though? We can never be sure because we cannot ask them. The REM sleep movements do not prove the animals are dreaming because the paw movements are not really like those of a dog or cat walking or running. The yelping is probably just the result of the irregular flow of air at the same time various airway muscles are twitching without any particular pattern. Thus, for example, a Labrador retriever makes sounds just like a hound, which it would never do while awake, suggesting that the sounds are more reflexive and unrelated to mental processes.

As a result of an experimental manipulation, however, it has been possible to gain some insights into what an animal's sleeping brain is "thinking" about. Damage (Figure 1, left) to a small part of the pons in the caudal brain of cats will eliminate the usual atonia. Other than experiencing periods of REM sleep without atonia such cats are essentially normal. They are perfectly healthy and have the alternation between NREM sleep and REM sleep that they had before the damage (Morrison, 1983).

With the pontine damage, however, behavior can be expressed during the altered REM sleep periods. Some cats are able to walk in REM sleep, although their postural support is not perfect (Figure 1, bottom right). The cats often appear

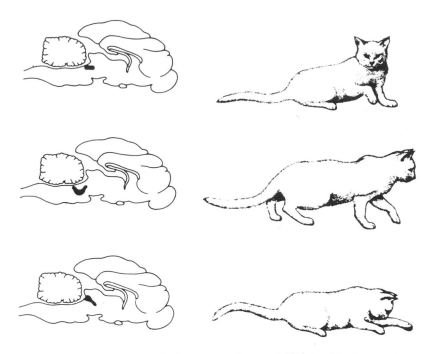

Figure 1. Three cats with damage in the caudal brain (black areas in left column) that permits elaborate behavior during REM sleep without atonia. *Reproduced from Morrison, 1983, with permission.* Copyright 1983 by Scientific American, Inc. All rights reserved.

to be looking around or searching. Because their third eyelids (nictitating membranes) are partially relaxed as in normal REM sleep, one can clearly see they are not awake. Furthermore, they will not react to an observer's movements but can be awakened by a hand clap.

The alertlike REM sleep behavior in these cats is consistent with the fact that brain activity in REM sleep is very much like that of alert wakefulness. One group of neurons, the locus coeruleus, is silent, however, which may mean that these neurons are very important in dictating whether the brain is awake or in REM sleep.

A condition in humans, REM SLEEP BEHAVIOR DISORDER, is like REM sleep without atonia in cats and was recognized because of earlier experimental work with cats (Mahowald and Schenck, 1989). People with this disorder will actually act out with appropriate movements the dream they are having. We might conclude that the cat in REM sleep without atonia is searching for an imagined, or "dreamt," object. We will never know for sure; but then, who ever knows what a cat is thinking?

REFERENCES

Mahowald MW, Schenck CH. 1989. REM sleep behavior disorder. In Kryger MH, Roth T, Dement WC, eds. *Principles and practice of sleep medicine,* pp 389–401. Philadelphia: Saunders.
Morrison AR. 1983. A window on the sleeping brain. *Sci Am* 248:94–102.

Adrian Morrison

ANIMALS IN SLEEP RESEARCH

Animals have been and will continue to be indispensable for the study of sleep and its disorders. Although the discovery of REM sleep, which caused the explosion in sleep research that has continued without letup for 40 years, was made in humans, many of the characteristics of REM sleep have been revealed by studies in animals.

This is because all mammals have sleep that is essentially similar to that of humans.

One example is the muscle paralysis, or ATONIA, that characterizes REM sleep. Atonia was first recognized in cats by researchers who were actually investigating an entirely different subject. They wanted to study the startle reflex in the absence of all but the hindmost or caudal brain. A transection that cut off much of the front part of the brain from the rest of the central nervous system (called a decerebration) allowed them to examine the effects of different stimuli on simple startle jerks in neck muscles. They happened to notice that the cats' muscles periodically become totally inactive. They then looked more carefully at the decerebrated animals and observed that their toes, vibrissae (whiskers), and eyes jerked as in normal REM sleep. This serendipitous observation led to all the later work showing that the part of the brain lying caudally to the transection level is a key structure for the occurrence of REM sleep (Jouvet, 1972). Science works this way: Nature often answers our questions in ways we do not expect.

To learn how different parts of the brain work during sleep as compared with wakefulness, especially to learn which nerve cells might be controlling sleep processes, it is necessary to record impulses from neurons deep within the brain for many hours or even days. This cannot be accomplished ethically in humans, although similar electrodes are also implanted in people for purposes of treatment or diagnosis.

By determining the neurons that have a particular role in sleep regulation, it will then be possible to identify the neurotransmitters they use to communicate with other nerve cells. This is a necessary step in the development of specific drugs to alleviate sleep problems, because in the brain all drugs either facilitate or impede the function of cells that operate as a result of specific transmitters. Such information could never be attained simply by studying humans with diseases—a false claim proposed by individuals in the animal rights movement.

Animals with naturally occurring sleep problems are useful for developing a greater understanding of the human counterparts to these diseases. There are currently two animal models available for sleep disorders. NARCOLEPSY, a condition in which a person suddenly experiences partial or complete paralysis like that of REM sleep or even enters REM sleep directly

from wakefulness, also occurs in dogs (see CANINE NARCOLEPSY). A colony of Doberman pinschers and Labrador retrievers is now providing valuable insights into what mechanisms are not working properly in humans with narcolepsy.

English bulldogs are afflicted with a disorder that occurs in humans: obstructive sleep APNEA. This problem occurs primarily in middle-aged men, who are often overweight. Any body feature that impedes the flow of air when the airway muscles either have reduced activity or are paralyzed as in REM sleep will cause difficulty in breathing during sleep. The short-snouted bulldog has many such features: distorted nasal passages, a big tongue in a short jaw, and thick extra tissues around the throat where the entrance to the trachea (windpipe) lies. These features add to the impairment of airflow when the muscles are relaxed, or atonic, in sleep, causing the dog to arouse briefly many times to get air. Their disturbed sleep causes bulldogs to be sleepy all the time, just as humans with sleep apnea are (Hendricks et al., 1987; see ENGLISH BULLDOGS AS AN ANIMAL MODEL OF SLEEP APNEA).

It is important to know that all work with animals is carefully regulated by federal agencies to ensure that research is conducted as humanely as possible. We are indebted to animals and owe them the very best of care.

REFERENCES

Committee on Care and Use of Laboratory Animals, National Research Council. 1985. *A guide for the care and use of laboratory animals.* Washington, D.C.: U.S. Department of Health and Human Services.

Hendricks JC, Kline LR, Kovalski RJ, O'Brien JA, Morrison AR, Pack AI. 1987. The English bulldog: A natural model of sleep disordered breathing. *J Appl Physiol* 63:1344–1350.

Jouvet, M. 1972. The role of monoamines and acetylcholine containing neurons in the regulation of the sleep-waking cycle. In *Ergebnisse der Physiologie: Neurophysiology and neurochemistry of sleep and wakefulness,* 64:166–307. New York: Springer-Verlag.

Adrian Morrison

ANTIDEPRESSANTS

Antidepressants include drugs from several different chemical classes that have potent effects on sleep, sleepiness, and performance (Table 1). Predicting the effects of any single antidepressant can be difficult, since each drug probably affects multiple neurotransmitter systems. In addition, these drugs may have distinct effects when given acutely versus chronically and when they are discontinued.

As their name implies, antidepressants are usually prescribed for the treatment of major DEPRESSION occurring in single or recurrent episodes, or of manic-depressive (bipolar) illness (see AFFECTIVE DISORDERS OTHER THAN MAJOR DEPRESSION). Antidepressants are also used in psychiatry for the treatment of anxiety disorders (such as PANIC DISORDER) and attention deficit hyperactivity disorder. Less frequently, they may be prescribed for chronic PAIN syndromes.

In sleep medicine, antidepressants are most commonly used to control the accessory symptoms of NARCOLEPSY, including CATAPLEXY, sleep-related HALLUCINATIONS, and SLEEP PARALYSIS. The more sedating antidepressants may be recommended for the treatment of acute or chronic INSOMNIA, particularly if there is a past personal or family history of mood disorder. The alpha-NREM sleep disturbance of fibromyalgia syndrome also responds to tricyclic drugs. Antidepressants (especially protriptyline) have been used for the treatment of sleep APNEA syndromes, although the degree of improvement with these medications is small and usually of limited clinical value. Similarly, nocturnal enuresis (see BEDWETTING) can be treated acutely with tricyclic antidepressants such as imipramine, but the medications do not cure the condition, and return of enuresis is expected with their discontinuation. Although one study found that imipramine may improve the nocturnal sleep of patients with periodic limb movements, antidepressants are generally not recommended for this disorder, since they appear to exacerbate the limb movements (see PERIODIC LEG MOVEMENTS).

Tricyclic Antidepressants

Tricyclic refers to the three-ring chemical structure common to all drugs in this class; they differ from one another in the various chemical side chains attached to the rings. At least some of the tricyclics have active metabolites. For instance, desmethylimipramine (desipramine) is a metabolite of imipramine, and both the parent drug and metabolite have antidepressant activity. The exact mechanism of antidepressant action is not known, but it most likely relates to these drugs' ability to block the presynaptic reuptake of serotonin and norepinephrine (see CHEMISTRY OF SLEEP: AMINES AND OTHER TRANSMITTERS). Changes in the number or sensitivity of postsynaptic receptors are also likely mechanisms of action. Sleep effects of the tricyclic antidepressants are related to the same mechanisms, but occur more rapidly than the clinical antidepressant response. Some of the drugs' properties, such as anticholinergic and antihistamine effects (see ANTIHISTAMINES; CHEMISTRY OF SLEEP: ACETYLCHOLINE), are not critical for the antidepressant effect but are important for their effects on sleep. Tricyclic antidepressants—and, indeed, all antidepressants—may also have a more nonspecific effect on sleep in depression: Since depression is often associated with insomnia, improvement in depression may lead to improvement in sleep.

Specific tricyclic drugs affect sleep very differently. They can be classified according to their sedative potency, which in general correlates with their anticholinergic and antihistamine effects. Thus, some tricyclics, such as doxepin and amitriptyline, clearly reduce nocturnal wakefulness; others, such as imipramine and nortriptyline, have more variable effects on wakefulness; and still others, such as clomipramine, actually increase nocturnal wakefulness. In general, tricyclics have only minor effects on *total* SLOW-WAVE SLEEP (SWS), although they may increase the amount of SWS *early* in the night and thereby alter the distribution of SWS across the night. Again, as a general rule, tricyclics suppress REM sleep, although there is a wide range in this property: Clomipramine suppresses REM sleep almost completely, whereas trimipramine has no REM-suppressing effect. It is also worth noting that drugs like clomipramine may "dissociate" sleep stages, so that rapid eye movements may occur in the absence of muscle atonia or during stage 2 NREM sleep.

In high enough doses, most tricyclic drugs can cause daytime sedation. For this reason, they are usually given in a single dose at bedtime. A smaller number of patients may experience drugs

Table 1. Antidepressant Drugs: Neurochemical and Sleep Effects

Drug	Neurochemical Actions[a]			EEG Sleep Effects[b]			Sedation[c]	Comments
	5-HT	NE	Ach	Contin	SWS	REM		
Tricyclics								
Amitriptyline	+++	++	++++	↑↑↑	↑	↓↓↓	+++	
Doxepin	++	++	+++	↑↑↑	↑↑	↓↓	++++	
Imipramine	+++	+++	+++	→↑	↑	↓↓	++	
Nortriptyline	++	+++	++	↑	↑	↓↓	++	Amitriptyline metabolite
Desipramine	++	++++	+	→	↑	↓↓	+	Imipramine metabolite
Clomipramine	++++	++	+++	↓→	↑	↓↓↓↓	−/+	Chlorinated imipramine
Trimipramine	+	+	++++	↑↑	↑	→	+++	Lack of REM suppression unique among tricyclics
Protriptyline	++	++++	++++	↓	↑	↓↓	−	Activating but very anticholinergic
Amoxapine	+++	+++	+	↑↑	↑	↓↓	++	Resembles antipsychotic drugs loxapine; dopamine receptor antagonist
Maprotiline	−	+++	++	↑↑	↑	↓↓	+++	Structure has four rings
Monoamine Oxidase Inhibitors								
Phenelzine				↓	→	↓↓↓↓	−	Irreversible monoamine oxidase inhibitor
Tranylcypromine				↓↓	→	↓↓↓↓	−	Structural, functional similarities to amphetamine
Other Drugs								
Trazodone	+++	−	−	↑↑↑	↑↑↑	↓	++++	Short elimination time
Fluoxetine	++++	+	−	↓	→↓	→↓	+/−	Alerting; appetite suppressant
Bupropion	−	+	−	↓	?	?	−	Risk of seizures at high dose; does not inhibit transmitter reuptake
Ritanserin	−	−	−	→	↑↑↑↑	→	−	Serotonin receptor antagonist; does not inhibit reuptake
Lithium				↑↑	↑↑↑	↓	++	Affects neuronal membranes

[a]Neurochemical actions refer to reuptake inhibition for serotonin (5-HT) and norepinephrine (NE) and antagonism of receptors for acetylcholine (ACh). Plus signs indicate degree of activity; minus signs indicate no significant activity. No neurochemical actions are listed for monoamine oxidase inhibitor (MAOI) drugs or lithium, as their mechanisms of action do not involve primarily reuptake blockade or receptor blockade.

[b]Electroencephalographic (EEG) sleep effects refer to relative degree of change in sleep continuity (Contin), slow-wave sleep (SWS), and rapid eye movement (REM) sleep with acute administration. ↑, degree of increase; ↓, degree of decrease; →, no change; ?, lack of objective data.

[c]Sedation refers to relative degree of subjective daytime sedation with acute administration. +, relative sedation; −, lack of sedation, or activation.

such as imipramine, desipramine, and protriptyline as activating and may prefer daytime doses. Although healthy control subjects usually demonstrate impaired psychomotor performance during treatment with tricyclics, depressed patients may actually *improve* their performance. This may be because depressed patients have impaired performance prior to treatment, or because tricyclics improve their nocturnal sleep and thereby influence daytime performance. Other side effects of tricyclic drugs include orthostatic hypotension (drop in blood pressure on standing), increased heart rate, abnormal heart rhythms, weight gain, dry mouth, constipation, increased sweating, and sexual dysfunction.

Monoamine Oxidase Inhibitors

The monoamine oxidase inhibitors (MAOIs) were originally discovered in the search for antituberculosis drugs. They act by inhibiting the monoamine oxidase enzyme, which normally metabolizes norepinephrine, dopamine, and other neurotransmitters. This inhibition may be relatively reversible (tranylcypromine) or irreversible (phenelzine), but has the net effect of increasing the amount of presynaptic norepinephrine available for neurotransmission. Subsequent changes in neuronal firing rate and postsynaptic receptor sensitivity are also observed. When monoamine oxidase is inhibited, the body loses its ability to degrade norepinephrine-like substances (such as tyramine) present in many aged foods, red wine, blood pressure medications, and over-the-counter cough and pain remedies. One of the systemic effects of these substances is to increase blood pressure to potentially dangerous levels. For this reason, patients being treated with MAOI drugs must adhere strictly to a tyramine-free diet during treatment and for several weeks afterward.

Monoamine oxidase inhibitor drugs (particularly tranylcypromine) are often experienced as being alerting, possibly because of their structural similarity to amphetamine (see AMPHETAMINES). For this reason, most patients prefer to take MAOI drugs in the morning or early afternoon. Paradoxically, some patients also complain of increased sedation several hours after their dose. MAOIs can increase nocturnal wakefulness on polysomnographic recordings; however, the most powerful effect of MAOIs on sleep is a rapid

and almost complete suppression of REM sleep. There is a compensatory increase in NREM sleep, but without any consistent effect on SWS. REM sleep REBOUND is often seen on abrupt discontinuation.

Other Antidepressants

This category includes drugs from several different chemical classes, but they share the common feature of having from one to four ring structures. For this reason, they are sometimes classified (with the tricyclics) as *heterocyclic* or *cyclic* antidepressants. Because they were developed after the tricyclic and MAOI drugs, and because they brought the hope of reduced side effects and toxicity, they are also sometimes referred to as *second-generation* antidepressants. Some of these drugs (trazodone, fluoxetine) share a common mechanism of action with tricyclics, the presynaptic reuptake blockade of amine neurotransmitters. Others (bupropion, ritanserin) do not block reuptake, and their exact mechanism of action is unknown. They are indicated for the same purposes as other antidepressants. These drugs have not been studied as thoroughly as the tricyclics, but appear to have widely divergent effects on sleep, sleepiness, and performance.

Trazodone is a very sedating antidepressant which is further distinguished by its relatively short elimination rate. Because of these properties, it is sometimes prescribed in low doses as a hypnotic in conjunction with other, more activating antidepressants, such as fluoxetine and MAOIs. Trazodone is one of the few antidepressants that clearly increases SWS. It improves sleep continuity, but has a relatively weak REM-suppressant action. Side effects include sedation and, in a very small number of cases, sustained and painful penile erections in men (priapism).

Fluoxetine is a specific inhibitor of serotonin reuptake with a very long duration of action. It differs from other antidepressants in several of its clinical properties, such as an alerting effect, interruption of sleep continuity, and anorectic (appetite suppressant and weight loss) effect. In high doses, fluoxetine can suppress REM sleep. It is often prescribed for hypersomnic depressed patients. Side effects can include agitation, anxiety, insomnia, and nausea. A small number of patients actually report sedation during fluoxetine use, which may be related to nocturnal sleep disruption. Other antidepressant drugs that are specific blockers of serotonin reuptake, such as fluvoxamine and zimelidine, have sleep effects similar to those of fluoxetine: in particular, "alerting" effects during the day, sleep continuity disruption at night, and little suppression of REM sleep at usual doses.

Bupropion is also a more alerting antidepressant, but it has a short elimination rate. Like fluoxetine, it can disrupt nocturnal sleep continuity. There are few objective studies of its sleep effects. Bupropion is free of many of the typical side effects of antidepressants, but high doses have been associated with an increased incidence of seizures.

Ritanserin is a potent antagonist of postsynaptic serotonin receptors, which may affect neuronal firing rate or numbers of receptors. It has been used for the treatment of anxiety and depression. Its most notable effect on sleep is a rapid and large increase in SWS, with no consistent effects on sleep continuity or REM sleep.

Lithium carbonate is a salt used for the treatment of mania and the prevention of depressive episodes in patients with manic-depressive illness. It is also used as an adjunct for other antidepressant medications in unipolar depression. Its most notable effects on sleep are an increase in SWS, mild suppression of REM sleep, and the appearance of atypical sleep stages. Subjectively, lithium is often somewhat sedating, particularly when it is first administered.

Daniel J. Buysse
Eric A. Nofzinger
Charles F. Reynolds III
David J. Kupfer

ANTIHISTAMINES

Among the most commonly used medications in the world are antihistamines taken for relief of colds, allergies, hives and other skin disorders, motion sickness, and ulcers. Antihistamines block the action of histamine, a chemical that occurs naturally in almost every organ and tissue in the body. Histamine works primarily through two types of receptors referred to as histamine-1 (H_1) and histamine-2 (H_2) receptors.

Just as there are two different types of histamine receptors, there are two different types of antihistamines. H_1 antihistamines block the actions of histamine at H_1 receptors and are used to relieve allergy and cold symptoms, as well as itching and skin disorders (Table 1). H_2 antihistamines, which are used to treat stomach disorders such as ulcers, block H_2 receptors and have no direct effect on sleep and wakefulness, because they do not easily enter the brain, where sleep and wakefulness are controlled.

Among H_1 antihistamines, there is a further distinction depending on whether the drug enters the central nervous system or acts only in peripheral tissue. To the degree that they enter the brain, H_1 antihistamines can affect sleep and wakefulness. First-generation or "classic" antihistamines act in the brain and in peripheral tissue; second-generation (the newer) antihistamines do not easily enter the brain and therefore have no significant effects on sleep and wakefulness. Because second-generation H_1 antihistamines do not enter the brain very readily, they have the beneficial effects of first-generation H_1 antihistamines without the primary side effect of sedation.

Table 1.   Antihistamines (Generic Names)

First-generation H_1 antihistamines	Second-generation H_1 antihistamines
brompheniramine*	astemizole
chlorpheniramine*	terfenadine
clemastine	
cyproheptadine	H_2 antihistamines
diphenhydramine*	cimetidine
hydroxyzine	famotidine
meclizine*	nizatidine
promethazine	ranitidine
pyrilamine*	
trimeprazine	
triprolidine*	

Also available over-the-counter.

Before the development of second-generation H_1 antihistamines, all available H_1 antihistamines entered the brain fairly readily and thus produced the most common side effect, sedation (although in a small number of persons, particularly children, nervousness and agitation occurred). When H_1 antihistamines are taken during the day to relieve a runny nose, for example, the feeling of drowsiness can be very unpleasant and sometimes dangerous. Studies show that cognitive and motor abilities such as driving are impaired, at times leading to accidents on the road or on the job. Even when the sedation is unnoticed or seems mild, it can be significant enough to worsen a person's mood and ability to perform well. Because of this, warning labels tell consumers to exercise caution while driving or using heavy machinery when taking these H_1 products. Further, when alcohol is consumed together with classic antihistamines, the sedating effects are even more severe.

Although drowsiness during the day may be an unwanted side effect of classic H_1 antihistamines for those who suffer from allergies or colds, people who have trouble sleeping sometimes turn to antihistamines to induce sleep. In fact, the active ingredient in almost all OVER-THE-COUNTER SLEEPING PILLS is one of the first-generation antihistamines; however, there is little scientific evidence that these compounds at the available doses are effective in relieving insomnia, possibly because of the relatively slow onset of action of H_1 antihistamines. Further, the sedative effect of these antihistamines may not be sufficient to produce sustained sleep. Even worse, the effects of these medications are prolonged and often produce sedation through the next day, thus adversely affecting one's performance. There is little, if any, benefit in taking medication for sleep if the drug causes tiredness or lethargy when one should be alert, especially given that there is no evidence such medication actually improves one's sleep.

(See also CHEMISTRY OF SLEEP.)

REFERENCES

Meltzer EO. 1990. Antihistamine and decongestant-induced performance decrements. *J Occup Med* 32 (4):327–334.

Nicholson AN, Stone BM. 1986. Antihistamines: Impaired performance and the tendency to sleep. *Eur J Clin Pharmacol* 30:27–32.

Roehrs TA, Tietz EI, Zorick FJ, Roth T. 1984. Daytime sleepiness and antihistamines. *Sleep* 7 (2):137–141.

James K. Walsh
Christin L. Engelhardt

ANXIETY

[*Anxiety, whether defined in psychiatric terms as an intense fear or dread lacking a clearly defined cause, or in more commonplace terms as uneasiness and distress about life's uncertainties, can have a significant effect on sleep and dreaming. A chief contributor to* INSOMNIA *in certain individuals is anxiety related to a fear of being unable to fall asleep. Other insomnia-producing anxieties include those associated with apprehension about an upcoming event, such as a test, performance, surgery, and so forth.* DEPRESSION *and anxiety often occur together, a situation in which sleep may be significantly impaired, and* AFFECTIVE DISORDERS OTHER THAN MAJOR DEPRESSION *may also involve an anxiety component great enough to aggravate sleep-associated changes.* PANIC DISORDER *also includes a strong anxiety component; when panic attacks occur during sleep, the associated anxiety can intensify an insomnia complaint.*

Feelings of anxiety engender responses in the AUTONOMIC NERVOUS SYSTEM; *thus, anxiety may generate a level of physiological* AROUSAL *that is incompatible with sleep. The biochemical components of this interaction may have a direct influence on the brain's sleep mechanisms (see* CHEMISTRY OF SLEEP*).* TRANQUILIZERS, *which are often used to reduce patients' anxiety states, are known to produce sleepiness and to enhance sleep; compounds that can induce anxiety, such as* AMPHETAMINES *and other* STIMULANTS, *typically have a side effect of interfering with sleep.*

On occasion, CHARACTERISTICS OF DREAMS *and* CONTENT OF DREAMS *may reflect waking anxiety. One of the most profound connections between anxiety, stress, and dreaming is seen in* POST-TRAUMATIC NIGHTMARES. SLEEP TERRORS, *while not anxiety-provoking for the sleeper, often create anxiety in others such as the sleeper's parents. Many dream theories attempt to explain the relationship of anxiety to dreaming (see* ADLER'S DREAM THEORY; FREUD'S DREAM THEORY; JUNG'S DREAM THEORY; SENOI DREAM THEORY*); conversely, certain theories of the* FUNCTIONS OF DREAMS *relate to the role of dreaming in overcoming waking anxieties.*]

APNEA

When humans first began to come together at night to sleep, the sound of SNORING reverberating off the walls of the cave must have made it obvious that sleep affects breathing. How dramatically and adversely is something we have learned only recently. There are thousands of people who cannot sleep and breathe adequately at the same time. They suffer from sleep apnea.

Derived from the Greek word *pnoia* meaning "breath" and the Greek prefix *a-* denoting "want" or "absence," *apnea* means a transient cessation of breathing in which there is no airflow at the mouth and nose for 10 seconds or longer, a period longer than the usual pause between breaths. Two basic types of apnea, as well as a combination of the two, have been described (Gastaut, Tassinari, and Duron, 1966). A global cessation of all respiratory effort is called a *central apnea* (Figure 1); *obstructive apnea* is a cessation of airflow at the nose and mouth despite persistent efforts to breathe (Figure 2). A mixture of central and obstructive mechanisms can also occur, leading to what is termed a *mixed apnea* (Figure 3).

Types of Apnea

Central Apnea

Central apneas occur in a variety of clinical conditions and most commonly reflect a respiratory control system instability (see RESPIRATION CONTROL IN SLEEP). This type of central apnea, for instance, can be seen in normal persons at altitudes

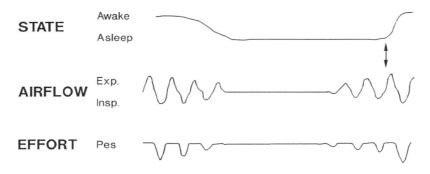

Figure 1. Central sleep apnea. Exp., expiration (breathing out); Insp., inspiration (breathing in); Pes, esophageal pressure.

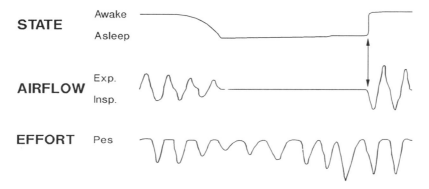

Figure 2. Obstructive sleep apnea. Exp., expiration (breathing out); Insp., inspiration (breathing in); Pes, esophageal pressure.

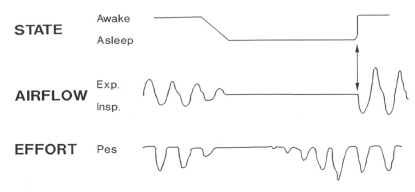

Figure 3. Mixed sleep apnea. Exp., expiration (breathing out); Insp., inspiration (breathing in); Pes, esophageal pressure.

where the hypoxemia-induced increase in ventilatory drive is destabilizing (see ALTITUDE). It can also frequently be seen at sleep onset, especially in patients who tend to hyperventilate for any reason, such as anxiety or pain. Heart failure, in which both increased respiratory drive and delay of transfer of information about arterial blood gases from lungs to sensors as a result of prolonged circulation time play a role, and some types of brain damage are frequently associated with repetitive central apneas. This type of apnea is also called *periodic breathing* or CHEYNE–STOKES RESPIRATION.

Another type of central apnea is very rare and reflects major damage to the portion of the brain controlling respiration. This results in something called ONDINE'S CURSE, a true failure of involuntary breathing leading hypoventilation in both sleep and wakefulness. During phasic REM sleep, breath holds that are apparently just part of the irregular breathing pattern of that state also may be seen.

Obstructive Apnea

Obstructive apnea is by far the most common type of clinically important apnea. It occurs because of a sleep-induced failure of the muscles of the pharynx to hold the airway open against the suction created by efforts to breathe. It is discussed in more detail below.

Mixed Apnea

A mixed apnea is one in which initially there is no breathing effort because the previous arousal-induced hyperventilation has driven the arterial

carbon dioxide level below the apnea threshold. Once the carbon dioxide rises above the apnea threshold, respiratory efforts resume, but the airway is closed, so the apnea becomes obstructive.

Hypopnea

A hypopnea is a decrease in airflow inappropriate to effort or metabolic needs, and may be just as important as a complete cessation of flow. Although there is no universally agreed-on definition of hypopnea, as a practical matter, any decrease in breathing that results in arousal should be considered a hypopnea. Usually hypopneas and apneas are accompanied by arterial blood oxygen desaturation, but this may be relatively minor. Figure 4 is a graphic representation of obstructive hypopnea.

The Obstructive Sleep Apnea Syndrome

The obstructive sleep apnea syndrome is a condition in which the pathogenic events, apneas occurring in sleep, can be observed at the bedside. Using this technique, Broadbent accurately described sleep apnea in 1877. Even earlier, Charles Dickens, in *The Pickwick Papers,* gave us the wonderful portrait of Joe, Mr. Wardle's immensely fat, snoring, hypersomnolent servant-boy. Over the years, a number of medical reports appeared noting the association of obesity, excessive sleepiness, cyanosis, pulmonary hypertension, and right-sided heart failure—a group of signs and symptoms that became labeled the *Pickwickian syndrome*. Although some of these articles mentioned noisy, irregular, or periodic

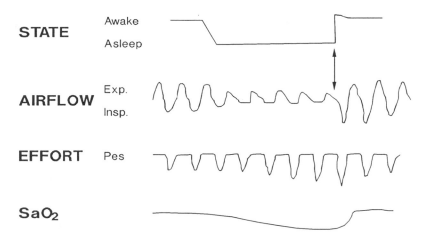

Figure 4. Obstructive sleep hypopnea. Exp., expiration (breathing out); Insp., inspiration (breathing in); Pes, esophageal pressure; SaO$_2$, arterial blood oxygen saturation.

respirations during sleep, their central role remained forgotten and unrecognized until 1966 when Gastaut reported the first polysomnographic study of a Pickwickian patient. He was able to show that this patient had repetitive apneas in sleep that led to brief, unremembered arousals.

The obstructive sleep apnea syndrome is fairly common. Estimation of prevalence ranges from 1 percent to 4 percent of the adult population. The prevalence in certain groups, for instance, obese, older males, is much higher. It is very uncommon in premenopausal females. It is the single most frequent problem seen in sleep disorder centers and is the most common cause of severe hypersomnolence in adult males.

In the vast majority of cases, the site of obstruction is the supraglottic airway, that is, the airway between the nasal openings and the voicebox. This tube is complicated, having to serve as both a passive passage for air and an active propulsive conduit for solids and liquids. To subserve swallowing and phonatory functions the tube has to be very compliant, but this makes it potentially collapsible. The airway here is relatively unprotected by bone or cartilage and depends on the coordinated action of a complex group of respiratory-linked muscles to hold it open during inspiration. In patients with obstructive sleep apnea (OSA) this critical portion of the airway is abnormal in configuration, in its compliance, or in both. Because the effective compliance depends in part on the activity of muscles that surround the airway, abnormalities of neuromuscular control have been postulated to be

responsible for obstructive sleep apnea. But evidence for abnormalities of neural input or timing is contradictory. On the other hand, almost all studies of pharyngeal size and shape during wakefulness show it to be smaller in patients with sleep apnea than in snorers, and smaller in snorers than in normal controls.

Inelegantly stated, obstructive sleep apnea appears to be a plumbing problem, that is, a problem of the flow of a fluid—air—through an abnormal tube. This concept is supported by the fact that most successful treatments have in one way or another increased the size or decreased the collapsibility of that tube.

Two cardinal manifestations of obstructive sleep apnea indicate the disturbance during sleep and the resulting alteration in wakefulness. The first is snoring that can typically be so loud as to cause the bed partner to move out of the bedroom. It is frequently of a crescendo variety, indicating increasingly severe narrowing of the airway. It can also be simply a series of snorts interspersed with an ominous silence (see SNORING). The daytime symptom is severe SLEEPINESS. Usually the patient shows evidence of falling asleep in all permissive situations. Unfortunately, driving is a permissive situation for a number of people, so patients with obstructive sleep apnea syndrome are at high risk for accidents. These two symptoms of loud, intermittent snoring and daytime sleepiness are so significant that any person having them should be considered to have the obstructive sleep apnea syndrome until proven otherwise.

Other clinical signs of obstructive sleep apnea are not seen in every patient and are listed as minor manifestations in Table 1. They include personality change, most likely as a result of severe sleepiness. Spouses often comment on the physically restless sleep of the sleep apneic patient. Patients with severe sleep disruption from sleep apnea may complain of morning confusion; this complaint may be more prominent in the subset of patients who develop carbon dioxide retention and may be accompanied by morning headaches. Intellectual deterioration is a complaint that may be difficult to measure objectively. A certain percentage of patients complain of impotence and a rare patient complains of bedwetting.

Almost all patients with obstructive sleep apnea have abnormalities involving the upper airway such as nasal obstruction, enlarged tonsils and adenoids, small and posteriorly displaced chins, and, of course, multiple chins as a result of obesity. The majority of patients with obstructive sleep apnea are obese. Other diseases associated with sleep apnea are hypothyroidism, acromegaly, and amyloidosis. High blood pressure is more frequent in patients with obstructive sleep apnea than in control populations. Most patients with obstructive sleep apnea have relatively normal pulmonary function while awake, but any coexistent abnormalities of the respiratory system will increase the risk of severe hypoxemia during the apneic episodes of sleep. It is only a small subset of patients with obstructive sleep apnea that develop daytime hypoventilation and the classic Pickwickian syndrome.

Table 1.   Clinical Signs of Obstructive Sleep Apnea in the Adult

Major
Snoring
Sleepiness

Minor
Physically restless sleep
Personality change
Cognitive impairment
Headache
Morning confusion
Nocturia
Nocturnal enuresis
Impotence

The polysomnographic (sleep recording) features of obstructive apnea are quite clear: repetitive apneas or hypopneas leading to arousals. Most patients with clinically important or symptomatic obstructive sleep apnea have at lease 20 apneas or hypopneas per sleep hour, and most spend at least 50% of their sleep time not breathing. The level of oxygen desaturation depends on a number of different variables, most importantly the apnea duration and the baseline oxygen saturation. The lower the starting saturation and the longer the apnea, the more severe the desaturation. The rate and depth of desaturation are also influenced by the oxygen stores in the lung, which are significantly less in obese individuals during sleep. Because the size of the lungs decreases even further during REM sleep, and apneas tend to be longer in that stage, the worst desaturation frequently occurs in REM sleep.

Apneas may be both position dependent and sleep stage dependent. Frequently, apneas are seen only when the patient is supine and disappear when the patient lies prone or on the side. Apneas may also occur only in stage 2 sleep and disappear or be replaced by severe obstructive hypoventilation and snoring during stage 3 and 4 sleep. In some patients, apneas are seen only in REM sleep.

In symptomatic sleep apnea, sleep continuity is severely disrupted. There is a decrease in stage 3 and 4 sleep, and a marked decrease in REM sleep. The other important phenomena are cardiac dysrhythmias, which can occasionally be life-threatening.

With each episode of apnea, there is a rise in systemic and pulmonary arterial pressures, which usually return to control levels when breathing resumes. Heart rate falls during the apneas and then increases at, or just before, the termination of apnea. Clinically important cardiac arrythmias are not common. The most serious, ventricular tachycardia, occurs only in 3 percent or less of reported cases. Serious ventricular arrythmias during sleep are more likely to be seen with oxygen saturation levels below 60 percent.

The long-term consequences of obstructive sleep apnea are just beginning to be understood. The frequent arousals to breathe lead to sleep fragmentation that ultimately results in diurnal hypersomnolence. This loss of alertness can cause a significant increase in the risk of accidents.

An increased risk for high blood pressure in

persons with sleep apnea has been reported in a number of studies, and patients with sleep apnea appear to have more hypertension than do controls. Sleep apnea has also been associated with an increased incidence of myocardial infarction.

Recently published retrospective analyses of long-term mortality in OSA show cumulative mortality rates of 11 percent and 13 percent. Both of these studies, as well as clinical experience, suggest the obstructive sleep apnea syndrome is a potentially lethal disorder.

Treatment

The treatment of obstructive sleep apnea can be conveniently divided into surgical and nonsurgical modalities, although these are not mutually exclusive. Nonsurgical therapy, in turn, can be categorized as behavioral, pharmacologic, or mechanical. Behavioral treatments include diet for weight loss in patients where obesity is playing a role in the sleep apnea, position restriction for those patients in whom the apnea occurs only in certain positions, and avoidance of alcohol and other central nervous system depressants. The patient should also avoid upper airway mucosal irritants, which may cause increased resistance to inspiratory air flow.

A variety of drugs have been tried for the treatment of obstructive sleep apnea, most with only limited success. Supplemental oxygen may be helpful in a small subset of patients, especially at altitude. Other types of drug therapy that have been tried are those that increase upper airway patency, such as nasal decongestants and anti-inflammatory agents; drugs that cause respiratory stimulation, such as progesterone and acetazolamide; and more generalized neuroactive drugs, such as protriptyline. For a time before the widespread introduction of nasal continuous positive airway pressure (nasal CPAP), there was almost a "drug-of-the-month" in treatment recommendations. Most of these have subsequently fallen into disuse. Protriptyline has been the most widely used, but it has only spotty and unpredictable success and suffers from poor patient tolerance of its side effects.

Mechanical devices aimed at altering the configuration or compliance of the upper airway include orthodontic devices, which hold the lower jaw forward, and tongue-retaining appliances, which hold the tongue forward. Both of these may be useful in selected patients. A nasopharyngeal tube may also help in certain patients. The major advance in treatment, however, is nasal CONTINUOUS POSITIVE AIRWAY PRESSURE (CPAP), described by Sullivan in 1981. It has largely replaced tracheostomy as the immediate and demonstrably effective therapy for obstructive sleep apnea. It simply acts as a pneumatic splint, holding the collapsible portion of the airway open with air pressure.

A surgical approach to obstructive sleep apnea provided the first "cure" when Kuhlo performed a tracheostomy to bypass the upper airway obstruction in 1969. Surgery to reconfigure the upper airway so that it remains patent during sleep continues to be a valid if not universally successful treatment goal. Tonsillectomy with or without adenoidectomy, nasal surgery, and UVULOPALATOPHARYNGOPLASTY are the most common procedures performed. More recently, anterior sagittal osteotomy of the mandible with hyoid myotomy and suspension, mandibular advancement (Le Fort type 1 osteotomy), and, most recently and aggressively, maxillomandibular and hyoid advancement have been performed by Riley and Powell (see MAXILLOFACIAL SURGERY), as well as laser midline glossectomy by Fujita and colleagues. Surgery can also be done to aid weight loss.

The treatment for central sleep apnea usually involves therapy of the underlying disorder that is tending to destabilize breathing. For instance, if central sleep apnea is an accompaniment to heart failure, then treatment of the heart failure would be the appropriate course of action. If there is a true failure of automatic control of breathing during sleep, then diaphragmatic pacing or controlled mechanical ventilation will be necessary.

REFERENCES

Gastaut H, Tassinari CA, Duron B. 1966. Polygraphic study of the episodic diurnal and nocturnal (hypnic and respiratory) manifestations of the Pickwick syndrome. *Brain Res* 2:167–186.

Guilleminault C, Partinen M, eds. 1990. *Obstructive sleep apnea syndrome: Clinical research and treatment*. New York: Raven.

Kuhlo W, Doll E, Franck MD. 1969. Erfolgreiche

Behandlung eines Pickwick-Syndroms durch eine Dauertrachealkanule. *Dtsch Med Wschr* 94: 1286–1290.

Riley R, Powell N, Guilleminault C. 1987. Current surgical concepts for treating obstructive sleep apnea syndrome. *J Oral Maxillofac Surg* 45: 149–157.

Sullivan CE, Berthon-Jones M, Issa FC, Eves L. 1981. Reversal of obstructive sleep apnea by continuous positive airway pressure applied through the nares. *Lancet* i:862–865.

Thawley SE, ed. 1985. *Symposium on sleep apnea disorders. The Medical Clinics of North America.* Philadelphia: Saunders.

Philip R. Westbrook

ARCHITECTURE OF SLEEP

See Cycles of Sleep Across the Night; Stages of Sleep

AROUSAL

In behavioral terms, *arousal* is awakening from sleep with mobilization of organism resources for adequate responses. Some regard the notion of arousal as applicable only to the short-lasting phase of transition from sleep to the enduring state of waking. During this brief period as well as during steady wakefulness, the sleepy unconscious brain becomes open to the outside world, thus allowing reception of sensory signals and, if necessary, providing quick adaptive motor responses.

Activation refers to a series of brain mechanisms underlying arousal. Thus, arousal is a behavioral term and activation a physiological term. Activation can be defined as a state of preparation in cerebral networks that brings the neuronal circuits closer to the point at which stimuli produce a response. While arousal refers to motoric and conscious processes during the awakening reaction, the brain is also very active during REM sleep, with dreaming episodes but absence of movements (see ATONIA). In many physiological aspects of brain functions, waking and REM sleep are similarly characterized by an enhanced excitability of the brain, and both these states are contrasted to NREM sleep when central nervous structures are less excitable (Steriade, 1991). Thus, activation can be considered as a response readiness of the brain, either to information from the external world (as in waking) or to internal drives (as in REM sleep).

Arousal Systems in the Brain

Some physiologists of the eighteenth and nineteenth centuries speculated that nervous centers in the brainstem (between the spinal cord and the diencephalon) and THALAMUS (between the brainstem and the cerebral cortex) are the substrates (underlying structural components) of arousal and consciousness. However, the first serious attempt to localize a brain structure involved in activation processes is credited to Moruzzi and Magoun (1949). They electrically stimulated a cat's reticular formation, which is the core of the brainstem, and observed that the electroencephalogram (EEG) showed signs of activity similar to those during behavioral arousal. These signs consist of the suppression of low-frequency (less than 15 cycles per second) high-amplitude oscillations and their replacement by waves having higher frequency and lower amplitudes (see ELECTROENCEPHALOGRAM).

Further studies have largely supported the findings of Moruzzi and Magoun. Moreover, recent investigations have shown that brainstem reticular neurons projecting to the thalamus and using acetylcholine as a neurotransmitter display increased activity, which reliably announces the most precocious (earliest) signs of transitions from NREM sleep to either arousal or REM sleep (Steriade et al., 1990). These cholinergic neurons are the best candidates for subserving brain arousal. They produce an enduring excitation of thalamic cells, which, in turn, facilitate cortical operations by releasing excitatory amino acids in the cerebral cortex (Figure 1).

When, however, investigators have lesioned (destroyed) the upper part of the brainstem reticular formation (including the cholinergic nuclei within it) and waited a sufficient length of time, arousal that was lost during the early postlesion days was recovered and the experimental animals began again to display awakening reactions. This result indicated that, although brainstem cholinergic neurons are very important for arousal, they are not the only neurons that induce and

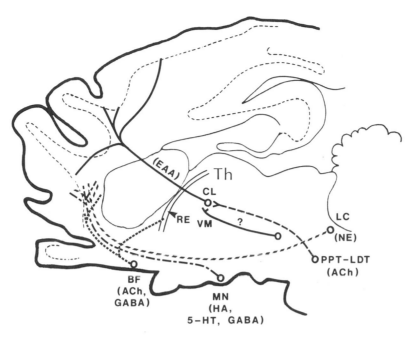

Figure 1. Diagram of different arousing systems shown on a parasagittal section of the brain of a cat, a species that was the subject of most experimental investigations in this field. The cerebral cortex is at left, and the upper part of the brainstem is at right; between them is the thalamus (Th) with two of its nuclei projecting diffusely and widely to neurons in the cortex (CL, centrolateral nucleus; VM, ventromedial nucleus). Thalamic cells use excitatory amino acids (EAA) as transmitters. The arousing systems are schematically drawn with just one cell. Neurons of the pedunculopontine tegmental and laterodorsal tegmental (PPT-LDT) nuclei use acetylcholine (ACh) as a neurotransmitter and project to neurons in the thalamus. In front of PPT-LDT nuclei, a brainstem reticular neuron with thalamic projection is also depicted; its transmitter is not known (?) but is thought to be EAA. Above these brainstem cholinergic nuclei is shown the locus ceruleus (LC), whose neurons use norepinephrine (NE) as their transmitter. At the ventral (lower) surface of the brain are located mammillary nuclei (MN) of the posterior hypothalamus. Near that region are located neurons using histamine (HA) as a transmitter, as well as other cells using serotonin (5-HT) or GABA (γ-aminobutyric acid). The basal forebrain (BF) area has neurons using ACh or GABA and projecting directly to the cerebral cortex. Some neurons in the BF also give rise to axonal collaterals (branches) to the reticular thalamic nucleus (RE).

maintain it. The consensus was recently reached that rather than being due to a single nervous system and a single neurotransmitter, arousal and activation processes are realized by a series of distributed systems using several neurotransmitters.

One of these multiple systems is located in the BASAL FOREBRAIN (Steriade and McCarley, 1990; see Figure 1) and its cholinergic neurons (neurons that use acetylcholine as a neurotransmitter) project directly to the cerebral cortex. Other systems are composed of monoaminergic neurons that also project directly to the cerebral cortex, such as the cells located in the locus ceruleus (not far from the brainstem cholinergic neurons), which use norepinephrine as a neurotransmitter, or the cells in the posterior hypothalamus, which use histamine as a neurotransmitter (Figure 1).

Surprisingly, many different transmitters of various arousing systems (such as acetylcholine, norepinephrine, and histamine) exert similar actions upon neurons in the thalamus and cerebral cortex. Essentially, they excite these cells by diminishing or suppressing special ionic conductances to potassium. So, why do we need so many arousal systems? Although this issue is not yet completely resolved, it has been suggested that this multiplicity provides compensatory systems when some arousal systems are lesioned or become inactive.

Brain-Activated States of Waking and REM Sleep

The externally generated perceptions and logical thought in waking contrast with the internally generated perceptions constituting the hallucinatory imagery during REM sleep. This dissimilar mentation occurs despite the fact that the brain is similarly active and there is no observable difference between its electrical activity in these two behavioral states. Indeed, the EEG has fast and generally low-voltage rhythms during both waking and REM sleep, thus standing in contrast to the EEG activity during NREM sleep (top traces in Figure 2). Even at the microphysiological level, waking and REM sleep are very similar. Thus, spontaneous discharges of thalamic neurons that project to the cortex, as well as of cortical neurons projecting at distant sites, are similarly tonic, as opposed to the spike bursts separated by long periods of silence in NREM sleep (middle traces in Figure 2). Tests of cellular excitability using various stimuli also show a similarly increased responsiveness of neurons during waking and REM sleep as compared with NREM sleep (bottom traces in Figure 2).

It thus appears that thalamic and cortical "gates" are closed during NREM sleep, whereas they are open during wakefulness, as well as during the aroused cerebral state of REM sleep. Although the central nervous system commands succeed in producing the motor acts required for adaptive reactions during waking, when such commands arise during REM sleep in a brain that is at least as highly excitable as in waking, they are blocked in the spinal cord because of the inhibition of motoneurons.

(See also CHEMISTRY OF SLEEP; MIDBRAIN; NICOTINE; NREM SLEEP MECHANISMS; PGO WAVES; REM SLEEP MECHANISMS AND NEUROANATOMY.)

REFERENCES

Steriade M. 1991. Alertness, quiet sleep, dreaming. In Peters A, Jones EG, eds. *Cerebral cortex*, vol 9, pp 279–357. New York: Plenum.

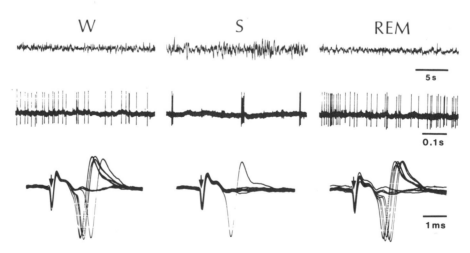

Figure 2. Similarity between two brain-activated behavioral states, waking (W) and REM sleep, both contrasted with NREM sleep (S). Upper traces in each show the EEG activity; middle traces show the spontaneous activity of a thalamic neuron projecting to the cerebral cortex; bottom traces show the responses of a thalamocortical neuron to a stimulus (at arrow) applied to prethalamic axons. See text for details.

Steriade M, Datta S, Paré D, Oakson G, Curró Dossi R. 1990. Neuronal activities in brainstem cholinergic nuclei related to tonic activation processes in thalamocortical systems. *J Neurosci* 10:2541–2559.

Steriade M, McCarley RW. 1990. *Brainstem control of wakefulness and sleep*. New York: Plenum.

M. Steriade

ART, SLEEP AND DREAMS IN WESTERN

In Western culture, sleep has been associated symbolically with vulnerability, susceptibility to evil, ignorance, sex, and death, and with the opportunity for wisdom and prophetic dreams. Whether used as props for loftier ideas, depicted as inherently important phenomena, or exploited as gateways to the unconscious and other worlds, representations of sleep and dreaming reflect these symbolic associations as well as changing social and cultural values.

The Christian Church and the Glory of God

Themes of sleep and dreaming are generally absent from classical Greek and Roman art, although sleeping satyrs, fauns, and hermaphrodites appear in bronzes and sculpture from the fourth century B.C. to the first century B.C. Images of sleep are also uncommon in Byzantine and Gothic art. By the early Renaissance, however, illustrations of biblical dreams appear. During the Middle Ages (roughly the fourth to the fourteenth century A.D.) and the Renaissance (roughly 1400–1600), the influence of the Catholic church on the arts was quite strong and art was meant to provide religious instruction. Holy men receiving divine wisdom through dreams was an acceptable subject matter for such instructional painting. In the mural *Joachim's Dream* by Giotto (1266–1336), the fresco *The Dream of Constantine* (ca. 1455) by Piero della Francesca (1416–1492), *The Dream of St. Joseph* by Georges de la Tour (1593–1652), and *The Vision of the Young Knight* (ca. 1502) by Raphael (1483–1520), the central figure sleeps at the bottom of the painting underneath the dream that floats above his head. This arrangement not only tells us that the action of the paint-

ing occurs within a dream, it also directs the eye (and the soul) upward—from the sleeper to the dream—toward God.

Classical Themes

Classical Greek and Roman themes reemerged in Renaissance art. The new Renaissance humanism broadened the range of acceptable themes in art and allowed for a wider range of subject matter; the human figure became more central to the focus of the picture as the distance between the viewer and the action of the painting was diminished. In this more intimate space, gods and goddesses from ancient Greek myths were revealed with a fuller human aspect: We see them sleeping not to dream God's will, but because gods and goddesses, like humans, must sleep. In *Venus and Mars* (ca. 1483) by Sandro Botticelli (1444–1510), *Antiope* by Correggio (1494–1534), *Apollo Asleep, and the Muses* by Lorenzo Lotto (1480–1556), *Venus and Adonis* by the Mannerist painter Paolo Veronese (1528–1588), and *The Dream of Aesculapius* by the Baroque painter Sebastiano Ricci (1659–1734), a female figure keeps watch over sleeping males. Themes of vulnerability during sleep appear: In Botticelli's *Venus and Mars,* Venus watches over her conquest, Mars, as he sleeps, and in *Samson and Delilah* by Francesco Morone (1471–1529), Delilah and her attendant are about to make the first cut into Samson's hair while he lies sleeping.

Social Change and Artistic Reaction

The spread of capitalism in the 1600s and the advent of the scientific revolution in the 1700s were two forces that greatly influenced Western art, as many artists made judgments about their changing world. Some viewed the acceleration of social change optimistically. They believed that painting should be objective and naturalistic; within this aesthetic there was little room for symbolism or allegory. In contrast to this position, other artists fought to keep the subjective and personal in art. This division might be reflected in a painter's decision to represent sleep objectively (i.e., to depict a sleeping person in a naturalistic way) or subjectively (i.e., to convey the experience of dreaming). By the nineteenth century, opposing schools of painting developed that explicitly addressed the antagonisms between spirituality and materialism and between subjectivity and objectivity.

From Everyday Life to the Fantastic

The rise of mercantile capitalism in Northern Europe and the expansion of themes in art beyond a religious canon paved the way for genre painting, or the illustration of scenes from everyday life. Paintings and drawings by Rembrandt van Rijn (1606–1669), Jan Vermeer (1632–1675), and Nicolaes Maes (1634–1693) show napping figures in household settings. Rembrandt's drawing *A Girl Asleep at a Window,* Maes's oil paintings *The Idle Servant* (1655) and *The Housekeeper* (1656), and Vermeer's *A Girl Asleep* (ca. 1657) illustrate a new attitude in figure painting. In Maes's paintings, a moral association between NAPPING and laziness, sloth, and the shirking of household duties is underscored. Dutch genre paintings of servants asleep at their jobs reflect not only the spread of the Protestant work ethic but also the increasing representation of daily activities, including napping, in seventeenth-century art.

The Swiss painter Henry Fuseli (Johann Füssli; 1741–1825) brought dreams and the "fantastic" into the visual arts. Fuseli, in contrast to the genre painters, was inspired by ancient poetry and literature. His works include the "Nightmare" paintings (ca. 1781), in which incubi terrorize their hapless victims (see INCUBUS ATTACKS). Fuseli's painted nightmares reinforce associations among sleep, sex, vulnerability, and death.

The English poet–painter William Blake (1757–1827) used sleep metaphorically in his art, much of which illustrated the Biblical book of Genesis, Milton's *Paradise Lost,* and his own *Marriage of Heaven and Hell.* Within Blake's personal mythology, there are two kinds of sleep: the shapeless, restless "sleep of Ulro," representing individuality and separation from community, and the fleeting, inspirational "sleep of Beulah." The sleep of Ulro is also associated with death and rebirth. When Albion, one of Blake's protagonists, awakens from the chaotic death-sleep of Ulro, his nightmare of individualistic selfhood is over, and he is reborn. The *Dance of Albion* (1794) portrays such an awakening.

Samuel Palmer (1805–1881) was a student of Blake and was impressed by Blake's spirituality and vision. Palmer claimed that "dreaming inspired him . . . and poetry set him dreaming." Palmer's childlike nightscapes *The Sleeping Shepherd* (ca. 1833) and *The Sleeping Shepherd, Early Morning* (1857) lack the terror of Fuseli's nightmares and the strange drama of Blake's underworld, yet Palmer aligned himself more with these artists than with genre painters whose patrons were wealthy aristocrats. Palmer's world is a safe haven where shepherds sleep restfully.

Artistic Reaction to Modernization

Throughout the nineteenth century, opposing schools of painting sprang up under the influence of the multiple social phenomena that characterized modernization: science and positivism, urbanization, and the growth of industrial capitalism. Whether they represented an escape from urban squalor or a desire to uplift the spirit, neoclassical works continued to celebrate the idealized human figure well into the nineteenth century. There was renewed interest in classical art, partly in response to archeological discoveries made in the mid-1700s. Such works as *The Sleeping Nymph* (1850) by the French painter Théodore Chassériau (1819–1856) reveal both the enduring influence of Greek art on European taste and the neoclassical nostalgia for an elegant and glorious past.

Realism brought to art scientific attitudes about the impartial observation of reality. The nineteenth-century fascination with physics and optics fed painters' interest in the light reflected from objects. In naturalistic paintings such as *Girls on the Banks of the Seine* (1856) by Gustave Courbet (1819–1877), the figures do not dream, they sleep. Much as in genre paintings, sleeping is seen as a natural daily activity without symbolic meaning.

The Late Victorian Poet-Painters

Other painters of the day did not share an equal faith in the merits of science and the objective depiction of reality. Reacting against the cultural values of materialism and scientific rationality, they turned their sights inward instead. Within this artistic category are found the works of Dante Gabriel Rossetti (1833–1898), Frederic Leighton (1830–1896), and Edward Burne-Jones (1833–1898). Like Blake and Palmer, Rossetti advocated renewed moral meaning and literary grounding in art. Late Victorian poet-painters could rely on a well-educated audience familiar with the popular Greek, Norse, Celtic, and Christian legends. Burne-Jones's paintings in the "Briar Rose" series (1871–1890) and his *Dream of Lancelot at the Chapel of the San Grael* (1896) and *A Dream, The Muses on Mount Helicon* (1871), *Dreamers* (1882) by Albert Moore (1841–1893), and *Saint Cecilia* (1895) by John W. Waterhouse (1849–1917) represent an idealistic and pseudo-medieval escape from the materialism of late Victorian urban society. Images of sleep and dreaming seem to stand for the moral slumber of modern humanity in the art of these nostalgic and utopian painters.

The Symbolists

Symbolist painters of the late 1800s also sought to put ideas and meaning back into painting. In reaction to the scientific emphasis of realism, the symbolist painters rejected mere visual analysis in favor of blending the spiritual and material worlds through emotional experience. Dreams were popular with symbolists for their personal and subjective nature as well as their potential for symbolic representation. Dream themes appear in the album of lithographs *In the Dream* (1879) by Odilon Redon (1840–1916) and in *The Dream* (1883) by Pierre Puvis de Chavannes (1824–1898). In *Night* (ca. 1889) by Ferdinand Hodler (1853–1918), multiple sleeping male and female figures are geometrically arranged as if to suggest social isolation in what should be an intimate setting.

Surrealism

Nowhere else in the history of Western art has a school or movement addressed itself so directly to dreams and the dream state as did surrealism in the early 1920s. Loosely borrowing from Freudian theories of dreams and the unconscious, surrealism was a reaction against the inherent scientism of naturalism and realism. According to the poet André Breton, the movement's self-appointed spokesman, surrealism opposed the "straitjacket of logic and rationalism" that had ultimately led to the carnage of World War I. Surrealism sought instead to tap an "absolute reality" found in the fusion of dream logic and waking experience. Paintings could draw on dream images or merely be reminiscent of dreams. These paintings are characterized by their "shorthand" visual representation; that is, objects are often stripped of their details. Additionally, surrealist images often appear either in a space that has no depth or in a space that seems to extend infinitely. Another hallmark of surrealist "hand-painted dream pictures" is the juxtaposition of objects that do not belong together.

The stripped-down imagery of Henri Rousseau (1844–1910; *Le Rêve,* 1910) appealed to the Surrealists, as did the somber plazas of Giorgio de Chirico (1888–1978) with their classical architecture and strange tailors' dummies. The irrational juxtaposition of forms in *Oedipus Rex* (1922) by Max Ernst (1891–1976) and *Personal Values* by René Magritte (1898–1967), the vast space and menacing figures in *Giraffe in Flames* (1935) by Salvador Dalí (1904–1989) and *Infinite Divisibility* (1942) by Yves Tanguy (1900–1955), and the odd creatures animating *The Tilled Field* (ca. 1923) by Joan Miró (1893–1983), all characterize the surrealist "dreamspace."

As a twentieth-century art movement, surrealism also directly influenced cinema. Cross-fertilization between surrealism and cinema included a collaboration between Salvador Dali and the film director Luis Buñuel; Dali also designed sets for the dream sequence in Alfred Hitchcock's film *Spellbound*. (See also MOVIES, SLEEP AND DREAMS IN.)

Sleep and dreaming appear both centrally and peripherally in Western art. At times, depictions of sleep and dreaming are laden with symbolic associations, as in early Renaissance dream imagery intended to teach the values of the Christian church, or Renaissance humanism brought the divine down to earth with figures of sleeping gods and heroes. In certain periods, sleep and dreaming were less imbued with symbolism. Genre painters naturalized figure studies by depicting scenes from everyday waking and sleeping life, and realists were more interested in objective documentation than in figurative meaning. Metaphysical painters like Fuseli, Blake, and Palmer and movements such as symbolism and surrealism took up the themes of sleep and dreaming most directly. Seen in historical perspective, all these works of art shed light on the changing cultural meanings of sleep and dreaming.

REFERENCES

Ades D. 1978. *Dada and surrealism.* New York: Barron's.

Gowing L. 1970. *Vermeer,* 2nd ed. London: Faber and Faber.

Grimes R. 1972. *The divine imagination: William Blake's major prophetic visions.* Metuchen, N.J.: Scarecrow.

Hughes R. 1980. *The shock of the new.* New York: Knopf.

Klonsky M. 1977. *William Blake: The seer and his visions.* New York: Harmony.

Pischel G. 1975. *A world history of art.* New York: Simon and Schuster.

Spalding F. 1978. *Magnificent dreams: Burne-Jones and the late Victorians.* New York: Dutton.

Joan Mancuso

ARTHRITIS AND OTHER MUSCULOSKELETAL DISORDERS

Musculoskeletal disorders are very prevalent in the general population. They are often associated with the complaints of disturbed nocturnal sleep and daytime sleepiness or fatigue. The complaint of fatigue is so prominent in some of the rheumatic disorders that it is actually used as an indicator of disease activity and response to therapy. Unfortunately, very little objective scientific evaluation of these important complaints has been carried out (McCarty, 1989).

The two most often cited complaints are poor quality of nighttime sleep and daytime fatigue or sleepiness. Most available studies addressing the quality and quantity of nighttime sleep have relied on subjective reports. It has been shown that even in normal individuals there may be striking discrepancies between the subjective and objective parameters of commonly employed indicators of sleep quality, such as time required to fall asleep, total sleep time, and number of awakenings. Such discrepancies are even more pronounced in individuals suffering from poor sleep. Caution must be used when interpreting such studies that use subjective reports, especially those dealing with change in sleep quality/quantity in different diseases and following various therapies (Mahowald et al., 1989).

Conventional wisdom and "common sense" have suggested that the sleep complaints in patients with musculoskeletal disorders are self-evident because of nocturnal pain. This relationship remains to be determined; however, preliminary studies indicate that pain may be a relatively minor cause of sleep disruption in these conditions.

The complaints of fatigue and daytime SLEEPINESS reported by patients suffering from musculoskeletal disorders may be extremely difficult to differentiate and are often confused, but actually refer to completely different phenomena. The complaint of "fatigue" is the seventh most frequent initial complaint in US medical offices and has a prevalence of 24 percent in primary care clinics. Fatigue is difficult to define, measure, and interpret, but probably represents different phenomena, including boredom, reduced motivation or vigilance, inattention, decreased enthusiasm or energy, or is a manifestation of depression (Solberg, 1984; Chen, 1986).

In contrast, the complaint of true "daytime sleepiness" refers to an inability to maintain wakefulness when desired during the day. Excessive sleepiness results in inappropriate sleep episodes that interfere with daily activities. Daytime sleepiness can be objectively measured in the sleep laboratory by the MULTIPLE SLEEP LATENCY TEST (MSLT), which demonstrates an abnormal tendency to fall asleep (physiological sleepiness). Unfortunately, most fatigue scales do not distinguish fatigue from sleepiness, undermining their clinical usefulness. Certain individuals complaining of fatigue may actually be hypersomnolent. There are important different diagnostic and therapeutic implications for these two groups.

Osteoarthritis is the most common of the rheumatic disorders. Its prevalence increases with age, being present in 20 percent to 50 percent of adults and in 85 percent of those over age

75. Sleep complaints are common in patients with osteoarthritis, and it has been speculated that these symptoms are caused by nighttime pain. No careful studies exist to confirm or refute this speculation.

Rheumatoid arthritis affects 0.3 percent to 1.5 percent of Americans. The onset of fatigue during the day is felt to be an important indicator of disease activity and response to therapy. Subjective fatigue affects 80 percent of patients with rheumatoid arthritis (but only 21 percent of a control population). Objective studies have indicated a variety of causes for "poor sleep" in patients with rheumatoid arthritis, including very frequent arousals. Some rheumatoid arthritis patients suffer from obstructive sleep apnea. This may be the result of anatomic arthritic changes in the upper airway and lower jaw. MSLT studies have shown that many of the "fatigued" patients actually experience significant daytime sleepiness.

The *fibrositis syndrome (fibromyalgia)* is a poorly understood condition characterized by complaints of muscular pain, stiffness, and fatigue. Nonrestorative sleep or sleep disturbance is one of the hallmarks, occurring in 60 percent to 90 percent of fibromyalgia patients. In 1975, a peculiar electroencephalographic sleep pattern termed the ALPHA–DELTA SLEEP pattern was described in association with this disorder. This phenomenon consists of the superimposition of alpha-frequency activity (8 to 13 cycles per second) on a background of NREM sleep patterns that contain delta-frequency activity (1 to 4 cycles per second). More recent, larger studies indicate that the alpha–delta sleep pattern is, in fact, nonspecific in nature and occurs in many individuals without musculoskeletal conditions. A genetic factor may be involved in its appearance. Its true relationship, if any, with fibrositis or any other medical condition remains to be determined before its significance can be established.

There are virtually no adequate population studies available that evaluate sleep and daytime alertness in other rheumatological conditions often associated with severe fatigue, such as *systemic lupus erythematosus, ankylosing spondylitis,* and *vasculitis.*

The effect of medications on sleep and daytime functioning in patients with musculoskeletal disorders is another important consideration. With the exception of corticosteroids (e.g., prednisone), which interfere with sleep continuity, the effects of arthritis medications on sleep and fatigue have not yet been studied.

The ubiquitous complaints of poor nighttime sleep along with daytime fatigue or sleepiness in patients with the musculoskeletal disorders need to be studied much more thoroughly. Sleep laboratory techniques are now available that will yield valuable, objective information regarding the quality and quantity of sleep and daytime sleepiness/alertness in these common conditions. Such information will undoubtedly reveal important new avenues of treatment.

REFERENCES

Chen MK. 1986. The epidemiology of self-perceived fatigue among adults. *Prev Med* 15:74–81.

Mahowald MW, Mahowald ML, Bundlie SR, Ytterberg SR. 1989. Sleep fragmentation in rheumatoid arthritis. *Arthritis Rheum* 32:974–983.

McCarty DJ (ed) 1989. *Arthritis and allied conditions,* 11th ed. Philadelphia: Lea and Febiger.

Solberg LI. 1984. Lassitude. *JAMA* 251:3272–3276.

Maren L. Mahowald

ASPIRIN

Throughout the Middle Ages, it was known that the tea made from willow bark was good for "curing anguish and intermitting disorders (fevers and pains)" (letter from Rev. Edmund Stone in Oxfordshire to the Right Honourable George, Earl of Macclesfield, president of the Royal Society, April 25, 1763). But it took until 1828 before Johann A. Buchner from Munich, Germany, could isolate the active ingredient in willow bark. Ten years later, Raffaele Piria of Pisa, working in Paris, called this active ingredient by the name we use today: salicylic acid. Aspirin is acetylsalicylic acid, a compound of salicylic acid and acetic acid.

Extracting salicylic acid from willow bark was costly. Luckily, in 1860 Kolbe in Marburg, Germany, learned how to synthesize this acid, making it from phenol, carbon dioxide, and sodium. In 1874 the first aspirin factory was built in Dresden, Germany, and today aspirin is one of the most often consumed drugs: Americans take

16,000 tons of aspirin tablets per year, or 80 million tablets.

A typical aspirin tablet contains 325 milligrams of medication. In low doses (one tablet or less per day), aspirin acts as a blood thinner, preventing heart attacks and cerebral thrombosis. Two to six tablets per day are useful to reduce pain or fever. Much higher doses (eight to twenty tablets per day) are useful to reduce the inflammation and swelling of joints in such disorders as rheumatic fever, gout, and rheumatoid arthritis. In addition, aspirin also dissolves corns on the toes, inhibits the clotting of blood, provokes loss of uric acid, and promotes fluid retention by the kidneys. If not buffered or diluted by considerable amounts of water, aspirin can also eat through the stomach wall and cause ulcers. It can also inhibit ion transport across cell membranes, interfere with the activation of white blood cells, and delay the production of the energy storage compound adenosine tryphosphate. There is an aspirin hypersensitivity syndrome called *Reye's syndrome* that has potentially fatal consequences, especially in children.

Patients have long reported that aspirin helps them sleep. Early studies were inconclusive, but in 1980 Hauri and Silberfarb published a double-blind study. They administered a placebo for the first 4 nights, then two tablets of aspirin (concealed in gelatin capsules) for 2 weeks, followed by 3 nights of placebo. On average, their eight insomniacs had significantly increased total sleep time and decreased wake time during the night when taking aspirin. This effect came mainly in the second part of the night. Three of the eight insomniacs showed improved sleep with aspirin over the entire 2 weeks, three showed the effect only in the first few nights, and two showed no effect. In some patients, aspirin was as effective as prescription SLEEPING PILLS.

How aspirin causes better sleep is currently unknown. John R. Vane, who received the Nobel Prize in 1982 for this work, showed that aspirin inhibits the synthesis of some prostaglandins (i.e., substances that are released when cells are injured or stimulated by other hormones). These prostaglandins may be involved in sleep. Others suggest that aspirin increases free tryptophan in the bloodstream, which is then available for transport across the blood–brain barrier and can increase serotonin (a sleep-inducing substance) in the brain. (See also CHEMISTRY OF SLEEP.) In any case, it is clear that the sleep-inducing properties of aspirin are not simple side effects of its pain- and fever-inhibiting properties; all subjects in the Hauri and Silberfarb study were carefully selected to be free of pain and fever.

On the basis of the Hauri and Silberfarb study, a trial with two aspirin tablets at bedtime may be recommended for some insomniacs, especially if the problem is intermittent. However, one should take aspirin only with a large glass of water. An aspirin tablet lying relatively dry on the stomach wall during sleep can cause a serious stomach ulcer by morning.

REFERENCES

Hauri PJ, Silberfarb PM. 1980. Effects of aspirin on the sleep of insomniacs. *Curr Ther Res* 28:867–874.
Weissmann G. 1991. Aspirin. *Sci Am* 264:84–90.

Peter Hauri

ATHLETICS

See Exercise; Sports and Sleep

ATONIA

[*Although the word* atonia *may not appear in most dictionaries, it is commonly used by sleep researchers. Atonia may be defined as the lack of muscle tone in sleep. While muscle tone is normally reduced during NREM sleep, during REM sleep there is a complete atonia of the muscles that maintain posture in waking, such as those in the back, neck, chin, and limbs. Atonia is discussed in the articles entitled* REM SLEEP MECHANISMS AND NEUROANATOMY *and* REM SLEEP PHYSIOLOGY. *Malfunction of the mechanism responsible for the suppression of tone in REM sleep is believed to cause* REM SLEEP BEHAVIOR DISORDER. *Hyperactivity of the muscle tone suppression system may contribute to sleep* APNEA. *See also* MOTOR CONTROL *for a discussion of brain mechanisms producing atonia. Related articles include* NARCOLEPSY, CATAPLEXY, ELECTROMYOGRAPHY, SLEEP PARALYSIS, *and* SLEEPWALKING.]

ATTENTION DEFICIT HYPERACTIVITY DISORDER

The history of the hyperactivity syndrome can be traced in the medical literature back to the early 1900s, when many features of the disorder were recognized and children with this symptom cluster were characterized as having defects in moral control. The terminology describing this disorder has changed over the years, varying with the prevailing views regarding suspected causes for the disorder (e.g., minimal brain damage syndrome, minimal brain dysfunction) or prominent symptoms of the disorder (e.g., hyperactive impulse disorder or attention deficit disorder). Currently, it is referred to as attention deficit hyperactivity disorder (ADHD), and children so classified are characterized by a core cluster of symptoms that may include extensive and often inappropriate activity, short attention span, distractibility, impulsivity, excitability, and, despite indications of normal performance on various intelligence measures, poor scholastic performance. Although there is disagreement about the precise prevalence of this disorder in the population (values range from 1 percent to 20 percent), there is a consensus that the symptoms clustered together to define this disorder can be found in a significant number of children.

Although various types of behavior therapy have been used in the treatment of these children, the most common form of treatment involves the administration of STIMULANT medications. The administration of stimulant medication commonly prescribed for children with this disorder, for example, d-amphetamine, methylphenidate, and pemoline, has been shown to improve attention and decrease restless behavior reliably in approximately 75 percent of these children. The quieting effects of such medication on the behavior of these children were at first thought to be paradoxical and unique; however, it has since been demonstrated that this medication also results in improvement in motor behavior and attention in normal children, so it is now recognized that the effects in ADHD children are neither paradoxical nor unique.

As sleep disruption has been associated with attentional and performance decrements similar to those noted in ADHD children, it would seem logical that many aspects of waking symptomatology in these children could result from disturbed sleep; however, the extent to which sleep disturbances are present in these children and, if present, whether they contribute to or result from these behaviors remains controversial. At one time, aspects of sleep disruption were considered among the characteristics of this disorder; however, in keeping with current research findings, sleep disturbance is not presently listed among criteria for ADHD. Indications of sleep disruption in ADHD have been derived from anecdotal clinical reports and survey studies. Such reports generally focus on the perception of parents and involve children referred for pediatric or child psychiatric consultation. For these reasons, the data generated may reflect characteristics of subpopulations and may not generalize to the larger ADHD grouping.

Laboratory studies using electrographic recording procedures have varied with respect to aspects of symptomatology of the subjects studied, study design, presence of stimulant medication, and when present, types and levels of such medication. Still, there is a remarkable consistency across these studies indicating the absence of marked differences in sleep patterns in ADHD children relative to those of normal children. Although stimulant medications are known to alter sleep patterns in adults, these medications have little effect on sleep in ADHD children. The absence of such effects may be attributable to several factors, including the scheduling of doses (generally 0.5 mg/kg) across the day at times that avoid sleep periods and the short half-life of these medications (approximately 2 hours for d-amphetamine and methylphenidate and 12 hours for pemoline). Considering theoretical arguments suggesting an arousal dysfunction in these children, it is notable that in these polygraphic studies neither the latency to sleep onset nor the total amounts of sleep are affected. The presence of slight increases in body movements reported during sleep in these children is suggestive of an arousal dysfunction, but certainly does not constitute a significant source of sleep disruption. (See DEPTH OF SLEEP.)

Another observation from polygraphic studies continues to surface: an extended latency to the onset of the initial REM sleep period. The interpretation of this finding remains unclear, but it is unlikely that it represents sleep disturbance, particularly occurring as it does in the absence of other signs of sleep disturbance or sleep curtailment.

Although the postulated arousal dysfunction in these children is not evident in their general sleep architecture, it was thought possible that this dysfunction might be reflected in variations in arousal threshold from sleep. Consequently, investigations have also been conducted examining sleep depth in these children. Again, however, the results of these studies underscore similarities between normal and ADHD children (medicated or unmedicated) on arousal-related variables; that is ADHD children awoke as often and in response to similar intensities of auditory stimulation as control children.

Given the acknowledged heterogeneity of the large population included under the ADHD classification, there can be little doubt that subpopulations of children with varying mixtures of symptomatology are present within this diagnostic category. Consequently, it is to be expected that experimental results will at times appear inconsistent and that sleep disturbances will be present in some of these children. The consensus of results from sleep studies conducted to date, however, argues for the absence of marked sleep disruption as a contributory factor or common correlate of this disorder.

REFERENCES

Barkley RA. 1981. *Hyperactive children: A handbook for diagnosis and treatment.* New York: Guilford Press.

Busby K, Firestone P, Pivik RT. 1981. Sleep patterns in hyperkinetic and normal children. *Sleep* 4: 366–383.

Busby K, Pivik RT. 1985. Auditory arousal thresholds during sleep in hyperkinetic children. *Sleep* 8:332–341.

Kaplan BJ, McNicol J, Conte RA, Moghadam HK. 1987. Sleep disturbance in preschool-aged hyperactive and nonhyperactive children. *Pediatrics* 80: 839–844.

Silver AA, Hagin RA. 1990. *Disorders of learning in childhood,* pp 383–421. New York: Wiley.

Simonds JF, Parraga. 1984. Sleep behaviors and disorders in children and adolescents evaluated at psychiatric clinics. *Dev Behav Pediatr* 5:6–10.

R. T. Pivik

AUDITORY AROUSAL THRESHOLD

See Depth of Sleep

AUTOMATIC BEHAVIOR

[*Automatic behavior is a phenomenon often reported by patients who suffer from excessive daytime* SLEEPINESS *or by individuals undergoing severe sleep* DEPRIVATION. *Many patients with severe untreated* NARCOLEPSY *or sleep* APNEA *syndrome report episodes during which they perform some relatively routine behavior and subsequently have no memory of the event. Examples of automatic behavior include driving a vehicle to an unintended destination, carrying on a conversation that is not remembered, or performing a routine task in a totally inappropriate manner, such as loading dishes into the clothes washer instead of the dishwasher. Similar behavioral anomalies can occur as a consequence of long-term, chronic insufficient sleep or total sleep deprivation.*

While such behavior may not necessarily be life threatening, it is quite discomfiting and disorienting to the individual. Furthermore, such behavioral manifestations of excessive sleepiness raise concerns for PUBLIC SAFETY IN THE WORKPLACE, *as well as* PUBLIC SAFETY IN TRANSPORTATION.

Current scientific data suggest that automatic behavior is related to the repetitive occurrence of MICROSLEEP *events. While such microsleep events may allow for continuing performance of certain rote behaviors in the absence of active* COGNITION, *they may also be associated with* AMNESIA, *or* MEMORY *failure, as a consequence of the effects of sleep on cognitive functioning.*]

AUTONOMIC NERVOUS SYSTEM

The autonomic nervous system controls a vast array of physiological systems ranging from the genitalia to the sweat glands to the pupils of the eye; all of these systems undergo major changes during different stages of sleep and wakefulness. Two components of the autonomic nervous system mediate these changes, the parasympathetic system and the sympathetic system, each component having separate structures within the brain that mediate control.

The actions of each component of the autonomic nervous system change with state. During NREM sleep, the PARASYMPATHETIC NERVOUS SYSTEM dominates; thus, heart rate slows, and beat-to-beat changes in heart rate reflect influences that alter parasympathetic outflow to the heart (see HEART REGULATION DURING SLEEP). Pupils become constricted, reflecting a reduction of SYMPATHETIC NERVOUS SYSTEM activity on the muscles that dilate the pupil. The genitalia become flaccid during NREM sleep, and the extent of sweating, which is mediated by the sympathetic rather than the parasympathetic component, is reduced. Thus, the galvanic skin response, which measures skin resistance and is heavily influenced by the amount of sweating, shows increased resistance during NREM sleep. Gut motility is enhanced, as the intestines are heavily innervated by parasympathetic fibers of the vagus, and actions of many digestive organ systems are enhanced.

The activity of organ systems innervated by the autonomic nervous system changes markedly during REM sleep. The primary change is one of episodic bursts of activity; in addition, increased sympathetic and parasympathetic activation occurs, with sympathetic outflow enhanced in particular portions of the body. The activation of sympathetic activity often occurs in transient bursts in REM sleep. Thus, peripheral manifestations of transient increases in sympathetic nerve discharge are apparent in this state; the pupils of the eye, for example, momentarily dilate in bursts from episodic sympathetic activation. Males undergo erections, and the genitalia of females become engorged (see ERECTIONS; NOCTURNAL PENILE TUMESCENCE; SEXUAL ACTIVATION). Observation of this last characteristic in males during REM sleep has been used as a diagnostic indicator to differentiate an inability to maintain an erection during waking from an inability to maintain an erection in any physiological circumstance.

Particular aspects of physiology that are dependent on integrity of the autonomic nervous system for expression change profoundly during sleep. Maintenance of body temperature, for example, depends on interactions between the anterior HYPOTHALAMUS, a structure in the forebrain, and the hindbrain sympathetic areas being functional; but these interactions between the two brain areas may be greatly disrupted during REM sleep.

A number of disorders of breathing during sleep can evoke autonomic nervous system activity to the level of an extreme response. Obstructive sleep APNEA, a syndrome of cessation of airflow through an obstructed upper airway with continued diaphragmatic movements, results in periodic loss of oxygen to body tissues. The brain senses this diminished oxygen (hypoxia) as well as the increased venous return to the heart from attempts to breathe against a closed upper airway, and initiates a response to preserve oxygen supply to vital tissues, such as the brain, and to adjust blood flow through the vessels. These responses include a pronounced sympathetic outflow to constrict the blood vessels of the periphery; sympathetic activation often results in profuse sweating as well. A marked blood pressure rise accompanies these events; rapid elevation of blood pressure initiates a reflex, called the baroreflex, that induces a pronounced parasympathetic response through the vagus to slow the heart. The heart rate slowing can be so pronounced that no beats occur for 5 seconds or more, and disturbed conduction of electrical signals across the heart muscle can appear. When the patient wakens from the airway obstruction, the release of the influences causing the transient elevation in pressure restores more normal heart rates. Repetitive obstructions, which are characteristic of this syndrome, result in characteristic slowing and acceleration of heart rate and multiple transient increases in blood pressure. In the morning, patients with obstructive sleep apnea are frequently drenched in sweat, as repetitive outpourings of sympathetic nervous activity accompany each obstruction.

REFERENCES

Orem J, Barnes CD. 1980. *Physiology in sleep.* New York: Academic Press.

Verrier R. 1989. Behavioral state and cardiac arrhythmias. In Lydic R, Biebuyck JF, eds. *Clinical Physiology of Sleep*, pp 31–51. New York: Oxford University Press.

Ronald M. Harper

B

BARBITURATES

The barbiturates are among the oldest sedatives currently in use, newer only than the venerable chloral hydrate. The first compound, barbituric acid, a cyclic structure that results from combining an organic acid (malonic acid) and urea, was made in 1864 by Adolf von Baeyer in Ghent (Mendelson, 1980). Von Baeyer was at the time a student of Friedrich August Kekulé, who himself occupies a famous place in the history of sleep, as he is said to have invented the benzene ring after a dream in which two snakes, biting each other's tails, formed a ringlike structure (see CREATIVITY IN DREAMS; PROBLEM SOLVING AND DREAMING). The barbiturate structure is also very similar to that of the anticonvulsant diphenylhydantoin (Dilantin), which is formed from the condensation of another organic acid (glycolic acid) and urea. Barbituric acid itself does not have sleep-inducing (hypnotic) properties; these are present only when two alkyl or aryl groups are added to the fifth carbon atom in the ring. This was first done by Fischer and von Mering in 1903. Following the reasoning that in another family of sedatives, the sulfonals, the addition of ethyl groups increased soporific properties, they began adding ethyl groups to similar structures. It is said that von Mering telegraphed the exciting news of success to the vacationing Fischer, who in turn coined for the new sedative barbital the trade name Veronal, after Verona, the restful city in which he received the good news. By 1912, Alfred Hauptmann introduced phenobarbital, a major medication for the treatment of epilepsy. Subsequently, roughly 2,500 barbiturate derivatives have been made, and perhaps 50 have been used medically.

Barbiturates, like the benzodiazepine sedative-hypnotics, are often classified by the time they remain active in the body (commonly expressed as the *half-life,* the time it takes for the body to metabolize and eliminate one half of the amount detected in the blood). The hypnotic barbiturates (amobarbital, secobarbital, and pentobarbital) are considered intermediate-duration agents, with half-lives of approximately 24 hours. They are broken down in the liver to inactive substances and excreted in the urine. In contrast, the much longer-duration phenobarbital, used as both an anticonvulsant and a daytime sedative, is much more water soluble and is excreted by the kidneys. One of the carbon atoms in the ringlike structure can be replaced by a sulfur atom, resulting in the thiobarbiturates, which leave the body in only a few hours and are used as intravenous surgical anesthetics (see ANESTHESIA).

Physiologically, the barbiturates have many different kinds of effects on various tissues. When applied locally to nerves, they have local anesthetic properties. They depress transmission across synapses in the central nervous system, in ganglia of sympathetic nerves in the AUTONOMIC NERVOUS SYSTEM, and at the junction of nerves and muscle cells. The exact mechanism by which they produce their effects on cells is not fully understood. One aspect of their action may be that they bind to one portion of the benzodiazepine receptor complex (see BENZODIAZEPINES), where they promote the flow of negatively charged chloride ions into the cell. It has been speculated that this may be a common feature of sedative compounds with many different chemical structures, including ALCOHOL and benzodiazepines.

Clinically, the barbiturates produce daytime sedation and, in higher doses, induce sleep. Unlike the gaseous anesthetics, they do not alleviate pain in an awake person, but do so only when they produce unconsciousness. They reduce the sensitivity of respiratory mechanisms that normally increase ventilation in response to lowered levels of blood oxygen or elevated levels of carbon dioxide. This can be of particular concern when these drugs are given to patients who already have compromised respiration, for instance due to chronic obstructive pulmonary disease or sleep APNEA (see also MEDICAL ILLNESS AND SLEEP). Although all barbiturates can inhibit convulsions when given in anesthetic concentrations, phenobarbital is alone among clinically used barbiturates in having a substantial anticonvulsant effect relatively independent of sedation.

Low doses of barbiturates may induce euphoria, accompanied by increases in fast activity on the electroencephalogram (EEG), which is sometimes known as *barbiturate activation*. At higher doses, slower EEG waves become prominent. During sleep, like most hypnotics, barbiturates induce SLEEP SPINDLES. They are potent hypnotics that decrease sleep latency and increase total sleep time. They have potent REM sleep–suppressing properties, and marked increases in REM ("REM REBOUND") occur on withdrawal (Buysse and Reynolds, 1990).

The major drawbacks of the barbiturates include their marked toxicity in overdose, which is made much greater yet by concomitant ingestion of alcohol (Mendelson, 1980). Roughly ten therapeutic doses can be fatal. In these situations, the EEG of the comatose patient is dominated by large, slow waves, and eventually death occurs as a result of respiratory or cardiac failure. The barbiturates also have substantial potential for the development of clinical tolerance and dependence. Indeed, "street" abuse of barbiturates was widespread for many years, although substantially less so than opiate abuse. The prominence of both as DRUGS OF ABUSE has now been largely supplanted by concern with COCAINE and its derivatives. Withdrawal from large doses of barbiturates taken for prolonged periods can cause severe withdrawal syndromes (Jaffe, 1987), which are characterized by hyperthermia and seizures and are often considered much more medically dangerous than even those induced by

opiate drugs. In recommended doses, the barbiturates also can stimulate enzymes in the liver that break down a variety of drugs; the result can be that many other medications, if taken simultaneously with barbiturates, can have reduced effectiveness.

Because of these many concerns, the barbiturates, which were by far the most widely used sedative-hypnotics since the turn of the century, underwent a rapid decrease in popularity with the introduction of the benzodiazepines in the 1960s. Although they clearly continue to have a useful role as anticonvulsants and intravenous anesthetics, their clinical utility as hypnotics is very limited.

REFERENCES

Buysse DJ, Reynolds CF III. 1990. Insomnia. In Thorpy MJ, ed. *Handbook of sleep disorders,* pp 373–434. New York: Marcel Dekker.
Jaffe JH. 1987. Pharmacological agents in the treatment of drug dependence. In Meltzer HY, ed. *Psychopharmacology: The third generation of progress,* pp 1605–1616. New York: Raven.
Mendelson WB. 1980. *The use and misuse of sleeping pills.* New York: Plenum.

Wallace B. Mendelson

BASAL FOREBRAIN

As its name implies, the basal forebrain is a region in the ventral, or basal, part of the front of mammalian and avian brains. This area contains a number of neuronal groups and fiber pathways including several nuclei of areas called the preoptic-anterior hypothalamus (POAH), the diagonal bands of Broca, the substantia innominata, and subpallidal areas (see HYPOTHALAMUS for a figure showing these cellular regions). The BF is a major hub of neuronal connections, with inputs and outputs to brainstem, hypothalamus, thalamus, limbic system, striatum, and neocortex (Swanson, 1987). It also regulates certain hormonal outputs of the pituitary gland and receives many of the afferent impulses from the adjacent SUPRACHIASMATIC NUCLEUS OF THE HYPOTHALAMUS, the site of the mammalian circadian clock

(Meijer and Rietveld, 1989; see also CIRCADIAN RHYTHMS). This very complex region plays a role in almost every vegetative and behavioral process in mammals, including control of sleep. Because of its strategic position as a hub among cortical, limbic, brainstem, circadian, and hormonal mechanisms, this area is viewed as an integrative center for regulation of physiology and behavior. It coordinates the circadian, vegetative, and hormonal regulatory processes of the medial hypothalamus and the emotional and memory processes of the limbic system with the sensory, discriminatory, and fine motor control functions of the thalamus, striatum, and neocortex.

The anterior hypothalamus was first implicated as a sleep-inducing area by von Economo (1930) on the basis of observations and neuropathological data from patients with insomnia after encephalitic infections. These patients were found to have lesions in the anterior medial hypothalamus. Nauta (1946) observed behavioral insomnia in rats with experimental lesions of the same region. Subsequently, several experimental lesion studies confirmed these observations with modern polygraphic monitoring techniques (e.g., McGinty and Sterman, 1968; Szymusiak and McGinty, 1986). In sharp contrast to the transient effects of lesions of lower brainstem regions implicated in arousal (e.g., Denoyer, Buda, and Jouvet, 1989), lesions in the basal forebrain have long-lasting effects on sleep. In addition, electrical stimulation of this region was found to induce sleep (Sterman and Clemente, 1962) and produce the autonomic and motor changes that normally accompany sleep (Hess, 1957). Moreover, both medial and lateral basal forebrain stimulation suppresses the activity of neurons in the midbrain reticular activating system (Szymusiak and McGinty, 1989). Certain neurons that are selectively active during sleep have been discovered in the lateral and anterior parts of the basal forebrain (Szymusiak and McGinty, 1986), and cells that increase discharge during sleep are also found in the medial preoptic area (e.g., Mallick et al., 1983). Such neurons may code a hypnogenic (sleep-inducing) drive. Finally, many chemical agents exert their hypnogenic effects when microinjected in this region. These include muramyl peptide (Garcia-Arraras and Pappenheimer, 1983), adenosine (Ticho et al., 1990), prostaglandin D_2 (Ueno et al., 1982), the serotonin precursor 5HTP (Denoyer, Buda, and Jouvet, 1989), and the hypnotic triazolam

(Mendelson et al., 1989). (See also CHEMISTRY OF SLEEP.)

The hypnogenic mechanism of the basal forebrain may have at least two components, the medial POAH and the lateral POAH and adjacent magnocellular BF. The hypnogenic effects of the medial POAH region are closely integrated with thermoregulation, the physiological regulation of body temperature. The medial POAH is well-known as a thermosensitive and thermoregulatory center of mammals; some neurons there are known to change their activity with changes in local brain temperature (Jell and Gloor, 1972). Local warming of this area also triggers sleep (Roberts and Robinson, 1969), and sleep deficits that occur after lesions of the medial POAH are linked to thermoregulatory deficits (Szymusiak, Danowski, and McGinty, 1991). Indeed, there is current speculation that the regulation of NREM sleep is closely integrated with thermoregulation (Obal, 1984; Rechtschaffen et al., 1989; McGinty and Szymusiak, 1990; see THERMOREGULATION).

The lateral basal forebrain area could have an integrative role, receiving signals about sleep regulation from the thermoregulatory elements in the medial area and conveying hypnogenic signals through long axons to distant brain areas. The sleep-active neurons in this area are known to project both to neocortex and to the midbrain electroencephalograph (EEG)-activating areas (Szymusiak and McGinty, 1989). Through these projections, basal forebrain neurons could orchestrate sleep through actions in brainstem and cortex. The chemical signatures of sleep-regulating neuronal types in the medial POAH are not yet known; this area contains a wide variety of neuronal types (Swanson, 1987). The projection neurons of the lateral basal forebrain include two intermixed types: acetylcholine (ACH) containing and gamma-aminobutyric acid (GABA) containing. Available evidence suggests that the GABA-ergic neurons convey hypnogenic information, while ACH-ergic neurons have electroencephalograph-activating effects (Buzaki et al., 1988; Szymusiak and McGinty, 1989).

REFERENCES

Buzaki G, Bickford RG, Ponomareff G, Thal LJ, Mandel R, Gage RH. 1988. Nucleus basalis and thalamic control of neocortical activity in the freely moving rat. *J Neurosci* 8:4007–4026.

Denoyer M, Buda C, Jouvet M. 1989. La destruction des perikaryas de la formation réticulée mésencéphalique et de l'hypothalamus postérieur n'entraîne pas de troubles majeurs de l'éveil chez le chat. *C R Acad Sci* 309:265–274.

Garcia-Arraras JE, Pappenheimer JR. 1983. Site of action of sleep-inducing muramyl peptide isolated from human urine: Microinjection studies in rabbit brains. *J Neurophysiol* 49(2):528–533.

Hess L. 1957. *The functional organization of the diencephalon.* New York: Grune and Stratton.

Jell RM, Gloor P. 1972. Distribution of thermosensitive and non-thermosensitive preoptic and anterior hypothalamic neurons in unanesthetized cats, and effects of some anesthetics. *Can J Physiol Pharmacol* 50:890–901.

Mallick BN, Chhina KR, Sundaram KR, Singh B, Kumar VM. 1983. Activity of preoptic neurons during synchronization and desynchronization. *Exp Neurol* 81:586–597.

McGinty DJ, Sterman MB. 1968. Sleep suppression after basal forebrain lesions in the cat. *Science* 160:1253–1255.

McGinty DJ, Szymusiak R. 1990. Keeping cool: A hypothcsis about thc mechanisms and functions of slow wave sleep. *Trends Neurosci* 12:480–487.

Meijer JH, Rietveld WJ. 1989. Neurophysiology of the suprachiasmatic circadian pacemaker in rodents. *Physiol Rev* 69:671–707.

Mendelson WB, Martin JV, Perlis M, Wagner R. 1989. Enhancement of sleep by microinjection of triazolam into the medial preoptic area. *Neuropsychopharmacology* 2(1):61–66.

Nauta WJH. 1946. Hypothalamic regulation of sleep in rats. An experimental study. *J Neurophysiol* 9:285–316.

Obal F. 1984. Thermoregulation and sleep. *Exper Brain Res* suppl 8:157–172.

Rechtschaffen A, Bergmann BM, Everson CA, Kushida CA, Gilliland MA. 1989. Sleep deprivation in the rat: X. Integration and discussion of the findings. *Sleep* 12(1):68–87.

Roberts WW, Robinson TCL. 1969. Relaxation and sleep induced by warming of the preoptic region and anterior hypothalamus in cats. *Exp Neurol* 25:282–294.

Sterman MB, Clemente CD. 1962. Forebrain inhibitory mechanisms: Cortical synchronization induced by basal forebrain stimulation. *Exp Neurol* 6:91–102.

Swanson LW. 1987. The hypothalamus. In Bjorklund A, Hokfelt T, Swanson L, eds. *Handbook of chemical neuroanatomy. Vol. 5: Integrated systems of the CNS, Part I,* pp 1–124. Amsterdam: Elsevier.

Szymusiak R, Danowski J, McGinty D. 1991. Exposure to heat restores sleep in cats with preoptic/anterior hypothalamic cell loss. *Brain Res* 541:134–138.

Szymusiak R, McGinty D. 1986. Sleep-related neuronal discharge in the basal forebrain of cats. *Brain Res* 370:82–92.

———. 1989. Sleep-waking discharge of basal forebrain projection neurons in cats. *Brain Res Bull* 22:423–430.

Ticho SR, Lekovic M, Vugrincic C, Dziennik E, Radulovacki M. 1990. Comparison of effects on sleep of adenosine and adenosine analogs microinjected to the striatum and preoptic area of rats. *Soc Neurosci Abstr* 15:242.

Ueno R, Ishikawa Y, Nakayama T, Hayaishi O. 1982. Prostaglandin D2 induces sleep when microinjected into the preoptic area of conscious rats. *Biochem Biophys Res Commun* 109:576–582.

von Economo C. 1930. Sleep as a problem of localization. *J Nerv Ment Dis* 71:249–259.

Dennis McGinty

BASIC REST–ACTIVITY CYCLE

The basic rest–activity cycle (BRAC) in the adult human has a periodicity of about 90 minutes. During sleep the BRAC is characterized by deep sleep and a lighter activity phase. The activity phase is represented by a brain wave frequency resembling that of wakefulness, an acceleration of respiration and heart rate, and contractions of the stomach, accompanied by rapid eye movements (REMs). Dreaming occurs during the activity phase. The BRAC has also been shown to be operative during wakefulness, with its activity phase involved in self-preservation via feeding and, at maturity, continuation of the species via reproduction.

At birth, sleep in humans is the dominant part of existence, accounting, with several interruptions, for about two-thirds of the time. At maturity, sleep takes up only about one-third of the time. Thus, the wakefulness capability of humans increases fourfold, as the sleep-to-wakefulness ratio changes from 2:1 to 1:2.

The length of the BRAC varies directly with the size of the animal and increases from birth to maturity. In human subjects, the BRAC increases from about 50 to 60 minutes in infancy to about 85 to 95 minutes in adulthood.

From birth on, wakefulness of necessity expresses itself in the need for nourishment, manifested by the hunger contractions of the stomach during the activity phase of the BRAC. In infants, on a self-demand schedule for nourishment, crying for feeding occurs at the end of the fourth or fifth cycle. Failure to get a response to crying in the middle of the night gradually leads to an unbroken night's sleep, the beginning of the infant's adjustment to the alternation of night and day (see INFANCY, NORMAL SLEEP PATTERNS IN).

Later in life, the call for nourishment may be interfered with by schedules for work, school, and recreation. Nevertheless, an individual in isolation, without a timing device but supplied with reading matter, food, and drinks, is likely to help himself to nourishment about every 90 minutes or so, at the same intervals as the lengths of the BRACs.

The activity phase of the BRAC also shows up in a variety of other functions, both motor and sensory, including, at puberty, sexual excitation. A similar periodicity has been observed in animals in line with their respective rest–activity cycles, which are usually shorter than those of humans. These are examples of the utilitarian functioning of the operation of the BRAC during wakefulness.

With growth and development, in addition to wakefulness of necessity, a wakefulness of choice depends on the interests of the individual and environmental happenings or on there being "something to do." For instance, as shown by Schaller (1964), gorillas in their natural habitat in the presence of an abundance of food generally spend only about 7 hours in wakefulness, with the remaining time devoted to 13 or 14 hours of night sleep and to several naps during the waking period. Similarly, a person left alone in the evening with little to do or otherwise bored may find it hard to keep awake, whereas the same individual, interested in what's going on at a party with friends, remains wide awake.

Dreaming, during the activity phase of the BRAC in sleep, involves a level of critical reactivity of the cerebral cortex lower than that in alert wakefulness. Thus, during dreaming, the level of consciousness may be compared to that of a very young child, a senile individual, or a normal adult under the influence of a large dose of alcohol. Reports of dream content may be of value for diagnostic and therapeutic purposes, but dreaming, as a process, is as inevitable in the activity phase of the BRAC during sleep as thinking is in wakefulness.

It should be noted that a number of other motor and sensory functions have been reported with cycles of a few minutes to several hours, but they in no way affect the significance of the BRAC.

After the 90-minute sleep–dream cycle was discovered, it was proposed that this might be a basic rest–activity cycle operating around the clock, in wakefulness as well as in sleep, and this proposal was confirmed in several observational and experimental studies.

REFERENCES

Kleitman N. 1982. Basic rest–activity cycle—22 years later. *Sleep* 5:311–317. Contains an exhaustive bibliography.

Schaller GB. 1964. *The year of the gorilla*. Chicago: University of Chicago Press.

Nathaniel Kleitman

BEDS

Most mammals seek out a specific site or nest for the purpose of sleep. The bed originates in the human equivalent of this behavior. From the earliest times of humanity, people created an area to be protected from the night as they slept. Beginning with piles of grasses, hides of animals, and leaves, a place to sleep developed into the crafted piece of furniture that has become the bed of today. The importance of the bed manifests itself in subtle ways and possesses a strong social link in everyday life. One-third of a person's life is spent sleeping in a bed. Currently, most people in our society are conceived, are born, and die in a bed. The bed achieves a place of importance in the household, being one of the few pieces of furniture with a room dedicated to it. The bed of today, however, had a long journey through history before reaching its place in the modern world.

The Egyptians created the first beds. While most of the people slept on the ground or narrow wooden planks, royalty enjoyed beds of rich workmanship. The piece of furniture that most resembles a modern bed remained a luxury of the upper classes throughout most of ancient civilization. Tutankhamen's tomb yielded a bed of carved ebony and chased gold. No matter how ornate the frame of the bed, it still had to be functional and support the lattice of palm reeds or leather thongs where people slept. The most enduring contribution of the Egyptians came about when the footboard was moved to the head of the bed, presumably to bolster cushions. The tradition of a headboard continues today.

The Assyrians, Babylonians, Phoenicians, and other peoples who followed Egypt in the rise of civilization continued to modify the bed. The ruling classes of Assyria and Babylonia possessed beds of bronze studded with gems. The common household had small troughs filled with straw, or just mats on the ground. In Greece, the wooden frame began to be tooled and lathed. Still very austere, the bed took on a couchlike appearance. Romans relied on wooden beds or a rock ledge in the home. In Rome, beds could be found large enough to hold six people comfortably and would be the centerpiece of banquets. At this point in history, the mattress became commonplace in the homes of the affluent.

With the collapse of the Roman empire and Western civilization's decline into the Dark Ages, the bed became nonexistent. The peoples of Europe remained on the ground at night. In the ninth century, the time of Charlemagne, the bed returned alongside other luxuries of the ancient world. Beds slowly became more and more aggrandized, gaining size and height off the floor. The eleventh century saw the return of the bedstead, a frame to support an ever larger bed. When the knights returned from the First Crusade, they brought curtains from the Muslim world. No bed was complete without folds of fabric. The thirteenth century saw the arrival of the tester, a full or partial canopy over the bed. This canopy was either suspended from the ceiling or held up by the bedposts. Throughout the Middle Ages the bed was the guarded property of the affluent; the poor slept in piles of straw on the ground.

The Italian Renaissance brought the bed out from beneath the curtains and into society. Kings would hold court from their beds, most notably Louis XIV. Beds became more common among the less wealthy. When the colonists left for America, they all slept on beds in the New World. The Americas pared the heavy designs of the European continent down to the basics of a frame and cushioning. Alongside industrialization in the eighteenth century came iron and brass beds. The MATTRESS also took shape, becoming hair-filled. The amorphous straw and feathers began to phase out. The 1920s saw the invention of the innerspring mattress. With all the pieces in place, the modern bed was created: metal frame, boxspring, and innerspring mattress. In combination, this accounts for the majority of the myriad designs of the bed in the modern Western world. The most recent innovation to the bed, the waterbed, appeared in the 1970s. The designs of a water-filled puncture-proof mattress or a series of water-filled cylindrical pouches are the most common.

As Western society became more and more industrialized, the bed became a stage for a large portion of many peoples' lives. Life became routinized. The bed, for many, became the only appropriate place for sex. Bouts of illness and pleasure occur in a bed. More than ever, the bed had achieved the power of a symbol in Western culture. It represented rest from the hectic pace of life, with promise of pleasure. A sick person recuperates in a bed. The familiarity of a bed lends security to the sleeper. Rituals associated with bed can be bizarre and extreme in some cultures. However, most everyone will admit an aversion to sleeping with the head at the foot of the bed.

The type of bed a person sleeps in can affect a night's rest if the sleeper feels unaccustomed to the bed. The right bed is the familiar one. Comfort and ease of mind have more effect on sleep than do innersprings versus a waterbed. There is no scientific evidence that innersprings, foam, or waterbeds will make sleep any more fulfilling. Even a strange or uncomfortable bed will not prevent a good sleep. Healthwise, a firmer bed surface is recommended for people with bad backs to keep the spine from sagging or from tiring back muscles. Those who have trouble with heartburn, choking, or breathing often benefit from elevating the head and trunk of the body by 6 inches.

(See also PILLOWS.)

REFERENCES

Dittrick M. 1980. *The bed book*. New York: Harcourt Brace Jovanovich.

Horne J. 1988. *Why we sleep*. New York: Oxford University Press.

Kleitman K. 1963. *Sleep and wakefulness*. Chicago: University of Chicago Press.

Lamberg L. 1984. *The American Medical Association guide to better sleep*. New York: Random House.

Luce GG, Segal J. 1966. *Sleep*. New York: Coward-McCann.

Jason Sullivan

BEDTIME STORIES

Bedtime stories told to children before they fall asleep are a common part of being "tucked in." Parents generally begin this custom when their child is old enough to understand a simple story, often at about 15–17 months of age. The telling of bedtime stories has a long and varied history and differs across cultures. Story formats range from fairy tales, fables, and folk tales to modern children's stories and original tales created by the caretaker. Storytelling styles also differ: Parents may elect to read from a book or to tell a story from memory, and the child may be encouraged to participate in the story or to lie quietly in bed. Although bedtime stories serve a variety of functions—as educational tools, part of a bedtime ritual, or rewards for desired behavior—perhaps caretakers of today have found them most useful in captivating the attention of young children while spending "quality time" with them.

Origin

Several theories have been proposed to explain the origin of the bedtime story. The ritual most likely has roots in storytelling traditions. In ancient times, adults entertained themselves after dark by telling stories around the fire, and the time for sleep naturally followed as the fire died. It is speculated that children present at these gatherings were lulled to sleep by the stories. Thus, storytelling eventually became ingrained as part of the bedtime ritual. Such behavior is also seen in adults, who often enjoy reading before bedtime. Perhaps, as some believe, bedtime storytelling originates in functional necessity. Parents, trying to prepare children for bed,

choose an entertaining yet soothing experience to help induce sleep. Another notion is that bedtime stories are a continuation of the ritual of singing lullabies to babies; as infants mature and begin to acquire speech and language, caretakers move from simple songs to more complex tales.

The stories themselves have varied origins. Many of the traditional fairy tales familiar to children in the Western world are rooted in European culture. These tales consist of fantasy worlds that capture a child's attention. Folk tales, on the other hand, reflect the lives and histories of everyday people, and were passed down through the oral tradition. Modern children's books draw upon these old tales as well as the creativity found in writer's imaginations. Many parents and babysitters also spontaneously invent bedtime stories incorporating daily events, fantasy figures, and images familiar to the child.

Cross-Cultural Practices

Cross-culturally, storytelling before bed varies in content and method. In certain cultures, such as India, bedtime rituals are not practiced, and therefore no custom of reading before bed exists. Different cultures, as might be expected, have their own histories of folk tales and popular stories, emphasizing different morals and values. The bedtime story ritual is one way to keep these alive for succeeding generations.

With regard to the literate versus oral traditions, the custom of reading the story is more prevalent in literate societies, whereas telling the story is a function of less literate societies. Wagner and Stevenson's (1982) study of cultural differences in child development found that mothers in Mexico were more likely to tell stories to their children and that mothers in the United States were more likely to read to their children from books. Accordingly, Mexican children exhibited earlier conversational skills and later reading skills than their counterparts in the United States.

Functions

The bedtime story functions primarily as a device to lull the child to sleep. It is not uncommon to find a child fast asleep during storytelling time. Besides its use as a sleep aid, reading at bedtime is a widely accepted opportunity for parents to interact with children and for children to learn from their parents. Parents can encourage psychological and intellectual growth while discussing emotional issues or developmental problems. Through stories at bedtime, parents may enhance family communication skills and promote their child's communicative skills.

The bedtime story can also be seen as a TRANSITIONAL OBJECT. White and colleagues (1990) found that hospitalized children who heard parent-recorded bedtime stories fell asleep sooner and used more self-soothing behaviors to cope with the separation than children who did not hear a bedtime story. Parental recordings of bedtime stories tailored around familiar imaginative figures and everyday interests have long been used by Porter (1965) as a treatment for childhood insomnia. Bedtime stories have been studied by Knight and McKenzie (1974) as rewards to motivate children to stop thumbsucking.

The bedtime story has also been researched as an educational tool. The act of reading together builds interest in books and enables the child to practice language skills. Most mainstream child development books tout bedtime reading as an early way to promote literacy. For example, Whitehurst and others (1988) found that vocabulary size and sentence construction were improved in children when their parents increased the amount of interactive reading and that open-ended questioning during story time was a more effective tool than straight reading alone. Story content is an important consideration for many parents: Much fun has been made of those who use science texts as bedtime stories, but even fairy tales can lead a child to discover insights about the world.

The custom of reading bedtime stories is found around the world as part of the bedtime ritual. In addition to helping children make the transition to sleep, these stories allow a parent to communicate with the child while improving reading and vocabulary skills. For many families, bedtime stories are an invaluable component of the sleep process.

REFERENCES

Bloome D. 1985. Bedtime story reading as a social process. *Nat Reading Conf Yearb* 34:287–294.

Coplon JK, Worth D. 1985. Parent–child communication through preschool books. *Soc Casework* 66(8):475–481.

Heath SB. 1982. What no bedtime story means: Narrative skills at home and school *Language Soc* 11(1):49–76.

Knight MF, McKenzie HS. 1974. Elimination of bedtime thumbsucking in home settings through contingent reading. *J Appl Behav Anal* 7(1):33–38.

Ninio A. 1983. Joint book reading as a multiple vocabulary acquisition device. *Dev Psychol* 19(3):445–451.

Pellegrini AD, ed. 1988. *Psychological bases for early education.* New York: Wiley.

Porter J. 1965. Guided fantasy as a treatment for childhood insomnia. *Aust NZ J Psychiatry* 9(3):169–172.

Shokeid M. 1982. Towards an anthropological perspective on fairy tales. *Sociol Rev* 30(2):223–233.

Trelease J. 1989. *The new read-aloud handbook.* New York: Penguin.

Wagner DA, Stevenson HW, eds. 1982. *Cultural perspectives on child development.* San Francisco: Freeman.

White MA, Williams PD, Alexander DJ, Powell-Cope GM. 1990. Sleep onset latency and distress in hospitalized children. *Nurs Res* 39(3):134–139.

Whitehurst GJ, Falco FL, Lonigan CJ, Fischel JE, et al. 1988. Accelerating language development through picture book reading. *Dev Psychol* 24(4):552–559.

Jenny Hua

BEDWETTING

Enuresis, or bedwetting as it is commonly known, is a childhood problem that has concerned parents and physicians for centuries. A review of the history of treatments that have been applied to children who wet the bed over the years reads like a description of cruel and unusual punishments. Tying a string tightly around the penis, having the child sleep on sharp objects, inflating vaginal balloons, and "stimulating" the sacral nerves by burning them—these and many other painful, punitive approaches have been recommended at one time or another. Although bedwetting is not inherently harmful, it can be associated with serious developmental problems for the growing child. Family life can be altered as too much attention is focused on the enuretic child through scapegoating, unpleasant treatment attempts, or the need to maintain a family secret. For the child, bedwetting may lead to chronic anxiety, impaired peer relationships, and lowered self-esteem. Today, enuresis continues to be a difficult problem for which complete medical understanding is still lacking.

A number of studies have demonstrated that enuresis is remarkably common. Up to 25 percent of 4-year-old children and up to 10 percent of 8-year-old children are still wetting the bed. It is by no means uncommon even in adolescence and young adulthood; 1 percent of 18-year-olds were found to be enuretic in one study. *Primary enuresis* refers to children who have wet the bed continuously all their lives, without a 6-month period of dryness. *Secondary enuresis* defines the symptom in children who have resumed wetting after a prolonged period of dryness; it is approximately one-third as common as primary enuresis. Spontaneous dryness occurs in 12 percent to 15 percent of the enuretic population in any given year. After the age of 6, older children are not more likely to become dry spontaneously in the subsequent year than are younger children.

Enuresis is most appropriately seen as a symptom (similar to fever) rather than a disease in itself. A number of known, specific causes of enuresis must be ruled out before a treatment is undertaken. Urological problems relating to congenital or acquired abnormalities of the urinary system can cause enuresis. Chronic urinary tract infections, serious constipation, diabetes, cerebral palsy, and some other uncommon medical conditions may present with enuresis as an early symptom. Many enuretic children show evidence of developmental immaturity (learning disability, immature social skills, etc.), and in these children enuresis is presumed to be another component of the delayed maturation; however, scientific evidence for this appealing concept is incomplete. Psychological stressors, such as family problems, acute illness or hospitalization, accidents, or the like, can lead to secondary enuresis. In the past, enuresis has been viewed as a specific sleep disorder. Except when enuresis is associated with sleep apnea, we now know that the wetting occurs in different STAGES OF SLEEP at different times of the night, roughly in proportion to the time spent in each sleep stage. An individual may wet the bed more than once in a night in different stages of sleep each time. The relationship of the enuresis to sleep architecture is an area badly in need of further study.

For a child who is wetting the bed and is older than age 6, a thorough diagnostic evaluation including a detailed history is needed that assesses important aspects of the symptom itself and its relationship to other aspects of the child's and family's life. A careful medical history and physical examination should be done, specifically looking for findings that are relevant to the specific causes mentioned earlier. Now we know that in addition to this evaluation, only a urine analysis and urine culture are routinely needed, although in the past many more complicated and invasive studies were typically ordered as part of the workup.

Once a diagnostic evaluation is complete, specific causes are treated individually. Urinary tract infections are treated with antibiotics, constipation is relieved with laxatives and enemas, sleep apnea may be treated with a tonsillectomy, urological problems receive surgical attention, and so on. When all specific causes are ruled out, a number of generally useful treatments are available to choose from for the child and the family. Some of these treatments could be described as common-sense approaches, but they can be much more effective when used in a systematic way with professional guidance. These common-sense treatments include keeping a diary or calendar, waking the child at intervals, and rewarding dry nights. Behavior modification techniques using conditioning with an alarm that is triggered by the first drops of urine have been found to be useful in approximately two thirds of the cases; however, recurrence occurs about 40 percent of the time and necessitates re-treatment with the alarm. A new, simplified device that is worn entirely on the child now usually replaces the old pad and alarm that have been available for the last 30 years, but the approach is basically the same and the results have changed little over the years. Some businesses have grown up that charge high rates to carry out the conditioning treatment without professional involvement. The other realm of generally applicable treatment consists of medications—imipramine and desmopressin acetate, or DDAVP. Imipramine is approximately as effective as the conditioning approach and is safe and well tolerated when taken under close monitoring by a knowledgeable physician. DDAVP is marketed as a nasal spray that alters the body's hormonal balance, which dictates fluid maintenance, and its arrival on the scene has generated considerable enthusiasm. Overall, however, definitive treatments based on a good understanding of the cause of the problem have yet to be discovered for the vexing symptom of enuresis.

REFERENCES

Fritz GK, Armbrust J. 1982. Enuresis and encopresis. *Psychiatr Clin North Am* 5:283–296.
Rockney R, Caldamone AA. 1990. The management of persistent primary enuresis. *Problems Urol* 4:9–23.

Gregory K. Fritz

BEHAVIORAL MODIFICATION

It is often extremely difficult to change long-standing habits or actions that are detrimental to health or well-being. One approach to altering the behavior associated with human problems is called *behavioral modification*. Its roots are in a school of psychological theory suggesting that our actions are regulated through our responses to external cues and information in the environment (Eysenck, 1960; Skinner, 1974; Wolpe, 1969). A certain cue that is normally neutral in the environment can evoke a particular, associated action once a relationship between the two is learned and reinforced. For example, a simple song played every time an ice cream truck drives down a street may not only make you feel hungry but also prompt you to go out and buy an ice cream. This particular behavior is reinforced every time you eat the delicious ice cream and associate the experience with the song and the truck. Although behavioral modification has dealt specifically with interactions between an individual and his or her environment, theories have expanded this approach to include a cognitive–behavioral perspective that acknowledges our responses to internal information such as thoughts and emotions (Meichenbaum, 1977). This approach emphasizes that how people view, interpret, and respond to internal processes (e.g., feelings, attitudes) is an important mediator of our actions. Many behavioral and cognitive–behavioral theories have been proposed to explain the complexities of human behavior.

Beyond theory, however, behavioral and cognitive–behavioral modification techniques have been used successfully to treat a wide range of maladaptive and problematic behaviors and habits, including headaches, eating patterns, smoking habits, communication patterns, assertiveness, children's behavioral difficulties, phobias/fears, and anxiety. An advantage of these approaches over more traditional forms of psychotherapy is that they are typically time-limited and focus on altering of a specific behavioral problem. The elimination or reduction of this specific behavioral difficulty clearly indicates the success or failure of the treatment. These theories and techniques have been successfully used to treat sleep problems, in particular nocturnal BEDWETTING and INSOMNIA. An often-cited example of an effective behavioral technique is the bell-and-pad method for reducing nighttime bedwetting in children (Mowrer and Mowrer, 1938). A pad is placed under a child, and a buzzer is sounded whenever moisture touches the pad. When a child begins to wet the bed, the buzzer will sound until the child awakens. Through repeated associations, this technique can teach children to relate their distended bladder to waking up (and hence a trip to the bathroom) rather than emptying their bladder during sleep.

One of the most effective approaches applied to disturbed sleep has been STIMULUS CONTROL FOR INSOMNIA (Bootzin and Nicassio, 1978). On the basis of behavioral and cognitive–behavioral principles, these psychologists believed that the bed and the bedroom could become associated with habits, physiological arousal, and thoughts that would disturb sleep, especially sleep onset. The stimulus control treatment of insomnia involves learning to associate the bed and the bedroom only with sleep-conducive and relaxing cues and activities. Thus, insomnia clients are not allowed to work, argue, or exercise in their bed or bedroom. Instead, the bed and the bedroom are used only for relaxation, preparation for sleep, and sleeping.

Another successful behavioral treatment of chronic insomnia involves the restriction of time in bed (Spielman, Saskin, and Thorpy, 1987). One factor that may perpetuate insomnia is spending an extended time in bed but not sleeping. Therefore, insomniacs are restricted to a time in bed that roughly equals how long they actually sleep, and are not allowed to stay in bed for prolonged periods awake. As their sleep becomes more consolidated and efficient, the time in bed is expanded and generally their sleep also increases and improves. (See also SLEEP RESTRICTION, THERAPEUTIC.)

Behavioral self-management also has been demonstrated to be an effective treatment for insomnia (Thoresen et al., 1980). In the self-management approach, a wide variety of factors that may relate to an individual's poor sleep are assessed, the information is used to apply specific treatment strategies, and generally, an individual's sense of control over those conditions and situations associated with poor sleep is enhanced. One important aspect of this approach is an emphasis on personal mastery over influences that can be altered to improve sleep.

Behavioral and cognitive–behavioral approaches and interventions can be very powerful and effective methods to improve maladaptive human behavioral problems. The application of such treatment strategies may result in more effective ways to improve many sleep disturbances.

REFERENCES

Bootzin RR, Nicassio PM. 1978. Behavioral treatments for insomnia. In Hersen M, Eissler RM, Miller PM, eds. *Progress in behavior modification.* Vol 6, pp 1–45. New York: Academic.

Eysenck HJ. 1960. *Behaviour therapy and the neurosis.* London: Pergamon.

Meichenbaum DH. 1977. *Cognitive-behavior modification: An integrative approach.* New York: Plenum.

Mowrer OH, Mowrer WA. 1938. Enuresis: A method for its study and treatment. *Am J Orthopsychiatry,* 8:436–447.

Skinner BF. 1974. *About behaviorism.* New York: Knopf.

Spielman AJ, Saskin P, Thorpy MJ. 1987. Treatment of chronic insomnia by restriction of time in bed. *Sleep* 10(1):45–56.

Thoresen CE, Coates TJ, Zarcone VP, Kirmil-Gray K, Rosekind, MR. 1980. Treating the complaint of insomnia: Self-management perspectives. In Ferguson JM, Taylor CB, eds. *The comprehensive handbook of behavioral medicine.* Vol 1, *Systems intervention,* pp 213–234. New York: Spectrum.

Wolpe J. 1969. *The practice of behavior therapy.* New York: Pergamon.

Mark R. Rosekind

BENZODIAZEPINES

The benzodiazepines are widely used as hypnotics, anxiolytics, anticonvulsants, and muscle relaxants. They were popularized in the mid-1950s by Dr. Leo Sternbach, who had first examined them at the University of Krakow in the 1930s. Benzodiazepine-like compounds had appeared in the German literature as far back as 1891. Sternbach first determined their true structure and found that these early compounds had relatively uninteresting pharmacological properties. He went on to enlarge the ring structure by treating a quinazoline derivative with methylamine, producing compounds with taming, sedative, and anticonvulsant properties in animals and anxiety-decreasing effects in humans. The first of these, chlordiazepoxide, was marketed as a tranquilizer in the 1960s, followed rapidly by the more potent diazepam. The first compound recommended specifically for sleep in the United States was flurazepam; sleep agents currently available in the United Stated include triazolam, temazepam, estazolam, and quazepam. The clinical use of these agents is discussed under SLEEPING PILLS.

Benzodiazepines are thought to produce their pharmacological effects via interaction with the benzodiazepine receptor complex (Mendelson, 1987), a protein structure in nerve cell membranes thought to have at least three moieties: recognition sites for benzodiazepines and the inhibitory neurotransmitter gamma-aminobutyric acid (GABA) as well as a chloride ion channel (ionophore). The two recognition sites interact with each other in a complex manner; when a benzodiazepine binds to its recognition site, the chloride channel opens up, allowing negative chloride ions to enter the nerve cell and reducing its tendency to generate an action potential (to *fire*). More recent work has shown that this receptor structure is an acidic glycoprotein, with at least two parts, designated alpha and beta, roughly corresponding to the recognition sites for benzodiazepines and GABA.

Benzodiazepine receptors are found near the junctions of neurons, implying a role in neurotransmission. The majority are located in "newer" parts of the brain, such as the cerebral cortex, with smaller numbers in the brainstem. These receptors are relatively new phylogenetically, going back only as far as the bony fish, which may imply that they are involved in relatively complex behaviors. Much research has been done to determine if there is an *endogenous ligand,* a naturally occurring substance in the body that might bind to these receptors and be a natural tranquilizing or sleep-inducing substance in normal physiology. So far, a number of candidates have been proposed, including nicotinamide and nucleosides such as the purines (Marangos et al., 1983), but no single compound has clearly been demonstrated to play this role. Evidence in such disease states as liver failure suggests that sleepiness and coma may result from the accumulation of substances that bind to the benzodiazepine receptor. It should also be mentioned that many sleep-inducing medications of other pharmacological classes may bind to, or alter the function of, various constituents of the benzodiazepine receptor complex. Included among these are BARBITURATES, ALCOHOL, and newer hypnotics including zopiclone and zolpidem. This evidence suggests, then, that interaction with this receptor complex may be a common mode of action for many of the wide range of compounds that can induce sleep.

The site(s) in the nervous system at which benzodiazepines act to induce sleep remains uncertain. Microinjections of benzodiazepines at various nuclei thought to be involved in sleep regulation have had little effect on sleep. One notable exception is the anterior HYPOTHALAMUS, where microinjection enhances sleep in animals (Mendelson et al., 1989). Such observations are consistent with studies going back many years that suggest the importance of the hypothalamus and the BASAL FOREBRAIN in the regulation of sleep and waking.

Benzodiazepines share a number of clinical pharmacological properties. They are relatively lipid-soluble substances that are absorbed from the stomach at different rates but cross the blood–brain barrier with relative ease. They are potent at inducing sleep and produce relatively small decrements in REM SLEEP but profound decreases in SLOW-WAVE SLEEP. Although benzodiazepines have substantially less respiratory suppressant effect than do BARBITURATES, they do

have this property to a limited extent, which may be important in administration to patients with compromised respiratory status. They do not stimulate the liver to alter the rate of metabolism of other drugs. (On the other hand, drugs such as barbiturates, which stimulate this system, may cause benzodiazepines to be metabolized more rapidly.) Benzodiazepines may alter memory function, primarily by reducing episodic memory, the ability to acquire and use new information. This property is generally fairly benign, but can potentially be accentuated by special circumstances, including when they are taken in combination with alcohol or in the context of the combination of sleep deprivation and circadian shifts that occurs during jet travel. As with all hypnotics, their sedative properties are also increased when they are taken by a previously sleep-deprived person. There has been some interest in animal studies suggesting that benzodiazepines might alter the hypothalamic circadian timing system that regulates the occurrence of sleep and waking (Turek and Losee-Olson, 1986). In humans, it seems more likely that they can aid sleep after travel to new time zones, with improved wakefulness during the new local daytime, but this probably does not actually involve resetting the circadian pacemakers. (See also CIRCADIAN RHYTHMS; JET LAG.)

The longer-acting benzodiazepines, such as flurazepam, are metabolized into other active compounds, and eventually are conjugated in the liver and excreted in the urine. Those with briefer durations of action, such as triazolam and temazepam, are metabolized to inactive substances, which are also passed as conjugated urinary substances. Clinically, the benzodiazepines are relatively benign when taken acutely in overdose by otherwise healthy individuals, but they may be very toxic when taken in combination with other drugs such as alcohol (Rango, Dumont, and Sitar, 1982). They have had relatively less popularity as drugs of abuse than have older hypnotics. On the other hand, as discussed under SLEEPING PILLS, tolerance can develop after their nightly use, and withdrawal sleep disturbance can occur when they are discontinued. It is also possible that the frequency of reliance, the tendency of patients to want to stay on medication without increasing dosage, is as great as with older hypnotics.

The number of benzodiazepine hypnotic prescriptions has remained relatively constant, near

20 million prescriptions per year, since the mid-1980s, and they are taken by about 2 percent of Americans every year. Perhaps twice as many people take benzodiazepines for their tranquilizing properties. Because of perceived concern about some aspects of benzodiazepine use, states have passed regulations to restrict their prescription by physicians. Thus, it seems likely that in the next few years we will see two types of changes: (1) the introduction of newer, nonbenzodiazepine agents, and (2) a possible rise in the use—and the complications—of the older hypnotics.

REFERENCES

Marangos PJ, Patel J, Skolnick P, Paul SM. 1983. Endogenous "benzodiazepine-like" agents. In Usdin E, Skolnick P, Tallman J, Greenblatt D, Paul SM, eds. *Pharmacology of benzodiazepines*, pp 519–527. London: Macmillan.

Mendelson WB. 1987. *Human sleep: Research and clinical care.* New York: Plenum.

Mendelson WB, Martin JV, Perlis M, Wagner R. 1989. Enhancement of sleep by microinjection of triazolam into the medial preoptic area of rats. *Neuropsychopharmacology* 2:61–66.

Rango RE, Dumont CH, Sitar DS. 1982. Effect of ethanol ingestion on outcome of drug overdose. *Crit Care Med* 10:180—185.

Turek FW, Losee-Olson S. 1986. A benzodiazepine used in the treatment of insomnia phase-shifts the mammalian circadian clock. *Nature* 321:167–168.

Wallace B. Mendelson

BIOFEEDBACK

It was once believed that the autonomic nervous system was literally automatic: through involuntary and unconscious processes the brain controlled important physiological functions such as heart activity, blood pressure, and brain and muscle activity. However, scientific research has demonstrated that people can learn to control these "automatic" physiological functions. In biofeedback, information about subtle or unconscious physiological activity (for example, heart rate or blood pressure) is provided to an individual so that it can be consciously controlled through learning. Through physical and mental activities an individual can learn to control physiological processes, for example, lowering blood pressure or decreasing muscle tension. An individual receives external information (i.e., feedback) about an internal biological process—hence the name *biofeedback*. Biofeedback has been applied successfully to control physiological factors related to a variety of health problems, such as blood pressure in hypertension, forehead muscle tension in headaches, skeletal muscles in rehabilitation, brain activity in epilepsy, and muscle tension in anxiety and related disorders (Basmajian, 1983).

The external information about internal physiological processes can be simple or highly sophisticated. Biofeedback devices typically use sensors or electrodes attached to the surface of the skin to translate the very small physiological signals (sometimes a millionth of a volt) produced by the body into an audio tone or visual image. By learning to manipulate the audio or visual signal, an individual can learn to increase or decrease the target physiological activity. A variety of health care professionals provide treatment with biofeedback and might see an individual for 30-to 60-minute sessions over a period of weeks or months for training (Schwartz, 1987). Scientific studies have demonstrated the effectiveness of biofeedback in treating many different health problems, including applications to three specific sleep disorders: INSOMNIA, TOOTHGRINDING, and BEDWETTING.

In 1967, Monroe found that poor sleepers had higher autonomic activity (e.g., higher temperature and heart rate) before and during sleep than did good sleepers. Although other studies have not consistently supported these findings, Monroe's study laid the foundation for the physiological-hyperactivity or somatic-arousal hypothesis of insomnia. This concept led to extensive applications of relaxation techniques to improve disturbed sleep (see RELAXATION THERAPY). Biofeedback to reduce muscle tension electromyographically measured from the forehead (frontalis muscle) has been used in several studies to treat insomnia effectively. Biofeedback for brain activity (electroencephalographic patterns) associated with quiet relaxed wakefulness (alpha) and the transition into sleep (theta) has been used to improve disturbed sleep. Another specific electroencephalographic biofeedback approach has used sensorimotor rhythm (SMR) from the sensorimotor cortex. Significant improvements in sleep were associated with SMR biofeedback when subjects were appropriately matched to the treatment (Borkovec, 1982).

Nocturnal toothgrinding or bruxism is a clenching or grinding of the teeth that can result in facial pain, wear on teeth, and other significant dental problems. Electromyographic biofeedback to reduce the activity of the masseter muscles, those that bulge when the teeth are clenched, has been used to treat nocturnal bruxism. Portable electromyographic biofeedback devices with sensors placed on the masseter muscles before sleep can be used so that treatment is conducted in the home. When the grinding either reaches a certain level of muscle tension or lasts for a specific length of time, an alarm awakens the individual. Usually the person gets out of bed, records the event, possibly uses a relaxation technique, and then goes back to sleep. Research on this treatment approach has provided inconsistent results. Some studies show a decrease in grinding activity, although these positive effects often disappear after treatment is discontinued. In the most successful studies, an auditory signal was used to awaken the subject, who then performed some task before going back to sleep (Mealiea and McGlynn, 1987).

A variety of treatments for bedwetting, or nocturnal enuresis, have been studied extensively (Doleys, 1980). Biofeedback is among the most effective interventions for bedwetting that is not related to a physical problem. The biofeedback treatment involves a sensing device (either a bedpan or a sensor placed in the underwear) that is activated by urine. A sound or light signal awakens the individual, who then gets up and completes the urination in the bathroom. After 5 to 12 weeks of this treatment, there is a 75 percent remission rate; 41 percent of these individuals relapse, but 68 percent of those who relapse respond when retreated.

REFERENCES

Basmajian JV, ed. 1983. *Biofeedback: Principles and practice for clinicians.* Baltimore: Williams & Wilkins.

Borkovec TD. 1982. Insomnia. *J Consult Clin Psychol* 50(6):880–895.

Doleys DM. 1980. Enuresis. In Ferguson JM, Taylor CB, eds. *The comprehensive handbook of behav-ioral medicine,* vol. 1: *Systems intervention,* pp 257–272. New York: Spectrum.

Mealiea WL, McGlynn FD. 1987. Temporomandibular disorders and bruxism. In Hatch JP, Fisher JG, Rugh JD, eds. *Biofeedback: Studies in clinical efficacy,* pp 123–151. New York: Plenum.

Monroe L. 1967. Psychological and physiological differences between good and poor sleepers. *J Consult Clin Psychol* 72:255–264.

Schwartz MS, ed. 1987. *Biofeedback: A practitioner's guide.* New York: Guilford. A good practical guide.

Mark R. Rosekind

BIOLOGICAL RHYTHMS

[*The term* biological rhythms *often refers to* CIRCADIAN RHYTHMS—*that is, those rhythms with a period of approximately 24 hours. In a larger time context, however, many other biological rhythms occur, and together they emphasize the importance of temporal organization in physiology. Across the scale of duration from seconds to years, organisms demonstrate sophisticated internal mechanisms for measuring and timing events. For example, the heartbeat is a carefully regulated biological rhythm with a period measured in tenths of seconds, coordinating contractions of the heart muscles in a precise sequence ensuring that an adequate blood supply reaches the body. This cardiac cycle is one of many* ULTRADIAN RHYTHMS, *as is the REM–NREM sleep cycle, which has a period of approximately 90 minutes in humans and marks the alternation between the two states of sleep. This 90-minute cycle may also persist during wakefulness as the* BASIC REST-ACTIVITY CYCLE.

As mentioned above, rhythms with a daily—approximately 24-hour—period are called circadian rhythms. Circadian rhythmicity is a characteristic of virtually all life processes on earth, presumably deriving from the profound changes in the external environment that occur across the day, which provided impetus for the development of internal clocks that allow organisms to adapt to and predict the state of the external world. The daily alternation of sleep and wakefulness activity is the most evident behavioral marker of circadian rhythms, whereas the BODY TEMPERATURE *cycle may serve as a physiological marker of internal timekeeping processes.*

Biological rhythms also occur with period lengths on the order of days or weeks; in mammals, most of these infradian rhythms are fertility cycles. For example, the estrus cycle of rodents has a period of 3 days or more, and the MENSTRUAL CYCLE *in humans typically lasts 28 days. Such cycles provide a balance between the biological advantages of high fertility rates and the disadvantages of maintaining more constant fertility. Many other biological rhythms have a duration of about a year; annual cycles allow adaptation to the changing seasons, and typically control such behaviors as breeding, hibernating, or nesting that are optimally performed at particular times of the year, or regulate other features of seasonal adaptation to environmental change, such as fur color. While* SEASONAL EFFECTS ON SLEEP *are usually minimal in humans, certain people suffer from* SEASONAL AFFECTIVE DISORDER, *which may reflect underlying annual rhythms.*]

BIRDS

Birds are related much more closely to reptiles than to any other creatures, but in some ways their sleep is more like that of mammals. The sleep systems of birds and mammals are thought to have evolved independently, so the similarities between them are perhaps more surprising than the differences. Comparisons between these parallel systems may eventually provide insight into basic questions about sleep.

Prior to the 1960s the study of avian sleep was largely neglected, but it has since become an active field of research.

Physiology

Quiet Sleep and Active Sleep

Episodes of quiet sleep in birds are interrupted by short bouts of active sleep, which is analogous to REM sleep in mammals.

In quiet sleep, the bird is usually motionless and the eyes show little movement; the eyes are usually, but not always, closed. Compared with wakefulness, the arousal threshold is raised, heartbeat and breathing rates are reduced, and muscle tone is generally reduced. Brain activity in quiet sleep shows an electroencephalographic pattern of high-amplitude slow waves. SLEEP-SPINDLES, common electroencephalographic features of quiet (NREM) sleep in mammals, have not been recorded in birds.

Active sleep, which always follows an episode of quiet sleep, is best characterized by a change in the electroencephalographic pattern to low-amplitude fast waves. Heartbeat and breathing rate may change from the condition of quiet sleep, but this is variable. Muscle tone may be reduced (a bird facing forward will often nod slightly at the onset of an episode of active sleep), but rarely do any of the muscles become totally relaxed. The eyes may or may not move; hence the term *REM (rapid eye movement)* is seldom used to designate this sleep state in birds.

Episodes of active sleep are very brief, averaging seven to ten seconds for most birds studied, rarely more than twenty seconds. Their length remains fairly constant: Later in the sleep cycle they may become more frequent, but not longer. Episodes of quiet sleep are also brief, generally lasting a few seconds to a few minutes. Quiet sleep may be interrupted by periods of wakefulness or by one of the intermediate stages described below. Young birds tend to have more total sleep time and more episodes of active sleep than adult birds.

Intermediate Stages

Birds show several arousal states intermediate between quiet sleep and wakefulness, and these have caused classification difficulties for researchers. Stages detected in some (but not all) species studied have been called quiet wakefulness, drowsiness, and gaze wakefulness. Another, vigilant sleep, often alternates with quiet sleep. Birds in vigilant sleep do not change posture, but their eyes are open, and their electroencephalogram (EEG) and arousal thresholds are intermediate between the levels of normal sleep and wakefulness.

Unihemispheric Sleep

Birds can be literally "half asleep," with the EEG showing sleep patterns for one hemisphere of the brain and patterns of wakefulness for the other hemisphere. In this state, usually only one eye is closed. Observations of unihemispheric sleep in birds from several different orders—chickens, quail, pigeons, and parakeets, to mention a few —suggest that this capability is widespread. The unihemispheric pattern has been observed only in quiet sleep.

Torpor and Hibernation

Birds from several groups have been found in a torpid state, with lowered heartbeat, breathing rate, body temperature, and metabolism. The reduced energy requirements of this torpid state apparently allow birds to survive periods of food scarcity. Some hummingbirds routinely become torpid at night; some swifts may become torpid for several days when bad weather prevents foraging. An extreme case involves a desert bird, the poorwill, which may enter an extended torpor (up to three months), effectively hibernating through the winter when food is scarce. Torpidity apparently may be induced by food deprivation, low temperature, or a combination of the two, but physiological details and its relation to normal sleep remain poorly understood. (See also ESTIVATION; HIBERNATION; TORPOR.)

Sleep Behavior

Roosting Sites

The verb *roost* may be used synonymously with *sleep* in birds, or it may be restricted to long periods of sleep at night (or by day, in nocturnally active species), excluding short episodes at other times. *Roost* as a noun is also applied to the site chosen for roosting.

Most birds roost in situations similar to those in which they forage or raise their young. The majority of species roost on elevated perches in vegetation; swimming birds, however, usually sleep afloat, and birds that forage exclusively on the ground usually sleep there as well. Species that nest in tree cavities or in ground burrows often roost in those sites.

Sleeping Postures

In the most common sleeping posture (see Figure 1), the bird's head is turned so that the bill

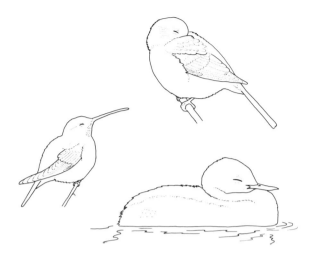

Figure 1. Three examples of sleeping postures in birds, characterized by the position of the bill in sleep. Top: head turned and bill tucked under scapular feathers on back (finch). Lower left: bill forward and slightly raised (hummingbird). Bottom: head pulled back, bill resting on chest (grebe).

points backward and rests on or under the scapular feathers. In the second most common posture, the head faces forward as in wakefulness, but may be nodded somewhat. Short-necked birds, such as owls and nightjars, may use the second posture exclusively; long-necked and long-billed birds may adopt variations of the first. Other uncommon postures among ostriches and their relatives include lying on the ground with the neck extended; a very few birds, including some Australasian parakeets, sleep hanging by their feet.

Sleeping While in Motion

Some birds can sleep while actively swimming, that is, paddling with their feet. Apparently such routine actions can be controlled by spinal reflexes, and the brain itself need not be awake.

The evidence is circumstantial, but some birds may sleep while flying; this has been suggested for swifts, swallows, and some seabirds, aerial species that forage on the wing. Sleep episodes in birds are often brief, so such sleep in flight is at least plausible, though difficult to prove.

Timing of Sleep and Wakefulness

With a few notable exceptions, the majority of bird species forage by day and sleep by night;

however, even strictly diurnal birds may have sleep episodes during daylight and many brief periods of wakefulness during the night. Many diurnal birds, including most North American songbirds, perform their migratory flights at night. In coastal environments, cycles of foraging and sleeping may be dictated more by tides than by light and darkness.

Communal Roosting

Some birds will fly many miles to spend the night in a large communal roost with others of their own kind or similar species. These aggregations sometimes number up to one million for such species as starlings and red-winged blackbirds. No complete explanation has been accepted, but two likely factors are defense against predators and sharing of information about food sources.

Bibliography

Amlaner CJ Jr, Ball NJ. 1983. A synthesis of sleep in wild birds. *Behaviour* 87:85–119.
———. 1988. Avian sleep. In Kryger MH, ed. *Principles and practice of sleep medicine.* pp 50–63. New York: Saunders.
Skutch AJ. 1989. *Birds asleep.* Austin: University of Texas Press. An extensive behavioral survey; no details on physiology.

Kenn Kaufman

BIZARRENESS

See Activation–Synthesis Hypothesis; Characteristics of Dreams

BLACK AND WHITE

See Color in Dreams

BLINDNESS

[*This composite entry consists of two articles:* Dreams of the Blind *by Nancy H. Kerr, and* Effects on Sleep Patterns and Circadian Rhythms *by Heinz Martens.*]

Dreams of the Blind

Because most people's dreaming seems dominantly visual, questions frequently arise about the dreams of the blind. How, for example, can dream settings, characters, and activities be apprehended without being visualized? Helen Keller, who was deaf as well as blind, was asked repeatedly about her dream experiences. Knowing that her questioners generally expected her dreamlife to be somehow impoverished, she once gave the following reply.

> My dreams do not seem to differ very much from the dreams of other people. Some of them are coherent and safely hitched to an event or a conclusion. Others are inconsequent and fantastic. All attest that in Dreamland there is no such thing as repose. We act, strive, think, suffer, and are glad to no purpose. We leave outside the portals of Sleep all troublesome incredulities and vexatious speculations as to probability. I float wraithlike upon clouds in and out among the winds, without the faintest notion that I am doing anything unusual. In Dreamland I find little that is altogether strange or totally new to my experience. No matter what happens, I am not astonished, however extraordinary the circumstances may be. (Keller, 1908, pp. 138–139)

Researchers who have studied the dreams of the blind largely corroborate Keller's personal observations. Except for the absence of visual imagery in clearly defined subsets of blind people, the dreams of the blind are fully elaborated simulations of life, complete with settings, characters, and storylines similar to those in the dreams of sighted people.

Systematic research began in the nineteenth century with studies by Jastrow and others that generally involved questionnaires administered to blind subjects. Although this research is relatively old by psychology's standards, these studies provided much normative data that still seem today to be generally reliable. In the first half of the twentieth century, research turned more to the individual case study and data obtained through interviews, often in a clinical setting. Kirtley's *The Psychology of Blindness* (1975) gives a useful review of these earlier questionnaire and case study approaches, as well as his own work based on dream diaries.

With the discovery in the early 1950s of REM sleep and of its association with vivid visual dreaming in sighted subjects, attention soon turned to using REM sleep monitoring and REM sleep awakening methods with blind subjects. For blind as well as sighted subjects, the new laboratory method of dream collection offered both the possibility of comparing physiological sleep variables with dream reports and the promise of more systematic sampling of a person's dreamlife under conditions least susceptible to biases introduced by the selective processes of waking memory. Thus, laboratory research has provided a more controlled means of testing the earlier findings based on less formalized observations.

Dreams of the Totally Congenitally Blind

The one respect in which the dreams of individuals with lifelong total blindness consistently differ from those of sighted people is the absence of visual imagery or visual experience. It is relatively unsurprising that individuals who have never seen in waking life report no experience of seeing in their dreams, but it does raise the question as to how their dreams are experienced. Totally congenitally blind people do report sensory experience in dreams that is auditory, kinesthetic, tactile, and occasionally olfactory or gustatory, but not any more frequently than do sighted people. The key to understanding the mode of dream experience in the blind is that they can "just know" about a spatial environment without directly sensing it. They may describe in detail a very elaborate dream setting in which they move about with perfect awareness of the locations and movements of other characters and objects in the surround, although they never touch them or sense them directly. This mode of experience is not unlike a sighted person's awareness of location when the lights go out or the eyes are closed, and it is entirely consistent with the waking experience of blind people: In familiar places, they generally have a good understanding of where they are and of where other people and objects are located.

Dreams of the Congenitally Partially Blind

Whether an individual who is born with partial sight experiences vision while dreaming depends, at least in part, on the degree and usefulness of the residual vision. People who are able to see only well enough to distinguish dark from light rarely, if ever, report awareness of seeing while dreaming. In contrast, people who are able to see some shapes and colors generally report frequent dream vision, although they never are able to see more clearly in dreaming than in waking life.

Dreams of the Adventitiously Blind

Age of onset of blindness is the critical variable in determining whether individuals who become blind after birth will experience visual dream imagery. In general, individuals who become totally blind within the first 5 years of life subsequently report dreaming without vision, and those who become partially blind during that time report only partial vision while dreaming. People who become totally or partially blind after the age of 7 generally continue to experience clear visual imagery in their dreams. People who become blind between the ages of 5 and 7 may or may not experience vision in dreaming. Some exceptions to these remarkably reliable findings have been reported, but the most credible of these involve children who became blind within a few years of the critical age boundaries and present no strong contradiction to the general principle. Evidence from sighted children's dreams also supports the idea that the period between ages 5 and 7 is in general a critical time for the development of autonomous dream processes in children (see CHILDREN'S DREAMS).

Although dream visualization in people who have become blind after the age of 7 is widely reported, there appear to be substantial individual differences in its pervasiveness, clarity, and longevity. Data from several studies suggest (1) that dream vision can be retained for very long periods following blindness after the age of 7, (2) that it is more likely to continue for people blinded when they are well past the 7-year marker, but (3) that dream vision for these people may, over time, become less frequent and less clear or vivid and may eventually cease altogether.

Adventitiously blind people can and do dream visually of people and places they have never seen, as well as of those with which they were familiar before their visual impairment. This finding is consistent with the fact that both blind and sighted people dream of novel settings and characters, and it provides additional evidence that dreaming involves active construction of scenes and events rather than passive perceptual replay.

Eye Movements and Dreams of the Blind

The discovery of the correlation between REM sleep and dreaming in the 1950s invited speculation that rapid eye movements corresponded to the mental activity of seeing in dreams. One implication of this was that totally congenitally blind people, who experience no visual imagery in dreaming, might also exhibit no eye movements in their REM sleep. Initial reports in the 1960s from sleep laboratories were mixed, with only some researchers reporting rapid eye movements during the background REM sleep of some blind subjects. In 1965, Gross, Byrne, and Fisher provided a plausible explanation for these discrepancies by showing that eye movements in blind subjects sometimes cannot be detected by traditional recording methods, but rather have to be observed directly or monitored by particularly sensitive recording techniques. They established that, although less easily detected in blind than sighted subjects, eye movements were present. Interest in eye movements during REM dreaming in the blind subsequently waned as other evidence disconfirmed the hypothetical link between rapid eye movements and seeing in dreams.

REFERENCES

Gross J, Byrne J, Fisher C. 1965. Eye movements during emergent stage 1 EEG in subjects with lifelong blindness. *J Nerv Ment Dis* 141:365–370.

Jastrow J. 1900. *Fact and fable in psychology.* Boston/New York: Houghton Mifflin.

Keller H. 1908. *The world I live in.* New York: Century.

Kerr NH, Foulkes D, Schmidt M. 1982. The structure of laboratory dream reports in blind and sighted subjects. *J Nerv Ment Dis* 170:286–294.

Kirtley DD. 1975. *The psychology of blindness.* Chicago: Nelson-Hall.

Nancy H. Kerr

Effects on Sleep Patterns and Circadian Rhythms

Millions of years of alternation between light and darkness—day and night—have left an imprint on all organisms, from unicellular algae to humans. In response to light and its absence, most higher organisms have developed a cycle of alternating activity and rest that is linked to the change from day to night. This cycle is regulated by an internal clock that keeps the organism "in rhythm" with the external environment. One situation in which we become aware of the existence of this internal clock is commonly known as JET LAG; when we cross several time zones at once, there is an abrupt shift in "time cues," and our internal clock is out of step with the outside environment.

The internal clock is set so that one complete cycle of rest and activity lasts a little longer than 24 hours. As the period covered by the cycle is approximately equal to a 24-hour day, the rhythmical patterns of alternating body functions are called CIRCADIAN RHYTHMS, from the latin *circa* ("about") and *dies* ("day").

The biological rhythms that are driven by the internal clock persist even when time cues, such as the change from daylight to darkness, are absent (Aschoff and Weaver, 1981). For example, a person living alone inside a completely dark cave without a watch would not be able to tell what time it was but would still sleep and wake on a cycle controlled by the internal clock. Suppose one cycle of his is completed in 24 hours, 30 minutes: on the second day in the cave he then would wake up 30 minutes later than he would in the presence of time cues (such as an alarm clock); on the third day, he would wake up 30 minutes plus 30 minutes later, and so on, according to the 24-hour, 30-minute cycle in this example. After 24 days, this person would be on a reversed schedule, sleeping during the day and awake during the night; after 48 days he would again be sleeping at night and awake during the day, but he would have "lost" one day. This phenomenon of continuously drifting body rhythms in the absence of time cues is called a *free run* (see also FREE RUNNING).

If daily biological rhythms in the human body are to stay in synch with the environment on a day-to-day basis, the internal clock must be able to "reset" itself to match the 24-hour day (as opposed to the "free-running" day of, for example, 24 hours, 30 minutes). Otherwise, we would feel sleepy a little later every "night" and wake up progressively later every "morning." The time cue that is most potent in resetting the internal clock every 24 hours is LIGHT (Czeisler et al., 1989).

Researchers have begun to study what happens to the internal clock and to the circadian rhythms it regulates in blind individuals, who cannot perceive light and whose internal clocks thus are not reset by this mechanism. These investigations have examined the most prominent manifestation of the internal clock, the sleep–wake cycle. Forty percent of blind persons suffer from recurrent sleep disturbances (Miles, Raynal, and Wilson, 1977). In the typical pattern, several days or weeks of undisturbed nighttime sleep are followed by a gradual transition into a phase of severely disturbed sleep and a subsequent gradual return to normal. For example, a blind teacher who adhered to a regular 24-hour schedule recorded his daily sleep duration over a period of 15 years. A typical alteration between disturbed and undisturbed nighttime sleep became evident; total nighttime sleep varied from about 4 to about 7 hours in a cycle that recurred approximately three times per year. During times when this man was unable to get more than 3 or 4 hours of nighttime sleep, he had to compensate for the loss with a prolonged daytime nap. What causes this kind of disturbance in blind individuals?

For the majority of blind persons with such sleep problems, the circadian rhythms (including the sleep–wake cycle) have been shown to be free-running; that is, they are not synchronized to the 24-hour day. In fact, the situation of a blind person is comparable to that of a person living in a cave because of the lack of exposure to bright light. In most cases, social and other time cues (other than light) are not adequate to synchronize the body rhythms of blind persons with the 24-hour day. The result is a free-running pattern of these rhythms with severe, recurring sleep disturbances in the case of the blind teacher. Likewise, many blind individuals have difficulties similar to those experienced by persons who travel across time zones or work a variety of shifts at their jobs (see SHIFTWORK). If the internal clock tells them that it is daytime, even though it is actually nighttime, they may have great difficulty falling asleep and staying soundly asleep; conversely, even though it is daytime, they may find it hard to stay awake and alert.

How can these sleep disturbances in the blind be prevented or cured? First, it is important to preserve even minimal vision, as even a very limited ability to perceive light can prove sufficient for resetting the internal clock. Even in "totally" blind persons who have no conscious light perception, the neuronal pathway from the eye to the biological clock, which is located deep in the brain, may still be intact and thus capable of inducing resetting of the clock by light signals. Preservation of this pathway together with timed exposure to bright light may keep some blind persons in synchrony with the 24-hour day. Conventional SLEEPING PILLS are not useful because these medications do not reset the clock. One possible approach to the problem would be to strengthen the impact of time cues other than light by minimizing some factors that disturb the circadian system; emotional stress, which might cause INSOMNIA and disturbed circadian rhythms, might be reduced either directly through changes in a person's life-style or indirectly through relaxation exercises. Another possibility would be to standardize the optimal timing of non-light-related time cues or to use artificial time cues. Finally, current studies are evaluating treatment with MELATONIN, a hormone that is involved with the control of the circadian system and that is secreted in the human body in the "subjective night," that is the "rest" part of the rest–activity cycle, which may or may not correspond to actual nighttime (Sack, Lewy, and Latham, 1991).

It becomes clear how vital timed exposure to light is to resetting the human biological clock. The findings from these studies in blind individuals may be applicable in sighted people who experience certain forms of sleep disturbances (so-called CIRCADIAN RHYTHM DISORDERS) that are related to nonsynchronized circadian rhythms and may be effectively treated by timed exposure to light. (See also LIGHT THERAPY.)

REFERENCES

Aschoff J, Wever R. 1981. The circadian system of man. In Aschoff J, ed. *Handbook of behavioral neurobiology: Biological rhythms*. New York: Plenum.

Czeisler CA, Kronauer RE, Allen JS, Brown EN, Jewett ME, Ronda JM. 1989. Bright light induction of strong (type 0) resetting of the human circadian pacemaker. *Science* 244:1328–1333.

Martens H, Klein T, Kronauer RE, Czeisler CA. 1991. Chronic non-24-hour sleep–wake disorder in a totally blind man: Evaluation of a 15-year sleep diary reveals remarkably stable period. *Sleep Res* 20A:548.

Miles LEM, Raynal DM, Wilson MA. 1977. High incidence of cyclic sleep–wake disorders in the blind. *Sleep Res* 6:192.

Sack RL, Lewy AJ, Latham J. 1991. A phase response curve for melatonin administration in humans. *Sleep Res* 20:461.

Heinz Martens

BLINKING

There are at least three kinds of blinking. One is reflex blinking, the rapid closure of the eyes in response to various stimuli such as bright light, objects suddenly approaching or threatening to approach the eyes, or air puffs or other stimuli touching the cornea. The function of this kind of blinking is obvious. It is to protect the eye. A second kind of blinking is the slow blinks that occur during drowsiness and are really the beginning of eye closure, which detaches the brain from the outside world in preparation for sleep. A third kind of blinking is spontaneous blinking—very brief closure of the eyes periodically throughout the day. This is the kind of blinking to be considered here.

What is the function of spontaneous blinking? "To irrigate the eyeball, to keep it from drying out, to wash away dust or other foreign material" will be the reply of most people asked this question. But this is probably not the whole story. Scientists studying this subject have found that each species of animal, including humans, has a characteristic blink rate that changes little from day to day, even under conditions of changing light, heat, and humidity. The blink rate remains remarkably constant for each species even when the cornea is anesthetized or cranial nerve V, which carries sensation from the surface of the eye to the brain, is destroyed (Hall, 1945).

In field studies, researchers have found that pigs, primates (including humans), cows, and horses were among the fastest blinkers (15–33/ minute), whereas rats, mice, rabbits, guinea pigs, and tree shrews hardly blink at all, at least if blink rates during the day are counted. Deer, antelopes, dogs, cats, and foxes fall somewhere in between—blinking around 2–4 times per minute. During blinking, not only does the eyelid suddenly come down (or up in ostriches) briefly and rapidly, but the eyeball moves slightly upward beneath the closed lid.

When blink rates of many species are examined, it appears that animals that are active in daytime, like cows, horses, monkeys, and other primates (including humans), have significantly higher blink rates than those normally active at night but asleep by day (for example, rats, mice, and cats). Curiously, the opposite is true for another spontaneous eye movement found in all mammals—the rapid eye movements (REMs) of REM SLEEP. Field studies have shown a roughly reciprocal relationship between the rate of spontaneous blinking and the duration of REM sleep. That is, animals that blink least have the longest duration of REM sleep, and vice versa (Stevens and Livermore, 1978). This observation led to the hypothesis that REMs and spontaneous blinking, both of which involve rapid movement of the eyeball beneath the closed lids, may serve similar functions. One such function could be to provide a series of pulses to the visual pathway, transmitted through the red filter of the eyelids and modulated by external light intensity. Experiments with cats having recording electrodes in various brain areas supported this hypothesis—each blink, or REM, is followed in a few milliseconds by a brain potential, the strength of which is related to the brightness of external light (Stevens and Livermore, 1978). This could mean that both blinks and REMs could be light transducers that evoke brain responses and thus modulate certain endocrine and activity functions in accordance with diurnal and seasonal rhythms related to the duration of light and darkness.

Spontaneous blinking is rare or even absent in the human infant, reaching adult rates near puberty and remaining relatively constant thereafter (Zametkin, Stevens, and Pittman, 1979). There are, however, a number of conditions that affect blink rate very profoundly. For example, drowsiness and emotional excitement both increase the blink rate. Certain neurologic and psychiatric disorders are also associated with a change in blink rate. There is a striking decrease in blink rate in patients with PARKINSON'S DISEASE, a disorder in which 80 percent or more of the dopamine-containing cells of the brain die. In contrast, individuals with schizophrenia, a common mental disorder of unknown cause, may blink two to three times as often as normal individuals (Stevens, 1978). Treatment with drugs that block central dopamine transmission in the brain relieve many symptoms of schizophrenia, slow the blink rate, and often give patients other side effects resembling Parkinson's disease (Karson, 1983). Treatment of Parkinson's disease with dopamine-augmenting drugs restores more normal blink rates and may cause paroxysms of rapid blinking. These observations suggest that spontaneous blinking is strongly affected by the availability of dopamine in brain synapses. (See also PSYCHOPATHOLOGY, NONDEPRESSION.)

Nearly all the dopamine in the brain is made by neurons darkly pigmented with melanin that lie in a long narrow strip of cells in the upper brainstem. Axons of these neurons innervate many parts of the brain, but the vast majority ascend to the basal ganglia deep in the forebrain (Fuxe, 1965). There is another cluster of dopamine cells in the hypothalamus. Other dopamine fibers, far fewer in number, extend to many brain regions including the cerebral cortex and limbic system. Which of these areas is responsible for the effects of central dopamine activity on blinking is unknown. Although there is still no definitive answer as to why all animals blink spontaneously at a more or less steady rate, blinking appears to have more uses than just cleansing the eyeball.

REFERENCES

Fuxe K. 1965. The distribution of monoamine terminals in the central nervous system. *Acta Physiol Scand* 64(Suppl 247):37–85.

Hall A. 1945. The origin and purposes of blinking. *Br J Ophthalmol* 29:445–467.

Karson CN. 1983. Spontaneous eye blink rates and dopaminergic systems. *Brain* 106:643–653.

Stevens JR. 1978. Disturbances of ocular movements and blinking in schizophrenia. *J Neurol Neurosurg Psychiatry* 41:1024–1030.

Stevens JR, Livermore A, Jr. 1978. Eye blinking and rapid eye movement: Pulsed photic stimulation of the brain. *Exp Neurol* 60:541–556.

Zametkin AJ, Stevens JR, Pittman R. 1979. Ontogeny of spontaneous blinking and habituation of the blink reflex. *Ann Neurol* 5:453–457.

Janice R. Stevens

BLOOD PRESSURE

See Apnea; Autonomic Nervous System; Heart Regulation during Sleep

BODY TEMPERATURE

[*Body temperature in mammals is maintained within a narrow range by a thermoregulatory system that balances rates of heat production and heat loss to keep brain and core body temperature within biologically functional limits. Within this range, body temperature varies across the day in a regular, rhythmic pattern. This circadian rhythm (see* CIRCADIAN RHYTHMS*) in humans normally shows highest temperature peaks in the mid-to late afternoon, and a trough in the early hours of the morning. The consistency of this variation, the evidence that it is directly linked to the circadian clock (the* SUPRACHIASMATIC NUCLEUS OF THE HYPOTHALAMUS*), and the relative ease of obtaining continuous measurements make body temperature an important and useful index of circadian clock function.*

The relationship between body temperature and sleep is complex. As a marker of the position of the circadian clock, the circadian rhythm of body temperature predicts daily modulations of sleep–wake tendency; thus, sleep during the body temperature peak in the late afternoon is usually disrupted and short, while sleep closer to the trough of the body tem-

perature curve is more restful (see TIMING OF SLEEP AND WAKEFULNESS).

Another direct effect of body temperature on sleep is suggested by studies of passive warming of human subjects with a warm bath, with resulting greater amounts of SLOW-WAVE SLEEP *(see* EXERCISE AND SLEEP). *Other* TEMPERATURE EFFECTS ON SLEEP *are seen in humans and other animals.* THERMOREGULATION *is significantly and profoundly altered as a function of specific sleep state. In small mammals and birds, sleep may also be a major influence or facilitating process for the thermal states involved in energy conservation;* HIBERNATION, TORPOR, *and* ESTIVATION *may all share some common physiological link to sleep. Finally, studies of the formidable impact of sleep* DEPRIVATION *on body temperature in rats indicate that sleep plays a crucial role in maintaining an animal's thermal balance.*]

BRAIN MAPPING

Brain electrical activity mapping (BEAM) and computed electroencephalographic topography (CET) are sophisticated, computer-based methods of displaying and analyzing large amounts of brain wave activity from an ELECTROENCEPHALOGRAM (EEG) during wakefulness or sleep. During wakefulness doctors are often concerned that a patient's EEG may be abnormal in a particular part of the brain. To determine which part of the brain might be affected, electroencephalographic activity is typically measured at eight to sixteen different locations on the scalp. These scalp locations are spaced apart in a pattern that provides representative samples of the EEG over the whole head. An electroencephalograph typically traces the brain's activity onto moving paper using rapidly moving pens to produce in eight to sixteen channels of EEG data. The resulting EEG consists of eight to sixteen squiggly lines that represent the brain's activity from moment to moment. Each line is analyzed visually for the basic EEG frequency (how fast the waves are, measured in cycles per second) and its amplitude (how high the waves are, usually measured in microvolts). Interpreting the EEG requires extensive experience, a practiced eye, and an ability to construct a mental map of how the EEG varies at each location on the scalp; this enables the doctor to determine where in the brain the problem is occurring. In practice, even the most experienced EEG experts have difficulty noting subtle differences in the frequency and amplitude of brain waves from channel to channel.

BEAM was created to assist the doctor in analyzing the EEG. Instead of being written out by a normal EEG machine, the data are stored in powerful computer. The computer then analyzes the data from each EEG channel for frequency and amplitude, usually every 2.5 seconds, for as long a period as the doctor specifies. Each frequency detected is assigned a specific color. The computer then "paints" the appropriate color at the right location on a model of the top of the brain displayed by a computer monitor. When each channel of the EEG has been analyzed and the correct color "painted" on a model of the brain, activity in all parts of the brain can be seen with a single glance (Figure 1).

Sleep researchers have long studied the brain during sleep using only a single channel of the EEG (see POLYSOMNOGRAPHY). This convention arose from technical limitations of old electroencephalographic equipment and because many scientists thought there was nothing of interest during sleep at other sites of the brain. BEAM and CET have only recently begun to be used and have already shown that electroencephalographic activity during sleep is much more complicated than was originally thought. Not only does the sleep EEG have certain frequencies and amplitude characteristics, but it has a certain topography or location that stretches over many different areas of the brain. An early study using brain mapping techniques during daytime naps showed an unexpected area of alpha wave activity in the frontal area of the brain when subjects were in deep sleep (Buchsbaum et al., 1982). Because alpha activity usually occurs with arousal or wakefulness, this finding was surprising; it suggested that the EEG of sleep stages is not the same in all parts of the brain (see STAGES OF SLEEP). Brain mapping may thus be useful in developing new ways of categorizing sleep stages. An additional study using brain mapping techniques was the first to demonstrate that PGO (ponto-geniculo-occipital) waves exist in humans (McCarley et al., 1983). PGO waves are one of the main characteristics of REM sleep in animals and typically occur just before rapid eye movements. They seem to be related to activation of the visual sys-

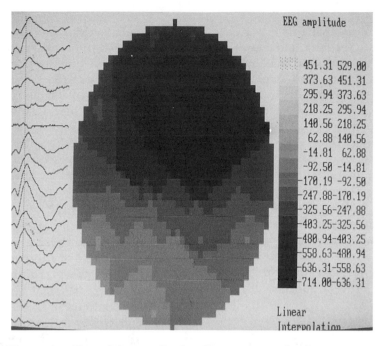

Figure 1. Map of the amplitude of a negative peak of a K-complex, with the raw EEG from which it was computed at the left.

tem and may be involved in the production of visual images during dreaming (see PGO WAVES; PHASIC ACTIVITY IN REM SLEEP). Thus, their demonstration by brain mapping techniques was very important and suggests a new way to study this REM sleep phenomenon in humans. BEAM and CET are newly developed techniques that are the sleep research tools of the future.

REFERENCE

Buchsbaum MS, Mendelson WB, Duncan WC, Coppala R, Kelsoe J, Gillin JC. 1982. Topographic cortical mapping of EEG sleep stages during daytime naps in normal subjects. *Sleep* 5(3):248–255.

Duffy FH, Burchfield IL, Lombroso CT 1979. Brain electrical activity mapping (BEAM): A method for extending the clinical utility of EEG and evoked potential data. *Ann Neurol* 5:309–332.

McCarley RW, Winkleman JW, Duffy FH. 1983. Human cerebral potentials associated with REM sleep rapid eye movements: Links to PGO waves and waking potentials. *Brain Res* 274:359–364.

Mark R. Pressman

BRAIN MECHANISMS

[*Sleep is generated by networks of cells within the brain. Many entries in this encyclopedia discuss aspects of the brain mechanisms involved in sleep. Those specifically dealing with this topic include* AMPHETAMINES; ANESTHESIA; ANTIDEPRESSANTS; ANTIHISTAMINES; AROUSAL; BASAL FOREBRAIN; CEREBRAL METABOLISM; CHEMISTRY OF SLEEP; COMA; HYPOTHALAMUS; LATERAL GENICULATE NUCLEUS; MEDULLA; METABOLIC CONTROL OF REM SLEEP; MIDBRAIN; NREM SLEEP MECHANISMS; PARASYMPATHETIC NERVOUS SYSTEM; PGO WAVES; PONS; REM SLEEP PHYSIOLOGY; REM SLEEP MECHANISMS AND NEUROANATOMY; REM SLEEP, FUNCTION OF; RESPIRATION CONTROL IN SLEEP; SYMPATHETIC NERVOUS SYSTEM; *and* THALAMUS. *Control of the rhythmic expression of behavior on a daily basis (*CIRCADIAN RHYTHMS*) is localized in mammals to two small clusters of neurons called the* SUPRACHIASMATIC NUCLEUS OF THE HYPOTHALAMUS.]

BRAIN TUMORS

It is estimated that approximately 35,000 people develop brain tumors in the United States each year. The majority of these patients experience symptoms of headaches, seizures, and neurological dysfunction such as weakness or numbness; however, many patients with brain tumors also develop alterations in sleep patterns and level of consciousness, especially late in the course of their illness.

Brain tumors may affect sleep and the level of consciousness in several ways. Direct growth of the tumor and increase in the amount of swelling (edema) around the tumor may exert pressure on surrounding brain structures, such as the brainstem, that are important in maintaining ALERTNESS. In addition, sleep may be affected by many of the treatments given to patients with brain tumors.

Direct growth of tumors can affect the level of consciousness through several mechanisms.

1. Patients with brain tumors frequently experience seizures. These may vary in severity from transient episodes of unresponsiveness lasting seconds, to grand mal seizures characterized by loss of consciousness, shaking of all four extremities, and often tongue biting and urinary incontinence. Following grand mal seizures there is often a postictal period during which the patient is initially unresponsive and then drowsy and confused. This may last from minutes to several hours, but can persist for more than a day.

2. As tumors enlarge and as the amount of surrounding edema increases, there is displacement of the surrounding brain, producing symptoms such as weakness. Because the volume inside the skull is fixed, the presence of an enlarging mass also increases the pressure inside the skull (the intracranial pressure). This may lead to symptoms such as headaches, nausea, and vomiting. As the tumor enlarges further, there is compression of the brainstem, which connects the cerebral hemispheres with the spinal cord. The brainstem contains many vital structures, including the reticular activating system, a loosely grouped network of nerve cells (neurons) important in maintaining wakefulness, as well as neurons important for maintaining normal respiration, heart rate, blood pressure, and muscle tone. Compression of the brainstem by the enlarging tumor may disrupt the re-

ticular activating system and lead to drowsiness, stupor, and eventually COMA. Other brainstem functions may also be affected, producing changes in pupil size and paralysis of eye movements, irregular respiration, changes in blood pressure and heart rate, abnormal posturing of the extremities, and eventually death. These changes occur in characteristic sequences and are termed *herniation*. Intracranial pressure can often be reduced by treatment with medications such as steroids, diuretics, and mannitol.

3. Tumors may obstruct the flow of cerebrospinal fluid, causing increased drowsiness. Cerebrospinal fluid is a clear, colorless fluid that provides nutrients and support for the brain and spinal cord. It is produced inside the brain in fluid-filled cavities called ventricles and flows through a specialized pathway before emerging to bathe the surface of the brain and spinal cord. A tumor growing near this pathway may obstruct the flow of cerebrospinal fluid, leading to enlargement of the ventricles (hydrocephalus) and increase in the intracranial pressure. The resultant downward compression or displacement of the brainstem can produce impairment of consciousness. Unless the hydrocephalus is relieved by an operation (shunting), coma and death can occur.

4. Tumors such as brainstem gliomas directly infiltrate or destroy the brainstem and the reticular activating formation, producing increasing drowsiness in addition to other neurological deficits.

In addition, sleep in people with brain tumors may also be altered as a result of treatment. To prevent seizures, most people with brain tumors are treated with anticonvulsant medications throughout their illness. These medications tend to produce sedation during the day and deeper sleep at night. These effects are especially prominent when the medications are first started and often diminish over the ensuing weeks as the body adapts to the medication. Of the anticonvulsants, phenobarbital has the greatest sedating action.

Many patients with brain tumors are also treated with steroids, such as dexamethasone, to reduce the amount of swelling surrounding the tumors. This frequently has a stimulant action and may interfere with the patient's ability to fall asleep at night.

The majority of patients with malignant brain tumors are treated by radiation therapy. This is usually administered in small doses (fractions) over a number of weeks to avoid significant injury to the surrounding brain. Despite this, there may be injury to normal brain, and this is often manifested in increased sleepiness. Several syndromes are recognized. Rarely, when large fractions of radiation are administered, an *acute reaction* is seen in the first few days. This occurs as a result of swelling around the tumor and leads to increased intracranial pressure with headaches, nausea, vomiting, and drowsiness. Steroids may be helpful in ameliorating these symptoms. More commonly, patients complain of increasing tiredness and sleepiness during the course of radiation. These symptoms generally reach a peak toward the end of radiation and rapidly improve once the radiation is stopped. The reason for these symptoms is unclear, but it has been suggested that the release of tumor necrosis factor may be partly responsible. A third syndrome that is occasionally observed a few weeks or months following irradiation is the *early delayed reaction*. This reaction is characterized by transient somnolence and lethargy, which resolve spontaneously after days or weeks. This syndrome was first described in children receiving radiation for scalp ringworm but has subsequently been seen in patients receiving radiation for leukemia and brain tumors. The cause is unknown but may be related to transient injury to oligodendrocytes, cells that make the myelin covering that surrounds neurons. A fourth syndrome results from long-term radiation injury and is seen in some patients who have survived several years after their treatment. This syndrome is characterized by dementia and occasionally increased sleepiness, gait unsteadiness, and urinary incontinence.

Finally, in common with other patients experiencing serious illnesses, patients with brain tumors frequently suffer from ANXIETY and depression. Anxiety may interfere with the patient's ability to fall asleep at night, whereas depression may lead to early-morning wakening.

REFERENCES

Adams RD, Victor M, ed. 1989. *Principles of neurology.* 4th ed. New York: McGraw-Hill.
Plum F, Posner JB, eds. 1980. *The diagnosis of stupor and coma,* 3rd ed. Philadelphia: Davis.

Patrick Wen

BRAIN WAVES

See Electroencephalogram; Elcctrocnccphalography; K-Complex; PGO Waves; Polysomnography; Sleep Spindles

BREATHING

See Allergies; Apnea; Autonomic Nervous System; Cheyne-Stokes Respiration; English Bulldog as an Animal Model of Sleep Apnea; Respiration Control in Sleep; Smell During Sleep; Snoring

BRUXISM

See Toothgrinding

C

CAFFEINE

Caffeine (Figure 1), a methylxanthine, is a central nervous system (CNS) stimulant derived from the seeds of the plant *Coffea arabica*. Chemically it is closely related to two other methylxanthine drugs, theophylline and theobromine, which also occur in common plants of the world (Ritchie, 1975). *Xanthine* is derived from the Greek word for "yellow," referring to the color of the residue left when these drugs are heated with acid. The three methylxanthines have similar pharmacological effects, all being stimulants, and differ only in the intensity of a given effect on a particular system.

Caffeine is present in a variety of common foods and drinks and is a component of a number of prescription and over-the-counter drugs, as well as some drugs sold on the street as "look-alikes" for AMPHETAMINES. (Pentel, 1984). A brewed cup of COFFEE contains about 100–150 milligrams of caffeine, a 12-ounce cola drink (see COLAS) 35–50 milligrams, and a CHOCOLATE bar as much as 25 milligrams per ounce (see Sawyer, Julia, and Turin, 1982, for listing).

Caffeine typically is consumed by mouth, and it is rapidly absorbed from the stomach, reaching peak plasma concentration in 30 to 60 minutes (Ritchie, 1975). It is equally distributed throughout the total body water, including the brain. Caffeine is metabolized primarily by the liver before it is excreted by the kidneys. The duration of caffeine activity is 3 to 5 hours in adults, although its effects sometimes are extended to 10 hours in some people. Smoking, use of other drugs, and repeated caffeine use generally accelerate caffeine metabolism and elimination, and

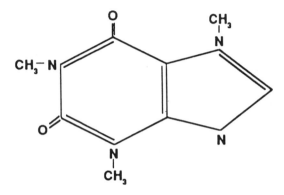

Figure 1. Structural formula of caffeine.

its metabolism and elimination are delayed in children and the elderly.

Caffeine is a CNS stimulant affecting a variety of functions in the brain, including respiratory and cardiac control and the focus of this article, sleep and wakefulness (Ritchie, 1975). When administered prior to nocturnal sleep (typically 30 minutes before lights out) it disturbs sleep (Karacan et al., 1976). In doses of 100 to 400 milligrams, sleep efficiency (sleep time per time in bed) for an 8-hour period is reduced by a factor of two to three, with sleep onset considerably delayed. In addition, the amount of wakefulness and the number of awakenings after sleep onset are increased. This dose range also increases the amount of light stage 1 sleep and reduces the amount of deep stage 3 and 4 sleep (see STAGES OF SLEEP). As a point of reference, the magnitude of sleep effects at these caffeine doses is similar to that of prescription stimulant medications such as methylphenidate and pemoline at their clinical doses (Nicholson and Stone, 1980; see STIMULANTS). Considerable individual variability in caffeine effects on sleep is reported, and the variability may relate to the age and history of caffeine use in the people being studied. How long these effects on sleep remain when the same caffeine dose is administered nightly has not been determined.

The effects of caffeine on waking function are consistent with its known stimulant properties (Sawyer, Julia, and Turin, 1982). Subjective assessment of alertness indicates that 100 to 400 milligrams of caffeine increases ratings of arousal and reduces ratings of fatigue. Objective assessment (using sleep laboratory technology) in which the latency to sleep onset (i.e., time it takes the subject to fall asleep) during the day is repeatedly tested also clearly indicates that caffeine has alerting effects (Zwyghuizen-Doorenbos et al., 1990; see MULTIPLE SLEEP LATENCY TEST). A systematic dose-related increase in the average latency to sleep onset is found (just as in the nighttime studies). Further, the degree of sleepiness before taking caffeine does not seem to alter the capacity of a given dose to increase alertness. But tolerance begins to develop quickly to the alerting effect of caffeine (i.e., the effect of a given dose decreases with repeated administration) in studies using these objective measurements of alertness.

Assessment of psychomotor performance, particularly tasks involving endurance, vigilance, and attention, shows that caffeine (100 to 400 milligrams) improves performance in such tasks (Weiss and Laties, 1962). Some studies with carefully selected subjects have shown improved performance even with small doses (35 to 75 milligrams) such as are found in foods, cola drinks, and OVER-THE-COUNTER STIMULANTS (Lieberman et al., 1987). Tasks involving simple arithmetic and coding have also shown improved performance with caffeine. How rapidly tolerance develops to the performance-enhancing effects of caffeine has not been clearly established.

Often the studies suggest that caffeine does not necessarily improve functioning, but rather restores degraded function under conditions in which there is fatigue (long periods on task) and increased sleepiness (prior sleep loss). For example, several studies have shown that caffeine (100 to 300 milligrams) maintains performance in simulated night shiftwork (Borland et al., 1986). On the other hand, in well-rested, alert subjects it has been difficult to show enhanced performance with caffeine.

Not all the evidence indicates that performance is improved and mood is enhanced with caffeine (Sawyer, Julia, and Turin, 1982). At high doses and at lower doses in persons relatively naive to caffeine (nonhabitual users), the drug is found to disrupt performance on some tasks. Subjectively, such individuals may report being jittery, anxious, and irritable and experiencing headache. Caffeine also appears to degrade performance on tasks that require dexterity or hand steadiness. It seems then that several factors, including caffeine dose, caffeine sensitivity (i.e., previous history of caffeine use), type of task, and level of alertness, all interact to determine the effects of caffeine.

Possible compensatory effects associated with caffeine have not been well characterized. Other drugs that affect sleep (e.g., ALCOHOL) show compensatory effects after the elimination of single doses and after discontinuation of regular and excessive use. Generally, these compensatory effects are opposite to the primary effect of the drug (e.g., increased wakefulness after ethanol). Recordings of the waking ELECTROENCEPHALOGRAM (EEG) in individuals to whom auditory or visual stimuli are presented yield a characteristic waveform termed an *evoked potential*. Some studies suggest an initial enhancement of the evoked potential with caffeine (300 milligrams) that is then followed by a depression of the potential 2 to 3 hours after the caffeine dose (Janssen et al., 1978). These findings suggest compensatory effects after single caffeine doses, as are found with ethanol. But the issue must be studied more carefully. Compensatory effects during the discontinuation of regular and excessive caffeine use are also reported. Among the prominent symptoms reported by individuals discontinuing excessive caffeine use (usually defined as more than five cups of coffee per day) are lassitude, drowsiness, fatigue, and decreased performance (Sawyer, Julia, and Turin, 1982). These symptoms are reversed by the administration of caffeine. Some scientists have suggested that people who are excessive caffeine consumers continue caffeine use to avoid these symptoms. Such a pattern of use suggests caffeine dependence.

The mechanisms by which caffeine produces its alerting effects are not clearly established (Snyder and Sklar, 1984). Caffeine, like other methylxanthines, is an adenosine antagonist at adenosine receptor sites in the brain. Adenosine is active in the CNS and has been shown to inhibit neuronal firing. Consequently, the current notion is that caffeine is alerting through an antagonism of adenosine inhibition. But caffeine also is known to be a phosphodiesterase inhibitor. This is an important enzyme in degrading cyclic adenosine monophosphate (AMP), a second messenger in the brain. The result of phosphodiesterase inhibition is increased cyclic AMP in the brain. Because the classic stimulant, amphetamine, also increases cyclic AMP, it is suggested that the stimulant effects of the methylxanthines may also occur through this mechanism. Caffeine also stimulates the release of epinephrine and norepinephrine from the adrenal gland. These hormones themselves are known to have stimulatory effects, and this may be another possible caffeine mechanism. (See also CHEMISTRY OF SLEEP: ADENOSINE.)

REFERENCES

Borland RG, Rogers AS, Nicholson AN, Pascoe PA, Spencer MB. 1986. Performance overnight in shiftworkers operating a day–night schedule. *Aviation, Space, Environ Med* 57:241–249.

Janssen RH, Mattie PC, Plooij-Van G, Werre PF. 1978. The effects of a depressant and a stimulant drug on the contingent negative variation. *Biol Psychol* 6:209–218.

Karacan I, Thornby JI, Anch M, Booth GH, Williams RL. 1976. Dose-related sleep disturbances induced by coffee and caffeine. *Clin Pharmacol Ther* 20:682–689.

Lieberman HR, Wurtman RJ, Emde GG, Roberts C, Coviella ILG. 1987. The effects of low doses of caffeine on human performance and mood. *Psychopharmacology* 92:308–312.

Nicholson AN, Stone BM. 1980. Heterocyclic amphetamine derivatives and caffeine on sleep in man. *Br J Clin Pharmacol* 9:195–203.

Pentel P. 1984. Toxicity of over-the-counter stimulants. *JAMA* 252:1898–1903.

Ritchie JM. 1975. Central nervous system stimulants: The xanthines. In Goodman LG, Gilman A, eds. *The pharmacological basis of therapeutics*, pp 367–378. New York: Macmillan.

Sawyer DA, Julia HL, Turin AC. 1982. Caffeine and human behavior: Arousal, anxiety, and performance effects. *J Behav Med* 5:415–439.

Snyder SH, Sklar P. 1984. Behavioral and molecular actions of caffeine: Focus on adenosine. *J Psychiatr Res* 18:91–106.

Weiss B, Laties VG. 1962. Enhancement of human performance by caffeine and amphetamines. *Pharmacol Rev* 14:1–36.

Zwyghuizen-Doorenbos A, Roehrs T, Lipschutz L, Timms V, Roth T. 1990. Effects of caffeine on alertness. *Psychopharmacology* 100:36–39.

Timothy A. Roehrs

CANCER

See Brain Tumors; Medical Illness and Sleep

CANINE NARCOLEPSY

Human narcolepsy is a lifelong neurological condition that affects roughly 0.1 percent of the general population. It involves both sexes and is seen in all races, although the percentage of affected individuals may vary substantially according to ethnic group. The disease is characterized by abnormal sleep tendencies, including excessive daytime SLEEPINESS, often disturbed nocturnal sleep, and pathological manifestations of REM sleep. These include an abnormal tendency to fall into REM sleep (sleep-onset REM periods), CATAPLEXY, SLEEP PARALYSIS (pathological equivalents of REM sleep ATONIA), and HYPNAGOGIC HALLUCINATIONS (pathological irruptions of dreamlike experiences). The causes of human narcolepsy are currently unknown, but likely involve a defect of the specific mechanisms regulating REM sleep and wakefulness.

Narcolepsy is of particular scientific interest because it is a disorder of sleep processes with a clear genetic basis in both humans (Honda et al., 1983; Guilleminault, Mignot, and Grumet, 1989; Singh et al., 1990) and animals (Baker and Dement, 1985; Mignot et al., 1992). Identifying the pathogenesis of narcolepsy may help unravel previously unknown aspects of sleep physiology. The task is a difficult one because human narcolepsy is a multifactorial and heterogeneous disorder involving several genes and environmental factors, making it difficult to study at the genetic level (Singh et al., 1990). One of the predisposing genetic factors is located on chromosome 6, within a group of genes involved in immune response: the HUMAN LEUKOCYTE ANTIGEN (HLA) genes. Because a number of disorders associated with specific HLA genes are autoimmune in nature, a similar mechanism has been proposed for narcolepsy. None of the results to date, however, substantiate this hypothesis (Parkes, Lock, and Langdon, 1986; Matsuki, Juji, and Honda, 1988; Rubin, Hajdukovitch, and Mitler, 1988; Frederikson et al., 1990).

The existence of an HLA-related susceptibility gene in human narcolepsy is also insufficient to explain the pathology. Ninety-five percent of Caucasian narcoleptic patients carry a specific sequence of HLA genes referred to as the HLA-DRw15 (DR2), Dw2, DQw6 haplotype, but 30 percent of normal control subjects also carry the same haplotype (Dupont, 1989). Since narcolepsy is relatively infrequent, other genetic and environmental factors are needed to induce the disease. This hypothesis is consistent with the canine narcolepsy model in which at least two types of narcolepsy expression are observed, one of which (in Dobermans and Labradors) is determined by a gene not related to the HLA system (Dean et al., 1989; Motoyama et al., 1989).

Clinical Aspects of Canine Narcolepsy

Narcolepsy–cataplexy has been observed in Doberman pinschers, Labrador retrievers, miniature poodles, dachshunds, beagles, and eleven other breeds (Mignot et al., 1992). It has also been noted in goats, donkeys, ponies and miniature horses, and possibly exists in bulls. The disorder has been studied extensively in Dobermans and Labradors, who transmit narcolepsy as an autosomal recessive trait with full penetrance. Symptoms first appear in these breeds between 3 and 18 weeks of age. (Baker and Dement, 1985; Mignot et al., 1992).

Canine narcolepsy is characterized by cataplexy and sleepiness. Cataplexy is defined as an abrupt loss of motor tone usually induced by such excitement as accompanies play, feeding, or sexual activity in the dogs. The loss of motor tone experienced during cataplexy in dogs can strike the entire body or only a few muscles (often the back limbs or the neck), thus defining a "complete" (Figure 1) or "partial" attack. Whether complete or partial, the cataplectic episodes can usually be reversed by a loud noise or direct body stimulation. As in human cataplexy, long attacks

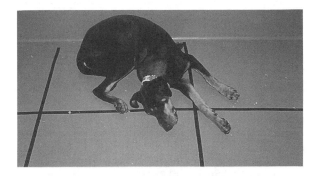

Figure 1. A narcoleptic Doberman pinscher in the midst of a cataplectic attack. Notice that the animal is lying in an awkward position, indicating muscle hypotonia.

may lead to actual REM sleep bouts (documented using electroencephalographic recordings and spectral analysis) with rapid eye movements and muscle twitches of the extremities (Mitler and Dement, 1977; Kushida, Baker, and Dement, 1985). Finally, canine cataplexy is often associated with a measurable increase in penile tumescence (J. Siegel, personal communication), a phenomenon associated with normal REM sleep.

Sleepiness has been demonstrated in narcoleptic animals with use of a modified version of the MULTIPLE SLEEP LATENCY TEST (Lucas et al., 1979). Animals are kept alert for 30 minutes and allowed to sleep for 30 minutes every hour throughout a 24-hour test. Electroencephalographic, electrooculographic, and electromyographic recordings are used to measure sleep latency. Sleep latencies are much shorter for narcoleptic canines than for control dogs (0.8 to 3.8 minutes and 6.5 to 28.5 minutes, respectively). Some of the narcoleptic canines also show typical drowsy attacks, sometimes induced by food. The animal will suddenly stop and wobble on its feet for 10 to 30 seconds. The loss of motor tone is not the most obvious symptom in these attacks, and the animal appears more sleepy than cataplectic.

A comparison of sleep patterns in narcoleptic and control dogs has been performed by several investigators in various breeds (Mitler and Dement, 1977; Kaitin, Kilduff, and Dement, 1986). These studies have shown that narcoleptic canines have more fragmented sleep than do normal animals of the same breed. The affected animals have more frequent sleep stage transitions and awakenings, but no major circadian rhythm abnormalities—trends that mirror sleep patterns of human narcoleptics.

Finally, narcoleptic canines have been studied to identify specific neuron groups involved in the control of REM sleep atonia. Siegel et al. (1991) reported the existence of a group of neurons located in the medial medulla that discharge at a higher rate during REM sleep and cataplexy. These cells may be involved in the control of REM sleep atonia. This finding illustrates how the animal model of narcolepsy is helping to uncover the mechanisms of normal human REM sleep.

Genetic Transmission of Narcolepsy in Animals

The first cases of narcolepsy in dogs were reported independently in 1973 by Mitler and Knecht. Mitler and Dement then tried unsuccessfully for several years to breed narcoleptic canines donated to Stanford in order to establish the genetic transmission of the disorder. All their attempts were unsuccessful until 1982, when several Dobermans and Labradors showing the symptoms of narcolepsy were born. It is now well established that although most cases of canine narcolepsy are multigenic and/or environmentally influenced (as in humans) Dobermans and Labradors transmit the disease as an autosomal recessive trait with complete penetrance (Baker and Dement, 1985).

Immunogenetic and Linkage Studies in Canine Narcolepsy

Pursuing the association between human narcolepsy and HLA-DR2, Stanford researchers first examined the possibility of a relationship between canine narcolepsy and the canine equivalent of the HLA system, the dog leukocyte antigen (DLA) system, with use of an association and a linkage study. Results indicate that narcoleptic canines do not share a unique DR antigen contrary to the human case, and that *canarc-1* is not located within the DLA complex (Dean et al., 1989; Motoyama et al., 1989; Mignot et al., 1991b, 1992). This result, however, does not exclude the participation of DLA in the pathophysiology

of the disorder. A permissive genetic background (of the DLA system or of non–DLA-related genes) in the canine population could allow the canine non-MHC narcolepsy gene, *canarc-1*, to be expressed in a fully penetrant fashion. It is also possible that the human equivalent of *canarc-1* is one of the factors underlying human narcolepsy, but that additional genetic and/or environmental factors are needed to express the disorder in humans. The discovery of human HLA-DR2–negative narcoleptic cases and the report of a non-DR2 narcoleptic family also provide an alternative to this model, demonstrating that HLA predisposition is not a requirement for the expression of narcolepsy.

The well-established mode of transmission of canine narcolepsy offers a unique opportunity to identify and isolate a high-penetrance gene responsible for the syndrome through reverse genetics. To do so, the Stanford team carried out a linkage study with use of various candidate genes and randomly distributed markers (Mignot et al., 1992). With this double approach, a unique gene related to a human μ-switch immunoglobulin gene (Sμ) genetically linked with *canarc-1* (Mignot et al., 1991b) was recently identified. When applied on canine DNA, this human gene probe detected several related genes at high stringency. At least three were found, two of them (strong hybridizing bands) in linkage with each other but not with *canarc-1,* and the third locus (weak hybridizing band) cosegregated with *canarc-1*.

Immunological switch genes are involved in a complex somatic recombination process allowing B-cells to switch immunoglobulin class upon activation (Essert and Radbruch, 1990). The band in linkage with *canarc-1* could be either a nonfunctional segment or involved in a somatic recombination process involving the immune system or another system. It could also be the narcolepsy gene or be in tight linkage with it. In humans and mice, most of the switch genes are clustered in only one region of a few hundred kilobases localized at the 3′ end of the immunoglobulin heavy chain locus (14q32 and 12, respectively) (Lai, Wilson, and Hood, 1989). The fact that the marker for *canarc-1* is not in linkage with the two other strong crosshybridizing loci detected with the probe suggests that *canarc-1* is not located within the canine immunoglobulin heavy chain cluster locus. A somewhat less likely explanation is that canine immunoglobulin switch genes are organized in unlinked clusters. Sμ-like genes located outside the main heavy chain complex have been isolated (Migone et al., 1983; Stockinger et al., 1986), and one marker could represent another example of this phenomenon.

The exact mechanism of action of *canarc-1* remains to be determined. Although novel, non-immunological functions could be proposed, the implication of immune genes in humans and canines (i.e., HLA haplotype association in human and Sμ linkage in dogs) suggests an immunopathology in both the narcoleptic canines and humans. The Stanford team has cloned the Sμ-like gene in linkage with *canarc-1* and will be using the clone as a probe in human narcoleptic patients to test for the involvement of *canarc-1* in the human pathology. They have also found that animals heterozygous for *canarc-1* display some degree of sleep abnormality. With use of a specific combination of drugs with cataplexy-inducing properties, the Stanford team was able to induce cataplexylike behavior in heterozygous animals but not in control dogs (Mignot et al., 1991a). This result tends to support the involvement of a *canarc-1*–like equivalent in some cases of human narcolepsy where predisposing genes seem to be autosomal dominant.

Pharmacological and Neurochemical Investigations in Canine Narcolepsy

Human narcolepsy is a disabling disorder only partially controlled by currently available medications—usually antidepressants and stimulants. The Stanford team has examined the effects of new pharmacological agents on narcoleptic canines in order to identify better treatments for human patients. In addition, these studies allow the Stanford group to determine neurochemical systems that are functionally important *in vivo* in the control of cataplexy and also, presumably, REM sleep. They have determined that the pharmacological control of cataplexy mainly involves two reciprocal systems: the cholinergic and adrenergic systems (Mignot et al., 1990). This result closely parallels what is known of the pharmacological and neurophysiological control of REM sleep.

The results of *in vivo* pharmacological experiments indicate the involvement of specific neurotransmitters (acetylcholine, norepinephrine) and receptors (M2 cholinergic, alpha-1 and alpha-2 adrenergic, and D2 autoreceptor) (for review see Mignot et al., 1990). The Stanford team is using neurochemical techniques to explore the possibility of a deficiency in these systems as a cause of narcolepsy with use of neurochemical techniques. To date, they have identified abnormalities in cholinergic systems in the PONS (Boehme et al., 1984; Kilduff et al., 1986), noradrenergic transmission in the preoptic HYPOTHALAMUS, and dopaminergic systems in the amygdala (Miller et al., 1990). They inject small doses of compounds acting on these systems in selected brain areas, record effects on narcolepsy and electroencephalographic recordings, and measure neurotransmitter levels in local brain structure perfusates (*in vivo* dialysis). These experiments may help establish a neuroanatomical and neurochemical map of the structures and neurotransmitters that control REM sleep and cataplexy. (See also CHEMISTRY OF SLEEP.)

Conclusion

Biochemical, physiological, and pharmacological studies of narcoleptic dogs will progressively enhance our therapeutic arsenal to treat human narcolepsy and our understanding of the neurochemical and neuroanatomical control of REM sleep. Also, the discovery of a genetic marker for *canarc-1* will allow us to explore the putative role of this gene in humans. This research may result in new diagnostic tools and ultimately the identification of genes underlying the pathophysiology of narcolepsy. The fact that both canine and human narcolepsy are associated with immune system–related genes may allow us to answer an even broader question: What are the links among sleep, the immune system, and narcolepsy?

Finally, we have emphasized that human and canine narcolepsy are clearly associated with abnormal control of REM sleep. We hope that understanding narcolepsy with use of the canine model will also shed light on the mechanisms and functions of the sleep process itself.

(See also DOGS; IMMUNE FUNCTION.)

REFERENCES

Baker TL, Dement WC. 1985. Canine narcolepsy-cataplexy syndrome: Evidence for an inherited monoaminergic-cholinergic imbalance. In McGinty DJ, Drucker-Colin R, Morrison A, Parmengiani P, eds. *Brain mechanisms of sleep,* pp 199–233. New York: Raven.

Baker TL, Foutz AS, McNerney V, Mitler MM, Dement WC. 1982. Canine model of narcolepsy: Genetic and developmental determinants. *Exp Neurol* 75:729–762.

Boehme R, Baker T, Meford I, Barchas J, Dement W, Ciaranello R. 1984. Narcolepsy: cholinergic receptor changes in an animal model. *Life Sci* 34: 1825–1828.

Dean RR, Kilduff TS, Dement WC, Grumet FC. 1989. Narcolepsy without unique MHC Class I antigen association: Studies in the canine model. *Hum Immunol* 25:27–35.

Dupont BO. 1989. *Immunobiology of HLA,* vol. 1 and 2. New York: Springer-Verlag.

Essert C, Radbruch A. 1990. Immunoglobulin class switching: Molecular and cellular analysis. *Annu Rev Immunol* 8:717–735.

Fredrikson S, Carlander B, Billiard M, Link H. 1990. CSF immune variable in patients with narcolepsy. *Acta Neurol Scand* 81:253–254.

Guilleminault C, Mignot WC, Grumet FC. 1989. Familial patterns of narcolepsy. *Lancet* 335: 1376–1379.

Guilleminault C, Passouant P, Dement WC. 1976. *Narcolepsy.* New York: Spectrum.

Honda Y, Asaka A, Tanaka Y, Juji T. 1983. Discrimination of narcolepsy by using genetic markers and HLA. *Sleep Res* 12:254.

Kaitin KI, Kilduff TS, Dement WC. 1986. Sleep fragmentation in canine narcolepsy. *Sleep* 9: 116–119.

Kilduff TS, Bowersox SS, Kaitin KI, Baker TL, Ciaranello RD, Dement WC. 1986. Muscarinic cholinergic receptors and the canine model of narcolepsy. *Sleep* 9:102–107.

Knecht CD, Oliver JE, Redding R, Selcer R, Johnson C. 1973. Narcolepsy in a dog and a cat. *J Am Vet Med Assoc* 162:1092–1093.

Kushida CA, Baker TL, Dement WC. 1985. Electroencephalographic correlates of cataplectic attacks in narcoleptic canines. *Electroencephalogr Clin Res* 61:61–70.

Lai E, Wilson RK, Hood LE. 1989. Physical maps of the mouse and human immunoglobulin-like loci. *Adv Immunol* 46:1–59.

Lucas EA, Foutz AS, Dement WC, Mitler MM. 1979. Sleep cycle organization in narcoleptic and normal dogs. *Physiol Behav* 23:737–743.

Matsuki K, Juji T, Honda Y. 1988. Immunological features in Japan. In Honda Y, Juji T, eds. *HLA and narcolepsy,* pp 58–76. New York: Springer-Verlag.

Mignot E, Guilleminault C, Dement WC, Grumet C. 1992. Genetically determined animal models of narcolepsy, a disorder of REM sleep. In Driscol P, ed. *Genetically defined animal models of neurobehavioral dysfunction,* pp 90–110. Cambridge, Mass.: Birkhäuser Boston.

Mignot E, Hunt Sharp L, Arrigoni J, Nishino S, Guilleminault C, Dement WC, Ciaranello R. 1991a. Gene dosage in canine narcolepsy: Induction of cataplexy-like behaviors in heterozygous dogs after drug challenge. *Sleep Res* 20:294.

Mignot E, Nishino S, Valtier D, Renaud A, Guilleminault C, Dement WC. 1990. Pharmacology of canine narcolepsy. In Horne J, ed. *Sleep 90,* pp 409–415. Bochum, Germany: Pontagenel.

Mignot E, Wang C, Rattazzi C, Gaiser C, Lovett M, Guilleminault C, Dement WC, Grumet C. 1991b. Genetic linkage of autosomal recessive canine narcolepsy with an immunoglobulin μ chain switch like segment. *Proc Natl Acad Sci U S A* 88: 3475–3478.

Migone N, Fefder J, Cann H, Van West B, Wang J, Takahashio N, Honjo T, Piazza A, Cavalli-Sforza LL. 1983. Multiple DNA polymorphisms associated with immunoglobulin μ-switch-like regions in man. *Proc Natl Acad Sci U S A* 80:467–471.

Miller J, Faull K, Bowersox S, Dement WC. 1990. CNS monoamine and their metabolites in canine narcolepsy: Replication study. *Brain Res* 509: 169–171.

Mitler MM, Boysen BG, Campbell L, Dement WC. 1974. Narcolepsy cataplexy in a female dog. *Exp Neurol* 45:332–340.

Mitler MM, Dement WC. 1977. Sleep studies on canine narcolepsy: Pattern and cycle comparisons between affected and normal dogs. *Electroencephalogr Clin Res* 43:691–699.

Motoyama M, Kilduff TS, Lee BSM, Dement WC, McDevitt HO. 1989. Restriction fragments length polymorphisms in canine narcolepsy. *Immunogenetics* 29:124–126.

Parkes JD, Lock C, Langdon N. 1986. Narcolepsy and immunity. *Br Med J* 292:359–360.

Rubin RL, Hajdukovitch RM, Mitler MM. 1988. HLA DR2 association with excessive somnolence in narcolepsy does not generalize to sleep apnea and is not accompanied by systemic autoimmune abnormalities. *Clin Immunol Immunopathol* 49: 149–158.

Siegel J, Nienhuis R, Fahringer HM, Paul R, Shiromani P, Dement WC, Mignot E, Chiu C. 1991. Neuronal activity in narcolepsy: Identification of cataplexy-related cells in the medial medulla. *Science* 252:1315–1318.

Singh SH, George CP, Kryger MH, Jung JH. 1990.

Genetic heterogeneity in narcolepsy. *Lancet* 335: 726–727.

Stockinger H, Schmidtke J, Bostock C, Epplen JT. 1986. Human DNA sequences isolated with an immunoglobulin switch region probe: Sequence, chromosomal localisation, and restriction fragment length polymorphism. *Hum Genet* 73: 104–109.

E. Mignot
W. C. Dement

CATAPLEXY

Cataplexy is a sudden spell of weakness due to a decrease in muscle tone triggered by external or internal stimuli. It is one of the most important symptoms in sleep disorders medicine because it occurs almost exclusively with NARCOLEPSY; no other sleep disorder causes cataplexy.

There is a wide range of severity of cataplexy. Mild attacks may cause slight weakness at the knees, drooping of the eyelids, sagging of the jaw or head, or inability to rise from a chair that lasts just a second or two. More severe attacks may last several minutes and cause the person to stagger briefly and then fall to the ground completely paralyzed. Patients are fully alert initially, but as the attack continues for a minute or more, the patient often passes into REM sleep with the appearance of rapid eye movements and brief facial twitches.

Many patients with narcolepsy have cataplectic attacks just a few times per year; others may have several attacks per day. On occasion, particularly after withdrawal of medications that suppress cataplexy, attacks may last hours or occur repeatedly over the course of a few days, a condition referred to as *status cataplecticus*.

Cataplexy usually begins within a few months of the onset of other symptoms of narcolepsy. Most commonly, sleepiness begins first, but some patients may develop cataplexy before sleepiness has become a serious problem. Although the peak age of onset is between 15 and 25 years, occasional patients do not develop cataplexy until middle or late life, decades after the onset of other narcoleptic symptoms. In about one third of narcoleptic patients, cataplexy improves with advancing age.

Precipitants of Cataplexy

One of the most striking features of cataplexy is its association with specific situations. The most common trigger is laughter; other common precipitants are anger, surprise, elation, excitement, and shock. Many people with cataplexy experience it during sports activities; for example, the excitement of a fish striking the line may be enough to make the fisherman too weak to reel in his catch.

Differential Diagnosis

Several medical disorders can cause sudden weakness, including inadequate blood flow to the brain, periodic paralysis associated with sudden changes in blood potassium levels, and some types of epilepsy. The association of cataplexy with laughter and other trigger factors helps to distinguish it from other medical disorders.

Pathophysiology

Cataplexy is closely linked to the REM sleep abnormalities characteristic of narcolepsy. The loss of muscle tone that occurs with cataplexy appears to be physiologically identical to the muscle ATONIA of REM sleep. The tendon reflexes, such as those elicited by tapping the quadriceps tendon at the knee or the Achilles tendon at the ankle, are reduced or absent during cataplexy, as they are during REM sleep; electrophysiological studies of the H-reflex, an electrical correlate of the tendon reflexes, have shown that the nerve cells leading to muscles are inhibited from firing during cataplectic attacks and during REM sleep.

Isolated Cataplexy

In rare instances, cataplexy can occur as an isolated symptom in patients without narcolepsy or sleep abnormalities, usually on a familial basis. In such persons, cataplexy appears to be identical to the cataplexy that occurs in narcoleptic patients, but no REM sleep abnormality is present.

Animal Models of Cataplexy

A disorder closely resembling the human narcolepsy–cataplexy syndrome occurs in several species of animals. In dogs, the disorder is sometimes inherited through recessive genes; by inbreeding these dogs, a colony of canine narcoleptics has been established. As all dog owners know, food is an exciting and emotional stimulus for dogs, and the number and severity of cataplectic attacks induced by food can be used to assess the effects of drugs or other experimental manipulations on cataplexy. Drugs that affect dopamine, noradrenaline, and acetylcholine—chemicals that act as neurotransmitters, or messengers between brain cells—have dramatic effects on canine cataplexy, and the number of receptors for these neurotransmitters is abnormal in certain areas of canine narcoleptic brain. These studies of canine narcolepsy have resulted in greater understanding of the brain abnormalities that are associated with narcolepsy and cataplexy and may ultimately lead to better treatments for this condition. (See CANINE NARCOLEPSY; CHEMISTRY OF SLEEP.)

REFERENCES

Guilleminault C. 1975. Cataplexy. In Guilleminault C, Dement WC, Passouant P, eds. *Narcolepsy,* pp 125–143. New York: Spectrum.

Parkes JD. 1985. *Sleep and its Disorders,* pp 289–294. London: Saunders.

Michael Aldrich

CENTRAL NERVOUS SYSTEM

[*The* central nervous system *comprises the brain and the spinal cord. The neurons located outside of the central nervous system make up the* peripheral nervous system. *The* AUTONOMIC NERVOUS SYSTEM, *which can be subdivided into sympathetic and parasympathetic divisions (see* PARASYMPATHETIC NERVOUS SYSTEM *and* SYMPATHETIC NERVOUS SYSTEM), *originates within the central nervous system and includes portions of the peripheral nervous system. See* BRAIN MECHANISMS *for a listing of entries related to the brain and the spinal cord.*]

CEREBRAL METABOLISM

Sleep has long been considered to be a time of "energy conservation," "rest," or "restoration." The discovery of REM sleep, however, required a revision of this older view. Whereas NREM sleep is, in a certain sense, less active than wakefulness, REM sleep was found to be paradoxically activated both psychologically and physiologically. REM sleep is associated not only with dreaming but with other measures of activation, including increased rates of single cell firing in most but not all areas of the brain, brain wave patterns similar to those seen in wakefulness, variability of autonomic activity such as breathing and heart rate, and increased overall oxygen consumption.

It is only relatively recently, however, that methods have been available to study brain energy expenditure during sleep. In recent decades, remarkable new methods have been developed for measuring localized brain function in living organisms. Unlike computerized axial tomography (CAT) and magnetic resonance imaging (MRI), which provide anatomic pictures of the brain, these new techniques provide pictures of brain function, demonstrating areas of the brain that are more or less active. Three major methods have been used to study sleep. First, local cerebral blood flow is measured, for example, by administering the inert radioactive gas Xenon 133, which is detected as it flows into and out of cortical areas by means of radioactivity detectors next to the skull (Greenberg, 1980). Second, localized glucose or sugar utilization is measured, for example, by administering the radioactive sugarlike compound deoxyglucose, which is taken up into the brain just like glucose, the major source of energy for neurons in the brain. The deoxyglucose method has been used during sleep studies both in animals (Kennedy et al., 1982; Ramm and Frost, 1986) and humans (Buchsbaum et al., 1989). In the case of humans, the deoxyglucose is tagged with a radioactive isotope of fluorine (^{18}F-deoxyglucose), and its radioactivity is measured by placing the subject's head in a large donutlike piece of equipment—a general method called positron emission tomography (PET). Finally, sleep is studied by measuring the brain's uptake of specialized radioactive tracers that can be imaged with single photon emission computerized tomography

(SPECT) (Madsen et al., 1991). All three methods assume that local neuronal activity is reflected more or less in real time by measurable changes in cerebral blood flow or glucose metabolism. That is, the "harder" a local area of the brain is "working," the more arterial blood flow it needs for the delivery of oxygen and the more fuel (glucose) it uses.

Studies of cerebral blood flow and glucose metabolism support the brain energy–conservation hypothesis for NREM sleep. For example, whole brain glucose utilization decreases in NREM sleep by about 23 percent to 35 percent compared with quiet wakefulness in the dark in both monkeys and humans. This is one of the largest decreases in cerebral metabolism occurring under normal physiologic conditions (Kennedy et al., 1982; Buchsbaum et al., 1989). Nearly all areas of the human brain show diminished glucose utilization during NREM sleep, with some of the largest decreases found in the frontal lobes, which are generally involved in attention and higher intellectual activities, as well as in the basal ganglia, structures beneath the cortex that are involved in the coordination of movement.

In contrast, whole-brain metabolic rate during REM sleep is similar to wakefulness, although showing a different pattern of brain activity. The normal waking pattern of higher metabolic rate in the right than left cerebral hemisphere, for example, is reversed during REM sleep, suggesting that the left side of the brain plays an important role in dreaming. This finding is somewhat surprising because many scientists assumed that dreaming takes place in the right side of the brain, which has been associated with nonverbal and artistic functions. Another area that shows significantly increased activity in REM sleep is the cingulate gyrus, a part of the limbic system of the brain that plays a major role in emotional activity. A recent study using SPECT showed that cerebral blood flow increases in the visual association areas during REM sleep (Madsen et al., 1991).

Preliminary studies relating certain features of dream recall in normal volunteers to regional metabolic rate have been carried out by Gottschalk and colleagues (1991a; 1991b). These investigators found significant positive correlations between the anxiety levels in dreams and localized glucose metabolism rate in the lateral parietal and medial frontal cortex.

Turning now from the effects of sleep on brain activity to the effect of sleep deprivation on waking cerebral metabolism, only one study using PET has been reported in humans before and after sleep deprivation (Wu et al., 1991). Subjects were studied while they performed a continuous performance task that required rapid responses to specific visual signals. After about 32 hours of total sleep deprivation, overall brain glucose metabolic rate was slightly but not significantly reduced. The metabolic rate in frontal areas compared with occipital (or visual) areas was significantly reduced. Poor performance on the task was associated with reduced metabolic activity in the frontal areas, suggesting that sleep deprivation may reduce normal mechanisms of attention. Metabolic rate was also reduced in thalamus and upper mesencephalon, presumably reflecting decreased activity in areas of the brain that maintain AROUSAL. These results suggest that sleep deprivation has both nonspecific effects on arousal systems and state-specific effects on different brain systems, depending on the demands placed upon the brain at the time of the study.

These studies with the new brain-imaging methods, which are only now beginning, promise exciting new vistas into the inner workings of the human brain during sleep and dreaming.

REFERENCES

Buchsbaum MS, Gillin JC, Wu J, Haslett E, Sicotte N, Dupont R, Bunney WE, Jr. 1989. Regional cerebral glucose metabolic rate in human sleep assessed by positron emission tomography. *Life Sci* 45: 1349–1356.

Gottschalk LA, Buchsbaum MS, Gillin JC, Wu JC, Reynolds CA, Herrera DB. 1991a. Anxiety levels in dreams: Relationship to localized cerebral glucose metabolism rate. *Brain Res* 538:107–110.

———. 1991b. Positron emission tomographic studies of the relationship of cerebral glucose metabolism and the magnitude of anxiety and hostility experienced during dreaming and waking. *J Neuropsychiatry Clin Neurosciences* 3:131–142.

Greenberg JH. 1980. Sleep and the cerebral circulation. In Orem J, Barnes CD, eds. *Physiology in Sleep*, pp 57–95. New York: Academic.

Kennedy C, Gillin JC, Mendelson W, Suda S, Miyaoka M, Ito M, Nakamura RK, Storch FL, Pettigrew K, Mishkin M, Sokoloff L. 1982. Local cerebral glucose utilization in non-rapid eye movement sleep. *Nature* 297:325–327.

Madsen PL, Holm S, Vorstrup S, Friberg L, Lassen NA, Wildschiødtz G. 1991. Human regional cerebral blood flow during rapid-eye-movement sleep. *J Cereb Blood Flow Metab* 11:502–507.

Ramm P, Frost BJ. 1986. Cerebral and local glucose cerebral metabolism in the cat during slow wave and REM sleep. *Brain Res* 365:112–124.

Wu JC, Gillin JC, Buchsbaum MS, Hazlett E, Sicotte N, Bunney WE, Jr. 1991. The effect of sleep deprivation on cerebral glucose metabolic rate in normal humans assessed with positron emission tomography. *Sleep* 14(2):155–162.

J. Christian Gillin
Monte S. Buchsbaum
Joseph C. Wu

CEREBROVASCULAR ACCIDENT

See Death; Stroke

CHARACTERISTICS OF DREAMS

The characteristics of dreaming are difficult to define, because dreaming is a private event. Unlike a chair or table, public objects, one cannot be certain that the private referents for *dream* are the same for all persons. Nevertheless, the fact that the neurophysiologically defined state REM sleep, as contrasted with NREM sleep, strongly matches the strength of reported dreamlike quality indicates that the subjective judgment of dreaming is a reliable one. *Dreaming* refers to a mixture of thought and emotional properties that are rare in normal waking, but common in sleep.

The dominant characteristics of dreams are a storylike sequence of bright, clear visual imagery that is sometimes bizarre and always regarded by the sleeper as perceptually "real." The strength of these characteristics varies greatly with stage of sleep, time of night, and the individual. Because different characteristics are produced by different physiological processes, the "causes" of dreaming are multiple and are best studied by examining each property independently (Antrobus, 1991).

By matching dream images to color photo-graphs of varying brightness and clarity, Antrobus and colleagues (1987) showed that the best images in any dream are typically three-quarters as bright as a waking perception, and the visual clarity of some dreams approaches that of a waking percept. On the other hand, many dream images, and certain entire dreams, have little color and image definition. Thus, sometimes the dreamer "knows" that she or he is in a particular place or with a particular person but cannot recall any specific visual image. Sometimes what the dreamer "sees" and "knows" are incompatible, as when the dreamer "sees" a girl but "knows" it is her brother. These incompatible identities suggest that the production of visual imagery is somewhat independent of the knowledge or interpretive process of dreaming.

The more detail can be resolved in an image, the more likely the sleeper will "see" it as strange, bizarre, or out of place, for example, false teeth that are too large to fit in one's mouth. This discrepancy implies that although part of the sleeper's mind/brain is producing the image, the image does not necessarily fit the dream context as established in another part of the mind/brain.

Much of the dream seems to consist of the sleeper's continuous interpretation of images and events that are in some way strange or unexpected (Antrobus, 1991). For example, "seeing" a strange man in one's kitchen may result in the dreamer trying to flee from the strange man. This brings us to a characteristic of dreaming that is confined to REM sleep, where there is strong inhibition of the motor system and feedback from the proprioceptive nervous system that conveys sensations from our muscles and joints (Antrobus, 1991). The dreamer tries to run but, because of the motor inhibition, cannot. This state of affairs may lead to a panic that results in the dreamer waking up. At that point the contrast between the person's familiar bedroom and the hallucinated escape scene becomes clear, and the fantasy is declared a dream.

Such dreams from which one awakens at home define the common characteristics of dreaming for most people. Laboratory dreams, however, are less dramatic and markedly less emotional. Laboratory dreamers may describe horrifying episodes that are devoid of any expression of pain, fear, or anger. The neurological pathways necessary for the experience of these emotions are apparently inhibited in REM sleep, but as the dreamer struggles toward wakefulness, the inhibition is overcome and the emotions appropriate to the dream are experienced. This struggle to awaken is more likely to succeed if the dreamer is sleeping late on a weekend morning at a time when she or he would normally be awake. In conclusion, the strongly felt emotions that are popularly associated with dreaming may be experienced more in the sleep–wake transition than in dreaming sleep itself.

The *Goblot hypothesis* that all dreams take place in the sleep–wake transition was widely accepted for many years (Goodenough, 1991). Although the hypothesis has never been properly tested, it lost its credibility when Dement and Wolpert (1958) showed that the time required to act out a dream in real life was approximately equal to the 30-second interval between when they stimulated the dreamer with a bell or fine spray of water and when they awakened the dreamer for a dream report (see INSTANTANEOUS DREAMING).

This association of dreaming with real-time experience, the continuity of dream themes over very long dream reports, and the association of dreaming with biological states such as REM sleep that are sustained for intervals sometimes longer than 60 minutes imply that dreaming is continuous over very long intervals. From this perspective, "the dream" typically refers only to a tiny fragment that is recalled from the end of a much longer sequence and that is not a meaningful unit within dreaming sleep. In this sense, it is appropriate to ask, How long do we dream each night? but not, as is often asked, How many dreams do we have per night?

The issue of dream continuity brings us to the most common kind of bizarreness: sequential discontinuities. In the course of describing a dream episode, dreamers frequently find themselves at a loss for a plausible transition and say, "and all of a sudden," followed by the introduction of a new character or scene. The dreamer accepts the transition because she or he "saw" it happen but, on waking, regards it as bizarre because it is improbable given the preceding context. One has the impression that dreaming involves a continuous string of visual scene changes, most of which the dreamer is able to interpret so that they appear to be reasonable. When an image is sufficiently out of context, however, the dreamer is at a loss to account for the shift and, at the point of the waking re-

port, can only say, "and all of a sudden my aunt from Timbuktu walked into the kitchen." From this perspective, sequential discontinuities are another example of how bizarre dream events are simply less-than-totally-plausible attempts of the dreamer to interpret visual transitions, transitions that are not under the control of the interpretive process. Often this interpretive process continues on awakening when the individual tries to name or explain an image that was "observed" less critically within the dream state.

These interpretive processes are precisely the same as those of waking visual perception, except that waking percepts originate with external stimuli, whereas dream "percepts" are created without sensory input. This phenomenon is one of the greatest puzzles about dreaming: How is it that the mind/brain can be surprised and unable to interpret what it itself has produced? Part of the answer requires that we assume that the part of the mind/brain that produces the imagery is not the same as or under the control of the part of the mind/brain that "perceives" or interprets the imagery. This dichotomy would account for the type of dream where the dreamer has the feeling of passively watching a movie or TV story. Yet when the dreamer is an active participant, she or he has the impression that the visual scenes follow his or her intention and actions. For example, when the dreamer turns and attempts to run from the strange person, the scene seems to be appropriate to the escape route. Antrobus (1991) has suggested that the interpretive part of the mind/brain may have intermittent control over the image-generating component of dreaming, and this control increases as the mind/brain becomes more activated, as is the case in the above example.

One must ask, Why is the dreamer so gullible? Why does the dreamer believe in the improbable events of the dream? If the perceptual information from the sleeper's bedroom could reach the mind/brain of the dreamer, the dream images and their interpretation would assuredly be rendered untenable; but the sensory thresholds in sleep are so high that very little information from the outside world ever reaches the perceptual portions of the sleeper's mind/brain. Therefore, there is nothing to contradict the internally produced dream "percepts." Moreover, the internally produced "percepts" may be generated in the same parts of the mind/brain that receive the waking percepts. Thus, both the perceptual and interpretive parts of the mind/brain may be doing what they do during waking perception, except that in sleep there is no sensory input to the perceptual portion of the mind/brain. Hence, dream and waking perceptions are indistinguishable to the interpretive portion of the mind/brain; the interpretive portion has no alternative but to believe what it "sees." This is the characteristic that makes the dream hallucinatory.

The ability of personally significant or intense (but not strong enough to awaken the sleeper) external stimuli to modify the course of the dream provides a way to study the interpretive process of the dreamer's mind/brain. Stimulated with a fine spray of water, the sleeper may report a dream in which it was raining; exposed to a ringing doorbell, the sleeper may dream that she or he is getting up to answer the phone; cool the sleeper's feet and he or she may dream of hiking in a blizzard. That is, certain features of the external stimuli are interpreted in a way consistent with the ongoing dream. One cannot but be impressed by the remarkable facility of the human mind/brain to interpret any kind of external stimulus in a way that is compatible with whatever dream it is producing at the moment.

Freud called the process of generating the dream *dream work*, which he distinguished from a postawakening interpretive process he called *secondary revision*. Freud attributed the bizarreness of dreams to the mental contortions required to camouflage the frightening thoughts and feelings that would awaken the sleeper. For Freud, the "incorporation" of external stimuli into the dream was further evidence of the function of the dream—to protect sleep. Hobson and McCarley (1977) have argued that the periodic occurrence of dreaming on a 90-minute REM/NREM sleep cycle controlled by subcortical structures (rather than the cortical site that holds frightening memories) argues against Freud's theory that psychic conflicts and wishes initiate dreaming. (See ACTIVATION–SYNTHESIS HYPOTHESIS; FREUD'S DREAM THEORY; INCORPORATION INTO DREAMS.)

People have been interpreting the meaning of dreams since the beginning of recorded history. Their strangeness, once taken as evidence of their supernatural origin, gives dreams a degree of ambiguity that invites a wide diversity of interpretations, many of which are quite compelling, but all of which are impossible to test in an unbiased manner. Dream interpretations generally also rest on elaborate belief systems or theories that are also difficult to test. Freud's interpretations were tied to his elaborate theory of neurosis, which is still accepted by psychoanalysts and their patients. Nevertheless, Freud's work deserves credit for emphasizing the role of nonconscious meaning and emotion in the production of thought.

Virtually everyone has experienced dreams that seem, in retrospect, clearly related to a recent or upcoming significant event in their lives, or to a particular personality characteristic, or to a strong personal desire or goal. For this reason, retrospective or post hoc interpretations of dreams seem rather satisfying. That two independent interpretations rarely agree and that no scientist has ever been able to test dream interpretations independently effectively discourages most dream researchers from indulging in this particular pastime. The mind/brain is a far more complex place than dream interpreters are willing to acknowledge. The process of dream production is just beginning to be understood, and it remains one of humanity's most fascinating intellectual puzzles.

Given this uncertain state of affairs, it is obviously difficult to answer with confidence such questions as, Do people dream about their problems? Do they solve problems in their dreams? Are they more creative in their dreams than in the waking state? As long as one accepts post hoc explanations, one can always find some dream that supports one's position.

In describing the dream as an interpretive process, I have implied that the colorful images produced by the visual part of the mind/brain make up a large part of what is interpreted; however, the dreams of people who have been blind from birth demonstrate that the dreaming process can get along quite well without the help of color, shading, perspective, and other visual qualities. A dream of the blind may consist of a perfectly typical family kitchen scene with everyone and everything located in the proper place. In this respect, their reports are indistinguishable from those of the sighted, except that they do not include vistas, objects, or persons that cannot be heard or touched (Kerr, Foulkes and Schmidt, 1982). As information about the locations is stored in the spatial portion of the mind/brain, we may speculate that this it the source of the images that make up the dreams of blind and sighted alike (see BLINDNESS AND DREAMING).

Relative to visual-spatial imagery, speech imagery is much less common in dreaming sleep. The dreamer often reports knowing what people are saying and thinking, but actual quotations are less frequent, and even these often seem to be paraphrases or the interpretations of the dreamer. Of course, people rarely recall actual quotations even in waking life. Dreams that describe specific acoustic qualities of speech are extremely rare, and they usually fail to resolve into specific words.

Dreams differ from most waking thought in that the former are more visual and the latter more verbal. Nevertheless, if fully awake people are left in bed in a dark quiet bedroom for more than 10 minutes, their imagery becomes as vivid and bizarre as when they are in REM sleep (Antrobus, 1991). Two differences remain, however. The awake individual does not confuse the imagery for reality, and the storyline theme of the waking dream is more frequently broken or disrupted by distractions from the outside world. Between these extremes everyone experiences brief intervals of daydreaming of varying degrees of imaginal vividness. But that is another story. (See also CONTENT OF DREAMS; INTERPRETATION OF DREAMS.)

REFERENCES

Antrobus J. 1991. Dreaming: Cognitive processes during cortical activation and high afferent thresholds. *Psychol Rev* 98:96–121.

Antrobus J, Hartwig P, Rosa D, Reinsel R, Fein G. 1987. Brightness and clarity of REM and NREM imagery: Photo response scale. *Sleep Res* 1958 16:240.

Dement WC, Wolpert EA. 1958. The relation of eye movements, body motility and external stimuli to dream content. *J Exp Psychol* 55:543–553.

Goodenough D. 1991. Dream recall: History and current status of the field. In Ellman S, Antrobus JS, eds. *The mind in sleep*, 2nd ed., pp 143–171. New York: Wiley Interscience.

Hobson JA, McCarley RW. 1977. The brain as a dream state generator: An activation–synthesis hypothesis of the dream process. *Am J Psychiatry* 1335–1348.

Kerr NH, Foulkes D, Schmidt M. 1982. The structure of laboratory dreams in blind and sighted subjects. *J Nerv Ment Dis* 170:286–294.

John Antrobus

CHEMISTRY OF SLEEP

[*Brain cells communicate by releasing chemicals. These chemicals, called neurotransmitters, are synthesized (put together) within the neuron. They are usually released when an electrical impulse travels down the axon. The arrival of the electrical impulse at the end of the axon causes ion channels in the axon to open. (Ions are charged particles of elements such as sodium $[Na^+]$, potassium $[K^+]$, chlorine $[Cl^-]$, or calcium $[Ca^{2+}]$.) The entry into the axon terminal of ions such as calcium then causes small containers of neurotransmitter within the axon tip, called vesicles, to release neurotransmitter through the membrane of the neuron and into a region where the neurotransmitter can interact with neighboring cells. Generally, this process happens at a specialized junction between the axon and the neuron that is capable of responding to the chemical. This junction is called a synapse, and the space between the two neurons is called the synaptic cleft. (See REM SLEEP, PHYSIOLOGY OF for a schematic illustration of a neuron and a synapse.)*

The neurotransmitters interact with receptors, which are specialized proteins embedded in the external membrane of neurons and other cells. When receptors are occupied by their specific transmitter, the transmitter/ receptor combination either causes channels to open in the cell membrane or causes the activation of various chemical pathways within the cell. These changes can excite or inhibit the cell. When excitation reaches a sufficient level, an action potential propagates down the cell's axon, causing the release process to start again.

After occupying the receptor, the neurotransmitter drifts away. It can be taken back up by the releasing cell or degraded by adjacent neurons or other brain cells. Chemicals that interfere with these uptake and breakdown processes produce major effects on neural function, since they increase the time the transmitter is present and able to join with the receptors.

A single chemical may have several types of receptors. For example, acetylcholine receptors can be divided into two general classes, called nicotinic (i.e., responding to nicotine) and muscarinic (responding to muscarine). The membranes of various cells have different proportions of each receptor type, and each receptor type produces different kinds of changes in each cell. In certain cases, chemicals can attach themselves to a receptor without activating it. For example, a chemical called atropine binds to muscarinic-type acetylcholine receptors. Chemicals that bind to receptors without activating them are called antagonists, since they block access to the receptor by its true transmitter and thereby prevent its activation.

A single neuron typically has receptors for a number of different chemicals. These receptors often interact with one another. In terms of sleep control, the interaction of transmitters such as acetylcholine, serotonin, and adenosine with other transmitters such as glutamate is as important as is the direct effect of these substances on membrane excitability. For example, only after acetylcholine depolarizes certain neurons can a different excitatory transmitter produce the prolonged excitation required for the waking activity pattern.

Receptors are not only located on the cell bodies of neurons but are also found on the axon terminals, where they can directly regulate transmitter release. For example, many cells have receptors for the transmitter they release. Such cells, called autoreceptors, are thought to function as a feedback loop reducing release of the transmitter. Autoreceptors can be selectively activated by certain drugs.

The sensitivity of receptors can change as a result of exposure to their transmitter. For example, receptors may become less sensitive to the transmitter, a process called desensitization. The number of receptors can also increase and decrease over time, presumably as a result of genetic control. Changes in receptor number have been implicated in many brain diseases, including sleep disorders such as narcolepsy (see NARCOLEPSY).

The complexity of these receptor interactions allows the subtle and complex information processing that characterizes states of consciousness. Not all of the transmitter and receptor mechanisms involved in sleep control are known, but great strides have been made in identifying a number of transmitter–receptor groups with major roles in sleep control. These are discussed in the entries that follow.]

Acetylcholine

The concept that states of wakefulness and sleep can be altered chemically is derived from more than 5,000 years of experience with ALCOHOL and plant extracts. Early humans understood that some exogenous substances blunt wakefulness and enhance feelings of sleepiness. Because sleep normally occurs at regular intervals without ingesting drugs, it was natural for scientists to postulate that sleep might be caused by the ebb and flow of some internally produced chemical. Acetylcholine (ACh) was one of the first endogenously synthesized chemicals hypothesized to be involved in the control of sleep and wakefulness. A large amount of recent experimental data shows that acetylcholine plays a key role in the generation and regulation of rapid eye movement (REM) sleep. The idea that chemical substances mediate communication between nerves and effector organs was firmly established at the beginning of the 1900s. Within 30 years, acetylcholine became the first chemical substance shown to be released from a nerve (the vagus) and to have a direct effect on an organ (the heart). Because we now know that acetylcholine is critically involved in generating the dreaming phase of sleep, it is interesting to note that the idea for the experiment establishing acetylcholine as the first neurotransmitter, performed by Otto Loewi, came to him in a dream.

The term *cholinergic* is used to describe neurons or neurotransmission involving acetylcholine. There is presently a good understanding of all the components of cholinergic neurotransmission, including acetylcholine synthesis, storage, release, and degradation. Of particular interest to neuroscientists studying brain mechanisms that generate sleep states are the enzymes that synthesize and degrade acetylcholine, as well as the receptors that recognize it once it has been released from nerve terminals.

Cholinergic neurons manufacture acetylcholine with use of the biosynthetic enzyme choline acetyltransferase (ChAT). The development of specific antibodies against choline acetyltransferase in the early 1980s has provided a powerful tool for the selective labeling of cholinergic neurons. Sleep researchers have shown that cholinergic neurons located in the dorsolateral PONS send projections to brainstem reticular formation regions known to be important for the generation of REM sleep. Pontine cholinergic neurons also send projections rostrally to the THALAMUS and the BASAL FOREBRAIN, other brain regions that are involved in generating sleep and wakefulness. (See REM SLEEP MECHANISMS AND NEUROANATOMY.)

Acetylcholine is released from cholinergic neurons into specialized regions of nerve cells called synapses, where it is recognized by cholinergic receptors and inactivated by acetylcholinesterase (AChE). Acetylcholinesterase is present in large quantities and is very potent. Thus, it has been difficult to study the cholinergic regulation of REM sleep using the acetylcholine molecule. Instead, two research strategies have been productively employed. First, scientists inject synthetic chemicals that are resistant to degradation by acetylcholinesterase and act at cholinergic receptors to either mimic the actions of acetylcholine (cholinergic agonists) or to block the actions of acetylcholine (cholinergic antagonists). Cholinergic agents most frequently used to study sleep include the agonists carbachol and arecoline and the antagonists atropine and scopolamine. A second strategy useful for studying cholinergic control of REM sleep involves administering compounds that inhibit acetylcholinesterase and allow for the accumulation of natural acetylcholine. Two such drugs are physostigmine and neostigmine.

For almost 30 years it has been known that direct administration of cholinergic agonists, such as carbachol, into certain brain regions of experimental animals causes a state that is remarkably similar to naturally occurring REM sleep. The ability to cause this REM sleep–like state has played a major role in advancing our understanding of the specific brain regions, neurons, and receptors that regulate REM sleep. This cholinergically induced REM sleep–like state is also unique in providing the only pharmacological model of REM sleep. In humans, intravenous administration of the cholinergic agonist arecoline has also been shown to induce REM sleep.

Perhaps the most convincing evidence that endogenously produced acetylcholine plays a key role in REM sleep generation comes from the finding that experimental animals will enter the REM sleep–like state if they receive a pontine injection of the acetylcholinesterase inhibitor neostigmine. Thus, an accumulation of endogenously released acetylcholine in the pons will produce the behavioral and polygraphic signs of REM sleep. A related compound, physostigmine,

will also produce REM sleep in humans if it is given intravenously during NREM sleep. In the presence of a small amount of the acetylcholinesterase inhibitor neostigmine, the release of endogenous acetylcholine from nerve terminals can be measured in specific brain regions in intact animals. Acetylcholine was recently the first neurotransmitter shown to increase in the pons during both natural REM sleep and during the carbachol-induced REM sleep–like state.

Whether acetylcholine excites or inhibits a neuron depends on which type of cholinergic receptor is present. There are two classes of cholinergic receptor proteins. One class, nicotinic receptors, will not be discussed here. Another class of cholinergic receptors is called muscarinic. Muscarinic receptors exist as three subtypes, identified pharmacologically through the use of specific antagonists. Investigators in several laboratories throughout the world are currently attempting to specify the roles of muscarinic M1, M2, and M3 receptor subtypes in REM sleep generation.

Although it is clear that no single neurotransmitter controls the generation of REM sleep, multiple lines of evidence have shown that acetylcholine is critically involved in producing REM sleep. Exciting opportunities exist in the use of pharmacological, anatomical, and electrophysiological techniques to continue specifying the role of acetylcholine in REM sleep generation.

REFERENCES

Baghdoyan HA, Lydic R, Callaway CW, Hobson JA. 1989. The carbachol-induced enhancement of desynchronized sleep signs is dose dependent and antagonized by centrally administered atropine. *Neuropsychopharmacology* 2:67–79. The findings reported in this paper are important because they help to establish the fact that muscarinic cholinergic receptors in the pons play a key role in REM sleep generation. This paper also contains references to earlier studies describing the cholinergically induced REM sleep–like state.

Baghdoyan HA, Monaco AP, Rodrigo-Angulo ML, Assens F, McCarley RW, Hobson JA. 1984. Microinjection of neostigmine into the pontine reticular formation of cats enhances desynchronized sleep signs. *J Pharmacol Exp Ther* 231:173–180. This is the first report showing that the REM sleep–like state could be produced by administering the ace-tylcholinesterase inhibitor neostigmine directly into the pontine reticular formation. These data imply that an accumulation of endogenously re-leased acetylcholine in the pons can cause the REM sleep–like state to occur.

Gillin JC, Sutton L, Ruiz C, Kelsoe J, Dupont RM, Darko D, Risch SC, Golshan S, Janowsky D. 1991. The cholinergic rapid eye movement induction test with arecoline in depression. *Arch Gen Psychiatry* 48: 264–270. This important study, conducted in humans, examines the relationship between cho-linergic mechanisms in affective disorders and sleep. This report also addresses the hypothesis that depressed patients may have a hypersensitive cho-linergic system. Many useful references can be found in the bibliography.

Steriade M, Biesbold D, eds. 1990. *Brain cholinergic systems.* New York: Oxford University Press. The chapters of this book describe the functional organ-ization, physiological aspects, and clinical impor-tance of the brain's cholinergic systems. This book is most appropriate for advanced students.

Steriade M, McCarley RW. 1990. *Brainstem control of wakefulness and sleep.* New York: Plenum. This monograph is a very useful resource for advanced students. The authors have integrated electrophysi-ological, pharmacological, anatomical, and behav-ioral data to provide the most complete summary to date of the neurobiological mechanisms underlying the generation of sleep and wakefulness.

Velazquez-Moctezuma J, Shiromani PJ, Gillin JC. 1990. Acetylcholine and acetylcholine receptor subtypes in REM sleep generation. *Prog Brain Res* 84:407–413. This review article provides a cur-rent, complete, and understandable summary of cholinergic mechanisms and REM sleep generation.

Helen A. Baghdoyan

Adenosine

A number of substances in the human body have been implicated in the regulation of sleep. One of them is adenosine, a nucleotide (or fragment of a nucleic acid) that is readily synthesized in cerebral tissue and other body organs. Being widely distributed in the organism, adenosine af-fects many biochemical and physiological sys-tems. Early experiments with the administration of adenosine into the brains of cats, fowl, and dogs indicated a possible hypnotic (sleep-inducing) role for adenosine. A decade later, Snyder et al. (1981) and Rall (1980) reported that stimulant effects of caffeine and theo-phylline, methylated dioxypurines, or xanthines, which occur naturally in plants, involve a block-ade of receptors for adenosine in the brain. Fur-thermore, the work of Phillis et al. (1979) showed that when adenosine was applied to rat brains it produced potent depressant effects on the responses of neurons in several brain areas, which indicated a general inhibitory role for adenosine that was in accordance with its ob-served hypnotic effect.

The structural formulas of adenosine and caf-feine (Figure 1) reveal that both of these com-pounds, although different, have a purine base in common. Because of this similarity, caffeine is able to attach to receptors for adenosine and thereby block the activation of these receptors. In this way, caffeine is an antagonist of adenosine receptors. As adenosine antagonists were hypoth-esized to produce behavioral excitation by re-moving the inhibition imposed by adenosine, the

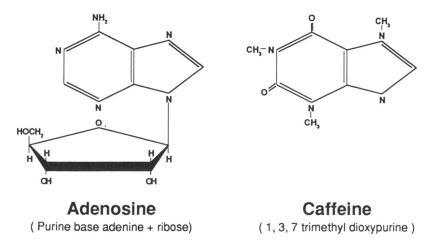

Adenosine
(Purine base adenine + ribose)

Caffeine
(1, 3, 7 trimethyl dioxypurine)

Figure 1.   Structural formulas of adenosine and caffeine.

hypnotic effect of adenosine was thought to be caused by stimulation of central adenosine receptors. This possibility was tested, and the results in rats showed an increase in slow-wave and REM sleep on administration of three adenosine receptor stimulants: N^6-L-1-methyl-2-phenylethyl adenosine (L-PIA), cyclohexyl adenosine (CHA) and 5′-N-ethylcarboxamide adenosine (NECA) (Radulovacki et al., 1984). When caffeine was given to rats before administration of L-PIA, the L-PIA failed to produce a hypnotic effect (Radulovacki et al., 1982). These experiments indicate that adenosine receptors may have a role in the regulation of sleep–wakefulness.

Hypothesis for Adenosine Hypnotic Action

Two types of extracellular adenosine receptors (A_1 and A_2) occur in the mammalian brain. Adenosine A_1 receptors mediate the *inhibition* of adenylate cyclase activity and are present in many areas of the brain. In contrast, adenosine A_2 receptors mediate the *stimulation* of adenylate cyclase activity and are present only in one brain area. (Adenylate cyclase is a chemical whose activity can affect the excitability of neurons.) Caffeine antagonizes both adenosine receptors, but has a slightly greater affinity and thus a stronger effect at A_1 than at A_2 adenosine receptors (Bruns et al., 1986).

As there are two types of adenosine receptors whose role in sleep is not yet clear, our hypothesis is that stimulation of adenosine A_1 receptors by adenosine leads to a suppression of calcium ion influx into nerve terminals, which may be a consequence of adenylate cyclase inhibition. This sequence of events then prevents the release of brain neurotransmitters that are critical for wakefulness (Dolphin, Prestwich, and Forda, 1985; Radulovacki, 1991).

REFERENCES

Bruns RF, Lu GH, Pugsley TA. 1986. Characterization of the A_2 adenosine receptor labelled by [^{3}H]NECA in rat striatal membranes. *Mol Pharmacol* 29: 331–346.

Dolphin AC, Prestwich SA, Forda SR. 1985. Presynaptic modulation by adenosine analogues: Relationship to adenylate cyclase. In Stefanovich V,

Rudolphi E, Schubert P, eds. *Adenosine receptors and modulation of cell function,* pp 107–117. Oxford/Washington, DC: IRL Press.

Phillis JW, Edstrom JP, Kostopoulos GK, Kirkpatrick JR. 1979. Effects of adenosine and adenine nucleotides on synaptic transmission in the cerebral cortex. *Can J Physiol Pharmacol* 57:1289–1312.

Radulovacki M. 1991. Adenosine and sleep. In Phillis, JW, ed. *Adenosine and the adenine nucleotides as regulators of cellular function,* pp 381–390. Boca Raton, Fla.: CRC Press.

Radulovacki M, Miletich RS, Green RD. 1982. N^6-(L-phenylisopropyl) adenosine (L-PIA) increases slow-wave sleep and decreases wakefulness in rats. *Brain Res* 246:178–180.

Radulovacki M, Virus RM, Djuricic-Nedelson M, Green RD. 1984. Adenosine analogs and sleep in rats. *J Pharmacol Exp Ther* 228:268–274.

Rall TW. 1980. Central nervous system stimulants: The xanthines. In Gilman AG, Goodman L, Gilman A, eds. *The pharmacological basis of therapeutics,* pp 592–607. New York: Macmillan.

Snyder SH, Katims JJ, Annau Z, Bruns RF, Daly JW. 1981. Adenosine receptors and behavioral actions of methylxanthines. *Proc Natl Acad Sci USA* 78:3260–3264.

Miodrag Radulovacki

Amines and Other Transmitters

Different chemicals are released in the brain during waking and during sleep. Each chemical neurotransmitter is synthesized by particular neurons and released by those neurons when they are active. Chemical transmitters can either excite or inhibit other target neurons in the brain and accordingly stimulate, prevent, or shape their activity. They can thus change and maintain the waking or sleeping state of the brain.

Waking

Chemicals maximally released during waking are synthesized by neurons that make up the activating system of the brainstem and forebrain. When functioning, these neurons promote activity in the rest of the brain, notably the cerebral cortex, where perception and awareness of the self and the environment and conscious thought occur (see AROUSAL). Several chemicals are contained in different subsets of reticular neurons that generate and maintain the state of waking.

First, catecholamines, including noradrenaline and dopamine, are contained in clusters of cells within the brainstem. Noradrenaline-containing neurons are localized in the locus coeruleus nucleus of the pons, and they send their axons to the entire forebrain and cerebral cortex, where they release noradrenaline. These noradrenergic neurons are active and secrete noradrenaline during waking and to the greatest degree during highly aroused periods, when they may enhance attention through an influence on the cerebral cortex. Dopamine-containing neurons are located in the substantia nigra and ventral tegmental area of the midbrain and project up to the basal ganglia, where they release dopamine. These neurons are also involved in waking but primarily in behavioral arousal that is manifest as spontaneous or elicited movements. As evident by the deficits associated with PARKINSON'S DISEASE, degeneration or destruction of dopamine neurons is associated with a loss of mobility and voluntary movement, termed bradykinesia. Drugs, such as amphetamine, that increase the release of catecholamines, including both noradrenaline and dopamine, greatly enhance and prolong waking, as evidenced by increased cortical activation and behavioral arousal.

Another chemical, acetylcholine (see "Acetylcholine" above), is contained in several clusters of neurons within the brainstem (laterodorsal and pedunculopontine tegmental nuclei) and BASAL FOREBRAIN. The basal forebrain cholinergic neurons send their axons to the cerebral cortex, where they release acetylcholine. Acetylcholine is maximally released when the cortex is activated, that is, during waking. In fact, this chemical can generate the fast, desynchronized pattern of electroencephalographic activity that underlies wakefulness and consciousness. Drugs that enhance cholinergic functions such as neostigmine, muscarine, or NICOTINE prolong and enhance waking and vigilance, and conversely, drugs that block cholinergic transmission, such as belladonna or atropine, diminish waking and vigilance. As evidenced in patients with ALZHEIMER'S DISEASE, degeneration or destruction of cholinergic neurons is associated with a loss of vigilance and memory.

A third chemical, histamine, is contained in neurons of the posterior hypothalamus that also send long axons up to the cerebral cortex. These neurons are active during waking, when they release maximal quantities of histamine. Drugs that block the action of histamine, notably the antihistaminergics, diminish vigilance and produce drowsiness.

Finally, large numbers of neurons through the reticular activating system of the brainstem, posterior HYPOTHALAMUS, and basal forebrain contain glutamate, a potent excitatory amino acid. The release of glutamate in the cerebral cortex is maximal during waking and in association with cortical activation. Drugs that block the effect of glutamate result in a loss of consciousness and have been used as anesthetics.

These multiple neurotransmitter systems function in concert, promoting and maintaining wakefulness under normal conditions or enhancing and prolonging vigilance under demanding or stressful situations.

Sleep

Certain chemicals may be released before the onset of sleep that by their actions promote its onset. Serotonin may facilitate the initiation of sleep by multiple actions, such as decreasing the reaction to stimulation, including painful stimulation. Serotonin may also be important for the production of peptides that promote sleep. A lack of serotonin is associated with hyperreactivity and a diminished tendency to fall asleep.

Gamma-aminobutyric acid (GABA), a potent inhibitory amino acid, has the capacity to dampen activity of neurons throughout the brainstem and forebrain. It is synthesized by neurons that are intermingled with neurons of the activating system. GABA is released in the greatest amount from the cerebral cortex during slow wave sleep. Depending on the activity of the particular neurons that release GABA, this inhibitory neurotransmitter may be responsible for shaping the electroencephalographic spindles and slow waves of sleep in the forebrain and for preventing sensory stimuli from reaching the cerebral cortex and thus interrupting or preventing sleep. Drugs that mimic or enhance the activity of GABA in the brain include the major anesthetics (barbiturates), tranquilizers (benzodiazepines), and hypnotics.

The normal alternation of waking and sleep entails a dynamic interaction between chemically specific systems. Those chemical neurotransmitter systems promoting waking or sleep, as already described, are in turn interlinked with peptide or hormonal systems that generate long-term changes in the brain (Jones, 1989). During the normal sleep–wake cycle, specific peptides (see "Peptides" below) or hormones may stimulate or promote the concerted activity of the activating chemoneuronal systems versus the deactivating chemoneuronal systems and thus generate the chemical milieu of a waking versus a sleeping brain.

REFERENCE

Jones BE. 1989. Basic mechanisms of sleep-wake states. In Kryger MH, Roth T, Dement WC, eds. *Principles and practice of sleep medicine,* pp 121–138. Philadelphia: WB Saunders.

Barbara E. Jones

Peptides

The term *peptide* refers to any biochemical compound formed by two or more amino acids. A considerable number of peptides regulate different functions in the body, such as cardiovascular function, kidney physiology, processes of digestion, and many others. Peptides are called *neuropeptides* when their effects are exerted in the central as well as in the peripheral nervous system. Neuropeptides produce their effects mainly by modulating the release of several neurotransmitters or by acting directly on the target nervous structure.

According to one theory, sleep generation and maintenance depend on the activity of a group of neuropeptides called *sleep factors* (see "Sleep Factors" below). These sleep factors can be obtained from the blood or the cerebrospinal fluid (CSF) of either sleeping or sleep-deprived animals. Some of these factors were named on the basis of their ability to induce SLOW-WAVE SLEEP (SWS), also called delta sleep: for example, delta sleep–inducing peptide (DSIP), factor S, and sleep-promoting substance. However, another

group of peptides has been described in parallel. Originally, these were not considered neuropeptides, since they were first discovered in the digestive tract and were related to processes of digestion. Three of these peptides also promote sleep, preferentially enhancing REM sleep. In the following list of neuropeptides, the first three were originally isolated from the digestive tract. Other neuropeptides from diverse origins are also described.

Vasoactive intestinal polypeptide (VIP). This peptide—first extracted from the small intestine and later from the brain of pigs—has shown potent REM sleep–promoting properties. It induces REM sleep in normal rats and cats and can also restore REM sleep in animals rendered insomniac by pharmacological treatment. Additional investigations have shown that antibodies against VIP block REM sleep when administered into the ventricles of the brain. These antibodies also block the REM sleep–promoting properties of the CSF obtained from sleep-deprived cats. Moreover, VIP antagonists also block REM sleep. The mechanism of action of VIP may be via activation of the acetylcholine (Ach) system and through the release of at least two hormones, GROWTH HORMONE (GH) and PROLACTIN. These two hormones as well as Ach promote REM sleep in several species.

Cholecystokinin-8 (CCK-8). There are several forms of CCK; only the octapeptide, however, appears to be active in the brain. A number of investigations have shown that the systemic administration of CCK-8 induces a syndrome of food satiety, which is normally followed by SWS. Because CCK-8 penetrates the blood–brain barrier poorly, the effect on sleep may be mediated by peripheral mechanisms. Nevertheless, CCK-8 administered into the brain ventricles induces REM sleep with no promotion of SWS. When CCK-8 is systemically administered, the mechanism of action on SWS may be mediated by insulin. However, when administered into the brain, CCK-8 may affect REM sleep by interacting with Ach and VIP.

Somatostatin (SS). Small quantities of SS administered into the cerebral ventricles also promote REM sleep in rats, whereas its inactivation by antibodies strongly reduces REM sleep. A potent SS analogue, octreotide, is also able to increase REM sleep in aged rats to amounts comparable to those found in young rats (REM sleep amount decreases with age). The mechanism of action of somatostatin may also include interactions with Ach and GH.

Corticotropinlike intermediate lobe peptide (CLIP). This neuropeptide, isolated from the PI-TUITARY GLAND, increases REM sleep in rats. However, the consequences for sleep stages of the inactivation of CLIP by antibodies or its blockade by antagonists are unknown. The mechanism of action of CLIP may depend on its interaction with serotonin (see section on "Amines" above).

Other neuropeptides. Growth hormone–releasing factor, isolated from the HYPOTHALAMUS, increases both SWS and REM sleep when administered into the brain ventricles of rats. Arginine-vasotocin, isolated from the pituitary gland, increases SWS and completely suppresses REM sleep. Incidentally, insulin (which is a protein but not a peptide) induces SWS.

Since VIP, CCK-8, SS, and most of the hormones mentioned above play a role in the processes of nutrition of the body tissues, the quality of the food ingested by a given subject may affect the characteristics of his sleep. For example, intravenous administration of amino acids increases REM sleep in rats, whereas undernutrition reduces the total amount of sleep in several animal species, including humans.

BIBLIOGRAPHY

Inoué S, Krueger JM, eds. 1990. *Endogenous sleep factors.* The Hague: SPB Academic Publishing.
Inoué S, Schneider-Helmert D, eds. 1988. *Sleep peptides: Basic and clinical approaches.* Berlin: Springer-Verlag.

Steven J. Henriksen
Oscar Prospero-Garcia

Sleep Factors

Sleep results from communication between cells within the brain. Although we do not know exactly which cells cause sleep, we do know that brain cells communicate with each other using chemical signals. These chemical interactions range from very short-lasting (milliseconds) signals confined to very precise anatomical locations (neurotransmitters) to long-lasting influences. For example, some sex steroids can affect behavior throughout the life of an animal. Recent discoveries have shown that relatively long-lasting (hours) chemical signals are involved in sleep regulation. Thus, certain substances that are produced by brain cells, when given to animals or humans, cause the individuals to sleep more than they normally would. These substances are called *sleep factors.*

The idea of chemical regulation of sleep is old, dating back to Aristotle's time. Two millennia later, modern approaches to the study of Aristotle's hypothesis of humoral regulation of sleep have resulted in the chemical identification of sleep factors. The common observations that the longer we stay awake the more sleepy we become and that after such deprivation we sleep longer than usual are fundamental to one approach used to identify sleep factors. They led to the work of Legendre and Pieron who, at the beginning of the twentieth century, described the accumulation of a sleep factor in the fluid that bathes the brain (cerebrospinal fluid) in animals deprived of sleep. In the late 1960s, a similar sleep factor was found in goat cerebrospinal fluid after sleep deprivation. Subsequently an indistinguishable sleep factor was isolated from rabbit brain and human urine; it was identified as a muramyl peptide. A few micrograms of this factor was isolated from 17,000 rabbit brains and from about 4,000 liters of human urine. It is very potent; one picomole (about 0.000000001 gram) is sufficient to induce excess sleep for 10 to 12 hours in recipient animals. This material increases NREM sleep to values about 50% percent greater than normal. In its chemical nature it is related to the substances that make up the cell walls of bacteria.

This latter fact is related to a second major approach to the study of sleep factors. It is based on the feelings of sleepiness that often occur during infectious disease. Such observations led to the hypotheses that sleep is altered during infection and microbial products drive those sleep responses. Despite the fact that health care providers have for centuries prescribed bed rest (sleep) as an aid for recuperation, it was not until the 1980s that sleep was documented over the course of an infection and there remains today no data indicating that sleep helps in recuperation. Nevertheless, sleep is enhanced during infection and recent studies have shown that specific microbial products are responsible. Bacterial muramyl peptides, closely related to that isolated from brains as a sleep factor, form one class of such microbial products capable of enhancing NREM sleep.

An important facet of sleep factor research is to determine how such substances affect the production or breakdown of other biochemicals in the cascade of events that ultimately lead to sleep. It seems that both the sleep factor from brain and the microbial products elicit their effects on sleep, in part, by increasing the production of another substance called interleukin-1. Interleukin-1 was first identified as a substance involved in the immune response. It and receptors for it are also found in normal brains. Its levels in cerebrospinal fluid vary in phase with sleep–wake cycles, and human blood levels of interleukin-1 peak at the onset of sleep. When given interleukin-1, animals spend about 50 percent more time in NREM sleep for several hours, and patients receiving interleukin-1 report excess sleepiness. These types of data provide evidence that interleukin-1 is one of the substances involved in the sleep induced by muramyl peptides and in normal sleep.

There is also much indirect evidence supporting this hypothesis; substances that inhibit interleukin-1 production, such as glucocorticoids (adrenal-gland steroid hormones), or that inhibit the actions of interleukin-1, such as adrenocorticotropin-releasing hormone (a brain peptide localized in neurons), inhibit sleep. Substances that enhance interleukin-1 production, for example, viral double-stranded ribonucleic acid, enhance sleep. Interleukin-1 also alters the firing rate of neurons in parts of the brain known to be involved in sleep regulation.

Additional biochemical steps involved in muramyl peptide/interleukin-1-induced sleep remain uninvestigated; however, the involvement of growth hormone-releasing hormone seems likely. This substance is found in neurons and, when released into blood, causes the release of growth hormone from the pituitary gland. Human growth hormone blood levels peak at the onset of sleep. Interleukin-1 also induces growth hormone release through a brain mechanism that seems to involve growth hormone-releasing hormone. Finally, growth hormone–releasing hormone induces sleep when given to animals, and neurons that contain it are connected to areas of the brain involved in sleep generation.

Although it seems that many of the proposed sleep factors may be involved in this or similar biochemical cascades, the timing of these events in the brain and their impact on sleep remain to be determined. We need to discover, for example, why some substances induce increases in NREM sleep and REM sleep, whereas others are selective for just one type of sleep; why some substances enhance sleep after low doses, but inhibit sleep after higher doses; exactly how and where in the brain the interactions between sleep factors take place; and just how many sleep factors there are. Indeed, it often seems that for every puzzle of sleep regulation we decipher, countless more are still concealed. Nevertheless, it seems likely that if humankind is ever to understand how the brain works, we must first determine what sleep does for the brain.

REFERENCES

Krueger JM, Johannsen L. 1988. Bacterial products, cytokines and sleep. In Lernmark A, Dyrberg J, Terenius L, Hökfelt B, eds. *Molecular mimicry in health and disease,* pp 35–46. Amsterdam: Elsevier.

Krueger JM, Majde JA. 1990. Sleep as a host defense: Its regulation of microbial products and cytokine. *Clin Immunol Immunopathol* 57:188–199.

Krueger JM, Obal F Jr, Opp M, Toth L, Johannsen L, Cady AB. 1990. Somnogenic cytokines and models concerning their effects on sleep. *Yale J Biol Med* 63:157–172.

James M. Krueger

CHEYNE-STOKES RESPIRATION

For several days his breathing was irregular; it would entirely cease for a quarter of a minute, then it would become perceptible, though very low, then by degrees it became heaving and quick, and then it would gradually cease again. This revolution in the state of his breathing occupied about a minute during which there were about 30 acts of respiration. (Cheyne, 1818, p. 216)

Cheyne-Stokes respiration (CSR) refers to the pattern of respiration, so well described by John Cheyne, in which a gradual rise and fall of ventilatory activity occur over approximately a minute. The characteristic pattern can be seen in Figure 1 and most typically consists of a period of breathing (*hyperpnea*) alternating with a period of no breathing (*apnea*). The cycle then repeats itself with a period of 30 to 60 seconds. During the hyperpneic phase it is primarily the volume of each breath that increases or decreases rather than the frequency of breathing. This disturbance in respiratory control is present in a variety of conditions and disease states including sleep, neurological disease, heart failure, altitude exposure, hypoxia, sedation, metabolic or acid–base disturbances (especially alkalosis), and prematurity. It is also more likely to be observed in elderly persons.

Cheyne-Stokes respiration represents instability in a control system similar to that observed with certain mechanical systems. Application of principles relevant to the latter has yielded insight into the pathogenesis of CSR. Imagine a thermostat (sensor) regulating the heater (effector) for a room. When the room temperature reaches a certain level that is detected by a sensor, the heater is turned off. When the room temperature has fallen to a preset temperature, the sensor detects this change and activates the heater once again. The stability of the temperature of the room is a measure of the success of this feedback system. Likewise the respiratory system has sensors (which detect changes in gas content and acid–base balance) that instruct the effectors (lungs and respiratory muscles) to modify their activity to restore the state of balance. For example, if the quantity of oxygen falls below a predetermined level, then the lungs are commanded to increase the amount of breathing to return the oxygen level to normal. A perfect system would maintain the amount of oxygen (or the room temperature) exactly at the predetermined level; however, no system is perfect and consequently the controlled variable oscillates about the preset level, sometimes being higher, sometimes lower.

Two factors that lead to instability in feedback control systems are a high gain in the sensors and a delay in information transfer. In the respiratory system sensors are present for both oxygen and carbon dioxide, the two gases of respiration. These sensors are present in the blood vessels and in the brain and are able to respond to changes in the concentrations of these gases. A *high gain* for these sensors means that a small change in the gas being measured elicits a strong response from the effectors. The oxygen sensor exhibits a higher gain than the carbon dioxide sensor. Consequently situations in which changes in oxygen have a greater effect on breathing and changes in carbon dioxide have a lesser effect lead to ventilatory instability and the possibility of CSR. The best example of this is exposure to high ALTITUDE where the amount of oxygen is diminished and, because of compensatory overventilation, the concentration (and therefore the influence) of carbon dioxide is less. The gain of the respiratory sensors is also influenced by the state of the nervous system. When one goes to sleep, an influence from the wakeful centers of the brain is removed from the respiratory controller and causes instability for a period. As many as 50 percent of normal individuals exhibit brief episodes of CSR during sleep. CSR is most likely to be seen in stage 1 and 2 sleep (see STAGES OF SLEEP) and least likely to occur during REM sleep. Likewise, patients with damage to their brains, in the form of a STROKE or other serious degeneration or injury to the brain, exhibit CSR during both wakefulness and sleep.

A time delay in information reaching the sensor can also lead to instability in the feedback system. Again the room and heater analogy may be invoked. If the thermostat were moved 20 feet away from the room being heated, then the room would have to be heated to a very high temperature for the remote thermostat to respond and turn down the heat. Likewise, the room would get very cold before that information would reach the sensor to engage the heater again. A wide swing in temperature would be observed. In the respiratory system it

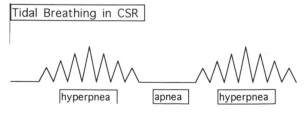

Figure 1. Tidal breathing in Cheyne-Stokes respiration.

is thought that conditions that slow down the circulation of blood from the heart and lungs to the sensors, such as heart failure, cause ventilatory instability from this mechanism. CSR is common in patients with a variety of heart diseases.

Several additional symptoms and signs are observed in association with CSR. Heart rate and blood pressure follow a similar pattern of rising and falling. Notably there is evidence of arousal or hyperarousal during the hyperpneic phase of CSR. Those patients in whom neurological disease is causing CSR may actually be alert during the hyperpneic phase and 30 seconds later totally unarousable during the apneic phase. During sleep (especially at altitude) the person exhibits lighter sleep during the hyperpneic phase of breathing and may even be awakened during this phase.

Treatment for CSR is aimed primarily at treating the underlying condition, if possible. At high altitude, breathing supplemental oxygen often abolishes CSR. Some medications have proved successful, most notably aminophylline, a drug with complex actions on the lung, circulation, and brain, and acetazolamide, a drug that influences acid–base balance and stimulates breathing. Although the gradual buildup of breathing characteristic of CSR usually occurs without any obstruction to breathing (as in the sleep apnea syndrome), this is not always the case. If obstruction is present, then treatments successful for sleep apnea can be applied, such as nasal CONTINUOUS POSITIVE AIRWAY PRESSURE (CPAP). With heart failure in particular, nasal CPAP has been successfully used for CSR.

(See also APNEA; RESPIRATION CONTROL IN SLEEP.)

REFERENCES

Alex CG, Onal E, Lopata M. 1986. Upper airway occlusion during sleep in patients with Cheyne-Stokes respiration. *Am Rev Respir Dis* 133:42–45.

Cherniack NS, Longobardo GS. 1973. Cheyne-Stokes breathing. *N Engl J Med* 288:952–957.

Cheyne JA. 1818. A case of apoplexy, in which the fleshy part of the heart was converted into fat. *Dublin Hosp Rep* 2:216–223.

T. Scott Johnson

CHILDHOOD, SLEEP DURING

Although the function of sleep remains a scientific mystery, there are a number of reasons to believe that one role of sleep is related to development. Normal early development is associated not only with changes in sleep patterns, but also with changes in the length and depth of sleep. In young animals, as well as young humans, the amount and depth of sleep gradually decline as they approach maturity. The issue of sleep depth is particularly interesting to consider with respect to development. In many ways, the feature that uniquely distinguishes *sleep* from *rest* is the lack of awareness and responsiveness to the external world that exists during sleep. Being relatively unaware and unresponsive to our immediate environment can be very dangerous. From an evolutionary or survival perspective, there is a need to balance the requirement for sleep with that for remaining aware of and responsive to potential predators or danger. Like other mammals, young humans, under the care of their parents for a relatively extended period, may have been endowed with the luxury of long, deep sleep patterns during the time their parents assume the primary role of watching for danger. Young children have large amounts of *very* deep sleep during which they are *very* unresponsive to sounds, light, movement, and so forth. In one experiment, children sleeping with headphones showed not a trade of arousal during deep stage 4 sleep despite extremely loud buzzing sounds (123 decibels, a sound level similar to that of a loud motorcycle) in both ears (Busby and Pivik, 1985). The researchers could not use louder sounds because of the concern that they might damage the hearing of the children.

Deep stage 4 sleep also gives rise to confused partial arousals, such as SLEEPWALKING, SLEEPTALKING, and SLEEP TERRORS. The amount and intensity of deep sleep appear to reach a developmental peak somewhere around 3 to 5 years of age and may be related to the child giving up daytime naps. That is, when children first begin to remain awake for extended periods, they are most likely to show the greatest and deepest stage 4 sleep. This demonstrates a general relationship between deep sleep and length of prior wakefulness: Anything that makes a child (or an adult) overly tired, such as being up very late, having disturbed sleep, or having an erratic schedule, causes a physiological response characterized by more and deeper sleep. As development progresses through later childhood and adolescence, there is a gradual but steady drop-off in the normal amount and depth of stage 4 sleep. Coincidentally, there is a reduction in stage 4-associated partial arousals (sleepwalking, sleeptalking, and so forth) with increasing age.

Sleep in the Toddler and Pre–School-Aged Child

One of the main areas of change at this age is the pattern of sleep with respect to daytime naps. Most young toddlers nap for an hour or more twice a day. Napping typically decreases to only once a day by age 3. By the age of 4 or 5, many young children have given up regular daytime napping. The total amount of sleep time is therefore decreasing for most children across this interval, from approximately 14 hours to only 11 or 12 hours a day, and by the end of this phase, there will generally be a single consolidated nighttime sleep period. Other developmental influences are also prominent during this phase of childhood. Bedtime problems (difficulties with falling asleep or child–parent struggles are reported to be very common, affecting as many as 50 percent of children 1 to 5 years of age. Issues of control and fearfulness appear to account for many of these problems. Nighttime awakenings are also common, and although brief awakenings are normal in all age groups, these appear to represent a problem in about 20 percent to 25 percent of 2-year-olds and 10 percent to 15 percent of pre-school-aged children (Richman, 1987).

It is important to stress that significant individual differences in sleep patterns emerge across this age range. Certain children will require much more sleep and multiple naps for a long period, whereas an occasional 2- or 3-year-old will give up napping completely and seem to get by on 10 hours of sleep at night. One of the most important, unanswered questions with respect to sleep in this age group is how to determine the "optimal" amount of sleep for a given child. For example, some of the children who seem to be getting by with less sleep might function better by getting more sleep. The symptoms of inadequate sleep in early childhood can be deceptive.

These children may not look sleepy, but may instead appear "hyperactive." Irritability, inattentiveness, impulsivity, and emotional changes are the most common symptoms of inadequate sleep in children. A general rule of thumb is that children should get enough sleep to be able to awaken easily in the morning without parental prodding. If there is any question that daytime irritability or fatigue is related to inadequate sleep, the family should try increasing the child's sleep time for 1–2 weeks and see if the situation improves.

Electrophysiologically (see POLYSOMNOGRAPHY), the young child descends into deep stage 4 sleep, usually within 10 minutes, and remains in slow-wave sleep for about an hour. At this point, the brain wave activity changes abruptly, reflecting a "mixed" state of sleep and arousal. The child moves about, changes positions, and may exhibit any number of behaviors, such as rubbing the face, blinking, whimpering, and even mumbling a bit. Some children may fully awaken briefly; however, most experience only a partial arousal lasting from a few seconds to a minute or two. After settling, the child again progresses into NREM sleep. There is often an attempt to enter REM sleep at this point; however, these early "REM attempts" are frequently not fulfilled in the young child. The child descends again into slow-wave sleep, remains there for another hour, and then moves about again in bed. At this point, the child usually experiences a brief (10–20-minute) REM sleep period. Thereafter, NREM and REM sleep cycle with one another at intervals of about 50–60 minutes. Children in this age range have seven to nine REM periods during a night. Overall, REM sleep occupies about 30 percent to 35 percent, and NREM slow-wave sleep about 20 percent to 25 percent, of the total amount of sleep. REM period duration increases from about 10 to 35 minutes until the middle of the sleep period, when REM period duration declines slightly to about 20–25 minutes. NREM stage 4 sleep is most prominent in the first half of the night in young children, lightens during the middle of night, and returns briefly during the final NREM sleep cycle of the night (Williams, Karacan, and Hursch, 1974; Ferber, 1985). Young children are almost impossible to awaken during deep slow-wave sleep, particularly in the early part of the sleep period. No consistent sex differences have been reported in the sleep of young children, although Williams and colleagues (1974) have suggested that girls may precede boys slightly in sleep changes during early childhood. (See also CYCLES OF SLEEP ACROSS THE NIGHT.)

Sleep in the Latency-Aged Child

From approximately age 6 to age 12 (or whenever puberty begins), the total amount of sleep shows a steady decline, particularly the amount of slow wave sleep. By this age, sleep is consolidated into a single nighttime sleep period and declines from about 10 hours in 6- and 7-year-olds to about 8 or 9 hours by the end of the latency phase. As with the younger child, however, there is again considerable individual variation: Questions regarding what is "optimal" sleep remain salient. The combination of late-night activities (television, games, music, homework, and some family interactions such as when parents are on late work schedules) and the need to get up early for school often restrict the time available to sleep for many children in this age group. Effects on mood and behavior are similar to those observed in the younger child. Evidence from one laboratory study suggests that 10 hours of sleep may be closer to the "sleep need" in 12-year-olds and even older adolescents (Carskadon and Dement, 1987).

Electrophysiological "norms" are more readily available for latency-aged than for younger children. Latency-aged children sleep 95 percent to 97 percent of the time they spend in bed. REM sleep occupies about 26 percent to 28 percent of the total sleep time among the younger children in this age range and declines to about 22 percent to 25 percent by the end of the latency period. Latency-aged children continue frequently to manifest a "missed" REM period during their first sleep cycle. Subsequent sleep cycle lengths are comparable to those in adolescents and adults, that is, about 90 minutes (see CYCLE OF SLEEP ACROSS THE NIGHT). The number of REM periods declines modestly from six in 6- to 8-year-olds to four or five in 10- to 12-year-olds. NREM slow-wave sleep (see STAGES OF SLEEP) continues to constitute 20 percent to 25 percent of the sleep period. Stage 4 sleep appears to be relatively stable between 6 and 10 years of age, after which time this deepest of the sleep stages begins to decline. Further and more striking changes in stage 4 sleep occur during adolescence (see ADOLESCENCE AND SLEEP). Consistent sex differences have not been demonstrated in the sleep of latency-aged children (Williams, Karacan, and Hursch, 1974; Coble et al., 1987; Carskadon, Keenan, and Dement, 1987).

REFERENCES

Busby K, Pivik RT. 1985. Auditory arousal thresholds during sleep in hyperactive children. *Sleep* 8:332–341.

Carskadon MA, Dement WC. 1987. Sleepiness in the normal adolescent. In Guilleminault C, ed. *Sleep and its disorders in children,* pp 53–66. New York: Raven.

Carskadon MA, Keenan S, Dement WC. 1987. Nighttime sleep and daytime sleep tendency in preadolescents. In Guilleminault C, ed. *Sleep and its disorders in children,* pp 43–52. New York: Raven.

Coble PA, Kupfer DJ, Reynolds CF, Houck P. 1987. EEG sleep of healthy children 6 to 12 years of age. In Guilleminault C, ed. *Sleep and its disorders in children,* pp 29–42. New York: Raven.

Ferber R. 1985. *Solve your child's sleep problems.* New York: Simon & Schuster.

Richman M. 1987. Surveys of sleep disorders in children in a general population. In Guilleminault C, ed. *Sleep and its disorders in children,* pp 115–127. New York: Raven.

Williams RL, Karacan I, Hursch CJ. 1974. *Electroencephalography (EEG) of human sleep: Clinical applications.* New York: Wiley.

Patricia A. Coble
Ronald E. Dahl

CHILDREN'S DREAMS

The development in the 1950s and 1960s of techniques for waking people up for immediate reports of REM dreaming has permitted more systematic and representative sampling of human dream life than previously had been possible. The results of such sampling have demolished many earlier stereotypes about typical dream life, including the idea that children's dream life is richly complex and/or highly disturbing.

Formal Properties

Instead, laboratory studies of REM dream samples from children age 3 and up indicate that children's dreaming is at no point any more complex than their waking reasoning and that dream content is typically mundane and benign from early to later childhood (Foulkes, 1982, 1989; Foulkes et al., 1990). Specifically, research suggests that the possibility of dreaming first occurs only after development of a stable system of conscious "representational intelligence," that is, the possibility of manipulating or operating on conscious representations of objects or events not currently present in the child's environment.

Accordingly, dream experience is largely or wholly absent as an accompaniment of REM sleep until at least the third year of life. REM periods in the preschool years are not consistently or even frequently associated with memorable dream experience. Those dreams that children do experience between ages 3 and 5 tend to have neither the formal properties of a story, from a narrative point of view, nor the formal properties of a movie, from a visual-representational point of view; rather, they can portray only momentary scenes or situations in static imagery. These scenes and situations are not inherently emotional and are not experienced with emotional accompaniment, nor are they experienced through the medium of an actively participating self character (that is, the child is not an active character in the dream).

Between ages 5 and 7, rudimentary narratives that employ kinematic or movielike visual imagery, are first experienced during REM sleep. It is not until after age 7, however, that dreams generally are experienced through the medium of an actively participating self character. By age 8 or 9, children's dreams have most of the narrative and visual-representational properties of adult dreams. Further, more subtle forms of dream representation (for example, simultaneous representation of self as participant and observer) may not occur until children approach adolescence. Emotions first become possible accompaniments of dream narratives only when active representation of self appears, but emotions are generally neither unpleasant in character nor inappropriate to their narrative context.

That the developmental progression described above is not merely a change in children's ability to remember or describe dreams is suggested by the research findings that children's waking memory or verbal skills are not reliably associated with the amount or kind of dream they describe when awakened from REM sleep. Rather, visual-spatial reasoning skills, that is, the kind of skills that presumably would be involved in actually creating dreams, are the best predictors of children's dream reporting and reports.

Thus, laboratory research suggests that dreaming is not an activity at which young children are particularly accomplished. Rather, as is the case with other (waking) mental activities, dreaming is something children access only gradually over the course of development. The observation that children's dreaming is correlated with—and constrained by—general intellectual development makes a very important point about the nature of dreaming: Dreaming is not a "perceptual" process, routinely accompanying REM sleep in any organism capable of perceptual processing; rather it is an "intellectual" process, accompanying the cortical activation of REM sleep (and other states) only in those organisms capable of representational intelligence, flexible mental imagery, and narrative simulation.

Content

The content of children's laboratory-sampled REM dreams, with several interesting exceptions, seems to draw largely on figures, settings, and actions familiar in their waking lives. Thus, parents and peers appear frequently as dream characters, home and outdoor recreational settings are common, and at least after age 5 or 6, friendly social interaction is a dominant theme. Among the exceptions are the preponderance of animal characters and of static body state (sleep, hunger, thirst) themes in the dreams of preschoolers. Based on obvious parallels with stories to which young children are exposed, it seems likely that animal figures may be a primitive form of self-representation, whereas body state themes may reflect young children's relative inability to shift attention from their own immediate needs or wants. Gender differences in dream content emerge in the early school years; for example, girls are more likely than boys to dream of female characters.

The generally realistic nature of children's

dream content, as sampled in the laboratory, is in contrast with a picture that may be generated by children's spontaneous reports at home (or by adults' elicitation, organization, and recollection of such reports). But the laboratory research indicates that the child's ordinary dream life (dreams that would be slept through and forgotten were the child not awakened) is far less remarkable than generally imagined.

Home Versus Laboratory

Anecdotal home observations and laboratory findings thus seem to disagree both about the prevalence of dreaming and about the nature of dream content in early childhood. Many parents think that they see signs of frequent dreaming as early as during their child's infancy and note a preponderance of unpleasant dream reports in their child's later preschool and early school years. Several factors are probably responsible for these home-versus-laboratory differences: (1) Parental impressions of frequent and early childhood dreaming may be based on motor activity (for example, fussing, talking) during sleep that has no known conscious accompaniment in dream experience. (2) Parental impressions of bad dreams in early childhood may be based on NREM night terrors (see SLEEP TERRORS) that do not arise out of dream experience. (3) Dreams spontaneously remembered by children at home constitute only a small proportion of the dreams they actually experience (but generally sleep through and forget), and these dreams probably are remembered precisely because they are different (that is, more disturbing) than the typical dream. (4) Children in laboratory studies are awakened quickly by an adult and directly oriented to the task of remembering a dream, whereas it is likely that children's spontaneously remembered dreams at home come from more gradual awakenings that permit intermediate confusional states to develop in which disturbing elaborations of the dream experiences, or wholly original fantasies, may occur.

In any event, it is known from control studies in which dreams from morning awakenings at home are compared with dreams from morning awakenings in the laboratory that the laboratory setting itself does not significantly influence the content of children's dreams. Thus, the representative sampling of children's dream life that laboratory monitoring permits is not purchased at the cost of altering that dream life. Therefore, laboratory dream samples give us by far the better view of children's ordinary or typical dream experience.

The distinction between typical dreams and typical spontaneously remembered dreams needs to be borne in mind when one encounters seemingly authoritative statements about children's dreams. Do such statements refer to representative samples of children's dream life or are they based on unsystematic samples of those few dreams sufficiently disturbing or out of the ordinary to distinguish themselves from the main body of that dream life? A recent encyclopedia of sleep, for example, states that "Young children tend to dream of unpleasant events, such as being chased. . . . By age five or six, the dreams include ghosts, physical injury, and even death." Such assertions may reflect certain dreams children are likely to recall spontaneously, but as applied to children's night-to-night ordinary dream life, they are wholly unsubstantiated and highly misleading.

REFERENCES

Foulkes D. 1982. *Children's dreams: Longitudinal studies.* New York: Wiley.
Foulkes D. 1989. Understanding our dreams. *The World and I* (12):296–303.
Foulkes D, Hollifield M, Sullivan B, Bradley L, Terry R. 1990. REM dreaming and cognitive skills at ages 5–8: A cross-sectional study. *Int J Behav Dev* 13:447–465.

David Foulkes

CHOCOLATE

Chocolate owes its flavor to cacao beans from the tree *Theobroma,* meaning "food of the gods." The Aztecs of pre-Columbian Mexico mixed roasted, ground cacao beans with water to make a brew resembling today's hot chocolate beverage. Women were forbidden to drink the cocoa because it was considered an aphrodisiac.

By 1518, the Spanish conquistadors had

learned of the wonders of chocolate and shipped it back to Spain, where a sweetened version of the Mexican drink became very popular among the nobility. The Spanish kept the recipe a national secret until Princess Marie Thérèse spilled the beans, after her marriage to Louis XIV of France in the mid-seventeenth century. Cocoa then spread to other parts of Europe, and in 1847 the British company Fry and Sons created the first chocolate bar by adding finely ground sugar to cocoa butter, a fatty extract of the cacao bean. The Swiss perfected the process of making solid milk chocolate, and soon chocolate began to appear in many different forms, such as candy, ice cream, cake, and mousse.

Today, Switzerland has the highest per capita consumption of chocolate in the world, averaging about 20 pounds per person annually. Americans eat more than 10 pounds per person each year. To produce 1 pound of chocolate requires approximately 400 cacao beans, which are imported from Africa, South America, and Mexico.

Chocolate contains various amounts of cocoa butter, sugar, and vanilla flavoring, heated together and poured into molds. Milk chocolate must contain at least 12 percent milk solids; gourmet brands often contain as much as 22 percent. White "chocolate" is not officially chocolate at all, because it does not contain enough of the liquid extracted from the cacao bean. In the United States, white chocolate must be labeled as "confectionary coating" instead.

Many people drink hot cocoa to relax before going to bed. Sugar in the chocolate causes the pancreas to release more insulin, which in turn stimulates the brain to release a neurotransmitter called serotonin (5-hydroxytryptamine). Serotonin has long been known to affect sleep processes. Chocolate also contains theobromine, however, which is a milder form of the stimulant caffeine (see CAFFEINE). Caffeine can disturb sleep and cause restlessness, although chocolate manufacturers claim that the low levels of caffeine contained in chocolate are not enough to produce these effects. Depending on the type of chocolate, a 1.5-ounce bar can contain 5 to 35 milligrams of caffeine (Table 1). A 5-ounce cup of hot cocoa may contain 2 to 20 milligrams of caffeine; many instant brands advertise that they are 99.9 percent caffeine free. Compared with coffee and nonherbal tea, both of which usually contain much more than 20 milligrams of caffeine, cocoa is often a less stimulating bedtime

Table 1.   Caffeine in Chocolate Products

Product	Milligrams of Caffeine
Dark chocolate (1.5 ounces)	31
Milk chocolate (1.5 ounces)	9
Hot chocolate prepared with unsweetened cocoa powder (5 ounces)	8
Nestle's Instant Hot Chocolate (5 ounces)	3
Chocolate milk (5 ounces)	1.25
Hershey's Kisses (1 kiss)	1.2
Chocolate fudge topping (2 tablespoons)	5
Semisweet chocolate chips (¼ cup)	33

All values are based on average amounts of caffeine in Hershey's products, with the exception of Nestle's Hot Chocolate.

drink. (See COFFEE; TEA; FOLK AND OTHER NATURAL REMEDIES FOR SLEEPLESSNESS.) In any case, chocolate lovers around the world agree that it makes life a little richer.

REFERENCES

Bernikow L. 1991. Death by chocolate. *Cosmopolitan,* December, pp 212–215.
Cavendish R. 1990. The sweet smell of success. *History Today,* July, pp 2–3.
Somer E. 1991. The jive on java. *Shape,* November, pp 35–41.
Stone J. 1988. Lifestyles of the rich and creamy. *Discover,* September, pp 81–83.
Tooley J. 1989. Oh, chocolate. *U.S. News World Rep,* 27 February, p 75.
Trager J. 1970. *The foodbook.* New York: Grossman.

Semra Aytur

CHOLINERGIC ACTIVITY

See Chemistry of Sleep: Acetylcholine; REM Sleep Mechanisms and Neuroanatomy

CHRONIC FATIGUE SYNDROME

Chronic fatigue syndrome (CFS) is a medical illness of unknown etiology that is characterized by profound physical fatigue and weakness. The fatigue is intensified by minimal physical activity and is not resolved with bed rest. These symptoms usually follow an acute "flulike" illness. According to diagnostic criteria of the U.S. Centers for Disease Control (Holmes et al., 1988), the patient has no previous history of similar symptoms, and the illness lasts longer than 6 months; the patient does not have any medical or psychiatric condition that would account for the illness. Symptoms may include disturbed, unrefreshing, or nonrestorative sleep, chronic headache, generalized muscle and joint pains, sore throat, painful swollen lymph nodes, a feverish sensation, unsteadiness, blurring of vision, irritability, depression and disturbances in concentration, memory, or speech. Physical examination results are often unremarkable, but patients may show a low-grade fever, an inflamed throat, or tender lymph nodes in the neck or axilla.

Approximately 5 percent of those with CFS also have neurological disorders, such as epileptic seizures, transient blindness, and acute loss of balance. Many of the symptoms are similar to those of fibrositis or fibromyalgia (a chronic disorder associated with pain, tenderness, and nonrestorative sleep) (Moldofsky, 1989). As a group, however, patients with CFS have fewer tender points over the body and less intense tenderness. Nevertheless, those patients who experience diffuse muscle pain show multiple tender points, as do patients with fibromyalgia. Thirty-five percent to 70 percent of CFS patients experience symptoms of depression. Psychological assessments reveal major difficulties in discerning whether the subjective complaints and emotional distress are features of a primary depressive disorder, are hypochondriacal preoccupations, or are the result of a viral illness (Abbey and Garfinkel, 1989). Various viruses have been implicated in CSF, such as Epstein–Barr, human herpesvirus-6, and enteroviruses. Immunological abnormalities have been reported in the blood; however, the specificity of any virus or immune system dysfunction and its significance for the illness are unknown.

Chronic fatigue syndrome affects young women more often than men. A prevalence of 37.1 cases per 100,000 people has been found in Australia, but sporadic epidemics variously affecting large numbers of people in communities or hospitals have been reported since the mid-1930s. The disorder may result in impaired work or school performance. The illness tends to persist, but may gradually improve after 3 to 5 years.

Historically, the symptoms of CFS have been given various diagnostic labels according to current scientific beliefs about the cause or some special feature of the illness. Diagnostic labels that have been ascribed include Icelandic disease, Akureyri disease, Otago mystery disease, Royal Free disease, epidemic neuromyasthenia, epidemic or benign myalgic encephalomyelitis (ME), sporadic postinfectious neuromyasthenia, postviral fatigue syndrome, chronic mononucleosis(-like) syndrome, and chronic Epstein–Barr virus syndrome. Because of the concern that the term *chronic fatigue syndrome* trivializes the illness, a patient support organization in the United States employs the term *chronic fatigue and immune dysfunction syndrome* (CFIDS). *Myalgic encephalomyelitis* is the term most commonly used in the United Kingdom.

Sleep symptoms and sleep physiology in CFS are similar to those of fibromyalgia (Moldofsky, 1989). The light, nonrestorative sleep is accompanied by a prominent alpha (7.5 to 11 cycles per second) electroencephalographic sleep anomaly known as ALPHA–DELTA SLEEP. There is exaggerated delay in falling asleep and poor sleep efficiency. Occasionally, patients show obstructive sleep APNEA, and some have periodic involuntary limb movements during sleep. Often patients complain of sleepiness and feel obliged to rest or nap during the day. However, the MULTIPLE SLEEP LATENCY TEST usually does not show irresistible daytime somnolence in CFS patients (Whelton, Salit, and Moldofsky, 1992).

As yet, no specific effective treatment for CFS is available. A gentle graded aerobic fitness program and psychological support are advocated. An unconfirmed study showed that certain CFS patients had low red blood cell magnesium, which improved along with other symptoms when these patients received intramuscular magnesium sulfate injections (Cox, Campbell, and Dowson, 1991). Another report described reduced symptoms with intravenous infusions of immunoglobulin (Lloyd et al., 1990). There are anecdotal reports of various medication including antidepressant drugs, but no systematic studies have demonstrated the effectiveness of any specific treatment for CFS.

(See also FATIGUE; MEDICAL ILLNESS AND SLEEP; NONRESTORATIVE SLEEP.)

REFERENCES

Abbey SE, Garfinkel PE. 1989. Chronic fatigue syndrome and the psychiatrist. *Can J Psychiatry* 35:625–633.

Cox IM, Campbell MJ, Dowson D. 1991. Red blood cell magnesium and chronic fatigue syndrome. *Lancet* 337:757–760.

Holmes GP, Kaplan JE, Grantz NM, et al. 1988. Chronic fatigue syndrome: A working case definition. *Ann Intern Med 108*:387–389.

Lloyd A, Hickie I, Wakefield D, Broughton C, Dwyer J. 1990. A double-blind placebo controlled trial of intravenous immunoglobulin therapy in patients with chronic fatigue syndrome. *Am J Med* 89:561–568.

Moldofsky H. 1989. Nonrestorative sleep and symptoms after a febrile illness in patients with fibrositis and chronic fatigue syndromes. *J Rheumatol* 16(Suppl. 19):150–153.

Whelton CL, Salit I, Moldofsky H. 1992. Sleep, Epstein–Barr virus infection, musculoskeletal pain, and depressive symptoms in chronic fatigue syndrome. *J Rheumatol* 19:939–943.

Harvey Moldofsky

CHRONIC OBSTRUCTIVE PULMONARY DISEASE

See Apnea; Medical Illness and Sleep

CHRONOBIOLOGY

[Chronobiology *is the study of the biological clocks used by living organisms to keep time. In most cases, this term refers to the study of* CIRCADIAN RHYTHMS, *which are the best-studied and most universal type of biological clocks. Time measurement is also used to organize cycles of other durations, ranging from tenths of seconds to years (see also* BIOLOGICAL RHYTHMS *and* ULTRADIAN RHYTHMS*).*]

CHRONOTHERAPY

Chronotherapy is a specific treatment method that was devised to correct the timing abnormality of sleep known as DELAYED SLEEP PHASE SYNDROME (DSPS). Those affected by DSPS fall asleep and wake up abnormally late and are unable to correct this timing abnormality simply by going to bed and waking themselves at earlier times of day.

The aim of treating DSPS is to shift sleep from the late time of day at which it tends to occur (for example, 4 A.M. to 11 A.M.) to a time that is early enough to accommodate conventional morning activities, such as 11 P.M. to 6 A.M. The target bedtime and waking time in this example are each 5 hours earlier than the current sleep times. Efforts by people with DSPS to "set the clock back" (see BIOLOGICAL RHYTHMS; CIRCADIAN RHYTHMS) by 5 hours are unsuccessful and result in both INSOMNIA (difficulty falling asleep) and sleep DEPRIVATION. Chronotherapy reverses this unsuccessful strategy by *delaying* sleep by the amount needed to place it at an earlier target time of day, in our example, 24 hours minus 5 hours, or 19 hours. The long delay of 19 hours is accomplished in steps of 3 hours a day, and the complete treatment in the example would require 19 hours divided by 3 hours per day, or 6.3 days.

The process is illustrated in Figure 1, which illustrates bedrest periods (rectangles) and sleep periods (black bars) of a hypothetical person with DSPS. Vertical lines are drawn at midnight

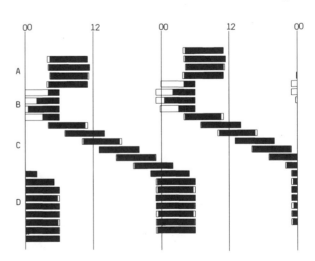

Figure 1. Bedrest and sleep periods of a hypothetical patient undergoing chronotherapy (see text for explanation).

("00") and noon ("12"). Twenty-two days are shown on consecutive levels starting at the top. To facilitate comparison, each bar appears twice on successive levels; each level represents a 48-hour period beginning 24 hours after the previous level. During the first four nights ("A"), the person sleeps on a comfortable ad-libitum schedule averaging around 4 A.M. to 11 A.M. During this period, there is no difficulty falling asleep, as shown by the brief (less than 20-minute) delays from retiring to sleep onset. On the next four days ("B"), attempts are made to fall asleep at 11 P.M. and get up at 7 A.M. The attempts are unsuccessful and result in severe insomnia, shown by the long delays from bedtime to sleep onset. Note that forced awakenings at 7 A.M. fail to shift sleep periods very far toward earlier times and only succeed in truncating the periods of sleep. On the ninth day, the person returns to the 4 A.M. to 11 A.M. sleep period, followed by progressive 3-hour delays of the bedrest period (chronotherapy, "C"). Seven daily shifts are required to reach the target sleep schedule of 11 P.M. to 7 A.M., which is then maintained for seven nights ("D") without further sleeping difficulty.

Chronotherapy should be carefully planned. First, a daily log should be kept of sleeping hours for a week or two. During this time, a regular schedule of normal sleep should be maintained to establish a stable sleep period. A target sleeping schedule should then be selected with the following considerations in mind: (1) the bedtime and rising time should be ones that can be followed every day, including weekends; and (2) the bedrest period should approximate the duration of sleep needed to maintain full daytime alertness. The chronotherapy schedule should provide adequate daily bedrest periods, delayed by up to 3 hours a day, until the target schedule is reached.

When properly carried out, chronotherapy usually succeeds, demonstrating that delayed sleep phase insomnia originated from attempts to sleep at times that were earlier than those at which sleep was biologically possible. Successful chronotherapy also provides direct evidence that the capacity of people with DSPS to shift sleep to earlier times of day is much smaller than the capacity to shift it to later times. It is likely that those not affected by DSPS are also more able to delay sleep than they are to advance it, but the difference is not as large. (See also PHASE RESPONSE CURVE.)

The capacity to advance the phase of sleep to earlier times of day is not entirely absent in people with DSPS. If it were, it would not be possible to synchronize the sleep–wake rhythm with the 24-hour day, because even small delays of sleep would be unopposed on subsequent nights, and the average interval between successive sleep periods would exceed 24 hours. The limited ability of people with DSPS to advance the timing of sleep means that the target schedule could be reached by corrective advances of sleep rather than delays. The steps must, however, be small (less than 30 minutes a day). This approach may not save time, because a 5-hour shift would require 10 days or longer to reach the target sleeping schedule; but the necessity of staying up for several nights and for sleeping through the day during the treatment period could be avoided.

Once the target schedule is reached, it is important to avoid late bedtimes and sleeping late; otherwise, sleep may again be delayed, making it necessary to repeat chronotherapy. The effects of chronotherapy may last several years. Additional methods of treating DSPS, including exposure to bright light soon after awakening in the morning (see LIGHT THERAPY), may be used in conjunction with chronotherapy to help prevent relapses.

In conclusion, the delayed sleep phase syndrome is a cause of insomnia that may be successfully treated without use of hypnotic drugs by progressively delaying the time of sleep until a socially appropriate target schedule is reached. This method avoids the severely limited ability of people with DSPS to advance the daily time of sleep and takes advantage of their unimpaired ability to delay it. Long-term control may be achieved, although repeated applications are required whenever sleep becomes severely delayed.

REFERENCE

Czeisler CA, Richardson GS, Coleman RM, Zimmerman JC, Moore-Ede MC, Dement WC, Weitzman ED. 1981. Chronotherapy: Resetting the circadian clocks of patients with delayed sleep phase insomnia. *Sleep* 4:1–21.

Charles P. Pollak

CIRCADIAN RHYTHM DISORDERS

[*The circadian system controlling the coordination and timing of diverse physiologic events and functions in humans is intricate, complex, and precise. Thus, it is not surprising that a breakdown in this system can cause a variety of circadian rhythm disorders, most of which will manifest a primary symptom of disrupted sleep. Only the timing is abnormal in circadian rhythm disorders—the rhythmic function itself is not affected. Sleep, however, is one function that must occur at its usual time to be experienced as "normal." Patients who are able to sleep only during the day and are alert only at night typically complain of* INSOMNIA, *reporting that normal sleep is not possible. Such patients often complain of excessive* SLEEPINESS *or daytime* HYPERSOMNIA *as well.*

Two well-known circadian rhythm disorders involving serious sleep complaints are the DELAYED SLEEP PHASE SYNDROME *(DSPS) and the* ADVANCED SLEEP PHASE SYNDROME *(ASPS). In DSPS, the timing of sleep is abnormally delayed, so patients complain of difficulty falling asleep at night until 3:00 A.M. or later and difficulty waking before noon or later. DSPS is more likely to occur in older adolescents and young adults, whereas ASPS is more likely to occur in the elderly. In ASPS, the timing of sleep is abnormally early, so patients cannot stay awake in the evening and cannot stay asleep beyond 1:00 to 2:00 A.M. DSPS and ASPS are thought to originate from either abnormally slow or fast intrinsic timing in the brain's clock, the* SUPRACHIASMATIC NUCLEUS OF THE HYPOTHALAMUS *(SCN) (see* CIRCADIAN RHYTHMS).

Infants and children with brain damage or MENTAL RETARDATION *may suffer sleep–wake schedule disorders due to underlying circadian rhythm problems, as do certain elderly patients with* SUNDOWN SYNDROME. *Aging may have direct implications for circadian functioning (see* AGING AND CIRCADIAN RHYTHMS). BRAIN TUMORS *affecting regions near the SCN are also associated with sleep complaints caused by malfunctions of circadian timekeeping. People who are entirely without light perception may also suffer circadian rhythm disorders such as* HYPERNYCHTHEMERAL SYNDROME, *in which the sleep–wake cycle continues as in* FREE RUNNING *with a clock period of 25 hours, causing episodic insomnia about every 2 weeks when the internal cycle goes in and out of phase with the external day–night cycle (see* BLINDNESS: EFFECTS ON SLEEP PATTERNS AND CIRCADIAN RHYTHMS).

JET LAG *involves a short-lived circadian rhythm disorder until the internal clock resynchronizes with the external environment by* ENTRAINMENT *to time cues—*ZEITGEBERS—*in the new time zone. People who do* SHIFTWORK *or those with an* IRREGULAR SLEEP–WAKE CYCLE *may also experience sleep–wake problems involving mismatches with their internal circadian clocks.*

Treatment of circadian rhythm disorders may incorporate a number of approaches. In the case of a brain tumor, treatment must address this underlying condition. Techniques used to reestablish synchrony between internal and external rhythms, particularly in DSPS and ASPS, include CHRONOTHERAPY *and* LIGHT THERAPY. *For many patients, a combination of these approaches with improved* SLEEP HYGIENE *is quite effective.*]

CIRCADIAN RHYTHMS

Regular daily variation is apparent in virtually every aspect of physiology. In mammals, such as humans, every measurable feature varies with the time of day. Perhaps the best-studied example is BODY TEMPERATURE; while everyone knows that "normal" body temperature is 98.6° Fahrenheit, fewer people realize that body temperature normally varies by 3 to 4 degrees over the course of a normal day. It is actively maintained near 100° at midafternoon and near 96° in the early morning hours before awakening. Similar rhythms can be seen in plasma levels of hormones such as CORTISOL, GROWTH HORMONE, and PROLACTIN as well as in urine production, heart rate, and blood pressure. Analogous daily variation can be seen in all eukaryotic organisms (i.e., organisms made up of cells with true nuclei), from single-celled algae to humans.

The consistent presence of this diurnal rhythmicity, both across species and within individual organisms, argues that such variation confers an important competitive advantage. One need only consider the outside environment to realize that most organisms evolved in a world that itself changes with time of day. By night, light intensity, temperature, and humidity are all significantly lower than by day; and for animals dependent on their senses to catch prey or avoid predators, or for insects whose larvae cannot survive in the mid-day sun, the environment presents very different challenges and opportunities at different times of day. From this "outdoor" perspective, it is not surprising that the functional organization of all organisms includes daily rhythmicity and that organisms are often remarkably accurate at keeping time and anticipating the daily changes in their environment. Nevertheless, for early students of circadian rhythms in biology, important questions remained unanswered by this survey of biology and physiology: Does rhythmic variation passively reflect the changing external environment? Or does the organism anticipate the predictable features of daily environmental variation through an internal timekeeping system?

The Search for the Circadian Clock

The answer to these questions has actually been available for some time. In the eighteenth century, Jean Jacques d'Ortous DE MAIRAN performed an experiment using a heliotropic plant, one that raises and lowers its leaves with a regular daily cycle. De Mairan observed that the diurnal leaf movements persisted even when the plants were kept in a dark closet, isolated from all environmental time signals. This finding and its implications were largely ignored until about 200 years later when a number of researchers began to study the activity patterns of rodents. In captivity, nocturnally active rodents such as mice vigorously run on running wheels, and they do so at a regular time of day (typically immediately after sunset). Several researchers noted that when mice and running wheels were placed in cages in light-proof, continuously dark chambers, the mice ran on their wheels with a regular almost-24-hour rhythm. Thus, despite the absence of any information about the time of day, these animals continued to exhibit daily rhythms of activity.

In the study of the activity patterns of rodents in TEMPORAL ISOLATION, two important principles were recognized. First, it was clear that rhythmic organization of activity persists in the absence of environmental time cues, collectively termed ZEITGEBERS. Second, the period of the activity rhythm (the time from one activity onset to the next) was no longer 24 hours. Instead (in mice) the period was significantly less than 24 hours. This non-24-hour period is a consistent feature of diurnal rhythms when observed in the absence of zeitgebers and is the origin of the term *circadian* (from Latin *circa* meaning "approximately" and *dies* meaning "day"). The precise circadian period is apparently under genetic control, and varies from species to species and between individual organisms within the species.

At this point in the study of circadian rhythm, it was clear that circadian rhythms originated within the organism, and an extensive effort was mounted to locate the source of circadian rhythmicity in mammals. Although it seemed clear that the circadian clock had to be within the brain, the exact location remained a mystery until a group of researchers realized that the important influence of light on circadian rhythms implied that the clock was linked to the visual system. In the early 1970s, researchers traced a path from the retina to a small nucleus of neurons in the anterior hypothalamus located immediately above the optic chiasm. These nuclei, called the *suprachiasmatic nuclei* (SCN; see SUPRACHIASMATIC NUCLEUS OF THE HYPOTHALAMUS), are now recognized as the source of circadian rhythmicity in mammals. Destroying them with small lesions eliminates an animal's ability to organize activities and behaviors within the day.

Circadian Rhythms in Humans

Despite evidence that diurnal variation in physiologic function also occurs in humans, researchers had several reasons to suspect that circadian organization might be different in humans than in other mammals. First, the advantages of an internal clock are less obvious for humans, because for the last several hundred years, humans have been able to control the heat and light of their environment by day and night. Second, humans are able to organize activity and behavior on a daily basis despite the conflicting influence of electric lights, which seemed to confound the zeitgeber role of sunlight. At very least, scientists suggested, humans clocks must depend on different environmental zeitgebers for entrainment to external time.

Studies of human volunteers in temporal isolation caves and in special apartments without windows or contact with the outside world for weeks or months showed that humans have internal clocks that continue to keep time. The free-running period of humans is typically greater than 24 hours, in contrast to less than 24 hours as in mice, but otherwise the principle is the same. Further, recent studies have shown that when LIGHT of sufficient intensity is used (equivalent to dim sunlight), the human circadian clock behaves exactly like those of other species. Studies of the human brain by neuropathologists have shown that humans also have suprachiasmatic nuclei, and the connections to the retina are similar to those seen in other mammals. (See also PHASE RESPONSE CURVE.)

Circadian Rhythms of Sleep and Wakefulness

The regular daily alternation between sleep and wakefulness is one of the most fundamental of mammalian circadian rhythms (see TIMING OF SLEEP AND WAKEFULNESS). The consolidation of human sleep into a single major episode makes it difficult for us to recognize the influence of the circadian clock under normal conditions. When we begin to feel sleepy at 11 P.M. or midnight (or 1:00 or 2:00 or 3:00 A.M), most people envision a "winding down," or exhaustion of available energy, rather than the ticking of an internal clock. But the body's internal clock plays a very important role in modulating sleepiness and alertness, facilitating sleep at one time of day and making sleep very difficult at others. Most people have had the experience of staying awake all night on at least one occasion. The hours from 3:00 to 6:00 A.M. are the toughest; it is extremely hard to stay awake, particularly if the activity is a quiet one like studying. After about 7:00 A.M., however, we get a "second wind," alertness returns, and it becomes relatively easy to stay awake. This waxing and waning of sleepiness reveals the impact of the circadian clock, facilitating wakefulness and inhibiting sleep. Thus, even though deprivation causes greater sleepiness due to a separate homeostatic effect (i.e., an effect related to the need to maintain internal stability)—we feel no-

where near as alert as if we had had a good night of sleep—the clock plays an important modulating role.

Disorders of Circadian Rhythms

The sophisticated and complex circadian timing system in humans occasionally malfunctions. The complete destruction of the suprachiasmatic nucleus by tumor or other pathologic processes, as mentioned above, produces complete loss of timekeeping and arrhythmicity of diurnal behaviors and functions. More subtle defects in the function of the circadian timing system can also produce pathology, and these problems manifest principally as disorders of sleep and wakefulness.

In DELAYED SLEEP PHASE SYNDROME (DSPS), the circadian system is shifted to a position markedly later than normal. The sleep propensity rhythm shifts with it, so that the patient with DSPS cannot fall asleep before 3:00 or 4:00 A.M. and cannot wake up before noon without extraordinary effort. An apparent defect in the circadian entrainment mechanism (see ENTRAINMENT) prevents normal corrective shifts to earlier hours while nevertheless allowing stable entrainment to the 24-hour cycle. This disorder is found more often in adolescents and young adults than in older adults; phase delay, though not necessarily DSPS, is quite common in college students. The opposite problem, in which the sleep–wake cycle is advanced to earlier hours, is termed ADVANCED SLEEP PHASE SYNDROME (ASPS). In ASPS, patients report overwhelming sleepiness at 7:00 or 8:00 in the evening, which makes it impossible to remain awake. At 3:00 or 4:00 in the morning they awaken and are unable to return to sleep. ASPS is more common in elderly than in younger adult patients. Studies suggest that shift in the prevalence of these sleep disorders reflects an age-dependent shortening of the circadian period. As the circadian period shortens, the entrained position moves earlier and earlier. Evidence from carefully controlled investigations suggests that older patients with severe ASPS have remarkably short internal circadian periods; some appear to have periods of less than 24 hours, similar to those seen in rodents.

Shiftwork syndrome is not really a disease, since most people who complain of this problem probably possess perfectly normal circadian timing systems. Instead, the root of this difficulty lies with the societal requirement that some people work nights, despite the daytime orientation of human circadian clocks. Although most shiftworkers are able to compensate for the increased sleepiness and poor day sleep imposed by the circadian clock, many shiftworkers do not adapt. Over time the resultant chronic sleep deprivation produces general stress and a host of secondary medical disorders. Comparisons of those who adapt and those who cannot suggest that shiftwork may be a very poor choice for some people, but an explanation for the difference in the ability to adjust is not yet available. (See also SHIFTWORK.)

Summary

Circadian rhythmicity is evident in virtually all physiological functions. These daily rhythms originate within the organism and are controlled by sophisticated internal clocks. In mammals, the circadian clock is located in the suprachiasmatic nucleus of the hypothalamus. The timing of this internal clock is set (entrained) by daylight for most species, including humans, and when entrained, the body's rhythms are said to be *synchronized*. The alternation of sleep and wake in humans is controlled in large part by circadian mechanisms, but also by homeostatic mechanisms that keep a balance between sleep–wake propensity. Abnormalities of circadian organization are apparent in several sleep disorders. (See also HYPERNYCHTHEMERAL SYNDROME; INTERNAL DESYNCHRONIZATION; IRREGULAR SLEEP–WAKE CYCLE.)

REFERENCES

Moore-Ede MC, Czeisler CA, Richardson GS. 1983. Circadian timekeeping in health and disease. *N Engl J Med* 309:469–476, 530–536.

Moore-Ede MC, Sulzman FM, Fuller CA. 1982. *The clocks that time us.* Cambridge, Mass.: Harvard University Press.

Czeisler CA, Johnson MP, Duffy JF, Brown EN, Ronda JM, Kronauer RE. 1990. Exposure to bright light and darkness to treat physiologic maladaptation to night work. *N Engl J Med* 322:1253–1259.

Gary S. Richardson

COCAINE

Cocaine is a drug extracted from the leaves of the coca plant, which is indigenous to South and Central America. People native to these regions have used the coca leaf for centuries as a mild stimulant and as sustenance while working under the harsh weather conditions of their environment. The coca leaf has also played a crucial religious and symbolic role in Andean society. Although it was once considered harmless enough for use in a soft drink (see COLA), cocaine is an addictive drug that is illegal in the United States, except for certain experimental and research uses. *Crack* is the common derivative of cocaine used by addicts today; known also as *rock* because of its rocklike formation, this is often a more potent form than cocaine powder.

Disturbed sleep patterns characterize addiction to these drugs (see DRUGS OF ABUSE). Cocaine and crack reduce the amount of total sleep, and of REM sleep specifically, but produce varied effects on daytime and nighttime arousal levels. Some individuals experience an increase in alertness, while others report an increase in drowsiness. The effects of cocaine also vary with dosage and length of time of ingestion. According to a manual of psychiatric diagnoses and classifications used by clinicians and other scientists, short-term withdrawal from cocaine produces noticeable sleep changes in addicts: insomnia, hypersomnia, and fatigue (American Psychiatric Association Staff, 1987).

REFERENCES

American Psychiatric Association Staff. 1987. *Diagnostic and statistical manual of mental disorders DSM-III-R.* 3rd ed. Washington, D.C.: American Psychiatric Press.

Beebe, DK, Walley E. 1991. Substance abuse: The designer drugs. *Am Fam Physician* 43:1689–1698.

Fischman MW. 1984. The behavioral pharmacology of cocaine in humans. *Nat Inst Drug Abuse Res Monogr Ser* 50:72–91.

Nicholi AM. 1984. Cocaine use among the college age group: Biological and psychological effects. *J Am Coll Health* 32:258–261.

Pacine D, Franquemont C, eds. 1986. *Coca and cocaine: Effects on people and policy in Latin America.* Peterborough, N.H.: Cultural Survival.

Weddington WW, Brown BS, Haertzen CA, Cone EJ. 1990. Changes in mood, craving, and sleep during short-term abstinence reported by male cocaine addicts. *Arch Gen Psychiatry* 47:861–868.

Jenifer Wicks

COFFEE

The first written reference to coffee is attributed to Rhazes, a physician of ancient Arabia, who called the coffee bean *bunchum* and recorded that coffee is "hot and dry and very good for the stomach . . . it fortifies the members, it cleans the skin and dries up the humidities that are under it, and gives an excellent smell to all the body" (Ukers, 1935). Some historians believe that he was writing about the root of a different plant; most agree that the coffee Rhazes described was a pastelike food rather than a beverage and that the Arabs began drinking coffee by A.D. 800. Venetian traders brought coffee beans to Europe from Constantinople beginning in the late 1500s, until the Dutch East India Company began importing directly from the African port of Mocha in 1616. At this time the Ottoman Empire held a monopoly on coffee cultivation, but European merchants eventually smuggled coffee seeds to establish plantations in the Dutch colony of Java. Coffee growing soon spread to the warmer climates of the Caribbean and Latin America, and the beverage became extremely popular throughout Europe and the American colonies. The word *coffee* reflects this history, deriving from the Arabic *qahwah,* the Turkish *kahve,* and the Italian *caffè*. More coffee is now consumed in the United States than in any other nation, at the rate of more than 535 million cups per day. Coffee also flavors a host of other products, from candy, ice cream, and yogurt to the "coffee milk" and "coffee syrup" favored by residents of the northeastern United States. Many American workers pause once or twice a day to take a "coffee break," a few minutes of relaxation that originally centered around this popular beverage.

Most of the coffee consumed today comes from the seed of the *Coffea arabica* plant, an evergreen shrub native to Ethiopia. (Coffee beans are also harvested from the African *Coffea robusta* plant, though robusta beans are thought to be of lower quality and harsher flavor than arabica beans.) Coffee plants produce fragrant white flowers that later form berries containing the coffee bean. After harvesting, two different methods are used to extract the bean from the berry. In the wet process, a pulping machine cleans off the skin and some of the pulp; the seeds are then soaked in water for 24 hours, while yeasts and bacteria remove more of the flesh; finally, the beans are washed and dried in the sun. In the dry process, which is less expensive but produces lower-quality beans, the berries are picked and allowed to dry in the sun for 2 or 3 weeks, and the dried skin and flesh of the berries are then easily removed. Both processes produce green coffee beans ready for roasting. Coffee beans are roasted in 260°C gases for up to 5 minutes: the longer they are roasted, the darker the beans, the higher the caffeine content, and the stronger the flavor. For example, the beverage espresso, which originated in Italy, is brewed from coffee beans that are roasted until black, and it has a much stronger flavor and more caffeine than an American-blend coffee made from beans roasted to a medium-brown color.

Dry coffee grounds made from arabica beans are approximately 1.1 percent caffeine by weight, whereas robusta beans are 2.2 percent caffeine by weight. Instant coffees, made by spray-drying or freeze-drying large batches of strong coffee extract, contain somewhat less caffeine as a result of processing. Though different brands have varying amounts of caffeine, the average 8-ounce cup of instant coffee contains about 65 milligrams. An 8-ounce cup of coffee freshly brewed from an average American blend (mostly arabica beans) contains about 80 milligrams of caffeine, though one study showed that the milligrams of caffeine per cup can range from 75 to 120 ("Coffee," 1991).

Three methods currently exist for decaffeinating coffee before it is roasted. In the most common process, organic solvent decaffeination, green coffee beans are soaked in hot water with methylene chloride to dissolve the caffeine; the caffeinated water is then precipitated out and sold to cola and drug companies. Alternatively, the coffee beans are soaked in water and the caffeine is removed from the water by charcoal filters or bubbles of carbon dioxide. Decaffeinated coffees have only trace amounts of caffeine; by law they must contain less than 5 milligrams per 8-ounce cup.

Research confirms that the caffeine found in coffee can affect sleep. Physiological reactions to caffeine can include an increase in the time a person takes to fall asleep, an increase in movement during sleep, a decrease in total sleep time, and a decrease in quality of sleep (see CAFFEINE).

REFERENCES

Coffee. 1991. *Consumer Rep* 56:30–50.
Gilbert RJ. 1986. Caffeine—The most popular stimulant. In *The encyclopedia of psychoactive drugs 18.* New York: Chelsea House.
Ukers WH. 1935. *All about coffee.* New York: Tea and Coffee Trade Journal Co.

Katherine M. Sharkey

COGNITION

One of the defining characteristics of sleep is that the individual becomes relatively unresponsive to external stimuli. Thus, if we fall asleep while the television is on, we do not appear to process what is being broadcast while we are asleep; we have no memory for having heard anything while asleep. In fact, if we remember hearing anything, we attribute that to waking up briefly during the program. Almost by definition, if we sleep, we do not expect to remember hearing anything.

Even though we cannot remember doing so, it is likely that we process information from our environment during sleep. For example, we almost never fall out of bed, despite turning over and moving often during sleep. How do we know where the edge of the bed is?

Considerable evidence exists to indicate that we can be awakened more easily by meaningful than nonmeaningful stimuli (see AROUSAL). The common observation that parents can sleep through a thunderstorm but wake to the cry of their child is true. We are also more easily awakened from sleep by hearing our own name than by hearing an equally loud, but meaningless sound. How do we know which sound to awaken to?

Many important questions about mental activity during sleep are just beginning to be understood: How much information from the environment can be processed by the sleeper? Why do we remember so little of what happens during sleep? What sorts of mental activities are associated with sleepwalking and sleeptalking? Are dreams meaningful, and if so, why aren't they better remembered? Can we become aware that we are dreaming during a dream, and can we control our dreams? What are the possibilities for learning during sleep?

An important theme of these questions is the lack of memory for events that take place during sleep (see AMNESIA; MEMORY). Individuals can be taught to respond to external stimuli in all stages of sleep, but they have little memory for doing so. In one study, sleepers were taught to take a deep breath whenever they heard a tone (Badia et al., 1985). In the morning, the sleepers were asked how many times they heard the tone. Despite taking deep breaths in response to a tone as many as 50 to 100 times during the night, the sleepers reported that they only heard and responded to the tone six or eight times during the night.

Research in other areas of cognitive psychology indicates that it is important to distinguish between explicit and implicit memory when dealing with issues of awareness. *Explicit memory* refers to the conscious recollection of recently presented information, whereas *implicit memory* refers to memories that are encoded and influence performance even though there is no awareness of them (Schacter, 1987). Thus, for example, if pairs of words are played through earphones for surgery patients while they are under anesthesia (Kihlstrom et al., 1990), the patients do not remember hearing the words (explicit memory) but are more likely to produce the paired word when asked to free-associate to the first word of each pair (implicit memory) than if the words had not been played.

Something similar may happen during sleep. Perhaps explicit memory for information during sleep is disrupted, but implicit memory remains. One recent experiment examined this hypothesis by evaluating the effect of sleep onset on memory. Pairs of words were played as individuals fell asleep (Wyatt et al., 1992), and participants were awakened after either 30 seconds or 10 minutes of sleep and tested for explicit and implicit memory of the words. Most participants who were allowed to sleep 10 minutes could not recall any of the words played during the 3 minutes just before they fell asleep; memory was not disrupted for participants who were only allowed 30 seconds of sleep. Even in the 10-minute condition, however, some types of memory for the words were still available as indicated by cued-recognition and implicit memory tests. In these tests, the first word of each pair was played and the participants had to respond either with the word they had heard paired with it (cued recognition) or with any word that came to mind (implicit memory). Although the patterns of memory performance on these two tests were different, both indicated that some memory remained even when participants could not initially recall hearing the words.

One usually experiences light sleep during the first 10 minutes of sleep. It is not surprising, therefore, that cognitive processing of external stimuli continues during the lightest stages of sleep. This study indicates, however, that even light sleep disrupts the conscious recall of events that immediately precede sleep.

How much processing of external stimuli takes place during later, deeper stages of sleep? Research on auditory EVOKED POTENTIALS during sleep indicates that stimuli are processed at the auditory cortex during sleep. Early components of the evoked potential (the first 100 milliseconds) are observed in all stages of sleep; the later components, however—those usually associated with more elaborate cognitive processing—are either delayed or absent.

Studies of cognitive processing during sleep have typically found a lack of memory for information presented during sleep unless the presentation was immediately followed by physiological arousal. The longer the arousal, the better the memory. Attempts to distinguish between explicit and implicit memory for information presented during sleep later in the night have not been fruitful. Thus, although information during sleep may reach the auditory cortex so that meaningful stimuli can be identified and we can be awakened if necessary, we are not likely to remember the stimuli unless we wake up during or immediately after them. This phenomenon may also explain our poor memory for dreams.

We typically do not remember dreams unless we wake up during them. Thus, people are usually aware of dreaming only when they wake up in the morning, because they are more likely to wake up during a dream and stay awake for a long

enough time to consolidate the dream content. Attempts to help individuals become aware of their dreams while still dreaming (called LUCID DREAMING) indicate that it is possible to become aware of some cognitive processes during sleep.

Overall, the evidence indicates that cognition does not stop during sleep, just our awareness of it. The relationship between cognition and sleep is one of the most exciting and challenging topics in sleep research.

(See also PERCEPTION DURING SLEEP; SENSORY PROCESSING AND SENSATION DURING SLEEP.)

REFERENCES

Badia P, Harsh J, Balkin T, O'Rourke D, Burton S. 1985. Behavioral control of respiration in sleep and sleepiness due to signal-induced sleep fragmentation. *Psychophysiology* 22:517–524.

Bootzin RR, Kihlstrom JF, Schacter DL, eds. 1990. *Sleep and cognition.* Washington, D.C.: American Psychological Association.

Ellman SJ, Antrobus JS, eds. 1991. *The mind in sleep,* 2nd ed. New York: Wiley.

Kihlstrom JF, Schacter DL, Cork RC, Hurt CA, Behr SE. 1990. Implicit and explicit memory following surgical anesthesia. *Psych Sci* 1:303–306.

Schacter D. 1987. Implicit memory: History and current status. *J Exper Psych Learning Memory Cognition* 13:501–518.

Wyatt JK, Bootzin RR, Anthony J, Stevenson S. 1992. Does sleep onset produce retrograde amnesia? *Sleep Res* 21:113.

Richard R. Bootzin
John F. Kihlstrom

COGNITIVE DREAM THEORY

Cognitive dream theory proposes that dreaming can best be understood in terms of the same concepts used in the systematic empirical study of the waking mind (*cognitive psychology*). Cognitive psychology, and the "cognitive sciences" more generally (e.g., artificial intelligence, psycholinguistics, neuropsychology), arose in the late 1950s and early 1960s as a concerted effort to bring the same objectivity to the study of the human mind that behaviorism earlier had introduced to the study of animal learning. One central metaphor underlying much of this effort was that of the mind as an *information processor.* By the 1970s, several dream psychologists began conceptualizing dreaming as a reprocessing of memories and knowledge that otherwise conformed to many principles of the waking processing of perceptual information. A number of different versions of cognitive dream theory have appeared (e.g., Antrobus, 1978, 1991; Foulkes, 1982, 1985), and many other realizations of it are theoretically possible, depending on which cognitive-psychological concepts or principles are chosen to map onto which dream phenomena.

Unlike dream theories arising from neurobiology, cognitive dream theory tends not to be reductionist: It holds that dreaming must be explained at a purely (cognitive-) psychological level (for a qualification, see Antrobus, 1991). Unlike most dream theories derived from clinical observation, cognitive dream theory does not routinely assume that a motivational unconscious organizes spontaneous mental acts like dreaming. Therefore, it tends not to hold that dreams have hidden meanings that can be arrived at only through "deep" interpretation. In fact, like cognitive psychology more generally, cognitive dream theory is relatively uninterested in specific mental contents, their derivation, and their significance. It is process oriented, seeking to characterize the generalized psychological conditions in which, and the generalized psychological means by which, dreams are produced. In addition, it seeks to understand differences between dreaming and other conscious states in terms of functional differences in the organization of mental processing.

One point of departure for several cognitive theories (e.g., Antrobus, 1991; Foulkes, 1985) is specification of differences in the mental "fields" in which dreaming, as opposed to ordinary waking mentation, is generated. The dreaming mind lacks regulation either by patterned world stimulation or by deliberate self-control. Hence, it is processing its own information, and this information is more diffusely and dissociatively active than most often is the case in waking life. In one recent statement of cognitive dream theory (Foulkes, 1990), it is proposed that the general function of waking consciousness is to produce models of currently available information that are coherent (facilitating effective action) and consistent with recently processed information

(guaranteeing stability over time), but also sensitive to major discrepancies from pattern or expectation. Dreaming is viewed as consciousness trying to implement these same goals, but in a context that is relatively unusual by waking standards—a diffusely active field of sometimes unrelated mental representations induced by lack of world- or self-regulation. In the dream, consciousness is providing a momentarily coherent synthesis of currently active information; it is doing so in the narrative format that also orders waking experience; but it is also generating scenarios that, in order to do justice to their various and sometimes unrelated sources, may seem somewhat odd to the dreamer upon later waking reflection.

As this example indicates, cognitive dream theories tend to see dreaming as a slightly special case of more generalized mental phenomena, that is, as waking information processing proceeding in cases where there no longer is standard waking informational input. A central problem for these theories is the characterization of the bases on which particular memories and knowledge are activated, and hence eligible for inclusion in consciousness, in states of relaxed external and internal direction of mentation. Useful research drawing on current cognitive-psychological models of memory has been directed to just this problem (e.g., Cicogna, Cavallero, and Bosinelli, 1986). The cognitive approach is supported both by general theoretical considerations (a unified mind theory across states) and by the specific evidence of dream psychology (the general plausibility and/or mundaneness of representatively sampled REM dreaming, i.e., its "wakinglike" quality). Moreover, the implication of cognitive dream theory that dreaming is more of an intellectual than a perceptual act, and thus that it is subject to much development in early childhood, has found substantial support in studies of children's REM dreaming (see CHILDREN'S DREAMS).

REFERENCES

Antrobus J. 1978. Dreaming for cognition. In Arkin AM, Antrobus JS, Ellman SJ, eds., *The mind in sleep: Psychology and psychophysiology,* pp 569–581. Hillsdale, N.J.: Erlbaum.

———. 1991. Dreaming: Cognitive processes during cortical activation and high afferent thresholds. *Psychological Rev* 98:96–121.

Cicogna P, Cavallero C, Bosinelli M. 1986. Differential access to memory traces in the production of mental experience. *Int J Psychophysiol* 4:209–216.

Foulkes D. 1982. A cognitive-psychological model of REM dream production. *Sleep* 5:169–187.

———. 1985. *Dreaming: A cognitive-psychological analysis.* Hillsdale, N.J.: Erlbaum.

———. 1990. Dreaming and consciousness. *Eur J Cognitive Psychol* 2:39–55

David Foulkes

COLA

The original cola is Coca-Cola, first produced in 1885 by John Pemberton, a pharmacist in Atlanta, Georgia. It was first marketed as the "French Wine Kola," the "ideal nerve and tonic stimulant." The first colas contained COCAINE as well as wine. After a year of marketing the colas, Pemberton took the wine out of his formula and added a flavorful extract of the kola nut. His marketing scheme also included changing the spelling of *kola* to *cola,* to go with *coca,* and incorporating the Spencerian script popular at the time as part of the product's logo.

Asa Candler bought the rights to the Coca-Cola formula in 1889 and started selling the syrup wholesale for use with carbonated water at soda fountains. Candler also introduced the shapely glasses associated with the Coca-Cola brand name. In 1889, Benjamin Thomas and Joseph P. Whitehead bought the rights to bottle the soda for a mere $1, inspired by bottled drinks that they had seen in Cuba. By subsequently selling rights to other businessmen, the partners created a network of independent bottlers who purchased Coca-Cola syrup from the company and held exclusive contracts to produce the carbonated soda in their respective territories in perpetuity. During World War I, when production of other sodas increased, "It's the real thing" was introduced as an advertising slogan to distinguish Coca-Cola from its competition.

The main effect that colas have on sleep is due to their CAFFEINE content. *Consumer Reports* (1981) has published the caffeine content of various sodas, including those listed in Table 1.

Table 1.   Caffeine Content of Soda Drinks

Brand of Soda	Caffeine (milligrams per 12 ounces)
Mountain Dew	52
Tab	44
Sunkist Orange	42
Dr. Pepper	38
Diet Dr. Pepper	37
Pepsi Cola	37
Diet Rite	34
Diet Pepsi	34
Coca-Cola	34
7-up	0
Sprite	0
Diet 7-up	0
Fresca	0
Hires Root Beer	0
Diet Sunkist Orange	0

Jolt Cola, a soft drink introduced during the late 1980s, was advertised as having twice the caffeine of regular colas (and all the sugar), for a total of 71.2 milligrams of caffeine per 12 ounces of soda, seemingly to appeal to those who seek its stimulating effects.

Interestingly, in 1911 a suit was filed against Coca-Cola by the federal government for marketing a beverage with a "deleterious ingredient," namely caffeine. Using what is today considered a rather sophisticated experimental design, Harry Hollingsworth investigated the behavioral effects of caffeine in connection with this lawsuit, although his results were not published (Benjamin, Rogers, and Rosenbaum, 1990).

REFERENCES

Benjamin LT Jr, Rogers AM, Rosenbaum A. 1990. Coca-Cola, caffeine, and mental deficiency: Harry Hollingsworth and the Chattanooga trial of 1911. *J History Behavioral Sci* 27:42–55.

Consumer Reports. 1981. Caffeine: How to consume less. Oct, pp 595–599.

Oliver T. 1986. *The real Coke, the real story.* New York: Random House.

Jenifer Wicks

COLIC

Colic affects one out of five infants each year in the United states, or 700,000 infants per year. Colic has been defined as crying longer than 3 hours per day for at least 3 days a week over 3 consecutive weeks (Wessel et al., 1959). It generally starts about the second month of life and lasts for 1 to 3 months, although some babies may start having colic earlier and some later. Furthermore, certain babies continue to have colic as they get older. Boys and girls are equally likely to develop colic, and it is equally common in first- and later-born children. Some babies with colic cry throughout the day; others are more likely to cry inconsolably at particular times of day, for instance, late in the afternoon or early in the evening (Weissbluth, 1984; Pinyerd and Zipf, 1989).

Babies with colic cry more intensely than other babies and appear to be in real discomfort. In the midst of a colic spell, a baby's body is tense, the legs may be drawn up, fists clenched, and face grimacing. Often the infant acts as if suffering from stomach cramps, and excess gas may be a problem. When colicky babies are worked up and crying, they are exceedingly difficult to soothe. Many babies with colic seem sensitive to noises and lights in their environment, and they can get worked up quite easily. Having a colicky infant can be very demanding for parents (Lester et al., 1990).

Along with intense and hard-to-soothe crying spells, babies with colic have disrupted sleep patterns. They tend to sleep less during the night than babies without colic, and they wake up more frequently. Sleep is more restless in babies with colic; when asleep during the day or night, they can be more easily disrupted and awakened. At night, parents often find this very difficult as they are awakened frequently by the crying, stay up trying to soothe the baby, and therefore lose valuable hours of sleep. During the day, easily disrupted sleep makes the baby's nap times less predictable, and parents are less certain of being able to do other things while the baby is sleeping. Furthermore, depending on where the baby sleeps, he or she can wake up other children. Thus, the sleep of the whole family may be disrupted by a baby with colic. (See also NIGHT WAKING IN INFANCY.)

There are many possible explanations for colic, and doctors do not yet fully understand the condition. When parents bring a colicky baby to a pediatrician, the baby is checked to see if an infection or other medical condition is causing the baby's discomfort. Certain babies with colic seem to be reacting to lactose, a sugar found in cows' milk; this digestive problem is called lactose intolerance. Thus, the pediatrician may suggest a change in formula (to a soy-based formula or a synthetic casein hydrolysate formula) or ask breastfeeding mothers to cut down on eating dairy foods (see also MILK ALLERGY AND INFANT SLEEP). Physicians once thought that colic was caused by anxious first-time parents who did not know how to handle the baby's crying; however, colic is equally likely in later-born children who have more experienced parents. Nevertheless, having a colicky baby who is difficult to soothe can make parents feel anxious and inadequate to the task of caring for their baby.

There are four main ways to treat colic: dietary change, medications, parental counseling, and changing soothing strategies. Dietary change involves changing the baby's formula or having breastfeeding mothers alter their diet to provide a type of milk or nutrition that is easier for the baby to digest. Certain medications help to soothe the baby's stomach, aid in digestion, and help to eliminate gas. Parent counseling involves helping parents to understand more about their baby's crying, temperament, and sensitivities, and to develop new strategies for managing their baby's care. Parent counseling also involves supporting parents during this difficult time, and support groups exist to help parents who have babies with sleep and crying problems (Boukydis, 1986). Changing soothing strategies may involve ways to soothe the infant directly (i.e., carrying, holding, or massaging) as well as indirectly (changing the baby's environment by cutting down on unwanted noise or stimulation; providing soothing, rhythmical stimulation through music or mechanical aids such as swings and rockers). Most of these methods of treating colic are used in combination. In addition, families may devise their own special remedies for colicky infants, for example, taking the baby for a walk or drive late at night or feeding the baby a weak solution of peppermint tea.

(See also INFANCY, NORMAL SLEEP PATTERNS IN; INFANCY, SLEEP DISORDERS IN.)

REFERENCES

Boukydis CFZ. 1986. *Support for parents and infants: A manual of parenting organizations and professionals.* New York: Routledge & Kegan Paul.

Lester BM, Boukydis CFZ, Garcia-Coll CT, Hole WT. 1990. Colic for developmentalists. *Infant Ment Health J* 11(4):321–333.

Pinyerd BJ, Zipf W. 1989. Colic: Idiopathic, excessive infant crying. *J Pediatr Nurs* 4:147–161.

Weissbluth M. 1984. *Crybabies: Coping with colic.* New York: Berkley.

Wessel MA, Cobb SC, Jackson EB, et al. 1959. Paroxysmal fussing in infancy: Sometimes called "colic." *Pediatrics* 14:421–424.

C. F. Zachariah Boukydis

COLOR IN DREAMS

Laboratory research has shown that most dreams recalled from REM sleep awakenings contain some color. Memories of dreams more distant in time are more ambiguous with respect to the presence of color. Because dreams can be known only indirectly through their recall, questions as basic as the presence or absence of color remain.

Nevertheless, electroencephalographic dream research has allowed the following conclusions: (1) most REM dreams (here the term *dream* refers to REM sleep recall) reflect the colors of the everyday world; (2) the distribution of colors is similar to that seen in waking perception; (3) dreams seem to be a bit darker and more out of focus than waking life; (4) the better the dream recall, the more likely color will be reported; (5) many people confuse a dream lacking color with a dream actually recalled as black and white; (6) REM dreams are described with more color than NREM dreams; and (7) color in dreams is based on recent perceptual experience and can be modified by having a subject wear colored goggles for as little as 1 day.

The study of color in dreams is a window into the nature of dream perception, or how the mind transforms the visual memories of waking images in the process of creating the dream. In a sense, the question is not so much of color but of the mental processes involved in the creation of dreams.

The probability that color will be reported in a dream is related to the length and detail of the dream report. As length of report increases, so does the clarity of the dreamed image and the richness of perceptual detail in the scene, including color. The reporting of color may be regarded as one indicator of the quality of dream recall and, therefore, is more likely to be present in REM dreams than in recall from NREM sleep, as REM dream narratives are typically longer.

Rechtschaffen and Buchignani (1983) awakened twenty-two subjects from REM sleep and asked them to select which of 129 versions of a single photograph best matched their dream images in visual quality (not content). The photographs varied along dimensions of color saturation, illumination, clarity of foreground and background, and color balance. The most frequently selected photographs (about 40 percent) were those that resembled waking visual perception in most respects. To judge from the other photographs selected, there is some tendency in dreams for color to be somewhat desaturated (i.e., less intense). Although the clarity of the central figure is fairly well preserved, there is some loss of clarity of the background, mostly because of diffusion or low brightness. Photos selected to match the first REM period dreams differed most from waking perception.

Another laboratory awakening study reported that color was present after 82.7 percent of REM awakenings with recall (Snyder, 1970). Herman and colleagues (1968) found color in at least one REM awakening from each of eight subjects and concluded that the capacity to dream in color is extremely prevalent. In this study, color was present in 75 percent of REM reports but only 25 percent of NREM reports. As the night progresses, the number of colored objects recalled in each awakening increases, as does the ratio of colored to uncolored objects and the saturation of object colors. Clearly, the frequency and intensity of color recall is affected by the quality of dream recall. If a subject has no recall of imagery after a REM awakening, is this an instance of color being absent, or should such an awakening be excluded from an analysis of color in dreams?

In contrast to the above studies, Rechtschaffen (personal communication) has described a small number of subjects who distinctly described their dreams as being in black and white. To these subjects, black-and-white dreams were clearly distinct from those lacking any color recall. Other scientists who have studied this question have not reported similar black-and-white dreams.

In a study by Roffwarg and colleagues (1978) that attempted to manipulate color in dreams experimentally, nine subjects wore red goggles continuously for 5 days. These goggles excluded all hues but red and did not allow any light to leak in around the rims. The authors found that the colors reported after REM awakenings changed from the baseline, in which normal color distributions were reported, to colors mimicking the visual images seen through the goggles. Thus, the color the subjects reported most frequently was a replica of the goggle experience, that is, a washed-out monochromatic red that they could describe only as "goggle color." There was a dramatic decrease in the frequency of nongoggle colors in the REM dreams. This transformation began in the very first REM–NREM sleep cycle after the goggles were worn for only 1 day, and penetrated into later REM–NREM cycles as the number of days wearing the goggles increased. Dream scenes similar to the visual field viewed through the goggles were reported frequently from REM, NREM, and sleep onset awakenings.

This study showed that recent waking perceptual experience strongly affects the appearance of dreamed scenes, influencing REM periods early in the night more than later ones. Color may be thought of as one element of the perceptual material on which the dream landscape is constructed. Although it would be difficult and fruitless to argue that color is universal in dreams or that everyone dreams in color, it is safe to say that color is a normal aspect of the dream process.

REFERENCES

Herman J, Roffwarg H, Tauber ES. 1968. Color and other perceptual qualities of REM and NREM dreams. *Psychophysiology* 5:223.
Rechtschaffen A, Buchignani C. 1983. Visual dimensions and correlates of dream images. *Sleep Res* 12:189.
Roffwarg HP, Herman JH, Bowe-Anders C, Tauber ES. 1978. The effects of sustained alterations of waking visual input on dream content. In Arkin AM, Antrobus JS, Ellman SJ, eds. *The mind in sleep: Psychology and psychophysiology,* pp 295–349. Hillsdale, N.J.: Erlbaum.
Snyder F. 1970. The phenomenology of dreaming. In Meadow L, Snow LN, eds. *The psychodynamic implications of the physiological studies on dreams,* pp 124–151. Springfield, Ill.: Thomas.

John H. Herman

COMA

Coma is a state of behavioral unarousability in which there is complete absence of conscious thought or purposeful behavior. A comatose person cannot respond to external stimulation such as sound, light, or touch in a meaningful way, although reflex behaviors such as withdrawal from pain often persist. By definition, the eyelids of a comatose person are closed. In coma, sleep–wake cycles are absent, as is REM sleep (and presumably dreaming). Coma is a pathological (i.e., abnormal) state caused by severe damage to brain structures above the level of the lower brainstem. Coma may be permanent or reversible and may last hours to weeks.

True coma never persists longer than a few weeks. Over extended periods, comatose patients spontaneously open their eyes and move them in episodic bursts. Over time, sleep–wake cycles also return, along with the reappearance of REM sleep. These behaviors are automatic brainstem responses and do not signify a return of consciousness. These people are said to be in a vegetative state rather than strictly comatose. People can remain in a vegetative state many years without demonstrating signs of conscious behavior.

Electrographic Features of Coma

The ELECTROENCEPHALOGRAM (EEG) measures and charts electrical activity on the surface of the brain (cerebral cortex), which in turn reflects the discharge of the millions of nerve cells (neurons) that make up the cortex. When there is a reduced amount of cerebral cortex activity, the EEG is slow and rhythmic. When activity increases, the EEG becomes faster and of smaller amplitude. In awake persons, the EEG is very fast (more than 15 cycles per second [CPS]) and varies from moment to moment in different brain regions, reflecting continuous change in sensory input, motor output, and information processing. When a person closes his or her eyes and relaxes into a state of quiet wakefulness, the EEG changes to a rhythmic 8- to 13-CPS pattern of "alpha" waves (see ALPHA RHYTHM). As a person drifts into deep NREM sleep, the EEG slows even further, and becomes dominated by large amplitude 1- to 2-CPS "delta" waves. Delta waves are the hallmark of stage 3 and 4 NREM sleep, and signify that the information processing capacities of the brain are greatly reduced.

In coma, the typical EEG pattern is composed of 1- to 4-CPS delta waves. As in deep NREM sleep, these waves signify that the information processing capabilities of the cerebral cortex have been severely impaired. Stage 4 sleep is the stage of sleep most like coma, although it should be emphasized that these two states are very different entities.

Not all patients in a coma produce a delta wave pattern on an EEG. An alpha rhythm ("alpha coma") similar to that in quiet wakefulness is seen in some cases. This pattern is distinguished from the alpha rhythm of quiet wakefulness by the observation that when a comatose person is stimulated, the EEG tracing usually does not change, whereas the EEG of an awake person will react to the stimulus and will change to the fast, desynchronous pattern characteristic of AROUSAL. This observation is useful in determining if a person is faking a coma ("psychogenic coma").

Other forms of coma, including "theta" (3 to 7 CPS) and "spindle" (12 to 18 CPS) coma have also been identified, and researchers are determining if any of these EEG patterns are predictive of recovery. In general, patients with "nonreactive" alpha coma and delta coma carry the worst prognosis for survival or recovery, and patients with "reactive" alpha coma have the best chance for recovery.

Causes of Coma

Coma may be caused by a wide variety of injuries to the brain. Plum and Posner divide these into two broad groups: (1) injuries that cause widespread damage to both cerebral hemispheres and (2) injuries that damage the core of the upper brainstem, specifically the structures contained in the pontine and midbrain portions. (See also HEAD INJURY.)

For coma to be caused by injury to the cerebral hemispheres, the injury must be very large. There does not seem to be one specific area of cerebrum that, if damaged, results in coma. In these cases, coma is likely caused by the destruction of massive amounts of neurons in the cerebrum, thereby thwarting the ability to carry out conscious behaviors, which require the interaction of a variety of cortical areas and communication between these areas. Widespread injury may be caused by trauma, which usually results in the tearing of nerve fibers (axons) rather than the destruction of nerve cell bodies. A second cause of cortical coma is inadequate oxygen delivery to the brain. Lack of oxygen to the brain is usually caused by failure of the heart to pump blood into the brain, as occurs in cardiac arrest, or by blockage of blood flow by a clot or bleeding blood vessel, as in a stroke. Drug overdose, including alcohol, is another common cause of damage to both cerebral hemispheres, causing coma. A variety of other agents, such as viruses and uncontrolled blood sugar, can cause coma.

For coma to be caused by damage to the brainstem, much more specific injury may occur. Injury to a rather small and well-circumscribed area of the upper pons and midbrain will result in coma. These parts of the upper brainstem contain neurons that are collectively referred to as the brainstem reticular activating system (RAS), which are critical in controlling arousal as well as sleep cycles. These neurons exert control over large areas of the cerebrum and facilitate or activate information processing mechanisms in the entire brain. Damage to these structures results in coma, and permanent damage to these structures causes irreversible coma or death in almost every case.

The most common mechanism of damage to the RAS is compression and/or twisting of the upper brainstem by the cerebral hemispheres' pressing downward on the brainstem. This is usually caused by increasing pressure from a growing mass on the skull such as blood or a tumor. Direct damage to the RAS, the result of either bleeding, tumor growth, or trauma, can also induce coma by compressing or destroying these cells.

Other Persistent Alterations in Consciousness

It is important to distinguish coma from other states of altered consciousness. Coma is a state of prolonged loss of consciousness and absence of purposeful behavior, from which it is impossible to be aroused. Stupor is a state of depressed consciousness. A stuporous person has a diminished level of arousal and may wax and wane in attentiveness, but is arousable and able to carry out conscious activities at all times. A classic example of a stuporous person is someone who is intoxicated by alcohol ("alcoholic stupor"). Obtundation is a state of even deeper somnolence from which it is very difficult to be aroused. An obtunded person lapses into and out of consciousness, but with effort can always be aroused for brief periods. Obtundation is often a warning sign that a person is progressing into coma.

Coma, stupor, and obtundation represent a continuum of pathological alterations in consciousness. These states should be distinguished from sleep, which is a physiological and normal state of unconsciousness. Sleep is a natural component of mammalian behavior containing both REM and NREM components. In sleep, conscious behavior is temporarily suppressed but the subject is arousable at all times. In coma, sleep–wake cycles are absent as is REM sleep. Sleepwalking and sleeptalking, both sometimes observed in stage 4 NREM sleep, are not observed in coma.

Coma should also be distinguished from brain death. Brain death refers to a state in which both cortical and vegetative functions such as control of breathing have been permanently destroyed. A brain-dead person is kept alive only by artificial support devices, such as a mechanical ventilator to control breathing, and the EEG demonstrates almost complete absence of electrical activity in the brain. This is in sharp contrast to coma patients, who have active EEGs and are often able to maintain basic vegetative functions with minimal support. There is presently no chance of recovery from brain death.

Prognosis in Coma

Predicting which patients will awaken from coma is a complex subject. The mechanism of coma and site of injury are probably the most important factors. The patients with compressing masses detected and removed early have a relatively good chance of recovery, as do patients with drug overdoses or metabolic problems treated quickly. Patients with direct injury to the RAS have a very

poor prognosis and rarely, if ever, recover. Patients that remain in coma longer than 24 hours have a significantly worse chance of recovering than those who begin to awaken shortly after coma begins. At present, supportive therapy remains the mainstay of treatment for comatose patients. Experimental treatments offer promise for improving outcomes in the future.

REFERENCES

Black PM. 1978. Brain death. *N Engl J Med* 299:338–344, 393–401.

Fisher CM. 1969. The neurological exam of the comatose patient. *Acta Neurol Scand Suppl* 36:1–56.

Jennet WB, Teasdale G. 1977. Aspects of coma after severe head injury. *Lancet* 1:878–881.

Plum F, Posner JR. 1980. *The diagnosis of stupor and coma.* Philadelphia: FA Davis.

Synek VM. 1988. Prognostically important EEG coma patterns in diffuse anoxic and traumatic encephalopathies in adults. *J Clin Neurophysiol* 5(2):161–174.

Adam N. Mamelak

CONDENSATION

Sigmund Freud developed condensation as an important part of his theory of dreaming, and the concept has become an important part of other dream theories as well.

To Freud, the dream we can recall and can tell to others is far removed from its "real" meaning (SEE FREUD'S DREAM THEORY). Freud called the remembered dream—its characters, objects, and events—the *manifest content*. The underlying meaning of the dream out of which the characters, objects, and events were created is the *latent content*. Freud called the process of creating the manifest content out of the latent content *dream work*. Together with displacement and other processes, condensation is an important aspect of dream work.

Condensation occurs when two or more unconscious thoughts merge together into a single image or event in a dream. For example, a person might dream of having an overbearing boss. This character might represent an aspect of an actual boss and also some aspect of the dreamer's father, the dreamer's former teacher, and the dreamer's relationship with a good friend. Freud talked about the elements of a dream being over-determined as a result of condensation. That is, a single symbol in a dream may convey several meanings, with each meaning having had a role in its determination.

REFERENCES

Freud S. 1901/1980. *On dreams.* New York: Norton.
Moorcroft WH. 1989. *Sleep, dreaming, and sleep disorders. An introduction.* Lanham, MD: University Press of America.

William H. Moorcroft

CONSCIOUSNESS

[Consciousness *can be defined as a state in which one is capable of having subjective experiences and responding to sensory stimuli. States of consciousness can be defined on the basis of physiological variables and posture. The major states of consciousness so defined include waking and sleep. Waking can be subdivided into aroused and quiescent states. Sleep can be subdivided into NREM sleep and REM sleep. Further subdivisions of NREM sleep have been made on the basis of the characteristics of the brain waves present. Consciousness can be altered and interrupted by sleep and can also be suspended in coma and drug-induced states. These issues are discussed in the following entries:* ALPHA RHYTHM; ALTERED STATES OF CONSCIOUSNESS; AMNESIA; ANESTHESIA; ANIMALS' DREAMS; AROUSAL; BIOFEEDBACK; CHARACTERISTICS OF DREAMS; COGNITION; COMA; HALLUCINATIONS; HYPNAGOGIC HALLUCINATIONS; LUCID DREAMING; MEDITATION AND SLEEP; NIGHTMARES; REM SLEEP; *and* STAGES OF SLEEP.]

CONSTANT ROUTINE

In humans, daily variations have been described in a number of physiological functions, includ-ing cardiac, pulmonary, renal, thermoregulatory, endocrine, and cognitive functions. The daily cycles of some variables, such as heart rate and blood pressure, are principally associated with periodic variations in human activity patterns (i.e., both heart rate and blood pressure tend to be higher during the day, when people are awake and active, and they are, on average, lower at night when people are at rest and supine). Other daily cycles, such as that of cortisol secretion, are generated relatively independently of the individual's behavior by an internal biological clock (the circadian pacemaker; see CIRCADIAN RHYTHMS). The circadian pacemaker that generates these endogenous rhythms in mammals is located in the SUPRACHIASMATIC NUCLEUS OF THE HYPOTHALAMUS. It is not possible to study this pacemaker directly in humans, and therefore physiological rhythms that are driven by the pacemaker are used as markers of the status of the circadian system.

Rhythms that are strongly influenced by the circadian pacemaker include core body temperature; secretion of MELATONIN, CORTISOL, and THYROID-STIMULATING HORMONE; urine output; and REM SLEEP propensity. Even though these variables are strongly influenced by the circadian pacemaker, all are also affected by exogenous stimuli and behavioral changes. Examples of such stimuli include the increase in BODY TEMPERATURE in response to heavy exercise or in response to a change from the supine to the upright posture; the suppression of cortisol and thyroid-stimulating hormone that occurs at sleep onset; the inhibition of REM sleep by extremely high or low ambient temperatures (see TEMPERATURE EFFECTS ON SLEEP); and the suppression of melatonin secretion by bright light. Obscuring of the endogenous (or internally generated) component of a rhythm by such exogenous or behavioral stimuli is referred to as *masking.*

To study markers of the circadian system relatively free from masking effects, Mills, Minors, and Waterhouse (1978) proposed the constant routine procedure. The purpose of a constant routine is to eliminate or distribute evenly across the day as many exogenous and behavioral stimuli as possible. By studying physiological rhythms under constant routine conditions, one can observe the underlying endogenous component of those rhythms. Unfortunately, the term *constant routine* has been adopted by a number of research groups to describe procedures that

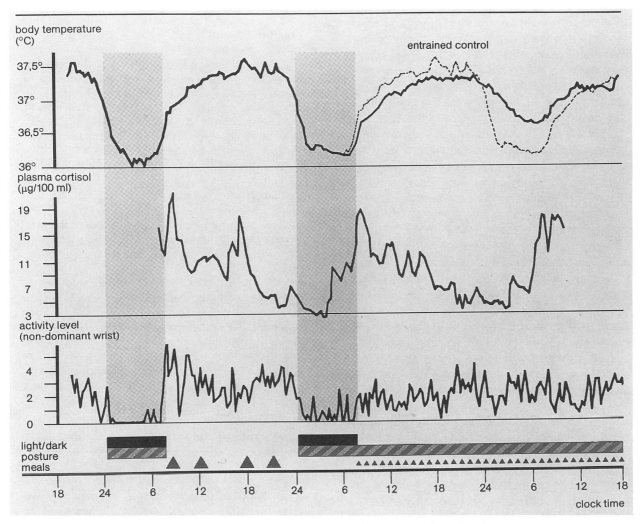

Figure 1. Patterns of core temperature, plasma cortisol, and wrist activity level during 36 hours of a normal schedule, followed by 36 hours of constant routine. Meals are indicated by triangles, recumbent posture by hatched bars, time of lights out by black bars. Activity level varies markedly between day and night during the normal schedule, but is maintained at an even level throughout the constant routine. Temperature begins to drop just before habitual bedtime, reaches its nadir just after the middle of the sleep episode, and then begins to rise, cresting during the latter half of the waking day. The scheduled day temperature pattern is superimposed on the constant routine temperature pattern for comparison. Oscillation of temperature continues even when posture and activity are held constant, but amplitude of oscillation is reduced, and the minimum of the rhythm appears to occur at a slightly later time. *Reproduced with permission from Czeisler CA (1986):* Circadian rhythmicity and its disorders, *p 17. Ingelheim, Germany: Boehringer Ingelheim Zentrale.*

are really quite different. For example, one group controls posture while allowing subjects to sleep when they wish, whereas another group requires subjects to remain continuously awake while allowing them to change posture and activity level. As both sleep and changes in posture and activity have been shown to mask endogenous circadian rhythms, results obtained under such varying conditions are not comparable. The constant routine described here attempts to control for all of these masking effects, thus unmasking the underlying endogenous circadian rhythms.

A constant routine should be carried out for at least one to one and one-half circadian cycles (i.e., 24 to 36 hours). Subjects undergoing a constant routine should remain awake for the entire constant routine, thus eliminating the influence of sleep on the rhythms being monitored. Subjects should be kept in a constant posture (usually semirecumbent), maintaining a low level of activity. Food and water intake should be distributed evenly throughout day and night. Ambient lighting and temperature should also be kept constant.

One drawback to the constant routine procedure is that it requires subjects to be deprived of sleep. Thus, when variables that are affected by sleep DEPRIVATION (such as performance) are studied, care must be taken in interpreting the results.

The constant routine procedure estimate of circadian phase has been validated against other prior estimation methods, including the method of monitoring core temperature during INTERNAL DESYNCHRONIZATION between the core temperature cycle and the sleep–wake cycle. Use of the constant routine procedure has made it possible to observe the endogenous rhythms of a number of physiological and behavioral variables (Figure 1). In addition, the ability of the constant routine to assess rapidly the phase of the circadian system has allowed experimenters to chart the response of the human circadian system to specific stimuli.

REFERENCES

Benoit O, Foret J, Merle B, Reinberg A. 1981. Circadian rhythms (temperature, heart rate, vigilance, mood) of short and long sleepers: Effects of sleep deprivation. *Chronobiologia* 8:341–350.

Czeisler CA, Brown EN, Ronda JM, Kronauer RE, Richardson GS, Freitag WO. 1985. A clinical method to assess the endogenous circadian phase (ECP) of the deep circadian oscillator in man. *Sleep Res* 14:295.

Czeisler CA, Johnson MP, Duffy JF, Brown EN, Ronda JM, Kronauer RE. 1990. Exposure to bright light and darkness to treat physiologic maladaptation to night work. *N Engl J Med* 322:1253–1259.

Czeisler CA, Kronauer RE, Allan JS, Duffy JF, Jewett ME, Brown EN, Ronda JM. 1989. Bright light induction of strong (type O) resetting of the human circadian pacemaker. *Science* 244:1328–1333.

Mills JN, Minors DS, Waterhouse JM. 1978. Adaptation to abrupt time shifts of the oscillator[s] controlling human circadian rhythms. *J Physiol (Lond)* 285: 455–470.

Minors DS, Waterhouse JM. 1984. The use of the constant routine in unmasking the endogenous component of human circadian rhythms. *Chronobiol Int* 1:205–216.

Moog R, Hildebrandt G. 1986. Comparison of different causes of masking effects. In Haiderm M, Koller M, Cervinka R, eds. *Night and shiftwork: Longterm effects and their prevention,* pp 131–140. Frankfurt: Peter Lang.

Jeanne F. Duffy

CONTENT OF DREAMS

Suppose a friend approached you and wanted to share an interesting dream from last night. If you agreed to listen to your friend, what kind of dream might you hear? What sorts of things do most people dream about?

Typical Dream Themes

One approach to discover common or typical dreams has entailed administering questionnaires to a large number of people and asking them if they have ever experienced certain types of dreams. The most frequently acknowledged type involves the dreamer being chased, pursued, or attacked by some threatening figure. As with all dreams, this type of dream may have different meanings for different individuals, depending upon their own life experiences and psychological characteristics. For example, such dreams might be expected from an individual who resides in a hostile environment such as a high-crime area; but people who live in affluent, secure neighborhoods also have this type of dream fairly frequently. One possible interpretation is that the external threatening figure may represent some internal fears that the dreamer is unwilling to confront directly and is attempting to run away from.

Dreams of falling are also extremely common; over 80 percent of college students report having had them. Such dreams may occur if the dreamer feels insecure or is afraid of losing emotional balance or of possibly "falling down" in performance on the job, in school, or some other setting where accomplishments are important. As before, the specific emotion reflected in the dream must be understood within the context of the individual dreamer's emotional life.

The ability to fly in dreams is claimed by about one-third of people, who almost always associate very positive feelings with them. The dreamer may soar through space with arms straight ahead in Superman style, at right angles in swan dive fashion, or sometimes flapping them up and down like birds' wings. The individual appears to "rise above" problems in flying dreams and get a larger aerial perspective of the situation. The elated feeling of achievement may arise because the dreamer successfully uses his or her own power and can control shifts in the direction, height, or speed of dream flight, rather than relying on anyone else or a mechanical vehicle for assistance. (See also FLYING IN DREAMS.)

Embarrassment generally accompanies dreams in which the dreamer appears nude or wearing inappropriate clothing such as only underwear in a crowded public place. The dreamer expects others to be shocked or critical because of the dreamer's skimpy or absent attire, but they typically don't notice or pay any attention to the dreamer's appearance. Because clothing is used to indicate whether one is a doctor, judge, or Indian chief, social class identity or rank cannot be identified when clothing is missing. The dreamer may have concerns regarding what other people would think about him or her if the dreamer were seen "the way I really am," with nothing concealed or disguised. The dreamer is therefore surprised to be found still acceptable in "psychologically naked" condition. (See also NUDITY IN DREAMS.)

Another common type of dream is the "exami-nation dream." The classic example of such a dream involves a setting where a student is attempting to complete an exam and has a pen that won't write, questions that are illegible, or only a few moments to answer an extremely long test. Other variations involve situations where the dreamer starts to address an audience and is speechless, is in a play and can't remember the lines, or is attempting to play in public a piano whose keys will not move. The common denominator underlying examination dreams involves the dreamer being subjected to a public evaluation of his or her skills by judgmental authorities who may find that the dreamer's performance fails to satisfy their standards.

Closely related to examination dreams are frustration dreams. The source of the frustration may be the dreamer's inability to handle a piece of equipment, the presence of a wall or fence that prevents the dreamer from making progress toward an intended goal, or the malfunctioning of such equipment as a telephone that keeps giving the dreamer wrong numbers. Some dreams may arise when the dreamer feels frustrated in waking life with his or her attempts to overcome a situation that seems difficult to resolve. When feeling excessive time pressures, a person may experience dreams of missing buses or trains, or arriving late for important appointments, which results in being fired or expelled, or in missing out on some opportunity.

With the exception of flying dreams, "typical" dreams deal primarily with negative emotions. In large-scale studies involving thousands of recently recalled dreams, it has been found that two-thirds of them contain material that is unpleasant. The dreamer is engaged in aggressive activities, rejected, lost, confused, unable to communicate with others, or threatened by a natural disaster such as an earthquake, tidal wave, or tornado.

Content Analysis of Dreams

Rather than using questionnaires that ask about overall themes, another way of answering the question "what's in a dream?" is to examine and systematically classify the individual items that appear in dreams. This systematic categorization of the elements found in written records is known as "content analysis." The person who pioneered the technique of content analyses of dreams was Dr. Calvin Hall, who established the Institute for Dream Research around 1960 and continued his studies of dreams until his death in 1985.

Hall collected several thousand dream reports from normal individuals, primarily college students. Five dreams each were randomly selected from the dream files of 100 male and 100 female American college students to create a normative standard for dreams. These 1,000 dreams, ranging in length from 50 to 300 words, were then scored on various content scales that had been developed to enable tabulation of the incidence of selected dream items. A description of the scoring scales and the results from applying them to the normative group are presented in *The Content Analysis of Dreams,* a book published by Calvin Hall and Robert Van de Castle in 1966. A large number of content differences were found between male and female dreamers in the Hall and Van de Castle study.

Gender Differences in Dreams

A man is more likely to dream about being in an outdoor setting that is unfamiliar to him such as a city street, while women more often dream about being in a familiar indoor setting involving their home, dormitory, or classroom. Men's dreams contain more references to automobiles and auto parts (e.g., engines) and to weapons such as guns and knives, while women report more household objects such as furniture. Women notice the appearance of others, describing the clothing and jewelry they wear and making references to their face, eyes, and hair style.

With regard to dream characters, men more frequently encounter groups of people who are unfamiliar to them or are identified on the basis of their occupational role. More people are present in women's dreams, but they are frequently known to the dreamer, who interacts with them on an individual basis. More children and babies as well as family members appear in women's dreams. Men dream much more often about other male characters; they have twice as many male as female characters in their dreams. In women's dreams, the gender ratio is more evenly distributed; they dream almost equally as often about

male and female characters, with slightly more female than male characters being present.

Although dreams with aggression are almost equally frequent for the two sexes (235 of 500 dreams for men; 222 of 500 dreams for women), the aggressive interactions are different in nature. When aggression is reported in dreams, physical demonstrations (killing, hitting) are involved for 50 percent of the men but only 34 percent of the women. Men are more likely to initiate aggression, whereas women are more prone to be the victim of others' aggressions. When men initiate aggression in dreams, it is generally directed toward other men and to characters who are unfamiliar to them. When women initiate aggression, it equally often involves men as women, but the characters are more than twice as likely to be familiar than unfamiliar to the dreamer. When the dreamer is the victim of another's aggression, the attacker is more than twice as likely to be a male, regardless of whether the dreamer is male or female. The attacker is twice as likely to be unfamiliar for male dreamers, but slightly more likely to be a familiar character for female dreamers.

More friendly acts (308) occur in women's dreams than in men's dreams (250). The recipient of this friendliness is more likely to be a female character regardless of the dreamer's gender. Both men and women generally extend friendliness to characters who are familiar to them.

Sex dreams are more frequently reported by males; their partners are usually attractive women whom the dreamer does not know. Women, in contrast, make love to male sexual partners who are very familiar to them, such as their boyfriends. Women's sexual dreams have a more romantic quality; for male dreamers, the sexual dream seems rather to involve an issue of conquest.

Not only in sexual dreams, but in all their dreams, men are more active. They engage in more physical than verbal activities, whereas the situation is reversed in women's dreams. Women report more emotions in their dreams, but for both genders, apprehension and confusion are the most frequent emotions experienced by the dreamer. Women use more adjectives (1,458) to describe features of their dreams than men do (1,110). Women are more likely to comment on attractiveness (pretty or ugly), moral qualities (good or bad), and colors. Men more frequently use adjectives referring to largeness or fastness.

Although the Hall and Van de Castle normative tables are based on dreams reported in the 1940s, the gender differences reported in their tables are similar to those found for college students reporting dreams in 1980. Gender is not the only variable that influences drea content. Other studies have shown that factors such as age, social class, family structure, physical health, and various personality patterns also play a role in shaping the content of dreams.

(See also PERSONALITY AND DREAM RECALL.)

REFERENCES

Griffith RM, Miyago O, Tago A. 1955. The universality of typical dreams: Japanese vs. Americans. *Am Anthropol* 60:1173–1179.

Hall CS, Domhoff B. 1963. A ubiquitous sex difference in dreams. *J Abnorm Soc Psychol* 66: 278–280.

Hall CS, Domhoff B, Blick K, Weesner K. 1982. The dreams of college men and women in 1950 and 1980: A comparison of dream contents and sex differences. *Sleep* 5:188–194.

Hall CS, Van de Castle R. 1966. *The content analysis of dreams.* New York: Appleton-Century-Crofts.

Rubenstein K. 1990. How men and women dream differently. In Krippner S, ed. *Dreamtime and dreamwork,* pp 135–142. Los Angeles, Calif.: Tarcher.

Ward C, Beck A, Rascoe E. 1961. Typical dreams: Incidence among psychiatric patients. *Arch Gen Psychiatry* 5:606–615.

Winget C, Kramer M. 1979. *Dimensions of dreams.* Gainesville: University of Florida Presses.

Robert L. Van de Castle

CONTINUOUS POSITIVE AIRWAY PRESSURE

Prior to 1981 the only effective treatments for sleep APNEA syndrome were surgical. TRACHEOSTOMY, although always an effective treatment, is repugnant to many patients. Alternative surgical treatments that were being developed at about the same time lacked (and still lack) the certain efficacy of tracheostomy. There was, therefore, reason to look for other treatments that might be more acceptable to patients than surgery.

Colin Sullivan in Australia reasoned that air blown into the nose should prevent the throat from collapsing. In 1981 he published a paper describing a method of doing this that actually worked. His device involved a plastic plug that fit into the nostrils and had holes through which air could be blown by a special blower. Wearing this device, patients who had had hundreds of obstructive sleep apneas every night were able to fall asleep and breathe without interruptions. Their snoring stopped, and their daytime sleepiness decreased dramatically. Even though these early prototype blowers worked, a few years passed before practical commercial devices were developed that could be used easily without the individual custom fitting of the early method (Figures 1 and 2). Nasal continuous positive airway pressure (CPAP) has gained wide acceptance since then. It is now the most commonly prescribed treatment for sleep apnea syndrome.

Continuous positive airway pressure works by preventing the negative pressure (suction) that causes the throat to collapse during sleep in patients whose loud snoring is already an indication that the airway is too small for normal airflow. A mass-produced plastic mask with soft edges is fitted over the nose, sealing against the skin of the cheeks, upper lip, and brow. Air is blown into this mask, and thereby into the nose, at the lowest pressure necessary to hold the throat open and stop the patient's snoring. This pressure can be determined only by having the patient sleep a second time in the sleep laboratory (the first time was to diagnose the obstructive sleep apnea and measure its severity) wearing the CPAP equipment. The pressure starts low and is turned up until there is no more apnea and no more snoring. When this pressure is reached, the patient starts to sleep better than she or he has since developing the disease years before, often launching into a long period of delta sleep or REM sleep. It is as if the patient is suddenly recovering from a long time without real sleep.

Indeed, once the sleep apnea is eliminated, the patient's recovery of normal daytime alertness follows a time course similar to recovery from severe sleep deprivation. Daytime alertness is significantly improved after just one night and is back to normal in less than 2 weeks.

Continuous positive airway pressure does have problems. The basic one is that the apparatus is uncomfortable for some people. People whose noses are blocked may require surgery on the nose before they can even be fitted successfully.

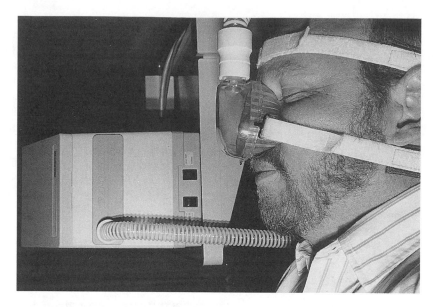

Figure 1. A typical continuous positive airway pressure apparatus. The blower unit is placed at the bedside and delivers air to the nasal mask.

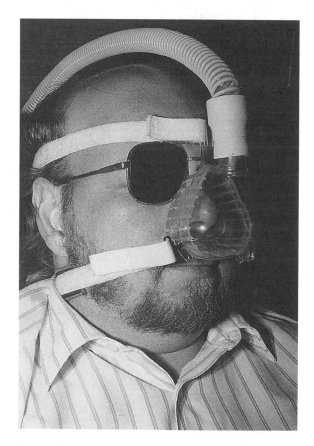

Figure 2. Continuous positive airway pressure device designed to prevent excessive sleepiness while driving. The unit is powered by plugging into a dashboard cigarette lighter.

People without upper teeth cannot support the mask on their upper lips and may have to be fitted with dentures before they can use CPAP. CPAP also produces side effects, among which nasal and sinus congestion is the most common. Sometimes these problems can be treated easily, and sometimes they bother patients enough to make them stop using CPAP entirely. With time the number of patients still using CPAP regularly drops off, so that after 6 months it is being properly used by 73 percent of those to whom it was prescribed. By 18 months this figure is down to 60 percent. In the best institutions supportive interaction with health care providers can help somewhat, but with time the usage of nasal CPAP declines, just as with other medical treatments that depend on people to persist.

Early studies comparing the mortality rates of patients with untreated sleep apnea with the rates for patients treated with tracheostomy, other surgery, or nasal CPAP showed tracheostomy and CPAP to be the most effective treatments. As time passes and the number of patients using (or having but not using as prescribed) CPAP increases, studies can be expected to show whether its early promise of increased longevity comparable to that with tracheostomy is being fulfilled or not.

If patients have irregular life-styles with erratic sleep times or ALCOHOL drinking habits that vary widely from day to day, good results may be hard to achieve. Alcohol influences muscle tone during sleep and raises (with drinking) or lowers (without) the CPAP pressure required to eliminate apnea and snoring. Because of this, some doctors recommend having the patient drink his or her usual amount (if there is a usual amount) prior to the night on which the CPAP pressure is adjusted. The early plastic masks had an additional problem: They deteriorated faster, becoming stiff and hard because of reactions that occurred with the alcohol vapor on the breath of some heavy imbibers. The result was a loss of the airtight seal, not always detected in a timely manner by such patients.

Sometimes a patient has more than one sleep disorder, and the problems connected with the added disorders make it hard for the patient to use CPAP. Examples are the restless leg syndrome or any other disorder associated with chronic insomnia. Insomnia makes it difficult to lie in bed wearing CPAP. In such cases the cause of the insomnia (assuming apnea is not the cause) must be addressed. If the insomnia cannot be treated effectively, or if the patient cannot tolerate CPAP for any other reason, alternative ways to treat the apnea have to be found.

Used alone, CPAP may be inadequate for a patient with lung or heart disease in addition to obstructive sleep apnea. If a patient is unable to get sufficient oxygen even when CPAP has eliminated sleep-related upper airway obstruction, oxygen may have to be added. Fortunately this is easy to do. Oxygen can be delivered into the CPAP mask with a small tube as easily as it can be given to someone who does not need the CPAP.

Nasal CPAP is a valuable addition to the selection of treatments doctors can offer to those who suffer with sleep apnea syndrome. An effective treatment can usually be found from among the options of CPAP, surgery, weight loss, and behavior modification. Some may be able to lose sufficient weight or alter life-styles to lessen the severity of sleep apnea. Surgical treatments ranging from specific corrective procedures (e.g., UVULOPALATOPHARYNGOPLASTY, MAXILLOFACIAL SURGERY) to tracheostomy can be done. It is now rare to encounter a patient with obstructive sleep apnea for whom an acceptable treatment cannot be found.

REFERENCES

He J, Kryger MH, Zorick FJ, et al. 1988. Mortality and apnea index in obstructive sleep apnea: Experience in 385 male patients. *Chest* 94:9–14.

Jenkins NA, Mrad R, Walsh JK. 1990. Long term CPAP use and follow-up care. *Sleep Res* 20:264.

Lamphere J, Roehrs T, Wittig R, Zorick F, Conway WA, Roth T. 1989. Recovery of alertness after CPAP in apnea. *Chest* 96(6):1364–1367.

Sullivan CE, Issa FG, Berthon-Jones M, Eves L. 1981. Reversal of obstructive sleep apnea by continuous positive airway pressure applied through the nares. *Lancet* i:862–865.

Robert Wittig

CORTISOL

Cortisol is a steroid hormone produced by the cortex of each of the two adrenal glands, located above the kidneys. Cortisol is a member of the glucocorticoid family of hormones (so-called because of their important effects on blood glucose) and is the most important glucocorticoid in humans. Like other steroids, cortisol is derived from cholesterol. It is transported in the blood to its target tissues primarily by the protein cortisol-binding globulin. Cortisol is degraded mainly in the liver and is excreted in the urine and feces. (See also ENDOCRINOLOGY.)

Major Functions in the Body

Cortisol has several major functions affecting metabolism, the response to stress, and inflammation.

Effects on Metabolism

Cortisol is involved in carbohydrate, protein, and fat metabolism. In the liver, cortisol stimulates gluconeogenesis, which is the production of glucose and glycogen, a carbohydrate, from other substances such as amino acids. Two major steps are required for this function: (1) stimulating enzyme synthesis in liver cells, and (2) mobilizing amino acids from tissues other than the liver. When amino acids are converted to glucose, glycogen is then produced and stored in the liver.

Cortisol affects protein metabolism by reducing protein synthesis and stimulating the breakdown of proteins. In addition, the uptake of amino acids from blood into tissues such as muscle decreases under the influence of cortisol. Thus, amino acids become available for glucose synthesis.

Fat metabolism is also influenced by cortisol. Cortisol leads to the release of fatty acids from adipose (fat) tissue as well as to their oxidation in cells for energy.

Response to Stress

Cortisol is released within minutes of a stressful event—mental or physical—including trauma, surgery, infections, and many others. Because cortisol mobilizes amino acids and fatty acids for energy, it makes sense that this hormone would be released during conditions when the survival of the individual may be at risk.

Response to Inflammation

Cortisol is known as an anti-inflammatory agent and can be found in over-the-counter ointments and prescription preparations for this purpose.

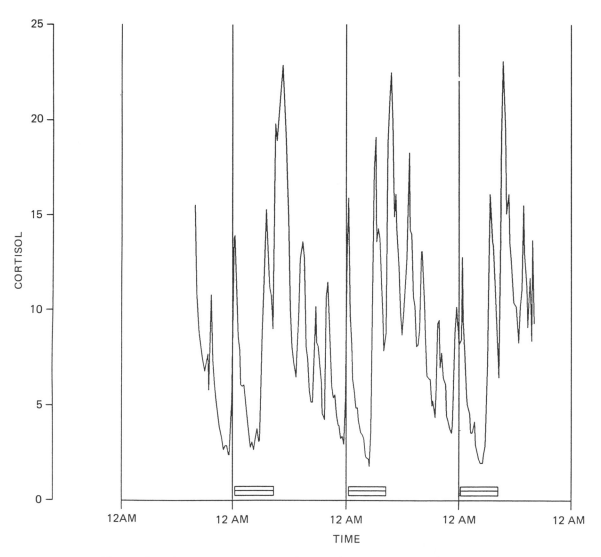

Figure 1. Plasma concentration of cortisol over time in a 26-year-old woman. Rectangles at bottom indicate sleep.

Cortisol interferes with the beginning and course of the inflammation process and then increases the rate of healing.

Control of Secretion

Cortisol is released from the adrenal glands in response to the anterior pituitary hormone corticotropin (or adrenocorticotropic hormone [ACTH]). Control of ACTH secretion, in turn, is a role of the HYPOTHALAMUS. This is an area of the midbrain that secretes releasing hormones, or factors, into a special set of capillaries (portal system) to the pituitary. Corticotropin-releasing factor (CRF) is the peptide hormone that stimulates the release of ACTH. Like other steroids, cortisol influences its own secretion by means of a negative feedback on the hypothalamus and anterior pituitary.

Rhythm of Secretion

Cortisol is secreted in pulses throughout the day, so that its plasma concentration is relatively unstable. Thus, to characterize the secretory pattern, samples must be obtained at frequent intervals, and time of day is especially important.

When frequent samples are taken over several days a daily pattern emerges. Such patterns (see Figure 1) are called CIRCADIAN RHYTHMS. One can see that cortisol decreases during the afternoon and is lowest during sleep. The concentration of hormone rises late in the sleep period before the person awakens.

The circadian rhythm of secretion is controlled by the biological clock located in the brain, probably also in the hypothalamus. How this "clock" sends timing signals to the CRF-ACTH-cortisol system is not yet understood. The rhythmic secretory pattern is modified by activities such as the sleeping and waking, but persists even when people stay awake for long intervals (more than 24 hours). Sleeping per se decreases cortisol secretion, but ordinarily cortisol begins to increase during the latter half of the sleep period so that blood levels are already elevated by the time the person awakens, as seen in Figure 1.

REFERENCES

Weitzman ED, Zimmerman JC, Czeisler CA, Ronda J. 1983. Cortisol secretion is inhibited during sleep in normal man. *J Clin Endocrinol Metab* 56: 352–358.

Margaret L. Moline

CO-SLEEPING

Co-sleeping is a relatively new term that describes the extremely old human practice of infants and children sleeping in contact or close proximity to their parents. The most obvious form of co-sleeping is an infant or child sleeping in the same bed with her or his parent(s). From the child's perspective, co-sleeping also occurs when the child is rocked or held while sleeping or when the parent and child are close enough to hear, feel, or smell one another. Although co-sleeping can also occur among siblings, the term generally means sleep contact between parents and children.

How Widespread Is Co-Sleeping?

The practice of infants and children sleeping beside their parents is found in the great majority of contemporary world cultures. In fact, parents and children sharing the same sleeping place was common for all peoples, including all industrialized countries, up until about 200 years ago (Thenevin, 1987). Most people in the world today live in one-room shelters, and mothers nurse their infants on demand throughout the first 2 years of life. This context virtually guarantees co-sleeping.

Where and exactly how infants sleep with their parents vary from one culture to another. In preindustrial societies, co-sleeping more often takes the form of infants sleeping on floor mats or on animal skins next to or between their parents, or at least within reach, sometimes as they sleep in baskets hanging above their parents' heads. Among a variety of Native American, East European, and Asian cultures infants either sleep alongside their mothers in physical contact or within a few meters in cradleboards, nets, hammocks, or baskets made of roots, twigs, grasses, and/or plant fibers.

Preindustrial and non-agriculturally based societies are not, however, the only ones that practice parent–infant co-sleeping. In Japan, parent–infant co-sleeping on a mat or *futon* is common. In the United States among most members of La Leche League, an organization composed of mothers committed to breastfeeding, late weaning, and close parent–infant physical contact, co-sleeping is advocated and practiced. A study by Elias, Nicolson, and Konner (1986) shows that between 60 percent and 70 percent of La Leche League infants aged 2 to 13 months regularly sleep with their mothers.

Co-sleeping is also common in both urban and rural areas throughout the Near and Middle East as well as in India, Pakistan, and Bangladesh. Hundreds of diverse cultures in China, Vietnam, Thailand, Burma, and Java also co-sleep, although the characteristics of the bed and bedding materials vary a great deal across cultures (Table 1).

Most infants around the world not only co-sleep at night, but also nap in a pouch, sling, or shawl tied to their mother's back or chest. Infants sleep sporadically as mothers walk to water holes, dig for roots, work in garden plots, prepare food, or collect berries. In many societies, the mother's economic role as food collector is critical. But unlike industrialized societies where alternate forms of child care may permit some mothers to leave the infant at home for lengthy periods, most infants in the world today accompany their mothers wherever they go; mother and child are necessarily linked by the infant's need to breastfeed. Hence, even daytime sleep is social sleep.

Parent–Infant Sleep Arrangements and Cultural Values: What's the Connection?

The idea that cultures guide the ways children are raised, including the way children sleep, is illustrated by considering Japan and the United States. Social interdependence and group harmony are two values rigorously enforced in Japan. Parents there sleep with their infants partly to encourage this interdependence. In contrast, the qualities Japanese parents hope to instill in their children are the very ones that Americans attempt to inhibit or suppress.

American parents want their children to learn how to be self-reliant and display their individu-

ality. They teach their infants to sleep alone. Japanese children are taught to "harmonize with the group," so sleeping with their parents is no coincidence. Sleeping arrangements reflect larger social values and goals.

Co-Sleeping in the United States

In societies such as the United States where co-sleeping is discouraged, the task of collecting reliable data on how many families actually practice it is difficult. Many parents are reluctant to admit to taking their infants or children to bed with them. Lozoff, Wolf, and Davis (1984) overcame the research difficulties to find that 29 percent of 150 Cleveland, Ohio families practiced some form of co-sleeping during the month prior to the interview. Although 65 percent of the mothers disclosed that they did not have any body contact with their child at bedtime, fewer than 35 percent of these mothers indicated that they always avoided co-sleeping, especially if the child continued to wake up during the night or was ill or frightened.

Schachter and colleagues (1989) found that among Hispanic-Americans in Harlem over 20 percent of the families slept with their children all night at least three times a week, whereas only 6 percent of the white families did so. Moreover, only one fourth of the white families but nearly half of the black families in Lozoff and colleagues' (1984) study in Cleveland regularly co-slept at least three nights a week.

In a different survey conducted near Boston, Massachusetts, Madansky and Edelbrock (1990) confirmed differences between black and white families in how they manage childhood sleep. These researchers report that 76 percent of black families reported co-sleeping compared with only 53% of white families. Black families in this area were more than twice as likely as white families to co-sleep more than once a week.

Among Hispanic-Americans, Schachter and colleagues (1989) found co-sleeping occurred more frequently with first-born or only children, with infants past the age of 12 months, and among households with extended families. In non-Hispanic populations it appears that co-sleeping occurs more regularly in single-parent households; and although infants from poor families are found sleeping with their parents more often than are infants from more affluent families, co-sleeping does not appear to be related to the number of bedrooms available. In most cases, and regardless of family income and ethnicity, co-sleeping children were reported to have had available to them another bed or another sleeping place.

Why Co-Sleeping Is Discouraged in European and Western Urban Societies

In most Western industrialized cultures, co-sleeping, or sharing the "family bed" as Tine Thenevin called it, is not usually recommended by pediatricians. They worry about the accidental suffocation of infants sleeping in soft modern beds where infants potentially could roll under a sleeping parent, especially if the parent is drunk, obese, or desensitized by drugs. Pediatricians and sleep experts suggest that co-sleeping may create excessive infant/child dependence on parents, retard the infant's social maturation, or possibly interfere with the husband–wife relationship, although no data have ever demonstrated these contentions. They maintain that even at a very young age infants are more than capable of sleeping alone and should do so. If infants and children cry and continue to resist sleeping alone, they argue, parents can implement on a gradual basis steps to distance themselves from their children to condition them to sleep alone (Ferber, 1985).

Most parents who elect to co-sleep will admit that in our culture sleeping with an infant or child confronts parents with new experiences and special challenges, especially for those parents used to getting an uninterrupted night's sleep and who work on schedules typical of Western urban life. The fact that sleep may be more fragmented when co-sleeping leads health professionals to worry that tired parents may prove less attentive or sympathetic caregivers during the day. Kung Bushman mothers of the Kalahari Desert in South Africa who sleep with their children regularly, however, insist that it is natural for infants to awaken during the night; hence, night waking is not regarded as a problem or a concern. They do not define their own sleep as "disturbed." When a Kung mother awakens to the stirring of her infant lying next to her she returns immediately back to sleep or she nurses her baby;

in this case even if the infant were sleeping in a different place, the mother would still have to awaken. Cultural expectations and needs of both parents and infants cannot be disregarded in the attempt to understand the benefits or disadvantages of parent–infant co-sleeping.

How and where we expect infants and children to sleep are clearly learned. Parents from different backgrounds and cultures typically think their method of child care is natural. For example, just as many American parents seem to be surprised, if not horrified, at the prospects of infants and children sleeping in their beds, as Kung Bushman parents are shocked when told of how Western parents make their infants sleep alone, a practice unheard of and unthinkable in Kung culture. As all Kung mothers slept as children with their own mothers, co-sleeping is familiar and expected, but not to American parents. Moreover, because bottle feeding and cow's milk is not an available option for Kung mothers, as it may be for mothers elsewhere in the world, infants must be close to the mother during the night for feeding.

Co-Sleeping and Evolution: How "Natural?" How Old? How Do We Know?

Despite all of these cultural complexities, in many ways co-sleeping makes good biological sense. From an evolutionary perspective, protection from predators and the access to food that nighttime co-sleeping provides are beneficial to infants, especially the human infant who develops more slowly than any other mammal and who begins life with the least developed nervous system and brain—only 25 percent of its adult brain volume. Moreover, purely from a biological point of view, the human infant "expects" to be in physical contact with his or her parent throughout the night. The infant's body temperature, heart rates, and growth patterns are now known to be affected by forms of physical and social contact with a caregiver (McKenna, 1986; McKenna and Mosko, 1990).

Because infants are unable to locomote on their own for months or sometimes years, or unable to digest anything but milk for the first few months of life, all primate infants are carried on their mothers' bodies day and night and never left alone. Even today not all human infants live in

Table 1. Cross-Cultural Survey of Infant Sleeping Arrangements: With Whom and on What Do Infants Sleep?

Culture	Geographic Location	Subsistence Pattern	With Whom Baby Sleeps	On What Baby Sleeps
Ainu	North Hokkaido, Japan	Gathering, fishing, animal husbandry	First month with mother	First month—floor mat; afterward—hanging cradle
Bemba	Central Africa	Gardening, horticulture, tribal-level society	With parents first 3 years	Wood beds
Bhil	Eastern Rajasthan and western Pradesh, in western Ghats	Market economy mixed with crops, animal husbandry	With mother	Soft blanket on floor
Cuna	Panama	Gardening, cash crops, gathering, fishing, crafts	With mother	On mother's hammock or hard mats made of cibu tree covered with plantain leaves
Flores	Indonesia	Gardening, fishing	With parents	Bamboo sleeping bench
Gund	Manchuria, northern China	Gardening	With mother	Fiber mats
Gusii	Kenya	Gardening, gathering, animal husbandry, maize/coffee cultivation, wage labor in urban areas	First month with mother	On blankets
Ifugao	Northern Philippines	Gardening, gathering, trade	With parents	Raised woven blanket on floor
Maori	New Zealand	Cash crops, wage labor, gardening, gathering, animal husbandry	With parents	Summer—scooped-out earthen hut; winter—sleeping huts
Nahaue	Pradash State, northwestern India	Hunting, gathering, small crops, gardening	With parents	In skin hammocks hung within mother's reach
Navaho	Southwestern United States	Mixed: traditional pastoralists, business (trade), wage labor	Next to parents, swaddled in cradleboard	
San Kung	Southern Africa (Kalahari Desert)	Gathering, hunting	With mother	Blankets, mats
Santal	India	Agriculture, trade, pastoralism; caste society	With parents until 13	String beds
Semang	Malaysia	Gardening, trading, fishing	With parents	Mattress of split bamboo

Table 1. *(Cont.)*

Tarahumara	Northern Mexico	Collecting, gathering, hunting, small gardens; tribal-level state	With parents	Summer—open canvas; winter—wood beds
Tiwi	Northern Australia	Hunting, gathering, fishing, gardening, wage labor	With parents	Mats of paper bark
Trobrianders	Northeastern New Guinea	Gardening, fishing	With mother	Raised bedstead with small fire underneath
Turadja	Indonesia	Small crops, gardening, gathering, trade	Between parents	Mats of reeds or cloth, and pillows
Tzeltul	Central America		With parents	On mats of leather or bark
Yapese	Pacific Micronesia	Horticulture, fishing	With mother	Hanging baskets

predator-safe environments. Just as nonhuman primate infants can be and sometimes are eaten by leopards, tigers, hyenas, or other predators, human infants are potential prey of the large and medium-sized predator cats, dogs, and hyenas in Africa and many other parts of the Old World, especially at night. For both human and nonhuman primates constant maternal monitoring reduces the chances of infant mortality.

What factors led to the increased neurological immaturity of the human newborn in the first place that made parent–infant co-sleeping necessary? The answer is quite surprising. Anthropologists have learned that as upright posture, that is, bipedalism, became more and more useful to early human beings, the pelvis had to change its shape to accommodate this form of walking. Unfortunately for mothers and infants, these physical changes made it much more difficult for babies to be born quickly, safely, and easily.

The fossil records from Africa some 4 to 5 million years ago indicate that as our ancestors descended from the trees to live on the ground, the hip (pelvis) bones of the first representatives of the human lineage, the Australopithecines (also referred to as the first hominids), rotated forward and broadened. This structural change was necessary so that the abdominal muscles can attach to bony structures to prevent our organs and intestines from jostling about when we stand up and

walk. At the same time, though, the bottom of the pelvis, the ischium, pushed up and shortened to stabilize these broadening hips and to permit the muscles of the legs and buttocks to work efficiently as we walk. The overall result of these bipedal adaptations, however, was the reduction of the size of the birth opening relative to the size of the head.

These changes alone were enough to make birth difficult for our evolving ancestors; but to make matters even worse, at the same time as the pelvic (birth) opening was diminishing because of the usefulness of bipedalism, natural selection was also favoring increased fetal head size. Fetuses and infants were fast acquiring larger brains providing the potential for more complex learning and postnatal sociality—two major adaptive characteristics of our species. The adaptive compromise to this potentially disastrous evolutionary dilemma was, and continues to be, the birth of exceedingly neurologically immature infants for whom the vast majority of this added brain growth occurs after birth, not before.

In short, increased parental contact and care including co-sleeping emerged early in human evolution. Some 4 to 5 million years ago as our evolving hominid ancestors left the trees, so too, and somewhat early, did hominid infants have to leave their wombs. Completion of a gestation process that could not be completed safely in utero was at stake.

Is Co-Sleeping Adaptive?

Whiting (1981) studied cultural data from over 180 societies. Most but not all of these were smaller traditional societies and less technologically advanced than Western industrialized societies. He found that infant care practices including where and how infants sleep to a large extent depend on the challenges imposed by the physical environment, especially the average winter temperature. In cold climates, for example, where the temperature in the winter averaged below 50° F, in the majority of the cultures studied mothers swaddled their infants heavily; that is, they wrapped them tightly in thick blankets and strapped them into cradleboards to minimize heat loss. Infants slept in proximity (same room) to mother but tended not to sleep in skin-to-skin contact. In this way babies could be kept warmer.

In warmer climates, however, where winters averaged above this mean temperature, infants slept next to the mother's body, skin-to-skin. Rather than being carried in cradleboards in these milder and warmer environments, mostly infants were carried in shawls, nets, or baskets. Whiting argues that in addition to reflecting cultural values, different sleeping arrangements around the world reflect responses to different environmental pressures and the strategies by which parents best protect infants from cold temperatures.

The idea that parent–infant co-sleeping may contribute to infant well-being in yet other ways and possibly offset other human infant vulnerabilities is proposed by McKenna and colleagues (McKenna, 1986; McKenna and Mosko, 1990; McKenna et al., 1990). Their data show that when mothers and their infants sleep together in the same bed in a sleep laboratory, they exhibit overlapping, partner-induced arousals. These interruptions are thought to give infants practice in arousing. Such practice may be important because of the suspected relationship between infantile arousal deficiencies and the SUDDEN INFANT DEATH SYNDROME (SIDS). McKenna (1986) also suggests that the co-sleeping environment represents the infant's "natural ecological setting" for sleep, and that co-sleeping may change the breathing and the unfolding nighttime pattern of deep and light sleep of the infant in ways that make it more difficult for deadly arousal

deficits to find expression in SIDS. Though not a preventive measure for all potential SIDS victims, McKenna suggests that co-sleeping may help some. Co-sleeping may help certain infants with unspecified deficits to override the deficits and to avoid potential life-threatening events. But much work must be done to test this assertion.

(See also CHILDHOOD, SLEEP DURING.)

REFERENCES

Elias MF, Nicolson NA, Konner M. 1986. Two subcultures of maternal care in the United States. In Taub DM, King FA, eds. *Current perspectives in primate dynamics,* pp 37–50. New York: Van Nostrand Reinhold.

Ferber R. 1985. *Solve your child's sleep problem.* New York: Simon & Schuster.

Lozoff B, Wolf AW, Davis NS. 1984. Cosleeping in urban families with young children in the United States. *Pediatrics* 74:171–182.

Madansky D, Edelbrock C. 1990. Cosleeping in a community of 2- and 3-year-old children. *Pediatrics* 86:1987–2003.

McKenna JJ. 1986. An anthropological perspective on the sudden infant death syndrome (SIDS): The role of parental breathing cues and speech breathing adaptations. *Med Anthropol* 10:8–92.

McKenna JJ, Mosko S. 1990. Evolution and the sudden infant death syndrome (SIDS). Part III. Infant arousal and parent–infant co-sleeping. *Hum Nature* 1:291–330.

McKenna JJ, Mosko S, Dungy C, McAninch J. 1990. Sleep and arousal patterns of co-sleeping human mother/infant pairs: A preliminary physiological study with implications for the study of sudden infant death syndrome (SIDS). *Am J Physical Anthropol* 83:331–347.

Schachter FF, Fuchs ML, Bijur PE, Stone RK. 1989. Cosleeping and sleep problems in Hispanic-American urban young children. *Pediatrics* 84:522–530.

Shand N. 1985. Culture's influence in Japanese and American maternal role perception and confidence. *Psychiatry* 48:52–67.

Thenevin T. 1987. *The family bed.* Wayne, N.J.: Avery.

Whiting J. 1981. Environmental constraints on infant care approaches. In Munroe RL, Whiting BB, eds. *Handbook of cross-cultural development,* pp 155–179. New York: Garland STPM Press.

James J. McKenna

COUNTING SHEEP

Although it would be difficult to find out who first conceived of counting sheep as a means of putting oneself to sleep, this method appeared in the literature of sleep as early as 1911. In *The Gift of Sleep*, Bolton Hall wrote of the common practice of creating an image in one's mind of sheep jumping over a gate and counting them as they go (Hall, 1911). It seems that people have passed such time-honored remedies for insomnia from generation to generation. Another repetitive visualization technique is to imagine counting beads up to a hundred on a strand of beads. Other repetitive stimuli known to have similar soothing effects include rocking a baby to sleep or silently repeating a mantra (see MEDITATION AND SLEEP). Mark Twain was reputed to overcome problems getting to sleep by lying down on the bathroom floor after taking a warm bath (see TEMPERATURE EFFECTS ON SLEEP). Hall (1911) also spoke of a friend of his, Willard Moyer, whose technique for sleep inducement was to eat a small snack, which presumably induced sleep by bringing blood from the brain to the stomach (see FOLK AND OTHER NATURAL REMEDIES FOR SLEEPLESSNESS).

REFERENCES

Hall B. 1911. *The gift of sleep.* New York: Moffat Yard.

Jenifer Wicks

CREATIVITY IN DREAMS

Scientists often characterize creativity and problem solving by four distinct stages (LaBerge, 1985, p 188). First is preparation, during which data and background information are gathered; next is a passive stage that involves abandoning any active attempt to solve the problem; then with inspiration, a novel method of solving the problem presents itself; finally, the fourth stage involves verifying that the creative solution indeed works. Although most stages of this process can be performed at will, the stage of inspiration is less controlled and is not necessarily subject to the problem solver's conscious desires. Sleep implies abandoning this conscious effort to solve problems: Dreams can impart clues, novel approaches, or even solutions that may elude us in the daytime. History is filled with anecdotes of creative works conceived and scientific problems solved through dreaming.

Dreams have often been the source of artistic creations, producing themes and plots as well as actual finished works. Giuseppe Tartini dreamed that he sold his soul to the devil, who then played an incredibly beautiful piece of music. When he awoke, he immediately took up his violin and attempted to reproduce the music from his dream. Although Tartini felt his own piece was much inferior to the devil's, the "Trillo del Diavolo" or "Devil's Trill Sonata" is now one of his most famous works. Beethoven, Mozart, and Wagner also credited dreams with inspiring many of their compositions.

Many authors have acknowledged dreaming as a source of literary inspiration. The poet A. C. Benson composed "The Phoenix" entirely during sleep, but did not claim to understand his dream creation. Robert Louis Stevenson reported that literary ideas came to him during sleep, most notably the plot for *Dr. Jekyll and Mr. Hyde*. Perhaps the most famous example is that of Samuel Taylor Coleridge, who fell asleep one afternoon in 1797 after reading about Kubla Khan's palace in *Purchas' Pilgrimage* and dreamed over 200 lines of a new poem; on awakening, he began at once to write it down, but unfortunately was interrupted by a visitor before reaching the end. Although "Kubla Khan" remains one of Coleridge's finest and most respected works, it is unfinished because, after the visitor's departure, Coleridge could not remember the last lines he had composed during his sleep. The genesis of this poem in normal dreaming sleep is somewhat suspect, however, because Coleridge had ingested an opium-based substance shortly before falling asleep. Thus, "Kubla Khan" was perhaps induced as much by drugs as it was by dreams. Nevertheless, studies of drug-induced sleep in habituated users (which Coleridge certainly was) have shown that many aspects of sleep remain substantially the same as in normal sleep (Dement, 1972). In any case, Coleridge also published poems he created during sleep that was not drug induced.

Problem Solving in Dreams

Scientists and inventors have benefited similarly from the thoughtful interpretation of a creative dream, often after a long and fruitless search for the solution to a problem. One of the most revolutionary findings in organic chemistry was reportedly made during sleep by Friedrich Kekule, who had worked for years to discover the atomic structure of the benzene molecule (C_6H_6). One night he dreamt of many snakes flitting about together, which finally coalesced into a ring of six snakes chasing each others' tails, whirling around in a circle. When he awoke, he correctly interpreted the snake hexagon as the elusive structure of the benzene ring.

Elias Howe had been trying for years to invent an automated sewing machine that could revolutionize the sewing industry. Exhausted by his work, he fell asleep one night and dreamed he had been captured by a tribe of savages who demanded that he produce a working sewing machine. He failed, of course, so they determined to cut off his head. When he managed to escape, the natives pursued him, lobbing spears as they ran: Howe noticed that the spears each contained a hole in the spearhead. On awakening, Howe realized that the hole should not be in the dull end of the needle (as for sewing by hand), but in the sharp end. Before long, he developed a working model of a sewing machine.

A famous archaeological riddle was solved one night in 1893 by Hermann Hilprecht, who was attempting to classify and date two stone fragments with an Assyrian inscription. After making his best guess, Hilprecht fell asleep. He dreamt that an Assyrian high priest approached him in his sleep and told him that he had classified the fragments incorrectly, that they belonged together as part of a dedication to the god Ninib, and that a third fragment completing the dedication would never be found. When Hilprecht awoke and reexamined the fragments, he found that the dream was accurate in every detail for which verification was possible. The third fragment has never been found.

The creative solutions that dreams hold are not always so obvious as in Hilprecht's case, nor are they often interpreted so ingeniously as Howe's dream. Perhaps many such dreams are wasted when people who are not attuned to their dreams ignore the suggestions they offer. If James Watt had dreamt of a molten lead shower only once and not three times, he might never have invented the shot tower (see PROBLEM SOLVING AND DREAMING).

Dreams in Everyday Life

Although historical examples abound of dreams revolutionizing a field or producing a great work of art, these reports probably underestimate the frequency of creative dreaming. Although most lives do not become part of the historical record, they can still benefit considerably from creative dreaming. For example, Faraday (1972) writes of a gynecologist who reported learning a new surgical technique in a dream. Dement (1972) asked 200 college students, "During sleep have you ever pursued a logically connected train of thought upon some topic or problem in which you have reached some conclusion, and the steps and conclusion of which you remembered upon awakening?" A full third of the students answered that they had. This suggests that the creative solutions that dreams may contain are available to many people, not just to a limited set of brilliant minds.

Unfortunately, the power of creative dreaming, like creativity itself, is somewhat unpredictable. Nevertheless, certain factors are common to all the cases of creative dreaming cited above. The dreamers were all well prepared with background knowledge about the issue, devoted extensive daytime activity attempting to solve the problem, and through all their work became emotionally involved in the problem. Although such factors cannot guarantee that a solution will be offered through a creative dream, they certainly seem to increase the likelihood. In addition certain researchers claim that a technique to affect consciousness during REM sleep offers a way to harness the creative power inherent in dreams (LaBerge, 1985) (see LUCID DREAMING).

The mechanism by which dreams offer creative solutions to problems is unknown, but it may be that the looser cognitive associations that occur during sleep lead to the exploration of alternate possibilities not examined in the daytime (Borebly, 1984). Intense conscious efforts made along paths doomed to failure can be unshackled and released to pursue new possibilities. When the dreamer awakens, old information may have been processed in new ways, and alternate solutions may be available. Possibly the old adage concerning a problem that cannot be solved—"sleep on it"—is correct.

REFERENCES

Borbely AA. 1984. *Secrets of sleep.* New York: Basic Books.

Dement WC. 1972. *Some must watch while some must sleep.* San Francisco: San Francisco Book Co.

Faraday A. 1972. *Dream power.* London: Hodder and Stoughton.

LaBerge S. 1985. *Lucid dreaming.* New York: Ballantine. 1985.

Van de Castle RL. 1971. *The psychology of dreaming.* Morristown, N.J.: General Learning Press.

Max D. Stone

CULTURAL ASPECTS OF DREAMING

The emphasis on dreams and beliefs about them differ considerably across cultures. In certain societies, dreams are generally dismissed as unreal figments irrelevant to the important concerns of day-to-day life. In other cultures people consider dreams important sources of information—about the future, about the spiritual world, or about oneself. In some, dreams are considered to be a space for action like waking life, or a means for communication with other people or with the supernatural. Certain societies attribute such importance to dreams that they have been designated (by Alfred Kroeber) *dream cultures.*

Cultures in which dreams are taken seriously accumulate a depth of observations of their dreams, so their beliefs may be of value to understand dreaming. Freud appealed to such folk wisdom for confirmation of his theory of dreams as wish fulfillment (SEE FREUD'S DREAM THEORY).

How dreams are dealt with in different cultures may be examined from four perspectives: beliefs people hold about the nature of dreaming; conventional systems by which people interpret particular dreams; the social context in which dreams are shared (or not shared) and discussed; and the ways in which dreams are used in practice, especially in curing. In addition, a number of anthropologists have interpreted dreams psychodynamically, as expressing the dreamer's inner wishes, fears, and conflicts.

Dream Space and the Space of Waking Life

A dream takes place in a subjective space, different from the space of waking life. The relationship between these two spaces is problematic. We consider one "imaginary," the other "real," but both have the same kind of subjective existence. In certain cultures, both spaces are considered real, though they may or may not overlap. For some, dreaming is just a different way of acting in life space: an Ojibwa Indian, coming to a spot for the first time, said he had visited it in a dream. In other cultures dreams are an entry into a different level of reality. Yet no culture confuses dreams with waking reality or fails to make a distinction.

Dreams in some cultures may be considered real acts or channels of communication. The story is often told of the missionary who was astounded at the frequency of adultery confessed by his converts, until he discovered that they were confessing, as sins actually committed, acts of adultery they had carried out in dreams. Many cultures hold that dreams involve direct communication between the dreamer and the person dreamed of, who may be held to have dreamed the same dream. To dream of someone erotically may mean that person is thinking about the dreamer with desire (among the Parintintin of South America), or may even be considered an intimate contact (Arapesh of New Guinea). The effects of love magic may show up in the dreams of the man or woman targeted with the magic (Trobriand Islands). Sufi disciples in Pakistan may be called by their *pir* (holy man) in a dream.

Dreams may be unique windows into the "other side of reality"—sources of *super*natural knowledge. The religious figures called *shamans,* who go into trance and contact spirits for healing, are often called to their role by "initiatory dreams." Priests, mediums, or shamans may communicate with spirits in their dreams; but in some cultures, ordinary people can enter into contact with supernatural beings through dreams. "Anyone who dreams has a bit of shaman," the Parintintin say. The Azande of Central Africa perceive the process of being bewitched through bad dreams, and Parintintin dreamers sense the presence of demons by nightmares: The feeling of anxiety betrays the demonic presence.

Dreams may also serve as a domain for real action. In some South American groups dreams are a medium for shamans to exercise their power: Parintintin, Tapirapé, and Ye'cuana shamans cause events by dreaming them (Kracke, 1991, pp. 205–206). In the first two, shamans' dreams play an important role in the conception of children: The soul to be born appears in a dream to a shaman, who directs it to a woman's womb. In the Trobriands, the spirit of an ancestress appears to a woman herself to announce conception. Jivaro (Shuar) men in Ecuador acquire their *arútam*—a soul essential for success in hunting and warfare—in dreams or visions.

In many cultures, then, the world in dreams claims a reality as great as the world in which one wakes. The question has been raised, Which is *more* real? The Chinese philosopher Chüang Tzu raises it in the form of a now well-known parable: If I wake from a dream that I am a butterfly, am I a man who has dreamed he was a butterfly, or a butterfly dreaming that I am a man? For the Ye'cuana and Tapirapé of South America, major parts of creation took part in dreams of the culture heroes. In India, the reality of dreams may be considered equal to that of waking, and the Upanishads hold that the world is itself a kind of dream (O'Flaherty, 1984).

Cultural Beliefs About the Nature of Dreaming

Cultural beliefs about dreaming are varied and complex. A frequently encountered concept is that dreams are the experiences of the soul of the sleeping person that wanders during sleep. The nineteenth-century anthropologist E. B. Tylor considered this to be the most typical primitive conception of dreams, and in fact argued that the first concept of soul grew from such a belief. The Mehinacu of Brazil identify such a soul with the "eye soul," which is visible in the inverted human image one can see in someone's eye (Kracke, 1991, note 76). The Andaman Islanders see dreams as related to a soul manifested in one's smell (see below).

People in many cultures—even in some of those in which dreams are seen as existing in some kind of real space—at the same time recognize that dreams are a kind of thought process. Quite common, in fact, is the observation that dreams are a continuation or transformation of a train of thought one was following as one went to sleep. Barbadians attribute their dreams to "studying"—thinking about something intensely. These beliefs implicitly recognize what Freud called the *day residues,* memories from the prior day that go into the dream.

Interpretation of Dreams as Predictions of the Future

In many cultures, dreams are held to provide knowledge of the future—either literally or, more often, metaphorically, through symbolic references to future events (like the dreams interpreted by Joseph in the Bible) or by certain rules (such as "dreams mean opposite"). The interpretation of dreams as omens is very nearly a universal tenet of dream lore. Descriptions of such systems of dream interpretation abound in the anthropological literature on dream beliefs (Kracke, 1991, pp. 206–208). Barbara Tedlock (1981, 1991) and her husband Dennis were apprenticed to a Quiché Maya dream interpreter in Guatemala and earlier studied dream interpreting among the Zuñi.

Why are such systems of dream interpretation so common? Certain conventional interpretations may help dreamers allay anxiety from a disturbing dream. In many systems of dream augury, emotion-laden dreams (violent, sexual, or frightening) are given relatively neutral or benign and positive interpretations: They foretell good hunting, for example, or general "good luck" or "bad luck." In Corsica and in Portugal, to dream of someone's death gives that person longer life. To explain disturbing dreams as "really" meaning something quite different may be reassuring.

Social Embeddedness of Dreams

Telling a dream may be a significant social disclosure, and there are social rules that govern appropriate settings and the kind of dreams that may be told. The context in which a dream is imparted may itself add something to its meaning, which may be conscious and intended (as when a man tells a woman he has dreamt of her) or may be unconscious (as is the transference message of a dream told in an analytic hour). Dreams in some cultures may provide important political arguments (as in ancient Rome according to Shakespeare's play *Julius Caesar*). In such a culture, for example, among the Sambia of New Guinea (Tedlock, 1987), the way a dream is told in a public, political context may be quite different from how it is told in private and may have a different meaning. Cultures differ, too, in the degree to which dreamers are held responsible for their activities in dreams. An erotic dream, among the New Guinea Arapesh, may be considered an adulterous act; the Sambia hold the dreamer accountable only for a dream he has told publicly. Dreams in some cultures contribute to the identity of the person: In Plains cultures one acquires one's guardian spirit and life path in a dream or vision; among the Jivaro of Ecuador, one acquires one's soul; and Pakistani Sufis may be led by a dream to their spiritual masters.

Therapeutic Use of Dreams

Dreams are important in a number of cultures for activities that some observers have called psychotherapeutic. Various rituals have been treated as therapy, from peyote rituals among the Ute Indians to elaborate systems of dream interpretation by specialists among the Diegueño Indians (Bourguignon, 1972). The seventeenth-century Iroquois had a ritual, perhaps cathartic in nature, in which a dreamer told his or her dream and others fulfilled it (Wallace, 1959). A major distinction is between those cultures in which it is the dreams of the *patient* that are used in therapy (the Iban of Borneo, the Ute, ancient rabbinical cures, Euro-American psychotherapy); those in which it is the dreams of the curer or shaman that are important (Makiritare, Tapirapé, and Parintintin of South America); and those in which both are used, such as the Diegueño.

Anthropological findings about uses of dreams in other societies have led to some developments in therapeutic practice in the United States. Kilton Stewart (1962) described a supposedly therapeutic use of dreams among the Senoi in the Malay tropical forest. This account stimulated the development of dream groups in the 1960s to experiment with such practices, but recent evidence marshalled by Dentan (1985) and Domhoff (1985) has called Stewart's description into question. (See also SENOI DREAM THEORY.)

A particularly interesting and valuable contribution is that of George Devereux (1951), an anthropologist who was also trained as a psychoanalyst. Working as a therapist with a Plains Indian patient, Devereux worked out a process of psychotherapy based on Plains Indian dream beliefs and practices.

Personal Meaning of Dreams

Dreams reflect the dreamer's feelings about events and relationships. If they are understood in terms of the very private code of expression that can only be unraveled through the dreamer's own associations to the dream, dreams can be used to get at a person's unconscious wishes, feelings, and fantasies about people and relationships. The wishes and fantasies may be incompatible with the person's cultural norms and values, although those values are not at all irrelevant to understanding the feelings and why they are repressed.

Some of the most sensitive interpretation of dreams of North American Indians has been done by the anthropologist Dorothy Eggan. Eggan got several Hopi Indians to tell their dreams and their free associations to them. In a series of finely crafted articles, she uses the dreams to get at their inner subjective experience of their cultural beliefs and values. Her premature death in 1965 left much rich material untapped. (For references to her work, see Eggan, 1961; von Grunebaum and Caillois, 1966.)

Sometimes culturally specific beliefs about dreams are essential in understanding what a dream means for an individual dreamer. Eggan wrote about the general meaning for Hopi dreamers of a particular mythical serpent that appears in their dreams. In Moroccan culture, some men are plagued with a possessive female spirit, Aisha Qandisha, who appears in their dreams and has sexual encounters with them and then demands their absolute faithfulness to her as her husband. Such dream elements, which can express various conflicts over sexual wishes, are termed by Vincent Crapanzano (1975) "symbolic-interpretive elements for the articulation of conflict."

Cultural Differences in the Dreams Themselves

Naturally, dreams in different culture have different subject matter, simply because people's experiences are different. But are there deeper differences in the *kinds* of dreams people have, or in *how* people dream?

Certain typical dreams (such as dreams of falling, flying, examinations, or being rooted to the spot when trying to run) seem to occur in all cultures, though some studies suggest they vary in frequency. Other dreams may be frequent in a culture because of that culture's beliefs about the meaning of dreams: In a culture where a "falling down house" is believed to predict death, it may become a typical dream in that culture.

There are also clear cultural differences in recall of dreams. In modern Western cultures, many people rarely remember their dreams. In some, such as that of the Parintintin, most people remember several dreams every night. Furthermore, in some cultures people dream quite openly of the sort of childhood memories and fantasies we rarely are in touch with: dreams of learning sexuality from watching parents, for example, or dreams that reproduce childhood ideas about childbirth. In psychoanalytic terms, dreams in these cultures tend to be less *disguised* than in ours (though there are no cultures where dreams are completely undisguised).

Reports from many cultures suggest the possibility of learning to *control* one's own dreams. If shamans are believed to be able to cause things to happen by dreaming about them, either directly or in symbols, then they must be able to dream at will of what they want to cause (or of its symbol). In the training of Quiché Maya dream interpreters, a novice may be instructed to await the recurrence of a certain dream on a given date and to complete an action in this dream that was left incomplete in the first (Tedlock, 1981, 1987). Stewart reported that the Senoi taught their children to change their dreams. Under the name of LUCID DREAMING, the notion of awareness and control of one's own dreams while in them has

been a source of controversy in modern dream research.

Dream Beliefs as Theories of Dreaming

To recognize a set of cultural beliefs about dreams as constituting a theory of dreaming requires a very close understanding of the native theory itself and of the precise aspect of the dream to which each specific term or belief refers. Few anthropological studies of dreaming have achieved this level of precision as yet, though a few anthropologists have noted parallels with the dream theories of our own culture, especially with Freud's.

The notion that one's thoughts continue into sleep and turn into a dream recalls not only Freud's notion of day residues, but also the dream-laboratory observation of a continuous train of thought that develops through dreams and the nocturnal thoughts between REM periods. The idea that dreams are wish fulfillments also recurs in many cultures.

An especially interesting dream theory comes from a hunting culture of the Little Andaman Island. The Ongis believe that a vital constituent of the person is one's personal smell, which tends to disperse and must be conserved to avoid depletion and consequent illness. During sleep, the spirit or soul associated with the person's smell comes out and goes to each spot the sleeping person has visited during the day, collecting the smell the person left there and bringing it back to the sleeper's body. One must not awaken a sleeping person lest this dreaming process be interrupted, exposing the person to grave danger of illness.

This idea of part of us wandering and visiting in dreams the places we have been during the day can readily be recognized as the day residues that go into the composition of a dream. But the reintegrating process described in this theory may be compared with recently proposed theories that dreams serve the function of sorting through the experiences of a day and integrating them with past experiences stored in memory. The Ongi speak of the process of reintegrating the smells with the body as *dane korale,* "spider home," suggesting how the dream weaves the past day's experiences back into the web of the self.

Careful study of such theories of dreaming in other cultures may lead us to new ideas about the nature of dreaming.

REFERENCES

[*Note:* Many articles on cross-cultural study of dreams may be found in the journal *Dreaming: Journal of the Association for the Study of Dreams.*]

Bourguignon E. 1972. Dreams and altered states of consciousness in anthropological research. In Hsu FLK, ed, *Psychological Anthropology,* 2nd ed, pp 403–434. Cambridge, Mass.: Schenkman.

Crapanzano V. 1975. Saints, *jnun* and dreams: An essay in Moroccan ethnopsychology. *Psychiatry* 38:145–159.

Dentan RK. 1985. A dream of Senoi. Buffalo, N.Y.: SUNY Buffalo Council on International Studies.

Domhoff GW. 1985. The mystique of dreams: A search for Utopia through Senoi dream therapy. Berkeley: University of California Press.

Devereux G. 1951. *Reality and dream: Psychotherapy of a Plains Indian.* New York: International Universities Press.

Eggan D. 1961. Dream analysis. In Kaplan B, ed, *Studying personality cross culturally,* pp 551–577. New York: Harper & Row.

Hollan D. 1989. The personal use of dream beliefs in the Toraja Highlands. *Ethos* 17:166–186.

Kracke W. 1979. Dreaming in Kagwahiv: Dream beliefs and their intrapsychic uses in an Amazonian indigenous culture. *Psychoanalytic Study of Society* 8:119–171.

———. 1991. Languages of dreaming: Anthropological approaches to the study of dreaming in other cultures. In Gackenbach J, Sheikh A, eds, *Dream images: A call to mental arms,* pp 103–224. Amityville, N.Y.: Baywood.

Lincoln JS. 1935. *The dream in primitive cultures.* London: Cressett.

O'Flaherty WD. 1984. *Dreams, illusions and other realities.* Chicago: University of Chicago Press.

O'Nell CW. 1976. *Dreams, culture and the individual.* San Francisco: Chandler & Sharp.

Stewart K. 1962. The dream comes of age. *Mental Hygiene* 46:230–237.

Tedlock B. 1981. Quiché Maya dream interpretation. *Ethos* 9(4):313–350.

———. 1987. *Dreaming: Anthropological and psychological interpretations.* New York: Cambridge University Press.

———. 1991. The new anthropology of dreaming. *Dreaming* 1:161–178.

von Grunebaum GE, Caillois R, eds. 1966. *The dream and human societies.* Berkeley: University of California Press.

Wallace AFC. 1959. The institutionalization of cathartic and control strategies in Iroquois religious psychotherapy. In Opler MK, ed. *Culture and mental health,* pp 63–96. New York: Macmillan.

Waud H. Kracke

CULTURAL ASPECTS OF SLEEP

Cultural aspects refers to constant ways of believing and behaving that differ between groups of individuals throughout the world. Cultural factors have a range of effects on the modes of sleep, the process of sleep, and the patterns of sleep.

By modes of sleep we mean the activities associated with preparing for sleep, sleeping, and awakening. A casual consideration of the modes of sleep displayed through history and across cultures makes apparent the wide range of sleep customs. Bed structures range from bare earth to highly elaborate and artistic creations such as those seen in Egyptian tombs. They may take the form of single pallets to enormous areas. They may be portable cots or may be niches such as found in Roman Pompeii. Head rests vary from carved head supports to feather pillows (see PILLOWS). Some cultures and groups within cultures emphasize sleeping alone; others may involve entire families or more extended groupings sleeping together. These arrangements may be based on complex age groupings and mating customs. Children may sleep with parents for extended periods (see CO-SLEEPING) or may be isolated quickly. Preparatory activities may involve communal storytelling (see BEDTIME STORIES) or group or private prayers, and awakening may be dictated by a variety of living arrangements, ritual recitals, and dream reporting. Modern societies have elevated the ALARM CLOCK.

Sleep research has given limited attention to these various customs. This reflects the perspective that sleep is a stable, adaptive biological process like, say, digestion. Although cultural factors may determine how we select, prepare, and serve our food, the physiological processes themselves will function, as a system, within these variations. Some justification of this viewpoint is found in the one area of sleep customs that has been studied: bed surfaces. Bed surfaces, by custom, range from hard surfaces to very soft surfaces and contemporary customs have extended these to various supports such as innersprings and water beds. Physiological measurements show the sleep surface has little effect on the sleep process (see BEDS.) From a cultural perspective, then, it seems likely that, from its onset to its termination, sleep maintains a common biological form regardless of the preparatory, interpersonal, or physical arrangements.

There is evidence that indicates that cultural factors influence the patterning of sleep. Patterning of sleep refers to the total amount of sleep obtained and the timing of sleep. At the outset, it should be recognized that these variables are difficult to measure and therefore the data available are limited (see INDIVIDUAL DIFFERENCES).

A carefully conducted survey of the sleep of 2,600 school children in California in 1910–1912 makes apparent the effect of cultural change on sleep amounts. This survey of sleep amounts was compared with a similar survey conducted on Florida schoolchildren in the 1963–1964 school year. The average amount of sleep of 8- to 12-year-old children for the California sample was 600 minutes per night, compared with 540 minutes for the Florida sample. The 13- to 17-year-old averages were 550 and 450 minutes, respectively (Webb, 1969). Assuming that sleep physiology remained unchanged from 1912 to 1964, cultural differences across this 50-year gulf may account for the sleep differences.

Further evidence of a cultural effect on sleep length amounts in our contemporary society is seen in the workday/day off patterning of sleep. The most extensive data on this topic were obtained from an analysis of sleep behavior obtained from a large daily time budget study of more than 30,000 adults in eleven industrial countries (Webb, 1985). The average amounts of sleep on workdays, across all subjects, were 453 minutes for males and 449 minutes for females. On "days off" the average for males was 547 minutes; for females it was significantly less, 533 minutes. Additional evidence of a generalized cultural effect on total sleep amounts was also found in this analysis. Two countries, France and Belgium, had significantly fewer individuals sleeping in the low sleep levels (less than 6 hours per day). Another apparent but often overlooked cultural effect on total amount of sleep is the en-

demic presence of shift work. There are consistent reports of reduced sleep amounts under shift work conditions (see SHIFTWORK).

Indeed there is scattered but strong evidence that our contemporary industrialized culture is placing strong pressures on total sleep. Surveys indicate that as many as 60 percent of working adults use alarms or other assists to terminate their daily sleep. The fact that workday sleep is typically 1 hour less than non-workday sleep adds evidence. A recent study (Roehrs et al., 1989) found that extension of normal sleep reduced daytime sleepiness.

With regard to the placement or timing of sleep, the nap has been subjected to a cultural analysis (Webb and Dinges, 1989, pp. 247–265). Webb and Dinges examined the Human Relations Area File (Murdoch, 1972), which describes more than 1700 worldwide cultures, and four studies of siesta cultures (Italy, Greece, Mexico, Peru). They concluded that the presence of systemic napping or the siesta was generally confined to tropical regions. Factors that inhibit napping in such cultures are nomadic and unstable domestic settings and irregular food supplies associated with fishing and hunting. In our increasingly industrialized setting, production demands serve as strong inhibitors. It was surprising to find that even in older and traditional settings, systematic napping was the exception rather than the rule. A particular example of the effect of a subculture on napping is seen in the presence of napping in college students. Two-week sleep diaries of students found that only 16 percent reported no naps; 42 percent reported five or more naps during the 2 weeks. The high level of napping probably reflects a combination of reduced nighttime sleep and a permissive naptime schedule. (See also NAPPING.)

One of the most apparent cultural influences on the placement of sleep has been the growing presence of SHIFTWORK in our contemporary society. Large numbers of individuals are being required to change the timing of their sleep from the regular "cocoon of darkness" that was once the sole domain of sleep.

Cultural factors have determined a wide range of activities and surrounds associated with preparing for, engaging in, and terminating sleep. This review also indicates that cultural factors of our industrial society are pressing on the total amount of sleep that is obtained. It also indicates that cultural factors are determinates of the timing of sleep. The presence of naps is strongly determined by cultural factors, and the presence of shiftwork markedly affects the timing of sleep.

REFERENCES

Murdoch GP. 1972. *Outline of world cultures,* 4th ed. New Haven, Conn.: Human Relations File. This introduction to a cross-cultural file is coded for sleep and dreams of 1,700 cultural units.

Roehrs T, Timms V, Zwyghuizen-Doorenbos A, Roth T. 1989. Sleep extension in sleepy and alert normals. *Sleep* 12:449–457.

Soldatas CR, Madianos MG, Vlachonikolis IG. 1983. Early afternoon napping: A fading Greek habit. In Koella W, ed. *Sleep 1982,* pp 202–205. Basel: Karger.

Webb WB. 1969. Twenty-four-hour sleep cycling. In Kales A, ed. *Sleep: Physiology and pathology,* pp. 53–65. Philadelphia: Lippincott.

——. 1985. Sleep in industrialized settings in the northern hemisphere. *Psychol Rep* 57:591–598.

Webb WB, Dinges DF, eds. 1989. *Cultural perspectives on napping and the siesta.* New York: Raven.

Wilse B. Webb

CYCLES OF SLEEP ACROSS THE NIGHT

That the human sleep ELECTROENCEPHALOGRAM (EEG) changes across the night was apparent from the first all-night recordings by Loomis, Harvey, and Hobart (1935). Not until the discovery of REM sleep by Aserinsky and Kleitman (1953), however, was it known that these fluctuations result from cyclic alternation of two qualitatively different kinds of sleep (NREM and REM), as well as from systematic EEG changes across successive cycles.

Early studies measured EEG changes across sleep by arbitrary units, such as hours or fractions of the sleep period. Quantitative descriptions of the durations and EEG characteristics of the physiological units of sleep (NREMPs and REMPs) were reported in 1967 and 1974 (Feinberg, Koresko, and Heller, 1967; Feinberg, 1974). These descriptions included statistical analyses of these cycle components within sleep and across age.

Figure 1 presents visually scored NREM–REM sleep period patterns for baseline sleep of children, young adults, and elderly. NREM period 1 (NREMP1) duration (REM LATENCY) declines steeply across adolescence (but see later) and shows a much smaller but statistically significant decline between young adulthood and normal old age. The absolute durations of NREMPs 2 through 5 and their declining trends across the night are similar for all age groups, beginning in early childhood. Time occupied by stage 4 EEG (see STAGES OF SLEEP) decreases in a quasi-exponential fashion across successive NREMPs; this declining pattern, along with other characteristics of high-amplitude dense delta (waves between 0.5 and 3 cycles per second in frequency) gave rise to the original homeostatic model of delta sleep by Feinberg (1974). (See also SLOW-WAVE SLEEP.)

Figure 1 also shows the powerful effects of age on visually scored delta sleep (stages 3 and 4); this age-related change also has been documented with computer analysis (Coble et al., 1987; Feinberg et al., 1983, 1990). In children and young adults, the first REMP is markedly shorter and has a lower density of eye movement than the second (and subsequent) REMP. These across-REMP differences are absent in the elderly, whose first REMP is longer and has a greater density of eye movements than in the younger groups. For children and young adults, successive REMPs increase in duration through REMPs 3 and 4 and then decline. There is only a slight tendency for eye movement density to increase across REMPs after the first; however, young adults show a striking increase in eye movement density when sleep is extended well beyond its habitual length (e.g., to 10.5 hours; Aserinsky, 1969).

Statistical analyses of complete cycle durations (NREMP + REMP and REMP + NREMP) have also been reported (Feinberg and Floyd, 1979). These measures, which tend to average around 90 minutes, have been difficult to interpret. The reader can compute average values for each age group by summing the component NREMP and REMP durations in Figure 1.

Since the mid-1970s, both period/amplitude (i.e., the duration of the individual waves of the EEG) (Feinberg and Floyd, 1979) and spectral analyses with the fast Fourier transform (i.e., the amount of electrical energy contributed by each frequency within a time interval; Borbely et al., 1981) have been applied to measure EEG

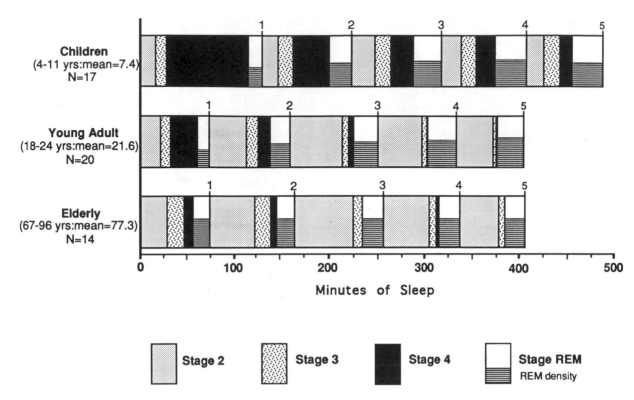

Figure 1. Durations of visually scored NREMPs and REMPs for three age groups; average sleep stages within NREMPs and REM eye movement density are also shown. Numbers designate the ordinal NREMP–REMP cycles. The first NREMP in children appears to be twice as long as that of young adults and the elderly, but this appears to be an artifact of a "skipped" first REMP (see text). Cycle durations in adults and elderly are strikingly similar despite the extensive awakenings (subtracted) in the elderly.

changes across NREMPs. This work has focused on delta frequencies for several reasons: (1) delta EEG plays a key role in the homeostatic model of sleep; (2) it contains the dominant energy of the sleep EEG; and (3) it manifests the most obvious changes across cycles and across age. Figure 1 shows the changes in delta wave amplitude and incidence across visually defined NREMPs for normal adults and elderly. Figure 2 presents computer measurement of the differences in the average amplitude and in the rate of production of 0.5-to 3-cycle-per-second EEG between young adulthood and normal old age. It is assumed that these age changes are related to declining brain plasticity; however, clear-cut experimental support for this belief does not exist.

Although it was long known that continuous measurement of sleep EEG across time (dynamic analysis) reveals cyclic patterns (Koga, 1965),

only recently were these cycles implemented as measures independent of visually scored REM and NREM sleep. An example of dynamic patterns is shown in Figure 3. These patterns overlap but are not identical to results obtained with visual scoring: early delta peaks generally correspond to visually scored stage 4, and stage REM is generally scored in delta troughs. Figure 3 also shows that cyclic oscillations are not limited to delta frequencies, but occur in fast (beta) frequencies as well. The beta oscillations are out-of-phase with those of delta across both NREM and REM sleep.

Application of dynamic analysis has shed new light on the phenomenon of the "skipped" first REM period—an absence of visually scored REM sleep at about the time the first REMP would be expected. This phenomenon had been described anecdotally in the baseline sleep of children and

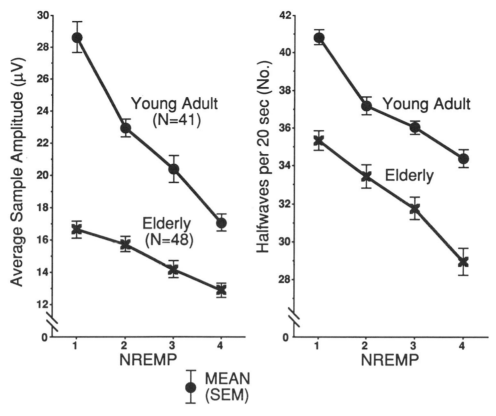

Figure 2. Delta (0.5–3 cycles per second) average sample amplitude (integrated amplitude/time in band) and half-waves per 20 seconds plotted by NREMP for normal young adults (mean age 24.5 years; range 20 to 29 years) and elderly (mean age 71.8 years, range 67 to 78 years). Linear trends were highly significant for both measures ($F = 378$ and 311, respectively, $p < 0.0001$). F's for curvature (quadratic trend) were not significant for either measure, arguing against an exponential decline. Mean levels of average sample amplitude and half-waves per 20 seconds of NREM were significantly lower in the elderly ($F = 91$ and 55, respectively, $p < 0.0001$). Thus, normal aging reduces both delta wave amplitude and the rate of delta wave production during sleep.

also in young adults after total sleep deprivation. As the onset of REM defines the end of each NREMP, a skipped first REMP results in a very long apparent first NREMP (as in Figure 1).

Dynamic analysis of children's sleep with automatic detection of peaks and troughs in delta activity reveals that the first delta (NREM) peak is not delayed in children or in young adults after sleep deprivation (Feinberg et al., 1988, 1990). It is simply not recognized visually that REM sleep has occurred, probably because eye movements are absent in these conditions of very low brain arousal. Thus, if delta peaks and troughs are considered the appropriate measures of cyclic patterns (irrespective of their visual scoring), dynamic analysis shows that the first cycle is not longer in children than in young adults.

Cyclic patterns viewed with dynamic analysis have also altered our conceptualization of the underlying mechanisms. We believe that these patterns more resemble those produced by a pulsatile process than by the systematic metabolic consumption of a substrate (as was hypothesized in the original homeostatic model of delta sleep). This altered view led us to propose the following mechanism: a NREM-producing pulse (perhaps driven by NEUROENDOCRINE HORMONES) occurs periodically across sleep. This pulse

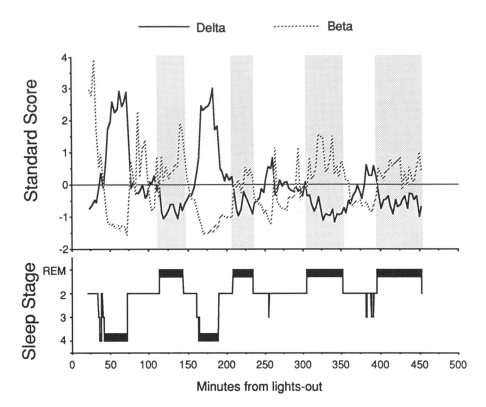

Figure 3. Integrated amplitude of delta waves (0.3–3 cycles per second) and derivative curve length of beta waves (23–30 cycles per second) plotted continuously across baseline sleep for a young adult. Both measures were converted to standard (*z*) scores so that they could be displayed on the same scale. Independent visual sleep stage scoring is plotted below. Beta and delta EEGs both show clear-cut, out-of-phase oscillations across sleep. REM sleep (shaded) occurs when delta activity is low and beta activity is high. These cyclic patterns can be quantified automatically and objectively and, although they overlap with visual scoring, such data might prove more predictive of physiology and behavior than traditional sleep stage measures. We propose that cyclic activity when viewed by dynamic analysis is more suggestive of a pulsatile than a metabolic homeostatic delta mechanism (see text).

produces EEG slowing and suppression of fast waves. These EEG changes are associated with neural inhibition, functional deafferentation, and a relative shutdown of MEMORY consolidation systems. When the effectiveness of the pulses wanes below a critical level, partial escape occurs. This escape from cortical inhibition is REM sleep, which we propose (as in the original homeostatic model) serves a function intrinsic to sleep rather than directed to reverse the effects of waking brain activity (for details, see Feinberg et al., 1990). (See also SENSORY PROCESSING AND SENSATION DURING SLEEP.)

REFERENCES

Aserinsky E. 1969. The maximal capacity for sleep: Rapid eye movement density as an index of sleep satiety. *Biol Psychiatry* 1:147–159.

Aserinsky E, Kleitman N. 1953. Regularly occurring periods of eye motility, and concomitant phenomena during sleep. *Science* 118:273–274.

Borbely AA, Baumann F, Brandeis D, Strauch I, Lehmann D. 1981. Sleep deprivation: Effect on sleep stages and EEG power density in man. *Electroencephalogr Clin Neurophysiol* 51:483–493.

Coble PA, Reynolds CF III, Kupfer DJ, Houck P. 1987. Electroencephalographic sleep of healthy children.

Part II: Findings using automated delta and REM sleep measurement methods. *Sleep* 10:551–562.

Feinberg I. 1974. Changes in sleep cycle patterns with age. *J Psychiatr Res* 10:283–306.

Feinberg I, Baker T, Leder R, March JD. 1988. Response of delta (0–3 Hz) EEG and eye movement density to a night with 100 minutes of sleep. *Sleep* 11(5):473–487.

Feinberg I, Fein G, Floyd TC, Aminoff MJ. 1983. Delta (.5–3 Hz) EEG waveforms during sleep in young and elderly normal subjects. In Chase MH, Weitzman ED, eds. *Sleep disorders: Basic and clinical research,* pp 449–462. New York: Spectrum.

Feinberg I, Floyd TC. 1979. Systematic trends across the night in human sleep cycles. *Psychophysiology* 16(3):283–291.

Feinberg I, Koresko RL, Heller N. 1967. EEG sleep patterns as a function of normal and pathological aging in man. *J Psychiatr Res* 5:107–144.

Feinberg I, March JD. 1988. Cyclic delta peaks during sleep: Result of a pulsatile endocrine process? *Arch Gen Psychiatry* 45:1141–1142. Letter.

Feinberg I, March JD, Fein G, Floyd TC, Walker JM, Price L. 1978. Period and amplitude analysis of 0.5–3 c/sec activity in sleep of young adults. *Electroencephalogr Clin Neurophysiol* 44:202–213.

Feinberg I, March JD, Flach K, Maloney T, Chern W-J, Travis F. 1990. Maturational changes in amplitude, incidence and cyclic pattern of the 0 to 3 Hz (delta) electroencephalogram of human sleep. *Brain Dysfunct* 3:183–192.

Haustein W, Pilcher J, Klink J, Schulz H. 1986. Automatic analysis overcomes limitations of sleep stage scoring. *Electroencephalogr Clin Neurophysiol* 64:364–374.

Koga E. 1965. A new method of EEG analysis and its application to the study of sleep. *Folia Psychiatr Neurol Jpn* 19:269–278.

Loomis AL, Harvey EN, Hobart G. 1935. Potential rhythms of the cerebral cortex during sleep. *Science* 81:597–598.

Irwin Feinberg
Sunao Uchida

D

DALI, SALVADOR

See Art, Sleep and Dreams in Western

DAYLIGHT SAVING TIME

It should come as no surprise that Benjamin Franklin, who coined the maxim "Early to bed and early to rise, makes a man healthy, wealthy, and wise," first proposed what has come to be known in the United States as Daylight Saving Time (DST). While living in France in 1783, he noted that although the sun rose much earlier in the summer, Parisians still began their day at the same clock time as they did in winter. The net effect was that the hours between sunset and bedtime were longer than they needed to be, at least in the larklike Franklin's opinion, and this fact required what he thought was a wasteful overuse of candles.

The French did not leap to adopt Franklin's suggestion, but in the twentieth century the United States, Great Britain, Germany, and other countries have at various times instituted a 1-hour time adjustment in order to allow a more economical use of the hours of available daylight. This was first done in Germany in 1916, and soon afterwards by the British, who called it Summer Time, as a conservation measure during World War I. A year later, the United States followed suit, and the practice continued until 1918. Both Britain and the United States adopted a 1-hour advance year-round during the World War II years of to 1945, with minor variations, and in Britain

there was even an additional 1-hour advance during those years, which was known as Double Summer Time.

Since the war there have been variations, but in most years the countries that have observed a time shift used the scheme of a spring clock advance and a fall clock delay, each of 1 hour. The starting and ending dates have been variable from year to year and from country to country. As of 1986, U.S. law specifies that DST should start on the first Sunday in April and end on the last Sunday in October. Some states have been exempted from the law and do not observe Daylight Saving Time, especially those that are usually split between two time zones. In Western Europe the adjustment usually begins on the last Sunday in March and ends on the last Sunday in September. Ireland, Paraguay, and the Dominican Republic make their time adjustment in winter, calling it Winter Time.

Using the mnemonic "Spring forward, fall back," Americans reset their clocks officially at 2 A.M. on the specified Sunday morning. The effects of the autumn clock delay on sleep and mood are generally positive, researchers have found, but the spring advance can cause problems. In either case it takes about a week for one's internal clock to adjust completely to the shift. The process is analogous to JET LAG: A fall clock delay is equivalent to traveling westward one time zone, and a spring advance is equivalent to traveling eastward one time zone. Studies have shown that a spring clock advance is associated with a significant (11-percent) rise in traffic accidents during the following week (Monk, 1980) and that traumatic injuries and outpatient hospital visits are also higher (Pfaff and Weber, 1982).

REFERENCES

Monk TH. 1980. Traffic accident increases as a possible indication of desynchronosis. *Chronobiologia* 7:527–529.

Monk TH, Aplin LC. 1980. Spring and autumn daylight saving time changes: Studies of adjustment in sleep timings, mood, and efficiency. *Ergonomics* 23(2):167–178.

Monk TH, Folkard S. 1974. Adjusting to and from Daylight Saving Time. *Nature* 261:688–689.

Pfaff G, Weber E. 1982. [More accidents due to daylight saving time? A comparative study on the distribution of accidents at different times of day prior to and following the introduction of Central European Summer Time (CEST). Published in German.] *Int Arch Occup Environ Health* 49(3–4):315–323.

Boyd Hayes

DEAFNESS AND DREAMING

Deaf persons show the same cycle of NREM and REM sleep as the hearing. Similarly, their rate of dream recall from REM sleep is about the same as in the hearing (Stoyva, 1965).

Unfortunately, the amount of systematic, all-night experimental work on sleep and dreaming in the deaf has been limited. Two such studies that do exist were stimulated by the motor theory of thinking—the idea that certain minimal motor (muscular) activities in the speech apparatus are closely associated with thinking. Since the deaf "speak" by means of finger and hand movements, scientists conjectured that any mental activity during sleep might be reflected in greater activity in finger and hand muscles than would be the case for hearing subjects.

Support for this theory was provided by Max (1935), who used surface electromyogram (EMG) sensors to detect bursts of forearm muscle activity associated with finger movements during sleep. Max reported that deaf persons showed a great deal more finger EMG activity during sleep than did hearing subjects. He also reported that the finger EMG bursts of deaf subjects during sleep were associated with dreaming. These intriguing early observations by Max have often been cited in support of a motor theory of thinking.

A subsequent study by Stoyva (1965), however, used more sophisticated instrumentation, and the results cast doubt on Max's conclusion that finger EMG bursts are a specific sign of dreaming in the deaf—any more than they are in hearing individuals. In the Stoyva experiment, eye movements, EEG brain waves, and finger EMG activity from the forearm were monitored. All subjects were either congenitally deaf or had become deaf younger than 2 years of age. Contrary to Max, this study found that hearing persons showed just as much finger movement activity (forearm EMG bursts) as did the deaf in all phases of sleep including REM sleep. Furthermore, both hearing and deaf subjects showed a large and comparable increase in finger EMG bursts during REM sleep. When they were awakened from REM sleep, deaf subjects showed about the same percentage of dream recall as is typical of hearing persons. In neither deaf nor in hearing persons, moreover, was finger EMG activity during NREM sleep particularly associated with recall of mental activity.

As regards the nature of dream content in deaf persons, the scientific literature remains sparse. Singer and Lenahan (1976) studied fantasy and imagination in twenty deaf 12- and 13-year-old children using material from storytelling, fantasies, and recall of (home) dreams. In general, the fantasy material of these children seemed more concrete and unimaginative than that of their hearing peers. At the same time, their dreams often dwelt on themes of trauma, pain, and loss (e.g., "going to the hospital to have my tonsils out" or "my sister going to the hospital and losing her baby").

Indeed, the topic of dreams in the deaf could be further investigated. It is now known, for example, that both the mental and emotional development of deaf persons can be profoundly affected by whether or not they learn a language early in life, such as American sign language or signed English (Sacks, 1990). Does the presence or absence of language, and the many intellectual attainments that go with it, also have an impact on the mental activity we call dreaming?

We might also ask whether the finger movements of deaf subjects during sleep could be interpreted by someone familiar with sign language. That is, are these finger movements the equivalent of SLEEPTALKING in hearing individuals? There remains the possibility that, even though the overall rates of finger movement activity (forearm EMG bursts) are about the same in the deaf and the hearing, the visible finger movements of the deaf are linguistic utterances, whereas those of hearing persons are more or less random activity without linguistic significance. Anecdotal evidence suggests that this may be the case. Sacks (1990, p. 35), for example, mentions the case of an elderly deaf woman on Cape Cod. Her daughter, who understood sign language, reported that she had often observed her mother making partially intelligible finger movements ("fragmentary signs") as she lay with her hands on the counterpane during afternoon naps.

REFERENCES

Max LW. 1935. An experimental study of the motor theory of consciousness. III. Action–current responses in deaf-mutes during sleep, sensory stimulation, and dreams. 19:469–486.

Sacks O. 1990. *Seeing voices: A journey into the world of the deaf.* New York: Harperperennial. The language and thought of the deaf engagingly described by a well-known neurologist.

Sarlin MB. 1984. The use of dreams in psychotherapy with deaf patients. *J Am Acad Psychoanal* 12: 75–88.

Singer DG, Lenahan ML. 1976. Imagination content in the dreams of deaf children. *Am Ann Deaf* 121:44–48.

Stoyva JM. 1965. Finger electromyographic activity during sleep: Its relation to dreaming in deaf and normal subjects. *J Abnormal Psychol* 70:543–549.

Johann Stoyva

DEATH

Human beings have expressed concern about morbid and mortal events during the night since recorded history. The Bible states that Solomon's bed was guarded by "sixty valiant men for fear of the night." In the Aeneid, Virgil called sleep "the kinsman of death." In the sixteenth century, St. John of the Cross also referred to the relationship among death, fear, and night. F. Scott Fitzgerald wrote: "In the real dark night of the soul it is always three o'clock in the morning." Ray Bradbury used the term "the soul's Midnight" to refer to the clock time 3 A.M. There is good scientific justification for such age-old concerns. Studies have found important physiological relationships between sleep and death.

Abnormally short or long sleep is a risk factor. In a nationwide study by the American Cancer Society, adults who said they slept less than 7 hours or more than 8 hours were 10 percent to 150 percent more likely to die over a 6-year follow-up period than adults who slept 7 to 8 hours. There is no clear answer as to why such people are more prone to die. They certainly did not all succumb to cancer; however, the finding of increased mortality in very short and very long sleepers has been corroborated by other studies and by polysomnographic recordings to measure actual sleep times. The most promising research on this issue is testing whether the many 24-hour cycles in human physiological functions, such as energy metabolism, sleep, and heart rate, may create windows in time when lethal events are more likely to happen; however, this research is slow and difficult because most people succumb to disease in circumstances that make it difficult to determine the precise time and sequence of the physiological events that actually caused the death.

Diurnal Rhythm of Death

There is a pattern of low points and high points throughout the 24-hour day in disease-related mortality that fits the diurnal low points and high points in the human tendency to fall asleep and to have sleep-related lapses in attention. Medical statistics dating to the late 1800s indicate that human mortality rises from a low between 12 midnight and 2 A.M. to a peak between 6 and 8 A.M.. Mortality data show a 60 percent increase in death from a nadir at about 2 A.M. to an apex at about 8 A.M. There is also a smaller peak at about 2 P.M. Figure 1 displays the temporal distribution around the 24 hours of over 437,000 disease-related mortalities. The large peak at 6 A.M. and the smaller peak at 2 P.M. coincide with known peaks in physiological tendency to fall asleep. Most of these deaths were due to ischemic heart disease. There is a similar two-peak pattern in nonlethal heart abnormalities as seen on electrocardiograms. Generally, the same 24-hour curve is also seen in the occurrence of lethal and nonlethal heart attacks documented by the presence of enzyme level changes characteristic of heart attack. Stroke or cerebrovascular accident (CVA) is another important cause of death that has its greatest effect during the usual hours of sleep. It

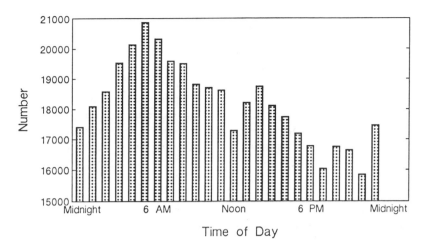

Figure 1. Temporal distribution for over 437,000 disease-related deaths.

appears that the two-peak temporal patterns observed in both sleep tendency and susceptibility to disease constitute a fundamental property of the human body.

The physiological changes that occur during REM sleep are thought to play a role in the timing of many lethal disease-related events. REM sleep, particularly in people with cardiovascular and pulmonary disease, is a time of increased risk for cardiac arrhythmias, respiratory insufficiency, and susceptibility to the toxic effects of sedative drugs and alcohol. (See SUDDEN DEATH IN ASIAN POPULATIONS; SUDDEN INFANT DEATH SYNDROME.)

REFERENCES

Baron RC, Thacker SB, Gorelkin L, Vernon AA, Taylor WR, Choi K. 1983. Sudden death among Southeast Asian refugees. An unexplained nocturnal phenomenon. *JAMA* 250:2947–2951.

Kripke DF, Simons RN, Garfinkel L, Hammond EC. 1979. Short and long sleep and sleeping pills. Is increased mortality associated? *Arch Gen Psychiatry* 36:103–116.

Mitler MM, Hajdukovich RM, Shafor R, Hahn PM, Kripke DF. 1987. When people die: Cause of death versus time of death. *Am J Med* 82:266–274.

Muller JE, Stone PH, Turi ZG, Rutherford JD, Czeisler CA, Parker C, Poole WK, Passamani E, Roberts R, Robertson T, et al. 1985. Circadian variation in the frequency of onset of acute myocardial infarction. *N Engl J Med* 313:1315–1322.

Merrill M. Mitler

DEEP SLEEP

See Depth of Sleep; NREM Sleep Mechanisms; Slow-Wave Sleep; Stages of Sleep

DELAYED SLEEP PHASE SYNDROME

OVERSLEEPING in the morning is common. It often follows a late night in which sleep was delayed for social or work-related reasons or after a trip to an easterly time zone. In such cases, the problem lasts only a few nights. For some people, however, it is never easy to get up in the morning (see EARLY BIRDS AND NIGHT OWLS).

Delayed sleep phase syndrome (DSPS) is a sleep disorder characterized by the inability to fall asleep and awaken according to ordinary schedules. Once asleep, REM/NREM sleep patterns are normal and not associated with sleep interruptions or early termination of sleep. Typically, the affected person is unable to fall asleep until 3 or 4 A.M. or later and finds it difficult or impossible to arise earlier than 10 or 11 A.M. Not surprisingly, severely affected persons have had difficulty in school or work, with a history of frequent tardiness and absenteeism. Those who work find that they cannot hold a "9 to 5" job and gravitate toward occupations with late working hours (restaurant, entertainment, hospital night-shift) or flexible hours (sales, writing, computer programming).

DSPS should be understood as a disorder of the timing of sleep, which is delayed to a relatively late time or phase of the 24-hour day (see TIMING OF SLEEP AND WAKEFULNESS). This is demonstrated by the success of a method of treatment called CHRONOTHERAPY, which progressively shifts the time of sleep.

Sleep in patients with DSPS occurs late, not only in relation to the time of day but also in relation to the BODY TEMPERATURE rhythm and probably additional CIRCADIAN RHYTHMS. It is therefore likely that DSPS results from an abnormality in the timing mechanism that governs sleep and wakefulness. Several abnormalities of the biological clock (see BIOLOGICAL RHYTHMS) have been hypothesized to explain DSPS. First, it is possible that the circadian clock may be unresponsive to stimuli, such as bright light, that normally shift sleep to an earlier time of day when given in the morning (see ZEITGEBERS; PHASE RESPONSE CURVE). Alternatively, the period of oscillation may be long, causing scheduled sleep periods to be delayed. Finally, it is possible that the morning stimuli that normally prevent delay of waking time, or the pathways of the brain by which the stimuli exert their effects, may be deficient.

Sleeping and waking are characteristically normal when people with DSPS do not follow an imposed sleeping schedule, as on vacations for example. Patients with DSPS who attempt to conform to a conventional sleeping and waking schedule report severe difficulty falling asleep, often resulting in futile attempts to reduce the delay in falling asleep with SLEEPING PILLS or ALCOHOL. They often seek psychiatric help to deal with the worries and ruminations that trouble them as they struggle to fall asleep and that they blame as the cause of their sleeplessness (see INSOMNIA). Further, people with DSPS must sometimes go to elaborate lengths to conform to an ordinary wake time, such as setting multiple ALARM CLOCKS or having family members drag them out of bed or throw cold water on them. Family strife may develop if the difficulty is assumed to reflect poor motivation. (Motivational problems associated with getting up in the morning such as school phobia do exist, however, and must be distinguished from DSPS.) Strongly motivated people with DSPS often succeed in waking and rising early but still cannot fall asleep until late, becoming increasingly sleep deprived until the weekend arrives, when they recover by sleeping long and late. It is remarkable that those with DSPS are unable to fall asleep before midnight despite multiple nights of sleep DEPRIVATION.

DSPS usually appears during late childhood or adolescence, but cases dating to infancy have been reported. Once established, it persists for many years and may be more severe in the autumn-winter months. It may affect 15 percent 20 percent of university students, resulting in lower academic performance.

Some may recognize in themselves a similar tendency to fall asleep late at night during the week and to sleep late on weekends. In contrast to DSPS, however, this tendency toward "eveningness" (see MORNINGNESS/EVENINGNESS) is not disabling. Eveningness is explained by the nearly universal tendency of human biological clocks to run more slowly than 24-hour clocks, tending to lengthen the subjective day. Rare individuals are unable to synchronize their periods of sleep and wakefulness with the 24-hour day at all. As a result, sleep periods tend to occur later everyday. Instead of being considered a sharply defined abnormality, then, DSPS may be thought of as lying near the middle of a spectrum ranging from eveningness, with its mild tendency to lengthen the day, to sleep patterns in which the day length cannot be limited to 24 hours (see HYPERNYCHT-HEMERAL SYNDROME).

REFERENCE

Weitzman ED, Czeisler CA, Coleman RM, Spielman AJ, Zimmerman JC, Dement W, Richardson G, Pollak CP. 1981. Delayed sleep phase syndrome: A chronobiologic disorder associated with sleep onset insomnia. *Arch Gen Psychiatry* 38:737–746. The first and most complete description of DSPS; includes case descriptions.

Charles P. Pollak

DELIRIUM TREMENS

Delirium tremens (DTs) is a very serious psychiatric/medical syndrome that occurs with acute ALCOHOL withdrawal and is characterized by extreme autonomic arousal manifested by tremors, fast heart rate, sweating, and subjective anxiety that can progress to extreme agitation and seizure. The syndrome frequently includes signs of dehydration, including fever, much evidence of perceptual distortion such as illusions and hallucinations, and psychosis; that is, the patient is delirious and is unable to remain oriented as to time, place, and person.

Perceptual distortions include HALLUCINATIONS such as seeing pink elephants or tactile hallucinations such as insects crawling all over the room and on or under the skin of the patient. The condition is very frightening to the patient and has about a 15 percent mortality untreated.

Delirium tremens is now most often treated with BENZODIAZEPINES. The main parameters of treatment effectiveness are a decreased pulse rate and the restoration of sleep.

Sleep disturbances are profound in DTs; some studies indicate that there is an alternation between hallucinations and rapid eye movement (REM) sleep which greatly contributes to the patient's delirium. Most patients with the DTs are nutritionally compromised in addition to being dehydrated, so vitamin B and magnesium deficiencies may play a part in the extreme agitation and lower seizure threshold as well as the disturbances in sleep.

In some patients, DTs end with what is called the *terminal sleep,* which may last up to 24 hours. REM sleep appears to be abnormal during this phase of recovery and sleep may in fact be a mixture of REM phenomena and stages 1 and 2. As the recovery process continues over the next 3 or 4 days, enormous REM rebounds (see REBOUND) may occur; however, REM sleep may continue to be abnormal because of partial failure of electromyographic suppression and fragmentation. SLOW-WAVE SLEEP may or may not recover after heavy drinking episodes that end in the DTs.

REFERENCE

Anch AM, Browman CP, Mitler MM, Walsh JK. 1988. *Sleep: A scientific perspective.* Englewood Cliffs, N.J.: Prentice-Hall.

Vincent P. Zarcone, Jr.

DELTA SLEEP

See Alpha-Delta Sleep; Slow-Wave Sleep

DELTA SLEEP–INDUCING PEPTIDE

See Chemistry of Sleep: Peptides

DE MAIRAN, JEAN JACQUES D'ORTOUS

Jean Jacques d'Ortous de Mairan (1678–1771), a French scientist, is credited by present-day biological rhythm researchers (chronobiologists) with the first experiment involving the isolation of an organism from daily time cues. Androsthenes, the ancient Greek chronicler of the marches of Alexander the Great, observed that the leaves of certain plants droop markedly during the night. For the next several thousand years everyone assumed that such "sleeping movements" of plants were simply due to the absence of sunlight and that the raising of a plant's leaves in the daytime was a simple reflex phenomenon. De Mairan apparently decided to see whether this was true. He placed a mimosa plant in a closet and peeked at it every so often for several days and nights. Like any good scientist, he repeated the experiment with more than one plant. What he found was that the plants continued to raise and lower their leaves on a daily basis despite the lack of sunlight.

De Mairan was reluctant to take the time to report his findings to the scientific world, being more occupied with his research on the physics of heat, motion, and the aurora borealis. However, as was customary at the time, a friend and colleague, M. Marchant, described de Mairan's observations on leaf motion in a paper to the French Royal Academy of Sciences in 1729. It is not known whether it was de Mairan or Marchant who reached the erroneous conclusion that the plant sensed the sun's movements. Almost 30 years later, another Frenchman, Henri-Louis Duhamel, confirmed de Mairan's observations and also showed that the movements were independent of temperature. More than 100 years passed before the Swiss botanist Augustin de Candolle showed that similar plants kept in constant light would continue to raise and lower their leaves about every 22 hours. This proved that the plants were not sensing the sun at all, because if they were, they should have "slept" every 24 hours. Instead, plants must contain some internal mechanism for telling time—in other words, a living biological clock. A multitude of experiments in the twentieth century, all using de Mairan's basic technique of time isolation, have shown beyond doubt that virtually all living organisms contain such biological clocks.

REFERENCES

Bunning E. 1973. *The physiological clock, circadian rhythms and biological chronometry,* 3rd ed. London: The English Universities Press.
Moore-Ede MC, Sulzman FM, Fuller CA. 1982. *The clocks that time us.* Cambridge, Mass.: Harvard University Press.
Ward RR. 1974. *The living clocks.* New York: Alfred A. Knopf.
Winfree AT. 1987. *The timing of biological clocks.* New York: Scientific American.

Daniel R. Wagner

DEMENTIA

Dementia refers to a generalized, progressive, and usually irreversible deterioration of the intellect. The progression may be rapid (over a period of weeks or months) or slow (over a period of years). Dementia is not an inevitable consequence of aging. Many elderly persons reach their seventies and eighties with only minimal decline in certain kinds of mental abilities. As such, dementia must be differentiated from *benign senescent forgetfulness* or so-called *age-associated memory impairment,* which are a normal part of growing old. It should also be pointed out that dementia may occur at any age. For example, patients with acquired immune deficiency syndrome (AIDS) often develop dementia when the virus enters the brain and destroys nerve cells.

Some dementias in old age are reversible. This means that if the condition causing the dementia is treated, the dementia will improve. Infections, metabolic derangements, and vitamin deficiencies are examples of such conditions, and they probably constitute about 10 percent to 15 percent of all dementias in old age. Another apparent type of dementia is called *pseudodementia* or *masked depression.* In this condition, individuals have symptoms of memory loss and cognitive

decline but when their DEPRESSION is treated, these symptoms improve. The largest proportion of elderly individuals with dementia have Alzheimer's disease, a progressive, invariably fatal condition characterized by distinctive changes in brain cells (see ALZHEIMER'S DISEASE for a more complete description of this disease). In the description of sleep disturbance that follows, the term *dementia* is meant to include both Alzheimer's disease and other dementias of old age as well. The reader interested in differences in sleep patterns and other phenomena among dementia syndromes is referred to references at the end of this article.

Often the most revealing descriptions of the tremendous disruption in normal sleep that occurs in dementia come from the caregivers (spouse, children) who take care of the patient. Typically, during the daytime hours, the patient appears docile and tranquil and may even doze. As evening approaches, however, the patient may become belligerent, hostile, and difficult to handle. The worst behavior may occur during the night, as the other family members try to sleep. The demented patient may become even more confused; he or she may wander outside or turn on the kitchen stove and leave the room. It is often at this point, when the family can no longer cope with the patient's behavior, that institutionalization often becomes neccessary. These types of behaviors are often lumped together under the more general term SUNDOWN SYNDROME. Most researchers typically define sundowning as agitation occurring concurrent with darkness; others prefer the term *nocturnal delirium* to describe this state. Sundowning differs from SLEEPWALKING and the REM SLEEP BEHAVIOR DISORDER. It probably occurs in about 30 percent of all demented patients at some point in their illness.

The mechanisms that cause sundowning are unknown. Because there appears to be some reversal of day/night functioning, researchers have speculated that sundowning occurs when certain areas in the brain controlling CIRCADIAN RHYTHMS (see SUPRACHIASMATIC NUCLEUS OF THE HYPOTHALAMUS) lose cells. If this hypothesis is correct, many physiological functions that show diurnal variation (body temperature, various hormones) should show abnormal rhythms in demented patients. Evidence to date does not support this hypothesis though it is an area of active research. One problem in studying sundowning physiologically is that it is extremely difficult to do studies on such patients, as they usually have difficulty tolerating the laboratory procedures.

When those demented patients who can tolerate the procedures are studied in the laboratory, the results are somewhat consistent. There is a virtual absence of SLOW-WAVE SLEEP (stages 3 and 4) and reduced sleep efficiency (time in bed actually spent asleep) relative to subjects of similar age who are not demented. Changes in REM sleep are complex. In normal aging, REM probably changes very little (see AGING AND SLEEP). Because REM sleep may partially depend on the neurotransmitter acetylcholine (see BRAIN MECHANISMS) and Alzheimer's disease has been linked to decreased levels of acetylcholine in the brain (see ALZHEIMER'S DISEASE; CHEMISTRY OF SLEEP), one might expect very little REM sleep in dementia. There is some evidence to support this hypothesis but because less REM sleep also occurs whenever there are many awakenings and arousals, this may simply be secondary to poor sleep. Some studies have even suggested elevated REM sleep in dementia.

One intriguing possibility that is the subject of much research is the possible role of sleep APNEA in dementia. If elderly persons have experienced years of repetitive nightly awakenings and drops in oxygen, might that eventually affect brain function? The answer to this question is not yet known. Some, but not all, studies have shown that sleep apnea does relate to some aspects of lower mental function, even separate from daytime sleepiness. There is no evidence at this time that treating sleep apnea has any effect on the progressive course of the dementia, though younger sleep apnea patients undergoing treatment often report better concentration, memory, and alertness.

Treatments for the sleep disturbance and nocturnal agitation (sundowning) accompanying dementia are generally poor. Many physicians use various kinds of medications. These range from typical SLEEPING PILLS (Halcion, Dalmane) to powerful TRANQUILIZERS (Haldol, Mellaril) to other medications affecting brain neurochemistry (Inderal, Catapres). Often the medications produce temporary improvement in the disruptive behaviors, but the effects seldom last. Additionally, some of these medications have side effects almost as bad as the sundowning itself (uncontrollable body movements, severe drops in blood pressure). A number of other nondrug treatments should at least be considered. One of the simplest (though often labor intensive) is the pre-vention of daytime dozing. There is good reason to believe that if the elderly, demented patient sleeps during the day, he or she is likely to be awake at night. This may require near-constant vigilance from the caregiver, who must constantly talk and, in some cases, gently move the patient to prevent dozing. Exposure to outdoor sunlight during the daytime may also be helpful not only in preventing daytime sleep but also in reinstituting a strong circadian sleep–wake cycle. For families caring for a demented family member, sundowning is a devastating condition with which to deal and often the family themselves need counseling and support.

REFERENCES

Bliwise DL. 1989. Dementia. In Kryger MH, Roth T, Dement WC, eds. *Principles and practice of sleep medicine,* pp 358–363. Philadelphia: Saunders.

Cummings JL, Benson DF. 1983. *Dementia: A clinical approach.* Boston: Butterworths.

Mace N, Rabins P. 1981. *The 36 hour day.* Baltimore: Johns Hopkins University Press.

Sleep disorders in the elderly. 1989. In *Clinics in geriatric medicine,* vol 5, No. 2. Philadelphia: Saunders.

Zarit S, Orr N, Zarit J. 1985. *The hidden victims of Alzheimer's disease: Families under stress.* New York: New York University Press.

Donald L. Bliwise

DE MANACÉINE, MARIE

See Deprivation, Total

DEPRESSION

Troubled minds have troubled sleep. It has long been recognized that the sleep patterns of patients with depression and other mood (affective) disorders are frequently disturbed, suggesting that sleep disturbance may be an integral part of these conditions. Most students recognize that sleep disturbance, such as the occasional ALL-NIGHTER, will also cause some disturbance in mood and performance. However, it turns out that the connection between mood and sleep is not a simple bidirectional one. For, whereas healthy adults often feel sluggish and slightly dysphoric the day after sleep DEPRIVATION, the same procedure results in clear (if short-lived) *improvements* of mood in depressed patients. Thus, while mood and sleep clearly interact with each other, they appear to interact differently in depressed patients and healthy subjects.

The study of sleep and depression in mood disorders holds interest for another reason as well: Many of the neurochemical and physiological processes involved in the regulation of sleep are also involved in the regulation of mood. Therefore, understanding sleep patterns in depressed patients may help in understanding the pathophysiology of depression itself.

What Are the Sleep Characteristics of Depression?

Before examining the sleep characteristics of depressed patients, it is important to identify what is meant by "depression." Unfortunately, this word has many meanings, ranging from a normal blue mood to a psychiatric disorder of major public health significance. In this discussion, "depression" will be used to denote the concept of *major depressive episode* as defined in the *Diagnostic and Statistical Manual* (DSM-III-R) of the American Psychiatric Association (Table 1). Depression defined in this way is a syndrome that includes not only mood disturbance, but distur-

Table 1.   Diagnostic Criteria for Major Depressive Episode

A. At least five of the following symptoms have been present during the same 2-week period and represent a change from previous functioning; at least one of the symptoms is either (1) depressed mood or (2) loss of interest or pleasure.

   (1) depressed or irritable mood most of the day, nearly every day, as indicated either by subjective account or observation by others

   (2) markedly diminished interest or pleasure in all, or almost all, activities most of the day, nearly every day

   (3) significant weight loss or weight gain when not dieting, or decrease or increase in appetite nearly every day

   (4) insomnia or hypersomnia nearly every day

   (5) psychomotor agitation or retardation nearly every day

   (6) fatigue or loss of energy nearly every day

   (7) feelings of worthlessness or excessive or inappropriate guilt nearly every day

   (8) diminished ability to think or concentrate, or indecisiveness, nearly every day

   (9) recurrent thoughts of death (not just fear of dying), recurrent suicidal ideation without a specific plan, or a suicide attempt or a specific plan for committing suicide

B. (1) It cannot be established that an organic factor initiated and maintained the disturbance.

   (2) The disturbance is not a normal reaction to the death of a loved one (uncomplicated bereavement).

C. At no time during the disturbance have there been delusions or hallucinations for as long as 2 weeks in the absence of prominent mood symptoms.

D. Not superimposed on schizophrenia, schizophreniform disorder, delusional disorder, or other psychotic disorders.

Adapted from the Diagnostic and Statistical Manual of Mental Disorders, Third Edition, Revised (DSM-III-R) of the American Psychiatric Association.

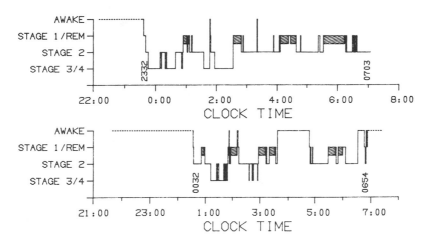

Figure 1. Representative sleep stage histograms for a young adult healthy control subject (top) and a young adult depressed patient. Compared with the control, the depressed patient has reduced REM latency (interval between stage 2 onset and REM onset), decreased stage 3 or 4 sleep, increased wake time, and a "flat" temporal pattern of REM sleep durations (i.e., all REM periods are about the same length in contrast to the lengthening of REM period durations in the control subject). The time axes are not identical for the two examples.

bance of other biological functions as well. The exact definition of depression is important in considering sleep research because sleep electroencephalographic findings are often compared to a "gold standard" diagnosis. In the case of depression, this gold standard is a clinical diagnosis based on signs and symptoms. Because the clinical diagnosis is itself imperfect and includes patients with various symptoms, one cannot expect sleep electroencephalographic studies to diagnose patients more accurately than this gold standard.

Subjectively, patients with depression complain most often of fragmented sleep, with difficulty falling asleep and frequent middle-of-night awakenings. The hallmark sleep disturbance in depression is EARLY MORNING AWAKENING: spontaneous awakening before the desired wakeup time and inability to fall back asleep. Depressed patients may also have increased dream activity, often with themes of pursuit, abandonment, or physical harm.

Electroencephalographic sleep studies in depressed patients have identified a fairly consistent constellation of findings that differentiate depressed patients from healthy control subjects. These findings include disrupted *sleep continuity* (such as prolonged sleep latency, increased number of awakenings, and early morning awakening); alterations of *sleep architecture* (includ-

ing decreased NREM stages 3-4 and small increases in REM sleep percent); and specific *REM sleep* findings (increased amount of REM sleep early in the night and increased phasic REM activity) (for review, see Reynolds and Kupfer, 1987). However, the hallmark sleep electroencephalographic finding in depression is a shortening of the first NREM period, also known as REM LATENCY. Representative "sleep histograms" for young control and depressed subjects are shown in Figure 1.

More sophisticated analytic techniques, such as period and amplitude analysis of the sleep electroencephalographic and electrooculographic signals, also show decreased amounts of SLOW-WAVE SLEEP (SWS) and increased REM activity in depressed patients. Similar findings have also been identified using power spectral analysis. These techniques further indicate that, not only are the absolute amounts of SWS and REM sleep activity altered in depression, but their temporal distribution across the night is also altered. Specifically, depressed patients show a decreased amount of SWS activity in the first NREM period and an increased amount of phasic REM activity early in the night. (See also TIMING OF SLEEP AND WAKEFULNESS.)

There is some controversy regarding the relationship between sleep electroencephalographic measures and severity of depression. Several early studies found direct relationships between severity and electroencephalographic findings such as REM latency. Other studies have not found as close a relationship. However, it remains clear that patients with psychotic depression (a particularly severe form of depression characterized by hallucinations or delusions) and patients who are hospitalized for their depression tend to have the most severe sleep disturbances.

Several investigators have examined various subtypes of major depression. The most robust findings have involved comparisons of patients with "endogenous" versus "nonendogenous" major depression. Endogenous refers to a specific symptom pattern with many biological symptoms, such as weight loss, loss of pleasure, and severe subjective sleep disturbance. When these two groups are compared, patients with the endogenous disorder have been found to have more severe electroencephalographic sleep abnormalities. Findings on distinctions, such as comparisons of patients with depression after medical illness versus those with "primary" depression, have been less consistent (see AFFECTIVE DISORDERS OTHER THAN MAJOR DEPRESSION; MEDICAL ILLNESS AND SLEEP).

Do Age or Gender Affect Sleep Electroencephalographic Findings in Depression?

Aging affects virtually all sleep electroencephalographic variables, even in healthy individuals. In general, the age-related findings of healthy individuals are mirrored by those in depressed individuals. In other words, the sleep electroencephalographic differences between healthy and depressed people remain across the adult life span. However, more recent evidence indicates that sleep electroencephalographic findings are more difficult to identify in children or adolescents with depression, whereas elderly depressed, demented, and control subjects are readily discriminated by the same measures. A recent metaanalysis of sleep electroencephalographic findings in depressed patients substantiates the impression that age-related changes may interact with depression, such that differences between depressed patients and healthy control subjects increase with age (Knowles and MacLean, 1990). (See also AGING AND SLEEP.)

There is much less evidence regarding gender differences in depression. In healthy adults, elderly women generally have better sleep continuity and more SWS than men. This same trend appears to be evident across the adult life span in depressed subjects, with depressed women experiencing much more SWS than depressed men (Reynolds et al., 1990).

Are Sleep Electroencephalographic Findings Related to an Episode of Depression or the Illness of Depression?

This question might also be phrased, "Are the sleep electroencephalographic changes in depression episodic (statelike) or persistent (traitlike)?" This has become an important question for researchers because it helps to define whether the sleep electroencephalographic changes seen in depression are a temporary phenomenon—a sign of predisposition to depression or a sign of "scarring" from the illness.

Several cross-sectional studies have suggested that the REM sleep findings in depression may improve after the individual recovers. Recent evidence also indicates that REM sleep findings may be more abnormal early in the episode, although once an episode is established, findings such as REM latency tend to remain stable. Cross-sectional studies have also indicated that some of the sleep continuity disturbance of depression seems to remain after remission.

There are actually very few longitudinal studies of sleep in depression. Available evidence suggests that most sleep electroencephalographic findings in depressed patients remain abnormal even after they are no longer depressed. This conclusion is also supported by a comparison of sleep electroencephalographic findings in patients who have experienced a single episode of depression versus those who have suffered numerous episodes during the course of their lifetime. These two groups tend to show very similar sleep electroencephalographic findings.

Another way of examining the question of episodic versus persistent changes is to perform family studies of depressed patients. Because a substantial portion of sleep electroencephalographic patterns are inherited (Linkowski et al., 1989) and because depressive illness clearly has a familial component, one might expect to see "depressive" sleep changes in the family members of depressed patients. In fact, this is just what has been found by Giles et al. (1988). In this study, family members of depressed patients who also had short REM latencies were more likely to have a past history of depression themselves.

How Do Sleep Findings in Depression Compare with Those in Other Psychiatric Disorders?

Given the large amount of research invested in the study of sleep and depression, it would be reasonable to ask whether these findings are characteristic of all psychiatric patients or only those with depression. The findings on this question have been contradictory, and are often difficult to interpret. For instance, a number of investigators have found similar shortening of REM sleep latency and decreases in the amount and temporal pattern of SWS in patients with schizophrenia (see PSYCHOPATHOLOGY). There appears to be better separation of depressed patients from those with anxiety disorders, eating disorders, and ALCOHOLISM. One of the main problems in comparing depressed patients with those with other psychiatric disorders is that many psychiatric patients may have more than one diagnosis. Alternatively, they may have family histories of another disorder. Thus, if a patient with schizophrenia has a personal or family history of depression, his or her sleep electroencephalographic characteristics may be determined in part by these factors, rather than purely by the illness of schizophrenia. The same situation is clearly true in patients with personality disorders.

Given these numerous complications and the difficulty with "gold standard" diagnoses noted earlier, it is not surprising that sleep electroencephalographic studies cannot be used very effectively as tools for diagnosis of specific mental disorders. For a further discussion of these issues, refer to Buysse and Kupfer (1990).

What Do Sleep Findings Tell Us About the Causes of Depression?

A number of theories have been advanced to explain the sleep electroencephalographic findings in depression and, at the same time, to comment on the causes of depression itself. A full discussion of this topic is clearly beyond the present discussion; refer to Wehr (1990) for further discussion.

One theory suggests that the sleep electroencephalographic findings in depression are consistent with increased activity of the neurotransmitter acetylcholine. According to this theory, depression may be caused in part by overactivity of cholinergic systems relative to systems driven by neuroenephrine, serotonin, and other neurotransmitters. This theory fits in nicely with findings of short REM sleep latency in depression, because REM sleep is thought to be driven mainly by cholinergic mechanisms (McCarley, 1982). Early studies examining the effects of infusion of cholinergic agents seem to support this hypothesis. Specifically, cholinergic drugs infused into depressed patients cause an earlier onset of REM sleep than a similar infusion in healthy control subjects. However, these studies have proven difficult to replicate. (See also CHEMISTRY OF SLEEP.)

Circadian rhythm theories postulate an abnormality in the 24-hour rhythms that govern sleep and wakefulness in depressed patients. An early version of this theory postulated that CIRCADIAN RHYTHMS governing REM sleep might be "phase advanced" in depressed patients (i.e., the peak in REM sleep propensity might occur earlier in depressed individuals) (Wehr and Wirz-Justice, 1981). While attractive in its simplicity, this theory has generally not been supported by empirical evidence in most groups of depressed patients. Another type of circadian rhythm theory has been set forth in the "Two-process" model of sleep regulation by Borbely and Wirz-Justice (1982). According to this theory, depression may be characterized by a deficient buildup in the homeostatic sleep factor, termed *Process S*. Evidence from sleep deprivation studies lends support to this theory, but it is less satisfactory at explaining the REM sleep abnormalities seen in depression.

Although less specific, a "sleep–mood" theory is suggested by results of sleep DEPRIVATION experiments. A variety of manipulations of the sleep–wake cycle seem to have directly beneficial effects on the mood of depressed patients. For instance, one night of total sleep deprivation, sleep deprivation in the second half of the night, or selective deprivation of REM sleep over a period of days or weeks can all lead to improvements in mood of depressed patients. While total and partial sleep deprivation have fairly short-lived effects, REM sleep deprivation may produce long-lasting benefits, as demonstrated by the elegant experiments of Vogel and colleagues (e.g., Vogel et al., 1980). These findings suggest that sleep itself may be "depressogenic" (Wu and Bunney, 1990) and that REM sleep in particular may be the cause. However, it is also possible that sleep deprivation has some effect on factors such as body temperature, circadian rhythms, hormones, or balance of various neurotransmitters (Wehr, 1990).

Sleep findings in depression have also been related to neuroendocrine changes in depression (see NEUROENDOCRINE HORMONES). These observations are important because sleep and various hormones may be regulated by similar neurochemical systems. Sleep–endocrine associations are suggested by the decrease in SWS and the decrease in sleep-associated GROWTH HORMONE secretion observed in depression. There is also evidence that the circadian rhythm of cortisol may be advanced in a similar manner to the advance of REM sleep relative to sleep onset. The sleep and endocrine changes characteristic of depression can be conceptualized in a model of episodic and persistent biological abnormalities in depression (Ehlers and Kupfer, 1987).

What Do Sleep Electroencephalographic Findings Tell Us About the Outcome of Depression?

Although sleep electroencephalographic studies have not emerged as important diagnostic tools in depression, they may tell us important information about the outcome of depression. A number of early studies indicate that early sleep changes in response to ANTIDEPRESSANT medication may presage favorable outcomes. Several other studies have confirmed this. Less information is available regarding sleep electroencephalographic measures and outcome during treatment with psychotherapy. However, recent studies appear to indicate that REM latency and other sleep measures do not predict success using cognitive-behavioral or interpersonal psychotherapy. Sleep electroencephalographic responses to one night of total sleep deprivation have yielded inconsistent findings. In one study of elderly adults, sleep electroencephalographic patterns during "recovery" sleep helped to predict ultimate outcome,

but in a study with middle-aged adults, sleep deprivation responses were not strongly connected to final medication treatment outcome.

Baseline sleep electroencephalographic findings, regardless of the type of treatment, may still be helpful for predicting ultimate outcome. For instance, both reduced REM sleep latency and reduced delta sleep in the first NREM period seem to predict earlier recurrences in patients with depression.

What Are the Future Directions in Sleep-Depression Research?

A number of advances have been made in sleep electroencephalographic studies in psychiatric illness over the past 20 years. These improvements include increased diagnostic precision, standardization of terminology and techniques, and increased attention to comorbid psychiatric and medical disorders. In the future, there will likely be further emphasis on "nonspecific" factors, such as the timing of the sleep period, social and physical time cues (ZEITGEBERS) that may affect sleep, and laboratory effects, which may be minimized by the use of in-home studies.

Further sophistication in sleep electroencephalographic analysis is also likely. For instance, increased attention will be paid to concepts such as nonlinear dynamics and "dimensionality" of sleep electroencephalographic signals. This type of technique can examine aspects of the electroencephalogram, such as its degree of complexity, that current analytic techniques do not examine.

It is also likely that there will be increased emphasis on the use of behavioral and neurochemical probes to examine the dynamic response of the sleep system in depressed patients. Specifically, the use of serotonergic and cholinergic agents, as well as more specific antidepressants, will continue. Behavioral probes such as phase shifts and sleep deprivation will also be used in longitudinal studies and studies examining treatment outcome.

A final trend is likely to involve the use of brain imaging techniques during sleep or sleep deprivation. For instance, positron emission tomography (PET) and nuclear magnetic resonance imaging (MRI) can be used to give functional "pictures" of the brain during sleep or sleep deprivation. The use of these techniques in depressed patients will contribute not only to our knowledge of sleep itself, but to the sleep changes characteristic of depressed patients.

Conclusions

Subjective and objective measures of sleep are disturbed in patients with clinical depression. Most evidence suggests that these findings are rather persistent and that they are most characteristic of patients with severe depression. There is emerging evidence for familial and perhaps even genetic aspects of the sleep changes in depression. An examination of sleep will contribute to our understanding of depression itself, as well as to our understanding of sleep regulation.

REFERENCES

Borbely AA, Wirz-Justice A. 1982. Sleep, sleep deprivation and depression: A hypothesis derived from a model of sleep regulation. *Hum Neurobiol* 1:205–210.

Buysse DJ, Kupfer DJ. 1990. Diagnostic and research applications of electroencephalographic sleep studies in depression: Conceptual and methodological issues. *J Nerv Ment Dis* 178:405–414.

Ehlers CL, Kupfer DJ. 1987. Hypothalamic peptide modulation of EEG sleep in depression: A further application of the S-process hypothesis. *Biol Psychiatry* 22:513–517.

Giles DE, Biggs MM, Rush AJ, Roffwarg HP. 1988. Risk factors in families of unipolar depression. I. Psychiatric illness and reduced REM latency. *J Affective Disord* 14:51–59.

Knowles JB, MacLean AW. 1990. Age-related changes in sleep in depressed and healthy subjects: A meta-analysis. *Neuropsychopharmacology* 3:251–259.

Linkowski P, Kerkhofs M, Hauspie R, Susanne C, Mendlewicz J. 1989. EEG sleep patterns in man: A twin study. *Electroencephalogr Clin Neurophysiol* 73:279–284.

McCarley RW. 1982. REM sleep and depression: Common neurobiological control mechanisms. *Am J Psychiatry* 139:565–570.

Reynolds CF, Kupfer DJ. 1987. State-of-the art review—sleep research in affective illness: State of the art circa 1987. *Sleep* 10:199–215.

Reynolds CF, Kupfer DJ, Thase ME, Frank E, Jarrett DB, Coble PA, Hoch CC, Buysse DJ, Simons AD, Houck PR. 1990. Sleep, gender, and depression: An analysis of gender effects on the electroencephalographic sleep of 302 depressed outpatients. *Biol Psychiatry* 28:673–684.

Vogel GW, Vogel F, McAbee RS, Thurmond AJ. 1980. Improvement of depression by REM sleep deprivation. *Arch Gen Psychiatry* 37:247–253.

Wehr TA. 1990. Effects of wakefulness and sleep on depression and mania. In Montplaisir J, Godbout R, eds. *Sleep and biological rhythms: Basic mechanisms and applications to psychiatry*, pp 42–86. New York: Oxford University Press.

Wehr TA, Wirz-Justice A. 1981. Internal coincidence model for sleep deprivation and depression. In *Sleep 1980, 5th European Congress on Sleep Research*, pp 26–33. Basel: Karger.

Wu JC, Bunney WE. 1990. The biological basis of an antidepressant response to sleep deprivation and relapse: Review and hypothesis. *Am J Psychiatry* 147:14–21.

Daniel J. Buysse
Charles F. Reynolds III
David J. Kupfer

DEPRIVATION

[*The effects of sleep deprivation are of interest from several perspectives. First, they can provide information about the function or functions of sleep; that is, what goes wrong when we don't sleep? A second major focus is the practical consequences of sleep loss. How does sleep loss interfere with mental or physical work? Which activities are affected most by sleep loss? A third focus is the consequences for mental and physical health.*

Because the effects of sleep deprivation are diverse and several kinds of sleep deprivation are possible, the topic is divided into a number of entries, including the topics that follow. A first obvious division is reflected in the two articles making up the entry on DEPRIVATION, TOTAL: PHYSIOLOGICAL EFFECTS *and* BEHAVIORAL EFFECTS. *In everyday life, however, partial deprivation of sleep is a much more common occurrence than total deprivation. Also included, therefore, is an article entitled* DEPRIVATION, PARTIAL. *Throughout the volume are other entries relevant to partial deprivation:* GRADUAL SLEEP REDUCTION; SLEEP RESTRICTION, THERAPEUTIC; *and* FRAGMENTATION. *Sleep may be partially reduced not only in total amount, but also by the selective elimination or restriction of specific sleep stages; accordingly, articles on selective deprivation of REM sleep and of NREM sleep appear under* DEPRIVATION, SELECTIVE.

Sleep reduction that results from pathological processes is covered in INSOMNIA *and* FATAL FAMILIAL INSOMNIA. *Sleep reduction voluntarily induced is covered in* OVER-THE-COUNTER STIMULANTS, SHIFTWORK, ADOLESCENCE, *and* ALL-NIGHTERS. *The article on* LONGEVITY *notes a possible serious consequence of chronic sleep deprivation. The article on* SHORT SLEEPERS IN HISTORY AND LEGEND *may also have relevance to the issue of sleep deprivation; however, it is generally not clear whether such individuals were sleep deprived or simply needed little sleep.*]

DEPRIVATION, PARTIAL

Partial sleep deprivation refers to a simple reduction in the amount of total sleep allowed per day. It is certainly the most common form of sleep deprivation seen. As might be expected, the behavioral effects from partial sleep deprivation when it is severe are very similar to those seen during total sleep loss (see DEPRIVATION, TOTAL: BEHAVIORAL EFFECTS).

Many studies have examined the effect of one or more nights of reduced sleep on performance and sleep variables. For example, Wilkinson (1968) varied sleep by allowing either 0, 1, 2, 3, 5, or 7.5 hours in which to sleep. Decreases in performance were found the following day when sleep was reduced below 3 hours for one night or was set at 5 hours for two consecutive nights. Increased sleepiness as measured by how quickly subjects can fall asleep has been observed when 5 hours of sleep per night was maintained for 4 nights. When the time available for sleep was reduced to 6 hours for 42 days, differences were not found for any daytime measures; however, when the time available for sleep was reduced to 5.5 hours for 60 days, a decrease in performance was found in the final 2 weeks.

In a different experimental paradigm subjects had their available sleep time shortened in 30-minute steps every 2 to 4 weeks from 8 hours until the subjects were unwilling to continue sleep reduction. The mean level of time in bed that both 8- and 6.5-hour baseline sleepers were able to reduce to was 5.0 hours. During sleep reduction, subjects reported having less difficulty in falling asleep and feeling less rested. Subjects began to complain of discomfort (fatigue and falling asleep in class and difficulty remaining

vigilant while driving) between 6 and 6.5 hours of time in bed. Although significant performance decline was not found on psychomotor tests, subjects nonetheless felt impaired. One said, "I am noticeably less efficient, less energetic; e.g., I can't seem to study as long as I used to, I get discouraged more easily, slightly depressed about overcoming difficulties, very much like I feel when I am sick with a cold" (Freidmann et al., 1977). The 6.5-hour sleepers returned to their baseline sleep levels at the end of the experiment; however, the original 8-hour sleepers reported on sleep logs that they were sleeping between 6.1 and 6.4 hours per night throughout a 1-year follow-up period.

Most partial sleep deprivation designs allowing more than 3 hours of sleep result primarily in reductions in REM and stage 2 sleep because of the distribution of sleep stages across the night (see STAGES OF SLEEP; DEPRIVATION, SELECTIVE). However, the acute partial sleep deprivation studies suggest that all stages of sleep except stages 3 and 4 are reduced during sleep restriction. Recovery sleep following a night of sleep reduced to 2 to 4 hours may differ very little from baseline if the recovery sleep period is held to 8 hours. If subjects have no set awakening time, the increased total sleep consists primarily of stage 2 and REM sleep (Webb and Agnew, 1975). In terms of sleep stages, amounts of all stages except stages 3 and 4 remained reduced as the number of partial deprivation nights was increased. In some cases, the amount of stage 4 sleep even increased during chronic sleep reduction; however, even after 8 nights on a 3-hour sleep schedule, no increase in stage 3 and 4 sleep was seen during the recovery sleep night.

Reduced sleep, usually in a chronic sense, is seen in many important groups, including doctors, soldiers, shiftworkers, mothers, and cross-country truck drivers. A number of studies have examined sleep, mood, and performance in doctors at various levels of training during their "on-call" work nights. Ninety percent of studies that examined various types of performance or mood in doctors who had slept an average of 2.8 hours, compared with recent baseline sleep amounts of 7.1 hours, reported significantly worse performance on at least one test or mood scale (Bonnet, 1991). As might be expected, performance decrement was more likely in doctors with less experience, on reasoning tasks, or on nonstimulating tasks. The performance impact was less than accompanying changes in mood. Even the reported baseline sleep amounts in doctors were about an hour reduced from prehospital baseline sleep amounts in the same doctors. This implies that most of these doctors continued to be partially sleep deprived even when they were not in the acute "on-call" situation.

Several sleep and circadian influences, situational characteristics, individual traits, and task characteristics influence the degree to which partial sleep loss affects behavior (see DEPRIVATION, TOTAL: BEHAVIORAL EFFECTS). Partial sleep loss may also be precipitated by frequently disturbed sleep (see FRAGMENTATION). Most normal young adults who sleep 8 hours can probably tolerate a 2-to 3-hour chronic reduction in their daily sleep amount without the accumulation of significant daytime functional compromise. It could, however, be argued that 2-to 3-hour reductions in total sleep produce mild decrements that cannot be shown statistically or that can be overcome by subject motivation in the laboratory test situation. Other scientists believe that human beings have a "core" sleep requirement of approximately 4 to 6 hours per day (Horne, 1987). In nutrition, there is a difference between the absolutely required calories, vitamins, and minerals and the meals that we eat. Similarly, for sleep, it is possible that the core 4 to 6 hours of sleep may maintain us without accumulating sleep debt. Like dessert after dinner, however, those last few hours of sleep seem particularly sweet.

REFERENCES

Bonnet MH. 1991. Sleep deprivation. In Kryger M, Roth T, Dement WC, eds. *Principles and practice of sleep medicine,* 2nd ed. Philadelphia: Saunders.

Freidmann J, Globus G, Huntley A, Mullaney D, Naitoh P, Johnson L. 1977. Performance and mood during and after gradual sleep reduction. *Psychophysiology* 14(3):245–250.

Horne J. 1987. *Why we sleep.* New York: Oxford University Press.

Webb WB, Agnew HW Jr. 1975. The effects on subsequent sleep of an acute restriction of sleep length. *Psychophysiology* 12(4):367–370.

Wilkinson RT. 1968. Sleep deprivation: Performance tests for partial and selective sleep deprivation. *Prog Clin Psychol* 8:28–43.

Michael H. Bonnet

DEPRIVATION, SELECTIVE

[*This composite entry comprises an article by Elizabeth B. Klerman on studies in which subjects are deprived of NREM sleep alone, and a discussion by Gerald Vogel of selective REM sleep deprivation.*]

NREM Sleep

NREM sleep constitutes the majority of mammalian sleep patterns (see NREM SLEEP MECHANISMS). Many studies have sought the relative importance and purposes of REM sleep and NREM sleep by comparing the effects of REM and NREM sleep deprivation (SD). By depriving subjects of only NREM sleep, experimenters hope to learn about NREM sleep's function and relative importance. Specifically, what are the changes in the subject's physiology, performance, and mood during and after NREM SD? Also, in the undisturbed sleep after the SD, is there more NREM sleep than usual, and if so, is the increase proportional or equal to that "missed"? Is there less of some other sleep stage during recovery? What other changes are seen on the electroencephalogram (EEG)?

There are several complications in doing a selective NREM sleep deprivation study. First, it is impossible to have NREM SD without REM SD. Because REM sleep rarely occurs before NREM sleep within a sleep episode, eliminating NREM sleep also prevents REM sleep from occurring. Therefore, most NREM SD studies only deprive the subject of the part of NREM sleep known as SLOW-WAVE SLEEP (SWS, or sleep stages 3 and 4 in humans) or stage 4 sleep alone (see STAGES OF SLEEP). If relative NREM SD is desired, then sleep restriction regimens in which subjects sleep less than usual can be used. Second, the subject must spend some time in the sleep state before the researcher recognizes that the subject is in that sleep state and intervenes. Therefore, deprivation is not complete, although much lower levels than usual of the sleep state are achieved. Third, the subject's EEG can still have delta frequency waves (the postulated important component of SWS) in other stages of sleep but not at the level which defines stage 3 or stage 4 sleep. Finally, although studies differ as to whether the intervention causes arousal or just a switch into another stage of sleep, the SD procedure causes sleep disruption, in addition to deprivation, and therefore causes changes in sleep architecture. The disruptions occur even if the procedure does not cause arousals or a significant loss of total sleep time.

There are few or no performance or mood effects of SWS deprivation. Agnew, Webb, and Williams (1964, 1967) noted that the subjects were "physically uncomfortable, withdrawn, less aggressive and manifest(ing) concern over vague physical complaints and changes in bodily feeling." However, other studies have not found this as a consequence of stage 4 SD alone. Instead, the changes seen are the same after SWS deprivation, REM SD, or a sleep episode with the same number and timing of disruptions. Therefore, any changes in performance and subjective measures are probably a result of sleep disruption rather than SWS deprivation. Some studies, however, may have found slight decreases in long-term memory or a specific type of recall after stage 4 SD that continued through the recovery nights.

A study of NREM SD in animals was done to determine whether NREM sleep is physically necessary. Rats were deprived of high-amplitude NREM sleep, a sleep stage that is similar to human SWS. After several weeks of SD, the animals died. Some REM SD also occurred during the high-amplitude NREM SD. Therefore, a combination of NREM and REM sleep is required to survive. During the experiment, the animals ate more, but they still lost weight and had changes in body temperature. These observations are consistent with current hypotheses of the role of NREM sleep in temperature and energy homeostasis. More studies are needed to replicate in part these results in humans and other species.

The timing of interventions to interrupt the sleep stage changes during the SD. SWS deprivation or stage 4 SD requires more interventions in the beginning of the sleep episode (early evening) than later in the episode. This differs from selective REM sleep deprivation in which more interventions are required late in the sleep episode (which corresponds to the early morning). If the deprivation is for an entire night's sleep episode, more interventions are required for stage 4 SD than for REM SD.

After NREM SD ends, subjects have more NREM or stage 4 sleep than usual. However, as after total sleep deprivations (see DEPRIVATION, TOTAL), not all of the minutes of stage 4 sleep lost during the deprivation are recovered and total sleep time is not prolonged. The amount of stage 3 sleep in the first recovery sleep may decrease as stage 4 sleep increases—the difference between stage 3 and stage 4 sleep is in the quantity of high-amplitude delta frequency waves—or both stage 3 and stage 4 sleep may increase. There is usually less Stage 2 sleep. REM sleep is increased on first or later recovery nights in some but not all studies.

The frequencies of the waves in the EEG also change during and after deprivation. During stage 4 SD, some researchers have found decreases in electroencephalographic activity not only in the delta frequency range (0.5 to 5 cycles per second), but also in the theta frequencies (4 to 7 cycles per second). Activity in the delta frequency range is usually associated with stages 3 and 4 and activity in the theta frequency range with REM sleep. During recovery sleep, either during the second half of the night or during the following morning, there were increases in delta and theta frequency activity, with decreases in spindle activity (12 to 14 cycles per second).

In conclusion, selective deprivation of SWS or stage 4 sleep is followed by increases in delta frequency activity in and duration of SWS, but no specific psychological or performance changes, except possibly a change in some memory tests.

REFERENCES

Agnew HW Jr., Webb WB, Williams RL. 1964. The effects of stage four sleep deprivation. *Electroencephalogr Clin Neurophysiol* 17:68–70.

——. 1967. Comparison of stage four and 1-REM sleep deprivation. *Percept Mot Skills* 24:851–858.

Bonnet MH. 1986. Performance and sleepiness following moderate sleep disruption and slow wave sleep deprivation. *Physiol Behav* 37:915–918.

Gilliland MA, Bergmann BM, Rechtschaffen A. 1989. Sleep deprivation in the rat: VIII. High EEG amplitude sleep deprivation. *Sleep* 12:53–59.

Elizabeth B. Klerman

REM Sleep

In humans and most mammals two different kinds of sleep, NREM and REM sleep, cyclically alternate with each other. REM sleep deprivation (RSD) is a condition in which only REM sleep is reduced, without a marked reduction of NREM sleep. Effects of RSD have suggested prominent theories about the function of REM sleep: that REM sleep plays a prominent role in mental health and in behaviors related to mental health, in learning and memory consolidation, and in regulation of body temperature and energy exchange. REM sleep deprivation is artificially produced by 1-to 3-minute awakenings when the onset of REM sleep is identified. Because NREM sleep necessarily follows wakefulness, the awakened subject returns to NREM sleep. After a period of NREM sleep, REM sleep begins and another awakening is made. This sequence is repeated for the duration of the RSD experiment. Both humans and animals have been REM sleep deprived, and several different methods have been developed for awakening animals from REM sleep.

Original Studies of REM Sleep Deprivation in Humans

The first studies of RSD were done for 3 to 7 consecutive nights in human subjects (Dement, 1960). Three effects of the RSD procedure were reported: (1) On consecutive nights of RSD, the number of awakenings required progressively increased. (2) More REM sleep occurred on nights immediately after RSD than on nights immediately before RSD. This increase in REM sleep after RSD was called REM REBOUND. The amount and duration of REM rebound were roughly proportional to the number of nights of RSD. Hence, in proportion to its debt, REM sleep loss stimulated REM sleep, not NREM sleep. This selective rebound suggested a specific need of the body or brain for REM sleep. Historically, this finding was the first indication that REM sleep was an autonomous state, different from NREM sleep. An implication was that REM sleep and NREM sleep have different functions. Much of the subsequent work on REM sleep was based on this implication of the early RSD experiments. (3) The original studies also reported that nocturnal RSD produced daytime psychological harm, such as anxiety, irritability, and difficulty concentrating. These symptoms disappeared as soon as the RSD stopped on the day after the first night of REM rebound.

The dramatic report that RSD caused psychological harm was theoretically related to the original view that dreaming occurred only during REM sleep. Hence, RSD was considered the equivalent of dream deprivation. The theory held that dreams "discharged" psychological tensions accumulated during the day. According to the theory, dream deprivation caused harm by preventing tension discharge. It was speculated that long-term dream deprivation would cause dreamlike mentation to spill over into waking life and produce hallucinatory psychosis including schizophrenia. Conversely, this theory claimed that dreaming protected mental health.

Later laboratory results refuted these speculations. RSD was not dream deprivation, because dreaming frequently occurred during sleep onset and during NREM sleep. In later studies, RSD produced no psychological harm (Vogel, 1975). Re-examination of the earlier RSD studies indicated that the subjects may have reported psychological symptoms because the experimenters suggested to them that "dream deprivation" had harmful psychological effects. When the suggestion was not made, no harm was reported. Waking schizophrenics who hallucinated showed no concurrent signs of REM sleep, and RSD in schizophrenics did not intensify their symptoms. Hence, schizophrenia was not an intrusion of dreaming into waking life. The ancient hypothesis of a relation between dreaming and madness was not supported.

Original Studies of REM Sleep Deprivation in Animals

In laboratory animals, RSD induced by awakenings for two to four 24-hour periods had the same effects on REM sleep as it did in humans. The number of awakenings during RSD steadily increased with the duration of the procedure. After the RSD, a REM rebound occurred that was proportional to the amount of prior RSD. In animals, RSD increased brain excitability. For example, the brain's electrical amplification of sensory signals was increased by RSD. Also, RSD reduced the amount of electrical current required to produce convulsions. RSD in animals also increased certain behaviors, including aggressive, sexual, locomotor, pleasure-seeking, and feeding behaviors. One theory about these findings is that RSD increases the excitability of the brain substrate responsible for drive-related behaviors.

Antidepressant Effects of REM Sleep Deprivation

The conclusion that RSD was psychologically harmless set the stage for considering noninjurious effects of RSD on mental health. Several findings led to the idea that RSD would improve endogenous DEPRESSION, a very severe kind of depression. (1) ANTIDEPRESSANT drugs that improved endogenous depression also decreased REM sleep much more than nonantidepressant drugs. (2) Drugs that increased REM sleep produced depression. (3) Prominent symptoms of endogenous depression (e.g., decreased aggressive, sexual, feeding, and pleasure-seeking activities) were opposite to the behavioral effects of RSD in animals. In an empirical test, RSD for 3 to 10 weeks improved patients' endogenous depression for months to years, much the same as antidepressant medications.

REM sleep deprivation was too laborious to be a practical treatment for depression. The main implication of its beneficial effect was the suggestion that antidepressant drugs work by producing RSD. In support of this hypothesis, 22 of 25 current antidepressant drugs were shown to produce (like REM sleep deprivation by arousals) large persistent RSD followed by a REM rebound. Nonantidepressant drugs did not have this effect. Yet, the theory cannot easily explain the three exceptional antidepressant drugs that do not decrease REM sleep, and hence it remains controversial.

Cognitive Effects of REM Sleep Deprivation

In animals, RSD impaired memory for tasks learned before RSD. For example, prior to RSD, rats learned that unless they moved to another part of their cage after a sound signal, they received a mild electric foot shock. After RSD, the memory of rats for the avoidance procedure was impaired. Subsequent animal studies indicated that RSD impaired new LEARNING rather than MEMORY. For example, after RSD, rats did not learn to avoid a painful stimulus as well as they learned

before RSD. The conclusion that in animals RSD impairs either memory or new learning remains unsettled because of technical or methodological problems in these studies. In humans, RSD for a single night did not impair learning. Thus, the implication that REM sleep functions to consolidate memory or to facilitate learning remains unproven.

Effects of REM Sleep Deprivation on Energy Regulation

Long-term RSD in rats resulted in a decline in body temperature in spite of an apparently compensatory increase in heat production. The implication for normal function is that REM sleep functions to prevent excessive heat loss (see THERMOREGULATION). In these experiments on energy regulation of rats, RSD for about 5 weeks was fatal. No structural changes in the brain were found on autopsy. The cause of death in the RSD animals remains unknown.

Summary

In humans, RSD is not dream deprivation, does not cause psychological harm, improves endogenous depression, and may be related to how antidepressant drugs work. In animals, RSD increases drive-related behaviors, may impair learning, increases bodily heat loss, and over several weeks is fatal.

REFERENCES

Dement WC. 1960. The effect of dream-deprivation. *Science* 131:1705–1707.

Ellman SJ, Speilman AJ, Luck D, Steiner S, Halperin R. 1991. REM deprivation: A review. In Arkin AM, Antrobus JS, Ellman SJ, eds. *The mind in sleep: Psychology and psychophysiology,* 2nd ed, pp 329–368. New York: Wiley.

Vogel GW. 1975. A review of REM sleep deprivation. *Arch Gen Psychiatry* 32:749–761.

Gerald Vogel

DEPRIVATION, TOTAL

[*In this composite entry, the effects of total sleep deprivation are discussed from a behavioral point of view by Michael H. Bonnet, and from a physiological point of view by Bernard Bergmann.*]

Behavioral Effects

In 1965, Randy GARDNER, a 17-year-old high school student, chose to remain awake for 264 hours as the topic of his science fair project (Dement, 1976). Randy was carefully monitored by sleep researchers and was quite successful in maintaining wakefulness. He had difficulty staying awake during the night and objected when observers would not allow him to close his eyes for long periods; however, he was able to play an arcade baseball game sufficiently well during his last night of sleep deprivation to beat the observer watching him consistently, and he was able to conduct himself well at a nationally attended press conference at the end of his vigil. Randy also recovered from his period of sleep deprivation by having one period of 14 hours and 40 minutes of recovery sleep. Randy's story is exceptional in that he was able to maintain a high level of physical activity and received national television coverage during his sleep deprivation. These factors certainly helped him stay awake.

In more normal circumstances, Kleitman (1963) asked research subjects to lie in bed at night and stay awake. Subjects had much difficulty remaining awake between 3:00 and 6:00 A.M. on the first night. During a second night of sleep deprivation, subjects had to get up and move around to maintain wakefulness. Even then, some could not stay awake. Following each night of sleep loss, the sleepiness diminished and subjects could perform more routine activities for at least short periods. If subjects were sitting or lying down, however, sleepiness would return with increasing rapidity so that they would be unable to take comprehensible lecture notes or a pulse reading because they lost concentration after 15 to 20 seconds.

These two examples illustrate some of the many factors that control our ability to remain awake (Bonnet, 1991). The contrasts in these examples also imply that one can do several things to exacerbate or diminish the effects of sleep loss The following sections explore several of the major factors that control the response to sleep loss.

Sleep/Circadian Influences

How an individual responds to sleep loss depends on when and how much he or she last slept. Performance during a period of sleep loss also depends on the time of day. Figure 1 shows how the ability to perform addition problems correctly declines over 64 hours of sleep loss. Performance declines over the first night but then improves on the second evening (time of day effect) before dropping again on the second night. Thus, CIRCADIAN RHYTHMS of performance influence the effects of sleep deprivation.

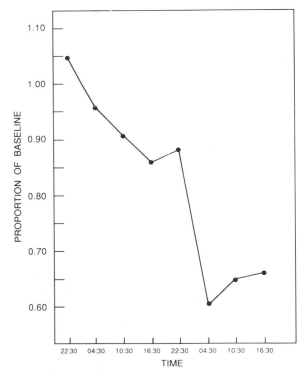

Figure 1. Proportion of the baseline number of correctly completed addition problems in repeated 1-hour test sessions over a period of 64 hours of sleep deprivation.

Situational Characteristics

The effects of sleep loss, particularly in early stages, are highly dependent on external influences including noise, exercise, temperature, and drugs. Some of these factors may briefly reverse all measurable decrements caused by sleep loss.

Noise It is generally assumed that NOISE increases arousal level, which may not be helpful during normal wakefulness, but will usually help during sleep loss.

Exercise A period of EXERCISE immediately before performing tasks provides transient reversal of some decrements secondary to sleep loss; however, more ambitious studies comparing relatively continuous high activity (eg, riding a stationary bike) and low activity continuing over 40- to 64-hour periods of sleep deprivation have shown no beneficial effects of exercise on overall performance (Webb and Agnew, 1973).

Temperature Although changing temperature is commonly used to help maintain alertness, there is very little research on how ambient (surrounding) temperature interacts with sleep loss. One study has shown that heat (92° F) was effective in increasing performance above baseline sleep deprivation levels on a vigilance task for the initial minutes of that test (Poulton, Edwards, and Colquhoun, 1974).

Drugs Many drugs have been studied in conjunction with sleep loss. Most studies have examined stimulants such as AMPHETAMINES and CAFFEINE. Although amphetamine typically does not improve performance in individuals who have had normal sleep, positive effects on mood, performance, and alertness have been found following sleep deprivation. In recent years, beneficial effects of caffeine during all-night work shifts (which involve only minor sleep deprivation) have been shown. The ingestion of 300 milligrams of caffeine at 11:00 P.M. significantly increased alertness for 7.5 hours (Walsh et al., 1990). Repeated use of caffeine was effective in maintaining performance near baseline levels for 24 hours of sleep loss but was unable to overcome the profound drop in performance characteristically seen during the second night of total sleep loss.

Subject Characteristics

The impact of sleep loss on a given individual depends on several characteristics that each participant brings to the sleep loss situation. Because sleep loss effects accumulate slowly, brief increases in motivation or interest may temporarily overcome them. Other characteristics, such as age and personality, may also modulate the effects of sleep loss.

Interest and Motivation All-night poker or video games demonstrate how an interesting task arouses individuals and can help them maintain performance for as long as 50 hours of sleep loss. Knowledge of results, for example, the publication of daily test results for all subjects to see, was sufficient motivation to remove the effects of one night of sleep loss. Even the knowledge that a prolonged episode of sleep deprivation was going to end in a few hours was sufficient incentive for performance to improve by 30 percent.

Repeated Periods of Sleep Loss Performance loss increases with the number of exposures to sleep loss (Webb and Levy, 1984). Increasingly poor performance may be secondary to decreased motivation or secondary to familiarization with the sleep deprivation paradigm (reduced stress resulting in decreased arousal).

Age Age appears to play a relatively minor role in the response of humans to sleep loss. Performance and alertness tests in normal older subjects undergoing sleep loss reveal a decrease in performance and alertness similar to that seen in younger individuals. (See AGING AND SLEEP.)

Good Versus Poor Sleepers Sleep loss had no greater impact (and perhaps less impact) on insomniacs than on matched normal sleepers. This implies that insomniacs do not suffer from chronic partial sleep deprivation (see INSOMNIA).

Personality and Psychopathology Mood changes, including increased sleepiness, fatigue, irritability, difficulty in concentrating, and disorientation are commonly reported during periods of sleep loss. Illusions and HALLUCINATIONS, primarily of a visual nature, occur in a significant number of normal individuals. Visual misperceptions increase if highly visual tasks are required. Such visual misperceptions are normally quite easy to differentiate from the primarily auditory hallucinations of a schizophrenic patient, but about 2 percent of normal individuals undergoing 112 hours of sleep loss expressed significant paranoid thoughts (Tyler, 1955). Some predisposition toward psychotic behavior existed in individuals who experienced significant paranoia during sleep loss. The paranoid behavior tended to become more pronounced during the night, partially recover during the day, and disappeared after recovery sleep. Sleep deprivation combined with social isolation and disinformation was used on American prisoners in the Korean conflict as a means of obtaining false confessions.

Test Characteristics and Types

The response to sleep deprivation is critically dependent on the characteristics of the test used. Several specific characteristics of psychomotor tests, including length of task, availability of results, task pacing, task complexity, and short-term memory requirement have been identified as factors that determine the effect of sleep loss (Bonnet, 1991). Ability to perform during sleep loss decreases as a task becomes longer, when outcome information is not given, when the task is timed, when the task is complex or performed under time pressure, when the task requires the use of short-term memory, or when the task involves newly learned skills. Responses during sleep loss may occur as rapidly as before, but those responses tend to be more stereotyped and less creative. Mood changes, such as increased fatigue and sleepiness, are some of the earliest indicators of sleep loss. The interaction of situational and test characteristics predicts that it should be relatively easy to remain awake playing a stimulating game but difficult to memorize a large number of Latin words under time pressure or to write an original play.

Recovery from Sleep Loss

As indicated by the Randy Gardner story, humans recover from even long periods of total sleep deprivation very rapidly and do not require nearly as much recovery sleep as they lost during deprivation. Young adults appear able to return to baseline levels after as much as 64 hours of

sleep loss with just one 8- to 10-hour sleep period, though full recovery may be delayed until 6 to 10 hours after waking up.

Other Types of Sleep Loss

It is much more usual that we will lose part of a night of sleep rather than being required to remain awake all night. The effects of partial sleep deprivation and selective sleep deprivation are covered in other entries. Individuals who have frequently disturbed sleep also behave as if they have been sleep deprived (see DEPRIVATION, PARTIAL; DEPRIVATION, SELECTIVE; FRAGMENTATION).

REFERENCES

Bonnet MH. 1991. Sleep deprivation. In Kryger M, Roth T, Dement WC, eds. *Principles and practice of sleep medicine,* 2nd ed. Philadelphia: Saunders.

Dement WC. 1976. *Some must watch while some must sleep.* San Francisco: San Francisco Book Company.

Kleitman N. 1963. *Sleep and wakefulness,* 2nd ed. Chicago: University of Chicago Press.

Poulton EC, Edwards RS, Colquhoun WP. 1974. The interaction of the loss of a night's sleep with mild heat: Task variables. *Ergonomics* 17(1):59–73.

Tyler DB. 1955. Psychological changes during experimental sleep deprivation. *Dis Nervous System* 16:293–299.

Walsh JK, Muehlbach MJ, Humm TM, Dickins QS, Sugerman JL, Schweitzer PK. 1990. Effect of caffeine on physiological sleep tendency and ability to sustain wakefulness at night. *Psychopharmacology* 101:271–273.

Webb WB, Agnew HW Jr. 1973. Effects on performance of high and low energy-expenditure during sleep deprivation. *Percept Motor Skills* 37(2):511–514.

Webb WB, Levy CM. 1984. Effects of spaced and repeated total sleep deprivation. *Ergonomics* 27(1):45–58.

Michael H. Bonnet

Physiological Effects

The term "total sleep deprivation" is used to describe both procedures for stopping all sleep in a subject (human or animal) and the nearly complete loss of sleep that results from such procedures. There are many ways sleep loss can occur, such as by taking drugs like amphetamines, which promote wakefulness, or as a result of diseases, such as sleep apnea. However, "total sleep deprivation" usually refers to researchers' deliberate elimination of sleep in subjects by arousing them whenever they get sleepy.

Why would researchers deprive humans or animals of sleep? Many researchers think that sleep has one or more important physiological functions (see FUNCTIONS OF SLEEP), but these functions are not obvious. Sleep deprivation can help reveal these functions by revealing what goes wrong when these functions are not performed. For example, if sleep restores some substance that is used up during waking, then sleep deprivation should cause the substance to become depleted. A basic problem with this scheme, however, is that any function that goes wrong may be a result, not of the sleep loss, but of the sleep deprivation procedure. For example, if an animal were kept awake by making it walk on a continuously moving treadmill and a substance were found to be depleted, the depletion could be due either to sleep loss or to some other effect of continuous walking.

This problem is more troublesome in depriving animals of sleep than in depriving humans. Animal researchers try to minimize procedural effects by making the arousal stimuli as brief and harmless as possible. They also try to give the same stimuli to "control" animals without inducing sleep loss, so that the other effects of the stimuli can be found. For example, one research group has a computer that monitors a rat that lives on a movable floor. When the computer detects that the rat is falling asleep, the computer causes the floor to move, which arouses the rat and forces it to move a few steps. A second rat living on the same floor is also forced to move, but the second rat can sleep whenever the deprived rat is not trying to sleep. This rat acts as a "control" for the moving floor stimulus.

The First Total Sleep Deprivation Experiments

The first total sleep deprivation experiment was performed in France in 1894 by Marie de Manacéine, who deprived puppies of sleep by handling and exercising them for four to six days until they died. The puppies had large decreases in body temperature before they died, and autopsies indicated changes in brain cells. Although details of these results have been disputed, de Manacéine's experiment provided the first evidence that sleep has a vital physiological function. Researchers have since repeatedly shown that prolonged sleep deprivation produces severe disability and even death in animals.

The first human sleep deprivation experiment was performed in the United States in 1896 by G. Patrick and A. Gilbert. They deprived three young men of sleep for four days and found increased nitrogen excretion (probably indicating increased protein metabolism), a slight decrease in body temperature, and a decrement in "performance" (i.e., poorer visual discrimination, poorer movement skills, poorer memory, and confusion). Such performance deficits obviously have some physiological basis but have been studied by researchers primarily as behavioral deficits (see "Behavioral Effects" above). On the whole, the subjects remained healthy. Perhaps the deprivation period was too short to produce major physiological deficits.

The Longest Human Total Sleep Deprivation

The longest documented total sleep deprivation time in humans is 11 days (264 hours). This record was established in 1964 by Randy GARDNER of California as a high-school science project. After 6 days on his own, Gardner's project came to the attention of sleep researchers, who monitored him for the rest of the deprivation and during his recovery. Late in deprivation he had a 1°C decrease in body temperature and a 10°C decrease in skin temperature, along with severe performance deficits. However, other physiological problems appeared mild, and after 1 or 2 days of recovery he seemed to be back to normal.

The longest planned human deprivation experiment, 8½ days (205) hours, was conducted by P. Naitoh, E. Kollars, and colleagues in California in 1966. Four men were subjected to a large array of physiological and behavioral measures before, during, and after deprivation. Once again, there were many small physiological changes but no obvious major health threats to the subjects.

The relatively weak effects of sleep deprivation

on human physiology are in contrast with the much more severe effects seen in animals. Are these differences because of the differences in the deprivation procedure, or does sleep function differently in humans than it does in other animals, or have humans simply not been deprived for a long enough period of time? One argument supporting the last viewpoint is that humans are much larger and have a lower metabolic rate per unit weight than the laboratory animals that have been sleep deprived, and thus humans may be better able to withstand extended sleep loss.

Physiological Effects of Total Sleep Deprivation

Sleep deprivation experiments have not provided a clear picture of the function of sleep. First, is sleep for recovery from exercise? Loss of muscle tone has been reported in sleep-deprived dogs. Sleep-deprived humans report fatigue sooner when exercising, but measurements of their muscle efficiency show no change. Second, is sleep for recovery of the brain? As noted above, de Manacéine found brain damage in sleep-deprived dogs. Other researchers have reported signs of brain abnormalities in sleep-deprived animals, but many researchers have reported no difference between sleep-deprived and control brains. One cannot, of course, directly study the brains of sleep-deprived humans, but their deficits in performance indicate neurophysiological problems. These problems may be no more than the brain trying to go to sleep. Sleep-deprived humans occasionally show brain wave patterns that resemble those of beginning sleep even while they are behaviorally awake. These patterns are called microsleeps (see MICROSLEEP), and they appear to be associated with performance deficits. Third, is sleep for recovery from the stress of waking life? Measurements of corticosteroid hormones, which are indicators of stress, have been made in sleep-deprived humans and rats. Increases have been reported, as might be expected with "stressful" deprivation procedures, but other reports indicate no change or even declines in corticosteroids. Fourth, is sleep for metabolic adjustment? Metabolism is adjusted by hormones such as thyroxine and catecholamines. In short-term sleep-deprived humans, thyroxine increases, but catecholamines do not. Metabolic rate is not greatly changed. Long-term sleep-deprived rats have decreased thyroxine but greatly increased catecholamines. Metabolic rate increases. Fifth, is sleep for thermoregulation? Sleep-deprived humans show small decreases in waking body temperature and, during exercise, decreases in sweating and in dry heat loss. In sleep-deprived rats, temperature increases and then decreases steadily, and there are large increases in overall heat loss. Sixth, is sleep for protection from infectious disease? Short-term sleep deprivation of humans has produced minor immune system deficiencies. Immune defects, however, were not observed in long-term sleep-deprived rats.

Recovery from Total Sleep Deprivation

After sleep deprivation, humans and animals have sleep that lasts longer and is more intense than normal baseline sleep. Patrick and Gilbert, in 1896, found that it took a much stronger electric shock to arouse a human subject from recovery sleep than from baseline sleep. Recovery sleep in rats and humans shows increases in high-voltage NREM sleep (NREM stages 3 and 4 in humans) and REM sleep. Stages 3 and 4 contain the most high-voltage slow waves (see STAGES OF SLEEP), which are sometimes used as a measure of NREM sleep "intensity." In humans, a large percentage increase in stages 3 and 4 occurs first, followed by a smaller percentage increase in REM sleep. In rats, the larger percentage increase early in recovery is in REM sleep, and periods of extended REM sleep are intermingled with periods of NREM sleep with increased slow-wave activity. In both species, the amount and timing of recovery sleep depend on the time in the circadian cycle when recovery begins (see CIRCADIAN RHYTHMS). In neither species does the recovery sleep time normally add up to the sleep time lost during deprivation. Like a skipped meal, some of the lost sleep is lost forever.

Because there is more "recovery" sleep after sleep deprivation, one can argue that sleep performs some important physiological function that must recover when deprivation ends.

REFERENCES

Borbely AA, Neuhaus HU. 1979. Sleep deprivation: Effects on sleep and EEG in the rat. *J Comp Physiol* 133:71–87.

Horne J. 1988. *Why we sleep.* New York: Oxford University Press.

Kleitman N. 1963. *Sleep and wakefulness.* Chicago: University of Chicago Press.

Rechtschaffen A, Bergmann BM, Everson CA, Kushida CA, Gilliland MA. Sleep deprivation in the rat: I. Conceptual issues. *Sleep* 12:1–4.

Bernard Bergmann

DEPTH OF SLEEP

The experimental study of sleep can be dated to 1862 when Kohlschütter, a student of the great German experimental psychologist Gustav Fechner, began the first systematic psychophysiological sleep experiment by using a sound pendulum to measure the depth of sleep. His apparatus allowed him to produce sounds of increasing intensity until his subject awakened. The sound pendulum intensity at awakening was defined as the subject's auditory arousal threshold (AAT) and served as an objective means of defining depth of sleep.

The initial data gathered by Kohlschütter were based on seventy-four arousals over eight experimental nights and indicated that awakening thresholds increased (that is, a higher-intensity sound was required to wake the subject) very rapidly shortly after sleep onset and then decreased in a logarithmic fashion across the night. This curve of decreasing threshold values was a good approximation of the previously described trend of "general unconsciousness" or "depth of sleep" proposed by Fechner yet failed to account for all the trials that were presented (Swan, 1929). Nevertheless, studies during the next 40 years included replication of these auditory threshold results, thresholds to electric shock in children, and an elegant study of pressure thresholds in which there was a clear 90- to 120-minute rhythmicity (De Sanctis and Neyroz, 1902).

In the 1930s, Kleitman and his students determined that sleep was "lighter" (that is, subjects could be awakened more easily) after a body movement and that movement time increased across the night; however, the movement factor could not explain all of the large threshold changes seen during the night. Other early investigators hypothesized that the "value" of sleep was related to its "intensity" (depth) and, in some cases, calculated the area under the depth-of-sleep curve as a measure of sleep effectiveness. The studies did not provide any scientific support for the idea that "deep sleep" was "better sleep," but the notion of deep sleep as especially beneficial has survived in theories of the function of sleep with electroencephalographic slow waves and in the myths that naps and sleep before midnight are "better."

During the 1930s, the electroencephalogram (EEG) was first used as a measure of sleep behavior by Blake and Gerard. They published the initial paper that validated electroencephalographic "stages" by showing systematic changes in auditory thresholds that corresponded to changes in the EEG (Blake and Gerard, 1937). In their study, they presented a 1,000-cycle-per-second tone of constant intensity for 1 minute during episodes of different brain rhythms, verbally asked subjects if they were awake, and measured response times. At a relatively high level of arousal (awake, resting) thresholds were low, and relatively fast electroencephalographic alpha rhythm was seen. When delta activity (slow-wave activity) was seen in the EEG, the increase in sleep depth was quite striking. A curve of data averaged from five subjects across ten nights showed an almost perfect correspondence between the predominance of delta in each hour of sleep and the response rate to a tone. Both curves corresponded well with the earlier studies. There was a smooth decline across the night and no secondary peak. Blake and Gerard did not convincingly deal with the low-voltage sleep EEG (presently associated with both stage 1 and REM sleep) but stated that it was to be considered a transition between the alpha and delta states, which had intermediate awakening thresholds.

A number of studies in ensuing years have examined threshold values during sleep in terms of stimulus variations, response characteristics, and variables such as sleep stage, drugs, prior wakefulness, time of night, circadian effects, and individual differences (Bonnet, 1982). The majority of depth-of-sleep studies have measured auditory thresholds during sleep. Several factors determine how readily one will respond to a sound during sleep. Those factors include how long the sound is presented, whether the sound is meaningful, how the sound varies in pitch, and the intensity of the sound. Tactile (pain, pressure, temperature), visual, olfactory, and vestibular sensory thresholds have been studied less completely than audition.

Many types of response have also been examined, and "depth of sleep" can be defined using any of these responses. Basic information input to the brain, as measured by monitoring sensory nerve signals going to the brain (EVOKED POTENTIALS), continues to occur with little change during sleep; however, the brain appears to ignore most nonmeaningful information during sleep. As sensory signals increase in intensity or meaningfulness, the sleep EEG may be interrupted for a few seconds by electroencephalographic alpha rhythms, heart rate will increase, and a body movement may occur. If the signal stops at this point, the individual will probably return to sleep with no memory for the event. If the signal continues to increase, the individual will awaken fully.

Variables that modify sensory thresholds during sleep include sleep stage, age, drugs, prior wakefulness, time of night, and individual differences.

1. *Sleep stage.* As noted above, many studies have focused on sleep stages as a threshold determinant. Depth of sleep consistently increases as we move from each stage of sleep to the next, that is, from stage 1 to stage 2 to stage 3 to stage 4. The thresholds in REM sleep are approximately equal to those in stage 2 sleep in humans. On the other hand, animal studies have consistently reported that sensory thresholds are higher during REM sleep than during NREM sleep.

2. *Age.* Sensory thresholds during sleep vary significantly as a function of age. Children have very high arousal thresholds (Busby and Pivik, 1983). It is often impossible to arouse them, even in stage 2 sleep, with pure tones of intensity as high as 123 decibels (a mean of successful arousal trials in one study was 111 decibels). Auditory thresholds decline as a function of age. One study showed that thresholds in stage 2 sleep at ages 22, 44, and 62 years decreased from an average of 82 to 70 to 60 decibels (Zepelin, McDonald, and Zammit, 1984).

The range of these intensities is from normal conversation (60 decibels) to an average car (70 decibels) to a noisy car or bus (80 decibels) to a rock concert or actual pain (123 decibels).

3. *Drugs.* Several studies have reported that auditory thresholds within given sleep stages are increased by sedatives, such as benzodiazepines or barbiturates, and decreased by stimulants such as caffeine (Bonnet, Webb, and Barnard, 1979). The normal dose of a commonly used sleeping pill (flurazepam) will increase auditory arousal threshold by 5 to 30 decibels, depending on the time elapsed since the pill was taken (which affects how much active medication is left in the body).

4. *Prior wakefulness.* Sleep deprivation increases sensory thresholds during all stages of recovery sleep. After 64 hours of deprivation, sleeping subjects' correct button-push responses to a tone 35 decibels above background noise decreased from a waking score of 25 percent to 4 percent in stage 2 and from about 10 percent to 1 percent in stage 4 (Williams et al., 1964). This implies that sleep is even deeper in stage 2 after sleep loss than it is in stage 4 before sleep loss.

5. *Time of night.* There are many reports that, even within a given stage of sleep, arousal thresholds decline later in the sleep period as compared with early in the sleep period. These findings may be based on the fact that arousal thresholds are lower for several minutes after a body movement or transient arousal and these events increase in frequency across the night.

6. *Individual differences.* The observation-to-observation and night-to-night reproducibility (reliability) of auditory threshold measurements taken during sleep has also been examined. Some individuals at each age level were consistently deep sleepers and others were consistently light sleepers. In addition to significant reliability from night to night and within the night, people who had high thresholds in stage 4 also tended to have high thresholds in stage 2 and REM sleep (Bonnet, 1982). However, auditory thresholds when awake were not significantly correlated with thresholds

when asleep. Personality differences have not been found in light versus deep sleepers. Individuals who are easily awakened during sleep tend to be more physiologically aroused during the night and to have more dreamlike mental activity throughout the sleep period.

7. *Subjective report.* Depth of sleep, as measured by sensory threshold, is not directly related to subjects' report of the depth of sleep. Subjective impression of deep sleep appears to be related primarily to the amount of time spent awake during the night. Although insomniacs usually report that they are "light" sleepers, as a group, their auditory arousal thresholds during sleep do not differ from those of normal sleepers.

The number of current studies examining depth of sleep with sensory threshold measures is small. This is primarily because EEGs can be recorded continuously during the night, can be obtained with minimal disturbance of the sleep process, and are generally correlated with threshold data. Regardless of the advantages of using EEGs versus threshold measures, sensory measures of depth of sleep do provide behavioral response data that are unobtainable by other means and that may differ significantly from results obtained by using only electroencephalographic criteria. For example, auditory threshold data lead one to doubt whether smoke alarms, which produce a standard 85-decibel sound, will be effective in arousing many people, especially younger people who have used sedatives or who are sleep deprived.

REFERENCES

Blake H, Gerard RW. 1937. Factors influencing brain potentials during sleep. *Am J Physiol* 119: 692–703.

Bonnet MH. 1982. Performance during sleep. In Webb WB, ed. *Biological rhythms, sleep, and performance*, pp. 205–237. New York: Wiley.

Bonnet MH, Webb WB, Barnard G. 1979. Effect of flurazepam, pentobarbital, and caffeine on arousal threshold. *Sleep* 1(3):271–279.

Busby K, Pivik RT. 1983. Failure of high intensity auditory stimuli to affect behavioral arousal in children during the first sleep cycle. *Pediatr Res* 17:802–805.

De Sanctis S, Neyroz U. 1902. Experimental investigation concerning the depth of sleep. *Physiol Rev* 9:254–282.

Swan TH. 1929. A note on Kohlschütter's curve of "the depth of sleep." *Psychol Bull* 26:607–610.

Williams HL, Hammack JT, Daly RL, Dement WC, Lubin AL. 1964. Responses to auditory stimulation, sleep loss, and the EEG stages of sleep. *Electroencephalogr Clin Neurophysiol* 16:269–279.

Zepelin H, McDonald CS, Zammit GK. 1984. Effects of age on auditory awakening thresholds. *J Gerontol* 39:294–300.

Michael H. Bonnet

DESYNCHRONIZED SLEEP

See Paradoxical Sleep; Phylogeny; REM Sleep

DEVELOPMENT

[Development, maturation, *and* aging *all designate a set of related processes that impact on sleep and related phenomena. If you could ask only one question to find out about someone's sleep, the best thing to ask would be how old the person is, since sleep patterns change in a marked fashion across developmental stages. A number of entries in this volume address the direct impact of maturation and aging on sleep processes:* FETAL SLEEP–WAKE PATTERNS, PREMATURE INFANTS, CHILDHOOD, ADOLESCENCE AND SLEEP, NORMAL SLEEP, INDIVIDUAL DIFFERENCES, MENOPAUSE, *and* AGING AND SLEEP *all describe the sleep–wake patterns that occur normally at different phases of life.*

The extremes of the lifespan also hold special interest in related areas, such as CHILDREN'S DREAMS. *The relationship between children and bedtime has promoted common cultural practices including* BEDTIME STORIES *and tales of the* SANDMAN, *as well as* TEDDY BEARS *and other* TRANSITIONAL OBJECTS, *for easing children to sleep. At the other extreme of life, we become concerned with* AGING AND CIRCADIAN RHYTHMS, *as well as the unusual sleep–wake patterns known as* SUNDOWN SYNDROME *in the very old, particularly those afflicted with* DEMENTIA.

A number of sleep-related phenomena also show developmental changes in their occurrence or appearance. NAPPING *is common among the very young and the very old.* NOCTURNAL PENILE TUMESCENCE *in males occurs throughout life, although the nature of sleep-related* SEXUAL ACTIVATION *varies significantly with age.* SNORING *also runs a developmental course, with much more snoring in older adults than younger individuals—though children with* TONSILLITIS *can be champion snorers.*

Certain medical disorders linked to developmental stages have important effects on sleep and wakefulness. Children with ATTENTION DEFICIT HYPERACTIVITY DISORDER, *for example, are reported to have disturbed nocturnal sleep. Sleep problems may also emerge in adult women who have* PREMENSTRUAL SYNDROME. *Elderly people with* ALZHEIMER'S DISEASE *or* PARKINSON'S DISEASE *often suffer concurrent sleep disruptions.*

Finally, several specific sleep disorders are associated with particular developmental stages. The incidence of SUDDEN INFANT DEATH SYNDROME, *a life-threatening condition thought to involve sleep, peaks at age 3 or 4 months.* BEDWETTING, SLEEPWALKING, *and* SLEEP TERRORS *are fairly common sleep-related disturbances in young children. Adolescence is the time of life when* NARCOLEPSY *is most likely to emerge, as are* KLEINE–LEVIN SYNDROME *and* DELAYED SLEEP PHASE SYNDROME. *Other sleep disorders such as* INSOMNIA *and* APNEA *also show developmental progression in their incidence and prevalence.*]

DEVIL'S TRILL SONATA

See Creativity in Dreams

DIAGNOSIS

See Sleep Disorders Centers (Appendix)

DISEASE

See Medical Illness and Sleep

DISPLACEMENT

See Freud's Dream Theory

DIURNAL RHYTHMS

See Biological Rhythms; Circadian Rhythms

DOGS

Given the close relationship between human and dog, dogs have been the subject of sleep studies both in the casual and in the deliberate sense. For example, one of the first sleep DEPRIVATION studies was performed in puppies. Currently, an effort is underway to map the chromosome patterns of dogs because of their species-specific behaviors and traits. For instance, the English bulldog, with its narrow and constricted airway, is being studied in an effort to understand more about sleep APNEA (see ENGLISH BULLDOGS AS AN ANIMAL MODEL OF SLEEP APNEA). Nervous or "gun-shy" dogs are noted to be poorer sleepers than their normal counterparts (Powell, Lucas, and Murphree, 1978) and perhaps represent a model for certain kinds of INSOMNIA. Dogs are also known to suffer a disease similar to NARCOLEPSY in humans (Mitler and Dement, 1977; see CANINE NARCOLEPSY). Although studied much less extensively than cats, mice, and rats, dogs do have a role in helping to understand more about sleep, particularly those disorders that tend to be inherited.

The sleep of dogs is very similar to that of humans and other warm-blooded animals, especially the cat (Lucas, Powell, and Murphree, 1977). Like cats, dogs approach sleep in a deliberate manner. They lay down, recline their heads, and close their eyes. After a variable period of drowsiness, sleep onset occurs. There is progressive relaxation, and they will usually turn to one side and extend their legs in sleep. About 20 minutes after sleep onset, an episode of REM (dream) sleep will usually occur lasting on average 6 minutes. It is often followed by a brief arousal and either more sleep or an awakening, depending on the time of day. The majority of sleep occurs during darkness in domesticated dogs. Little is known about the sleep of wild dogs. In a 24-hour period, dogs sleep about 8 hours. Like cats, the sleep of dogs is spread across most of the 24-hour period. It occurs in bouts of sleep averaging from 30 to 40 minutes in duration separated by wake episodes containing both alert and drowsiness of approximately equal length. This is like the frequent napping of cats and is similar to the sleep of humans for the first few weeks of life.

Of the 8 hours of daily sleep, about 2.5 hours is spent in dreaming (REM) sleep. It occurs in episodes lasting about 6 minutes, and these are usually 20 minutes apart during sleep. REM sleep in dogs is often preceded by very unstable sleep. This is in contrast to the very consistent and continuous sleep preceding the dreams of humans and cats. The sleep of dogs is more disrupted by drowsiness and brief wake episodes than is the sleep of cats. The old adage "Let sleeping dogs lie" is better understood in this light. Dogs are more easily alerted and take longer to return to sleep than cats do. Dogs spend about one-half of their day awake and alert. In addition, they are awake but relaxed with a drowsy electroencephalographic pattern for an additional 4 to 5 hours.

The brain wave patterns (ELECTROENCEPHALOGRAM, or EEG) of dogs associated with wake and sleep have several similarities to those of humans. Wake is identified by low-amplitude waves with faster frequency activity in both humans and dogs. In dogs, eye closure results in the development of wave patterns in the alpha range, and sleep onset is identified with the appearance of a unique brain wave pattern called SLEEP SPINDLES, very similar to those seen in humans. The dog, cat, and other lower animals do not develop special electroencephalographic waveforms called K-complexes seen in humans (see K-COMPLEX), and have less-pronounced slow-wave activity, which distinguishes deep slow-wave, or delta, sleep in humans. However, the electroencephalographic pattern of REM sleep in dogs is nearly identical to that of humans and other animals. In REM sleep, the electroencephalographic pattern changes to a very low amplitude, and faster frequencies appear, similar to wakefulness. At the same time, there are rapid eye movements, phasic twitches of the limbs, and inhibition of muscle tone. Studies in dogs of deep brain structures, including the hippocampus, show changes quite similar to those seen in humans and cats.

REFERENCES

Lucas EA, Powell EW, Murphree OD. 1977. Baseline sleep-wake patterns in the pointer dog. *Physiol Behav* 19:285–291.

Mitler MM, Dement WC. 1977. Sleep studies on canine narcolepsy: Pattern and cycle comparisons between affected and normal dogs. *Electroencephalogr Clin Neurophysiol* 43(5):691–699.

Powell EW, Lucas EA, Murphree OD. 1978. Influence of human presence on sleep-wake patterns in the pointer dog. *Physiol Behav* 20:39–41.

Edgar Lucas

DOLPHINS

See Mammals; Phylogeny

DOPAMINE

See Chemistry of Sleep: Amines and Other Transmitters

DOWN SYNDROME

Children with Down syndrome have an extra chromosome 21; instead of having the 46 chromosomes observed in cells of most human beings, persons with Down Syndrome have a total of 47 chromosomes. Because of the extra chromosome 21, children with Down syndrome often have some characteristic physical features, such as a small head, a flat face, slightly upward slanted eyelids, skin folds at the inner corners of the eyes, small nose and mouth, and small hands and feet. Most of these characteristics do not interfere with the child's overall functioning and are used by the physician primarily for diagnostic purposes. These physical features are variable; generally, children with Down syndrome are more similar to other children than they are different.

Individuals with Down syndrome also often have certain medical conditions, such as weak muscles, neurologic impairments, congenital heart disease, intestinal abnormalities, poorly functioning thyroid gland, eye abnormalities, hearing deficits, and skeletal problems. Nearly all children with Down syndrome are mentally retarded, frequently in the mild to moderate range; the degree of mental retardation varies considerably.

Children with Down syndrome frequently have somewhat smaller facial bones, particularly those of the midface. In addition, they may have enlarged tonsils and adenoids, or if they are overweight, they may have increased fat tissue in the throat. Moreover, children with Down syndrome often have a small mouth with a relatively large tongue that may fall back in the throat during sleep. All these factors result in a narrow upper airway, which may lead to such sleep problems as noisy breathing and snoring, restlessness, and even short episodes of breathing cessation (sleep apnea). During the daytime, these children may be lethargic and sleepy and may exhibit behavior problems. In the case of sleep apnea, less oxygen is supplied during sleep to various tissues of the body, including the brain, and increased blood pressure in the lungs with subsequent heart failure may be observed. These symptoms could cause serious health problems; therefore, children with Down syndrome should be evaluated for sleep apnea.

Several reports have been published during the past decade indicating that sleep-related upper airway obstruction is a frequently undetected complication of Down syndrome. In 1980, Clark, Schmidt, and Schuller first described three patients with Down syndrome who displayed sleep-induced breathing problems as a result of mechanical obstruction and central nervous system dysfunction. One year later, Loughlin, Wynne, and Victoria (1981) reported five children with Down syndrome who had pulmonary hypertension and sleep apnea. These researchers felt that the breathing disturbance was caused by anatomical factors in the midface of these children. Scientists at the University of Helsinki studied nineteen adults with Down syndrome and found nine with big tonsils or an enlarged tongue (Telakivi et al., 1987). Other investigators have also reported an increased prevalence of sleep apnea in persons with Down syndrome (Kasian et al., 1987; Levine and Simpser, 1982; Southall et al., 1987; Phillips and Rogers, 1988).

An unpublished study by a team including the present author found that parents could identify symptoms of sleep apnea in a high proportion of children with adenotonsillar enlargement and a moderate number of children with Down syndrome. Parents reported that 70 percent of their youngsters with Down syndrome were mouth breathers, 45 percent snored, and 15 percent were observed to hold their breath or stop breathing during sleep. In addition, a large number of children were difficult to arouse in the morning, had trouble staying awake during daytime, and often exhibited disruptive behaviors.

If sleep apnea is diagnosed in persons with Down syndrome, different treatments can be used to widen the narrowed upper airway. If tonsils and adenoids are significantly enlarged, a tonsillectomy and/or adenoidectomy may relieve some of the upper airway obstruction. If a person with Down syndrome is markedly overweight, a weight reduction program could also be helpful to decrease fatty tissue in the back of the throat. Surgical widening of the posterior nasal passages has been recommended by some physicians; others consider that the airway obstruction can be relieved only by tracheostomy. Because of the different facial bone structures often associated with Down syndrome, a routine tonsillectomy and adenoidectomy will not always relieve the upper airway obstruction; therefore, a modified pharyngopalatal surgical approach has been developed (Strome, 1986). Other doctors have suggested use of a special procedure called CONTINUOUS POSITIVE AIR PRESSURE, whereby air is pushed into the air passages through the nose.

Most persons with Down syndrome who have been diagnosed with sleep apnea can be treated effectively. Benefits of treatment include the prevention of oxygen deprivation in the brain, of increased blood pressure in the lungs, of heart failure, and even of some daytime behavior problems. Appropriate treatment of sleep apnea ultimately will improve the quality of life of persons with Down syndrome.

(See also APNEA.)

REFERENCES

Clark RW, Schmidt HS, Schuller DE. 1980. Sleep induced ventilatory dysfunction in Down's syndrome. *Arch Intern Med* 140:45–50.

Kasian GF, Duncan WJ, Tyrrell MJ, Oman-Ganes LA. 1987. Elective orotracheal intubation to diagnose sleep apnea syndrome in children with Down's syndrome and ventricular septal defect. *Canad Cardiol* 3:2–5.

Levine OR, Simpser M. 1982. Alveolar hypoventilation and cor pulmonale associated with chronic airway obstruction in infants with Down syndrome. *Clin Pediatr* 21:25–29.

Loughlin GM, Wynne JW, Victoria BE. 1981. Sleep apnea as a possible cause of pulmonary hypertension in Down syndrome. *J Pediatr* 98:435–439.

Phillips DE, Rogers JH. 1988. Down's syndrome with lingual tonsil hypertrophy producing sleep apnea. *J Laryngol Otol* 102:1054–1055.

Southall DP, Stebbens VA, Mirza R, Lang MH, Croft CB, Shinebourne EA. 1987. Upper airway obstruction with hypoxaemia and sleep disruption in Down syndrome. *Dev Med Child Neurol* 29:734–742.

Strome M. 1986. Obstructive sleep apnea in Down syndrome children: A surgical approach. *Laryngoscope* 96:1340–1342.

Telakivi T, Partinen T, Salmi L, Leinonen L, Härkönen T. 1987. Nocturnal periodic breathing in adults with Down's syndrome. *J Mental Deficiency Res* 31:31–39.

Siegfried M. Pueschel

DREAM-ENACTING BEHAVIOR

See REM Sleep Behavior Disorder

DREAMS AND DREAMING

[*Theories of why we dream and what dreams mean start with the article on* DREAM THEORIES OF THE ANCIENT WORLD *and continue with three articles on classical psychoanalytic theories of dreaming:* FREUD'S DREAM THEORY, JUNG'S DREAM THEORY, *and* ADLER'S DREAM THEORY. *More recent theories are reviewed in* COGNITIVE DREAM THEORY *and in* ACTIVATION–SYNTHESIS HYPOTHESIS.

What dreams are like (the manifest perceptual, cognitive, content, and stylistic features of dreams) is covered in articles on CHARACTERISTICS OF DREAMS, CHILDREN'S DREAMS, COLOR IN DREAMS, CONTENT OF DREAMS, HYPNAGOGIC REVERIE *(the sometimes dreamlike mental activity that occurs at sleep onset), and* HYPNAGOGIC HALLUCINATIONS. *Closely related topics are* RECALL OF DREAMS *and* COGNITION. *Specific kinds of dream content are covered in* FLYING IN DREAMS *and in* NUDITY IN DREAMS.

The psychological meanings and uses of dreams are covered in INTERPRETATION OF DREAMS, SYMBOLISM IN DREAMS, FUNCTIONS OF DREAMS, EXPERIENTIAL DREAM GROUPS (DREAM WORKSHOPS), CULTURAL ASPECTS OF DREAMING, SENOI DREAM THEORY, CREATIVITY IN DREAMS, UNCONSCIOUS, CONDENSATION, PICTORIAL REPRESENTATION, *and* SYMBOLISM IN DREAMS.

Special kinds of dreams are reviewed in articles on NIGHTMARES, POSTTRAUMATIC NIGHTMARES, RECURRENT DREAMS, *and* LUCID DREAMING *(in which we are aware that we are dreaming and may have a feeling of control over what we dream).*

Articles that are relevant to how sensory experiences affect dream content are INCORPORATION INTO DREAMS; BLINDNESS AND DREAMING; DEAFNESS AND DREAMING; *and* EYE MOVEMENTS AND DREAMING.

Articles directly relevant to the relationship between dreaming and physiological activity are PSYCHOPHYSIOLOGY OF DREAMING, ACTIVATION–SYNTHESIS HYPOTHESIS, MIDDLE EAR MUSCLE ACTIVITY, EYE MOVEMENTS AND DREAMING, *and* PHASIC INTEGRATED POTENTIALS. *Since dreams are most frequently reported on awakening from REM sleep, the articles* REM SLEEP, PHYSIOLOGY OF *and* DEPRIVATION, SELECTIVE: REM SLEEP *are of some relevance to this issue.*

Articles that reflect the attention paid to dreams in waking thought and culture are the following: ART, SLEEP AND DREAMS IN WESTERN; LITERATURE, SLEEP AND DREAMS IN; MOVIES, DREAMS IN; POPULAR MUSIC, SLEEP AND DREAMS IN.

Some believe that dreaming expresses special mental talents. Articles relevant to this topic are CREATIVITY IN DREAMS; PROBLEM SOLVING AND DREAMING; PSYCHIC DREAMS; *and* TELEPATHY AND DREAMING.

Additional articles on dreams are ANIMAL'S DREAMS; HYPNOSIS AND DREAMING; MYTHS ABOUT DREAMING; INSTANTANEOUS DREAMING; PREGNANCY AND DREAMING; *and* RELIGION AND DREAMING.]

DREAM THEORIES OF THE ANCIENT WORLD

In the writings of the ancient world, dreams are shown to occupy a prominent place in that world. The epics and philosophical, historical, and religious writings almost inevitably include dreams.

Dream interpretations are found in the Egyptian papyri from about 2000 B.C. There are long passages about dreams in the Upanishads of India from 1000 B.C. Message dreams are found throughout the legend of Gilgamesh and Homer's *Iliad*. The Old Testament has frequent references to important dreams, such as the explicit dreams of Abraham and Jacob and the interpretation of dreams by Joseph and Daniel. The Babylonian *Talmud*, compiled between 200 B.C. and A.D. 200, contains no fewer than 270 references to dreams. Historians such as Herodotus repeatedly recorded the guiding roles played by dreams in epic struggles for power.

Dreams were discussed by the Greek philosophers such as Pythagoras, Democritus, Plato, and Aristotle. Beliefs about dreams were elaborately developed in ancient Greece, where it was believed that sleeping in special temples provided access to dreams that foretold the future or prescribed cures for illnesses. More than 400 such temples have been found. A compilation of ancient dream beliefs was written by Artemidorus of Daldis in the second century. The Islamic religion, drawing heavily on its Near East heritage, emphasized spiritual revelation in dreams. For example, the legitimacy of the powerful Sunni sect is attributed to a dream of Mohammed. Finally, dreams have a significant place in the New Testament, leading to the continued struggle in the early Christian Church with the issue of dreams and their interpretation. Details of these beliefs about dreams can be found in Kelsey (1969), Von Gruenbaum and Callois (1977), and Webb (1981).

Underlying these beliefs in the importance of dreams was a central theme: there were powers higher than those present in the human domain. Dreams were thought to provide access to that power and, thus, guidance about worldly problems and the future. Many concepts about dreams contained the notion that sleep was a state in which the person was freed from worldly constraints and thus permitted easier access to the higher power.

The central problem, however, was receiving the message. Sometimes, particularly in the case of heroes, kings, or religious figures, the message was quite clear as the divine figure spoke directly to them. For example, Jacob responded directly to Yahweh's command; Assurbanipal invaded the Elamites on the command of Ishtar; and Joseph and Mary fled to Egypt on God's command. More often that not, however, there were problems of interpretation.

These problems shaped particular beliefs about dreams. First, it was possible that the dream was providing false information. Many, indeed most, of the early Near Eastern religions and pantheons of gods reflect a struggle between good and evil, light and darkness, gods and demons. The Mesopotamian and Sumerian records emphasized demonic dreams that required exorcisms. Second, there was the influence of the dreamer, who may distort or poorly receive the message. Third, the dream is likely to convey a symbolic message rather than a direct one. For example, Joseph was required to interpret the seven "fat kine" and seven "lean kine" as seven years of good harvest and seven years of famine. Finally, the interpreter may be incapable or even evil, as the prophet Jeremiah warned: "Let not your prophets and your diviners . . . deceive you, neither hearken to your dreams which you caused to be dreamed" (27:9).

Thus, the ancients developed a wide variety of methods for distinguishing good from evil dreams, rituals and procedures for preparing the dreamer, interpretations of the symbolic meaning of dreams, and means of designating the effective interpreter. These ranged from simple presleep incantations and preparations to elaborate temples for dreaming and interpretation. Books such as that of Artemidorus relative to symbols, the role of the dreamer, and methods of interpretation ran to many volumes.

Two remarkable exceptions to the notion of extrapersonal inspiration of dreams should be noted in the writings of Aristotle and Cicero. In the fourth century B.C., Aristotle wrote two chapters on dreams (Ross, 1931). He attributed them to "residual sensory impressions" from the person's past that present themselves without the controlling influences of the senses. Although dreams may relate to the future, Aristotle maintained that this is based either on coincidence or on our anticipation of the future. He said that dreams are not sent by the gods. Aristotle believed that the interpretation of dreams is based on the skillful interpretation of resemblances. Cicero also argued against the notion of god-given dreams on three grounds (Falconer, 1923). Most dreams are ignored, which implies that the god either is ignorant or is acting foolishly. If a god were trying to help us, he or she would do so when we were awake and better able to receive the information. And why would a god send false dreams with no distinguishing mark? Cicero is also concerned about ever establishing the relationship between dreams and the future, if this relationship even exists, because people dream an infinite variety of dreams that must be related to an infinite variety of subsequent results.

Although there were exceptions like the theories of Aristotle and Cicero, dream theories of the ancient world were concerned primarily with relationships between humans and higher powers. The importance of the dream in such theories rested on the assumption that the dream furnished access to these powers.

REFERENCES

Bonnusi L. 1975. About the origins of the scientific study of sleep and dreaming. In Lairy G, Salzarulo P, eds. *Study of human sleep: Methodological problems.* Amsterdam: Elsevier. Excellent review of the dream in early Greece.

Falconer WA, transl. 1923. Cicero's *De senectute, de amicitia, de divinatione.* Cambridge, Mass., Harvard University Press.

Kelsey MT. 1969. *God, dreams and revelation.* Minneapolis: Augsburg. A remarkable review of the role of dreams in the Christian Church.

Ross WD, ed. 1931. *The Works of Aristotle,* Vol. III. Oxford: Clarendon Press.

Von Gruenbaum G, Callois R, eds. 1977. *The dream in human society.* Berkeley: University of California Press. A collection of papers on dreams in primitive and ancient societies.

Webb W. 1981. A historical perspective on dreams. In Wolman B, ed. *Handbook of dreams.* New York: Van Nostrand.

Wilse B. Webb

DREAM WORK METHODOLOGY

See Adler's Dream Theory; Cognitive Dream Theory; Experiential Dream Groups; Freud's Dream Theory; Jung's Dream Theory

DREAM WORKSHOPS

See Experiential Dream Groups

DR. JEKYLL AND MR. HYDE

See Creativity in Dreams

DROCKLE

The word *drockle* was coined in 1968 by technicians at the Stanford University Sleep Research Laboratory, directed by William C. Dement. Its creators initially intended merely to concoct a frivolous expression describing the brief, so-called "drowsy" period between wakefulness and sleep. The term quickly gained acceptance among lab personnel and their acquaintances not only as a synonym for the verbs "to drowse" and "to nod off," but also as meaning to behave in a silly or foolish manner, as though addled by a semisleepy state (see SLEEPINESS).

The etymology of *drockle* is easy to trace, as it borrows its first three letters from the word *drowsy* and ends with a nonsense syllable designed to convey a whimsical impression. *Drockle* first came into usage when the drowsy state as depicted in sleep electroencephalographic recordings was being considered for separate status as an identifiable sleep stage immediately preceding stage 1 (see STAGES OF SLEEP). This idea was soon abandoned but the word had already caught on. Soon it was used to describe nodding off to sleep on a sunny day, with chin dropping toward the chest; daydreaming or falling into idle reverie; or passively killing time during slow or boring portions of a day. The nonsensical origin of the word has lent itself mainly to humorous applications, such as, "He drockled away the entire morning without listening to the lecture," or "I wasn't asleep, I was only drockling." The noun *drockler* can be used to describe a goofball, idler, or buffoon, as well as a drowsy nodder. An individual prone to napping could be said to have "drocklish" tendencies.

Current usage is limited to certain sleep researchers and their students, employees, and friends, and may vary from group to group. Because it is a relatively new word and lacks a precise, scientific definition, its meaning and usage will likely continue to evolve. The word *drockle* as described here is not, to the author's knowledge, found in other dictionaries, encyclopedias, or reference books.

Grant Hoyt

DROWSINESS

See Drockle; Sleepiness

DRUG DEPENDENCY

See Alcoholism; Cocaine; Drugs of Abuse

DRUGS OF ABUSE

A diverse collection of drugs from a number of different drug classes are used compulsively and excessively for nonmedical purposes leading to enormous personal and social harm. Given the diversity of the abused drugs, scientists have hypothesized that common biological mechanisms may explain the reinforcing effects of these drugs leading to their compulsive and excessive use. Interestingly, most of these drugs also have profound effects on sleep and wakefulness and on particular stages of sleep, typically REM sleep. It may be that sleep and wake changes, although not the primary reinforcing mechanisms, function as contributory factors in maintaining the excessive and compulsive drug use and as factors that increase the risk for relapse.

Drugs with an extremely high abuse liability are the STIMULANTS, drugs that produce arousal and excitation. The two most common are amphetamine and its derivatives (see AMPHETAMINES) and COCAINE. These drugs facilitate the activity of the neurotransmitters dopamine and norepinephrine (see CHEMISTRY OF SLEEP). The daytime alerting effects of amphetamine have been well documented using measures of mood and per-

formance and a direct physiological measure, the repeated test of the latency to electroencephalography-documented sleep onset (Mitler and Hajdukovic, 1991; see MULTIPLE SLEEP LATENCY TEST). When administered before sleep, amphetamine delays sleep onset, increases wakefulness during the sleep period, and specifically suppresses REM sleep (Rechtschaffen and Maron, 1964). Cessation of chronic amphetamine use is associated with an increase in slow-wave sleep on the first recovery night and, on subsequent nights, increased amounts of REM sleep and a reduced latency to the first episode of REM sleep, findings that have been termed *REM rebound.*

Cocaine, used medically as a local anesthetic, also has central nervous system (CNS) stimulant effects, which are the basis of its abuse. The effects of cocaine on the ELECTROENCEPHALOGRAM (EEG) were first studied in 1931 by H. Berger, the person who developed the EEG (Berger, 1931). Cocaine was found to increase fast-frequency EEG activity, suggesting an alerting effect such as that seen in the studies of the daytime effects of amphetamine discussed above. The self-reported use of cocaine during the late afternoon and early evening is associated with reduced nocturnal sleep time and REM sleep and an increased latency to REM sleep (Watson et al., 1989). Cessation of chronic cocaine abuse is followed by increased sleep time and REM rebound (i.e., reduced REM latency and increased REM sleep).

Drugs that reduce pain are called *analgesics,* and one class, the opiate analgesics (derived from the opium poppy), has a relatively high abuse liability. The opiates influence a number of different neurotransmitter systems in the brain, including those involved in sleep and wakefulness. Morphine, the primary active ingredient of opium, decreases the number and the duration of REM sleep episodes and delays the onset of the first REM period (Kay, Eisenstein, and Jasinski, 1969). It also increases awakenings and light sleep and suppresses slow-wave sleep. Heroin, a semisynthetic opiate, also suppresses REM sleep and slow-wave sleep and increases wakefulness and light sleep, producing a disruption of the usual continuity of sleep (Kay, Pickworth, and Neidert, 1981). Heroin appears to be more potent than morphine in its sleep effects. The synthetic opiate methadone has similar effects on sleep and wakefulness with a potency more comparable to that of morphine. Immediately after opiate administration before the onset of sleep, isolated EEG bursts of delta waves on the background of a waking EEG pattern are seen. Animal studies have correlated these delta bursts with the behavior of head nodding (a possible physiological correlate to the street term *being on the nod*).

Repeated administration of the opiates at the same dose leads to tolerance (a reduction in effect) to the sleep effects of these drugs, particularly the REM sleep effects (Kay, Eisenstein, and Jasinski, 1969). The cessation of opiate use leads to REM rebound, increased REM sleep, and shortened latency to the first REM episode.

Drugs that modify perceptions are called *hallucinogens,* and these drugs also are abused. The three classical hallucinogens are LSD (*d*-lysergic acid diethylamide), mescaline, and psilocybin. The state experienced following use of hallucinogens is somewhat similar to dreaming. As REM sleep is highly correlated with dreaming, scientists expected the hallucinogens to facilitate REM sleep. LSD is the only hallucinogen that has been studied for its effects on sleep. One study done in humans supported the expectation and showed that LSD prolonged REM sleep early in the night, although it did not alter the total amount of REM sleep for the night (Muzio, Roffwarg, and Kaufman, 1966); however, studies done in animals all indicate that LSD increases wakefulness and decreases REM sleep (Kay and Martin, 1978). Among other things, these contradictions could be due to species differences or to an inadequate number of human subjects. The frequency changes seen in the waking EEGs of animals (similar among all three hallucinogens) suggest an arousing effect, and the REM suppression in animals may be a nonspecific effect (Fairchild et al., 1979). Thus, it is difficult to reach a conclusion regarding the hallucinogens and REM sleep.

Another drug of abuse with hallucinogenic effects is MARIJUANA, its active ingredient being tetrahydrocannabinol (THC). The effects of THC on the waking EEG are quite distinct from those of the classical hallucinogens cited above (Fairchild et al., 1979). THC has sedating effects at lower doses and hallucinatory effects at higher doses. The acute administration of marijuana or THC to humans is associated with an increase in slow-wave sleep and a reduction in REM sleep (Pivik et al., 1972). When it is administered chronically, the effects on slow-wave and REM sleep diminish, indicating the presence of toler- ance. Discontinuing the use of marijuana is associated with increased wakefulness and increased REM sleep time (Feinberg et al., 1976).

Most of these drugs of abuse seem to alter sleep and wakefulness and, specifically, the amount and timing of REM sleep. Each affects chemicals in the brain that control sleep and wakefulness, and in chronic use some adaptation seems to occur. A characteristic REM rebound is seen on discontinuation, and in some studies the occurrence and intensity of the REM sleep rebound have been predictive of relapse. But how the sleep–wake changes and specifically the REM changes associated with these drugs contribute to their excessive use still needs further study.

REFERENCES

Berger H. 1931. Über das Elektrenkephalogramm des Menschen. *Arch Psychiatr Nervenkrankheiten* 94:16–60.

Fairchild MD, Jenden DJ, Mickey MR, Yale D. 1979. EEG effects of hallucinogens and cannabinoids using sleep–waking behavior as baseline. *Pharmacol Biol Behav* 12:99–105.

Feinberg I, Jones R, Walker JM, Cavness C, March J. 1976. Effects of high dosage delta-9-tetrahydrocannabinol on sleep patterns in man. *Clin Pharmacol Ther* 17:458–466.

Kay DC, Eisenstein RB, Jasinski DR. 1969. Morphine effects on human REM state, waking state, and NREM sleep. *Psychopharmacology* 14:404–416.

Kay DC, Martin WR. 1978. LSD and tryptamine effects on sleep/wakefulness and electrocorticogram patterns in intact cats. *Psychopharmacology* 58:223–228.

Kay DC, Pickworth WB, Neidert GL. 1981. Morphine-like insomnia from heroin in nondependent human addicts. *Br J Clin Pharmacol* 11:159–169.

Mitler MM, Hajdukovic R. 1991. Relative efficacy of drugs for the treatment of narcolepsy. *Sleep* 14:218–220.

Muzio JN, Roffwarg HP, Kaufman MD. 1966. Alterations in the nocturnal sleep cycle resulting from LSD. *Electroencephalogr Clin Neurophysiol* 21:313–324.

Pivik RT, Zarcone V, Dement WC, Hollister LE. 1972. Delta-9-tetrahydrocannabinol and synhexl: Effects on human sleep patterns. *Clin Pharmacol Ther* 13:426–435.

Rechtschaffen A, Maron L. 1964. The effect of amphetamine on the sleep cycle. *Electroencephalogr Clin Neurophysiol* 16:438–445.

Watson R, Bakos L, Compton P, Byck R, Gawin F. 1989. Cocaine use and withdrawal: The effect on sleep and mood. *Sleep Res* 18:83.

Timothy A. Roehrs

DRUGS FOR MEDICAL DISORDERS

It is well known that drugs whose target organ is the brain (i.e., psychotropics) have effects on sleep and daytime alertness (see ANTIDEPRESSANTS; SLEEPING PILLS; TRANQUILIZERS). It is becoming increasingly evident, however, that certain drugs whose target organ is not the brain (e.g., antihistamines, bronchodilators) also penetrate the brain and have an impact on sleep–wake function.

ANTIHISTAMINES of the H_1 type are drugs used for the treatment of allergy and are associated with sedative effects because they easily pass into the brain and affect neural structures associated with sleep (see CHEMISTRY OF SLEEP; NREM SLEEP MECHANISMS). In fact, the sedative potential of H_1 antihistamines has made them the most common ingredient of OVER-THE-COUNTER SLEEPING PILLS. Despite their sleep-inducing potential, overnight sleep studies on antihistamines do not typically show increased sleep times or decreased wakefulness. In contrast, daytime studies using the MULTIPLE SLEEP LATENCY TEST clearly demonstrate the sedative potency of these drugs, which also have been shown to impair daytime performance. The mechanism of this performance impairment is most likely related to the sedative effects of these compounds. Most recently, H_1 antihistamines (e.g., terfenadine and loratadine) have been developed that do not readily penetrate the CENTRAL NERVOUS SYSTEM and hence have minimal or no sedative effects.

Analgesics or pain killers are also known to affect sleep–wake function. Opioids such as morphine have been shown to produce sedativelike effects on waking EEGs (see NARCOTICS). Consistent with sedative effects, individuals taking these drugs also have impaired performance. The chief sleep-related effect of opioids is to decrease REM SLEEP. A commonly used nonopioid analgesic is ASPIRIN. Aspirin has mild hypnotic activity, as demonstrated by a slight reduction of wakefulness in patients with INSOMNIA. Its hypnotic activity, however, is not very great, and aspirin is not recommended as a sleep aid.

Anorectics—drugs used to suppress appetite—enhance central catecholamine activity and thus are central nervous system STIMULANTS. The appetite-suppressant action of these drugs is inseparable from the stimulant effects, so insomnia is a frequent side effect of therapy. Not surprisingly, drugs in this class are chemically related to AMPHETAMINES. (See also EATING DISORDERS.)

Bronchodilators are used to treat chronic obstructive lung disease and asthma (see MEDICAL ILLNESS AND SLEEP). While some drugs in this class (e.g., albuterol) have no effect on sleep–wake, other bronchodilators such as theophylline possess significant alerting effects. Theophylline belongs to a chemical class known as the xanthines, of which CAFFEINE is the most commonly used. Theophylline, like caffeine, increases alertness during the day but causes increased wakefulness and sleep FRAGMENTATION at night.

Finally, the effects of cardiovascular drugs have received increasing attention with regard to their central nervous system effects. Beta-adrenoreceptor antagonists, such as propranolol, metoprolol, and pindolol, are used mainly in the treatment of hypertension, cardiac dysrhythmias, and angina. Patients taking these drugs complain of difficulty falling asleep and an increased number of awakenings during the night. Some patients taking these compounds also report an increased frequency of dreaming, an experience due to the fact that dreams are more frequently recalled when awakenings are frequent, rather than to any effect of these drugs on REM sleep.

In summary, although a drug may be taken for its effect on the heart or lungs, the degree to which it penetrates the brain will determine the extent to which it affects sleep–wake function. Thus, drugs from a variety of therapeutic classes have the potential for disturbing sleep or producing daytime drowsiness.

Thomas Roth

D SLEEP

See Alpha-Delta Sleep

E

EARLY BIRDS AND NIGHT OWLS

The terms *early bird* and *night owl* have evolved as labels for people's sleep–wake preferences. *Early bird* denotes a person who is most alert and performs best in the morning hours. People who feel most active and alert during the evening hours, on the other hand, have been likened to night owls. The distinction of these diurnal types has been around for many years and in the scientific literature since the 1930s. More recently these labels have been identified using MORNINGNESS/EVENINGNESS or "Lark and Owl" self-assessment questionnaires designed to assess whether a person's sleep and activity patterns are more like those of the early-rising lark or the night-active owl (Horne and Östberg, 1976; Torsvall and Åkerstedt, 1980; Folkard, Monk, and Lobban, 1979; Smith, Reilly, and Midkiff, 1989). Several of these self-assessment questionnaires have been validated with physiological measures, such as BODY TEMPERATURE, which is a marker for the body's internal clock time. Thus, the peak of the daily body temperature cycle tends to occur earlier in people who are early birds than in night owls.

Perhaps the best known early bird is the lark, which awakens early to satisfy its thirst with the morning dew. The lark's preference for the early hours can be heard in its beautiful morning song or mating call. Morning is also important to another bird, the robin, which feeds on earthworms. Since earthworms surface only on cloudy days or at night, the robin must hunt for its food before the worms burrow back into the soil. Hence, this early bird does get the worm.

Owls are strictly nocturnal, unlike morning birds and also unlike other avian predators such as the hawk and the falcon, which are diurnal. Why, then, is the owl a bird of the night? According to the ancient Roman poet Ovid, the wren once attempted to become king of the birds by trickery, and was punished by being confined in a mousehole, with the owl assigned to guard the entrance; the owl fell asleep instead, and has been too ashamed to appear in the daytime ever since. A less poetic but more likely explanation is that the owl's senses are adapted to work in the darkness. The size and placement of their eyes give owls excellent binocular vision—a distinct advantage in judging distance—that, along with well-developed ears and nearly silent flight, allows them to take advantage of their prey. Thus, the owl is able to find food, defend its territory, and even woo a mate, all at night.

Both owls and morning birds are found in the literature, legends, and symbols of many cultures. Athena, the ancient Greek goddess of wisdom, adopted the night owl as her symbol. In Roman times, the hoot of an owl was a harbinger of death. The deaths of both Julius Caesar and Augustus were said to be foreshadowed by the owl's call; authors such as Chaucer and Shakespeare have also used the owl to foreshadow death in their works. Owls appear frequently in the Bible to depict destruction and devastation, often in the sinister company of ravens and vultures. The lark and other diurnal birds have cultural references with primarily positive connotations: *Lark* as a verb means to play or tease. One can also think of lovebirds, songbirds, and even "The Bluebird of Happiness." The dove has become the universal symbol for peace, and the soaring eagle is the American symbol for freedom. These examples demonstrate how culturally induced images have influenced attitudes about what it means to be an early bird or a night owl.

In actuality, there is no "good" or "bad" sleep preference. The merits of being an early bird or a night owl are different for everyone. Although Benjamin Franklin declared, "Early to bed, early to rise, makes a man healthy, wealthy, and wise," he might have withdrawn that statement had he lived to see how dramatically his discovery of electricity changed the world. Electricity has made it possible for people to be active by choice at any hour of the day or night.

Research has shown that our tendency to be owls or larks changes with age. Recent studies have confirmed that one of the biggest changes in sleep patterns occurs between high school and college. While most high school students are asleep by 12:30 A.M., the average bedtime for college students is later than 2:00 A.M. (Carskadon and Davis, 1989). The tendency to go to bed late, however, gradually changes with advancing age. The elderly become more larkish. Despite these documented age-related tendencies, the largest variation in our sleep-wake habits results from individual differences. Everyone's biological clock is different; people may be born with a tendency to be either owls or larks.

(See also AGING AND CIRCADIAN RHYTHMS; BIRDS; CULTURAL ASPECTS OF SLEEP; MORNINGNESS/EVENINGNESS; SLEEP AND DREAMING IN LITERATURE.)

REFERENCES

Carskadon MA, Davis SS. 1989. Sleep–wake patterns in the high-school-to-college transition. *Sleep Res* 18:113.

Folkard S, Monk T, Lobban M. 1989. Towards a predictive test of adjustment to shiftwork. *Ergonomics* 22:79–91.

Horne JA, Östberg OA. 1976. A self-assessment questionnaire to determine morningness-eveningness in human circadian rhythms. *Int J Chronobiology* 4:97–110.

Smith CS, Reilly C, Midkiff K. 1989. Evaluation of three circadian rhythm questionnaires with suggestions for an improved measure of morningness. *J Appl Psychol* 74(5):728–738.

Sparks J, Soper T. 1970. *Owls—their natural and unnatural history.* New York: Taplinger.

Torsvall L, Åkerstedt T. 1980. A diurnal type scale. *Scand J Work Envir Health* 6:283–290.

Pamela J. Bigler

EARLY MORNING AWAKENING

Early morning awakening or *premature awakening* refers to termination of sleep before the desired time. This type of sleep complaint is typically associated with either DEPRESSION or a phase advance syndrome (see CIRCADIAN RHYTHMS; ADVANCED SLEEP PHASE SYNDROME). In the case of depression, early morning awakenings occur in combination with other depressive symptoms, including mood changes, loss of appetite, loss of interest in sexual activities, and difficulty falling and staying asleep. Depressed individuals go to bed at a normal time, have difficulty falling asleep, and awaken prematurely. Thus, it is typical for an individual with depression to report going to bed at 11:00 P.M., taking an hour to fall asleep, waking up several times during the night, and waking up at 5:00 A.M. unable to return to sleep. Such an individual will get only 4 to 5 hours of sleep for the night. Patients with depression are typically treated with medications that reverse both the mood and sleep abnormalities (see ANTIDEPRESSANTS).

In contrast, individuals with early morning awakenings due to a phase advance syndrome also arise early in the morning but do not have difficulty falling asleep or staying asleep. A phase advance syndrome is a circadian rhythm disorder (see CIRCADIAN RHYTHM DISORDERS). That is, there is a mismatch between an individual's desired sleep time and his or her biological clock. For example, a common experience for an individual traveling from New York to Hawaii is to arise in the morning before the desired time. Such an individual gets sleepy early in the evening (bedtime in New York) and awakens early in the morning (arising time in New York). Thus, the desired sleep–wake times now that the individual is in Hawaii do not match the habitual sleep–wake times in New York (see JET LAG).

In the general population, the elderly are most likely to complain of early morning awakening. One hypothesis is that the biological clock speeds up as we age, and thus we go to sleep earlier and awaken earlier. In contrast to depressed patients who arise early and get only 4 to 5 hours of sleep, individuals with phase advance syndrome arise early in the morning but are generally able to get a normal amount of sleep during the night. The treatment for circadian rhythm disorders involves rescheduling the person's sleep–wake times (see CHRONOTHERAPY). More recently, research has been done demonstrating the value of bright light in resetting sleep–wake schedules. In people with phase advance syndrome, exposure to bright light in the evening delays bedtime and arising time (see LIGHT THERAPY).

Thomas Roth

EARLY SLEEP THEORIES

The earliest known theories regarding the physiological process of sleep and the function of sleep date back to the sixth century B.C. The Greek philosopher Alcmaeon, who was born in the second half of the sixth century, believed that sleep was caused by the retreat of blood from the vessels of the skin to those inside the body. In the fifth century Empedocles of Agrigentum theorized that sleep was brought on by a cooling of the warm element in blood; he believed that sleep served to make the body cold. Another philosopher of the fifth century B.C., Diogenes, thought that the presence of air in blood vessels was the principle of being and necessary for consciousness. Accordingly, he argued that sleep arises when air is replaced by blood in the vessels.

For each of these philosophers, sleep and death were founded on the same physiological process and were thought to differ only in intensity. Thus, for Alcmaeon, death was the complete retreat of blood from the periphery. Similarly, Empedocles thought that death was a result of the complete cooling of the blood, and Diogenes believed death to be the complete replacement of air by blood. This characteristic feature of early Greek theories concerning sleep may have taken root in Homer's *Iliad*, in which sleep and death (Hypnos and Thanatos) appear several times as twin brothers acting together.

Aristotle wrote extensively on the subject of sleep. According to him, sleep is the cessation of perception brought on by an excess of being awake. He believed that sleep was necessary to re-

cover perception, which was centered in the heart. The process of sleep was thought to be initiated by vapors generated by the digestion of food that were driven upward and caused drowsiness (see POSTPRANDIAL).

In the second century A.D., Galen, like Aristotle, related sleep to perception; however, Galen believed the brain to be the center of perception. The purpose of sleep, according to Galen, was the recovery of brain function and the renovation of innate warmth in the heart, which was thought to be the bearer of life.

Theories pertaining to sleep during the Renaissance period resembled those of Aristotle and Galen. Like Aristotle, writers of this period agreed that sleep was essentially the interruption of perception and that sleep depth and length were a function of the amount of vapors produced by digestion or physical exertion. Like Galen, however, Renaissance theorists thought that sleep was localized in the brain. Renaissance thinkers proposed many functions for sleep. Sleep was thought to enhance digestion, to create new animal spirits necessary for perception and motion, to increase natural warmth, and to boil the raw and possibly damaging humors. Sleep was also thought to free the soul of worry, anger, and mental derangement.

By the late nineteenth and early twentieth centuries, a greater understanding of brain physiology and a number of new ideas concerning the state of the brain during sleep were developed. Many authors offered new ideas to explain the loss of perception attendant upon the onset of sleep. Hill (1898) and Howell (1897) suggested that dilation of blood vessels in the skin causes an anemia of the brain. Purkinje, Osborne, and Mauther each offered separate mechanisms by which sensory input to the brain could be cut off by a swelling in another portion of the brain; Duval believed that sleep is initiated when contacts between neurons retract (see Kleitman, 1963).

Shepard (1914) proposed that as we go to sleep we become absorbed in sensations of fatigue that tend to inhibit other processes. Pavlov (1962) had a similar theory; he concluded that inhibition of any area of the cerebral cortex could be termed localized sleep and that sleep itself was a result of widespread inhibition.

Reminiscent of the Renaissance, it was widely believed during this period that sleep served to dissipate excess products of metabolism, or "hynotoxins," such as lactic acid or carbon dioxide. Such substances were thought to accumulate to dangerous levels during waking and to initiate sleep by virtue of their high concentration.

Early sleep theories progressed and changed as the understanding of physiology developed; however, certain themes such as the mechanisms underlying the loss of perception were maintained over many centuries.

REFERENCES

Hill L. 1898. Arterial pressure in man while sleeping, resting, waking, bathing. *J Physiol (London)* 22:26–29.

Howell WHA. 1897. A contribution to the physiology of sleep based upon plethysmographic experiments. *J Exp Med* 2:313–345.

Kleitman N. 1963. *Sleep and wakefulness,* 2nd ed. Chicago: University of Chicago Press.

Pavlov IP. 1962. *Essays in psychology and psychiatry, including a section on sleep and hypnosis.* New York: Citadel.

Shepard JF. 1914. *The circulation and sleep.* New York: Macmillan.

Wittern R. 1989. Sleep theories in antiquity and the Renaissance. In Horne JA, ed. *Sleep '88,* pp 11–22. Stuttgart/New York: Fischer-Verlag.

Douglas Nitz

EATING DISORDERS

Eating disorders may be associated with changes in total daily sleep time and sleep architecture. Eating disorders include anorexia nervosa and bulimia nervosa, which are both thought to have a significant psychiatric component, and obesity. Other problems with food may be important factors in the development or severity of some sleep disorders, such as food allergy insomnia, nocturnal eating syndrome, and narcolepsy (American Sleep Disorders Association, 1990).

Anorexia nervosa (from the Greek *an,* "no," and *orexis,* "appetite") was first described by Richard Morton in 1689. It is an eating disorder that occurs predominantly in females and that usually begins between the ages of 12 and 18. It is characterized by a refusal to maintain normal weight for one's age and height (i.e., total body weight less than 85 percent of expected body weight); intense fear of gaining weight or becoming fat, even though one is underweight; a distorted perception of one's own body weight, size, or shape; and (in females) loss of the monthly menstrual period. Weight loss usually is accomplished by a reduction in food intake, intense exercise, or the use of diuretics and laxatives, which promote urination and bowel movements (American Psychiatric Association, 1987). The effects of extreme cases of anorexia nervosa may be similar to those of chronic starvation. There may be both medical (e.g., low blood pressure, low body temperature, fluid retention) and psychiatric (e.g., depression, crying spells, obsessive thoughts, personality problems) components of the illness (Halmi, 1985).

Bulimia nervosa also tends to be more common in females than males and most frequently occurs between the ages of 15 and 30. It is characterized by recurrent episodes of binge eating, during which large amounts of food are consumed over a discrete period; self-induced vomiting after food intake; and the use of laxatives or diuretics. Like anorectic individuals, those suffering from bulimia nervosa may go to extreme lengths to prevent weight gain and may have a persistent overconcern with, or distorted perception of, body weight, size, or shape (American Psychiatric Association, 1987).

Crisp (1967) was among the first to report that patients with anorexia nervosa had disturbances of sleep. He showed that interruptions of sleep and early morning awakenings were likely to be associated with weight loss. Other investigators have since confirmed these early findings and also have reported that anorectic patients have more stage 1 sleep and less slow-wave sleep (SWS) than healthy control subjects (Levy, Dixon, and Schmidt, 1987, 1988; Walsh et al., 1985). All of these sleep abnormalities seem to recover with the normalization of body weight (Lacey et al., 1975). Patients with bulimia nervosa do not have sleep disturbances similar to those of anorectic patients. In fact, most studies have shown that the sleep of normal-weight bulimic patients is similar to that of healthy control subjects. There are exceptions. Some patients with bulimia may be prone to frequent awakenings and episodes of binge eating at night, which may result in sleep FRAGMENTATION. It also is known that patients who are *both* bulimic and anorectic may have sleep disturbances like those seen in anorexia nervosa alone. It has been suggested that extreme weight loss alone is responsible for the sleep disturbance seen in anorexia nervosa. This hypothesis is supported by studies of food deprivation and starvation in laboratory animals (see NUTRITION AND SLEEP).

It has been suggested that nutritional factors play a role in the sleep disturbances seen in people with problems other than anorexia nervosa. One large study of 375 patients has shown that weight loss occurring in the context of psychiatric illness is associated with decreased total daily sleep time and early-morning awakenings (Crisp and Stonehill, 1973). These disturbances are not seen exclusively in patients with depression, although they may be associated with increased awakenings from sleep when weight loss occurs as a symptom of severe depression. In addition, weight gain occurring in the context of depression can be associated with hypersomnolence and increases in total daily sleep time.

Some investigators have viewed the similarities between the sleep of anorectic and depressed patients as an indication that patients with anorexia nervosa may be depressed. This assertion was strengthened by reports that some patients with anorexia nervosa (alone or combined with bulimia nervosa) have a short latency to the first REM period of the night. Short REM LATENCY is seen in a large proportion of patients with endogenous depression (see DEPRESSION.) Therefore, it was thought that this finding might serve to validate the diagnosis of depression in anorectic patients (Katz, 1987). However, other studies of anorectic patients have failed to find disturbances of REM sleep that are consistent with depression. Trends showing disturbances of REM sleep like those seen in depression are seen only in eating disorder patients who *also* are clinically depressed, suggesting that eating disorders are not variants of depression.

It is well documented that obesity (being at least 20 to 30 percent above the expected average weight for one's age, sex, and height) is a complicating factor in sleep apnea (see APNEA), but very little is known about sleep in nonapneic obese individuals. One study suggests that the percentage of deviation from ideal body weight correlates with both total sleep time and the mean sleep cycle length, so that increasing weight is associated with longer total sleep time and sleep cycle length (Adam, 1977). Other studies have shown that obese patients who are losing weight sleep much less than when they are not dieting. Additional work needs to be done to confirm these findings and to determine if there are real similarities between the data obtained from obese laboratory animals and those obtained from obese humans.

Some eating disorders may be associated with sleep disorders. Food allergy insomnia is characterized by difficulty initiating or maintaining sleep because of an allergic response to certain foods. This disorder is most commonly seen in infants who are intolerant of cow's milk. They often cry, become agitated, or show other signs of allergy after repeated exposure to the offending food. Studies have shown that these infants awaken an average of five times per night and obtain an average of 4.5 hours of sleep per night (Ferber, 1987). Distraught parents often find that their attempts to soothe their babies are of no help in promoting sleep. Fortunately, the disorder can subside spontaneously between the ages of 2 and 4, and its symptoms may be resolved by substituting a hydrolyzed milk protein formula for cow's milk. (See also MILK ALLERGY AND INFANT SLEEP.) Food allergy insomnia also may occur in adults, some of whom will report allergic reactions to a variety of foods (e.g., eggs, fish). This disorder does not appear as an isolated incident but is identified when repeated exposures to a certain food consistently produce insomnia. Avoidance of the offending food(s) often is the best treatment.

Nocturnal eating (or drinking) syndrome is characterized by repeated awakenings during the night with the inability to return to sleep without eating or drinking. Approximately 5 percent of children between the ages of 6 months and 3 years are thought to suffer from this disorder. It may be a problem that arises from repeated nighttime feedings that actually "condition" the child to become hungry at these times. Elimination of nighttime feedings usually helps in resolving the sleep problem (Ferber, 1987). Recent evidence also suggests that some adults suffer from nocturnal eating (drinking) syndrome. Many awaken several times during the night to consume food or fluid, a factor that probably promotes repeated awakenings and that may contribute to total daily caloric intake and weight gain. At least one obese patient with this disorder has been known to consume during his nighttime awakenings more than twice his total daytime caloric intake.

Narcolepsy is a disorder characterized by

excessive daytime sleepiness, cataplexy, sleep paralysis, hypnogogic hallucinations, and sleep-onset REM periods (see NARCOLEPSY). Some people suffering from narcolepsy often experience sleep attacks during or after meals, and some report an increase in symptoms after the ingestion of certain foods. Starches (e.g., crackers, bread) and dairy foods (e.g., milk, cheese) were most often listed as offending foods. Elimination of these foods from the diet or the ingestion of small meals can result in an improvement in symptoms for certain people. Some narcoleptic people may avoid eating altogether until the evening hours, when sleepiness is least likely to be problematic. These data suggest that dietary factors can be important to some people in managing the symptoms of narcolepsy. Moreover, they highlight some of the interesting and important relationships between eating disorders and sleep disturbances.

REFERENCES

Adam K. 1977. Brain rhythm that correlates with obesity. *Br Med J* 2:234.

American Psychiatric Association. 1987. *Diagnostic and statistical manual of mental disorders, 3rd edition, revised,* pp 65–71. Washington, D.C.: American Psychiatric Association.

American Sleep Disorders Association. 1990. *The international classification of sleep and arousal disorders,* pp 98–104. Lawrence, Kans.: Allen Press.

Crisp AH, 1967. The possible significance of some behavioral correlates of weight and carbohydrate intake. *J Psychosomat Res* 11:117–131.

Crisp AH, Stonehill E. 1973. Aspects of the relationship between sleep and nutrition: A study of 375 psychiatric out-patients. *Br J Psychiatry* 122:379–394.

Ferber R. 1987. The sleepless child. In Guilleminault C, ed. *Sleep and its disorders in children,* pp 141–164. New York: Raven Press.

Halmi K. 1985. Eating disorders. In Kaplan HI, Sadock BJ, eds. *Comprehensive textbook of psychiatry,* pp 1731–1735. Baltimore: Williams & Wilkins.

Katz J. 1987. Eating disorder and affective disorder: Relatives or merely acquaintances? *Comp Psychiatry* 28:220–228.

Lacey JH, Crisp AH, Kalucy RS, Hartmann MK, Chen CN. 1975. Weight gain and the sleeping electroencephalogram: Study of ten patients with anorexia nervosa. *Br Med J* 4:556–558.

Levy AB, Dixon KN, Schmidt H. 1987. REM and delta sleep in anorexia nervosa and bulimia. *Psychiatr Res* 20:189–197.

———. 1988. Sleep architecture in anorexia nervosa and bulimia. *Biol Psychiatry* 23:99–101.

Walsh BT, Goetz R, Roose SP, Fingeroth S, Glassman AH. 1985. EEG-monitored sleep in anorexia nervosa and bulimia. *Biol Psychiatry* 20:947–956.

Gary K. Zammit
Sigurd H. Ackerman

ECHIDNA

The echidna is an Australian animal representing one of the earliest mammals in evolutionary history. Its ancient status has led it to be called a "living fossil." The importance of the echidna to sleep research has been in helping scientists to understand the evolution of sleep states along with the evolution of the mammalian brain (see PHYLOGENY).

The echidna is a member of an order of mammals called *Monotremata.* Monotreme simply means "single hole," and these very special mammals have a single outlet for their urinary, gastrointestinal, and reproductive tracts. The platypus is also a well-known member of this order. Another interesting feature of these animals is that they are egg-laying mammals; even so, they nurse

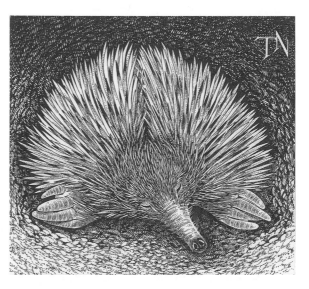

Figure 1.   An echidna. *Drawing by Trudy Nicholson.*

their young, just as all mammals do. The echidna is a burrowing insect eater, similar in that way to modern moles, yet the echidna has a very primitive brain. Sleep researchers found that the echidna experiences NREM sleep, but not REM sleep (Allison, Van Twyver, and Goff, 1972). Because of the echidna's status as a primitive mammal, this discovery led to the theory that in mammals NREM sleep evolved before REM sleep (see EVOLUTION OF SLEEP).

REFERENCES

Allison T, Van Twyver H. 1970. The evolution of sleep. *Nat Hist* 79:56–65.

Allison T, Van Twyver H, Goff W. 1972. Electrophysiological studies of the echidna *Tachyglossus aculeatus*. I. Waking and sleeping. *Arch Ital Biol* 110:145–184.

Kate B. Herman
Mary A. Carskadon

EEG

See Brainmapping; Electroencephalogram; Electroencephalography; Polysomnography

EKG

See Electrocardiogram; Polysomnography

ELECTROCARDIOGRAM

Electrocardiography, the recording of electrical activity associated with heart contractions, has been in use for over 70 years. The record produced by this technique is called an electrocardiogram (abbreviated ECG or EKG). Screening electrocardiography is currently done with twelve recording leads (electrode locations). Electrocardiographic monitoring during polysomnographic studies, however, uses only one lead. The polysomnographic electrocardiogram can be recorded with the same type of electrodes used to record the electroencephalogram or, alternatively, with special electrodes that are easier to fasten to and remove from the skin. The most typical location of the electrodes is the one known as lead II (right shoulder and left leg). The main purpose of including an electrocardiographic lead during routine polysomnographic studies is to assess the cardiac rhythm. This assessment is particularly relevant in polysomnographic studies of patients with obstructive sleep APNEA, who frequently have arrhythmias. The cardiac arrhythmia most often encountered in this group of patients is sinus arrhythmia (slowing or bradycardia during the respiratory event followed by speeding or tachycardia at the end of the respiratory event). Other cardiac arrhythmias that may be encountered include second-degree atrioventricular block, prolonged sinus pauses, paroxysmal tachycardia, and limited runs of ventricular tachycardia.

REFERENCES

Guilleminault C. 1982. Sleep and breathing. In Guilleminault C, ed. *Sleeping and waking disorders: Indications and techniques,* pp 155–182. Menlo Park, Calif.: Addison-Wesley.

Martin RJ, Block AJ, Cohn MA, Conway WA, Hudgel DW, Powles ACP, Sanders MH, Smith PL. 1985. Indications and standards for cardiopulmonary sleep studies. *Sleep* 8(4):371–379.

Leon D. Rosenthal

ELECTRODERMAL ACTIVITY

Electrodermal activity (EDA) is a general term for electrical activity of the skin and eccrine sweat glands. It can be measured in terms of a variety of quantities, including the GALVANIC SKIN RESPONSE (GSR). The electrical activity of the sweat glands is controlled by the sympathetic division of the AUTONOMIC NERVOUS SYSTEM (ANS) through an unusual mechanism. Control of the sweat gland is the only function of the autonomic nervous system involving the neurotransmitter acetylcholine, rather than noradrenaline. When body temperature is normal, changes in sweat gland

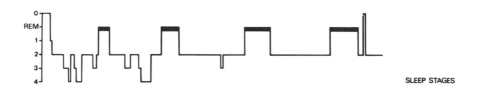

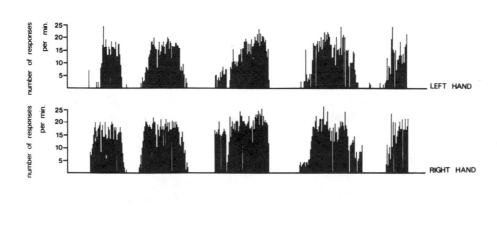

Figure 1. Histogram of sleep stages and electrodermal activity. *Modified with permission from Ware et al., 1984.*

activity are thought to reflect psychological events and are not due to efforts of the body to control internal temperature.

Electrodermal activity includes two general categories of measurements, exosomatic and endosomatic. *Exosomatic* refers to techniques such as GSR measurement, in which an external electrical current is passed through the skin and changes in skin resistance or conductance are measured. *Endosomatic* usually refers to measurement of spontaneously occurring electrical potentials of the skin.

Both of these techniques have been used to study sleep. The majority of research reports demonstrate that EDA is greater in NREM sleep than in waking and peaks during stage 4 sleep. The high levels of EDA activity have led some researchers to speak of "GSR storms" (McDonald et al., 1976). EDA is minimal in REM sleep, although some activity has been noted during phasic bursts of rapid eye movements (Broughton, Poire, and Tassinari, 1965; see PHASIC ACTIVITY IN REM SLEEP). Other studies have reported that presleep ANXIETY is correlated with

higher levels of EDA during sleep and lower levels of deep sleep (Lester, Burch, and Dossett, 1967).

Researchers have speculated that EDA occurs in NREM sleep because of a release of subcortical areas of the brain from inhibition by higher areas (Johnson and Lubin, 1966). Although this interpretation is thought to have some merit, it is not consistent with data showing that other sympathetic ANS activities related to cardiovascular function are low during NREM sleep and phasically higher during REM sleep.

REFERENCES

Broughton RJ, Poire R, Tassinari CA. 1965. The electrodermogram (Tarchanoff effect) during sleep. *Electroencephalogr Clin Neurophysiol* 18: 691–708.

Johnson LC, Lubin A. 1966. Spontaneous electrodermal activity during waking and sleeping. *Psychophysiology* 3:8–17.

Lester BK, Burch NR, Dossett RC. 1967. Nocturnal EEG-GSR profiles: The influence of pre-sleep states. *Psychophysiology* 3:238–248.

McDonald DG, Shallenberger HD, Koresko RL, Kinzy BG. 1976. Studies of spontaneous electrodermal responses in sleep. *Psychophysiology* 13(3): 128–138.

Ware JC, Karacan I, Salis PJ, Thornby J, Hirshkowitz M. 1984. Sleep related electrodermal activity patterns in impotent patients. *Sleep* 7(3):247–254.

Mark R. Pressman

ELECTROENCEPHALOGRAM

An electroencephalogram (EEG) is a recording of electrical signals generated by the brain. Luigi Galvani, an Italian physiologist working in the late eighteenth century, was one of the first scientists to demonstrate electrical properties of the nervous system with his observation that the leg muscle of a frog twitched when an iron wire in contact with the muscle touched a brass wire in contact with the nerve supplying that muscle.

In 1875, a British physiologist, Richard Caton, after performing experiments on the exposed brains of dogs and rabbits, reported that, "In every brain hitherto examined, the galvanometer has indicated the existence of . . . feeble currents of varying direction." After this first demonstration of brain electrical activity, more than 50 years passed before Hans Berger, an Austrian physician, showed that the human brain also produced electrical signals that could be recorded on paper, and the modern era of electroencephalography began. Modern EEG equipment, including highly sensitive amplifiers, signal analyzers and averagers, and imaging and storage devices, permits detailed analysis of virtually every aspect of brain electrical activity.

Berger noted a prominent 10-cycle-per-second rhythm in the surface EEG, which he designated as *alpha,* and faster frequencies, which he called *beta.* The EEG is now classified into four frequency bands: delta, 0 to 3 cycles per second; theta, 4 to 7 cycles per second; alpha, 8 to 13 cycles per second; and beta, above 13 cycles per second. The normal EEG varies in appearance depending on whether the subject is awake, in NREM sleep, or in REM sleep. In persons who are awake and resting quietly with eyes closed, the EEG is dominated by the ALPHA RHYTHM, a sinusoidal rhythm that is usually 9 or 10 cycles per second and most apparent over the posterior head regions. With eye opening or with active visual imagery, the alpha rhythm is replaced by a lower-voltage more irregular pattern with a mixture of frequencies. During sleep the EEG is dominated by slower frequencies in the theta and delta range.

Physiologic Basis

The EEG is generated by the nerve cells that line the surface, or cortex, of the brain. These cells, like all nerve cells, maintain a voltage difference between the inside and the outside of the cell called the *resting membrane potential.* Nerve impulses, called action potentials, arriving from other cells are of short duration and have very little effect on the surface EEG, but the fluctuations in the resting membrane potential induced by the arriving action potentials can be recorded at the scalp as EEG waveforms. Rhythmical EEG activity is thought to result from the effects of periodic trains of action potentials arriving from pacemaker nerve cells located deep within the brain.

Applications

The EEG is an invaluable tool for brain research because it provides a direct measure of electrical activity of brain cells, the means by which these cells communicate with each other. The EEG can be used to assess the effects of various drugs on the brain, and by implanting small electrodes within the brain, it is possible to examine the electrical activity of specific areas of the brain and to correlate the activity of the brain region in question with stimuli presented to the subject or with the activity of other brain areas.

In medicine, the EEG is used to assess the effects of a variety of disorders on brain function including strokes, brain tumors, and diseases that are associated with abnormal chemical constituents of bodily fluids. One of the most important uses of the EEG is in the diagnosis and management of EPILEPSY, a condition in which the pattern of abnormal EEG activity helps to define the type of epilepsy and the specific medications that are most likely to be beneficial.

(See also ELECTROENCEPHALOGRAPHY).

REFERENCES

Caton R. 1875. The electric currents of the brain. *Br Med J* 2:278.

Niedermeyer E. 1987a. The normal EEG of the waking adult. In Niedermeyer E, Lopes da Silva F, eds. *Electroencephalography. Basic principles, clinical applications and related fields*, 2nd ed, pp 95–118. Baltimore: Urban & Schwarzenberg.

———. 1987b. Sleep and EEG. In Niedermeyer E, Lopes da Silva F, eds. *Electroencephalography. Basic principles, clinical applications and related fields*. 2nd ed, pp 119–133. Baltimore: Urban & Schwarzenberg.

Michael Aldrich

ELECTROENCEPHALOGRAPHY

Electroencephalography is the method used to record brain wave patterns. The presence of electrical activity in the brain was first discovered in 1875 when Richard Caton, an English physiologist, observed activity from electrodes placed on the brain surfaces of cats and rabbits. To visualize this electrical activity, Caton set up an elaborate system of long strings connected to electro-encephalogram (EEG) electrodes. The strings moved in response to the electrical signal from the brain. A light source shining against these strings cast shadows on the wall and made the signal large enough to observe. Shortly after Caton reported his discovery, many European investigators began to evaluate EEGs in animals.

In 1929, Hans Berger, an Austrian psychiatrist, studied the first EEG in humans. He evaluated brain waves in patients who had suffered neurological accidents, and he was able to record the activity directly from the surface of the brain. The recordings were made using a pen attached to a mechanical system that scratched marks on a rotating drum. From these recordings, Berger discovered that the brain waves of alert and actively thinking subjects were noticeably different from the brain waves of sleeping individuals.

By the 1930s, the study of electroencephalography became increasingly scientific; over the years, EEG recording equipment has become more sophisticated. The first studies of EEGs during sleep were made by Loomis, Harvey, and Hobart (1937), who described several stages of sleep similar to what are now referred to as NREM sleep stages 1, 2, 3, and 4. In addition, they were the first to describe a special waveform during sleep known as a K-complex (see K-COMPLEX).

Standardized methods have been developed for recording the EEG; one of the most important has been the International 10–20 System of Electrode Placement, which emphasizes precise placement of EEG electrodes on the surface of the scalp (see Figure 1) (Jasper, 1958). The

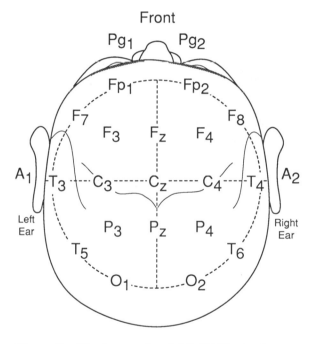

Figure 1. The International 10–20 Electrode Placement System emphasizes placing the electrodes very precisely on the surface of the scalp according to head measurements based on four standard landmarks: the front (nasion), back (inion), and both sides (left and right preauricular points) of the head. Using these landmarks to provide anterior/posterior and lateral planes, a "grid" of electrode placements can be made on any scalp. Placements most commonly used for polysomnography are labeled C_3, C_4, O_1, and O_2. C_3 and C_4 electrodes overlie the brain region called the central sulcus, and O_1 and O_2 electrodes overlie the occipital region of the brain.

central EEG electrodes (C_3 and C_4) are used for evaluating brain activity associated with different sleep stages. The occipital EEG leads (O_1 and O_2) are very useful for observing the transition from wake to sleep. They register the presence of alpha rhythm from the occipital cortex, which changes noticeably during the transition from the waking state to sleep (see ALPHA RHYTHM; STAGES OF SLEEP).

It has yet to be determined precisely what produces the electrical activity that is seen in the EEG. The most common explanations involve neurons in the cortex constituting the outer layers of the brain. The simplest of such models focuses on a particular type of neuron called a *pyramidal neuron*. This neuron gets its name from the shape of the cell body which is similar to a pyramid. This pyramidal cell neuron also has a long axon projecting from the bottom of the cell and elaborate dendrites at the top and lateral corners (Figure 2). Pyramidal cells are usually arranged with the apex, or top, pointing toward the surface of the cortex. This model of electrical activity views these neurons as simple dipoles, that is, elongated structures with different electrical field potentials on either end. Opposing charges change the electrical currents flowing around the pyramidal neurons, and that change is detected by electrodes on the surface of the scalp (Kooi, Tucker, and Marshall, 1978). Other models of electrical activity in the brain exist in which different types of neurons contribute to the EEG in a complex manner.

To understand sleep EEG patterns and why the EEG of the waking, active brain has a lower amplitude than the EEG of deep sleep, we must consider that the EEG activity represents the summation of many small electrical potential changes. Positive and negative potential changes are added together among hundreds and thousands of neurons so that, if the potential fields differ among these neurons, the additive quantity will be small. Thus, when a person is awake and actively thinking, the cortical neurons are differentially activated and have electrical charges that are desynchronized; when they sum, their additive quantity is low and exhibits lower-voltage EEG. In very deep sleep, by contrast, many neurons are simultaneously activated with similar potential shifts and their potentials add together to yield high-voltage, *synchronous* EEG activity. Such high-voltage (high-amplitude) activity is seen in SLOW-WAVE SLEEP.

(See also ELECTROENCEPHALOGRAM.)

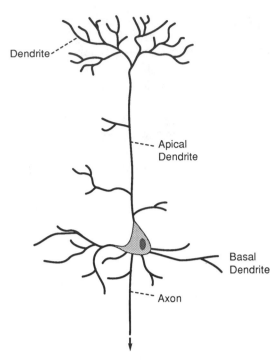

Figure 2. Schematic drawing of a pyramidal neuron in the cerebral cortex. One theory suggests that opposing charges in different parts of these cells change the electrical currents flowing around such neurons, producing the electrical activity that is measured by the electroencephalogram.

REFERENCES

Berger H. 1930. Über das Elektroenkephalogramm des Menschen. *J Psychol Neurol* 40:160–179.

Caton R. 1875. The electric current of the brain. *Br Med J* 2:278.

Jasper HH (Committee Chairman). 1958. The ten–twenty electrode system of the International Federation. *Electroencephalogr Clin Neurophysiol* 10:371.

Kooi KA, Tucker RP, Marshall RE. 1978. *Fundamentals of electroencephalography.* Hagerstown, Md.: Harper & Row.

Loomis AL, Harvey EN, Hobart GA. 1937. Cerebral states during sleep as studied by human brain potentials. *J Exp Psychol* 21:127–144.

Sharon A. Keenan

ELECTROMYOGRAPHY

Electromyographic recordings have been used routinely to measure sleep since the motor

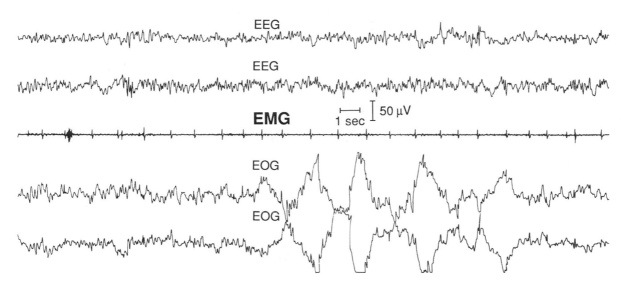

Figure 1. Electromyogram recorded during REM sleep.

paralysis of REM sleep was first described in the laboratory of Dr. Michel Jouvet in Lyon, France (Jouvet and Michel, 1959). For a standard polysomnographic recording (see POLYSOMNOGRAPHY), an electromyographic recording is required to monitor the activity of muscles, information that is essential for determining the presence of REM sleep.

The electromyogram (EMG) is recorded by measuring small electrical potentials created when muscle fibers contract. Each muscle contains many fibers and a section where the muscle connects with a nerve, which is called the motor end plate. At this point of connection, potentials are created by the flow of ions (charged chemicals). When many fibers contract, these ionic potential charges add up to give a larger electrical signal. Even when few fibers are contracting, which is the case in a resting muscle, a residual electrical potential can be recorded. During REM sleep, when motor neurons cease their firing entirely, the muscle fibers cease contracting (see ATONIA) and the electromyograph records electrical "silence," represented as a nearly flat line on the chart paper (see Figure 1). Figure 2, a NREM sleep sample, shows residual muscle tone with electrical activity of a moderate level. Figure 3 shows a body movement that is associated with the contraction of many muscle fibers; therefore, a large electrical potential ensues.

To record an electromyogram (EMG) for human polysomnography, electrodes are applied to the surface of the skin, usually on the chin (mentalis and submentalis muscles). These muscles are commonly used because they are conveniently located near the other electrodes used in polysomnography. Any skeletal muscle activity will change with the transition into REM sleep. Electromyographic electrodes may also be placed on the surface of the masseter muscle, the most important muscle for chewing, to allow for the detection of bruxism (teeth grinding) during sleep. Electromyographic electrodes may be applied to each leg, over the anterior tibialis muscle, and on the arms (extensor digitorum muscle) to detect movements that are associated with certain sleep disorders (see PERIODIC MOVEMENTS IN SLEEP and REM SLEEP BEHAVIOR DISORDER). In addition, recording electromyographic activity from the intercostal muscles between the ribs and from the diaphragm muscle in the thorax has been useful to assess breathing irregularities during sleep.

REFERENCE

Jouvet M, Michel M. 1959. Corrélations électromyographiques du sommeil chez le chat décortiqué et mesencephalique chronique. *CR Soc Biol (Paris)* 153:422–425.

Sharon A. Keenan

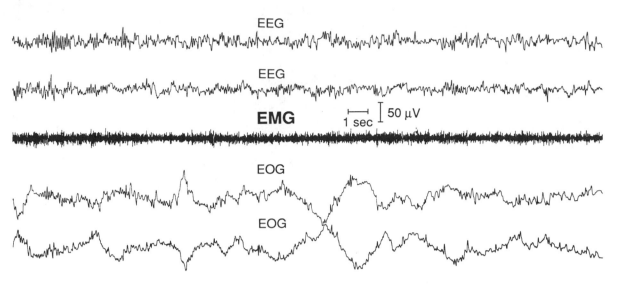

Figure 2. Electromyogram recorded during NREM sleep.

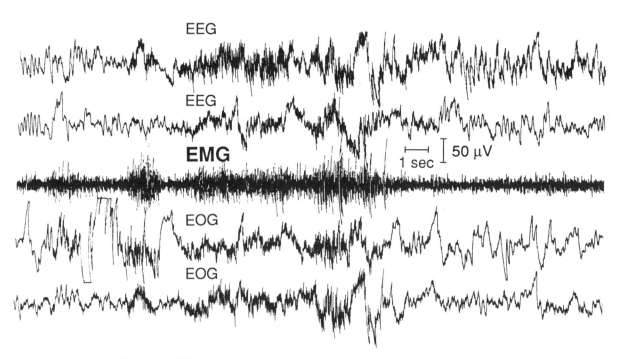

Figure 3. Electromyogram recorded during a body movement.

ELECTROOCULOGRAPHY

Electrooculography is the technique used to record eye movements in polysomnography. The important role of electrooculography in sleep recordings was first recognized in the laboratory of Dr. Nathaniel Kleitman at the University of Chicago, where REM sleep was first described (Aserinsky and Kleitman, 1953) (see REM SLEEP, DISCOVERY OF). Electrooculography measures the change in position of an electrical field that exists between the front of the eye (the cornea) and the back of the eye (the retina). This electrical difference is known as the corneo-retinal potential. The cornea is electrically positive with respect to the retina, and each eye sits in the skull, which acts as a volume conductor for this potential field. Changes in the orientation of this field are detected by electrodes placed on the skin, usually near the outer canthus (corner) of each eye. The right and left outer canthus electrodes are placed slightly off-center from the horizontal plane (see Figure 1) so that vertical as well as lateral eye movements can be observed. An amplifier receives the electrooculographic signal and enables the recording of eye movements. The output of the amplifier is the voltage change corresponding to the change in the position of the eye's corneo-retinal potential with respect to the monitoring electrode. When the subject looks to the left, the left outer canthus (LOC) electrode becomes more positive because, as the cornea moves closer to the electrode, the retina moves farther away from the electrode. At the same time, the right outer canthus (ROC) electrode becomes more negative as the retina moves closer to it and the cornea moves father away. The output

of the two eye channels are in opposite directions and therefore the two electrooculographic channels generate out-of-phase pen movements (see Figure 2).

Although vertical eye movements also produce out-of-phase tracings, the amplitude of the pens' deflections will be somewhat smaller for vertical eye movements if electrodes are placed as in Figure 1.

Electrooculography has a two-fold purpose in polysomnography. First, the electrooculogram (EOG) is useful for identifying the subtle transition from wakefulness to sleep. Slow eye movements often occur preceding and throughout this transition and are helpful in identifying the onset of stage 1 sleep (see STAGES OF SLEEP and SLEEP ONSET). The second and principal reason for including electrooculography in polysomnography is to monitor the bursts of rapid eye movements that characterize REM sleep (see REM SLEEP, PHYSIOLOGY OF).

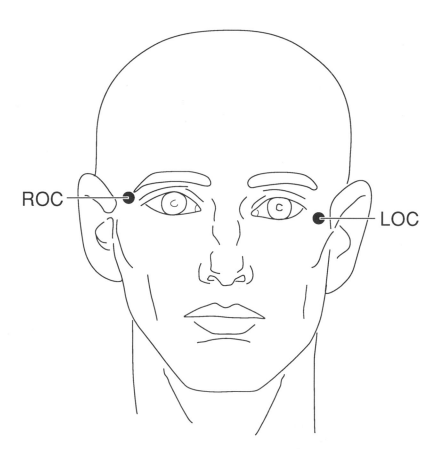

Figure 1. Placement of electrodes for electrooculography.

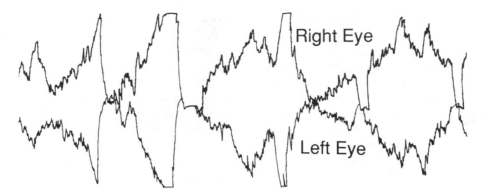

Figure 2.   A sample electrooculographic tracing.

REFERENCE

Aserinsky E, Kleitman N. 1953. Regularly occurring periods of eye motility, and concomitant phenomena, during sleep. *Science* 118:273–274.

Sharon A. Keenan

EMG

See Electromyography; Polysomnography

ENCEPHALITIS

Encephalitis is a general term describing any of a number of different infections of the central nervous system (CNS) that lead to tissue inflammation. These infections can be of a viral or bacterial origin. Representative examples of such infections include rabies, herpes, poliomyelitis, measles, mumps, Reye's syndrome, influenza, Guillain-Barré syndrome, and MONONUCLEOSIS. These infections are associated with a plethora of symptoms, including, for a few of the disease types, disordered sleep—either INSOMNIA or excessive sleepiness. Unfortunately, because of the scarcity of research in the area, little can be said with confidence about either the extent of the sleep disturbances in patients with encephalitis or the mechanisms underlying the sleep disturbances.

Routes of Entry and Neuronal Pathology

In general, the various types of viral encephalitis reach the CNS in different ways and cause different extents and types of damage. There are, however, a few general laboratory observations seen across the disease types. Viral infections appear to reach the CNS by moving along cells of the nervous system, by flowing through the circulatory system, or by a combination of the two. Once the viruses have reached their targets, they usually cause four types of damage: (1) alterations in the metabolic functioning of nerve cells that lead to cell death; (2) physical alterations of cells, such as the development of neurofibrillary tangles (an abnormal clustering of intracellular support fibers also seen in ALZHEIMER'S DISEASE); (3) evidence of cells edema (a gross inflammation of a cell caused by excess intracellular fluid); and (4) an immune system response, typically involving two types of glial cells (astrocytes and microglia) (see Booss and Esiri, 1986).

A Historical Note: Encephalitis Lethargica

One of the earliest observations of the association between encephalitis and sleep came from the work of the physician von Economo. His writings detailed the early outbreak of "encephalitis lethargica" in 1915, in Eastern and Central Europe. Within the next few years, the epidemic spread to the rest of mainland Europe, the United Kingdom, and eventually the United States. Typical symptoms included headache, muscle fatigue and weakness, fever, disordered oculomotor function, and either extreme drowsiness, or in rare cases, insomnia. Even after the disease had passed through the acute phase, clinicians reported that their surviving patients suffered numerous postinfection sequelae, such as PARKINSON'S DISEASE, sleep disorders, and abnormal motor tremors or twitches.

Areas of suspected neuropathology in the hypersomnolent encephalitis patients included midbrain regions, the THALAMUS, and the HYPOTHALAMUS. In those experiencing severe insomnia, damage to the preoptic area of the hypothalamus was found. Damage to this region has been shown to interfere with the maintenance of sleep—hence the complaint of insomnia (Broughton, 1971).

Recent Research on Encephalitis and Somnolence

In a recent study, Guilleminault and Mondini (1986) studied the nocturnal sleep, daytime sleepiness, and performance of twelve patients with either infectious mononucleosis (IM) or Guillain-Barré syndrome. In specific, all patients were thought to have been infected with the Epstein-Barr virus (EBV). Before undergoing recording in the sleep laboratory, all patients complained that the disease process had caused them to need both more nocturnal sleep and regular naps to offset persistent feelings of sleepiness.

Using POLYSOMNOGRAPHY, the authors found that the patients had unusually long total sleep times (versus normal control subjects) under both scheduled and *ad libitum* sleep conditions. However, no other abnormalities in the patients' sleep architecture or evidence of clinical sleep disorders (such as sleep APNEA or nocturnal myoclonus) were found. Assessments of their daytime sleepiness revealed two interesting findings. First, these individuals were profoundly sleepy during the day, despite their long sleep the preceding night. For example, if they were allowed to nap freely, they added another 1.5 to 3 hours to their sleep total per 24-hour period. If they were given the MULTIPLE SLEEP LATENCY TEST (MSLT), they only took an average of 6 minutes and 35 seconds to fall asleep. Second, the excessive daytime sleepiness was not caused by narcolepsy, as no sleep-onset REM periods were observed during the MSLT testing. (This propensity to fall asleep quickly during the day was not confined to the nap tests, however; the patients scored poorly on the performance tests as a result of repeated episodes of falling asleep).

Two years after the initial testing sessions, these patients reported continued long nocturnal total sleep times, regular napping, and unfortunately, an increase in daytime sleepiness. Based on the initial findings and the follow-up data, the authors concluded that patients with EBV-type encephalitis did in fact, on objective measures, exhibit chronic sleepiness (fatigue) despite increasing the total amount of sleep they obtained per 24 hours.

This clinical experience suggests that encephalitis can cause disruption of sleep–wake regulation, including both insomnia and HYPERSOMNOLENCE. Although the mechanisms are not clear, well-studied examples such as von Economo's encephalitis suggest that the hypothalamus may be involved.

REFERENCES

Booss J, Esiri MM. 1986. *Viral encephalitis: Pathology, diagnosis and management*. Boston: Blackwell Scientific.

Broughton R. 1971. Neurology and sleep research. *Canadian Psychiatric Assoc J* 16(4):283–292.

Guilleminault C. 1989. Idiopathic central nervous system hypersomnia. In Kryger MH, Roth T, Dement WC, eds. *Principles and practice of sleep medicine*, pp 347–350. Philadelphia: Saunders.

Guilleminault C, Mondini S. 1986. Mononucleosis and chronic daytime sleepiness. *Arch Intern Med* 146:1333–1335.

James K. Wyatt

ENDOCRINOLOGY

Endocrinology is the field of medicine and medical research devoted to the study of the function of hormones. The endocrine system includes the ductless glands, which synthesize and coordinate the action of hormones. Hormones are molecular messengers secreted into the blood circulation and transported to engage with appropriate receptor molecules on the surface of target cells where they exert a physiological effect. Since hormones may be cholesterol derivatives (e.g., sex steroids) or peptides (e.g., pituitary hormones), the mechanisms through which hormones exert their actions vary. Hormones influence a broad range of functions, including the rate of metabolic reactions, transport of nutritive substances through cell membranes, and regulation of water and electrolyte balances. On a cellular level, endocrine glands play a major role in the maintenance of homeostasis. Within this definition, other organs in the body such as the heart and kidneys can also be considered endocrine glands.

Endocrine Organization

Many endocrine systems are organized hierarchically with one gland (typically the PITUITARY GLAND) controlling the secretory action of another gland (e.g., the adrenals). This hierarchical organization facilitates integrated action across endocrine systems and interposes additional levels of control at which final action can be modulated for most endocrine systems. The pituitary gland, a center for such higher-order control, is directly governed by a region of the brain known as the HYPOTHALAMUS. The hypothalamus is the brain center responsible for monitoring homeostatic activities such as THERMOREGULATION, water balance, sexual activity, and sleep. It also contains the SUPRACHIASMATIC NUCLEUS OF THE HYPOTHALAMUS (SCN), the site of the circadian pacemaker in mammals. The pituitary is enlisted by the hypothalamus to control the adrenal and thyroid glands and the endocrine functions of the sexual organs. The proximity of the pituitary to the brain and its direct connections to the hypothalamus provide the principal pathway for information between the sensory and integrating functions of the CENTRAL NERVOUS SYSTEM (CNS) and the endocrine system. This pivotal function has earned the pituitary recognition as the body's "master gland."

Hormones whose release is orchestrated through hypothalamic influence are referred to as the NEUROENDOCRINE HORMONES, and their relationship to the state of sleep is further discussed below. While it is possible that sleep-related changes are mediated at nonhypothalamic CNS sites, the variety of hypothalamic–pituitary systems affected by sleep suggests that the hypothalamus is the mediating center for the sleep-related effects.

Hormonal Control

Like the nervous system, the endocrine network integrates the activities of various body systems, responding to the changing demands of exterior and interior environments through physiological adjustment and correlation. Many endocrine glands are activated to synthesize and release hormones in response to other hormones, changes in various metabolites, and/or specific stimuli. For example, the majority of GROWTH HORMONE released by the pituitary in adults is secreted in a long, nightly episode during the first hours or so following the onset of sleep. Human growth hormone is perhaps the best studied example of a hormonal process that is sleep dependent. During this nocturnal episode, plasma concentrations rise markedly and have a stimulating effect on systems controlling growth. Growth hormone's release is regulated by the opposing effects of growth hormone–releasing factor and somatostatin (growth hormone release inhibitor), both of which are released by the hypothalamus.

All pituitary hormones exhibit pulsatile secretion. The amplitude and frequency of these episodic pulses of hormone release, to a greater degree than mean hormone concentration, appear to be the regulated neuroendocrine parameters for the pituitary hormone systems. Target tissues sensitive to pituitary hormones respond to changes in these pulse parameters. Application of pulse recognition methods to the patterns of daily neuroendocrine secretion has demonstrated that diurnal variations in hormone concentration reflect underlying alterations in pulse frequency and/or amplitude, changes that can only occur at the level of the hypothalamic–pituitary unit.

Endocrine Function and Sleep

Sleep in humans is accompanied by prominent changes in the function of virtually every endocrine system in the body. Together these changes provide evidence of the variety and extent of physiological changes that occur during sleep, and the study of sleep-dependent endocrine changes can provide important insight into the nature and function of sleep itself.

Anterior pituitary neuroendocrine systems that undergo sleep-related changes include the anterior pituitary hormones, adrenocorticotropic hormone, THYROID-STIMULATING HORMONE (thyrotropin; TSH), GROWTH HORMONE, PROLACTIN, luteinizing hormone, and follicle-stimulating hormone. Also included is MELATONIN, the primary hormonal product of the PINEAL GLAND, secretion of which is principally under hypothalamic control. While other hormonal systems may be modulated by sleep, direct evidence of this relationship is not available. Most peptide hormones of the anterior pituitary, when subjected to rigorous analysis, have exhibited a tendency toward either circadian or sleep-dependent modulation, or both. Some hormones are inhibited by sleep, whereas secretion of others appears to be stimulated.

Sleep in humans and primates is monophasic, consolidated into one or two episodes per day, the timing of which is strongly modulated by the circadian pacemaker. By superimposing observed fluctuations of plasma concentrations of hormones upon known circadian rhythms of sleep, body temperature, and metabolism, researchers have begun to piece together the diurnal profile of neuroendocrine activity. Diurnal variation in pituitary hormones arises from two relatively distinct sources. First is the oscillatory signal from the body's internal biological clock known as CIRCADIAN RHYTHM. The second source of diurnal variation in neuroendocrine function is sleep itself. Among neuroendocrine parameters that are sleep related, sleep may have a stimulating or dampening role. For example, growth hormone and prolactin levels rise with sleep, whereas TSH shows a marked reduction in pulse amplitude during sleep.

In certain cases, the behavioral changes characteristically associated with sleep, such as supine posture or inactivity, are the proximal causes of altered physiologic function. A change in body position alters the demands placed on the heart and the rest of the cardiovascular system. For example, the renin–angiotensin–aldosterone hormone system, which links the kidneys and adrenal glands and helps to control blood pressure, exhibits reduced activity during sleep but

also any time we lie down, regardless of whether sleep occurs. Once behavior-influenced endocrine fluctuations are accounted for, the majority of oscillations in endocrine output may be divided among those influenced by circadian rhythmicity (non-sleep-dependent) and those linked to the state of sleep (sleep-dependent).

Circadian rhythms result from internal time keeping. Release of melatonin, which is synthesized by the pineal gland only in the absence of light, persists in the absence of external time information and independent of behavior changes such as posture, feeding, and sleep–wake cycles. Thus, melatonin release exhibits a circadian rhythm. In a sense, it may help the body keep track of time through its response to light–dark cycles, although the functional significance of melatonin rhythmicity is not clear and research is incomplete. Specific receptors for melatonin have been found in the SCNs of several species, including humans, and the hormone's influence on the hypothalamus–pituitary axis is under study. Melatonin's apparent link to the circadian oscillator, as well as the independence of melatonin secretion from modulation by other factors, makes the melatonin rhythm a useful marker of underlying clock function.

Unlike circadian rhythms, sleep-dependent changes are presumed to be adaptations to the altered physiologic conditions associated with sleep itself. Several endocrine systems with close links to the central nervous system demonstrate true sleep-related alterations in secretion and plasma concentration. In humans, the prolonged sleep episode, lasting 8 hours or more, presents special challenges for a number of regulatory systems, including glucose homeostasis, water balance, and thermoregulation. Although specific mechanisms involved are not yet clear, the sleep-dependent neuroendocrine changes may represent responses to (or preparations for) these extreme conditions.

As a consequence of circadian rhythmicity in sleep–wake organization, the sleep-dependent modulations in neuroendocrine function also occur on a regular daily basis. Unlike primary circadian rhythms in neuroendocrine function, however, sleep-dependent changes occur whenever sleep occurs; if sleep is prevented from occurring, the sleep-dependent neuroendocrine changes are also prevented (recall the example of growth hormone). As a group, these observed rhythms are said to represent *secondary* diurnal variation to distinguish them from rhythmic processes with direct links to the internal pacemaker. The importance of this subtle distinction lies in hypotheses about the functional significance of neuroendocrine modulation (see Figure 1).

Endocrine Disorders and Sleep

One consequence of the extensive interaction between endocrine function and sleep is that many endocrine disorders are associated with sleep disruption. For example, CORTISOL excess (Cushing's syndrome), arising as a consequence of either pituitary or adrenal overactivity, results in obesity and sleep APNEA syndrome. Excess cortisol itself may also disrupt sleep through a direct action on the brain. In another endocrine disorder, a tumor in the anterior pituitary gland causes increased secretion of growth hormone, which manifests as acromegaly. In addition to abnormal increase in the size of hands and feet, acromegaly

is characterized by growth of bones and soft tissues of the head and neck and is commonly associated with obstructive sleep apnea syndrome. Other tumors of the pituitary are also associated with sleep disruption. Although the specific mechanisms are unclear, it is currently thought that tumor growth disturbs the hypothalamic centers involved in regulating sleep and circadian rhythmicity (see NREM SLEEP MECHANISMS; REM SLEEP MECHANISMS AND NEUROANATOMY). Additionally, disorders associated with the thyroid axis, both hypo- and hyperthyroidism, are well-documented causes of sleep disturbances (see THYROID DISEASE AND SLEEP).

Summary

Despite the consistent finding of sleep-related changes in neuroendocrine function, the significance of this modulation remains unclear. Such changes may simply be passive reflections of changing neural activity in the brain. More likely,

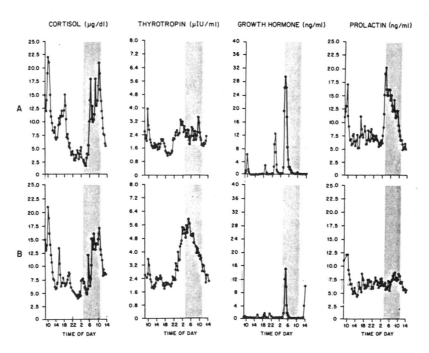

Figure 1.   Comparison of four anterior pituitary hormone profiles from one young male subject during sleep (A) and enforced wakefulness (B) over a 28-hour period. The shaded area depicts the usual sleep period of the subject. Assay values are for samples taken every 20 minutes via in-dwelling venous catheter for the entire duration of the study. μg, micrograms; μIU, micro–international units; ng, nanograms; dl, deciliter; ml, milliliter. *Source: G. S. Richardson, unpublished data.*

these sleep-related changes are important facilitators of physiological adjustments to the sustained reduction in physical activity inherent in sleep. For example, the growth hormone surge at sleep onset may serve to prevent hypoglycemia later in the night towards the end of an 8-hour fast. The observation that many of the sleep-related endocrine changes described here are unique to humans and primates with long uninterrupted sleep episodes, and are not seen in rodents with short, frequently interrupted sleep episodes, generally supports this hypothesis.

REFERENCES

Mendelson WB. 1987. *Human sleep: Research and clinical care.* New York: Plenum. See chapter 5, "Neuroendocrinology and sleep."

Shanahan TL, Czeisler CA. 1991. Light exposure induces equivalent phase shifts of the endogenous circadian rhythms of circulating plasma melatonin and core body temperature in men. *J Clin Endocrinol Metab* 73:227–235.

Weitzman ED, Boyer RM, Kapen S, Hellman L. 1975. The relationship of sleep and sleep stages to neuroendocrine secretion and biological rhythms in man. *Recent Prog Horm Res* 31:339–446.

Ellen Petro

ENERGY CONSERVATION

Energy conservation may have played an essential role in the evolution of sleep mechanisms in the groups of animals that are classified as *homeotherms*. Homeotherms are animals that regulate and maintain a constant body temperature; they include mammals and birds. Homeotherms have much higher basal metabolic rates (MRs) than *poikilotherms*. The latter are animals, including reptiles, amphibians, and fish, that do not increase their resting MRs to maintain a relatively constant body temperature. Metabolic rate measures the energy utilization of the animal. It reflects the use of food elements and stored reserves such as fat and glycogen to energize the cellular activities that are the basis of life. Because homeotherms have higher MRs, they must

eat more to survive. And because they must eat more, they are more dependent on food gathering, may be more exposed to predation, and are more susceptible to starvation when food is scarce. Thus, conserving energy reduces the need to find food and should contribute to survival. Because energy utilization is reduced during sleep, some researchers have speculated that the special features of sleep in homeotherms could be related to the adaptive advantages of conserving energy (Allison and Van Twyver, 1970; Zepelin and Rechtschaffen, 1974; Berger, 1975; see also FUNCTIONS OF SLEEP; METABOLISM).

This theory is supported by a comparison of sleep time across many mammals. Total daily sleep time is correlated with the weight-specific MR or with body mass (Zepelin and Rechtschaffen, 1974). Large animals with lower MRs, such as elephants, sleep less than 5 hours per day. Small mammals such as bats, moles, and tree shrews often sleep 15 or more hours per day, although there are some exceptions. Body size and MR are closely interrelated, and it is possible that body size is more closely related to sleep time than is MR (Zepelin, 1989).

MR is often estimated by measuring oxygen consumption, which accurately estimates MR under stable conditions. There is good agreement from several studies that oxygen consumption decreases during sleep. In humans, which have been studied most often, oxygen consumption decreases rapidly at sleep onset, then gradually decreases further to a minimal level in about the 4th hour of the night, rising again in the last hour (Kreider, Buskirk, and Bass, 1958; Shapiro et al., 1984; White, Weil, and Zwillich, 1985). The magnitude of the reduction in oxygen consumption from a presleep quiet waking to the minimal level is about 10–25 percent. Several studies have attempted to determine whether there are differences in MR among sleep stages, taking care to separate effects of sleep stages from the time of night. Although there have been some disagreements, most studies indicate that sleep stages 3 and 4 are associated with the lowest MRs; MRs during REM and stage 2 sleep are nearly equal, but lower than the waking rate (Brebbia and Altschuler, 1965; Shapiro et al., 1984). The rapid decrease in MR at sleep onset is due to sleep itself, not to a circadian influence or to fasting (Fraser et al., 1989). In rats, MR also decreases in NREM, but in contrast to humans, rat MR decreases further in REM sleep (Schmidek, Zachariassen, and Hammel, 1983; Roussel and Bittel, 1979).

Cerebral MR changes during sleep have also been measured in both experimental animals and in humans with use of radiologic techniques such as positron emission tomography. Cerebral MR decreases by about 30 percent during NREM sleep with some variations among specific brain regions (Kennedy et al., 1982; Ramm and Frost, 1986; Buchsbaum et al., 1989; see also CEREBRAL METABOLISM). In REM sleep, cerebral MR increases to waking levels or above. This factor may account for the relatively higher overall REM-related MRs in humans, in whom cerebral MR is a larger fraction of overall MR than in rats.

Because the decrease in overall MR during sleep is somewhat modest (about 10–25 percent), one could question whether the evolution of a phenomenon as complex, ubiquitous, and behaviorally specialized as sleep could be based on such a relatively small energy savings. Given that this calculation is based on a comparison of presleep basal MR at rest with overall sleep MR, however, sleep may also provide enforcement of rest, minimizing the much higher MRs associated with motor activity (Zepelin and Rechtschaffen, 1974). The actual savings produced by sleep would therefore depend on the MR in behaviorally active animals.

Another way to conserve energy is to minimize heat loss; behaviors such as seeking a warm nest serve this purpose. In rats studied under laboratory conditions, however, heat loss did not seem to be reduced during sleep (Schmidek, Zachariassen, and Hammel, 1983). The reduction in MR during sleep could serve a cooling function rather than energy conservation; this would explain the observation that heat loss is not minimized. On the other hand, cooling during sleep (see THERMOREGULATION) would help reduce MR because a wide variety of energy-consuming biologic processes proceed faster at higher temperatures.

The hypothesis that sleep functions to conserve energy by reducing MR has been studied in other ways. In support of this concept is the finding that states of HIBERNATION and TORPOR are entered as extensions of NREM sleep (Walker et al., 1977; see also ESTIVATION). Clearly hibernation and torpor serve energy conservation during seasons when food is scarce; their continuity with NREM sleep supports the energy conservation hypothesis. The transition to torpor may be induced

in doves by food deprivation; this manipulation also increases NREM sleep (Walker et al., 1983). Thus, in some species, increased NREM sleep can be a response to energy deficits. Other studies have examined the effect of increasing MR by administering the metabolic-stimulating hormone thyroxine (see THYROID-STIMULATING HORMONE). The best of such studies (Eastman and Rechtschaffen, 1979) did not find any change in sleep during periods of increased MR in rats. However, in humans with hyperthyroidism (excessive secretion of thyroxine), sleep stages 3 and 4 are increased, suggesting that sleep may compensate for increased metabolism (Dunleavy et al., 1974). One possibility is that energy conservation is one of two or more sleep functions and has greater importance in some species than in others. Energy conservation remains a viable and plausible hypothesis concerning the primary function of sleep, although additional hypotheses have not been ruled out.

REFERENCES

Allison T, Van Twyver H. 1970. The evolution of sleep. *Nat Hist* 79:56–65.

Berger RJ. 1975. Bioenergetic functions of sleep and activity rhythms and their possible relevance to aging. *Fed Proc* 34:97–102.

Brebbia DR, Altschuler KZ. 1965. Oxygen consumption rate and electroencephalographic stage of sleep. *Science* 150:1621–1623.

Buchsbaum MS, Gillin JC, Wu J, Hazlett E, Sicotte N, Dupont RM, Bunney WE, Jr. 1989. Regional cerebral glucose metabolic rate in human sleep assessed by positron emission tomography. *Life Sci* 45: 1349–1356.

Dunleavy DLF, Oswald I, Brown P, Strong JA. 1974. Hyperthyroidism, sleep and growth hormone. *Electroencephalogr Clin Neurophysiol* 36:259–263.

Eastman CI, Rechtschaffen A. 1979. Effect of thyroxine on sleep in the rat. *Sleep* 2:215–232.

Fraser G, Trinder J, Colrain IM, Montogomery I. 1989. Effect of sleep and circadian cycle on sleep period energy expenditure. *J Appl Physiol* 66:830–836.

Kennedy C, Gillin JC, Mendelson W, Suda S, Miyaoka M, Ito M, Nakamura RK, Sokoloff L. 1982. Local cerebral glucose utilization in non-rapid eye movement sleep. *Nature* 297:325–327.

Kreider MB, Buskirk ER, Bass DE. 1958. Oxygen consumption and body temperatures during the night. *J Appl Physiol* 12:361–366.

Ramm P, Frost BJ. 1986. Cerebral and local cerebral

metabolism in the cat during slow wave and REM sleep. *Brain Res* 365:112–124.

Roussel B, Bittel J. 1979. Thermogenesis and thermolysis during sleeping and waking in the rat. *Pflugers Arch* 382:225–231.

Schmidek WR, Zachariassen KE, Hammel HT. 1983. Total calorimetric measurements in the rat: Influences of the sleep-wakefulness cycle and of environmental temperature. *Brain Res* 288:261–271.

Shapiro CM, Goll CG, Cohen GR, Oswald I. 1984. Heat production during sleep. *J Appl Physiol* 56:671–677.

Walker JM, Glotzback SF, Berger RJ, Heller HC. 1977. Sleep and hibernation in ground squirrels (Citellus spp.): Electrophysiological observations. *Am J Physiol* 233:R213–R221.

Walker LE, Walker JM, Palca JW, Berger RJ. 1983. A continuum of sleep and shallow torpor in fasting doves. *Science* 221:194–195.

White DP, Weil JV, Zwillich CW. 1985. Metabolic rate and breathing during sleep. *J Appl Physiol* 59:384–391.

Zepelin H. 1989. Mammalian sleep. In Kryger MH, Roth T, Dement WC, eds. *Principles and practice of sleep medicine,* pp 30–49. Philadelphia: Saunders.

Zepelin H, Rechtschaffen A. 1974. Mammalian sleep, longevity and energy metabolism. *Brain Behav Evol* 10:425–470.

Dennis McGinty

ENGLISH BULLDOGS AS AN ANIMAL MODEL OF SLEEP APNEA

The human sleep apnea syndrome (see APNEA) was discovered in the late 1970s. It soon became obvious that this syndrome, defined as repeated pauses in breathing during sleep, is both serious and widespread, occurring in up to 15 percent of middle-aged men. Many questions about this disorder remain unresolved. For example, why are men more frequently involved than women? What is the relationship between snoring and the sleep apnea syndrome? One question is very difficult to resolve through the study of human patients: Is the neutral control of breathing (how the brain controls breathing) abnormal in sleep apnea? Investigating such problems in human patients is very difficult because treatment of the patient is the primary objective, thus leaving lit-

tle opportunity for experimentation with the disorder. Laboratory animals, on the other hand, can be bred, born, and raised under controlled conditions; genetic and environmental factors in disease can be manipulated; and studies can be much more thorough and conclusive. Therefore, animals showing signs that are similar to human diseases are sought by scientists and are termed *animal models* (see ANIMALS IN SLEEP RESEARCH).

Many humans with sleep apnea have changes in their nose, jaw, or throat that narrow the breathing passages. These changes are due to fat or fluid accumulation, trauma, or inherited features. It would seem logical to examine animal models that also have narrowed upper airway passages. The first candidate for examination was the English bulldog (see Figure 1). Veterinarians have long known that short-faced or *brachycephalic* dogs often develop breathing problems because their upper airways are partly blocked from birth. English bulldogs were chosen for study because, of all the brachycephalic breeds, they have the worst breathing problems.

Surgery to relieve this problem in the English bulldog was developed in the 1920s. This operation is similar to one commonly used for sleep apnea patients, the UVULOPALATOPHARYNGOPLASTY, which removes tissue from the back of the throat. This similarity of treatments suggested that the airway obstruction in English bulldogs might be similar to that in sleep apnea patients. If sleep apnea was found not to occur in these dogs, one could conclude there was a major difference in the control of breathing during sleep between humans and animals, as airway obstruction contributes to human sleep apnea.

Lewis Kline, a specialist in the treatment of sleep apnea, and Joan Hendricks, a veterinarian specializing in sleep research, had several owners volunteer to bring their English bulldogs in for a study at the Veterinary Hospital of the University of Pennsylvania. The dogs were taken into a quiet room and fitted with instruments to measure their breathing patterns and oxygen levels; then each dog was placed in a cage and the data were recorded. As predicted, these dogs showed the same kinds of problems as humans. First, they fell asleep quickly, generally within 10 minutes. (Normal dogs are unable to sleep under these conditions for several trials until they become used to the recording room and instruments.) This heightened sleepiness, or hypersomnolence, is a feature of human sleep apnea. Second, the bulldogs' breathing pattern was very irregular and they snored during sleep. Finally, during REM sleep, the dogs reduced or stopped breathing at least once every 3 minutes, and the oxygen saturation of their blood dropped dramatically. Even those dogs who appeared to be normal when they were awake showed disordered breathing during sleep. This, too, is similar to the pattern in humans, where no abnormality of breathing is seen during waking. In summary, English bulldogs shared several features of the human sleep apnea syndrome: hypersomnolence; disordered breathing, especially during REM sleep; oxygen desaturation; and normal respiratory function during waking.

The finding that English bulldogs were a useful animal model of sleep apnea led to other questions. First, do other nonhuman animals have sleep apnea? Many pet owners have called or written to Hendricks with complaints that their brachycephalic or extremely obese dogs snore and have difficulty breathing during sleep. It therefore appears likely that other dog breeds can have sleep apnea. Cats, even those with short faces like Persians, do not seem to have this problem. Second, what can we study in bulldogs that will help us treat human sleep apnea? No drug treatment has been successful for most patients. Alternative treatments for sleep apnea syndrome have been tested on dogs, and researchers have sought to discover whether changes in the central nervous system that lead to pauses in breathing during REM sleep can be altered. Finally, what can these dogs tell us about the development of sleep apnea in humans? Do eventual sufferers of sleep apnea show signs early in life that could alert them to the future problem? Study of these and other questions is under way.

(See also DOGS.)

REFERENCES

Sullivan CE, Issa FG. 1985. Obstructive sleep apnea. *Clin Chest Med* 6:633–650. A review of the syndrome.

Other Sleep Disorders Occurring Naturally in Animals

Baker TL, Mitler MM, Foutz AS, et al. 1983. Diagnosis and treatment of narcolepsy in animals. In Kirk RW, ed. *Current veterinary therapy VIII*, pp 755–789. Philadelphia: Saunders. Discussion of dogs with naturally occurring narcolepsy.

Hendricks JC, Lager A, O'Brien D, Morrison AR. 1989. Movement disorders during sleep in cats and dogs. *J Am Vet Med Assoc* 194:686–792. Presentation of animals with naturally occurring REM movement disorders.

Joan C. Hendricks

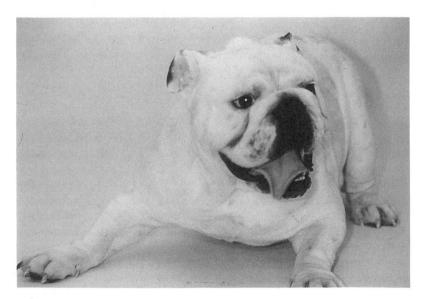

Figure 1.   An English bulldog.

ENTRAINMENT

In the absence of external information about the time of day, the physiology and behavior of creatures from algae to humans remains organized around a roughly 24-hour day. In most organisms, these circadian rhythms have periods near, but usually not exactly, 24 hours. In time cue–free conditions, such as caves or underground bunkers, humans adopt an approximately 25-hour day, while mice live on a nearly 23-hour day in the same conditions (see CIRCADIAN RHYTHMS). The period an animal's behavior adopts in the absence of time cues is called the FREE-RUNNING period. In the wild, however, animals maintain an exactly 24-hour day length. The environment provides one or more signals to the organism that synchronize its rhythms with the external world. This synchronization is called entrainment, and the external time cues that entrain the rhythm are called ZEITGEBERS (German for "time giver").

Many cues from the environment can act as

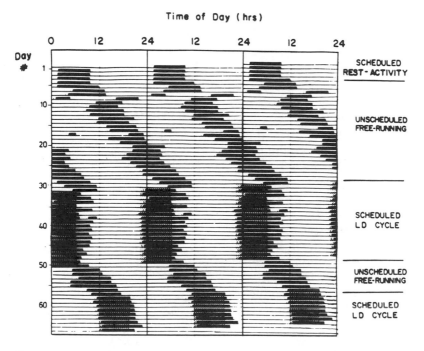

Figure 1.   The sleep-wake history of a human subject kept in time-isolated conditions for 67 days. The solid black lines indicate times of sleep. The data are presented in triplicate: The first full line represents days 1, 2, and 3; the second line, days 2, 3, and 4; the third days 3, 4, and 5; etc. Hours are read across the figure, and days vertically. In the top portion of the figure, the bedtimes for the subject were determined by the experimenter. In the section entitled "Unscheduled Free-Running," the subject was allowed to choose his own bedtime. Note that the subject wakes up about an hour later each day, on average. The free-running period is thus approximately 25 hours. Beginning at day 31, a fixed light–dark cycle of 8 hours' dark, 16 hours' light (with the stippling showing the dark period) was imposed on the subject. The light–dark cycle acts as a zeitgeber, and the rhythm entrains to a 24-hour period. Although the subject can choose his own bedtime, he sleeps and wakes with a 24-hour period. When the light–dark cycle is removed on day 51, the subject begins to free-run again. He is again entrained by a scheduled light–dark cycle beginning on day 58. *Reprinted with permission from Czeisler, Richardson, Zimmerman, Moore-Ede, and Weitzman. (1982)* Photochem Photobiol *24:239–247. New York: Pergamon.*

zeitgebers in mammals. For most species, LIGHT is the strongest entraining stimulus. Even weak 24-hour light–dark cycles can entrain rodent circadian rhythms to a 24-hour period. A regular 24-hour cycling of ambient temperature can likewise entrain the clock in some mammals. The availability of food can also entrain circadian rhythms in certain mammals. An animal fed at a regular time each day will adopt its circadian period to match the food stimulus, and will anticipate the feeding time. Access to exercise has also been shown to entrain the circadian rhythms of rodents. Giving a mouse access to a running wheel at the same time every day entrains the free-running rhythm.

Animals can also entrain each other. Pregnant mammals entrain the circadian rhythms of their fetuses with use of the hormone MELATONIN as the zeitgeber. Blind mice, which cannot normally entrain to a light–dark cycle, will entrain when caged with sighted mice, indicating that some sort of communication signal from one animal to another can entrain the clock. The identity of this signal is not known.

Humans also entrain their clocks via specific zeitgebers. For many years, researchers believed that the human clock was most sensitive to social cues and relatively insensitive to light. This has recently been disproved; the human circadian clock is very sensitive to light, and light–dark cycles can entrain the human clock. An example of entrainment of the human sleep–wake cycle to light–dark is shown in Figure 1.

Although circadian rhythms can be entrained to a range of different stimuli, they cannot entrain to a wide range of periods of these stimuli. A mouse cannot be entrained to a 40-hour light–dark cycle of 20 hours' light and 20 hours' dark, nor can it entrain to a 10-hour cycle. Although the range of periods capable of entraining a rhythm varies with the zeitgeber, very few stimuli can entrain circadian rhythms to new periods more than 2 or 3 hours different from the free-running period. Within this range, however, even very short stimuli can entrain the circadian rhythm. Light pulses as short as 10 seconds given once per day can entrain the activity of squirrel monkeys to a 24-hour period.

How zeitgebers entrain the circadian clock to adopt a new and different period length is not well understood. The physiological mechanism relies on the different effects of light in phase shifting the circadian clock (see PHASE RESPONSE CURVE). The biochemical mechanisms underlying this effect are not understood and remain an area of active inquiry.

REFERENCES

Aschoff J. 1982. Circadian rhythms in man. In Brady J, ed. *Biological timekeeping,* pp 143–158. New York: Cambridge University Press.
Moore-Ede MC, Sulzman FM, Fuller CA. 1982. *The clocks that time us.* Cambridge, Mass.: Harvard University Press.
Winfree AT. 1980. *The geometry of biological time.* New York: Springer-Verlag.

Russell N. Van Gelder

ENURESIS

See Bedwetting

EOG

See Electrooculography; Polysomnography

ENVIRONMENT

[*The environment can impinge upon sleep in a number of ways. Most individuals make some attempt to control the environment by their choice of* BEDS, MATTRESSES, PILLOWS, *and* PAJAMAS AND NIGHTWEAR. *These items often, however, follow fad and fashion as much as a concern for comfort in the sleeping environment. A number of environmental phenomena are known to affect such aspects of sleep–wake functioning as* SLEEP LENGTH *and* TIMING OF SLEEP AND WAKEFULNESS. *For example, the occurrence of* LIGHT *at specific phases of the day can help to entrain sleep–wake cycles and other* CIRCADIAN RHYTHMS; *this relationship is described by the* PHASE RESPONSE CURVE. NOISE *in the sleeping environment and* TEMPERATURE EFFECTS ON SLEEP *have been evaluated in a number of studies. Interestingly,* SENSORY PROCESSING AND SENSATION DURING SLEEP *are greatly suppressed, as evidenced by the reduced sense of* SMELL DURING SLEEP. *On the other hand, stimulus* INCORPORATION INTC DREAMS, *as well as findings pertaining to* COGNITION *during sleep, demonstrate that some sensory input is registered by the sleeper.*

The location of the sleeping environment can also have an effect upon sleep. Thus, mountain climbers or those who live at high ALTITUDE *show some changes in sleep and particularly in sleep-related breathing processes. Individuals who sleep under high* PRESSURIZATION, *such as personnel aboard submarines deep beneath the surface of the ocean, show other significant effects on sleep. Finally,* SPACE SHUTTLE SLEEPING ARRANGEMENTS *are designed with attention to the effects of* MICROGRAVITY AND SPACE FLIGHT *on sleeping in space.*

The most consistent effect of environmental disturbance on sleep is to produce sleep FRAGMENTATION *and consequent daytime* SLEEPINESS. *Furthermore, environmental disruption may be a cause of* INSOMNIA *in certain individuals.*]

EPIDEMIOLOGY OF SLEEP COMPLAINTS AND DISORDERS

Everyone has trouble sleeping at some point in life. Many surveys have tried to determine how common sleep complaints are in different groups of people. The disadvantage of these surveys is that the data collected are biased; that is, subjective reports of what is going on with a person's sleep are obtained, rather than objective records of sleep. The advantage of such surveys is that large numbers of representative people with different kinds of complaints can be studied. Results of different surveys differ because the studies ask different questions. "Do you have trouble sleeping?" will elicit a different response than "Do you have insomnia?"

Almost all surveys ask about "insomnia," that is, trouble falling asleep or trouble staying asleep. Insomnia is a complaint and not a sleep disorder. Insomnia can be caused by many different things. Most of these surveys therefore examine how common the complaint of insomnia is in the population, but not what causes these complaints.

The results of most surveys have shown that between 20 percent and 30 percent of the population report trouble sleeping. The complaint of insomnia is related to age and to sex, with women complaining more than men, older men and women complaining more than younger men and women, and older women complaining more than older men. Insomnia seems to be related to both mental health and physical health. People who report sleeping less than 7 hours or more than 8 hours a night have more health-related problems (such as coronary artery disease) and have a higher mortality rate. That does not necessarily mean that sleeping less than 7 hours will increase disease, but perhaps that people with physical illness sleep less than healthy people.

Survey Studies

One of the earliest surveys was done by McGhee and Russel in Great Britain in 1962, where 2,446 people, ranging in age from 15 to over 75 years, were interviewed. The results showed that 8 percent of those asked slept less than 5 hours each night. Difficulty falling asleep was found in 5 percent to 10 percent of men and 5 percent to 30 percent of women. Nearly 35 percent reported waking up often at night, 25 percent reported being tired in the morning, and 10 percent to 15 percent reported being sleepy during the day. Women were twice as likely to complain of trouble falling asleep. As people got older, they were more likely to report early-morning awakenings, frequent night awakenings, and being overall light sleepers.

In 1964, there was a report on over one million Americans, all over the age of 30 years, who had been interviewed by the American Cancer Society. Of the men, 16 percent complained of insomnia, and the complaint increased with age. Of the women, 31 percent complained of insomnia, and this complaint was stable once women turned 50 years old.

In 1974, sleep difficulties were surveyed in 1,006 households by Bixler and colleagues in Los Angeles, California. It was found that 32 percent of those asked had trouble falling asleep, and 42 percent had had a complaint of insomnia sometime during their life. Younger people (aged 18 to 29 years) complained of less insomnia than older people (aged 60 years and over). In all age groups, more women complained of insomnia than men.

Another large survey was conducted by Karacan and co-workers in 1976 in Alachua County, Florida. Of 1,645 people aged 16 years and over questioned, 45 percent reported trouble falling asleep or staying asleep during the night. Once again, sleeping difficulties were higher in women and complaints increased with age.

More recently, 5,713 people aged 3 to 94 years were surveyed by Lugaresi in the Italian republic of San Marino. Overall, 13.4 percent of the sample were "poor sleepers" (17 percent women and 10 percent men). Insomnia was hardly ever reported by those under 19 years of age; however, after 20 years, reports of insomnia increased, with most people reporting that their trouble sleeping was caused by worrying (43 percent) or physical discomfort (22.5 percent). Depression or anxiety was reported by 88 percent of poor sleepers; only 48 percent of good sleepers had such reports.

Insomnia is not the only sleep complaint surveyed. NIGHTMARES and SLEEP TERRORS are found in about 5 percent of the adult population and seem to be found equally in all adult age groups. Nightmares are reported more by women. Sleepwalking and enuresis (bedwetting) are reported by less than 1 percent of adults. All these disorders are primarily stress related in adults.

One survey examined sleep complaints of pregnant women. Most of the women reported waking up more at night and sleeping less overall than women who were not pregnant. The sleep disturbance was especially bad during the last trimester of pregnancy.

Complaints of daytime sleepiness (HYPERSOMNIA) are found in about 5 percent of the general adult population. Of the older adults, 35 percent had some daytime sleepiness (consistently falling asleep while reading or watching television) and 3–5 percent had severe daytime sleepiness (falling asleep while talking with friends or almost having a car accident because of sleepiness). The prevalence of the complaint of excessive daytime sleepiness is the same in men and women. This complaint can be associated with both mental problems (i.e., anxiety, depression, stress) and physical problems. A common psychological cause is insufficient sleep; one of the most common physical causes of this complaint is sleep APNEA.

A person with sleep apnea, or sleep-disordered breathing, periodically stops breathing during sleep. To start breathing again, the person wakes up. These apnea episodes can occur hundreds of times during the night, so that patients with sleep-disordered breathing wake up frequently during the night and, therefore, are sleepy during the day. Another symptom of sleep apnea is SNORING.

Snoring is caused by a partial obstruction of the airway, whereas apnea is caused by a complete obstruction of the airway. Occasional snoring is found in 16.8 percent of men and in 14.1 percent of women of all ages. Habitual snoring is found in 24.1 percent of men and in 13.8 percent of women. The prevalence of snoring increases with age, with 60 percent of men and 40 percent of women over 60 years of age reporting snoring.

Objective Studies

The prevalence of sleep apnea is higher in men than in women and is estimated to be around 1 percent to 5 percent in young adults. As people age, the prevalence increases. The prevalence of sleep-disordered breathing was objectively studied by recording sleep in older adults and found to be 24 percent in healthy elderly and closer to 27 percent to 39 percent in elderly with sleep complaints. The prevalence of sleep apnea is higher in older men (28%) than in older women (19.5%). It is estimated that the prevalence of sleep apnea is higher in postmenopausal women than in premenopausal women.

Another sleep disorder that increases with age is periodic leg movements in sleep (PLMS), or nocturnal myoclonus. People with this disorder kick or jerk their legs every 20 to 40 seconds for periods throughout the night, often waking themselves up. The prevalence of PLMS has been estimated to be 5 percent to 6 percent in the normal population (aged 18 to 74 years), 1 percent to 11 percent in patients with complaints of insomnia, and 13 percent to 18 percent in patients referred to sleep disorder clinics. In a study of 427 randomly selected elderly, 45 percent had PLMS.

(See also PERIODIC LEG MOVEMENTS.)

REFERENCES

Ancoli-Israel S. 1989. Epidemiology of sleep disorders. In Roth T, ed. *Clinics in Geriatric Medicine,* pp 347–362. Philadelphia: Saunders.

Ancoli-Israel S, Kripke DF, Klauber MR, Mason WJ, Fell R, Kaplan O. 1991a. Respiratory disturbances in sleep in community dwelling elderly. *Sleep* 14(6):486–495.

———. 1991b. Periodic leg movements in sleep in community dwelling elderly. *Sleep* 14(6): 496–500.

Bixler EO, Kales A, Soldatos CR, Kales J, Healey S. 1979. Prevalence of sleep disorders: A survey of the Los Angeles metropolitan area. *Am J Psychiatry* 136:1257–1262.

Karacan I, Thornby JI, Anch M, Holzer CE, Warheit GJ, Schwab JJ, Williams RL 1976. Prevalence of sleep disturbance in a primarily urban Florida county. *Soc Sci Med* 10:239–244.

Kripke DF, Simons RN, Garfinkel L, Hammond EC. 1979. Short and long sleep and sleeping pills: Is increased mortality associated? *Arch Gen Psychiatry* 36:103–116.

Lugaresi E, Zucconi M, Bixler EO. 1987. Epidemiology of sleep disorders. *Psychiatr Ann* 17:446–453.

McGhie A, Russel SM. 1962. The subjective assessment of normal sleep patterns. *J Ment Sci* 108:642–654.

Mellinger GD, Balter MB, Uhlenhuth EH. 1985. Insomnia and its treatment. Prevalence and correlates. *Arch Gen Psychiatry* 42:225–232.

Norton PG, Dunn EV. 1985. Snoring as a risk factor for disease: An epidemiological survey. *Br Med J* 291:630–632.

Schweiger MS. 1972. Sleep disturbance in pregnancy: A subjective survey. *Am J Obstet Gynecol* 114:879.

Sonia Ancoli-Israel

EPILEPSY

The word *epilepsy* is derived from Greek words meaning "to seize upon." The disorder has been recognized for thousands of years: The writings of Hippocrates and Galen contain detailed descriptions of various types of seizures. To the physicians of the Middle Ages, epileptic seizures suggested demonic possession, and the condition was called the *falling sickness* or the *falling evil.* The stigma associated with epilepsy has lessened in the modern era, although ignorance and fear still lead to prejudice against those afflicted.

Epilepsy, which affects approximately 0.5 percent of the world's population, is characterized by an intermittent disruption of brain function associated with a burst of abnormal brain electrical activity. Epileptic seizures, a consequence of the abnormal brain electrical activity, are classified into two main categories: partial seizures, initially affecting only one part of the brain; and generalized seizures, which affect both halves, or hemispheres, of the brain from the beginning. Although seizures usually last only a few seconds or minutes, they occasionally continue for hours or days, a condition called *status epilepticus.*

Partial Seizures

The clinical consequences of partial seizures depend on the portion of the brain affected. For example, seizures beginning in the occipital lobe, the area of the brain concerned with visual analysis, produce such symptoms as flashing lights or formed images; whereas seizures beginning in the motor portion of one of the frontal lobes may produce jerking movements of an arm or a leg. Partial seizures may progress to become generalized seizures; when this happens the initial partial seizure, for example, a sensory symptom such as an unpleasant smell, is often referred to as an *aura.*

Generalized Seizures

There are also a variety of types of generalized seizures. Generalized absence seizures, often called *petit mal seizures,* cause brief subtle episodes of staring that may be mistaken for daydreaming or that may pass entirely undetected despite occurring dozens of times each day. Generalized tonic–clonic seizures, also called *grand mal seizures,* produce convulsions of the entire body with stiffening and violent jerking movements that can last several minutes. The description by the poet Lucretius (95 to 55 B.C.) conveys the dramatic impact of a grand mal seizure:

> Oft too some wretch, before our startled sight,
> Struck as with lightning, by some keen disease
> Drops sudden:—by the dread attack o'erpowered
> He foams, he groans, he trembles, and he faints;
> Now rigid, now convulsed, his laboring lungs
> Heave quick, and quivers each exhausted limb.
> (Penfield and Jasper, 1954)

Seizures and Sleep

Although the occurrence of seizures during sleep has been recognized for centuries, William

Gowers, a British neurologist of the nineteenth century, was the first to perform systematic studies. He noted that seizures occurred exclusively during the night in more than 20 percent of epileptics and that another 32 percent had seizures during sleep as well as during wakefulness. Although the reasons why sleep facilitates the occurrence of seizures in some persons are not known, it is clear that most nocturnal seizures occur during NREM sleep, and it may be that the synchronous EEG activity of NREM sleep allows abnormal epileptic discharges to spread through the brain, while the desynchronized activity of REM sleep inhibits such spread.

Epilepsy and the Electroencephalogram

The ELECTROENCEPHALOGRAM (EEG) is one of the most valuable tools for the diagnosis of epilepsy because it is usually abnormal in patients with epilepsy and because the pattern of abnormality helps to define the type of epilepsy, the types of medications that are likely to be beneficial, and the prognosis. Because the occurrence of abnormal EEG activity is increased during sleep in many types of epilepsy, most electroencephalography laboratories attempt to obtain samples of EEG during sleep as well as during wakefulness. Sleep EEG recordings are especially useful in patients with seizures occurring exclusively during sleep, because EEGs during wakefulness are often normal. Sleep deprivation the night before a daytime EEG increases the likelihood that the patient will fall asleep during the recording and therefore increases the likelihood of finding an EEG abnormality.

Epilepsy Treatment

Treatment of epilepsy is determined by the type and frequency of seizures and by the underlying condition that caused the epilepsy. Some forms of epilepsy are associated with seizures only during childhood; other forms remain active throughout life. Medications used to treat epilepsy are highly effective in a majority of patients and, when taken regularly, permit many of them to lead essentially normal lives.

REFERENCES

Niedermeyer E. Epileptic seizure disorders. In Niedermeyer E, Lopes da Silva F, eds. *Electroencephalography. Basic principles, clinical applications and related fields,* 2nd ed, pp 405–510. Baltimore: Urban & Schwarzenberg.

Penfield W, Jasper H. 1954. *Epilepsy and the functional anatomy of the human brain,* p 8. Boston; Little, Brown.

Shouse MN. 1989. Epilepsy and seizures during sleep. In Kryger MH, Roth T, Dement WC, eds. *Principles and practice of sleep medicine,* pp 364–376. Philadelphia: Saunders.

Michael Aldrich

EPINEPHRINE

See Antihistamines; Autonomic Nervous System; Chemistry of Sleep: Amines and Other Transmitters

ERECTILE DYSFUNCTION

Erectile dysfunction, sometimes referred to as erectile failure or male impotence, afflicts approximately ten million men in the United States. Erectile dysfunction is the inability to obtain or maintain a penile erection sufficient for vaginal penetration (SEE ERECTIONS). Erectile dysfunction does not include decreased sexual desire (loss of libido), anorgasmia, and premature or retrograde ejaculation; however, these sexual problems may be associated with erectile impotence. In approximately 50 percent of the men suffering from impotence, the cause of the problem is organic. Common organic causes include diabetes, genital trauma, vascular disease, endocrine disorders, neurological dysfunction, and renal failure. Alcoholism and use of some medications can also impair erectile function. In contrast, psychogenic impotence may result from sexual performance anxiety, relationship problems, stress, or psychiatric problems.

Fortuitously, REM sleep is associated with episodic penile erections that occur in virtually all men who are sexually potent (SEE SEXUAL ACTIVATION). The observation that sleep-related erections fail to occur in some men complaining of impotence was noted by researchers in the early 1970s. Techniques for recording sleep-related erections developed as diagnostic indicators to differentiate organically caused impotence from erectile failure related to psychological or interpersonal factors. Partially because of its intuitive appeal, the NOCTURNAL PENILE TUMESCENCE (NPT) test quickly became the "gold standard" for indexing erectile capacity.

In general, a complaint of impotence in a man with normal sleep erections is thought to indicate psychogenic impotence (unless there is evidence of pelvic steal syndrome, Peyronie's disease, acute hypogonadism, or neurological lesions). By contrast, when tumescence is absent or decreased in the presence of reasonably undisrupted and intact REM sleep, an organic cause of impotence is suspected. Validation of the NPT test derives from numerous studies demonstrating decreased or absent sleep-related erections in groups of patients with diseases that are presumably associated with organic impotence.

(See also SEX AND SLEEP.)

REFERENCES

Segraves RT, Schoenberg HW. 1985. Diagnosis and treatment of erectile problems: Current status. In Segraves RT, Schoenberg HW, eds. *Diagnosis and treatment of erectile disturbances: A guide for clinicians,* chap 1, pp 1–21. New York: Plenum Press.
Ware JC. 1989. Monitoring erections during sleep. In Kryger M, Roth T, Dement WC, eds. *Principles and practice of sleep medicine,* chap 75, pp 689–695. Philadelphia: Saunders.

Max Hirshkowitz

ERECTIONS

Penile erections in men require coordination of psychological, endocrine, neural, and vascular mechanisms. The corpora cavernosum (erectile tissue forming the dorsum and sides of the penis) and the glans (cap-shaped tip of penis) have separate arterial supplies, differ structurally, and have different underlying physiological dynamics. Lue and Tanagho (1988) describe the glans as an arteriovenous fistula that acts essentially as a shock absorber, protecting the cervix from the thrusting impact of a rigid penile shaft. Discussion of erectile mechanisms characteristically focuses on the physiology of the corpora cavernosum.

During the initial phase of erection, arterial blood flow increases, causing the penis to elongate and slightly increase in girth. This phase, sometimes called the latent phase, is followed by the tumescence (swelling or T-up) phase. T-up is accompanied by continued arterial inflow and rising intracorporeal pressure. In the full or maximum (T-max) erection phase, arterial inflow may decline somewhat but remains higher than baseline. Expert opinion differs concerning the rate of venous outflow during the full erection phase; at the extremes, some investigators postulate equal inflow–outflow rates, whereas others argue for complete venous constriction. Animal studies indicate that electrical stimulation of the pudendal nerve during the full erection phase produces a "rigid erection phase." Muscle contraction, dramatically increased intracorporeal pressure, and cessation of blood flow occur. Although this phase may not be necessary in man, Lue and Tanagho report that it has been recorded during masturbation in humans. The detumescence phase, during which venous outflow increases and the circumference of the penis decreases, follows.

Neurologically, the initiation and maintenance of erection are under parasympathetic nervous system control. Smooth muscles relax and vascular mechanisms facilitate internal pudendal artery blood flow. The rigid phase, if and when it occurs, involves striated muscles under control of somatic nerves. Finally, detumescence is a sympathetic nervous system phenomenon associated with smooth muscle contraction and venous outflow.

The physiological mechanisms of erection during sleep are not known; however, they are thought to be similar to those of the awake state. This, however, is an assumption. Nocturnal erections (see NOCTURNAL PENILE TUMESCENCE) certainly have latent, ascending tumescence, full erection, and detumescence phases. Whether the rigid erection phase occurs needs further investigation. Bulbocavernosus and ischiocavernosus activity occurs during sleep erections, but their relationship to internal cavernosus pressure has not been measured. The REM sleep "autonomic storm" (see AUTONOMIC NERVOUS SYSTEM) can certainly supply the neural stimulation needed to initiate and maintain sleep-related penile erections. Penile blood flow increases during sleep-related tumescence have also been reported. The application of new and more sophisticated techniques will undoubtedly provide more detail about the physiology of nocturnal penile tumescence in the future.

REFERENCE

Lue TF, Tanagho EA. 1988. Hemodynamics of erection. In Tanagho EA, Lue TF, McClure RD, eds. *Contemporary management of impotence and infertility,* chap 2, pp 28–38. Baltimore: Williams and Wilkins.

Max Hirshkowitz

ESTIVATION

Unlike other animals, birds and mammals can maintain their body temperatures above environmental temperature by means of metabolic heat production. This adaptation, known as *endothermy*, is a metabolically expensive process for very small birds and mammals, which lose heat to the environment at a much greater rate than larger animals. To maintain a high and constant body temperature, some very small animals must consume an amount of food equal to their body weight each day! Because of their small body size, such animals have a limited ability to store energy in the form of fat. To combat this problem, some small birds and mammals allow their body temperature to decrease to close to that of the environment for periods of several hours or days. Certain animals allow this to occur on a daily basis and exhibit daily torpor cycles; others exhibit this adaptation on a seasonal basis in the winter (hibernation) or summer (estivation).

Estivation (or aestivation) is derived from the Latin word *aestivare* meaning to spend the summer. Like hibernation, estivation is a physiologic adaptation that enables an animal to avoid extreme environmental conditions. In the case of estivators, the extreme conditions are food shortage, lack of water, or high temperatures. In contrast to hibernation, the decrease of body temperature during estivation is relatively mild and animals therefore remain more alert and responsive to stimulation. Even a moderate decrease in body temperature, however, enables animals to conserve both water and energy because the rate of metabolism is decreased. Although the occurrence of estivation is correlated with hot, dry conditions, it is not clear whether estivation is a response to dehydration (and an adaptation for water conservation per se) or whether the onset of such environmental conditions indicates that suitable food will be limited in its availability in the near future. This is particularly evident from laboratory studies in which known estivating species can be maintained on a diet of dry seeds indefinitely without exhibiting estivation.

Among mammals, estivation has been observed in rodents, insectivores, and marsupials. Many estivators also hibernate. This combination of adaptations has helped ground squirrels become widespread in the Northern Hemisphere. In areas where the winters are cold, the resident ground squirrel species hibernate. In areas where there is prolonged drought, the squirrels estivate. In areas where rainfall is restricted to the winter and spring, the local squirrel species may both hibernate and estivate. In temperate or tropical areas with regular rainfall, neither hibernation nor estivation occur in the local squirrels. Electroencephalographic recordings in squirrels during entrance to estivation and during shallow torpor indicate that, as with hibernation, the entrance is mediated through slow-wave sleep at the expense of REM sleep and that slow-wave sleep and estivation may represent a continuum of adaptations that reduce energy expenditure.

REFERENCE

Hudson JW, Bartholomew GA. 1964. Terrestrial animals in dry heat: Estivators. In Dill DB, ed. *Handbook of physiology,* sec. 4, pp 541–550. Washington, D.C.: American Physiological Society.

Thomas S. Kilduff

ETHANOL

See Alcohol

EVOKED POTENTIALS

Evoked potentials (EPs) are the electrical activity that occurs in the brain following stimulation of one of the senses. For instance, when a sudden loud noise occurs, up to fifteen different electrical potentials may be evoked or elicited as the response to the sound. The sound stimulus starts at the ear, proceeds to the nerves of the ear, to the brainstem, to the subcortical areas of the brain, and finally arrives at the cortex or upper level of the brain. This pathway from the ear to the higher levels of the brain that recognize and interpret sounds is interrupted by many specialized groups of brain cells or nuclei. These nuclei are way stations or intersections in the nervous system pathway and give off an electrical signal or potential as the impulse passes them. Sometimes these evoked potentials are clearly visible in the brain wave activity or electroencephalogram (EEG) recorded at the scalp (see ELECTROENCEPHALOGRAM). However, evoked potentials are often too small to be clearly seen or are masked or distorted by the usually chaotic electroencephalographic activity of human beings.

Before computers became available to scientists, these hidden evoked potentials were impossible to study. It was the invention of a particular kind of computer, the averaging computer, that was most important in revealing evoked potentials. The averaging computer makes certain assumptions about the EEG and how the brain responds to stimulation of the senses. The first important assumption is that most of the EEG is random, having no particular pattern from moment to moment. The second assumption is that the brain's response to stimulation of the senses has a very specific pattern as the evoked potential moves along the sensory pathway, triggering potentials at important nuclei along the way. Evoked potentials should thus always occur at the same time (latency) after the sound is first heard, much as a train should arrive at certain stations on schedule. To unmask or uncover these very small potentials, the computer records the EEG immediately after the sound for a specific period of time, usually 1 second or less. Then another sound is presented to the ear and another second of EEG is recorded. The computer then adds these two pieces of EEG together. The computer then presents another sound and records another second of EEG and averages the third section with the sum of the first two. This may continue until as many as sixty-four to over 1,024 sections of EEG have been averaged. In principal, if a particular electroencephalographic wave is random and not related to the brain's response to the sound, it should be canceled out by repeated averaging with other waves. If a particular electroencephalographic wave is related to the brain's response to the sound, it should get bigger and be clearly visible as an evoked potential within the averaged segment of EEG.

Sleep and sleepiness have definite effects on the amplitude (height) and latency (time from the presentation of the stimulus to the wave of interest) of evoked potentials resulting from auditory, somatosensory (touch), and visual stimuli; of these, auditory evoked potentials (AEP) have been studied most during sleep. The response of the brain to single sounds was first noted by certain of the earliest EEG and sleep researchers in the 1930s, who reported that the amplitude and duration of the AEP waves increased as a person fell asleep (Davis et al., 1934). Researchers in the early 1960s were the first to use the averaging computer to study EPs during sleep (Clark et al., 1961). They used a loud speaker near the bed to make brief, but loud clicks every few seconds during sleep. They reported that certain later EP waves, thought to reflect cortical responses, underwent dramatic changes in shape. These EP waves were biggest during drowsiness or during light sleep and smallest during REM sleep (see Figure 1). These researchers believed that these EP changes indicated that sensory stimuli were blocked from reaching the brain during deep NREM stages of sleep, and especially during REM sleep. Later researchers have not always agreed with these findings, but consistently report that EP waves are smallest during REM sleep (Williams, Tepas, and Horlock, 1962). They give an alternative explanation, suggesting that the size of the waveforms is a result of the level of general activity of the neurons of the brain. When the brain is very active, neurons are busy and cannot respond to the new stimulus; when neurons are not busy, many are available to respond. Thus, a large waveform would indicate low levels of activity in the brain, suggesting that light sleep is not a very busy time for the brain, and a small waveform would indicate high brain activity suggesting that REM sleep is an extremely busy time for the brain.

These findings are only true for the electrical

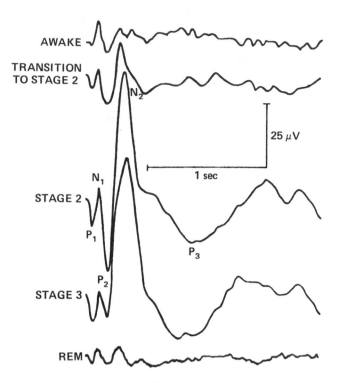

Figure 1.   The effect of sleep stages on EPs.

activity of the highest levels of the brain. Evoked potentials recorded from the brainstem and the midbrain usually do not show any changes at all during different types of sleep (Amadeo and Shagass, 1973).

Evoked potentials have also been used to study brain function in patients with sleep APNEA and with disorders that cause excessive daytime sleepiness, without conclusive results (Pressman et al., 1982). Nevertheless, the study of evoked potentials is a useful method of evaluating the activity of the brain during sleep. It is particularly of interest because it is noninvasive, can provide data on the function of the brainstem and subcortical areas of the brain, and can be used to study human sleep without waking the individual.

REFERENCES

Amadeo M, Shagass C. 1973. Brief latency click-evoked potentials during wakefulness and sleep. *Psychophysiology* 10:244–250.

Clark WA, Goldstein MH, Brown RM, Molnar CE, O'Brien DF, Zieman HE. 1961. The average response computer (ARC): A digital device for computing averages and amplitude and time histograms of electrophysiological responses. *Trans IRE* 8(1):46–51.

Davis H, Davis PA, Loomis AL, Harvey E, Hobart GA. 1934. Electrical reactions of the human brain to auditory stimulation. *J Neurophysiology* 2:500–514.

Pressman MR, Spielman AJ, Pollak CP, Weitzman ED. 1982. Long-latency auditory evoked responses during sleep deprivation and in narcolepsy. *Sleep* 5:S147–S156.

Weitzman ED, Kremen H. 1965. Auditory evoked responses during different stages of sleep in man. *Electroencephalogr Clin Neurophysiol* 18:65–70.

Williams HL, Tepas PI, Horlock HC. 1962. Evoked responses to clicks and electroencephalography of stages of sleep in man. *Science* 138:685–686.

Mark R. Pressman

EVOLUTION OF SLEEP

There are a number of questions regarding the history of sleep in the animal kingdom: When and why did sleep originate? Do all creatures sleep? Has sleep changed over time? Can it be explained as a product of natural selection for fitness and adaptation to the environment?

Wholly satisfactory answers to these questions are not yet available. Generalizations about sleep are risky when it has been studied in only two or three hundred of the million or more species in the animal kingdom and when most of the creatures studied have been mammals (Campbell and Tobler, 1984). Although common sense suggests that sleep is essential to sustain waking activity, precisely what sleep accomplishes has yet to be determined (see THEORIES OF SLEEP FUNCTION). Knowledge of sleep's purpose, when achieved, will do much to clarify its origin and history, but until then, understanding of its evolution will depend on expanded information about sleep in more animals of every type.

Evolutionary history is ordinarily derived from two sources: the fossil record of extinct forms and the diversity of living beings. A complication with respect to sleep is that, unlike body parts and plants, sleep leaves no fossil record. Its history must be inferred from its manifestations in living creatures, from available general knowledge about their phylogenetic relationships (i.e., evolutionary lines of descent), and from correlations between sleep and other traits. Guesswork and controversy are therefore unavoidable.

A most impressive clue to sleep's historical development is its similarity in birds and mammals, whose sleep is distinguished by the same behavioral features, by similar though not identical

electroencephalogram (EEG) changes (i.e., slowed waveforms at elevated amplitude), and, with minor exceptions, by the cyclical alternation of NREM and REM sleep, referred to as the sleep cycle or the NREM–REM cycle (see BIRDS; MAMMALS; REM SLEEP). Complexity of brain tissues, though not the same in birds and mammals, seems to account for the resemblance of their EEG patterns; the cyclical organization of sleep requires additional explanation. The sleep cycle was almost certainly *not* inherited from a common ancestor, but evolved independently in birds and mammals or in their extinct, immediate forebears (the dinosaurs and mammallike reptiles.) As indicated by the phylogenetic relationships shown in Figure 1, an explanation in terms of common ancestry requires the assumption that a similar cycle was present in the extinct stem reptiles, which, in turn requires evidence of a cycle in other descendants of the stem reptiles (turtles, snakes, lizards, or crocodilians). To date, convincing evidence of REM sleep or of a REM–NREM cycle is lacking in all of these animals (see REPTILES).

As with other multiple occurrences of evolutionary novelties (e.g., the eye, the powered flight of birds and bats), the repeated evolution of the sleep cycle emphasizes its adaptive significance. Of added importance is the sharing by birds and mammals of two additional, indepen-

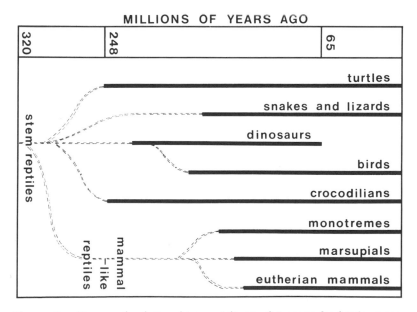

Figure 1. Temporal relationships and lines of descent for birds, mammals, and reptiles. Solid lines indicate availability of fossil record; dotted lines indicate still uncertain relationships.

dently evolved characteristics. One is the four-chambered heart, which improved on the circulatory efficiency of the three-chambered organ in reptiles; the other is *endothermy* (so-called warmbloodedness), the maintenance of a constant high body temperature with internally generated heat. The sleep cycle is thus part of a suite of characteristics that support a high activity level, equipping birds and mammals for survival in cold temperatures and climates. Endothermy, however, is very expensive in terms of food and energy requirements. The sleep cycle and its constituent states may have evolved to help cope with this cost, perhaps through some role in energy metabolism. Support for this inference comes from findings that prolonged experimental sleep deprivation or disruption of the sleep cycle in rats has fatal consequences preceded by lowered body temperature despite elevated metabolism (Rechtschaffen et al., 1989).

The REM–NREM cycle seems related additionally to the reproductive and maturational patterns of birds and mammals. Reptiles are fully mature at birth and receive little or no parental care, but elaborate parental care by birds and mammals permits the birth of altricial (immature) offspring. Relationship of REM sleep to this immature condition is indicated by its fetuslike lack of thermoregulatory capacity, by its prominence before and shortly after birth, and by the variation in daily REM amounts in mature mammals in proportion to the altriciality of the species. The sleep cycle amounts to the alternation of an early-maturing state (REM) with one that is endothermic and relatively late-maturing (NREM) (Zepelin, 1989).

Evaluation of sleep in the more ancient animals—reptiles, amphibians, fish, and invertebrates—brings to the fore problems regarding its definition. A question that arises is whether the criteria by which sleep's occurrence is judged should be uniform throughout the animal kingdom. Some writers take the view that EEG patterns like those found in birds and mammals are indispensable for sleep, but this is questionable because the less developed brains of other animals simply lack the tissue needed to produce comparable EEG activity. Invertebrates (animals without backbones), for example, have brains too small to generate any EEG activity but give other indications of sleep. Insistence on uniform EEG criteria arbitrarily limits sleep, by definition, to birds and mammals with no gain of in-

sight into its evolution. Furthermore, it is advisable to keep in mind the likely duality of sleep, consisting on the one hand of behavioral manifestations and, on the other, of a physiological essence. It is still too soon to say whether EEG activity is part of sleep's essence or just one of its manifestations. A stopgap solution to this dilemma is a distinction between electrophysiological sleep, defined by the presence of diagnostic EEG patterns in addition to behavioral signs, and *behavioral sleep,* defined solely by behavioral manifestations in the absence of diagnostic EEG patterns. The ultimate solution will come with clarity about sleep's purpose and essence.

The evidence of behavioral sleep in diverse branches of the animal kingdom indicates it is from the antecedent vertebrate state that the sleep of birds and mammals evolved (see AMPHIBIANS; FISH; REPTILES). Mammalian and reptilian sleep are also linked by an electrophysiological event that may be characteristic of vertebrate sleep in general. This event consists of spike potentials (fast, high-voltage activity) found in the brains of reptiles mainly during behaviorally quiescent periods, and also in certain fish and amphibians. Similar activity emanates from a primitive brain area in mammals, primarily during sleep. In both reptiles and mammals, experimental sleep deprivation and the consequent reduction of such spiking lead to a compensatory increase in spiking during recovery sleep. Pharmacological effects on the spiking are the same in the tortoise and in the cat. These findings point to an intermediate state between purely behavioral sleep and the electrophysiological sleep of birds and mammals, which appears to be an amalgam of behavioral sleep with subsequently evolved features. Some commonality of function in the sleep of vertebrates is suggested.

Because sleep, by any definition, is a state of rest, and because periods of rest are probably universal in living systems, a conclusion that sleep initially evolved from rest seems inescapable. If so, at what point did sleep evolve, and for what purpose? Consensus among scientists has yet to be achieved, but it can be argued that sleep first appeared in insects (classified as arthropods and invertebrates), as suggested by periods of neuronal insensitivity in the honey bee and reduced responsivity in moths. Additional support for this judgment comes from findings of compensatory reduction of activity in scorpions and cockroaches when deprived of rest, a reaction resembling the homeostatic self-regulation of sleep in mammals. The possibility that sleep evolved earlier, however, is suggested by the presence of endogenous CIRCADIAN RHYTHMS in various processes, even in unicellular organisms and plants. The concept of sleep may ultimately require broadening to incorporate phenomena at these levels.

The further back we go in evolutionary history, the more difficult it becomes to conceive of purposes of sleep particularly suited to each stage. But whatever else sleep is, it is everywhere a state of rest that prevents activity and limits energy expenditure. Perhaps this primitive characteristic is not just a manifestation of sleep but part of its essence.

REFERENCES

Campbell SS, Tobler I. 1984. Animal sleep: A review of sleep duration across phylogeny. *Neurosci Biobehav Rev* 8:269–300.

Radinsky LB. 1987. *The evolution of vertebrate design*. Chicago: University of Chicago Press.

Rechtschaffen A, Bergmann BM, Everson CA, Kushida CA, Gilliland MA. 1989. Sleep deprivation in the rat. X. Integration and discussion of the findings. *Sleep* 12:68–87.

Zepelin H. 1989. Mammalian sleep. In Kryger M, Roth T, Dement WC, eds. *Principles and practice of sleep medicine* pp 30–49. Philadelphia: Saunders.

Harold Zepelin

EXERCISE

A common assumption holds that exercise improves sleep. Exercise does not really make us sleep any better; however, if one is tense in the evenings, then some form of distraction and mental relaxation, as in a short jog, can help to avert INSOMNIA. But some forms of inactivity can be even more relaxing, especially lying in a warm bath. Both have interesting effects on SLOW-WAVE SLEEP (SWS) (stages 3 and 4).

Slow-wave sleep is particularly significant from the perspective of sleep function, as it is the type of sleep that has been linked to heightened tissue growth and repair ("restitution"), overcoming the wear and tear of wakefulness. If this is the role

for SWS, then there are implications for exercise and sleep: (1) deprivation of SWS, as in total sleep deprivation, would lead to impaired muscle restitution and a reduced efficiency for muscles to exercise; and (2) daytime exercise would produce greater muscle wear and tear, and the need for more restitution and SWS during sleep (see FUNCTIONS OF SLEEP).

Sleep Loss and Exercise

The most recent reviews (Horne, 1988; Martin, 1988) of this area indicate that there is little impairment to muscle efficiency during sleep loss and that subjects can continue exercising almost as normal. Because of the sleepiness, sleep-deprived subjects may give up more easily, but for psychological rather than physiological reasons. This relationship is thought to occur because the impact of sleep loss is greater on the brain rather than on the rest of the body. Thus exercised muscles can apparently recover quite adequately during relaxed wakefulness—a finding that runs counter to the body restitution hypothesis (Horne, 1988).

Nighttime SWS After Daytime Exercise

Certain functions indicate that lean people have more SWS than heavy people. Inasmuch as fit people tend to be leaner, the SWS increase may be related to fitness; however, the level of physical fitness itself does not seem to make much difference to the usual levels of SWS (Griffin and Trinder, 1978). On the other hand, when fit and unfit people have a bout of daytime exercise, the fit subjects often show a transient increase in that night's SWS, unlike the unfit subjects, who show no change. The total amount of energy expended during such exercise is not the explanation. Unfit subjects can walk or cycle for many hours without affecting sleep, whereas fit subjects who use up a quarter as much total energy in a half-hour burst of exercise can show a significant SWS increase.

A key difference between fit and unfit people in this respect is that the former can maintain a high exercise intensity for a much longer time. As a result they get hot. Because fit subjects can and will exercise for longer, they get hotter for longer, especially in a warm environment. The hotter they get, the greater the amount of ensuing SWS. A hot body also means a hot brain, and this may be the key behind SWS increases that can follow exercise or even a warm bath. A series of studies conducted at Loughborough University, England, helps to illustrate these latter points.

An initial experiment (Horne and Staff, 1983) used fit subjects who underwent three separate conditions during three afternoons: (1) intense exercise that made the subjects hot; (2) the same total exercise, but at half the rate for twice the time, which only led to a small rise in body temperature; and (3) replication of the body temperature increase under the intense exercise condition by sitting subjects in a bath of warm water ("passive heating"). Within half an hour after each procedure body temperature returned almost to normal; however, it remained higher by a few tenths of a degree Centigrade until bedtime, which may be a critical factor. Bedtime was at the usual time, and subjects had their sleep electroencephalograms (EEGs) recorded. The second condition of the experiment had no effect on sleep, except that subjects felt sleepier at bedtime and fell asleep faster. In contrast, the other two conditions both produced significant increases in SWS.

The extent to which the subjects were getting warm seems to be the key. This was further examined in another study in which fit subjects underwent the same high-intensity exercise as in the earlier study. One condition allowed them to get hot, and the other kept them cool in a blast of cold air, particularly to the face. This procedure reduces brain temperature selectively, as blood from the facial skin can cool the blood entering the brain via a special heat exchange system of blood vessels. The facial cooling almost nullified the potential brain temperature rise. Whereas SWS increased after the hot exercise, as before, the cool exercise left SWS unchanged.

To explore the body/brain heating effects on SWS in unfit subjects, a third study heated these people up without exercise in the warm bath. Body heating was a crucial factor, as SWS increased in a way similar to that of the fit subjects in the first study, who were heated by exercise or bath.

The brain can be heated separately from the body by blowing warm air onto the face. This procedure was done in a fourth study on unfit subjects who sat with a converted hair dryer hood on

their heads, with the drier set at a comfortable "hot." Brain temperature increased significantly (but harmlessly), leaving body temperature relatively unchanged. Again, SWS increased the following night.

Exactly why a warm brain leads to more SWS is still a matter for debate. Of the various possibilities, the two most popular are (1) increased brain temperature leads to rises in brain metabolism, accelerating the build-up of sleep factors that promote SWS; and (2) the remaining small elevation in brain temperature at sleep onset may be affecting other SWS control mechanisms.

The body restitution hypothesis can be discounted as an explanation for these findings. Given that SWS is produced by the brain, and not by muscle, SWS measured alone is no index of body/muscle restitution. None of the studies of sleep after exercise has looked at muscle restitution during sleep. Furthermore, the remaining evidence associating SWS with heightened tissue restitution does not bear up under close scrutiny (Horne, 1988).

See also BASAL FOREBRAIN; HYPOTHALAMUS; THERMOREGULATION.

REFERENCES

Griffin SJ, Trinder J. 1978. Physical fitness, exercise and human sleep. *Psychophysiology* 15:447–450.

Horne JA. 1988. *Why we sleep—The functions of sleep in humans and other mammals.* Oxford: Oxford University Press.

Horne JA, Reid AJ. 1985. Night-time sleep EEG changes following body heating in a warm bath. *Electroencephalogr Clin Neurophysiol* 60:154–157.

Horne JA, Staff LHE. 1983. Exercise and sleep: Body heating effects. *Sleep* 6:36–46.

Martin BJ. 1988. Sleep loss and subsequent exercise performance. *Acta Physiol Scand Suppl* 133 (1574):28–32.

J. A. Horne

EXPERIENTIAL DREAM GROUPS (DREAM WORKSHOPS)

An experiential dream group can be defined either broadly or narrowly. A broad definition would include any group outside of a formal clinical setting in which a leader orients the participants to "dream work" and encourages them to share one or more dreams at each session. The leader of such a group approaches dream work from one or another theoretical orientation—for example, Freudian, Jungian, or Gestalt—and the particular theoretical consideration plays a significant role in the group's interpretation of dream imagery. The leader, who functions as a facilitator or guide, presumably has had specialized training in the particular theory he or she espouses and is not obligated to share dreams of his or her own. The participants are generally in the group because of interest in their own dreams. If participants wish to carry on in the dream interpretation work on their own as group leaders, they are under an obligation to undergo whatever training might be needed to master the theory involved.

Many such broadly defined dream workshops have sprung up in recent years in the United States and abroad. The most popular have been those based on Jungian concepts that stress both the revealing rather than concealing nature of the manifest content of dreams (discarding the Freudian notion of dream content as disguised wish-fulfillment) and the manifestations of the collective unconscious through the appearance of archetypically derived imagery (that is, images that convey universal themes).

The experiential dream group may be defined more narrowly as an atheoretic approach, in which the leader teaches the group how to work with a dream in terms of its basic phenomenological features alone. These features may be defined with reference to form and content. This approach defines three distinct features of dream content:

1. Content begins with residual feelings, tension, or preoccupations that surface in the dreamer's life shortly (hours or days) before the appearance of the dream.

2. Content also includes memories from the past that are emotionally linked to the particular dreamer's current concerns. This information may reach far into the past and is not easily accessible while one is awake.

3. Content is a true reflection of the subjective state of the dreamer at the time. The honesty with which a dream discloses information that is not clearly known or felt in the waking state is its most important feature with regard to its potential for greater self-understanding.

The form of the dream is predominantly a sensory experience in which visual imagery appears. The experiential dream group considers these images not literal reproductions of reality, but rather symbolic representations of the life situation in the dream. The symbol most characteristic of dreaming is the visual metaphor. Such images are used to draw an implicit comparison to an aspect of the dreamer's life; for example, the image of coming upon a fork in the road might suggest the dreamer is coming to a decision point in waking life.

The foundation of this atheoretic approach is an understanding of these dream features and also the practice of certain skills essential to dream work. These include the capacity to listen to the dreamer, the art of putting questions to the dreamer that succeed in yielding the full range of associations needed to spark across the metaphorical gap between dream image and reality, and the sensitivity/delicacy to be helpful without being intrusive. Listening is a skill that requires acknowledging all that a dream says, including its emotional undercurrents, and, most important, avoiding premature conjectures about the meaning of any given image.

Questioning the dreamer requires respect for the dreamer as the gatekeeper of his or her own unconscious domain, so that control of the proceedings is never taken out of his or her hands. Thus, everyone including the leader avoids posing leading questions or making attempts to impose an interpretation on the dreamer. Skillful questioning also requires sensitivity to areas the dreamer prefers to remain private.

A flat structure prevails in a group of this kind; in other words, the leader has the same option to share a dream as everyone else. The social component of healing is stressed in the way that everyone, including the leader, is involved in sharing dreams and that once the basic skills are learned the process is carried on by everyone. The only special role played by the leader is to maintain a safe environment for the dreamer. By teaching the necessary skills (not theoretical concepts), the leader makes it possible for the group to help the dreamer get deep enough into his or her self to make the imagery come alive.

REFERENCES

Many books have appeared in recent years with the purpose of introducing the public to dream work. Most of these books describe techniques that can be of help to the general reader. In some, reference is made to group dream work, but the group approach is not the major focus. What follows is a small sampling of books that are devoted to group dream work and those in which group work receives significant attention.

Books Focusing on Group Dream Work

Neu ER. 1988. *Dreams and dream groups.* Freedom, Calif.: Crossing Press.

Shohet R. 1985. *Dream sharing.* Wellingborough, England: Turnstone Press.

Ullman M, Zimmerman N. 1979. *Working with dreams.* Los Angeles: Jeremy P. Tarcher.

Books Containing Reference to Group Dream Work

Delaney G. 1988. *Living your dreams.* New York: Harper & Row.

Faraday A. 1973. *Dream power.* New York: Berkley Medallion.

Kaplan-Williams S. 1988. *The Jungian-Senoi dream work manual.* Berkeley: Journey Press.

Maguire J. 1989. *Night and day.* New York: Simon & Schuster.

Morris J. 1985. *The dream workbook.* Boston: Little, Brown.

Taylor J. 1983. *Dream work.* Ramsey, N.J.: Paulist Press.

Montague Ullman

EXTERNAL STIMULI: EFFECTS ON DREAMS

See Incorporation into Dreams; Interpretation of Dreams: Methods; Noise; Perception

EXTERNAL STIMULI: EFFECTS ON SLEEP

See Altitude; Beds; Fragmentation; Pressurization; Sensory Processing and Sensation During Sleep

EXTRASENSORY PERCEPTION (ESP)

See Psychic Dreams; Telepathy and Dreaming

EYE MOVEMENTS AND DREAMING

In 1953, when researchers first discovered cycles of eye movements occurring regularly during sleep, they soon asked a question crucial to the relationship between mind and brain: Are the eye movements during sleep related to dreaming?

There are three phases in the study of the relationship between eye movements and dreaming: an early phase in which REM sleep eye movements were presumed to be directionally linked to the visual images of the dream (1953 to 1966), a middle phase in which the notion of such a relationship was dismissed with a great deal of skepticism (1967 to 1986), and a recent phase in which some degree of an association between eye movements and dreamed gaze is generally accepted (1987 to the present).

The eye movements of sleep constituted and remain one of the major mysteries confronting biomedical science; the question of their relationship to dreaming was pivotal to the rapidly expanding interest and research in this new field of sleep and dreams (see REM SLEEP, DISCOVERY OF).

The extraocular muscles that control eye movements, unlike the muscles that control body movements, remain active during REM periods. From the discovery of cycles of jerky eye movements during sleep comes the name *rapid eye movement (REM) sleep.* In the first electrographic study of eye movements and dreaming, Aserinsky and Kleitman (1953) considered the eye movements, and not the awakelike ELECTROEN-CEPHALOGRAM (EEG), to be the physiological counterpart of the dream image, as awakelike brain waves occur at other times during sleep (see STAGES OF SLEEP).

In 1953, Aserinsky and Kleitman awakened their subjects twenty-seven times following eye movements and twenty-three times when the EEG was similar to that accompanying eye movements but none were present. Twenty of the awakenings following eye movements resulted in vivid dream recall; only two of those when eye movements were absent produced dream reports. This study supported a relationship between the occurrence of eye movements and the experience of dreaming. Research soon went a step further to see if the direction of eye movements and the direction of gaze in the dream image are coupled.

Studies by Dement and Kleitman (1957) and by Roffwarg et al. (1962) reported a near-total agreement between the direction of eye movements and dreamed gaze. These studies went beyond Aserinsky and Kleitman's earlier findings demonstrating that transcripts of dream reports and eye movement recordings corresponded; however, these and other investigations that soon followed did not control the bias, or expectation, of the experimenter. They were not double-blind; that is, the experimenter knew which eye movement recording and dream report corresponded when evaluating the match.

Research with animals in the 1960s demonstrated that the eye movements of REM sleep are related to surges of electrical waves from the brainstem and MIDBRAIN that activate the cortex. These brain waves (see PGO WAVES) seem to link eye movements to dreaming because they signal that locations throughout the brain increase their activity when eye movements occur. REM sleep was divided into two components: phasic REM sleep, or the discontinuous, episodic flurries of activity, including eye movements and PGO spikes, and tonic REM sleep, or the continuous, long-lasting portions of this stage of sleep when eye movements and other indications of sudden change are absent (see PHASIC ACTIVITY IN REM SLEEP).

The tonic-phasic model proposed that vivid dreaming accompanied phasic REM sleep, especially eye movements. Tonic REM sleep was considered to be associated with thoughtlike mentation (Grosser and Siegal, 1971). In contrast to the eye movement-dream imagery hypothesis, which speculates that the eyes move in the same direction that the dreamer looks, the tonic-phasic model ignores the question of direction and speculates only that the presence of eye movements is a necessary biological indicator of vivid dreaming.

Newer observations and experiments began to spread doubt about the relationship between eye movements and dreaming (Berger and Ostwald, 1962). For example, Jouvet (1973) found that the "thinking" part of the brain, or the *cortex*, could be removed in animals and REM sleep, including eye movements, would continue. Sleep with rapid eye movements, similar to REM sleep

in adults, was found to be present in all newborn mammals, which obviously could not dream in a manner consistent with the normal definition of this term (see ONTOGENY; PHYLOGENY). Finally, it was discovered that the blind, who have few if any eye movements during REM sleep, have vivid (but nonvisual) dreams (see BLINDNESS: DREAMS OF THE BLIND).

The demonstration that detailed dreaming can occur in NREM sleep (Foulkes, 1962), although not as frequently as in REM sleep, showed that eye movements are not necessary for dreaming to occur. If REM sleep can occur without a cortex and dreaming can occur without eye movements, it was argued, how can dreaming and eye movements be linked? About this time, several studies that controlled for experimenter bias were unable to replicate the previously demonstrated relationship between the direction of recorded eye movements and the direction the subject reported looking in the dream.

The idea that eye movements and dreaming are linked so that their directions are the same is sometimes called *the scanning hypothesis*. This hypothesis predicts that during dreaming the direction of rapid eye movements is the direction that would be required to view the objects of interest in the dream. This theory speculates that the visual cortex contains a dream image that is "scanned" by brain centers that control eye movements, almost like a projection screen and a movie camera in the brain. Few researchers sophisticated in neuroscience ever supported this hypothesis, whether or not they believed in a link between eye movements and dreaming.

Some scientists thought that eye movements and dream images could still be linked in normal REM dreaming, despite the new evidence. An underpinning of this approach is the *pontine generation hypothesis*. This model maintains that information arrives simultaneously in the visual cortex and in the eye muscles by way of separate paths from a common stimulus-generating site in the brainstem. In this model, either pathway could be disrupted or severed, such as by blindness or removal the cortex, and the other would remain intact.

A recent study demonstrated that it is possible to predict the direction of the last eye movements before an awakening, on the basis of the subject's dream report (Herman et al., 1984). This study employed a double-blind design in an attempt to prevent experimenter bias. After awakening the sleeping subject from REM sleep according to a predetermined schedule, the technician connected an interviewer outside of the laboratory to the subject's room by means of a conference call hookup. The interviewer was isolated from the polygraph machine to prevent clues as to eye movement direction. The interviewer questioned the subject in detail before making a series of predictions. The interviewer knew that each awakening was performed after one to several horizontal or vertical eye movements. The interviewer was instructed to predict the direction of the last eye movement, the number of eye movements, the amplitude of the eye movements, and the prevailing direction of eye movements in the 10 seconds preceding the arousal (Figure 1).

These researchers found that the more confident the interviewer was of the predictions of eye movement direction and number, the more likely the predictions were to be correct. This finding supports the concept that the motor physiology of REM sleep and simultaneous dream mentation are two arms of a tightly coupled mind–brain event. In addition to demonstrating a relationship between the direction of eye movement and the direction of dreamed gaze, this study indicates that dream reports may be vivid and detailed in some cases, but not necessarily clear enough to predict recorded eye movement direction.

Another line of research has examined the eye movements in REM sleep to determine if the eye movement velocity is the same or different from that in the awake state. Aserinsky (1971) showed the eye movements in REM sleep to be slower then those in waking. He argued that this finding was evidence of a separate control mechanism for REM sleep eye movements, suggesting that eye movements and dreaming were not related in the same manner as eye movements and vision in waking. A subsequent study showed, however, that when eyes are closed, awake state eye movements have the same slowed velocities as REM sleep eye movements (Herman et al., 1984).

Subsequently, additional indirect evidence has emerged to support a coupling between dream imagery and eye movements, as well as other as-

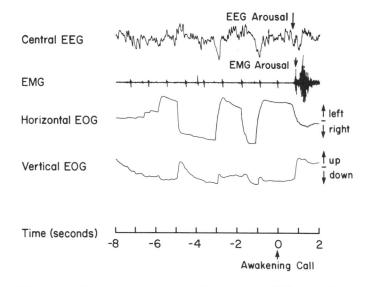

Figure 1. Awakening to obtain dream report following horizontal eye movements. The interviewer was uninformed with respect to the number and direction of the eye movements and was asked to predict them from listening to the dream report. The subject dreamed he was driving toward the Houston Astrodome; he looked at his father who was seated on his right, drove a bit further, looked straight ahead at the Astrodome 2 miles away, and finally glanced at joggers on his left, running from right to left. The interviewer predicted a moderate number of large horizontal eye movements followed by an interval of 3 seconds without eye movements.

pects of REM phasic muscle activity. Studies of lucid dreaming, or dreaming under conscious control, show that eye movements during REM sleep, executed according to instructions given before the onset of sleep, correspond to the direction of gaze in the dream (see LUCID DREAMING). Furthermore, studies of patients who act out during REM sleep (see REM SLEEP BEHAVIOR DISORDER) show their dream reports to be consistent with their actions observed while dreaming.

Both lucid dreaming and REM sleep behavior disorder permit validation of the relationship between dreaming and simultaneous eye or body movements. The demonstration of a relationship between eye movement direction and dreamed gaze indicates that the REM dream is different from other forms of fantasy. The body is involved as well as the mind in an attempt to carry out at least some of the actions portrayed in the dream images.

REFERENCES

Aserinsky E. 1971. Rapid eye movement density and pattern in the sleep of normal young adults. *Psychophysiology* 8:361–374.

Aserinsky E, Kleitman N. 1953. Regularly occurring periods of eye motility and concomitant phenomena during sleep. *Science* 118:273–274.

Berger RJ, Oswald I. 1962. Eye movements during active and passive dreams. *Science* 137:601.

Dement W, Kleitman N. 1957. The relation of eye movements during sleep to dream activity: An objective method for the study of dreaming. *J Exp Psychol* 53:339–346.

Foulkes D. 1962. Dream reports from different stages of sleep. *J Abnormal Social Psychol* 65:14–25.

Grosser GS, Siegal AW. 1971. Emergence of a tonic-phasic model for sleep and dreaming. *Psychol Bull* 75:60–72.

Herman JH, Erman M, Boys R, Peiser L, Taylor ME, Roffwarg HP. 1984. Evidence for a directional correspondence between eye movements and dream imagery in REM sleep. *Sleep* 7(1):52–63.

Jouvet M. 1973. Essai sur le rêve. *Arch Ital Biol* 111:564–576.

Roffwarg HP, Dement WC, Muzio JN, Fisher C. 1962. Dream imagery: Relationship to rapid eye movements of sleep. *Arch Gen Psychiatry* 7:235–258.

John H. Herman

F

FALLING ASLEEP

See Cycles of Sleep Across the Night; Sleep Onset; Microsleep; Stages of Sleep

FATAL FAMILIAL INSOMNIA

Fatal familial insomnia (FFI) is a heredofamilial disease transmitted as an autosomal dominant trait and characterized by loss of sleep and vegetative, endocrine, and neurological disturbances. The disease begins between the ages of 30 and 60 years and leads to death in 7 to 36 months.

The onset is characterized by progressive insomnia associated with neurovegetative disturbances (excessive perspiration, fever, rapid heartbeat, hypertension). Later neurological signs include incoordination, speech difficulties, and muscle spasms. Insomnia then becomes complete, although there occur stuporous episodes of increasing length with automatic gestures mimicking a dream (enacted dreams). Vegetative activation is associated with a marked and persistent increase in levels of plasma CORTISOL and catecholamines and a low adrenocorticotropin level. The circadian oscillations of body temperature, heart rate, blood pressure, and sleep-coupled (growth hormone, prolactin) and uncoupled (adrenocorticotropin, cortisol, melatonin) hormones are decreased or absent (see CHEMISTRY OF SLEEP; NEUROENDOCRINE HORMONES). The constant histopathological feature is the severe atrophy of the anterior and dorsomedian nuclei of the THALAMUS; other thalamic nuclei, cerebral cortex, and cerebellum are less consistently affected.

A protease-resistant prion protein has been found to be isoformed in the brain of patients with FFI; there is a mutation in the gene coding for the prion protein. Therefore, FFI is a prion disease.

The anatomoclinical findings in FFI provide evidence that the visceral (anterior and dorsomedian nuclei) thalamus intervenes in the regulation of the wake–sleep rhythm and in vegetative and endocrine homeostasis (maintenance of internal stability in the organism). The disease creates a lesion of the anterior and dorsomedian thalamic nuclei and thereby disrupts the circuitry between limbic cortex and hypothalamus. The hypothalamus is then freed from cortical control and becomes functionally imbalanced, with a prevalence of the activating (sympathetic or ergotropic) over the deactivating (parasympathetic, trophotropic) component, resulting in the worsening and eventually fatal symptoms.

(See also INSOMNIA.)

REFERENCES

Lugaresi A, Baruzzi A, Cacciari E, Cortelli P, Medori R, Montagna P, Tinuper P, Zucconi M, Roiter I, Lugaresi E. 1987. Lack of vegetative and endocrine circadian rhythms in fatal familial thalamic degeneration. *Clin Endocrinol* 26:573–580.

Lugaresi E, Medori R, Montagna P, Baruzzi A, Cortelli P, Lugaresi A, Tinuper P, Zucconi M, Gambetti PL. 1986. Familial insomnia and dysautonomia with selective degeneration of thalamic nuclei. *N Engl J Med* 315:997–1003.

Tinuper P, Montagna P, Medori R, Cortelli P, Zucconi M, Baruzzi A, Lugaresi E. 1989. The thalamus participates in the regulation of the sleep–waking cycle.

A clinico-pathological study in fatal familial thalamic degeneration. *Electroencephalog Clin Neurophysiol* 73:117–123.

Elio Lugaresi

FATIGUE

[*Fatigue is not the same thing as* SLEEPINESS, *although many people tend to confuse these words when describing how they feel. Scientists who study sleep and the* FUNCTIONS OF SLEEP *define sleepiness in direct relationship to factors that create a sleep debt (such as sleep* DEPRIVATION *or specific sleep disorders) and reserve the term* fatigue *to describe the detrimental physical and psychological effects of prolonged performance in any number of domains. For example, an individual who is sleepy will readily fall asleep, a fact that can be determined directly by the* MULTIPLE SLEEP LATENCY TEST; *on the other hand, a person who is fatigued may not be at all sleepy, but may be unable to perform a function at peak efficiency because of fatigue.*

One of the early models of the sleep–wake system, called the FATIGUE-RECOVERY MODEL, *hypothesized that a major role of sleep was to offset daytime fatigue. When fatigue and sleepiness occur simultaneously, the consequences for* PUBLIC SAFETY IN THE WORKPLACE *and* PUBLIC SAFETY IN TRANSPORTATION *are quite serious, as each factor may potentiate the other.*]

FATIGUE-RECOVERY MODEL

Why do we sleep? Virtually everyone's personal experience is that we sleep because we get sleepy and we cannot function during the day if we get too sleepy. This simple and yet profound answer is the basis of the *fatigue-recovery model* of sleep. According to this model, the duration of a period of wakefulness will determine the duration of the following period of sleep. Underlying the original formulation of this model was the assumption that certain chemicals, called *hypnotoxins* in the 1910s and 1920s, build up in our bodies during wakefulness (see EARLY SLEEP THEORIES). These hypnotoxins were thought to be cleared during sleep by sleep-specific metabolic processes. Research has identified several neurotransmitters, such as serotonin and adenosine, as well as molecules produced by the immune system, such as interleukin and tissue necrosis factor, that induce or promote sleep in experimental animals and may act as hypnotoxins in the fatigue-recovery model (see CHEMISTRY OF SLEEP; IMMUNE FUNCTION).

The fatigue-recovery model has some predictive value for sleep length but breaks down in explaining individual differences and time-of-day effects. The average amount of sleep for adult humans is 7–8 hours, and thus the model—on average—would predict a 2-to-1 ratio of wake to sleep. The range of nighttime sleep durations must be expanded, however, to include 6–9 hours in order to include most people. Furthermore, a few people feel fine with as little as 5 hours of sleep after 19 hours of wakefulness, while others require more than 10 hours of sleep after 14 hours of wakefulness (Hartmann, Baekeland, and Zwilling, 1972; Webb, 1979; see also DEPRIVATION, PARTIAL). In order to account for such individual differences, the model must be modified to postulate either individual rates of hypnotoxin build-up during wakefulness or individual rates of hypnotoxin catabolism during sleep.

Time-of-day effects on sleep duration are even harder to explain with the fatigue-recovery model. Typically, if someone goes to bed at 11:00 P.M. after 16 hours of wakefulness, he or she will sleep about 8 hours. Suppose, however, that someone skips a night of sleep and goes to bed at 11:00 A.M. after 28 hours of wakefulness. This person will not sleep proportionally longer (i.e., [28/16] × 8) as predicted by the fatigue-recovery model. In fact, he or she might sleep for only 2 or 3 hours and then have trouble falling asleep that night. (See also DEPRIVATION, TOTAL.)

The fatigue-recovery model, therefore, may help to explain certain characteristics of sleep, but is not sufficient to account for the wide variety of sleep patterns found in different individuals and in a number of common circumstances.

REFERENCES

Hartmann E, Baekeland F, Zwilling GR. 1972. Psychological differences between short and long sleepers. *Arch Gen Psychiatry* 26:463–468.

Webb WB. 1979. Are short and long sleepers different? *Psychol Rep* 44:259–264.

Merrill M. Mitler

FEAR

See Anxiety; Sleep Terrors

FEMALE SEXUAL RESPONSE

When a woman is awake and sexually aroused, a number of factors help to make the experience pleasant and fulfilling. There is the cognitive component, consisting of what she is thinking to herself and feeling emotionally; there is the behavioral component, consisting of the things she or her partner is doing to help her feel as aroused as possible; and there is the physical component, consisting of her bodily changes. Most research on female sexuality has focused on the physical component; sleep research has contributed to the knowledge of these bodily changes during sexual arousal.

An important study of the female sexual experience was published by Masters and Johnson in 1966. Through surveys and interviews of 700 people over the course of 10,000 sexual experiences, they defined female sexual arousal as comprising four phases: excitement, plateau, orgasm, and resolution (see Masters and Johnson, 1966, for a full description of these phases).

When awake, a woman can become physically aroused if her vagina is touched or if other parts of her body are caressed. The same bodily changes can occur in response to erotic or sensual audio tapes or videotapes or to sexual fantasy.

Much is now known about sexual arousal in women, although a number of questions remain. The physiological changes include an increase in blood flow to the lower third of the vagina; the deeper portions of the vagina show increased blood flow in some studies and decreased blood flow in other studies. These changes seem to be the most reliable indicators of the physical component of sexual arousal, rather than changes in blood pressure, waking electroencephalogram, or forehead temperature. Techniques used to measure vaginal blood flow during sexual arousal include the use of strain gauges around the clitoris, photoplethysmographs, heat cells attached to diaphragms, even thermography scanners. Certain researchers have attempted to measure volume and pressure within the vagina and uterus during sexual arousal; others have investigated the contractions of the vagina and anus (Bohlen and Held, 1979).

Sleep research has shown that changes in the vagina during REM and NREM sleep are similar to those of waking sexual arousal, and about one third of women surveyed report experiencing orgasms while asleep (Winokur, Guxe, and Pfeiffer, 1959). It does not seem that sexual thoughts are necessary to propel the female sexual response; if these physical changes are normal reactions to events within the brain's sleep system, then evaluation of sexual arousal during sleep can be a valuable means to identify and treat cases of physically based sexual dysfunction in women.

When a woman is experiencing sexual difficulties, it is important to assess whether the problems result from a physical inability (such as problems in blood flow, lubrication, or neuronal transmission of an impulse) or from psychological factors (such as relationship with her partner, fears related to sex, or concerns with herself and her performance). One way to differentiate a physical difficulty from a psychological one is to evaluate the patient while she sleeps. During REM sleep, a number of physiological changes typically occur at once; for example, breathing rate becomes variable, eyes move in rapid bursts, and temperature regulation is drastically reduced (see REM SLEEP, PHYSIOLOGY OF). In addition, it is well known that erections of the penis occur frequently during REM sleep in healthy men. These erections appear to be physiological events unrelated to erotic fantasy, dream content, stimulation of the penis in the daytime, or bladder pressure. In women, similar changes in the vagina occur before and during REM sleep. (See also ERECTIONS; NOCTURNAL PENILE TUMESCENCE; SEXUAL ACTIVATION.)

To determine whether a woman is physically capable of becoming aroused, the clinician must ascertain whether vaginal changes are occurring during sleep. Diagnostic sleep assessments utilize a number of the techniques used to measure daytime sexual arousal. In one of the first studies of female sexual arousal during sleep, Abel and his colleagues (1979) examined the vaginal signs of sexual arousal in eight women during

REM sleep, and found that increased pulse rate within the vagina was accompanied by decreased blood flow within the vaginal tissue. By comparison, when these women were asked to fantasize while awake about sexual experiences, increased vaginal pulse was accompanied by increased blood volume in the tissues. Thus, the researchers concluded that women's sexual response in sleep is more similar to the physiological changes of orgasm than to the engorgement of the excitement phase in waking sexual arousal. Fisher and his colleagues (1983), however, obtained different results using a temperature sensor attached to a vaginal diaphragm. An increase in blood flow to the vagina during REM sleep and, to a lesser extent, during the NREM sleep periods immediately preceding REM sleep periods was as great as that measured when the women were awake and sexually aroused, although their respiration and heart rates in sleep were much lower than in waking sexual arousal.

In another study, measurement of the sexual response in sleep was used to differentiate between women who reported having difficulty becoming sexually aroused and women who did not have such difficulty. The researchers found that nineteen of twenty subjects showed vaginal pulse rates during REM sleep that were as great as while they were awake and attending to erotic stimuli. Sleep measures of sexual arousal did not show differences between the women who described themselves as easily aroused and those who had difficulty becoming aroused (Rogers et al., 1985). One conclusion from this study is that the dysfunction reported by the women with low self-ratings of sexual arousability was not caused by a physical disorder.

It is not known whether the other physical components of the waking female sexual response (such as sex flushing and breast enlargement) or the cognitive and emotional changes that a woman experiences, are also typical components of sleeping sexual arousal. What is certain, though, is that many women report experiencing the sensation of sexual arousal or orgasm during sleep without direct stimulation of the vagina or other parts of the body. Kinsey and his colleagues (1953) reported that many women are awakened by the vaginal wetness and contractions of sleep-related orgasms; they also reported that 5 percent of women had an orgasm during sleep before experiencing an orgasm in waking life. In recent studies, more than one third of

women questioned have reported orgasms while asleep, and almost a third report that they have had a sleep-related orgasm within the past year. While studying the sleep-related sexual function of one woman, Fisher and his coworkers (1983) noted a large increase in blood flow to the vaginal tissues and extreme changes in heart and breathing for approximately 2 minutes during one REM sleep period; when awakened, the woman reported having experienced an orgasm.

BIBLIOGRAPHY

Abel G, Murphy W, Becker J, Bitar A. 1979. Women's vaginal responses during REM sleep. *Sex Marital Therapy* 5:5–14.

Bohlen J, Held J. 1979. An anal probe for monitoring vascular and muscular events during sexual response. *Psychophysiology* 36:318–323.

Fisher C, Cohen H, Schiavi R, Davis D, Furman B, Ward K, Edwards A, Cunningham J. 1983. Patterns of female sexual arousal during sleep and waking: Vaginal thermo-conductance studies. *Arch Sexual Behavior* 12:97–122.

Kinsey AC, Pomeroy W, Martin C, Gebhard P. 1953. *Sexual behavior in the human female.* Philadelphia: Saunders.

Masters WH, Johnson VE. 1966. *Human sexual response.* Boston: Little, Brown.

Rogers G, Van de Castle R, Evans W, Critelli J. 1985. Vaginal pulse amplitude response patterns during erotic conditions and sleep. *Arch Sexual Behavior* 14:327–342.

Weisberg M. 1984. Physiology of female sexual function. *Clin Obstetrics Gynecology* 27:697–705. Provides an excellent review of the work of Masters and Johnson as well as that of other investigators working in the field of female sexual response.

Winokur G, Guxe S, Pfeiffer E. 1959. Nocturnal orgasm in women. *Arch Gen Psychiatry* 1:180–184.

Mindy Engle-Friedman

FETAL SLEEP–WAKE PATTERNS

The frequent movements of the fetus in utero, which are first felt by the mother during the fifth month, are called quickening. These movements resemble those during REM sleep (active sleep) in infants. When these fetal movements were measured from the abdomen of pregnant women (Sterman and Hoppenbrouwers, 1971), and later when continuous fetal heart rates were recorded together with maternal sleep and waking states (Hoppenbrouwers et al., 1978), several discoveries were made. As early as 22 weeks of gestation, the fetus has an alternating pattern of activity and quiescence, termed the BASIC REST-ACTIVITY CYCLE (BRAC), which lasts about 40 to 60 minutes. Around 22 weeks there is only a faint resemblance between the BRAC and the REM–NREM sleep cycle of the newborn, but by 36 weeks there is great similarity (Nijhuis et al., 1982). The primitive BRAC is a forerunner of the adult REM–NREM sleep cycle, and the period of the fetal cycle is shorter than that of the mother, which ranges between 90 and 120 minutes.

In the mid-1960s, when the REM–NREM sleep cycle had been known for about a decade, scientists speculated that recurrent episodes of REM sleep might be caused by a hormone or other substance in the brain and the blood. Examining the mother/fetus sleep patterns was thought to shed light on this issue, because the mother and fetus share the same blood circulation through the umbilical cord. If such a circulating substance were involved in regulating sleep, then the pregnant mother and her fetus should enter REM sleep together. Such a synchrony, however, was clearly not present. Nevertheless, the mother and fetus seem to be communicating with each other, because often when the mother is falling asleep the fetus begins to move, an observation confirmed by increases in fetal heart rate, as well as by reports of the mother.

Is the fetus awake? The most modern equipment, such as ultrasound recordings, can visualize the fetus in utero, but cannot establish firmly whether the fetus is awake. Certain fetal heart rate and movement patterns, however, are remarkably similar to those in the same subjects while awake after birth (Hoppenbrouwers et al., 1978; Patrick et al., 1982). Moreover, as in the newborn, the arousal threshold of the fetus for auditory stimuli is lower during these episodes than during REM and NREM sleep. Thus, in utero, the fetus alternates between REM and NREM sleep and occasionally seems to "awaken." Close to delivery, "awake" episodes occur less than 5 percent of the time and are not random: They occur at 3- to 4-hour intervals and peak between 9 P.M. and 1 A.M. Several intriguing questions remain unanswered. Are these late-evening "awa-

kenings" the first evidence of the fetal circadian clock? If so, does the mother exert an influence on the formation and setting of this clock through her own sleeping pattern? Furthermore, even though the maternal circulation fulfills all fetal needs, "awakenings" have been observed at 3- to 4-hour intervals, which is approximately as often as newborns wake up for feeding. Does the fetus practice "awakenings" before needing them, in the same way as the fetus seems to practice breathing movements before they are needed?

REFERENCES

Hoppenbrouwers T, Ugartechea JC, Combs D, Hodgman JE, Harper RM, Sterman MB. 1978. Studies of maternal fetal interaction during the third trimester of pregnancy. I. Ontogenesis of the basic rest activity cycle. *Exp Neurol* 61:136–153.

Nijhuis JG, Prechtl HFR, Martin CB Jr, Bots RSGM. 1982. Are there behavioral states in the human fetus? *Early Hum Dev* 6:177–195.

Patrick J, Campbell K, Carmichael L, Natale R, Richardson B. 1982. Patterns of gross fetal body movements over 24-hour observation intervals during the last 10 weeks of pregnancy. *Am J Obstet Gynecol* 142:363–371.

Sterman MB, Hoppenbrouwers T. 1971. Development of sleep–waking and rest–activity patterns from fetus to adult in man. In Sterman MB, McGinty DJ, Adinolfi A, eds. *Brain development and behavior.* New York: Academic.

Toke Hoppenbrouwers

FIBROMYALGIA

See Arthritis and Other Musculoskeletal Disorders; Chronic Fatigue Syndrome; Nonrestorative Sleep

FISH

Fish are the most varied and largest class among the vertebrates (animals with backbones). Many species have well-defined daily rest–activity rhythms, and a majority of them are diurnal, that is, more active during the day. Nevertheless, several species such as some shark, tuna fish, saithe, and mackerel engage in continuous motion. Although many investigations of sleep in fish have been purely behavioral and did not involve continuous, long-term observations, the existence of sleeplike behavior in many fish is well established. The signs of sleep include preferred resting niches, specific sleeping positions, and decreased sensitivity to arousal stimuli. For example, several types of fish dive into the sand where they remain the entire night (e.g., many wrasses and trigger fishes). Moreover, certain fish change their color at night (many coral fish; e.g., doctor fish; barracuda), whereas others have been observed to float upside down in the water (e.g., some puffers). Fish may also lie flat in the sand or against a rock (wrasses, trigger fish), or they may wedge themselves into crevices, sometimes with their head pointing upward (some charasins). During the sleeplike behavior, the fins may be placed smoothly against the body or extended away from the body. One very peculiar adaptation is found in certain parrot fish and the cleaner wrasse, which secrete a mucous envelope in which they remain motionless all night (Lenke, 1988).

Whereas during the active phase of the day fish respond immediately to abrupt changes in their environment, in these quiescent states the fish react more slowly to sensory stimulation (e.g., trigger fish, Picasso fish). In a detailed observational study of a population of schooling fish, two states of rest were discriminated on the basis of the number of displacements in the tank per minute. These states occurred at distinct periods of the 24-hour cycle and differed in behavioral arousal threshold (Shapiro, 1976). When the fish were least active, the response to an electrical stimulus or to feeding was lowest. In preliminary studies of the rainbow wrasse, arousal threshold and oxygen consumption were measured to determine whether the fish that regularly dive into the sand during the dark engage in a sleeplike state. Arousal thresholds to tactile stimulation were higher and oxygen consumption lower in the dark compared with the light period, when fish sometimes spontaneously dive into the sand (Videler, 1988).

Although there is agreement that many fish exhibit sleep by behavioral criteria, the electrophysiological correlates of sleeplike behavior in fish have received little attention. Only two species have been investigated in electrophysio-

logical studies of sleep (see Tobler, 1984, for a review). There is no evidence for either mammal-like SLOW-WAVE SLEEP or REM SLEEP in fish. Although rapid eye movements were observed in several species of parrot fish, no such movements were identified in schooling fish or tench. Continuous electroencephalographic (EEG) recordings of tench for several days revealed no changes in the electroencephalogram that correlated with the change from behavioral activity to rest as defined by an activity meter, respiration rate, cardiac rate, muscle activity, and arousal threshold. On the other hand, spectral analysis (computer analysis of frequency components) of short EEG fragments in catfish showed a decrease in frequency and amplitude of the electroencephalogram as a correlate of rest (Karmanova, 1982). In the course of behavioral relaxation accompanied by a decrease in heart rate, more slow waves predominated and EEG spikelike activity increased in the catfish. Furthermore, the spikes increased after behavioral stimulation. Similar EEG changes have been described in some reptiles. Although such studies indicate that there may be EEG correlates of sleep in fish, further confirmation is required to substantiate these findings. In addition to the difficulties encountered in carrying out continuous physiological recordings in the water, sleep investigations in fish have been affected by a large effect of the electrode placement (Laming, 1980) and of the time of the year when EEG recordings are obtained (Hara, Ueda, and Goreman, 1965).

As a further attempt to determine similarities between mammalian sleep and rest in fish, the effect of rest deprivation was studied in perch (Tobler and Borbély, 1985), carp, and gudgeon (Inoue, 1989). Activation of perch during 6 or 12 hours of the normal rest period and of carp and gudgeon for 24 hours resulted in an increase in resting behavior during recovery in the three species. The effect depended on the length of the deprivation. Similarly, activation of schooling fish by continuous light was followed by a shorter delay to resting behavior than under control conditions of normal light and dark. These results could be interpreted as compensatory responses to the preceding deprivation of rest that are similar to those observed in other vertebrates.

In summary, on the basis of behavioral criteria, sleep has been found in many fish, but the experimental data on EEG correlates of sleep cannot be regarded as conclusive.

REFERENCES

Hara TJ, Ueda K, Goreman A. 1965. Electroencephalographic studies of homing salmon. *Science* 149: 884–885.

Inoue S. 1989. *Biology of sleep substances.* Boca Raton, Fla.: CRC Press.

Karmanova IG. 1982. *Evolution of sleep. Stages and the formation of the "wakefulness–sleep" cycle in vertebrates.* Basel: Karger.

Laming PR. 1980. Electroencephalographic studies on arousal in the goldfish (*Carassius auratus*). *J Comp Physiol Psychol* 94:238–254.

Lenke R. 1988. Hormonal control of sleep–appetitive behaviour and diurnal activity rhythms in the cleaner wrasse, *Labroides dimidiatus* (Labridae, Teleostei). *Behav Brain Res* 27:73–85.

Shapiro CM, Hepburn HR. 1976. Sleep in a schooling fish, *Tilapia mossambica. Physiol Behav* 16: 613–615.

Tobler I. 1984. Evolution of the sleep process: A phylogenetic approach. In Borbély A, Valatx JL, eds. *Experimental brain research*, Suppl. 8, pp 207–226. Berlin: Springer-Verlag.

Tobler I, Borbély AA. 1985. Effect of rest deprivation on motor activity in fish. *J Comp Physiol* 157: 817–822.

Videler JJ. 1988. Sleep under sand cover of the labrid fish *Coris julis*. In Koella W, Obàl F, Schulz H, Visser P, eds. pp 145–147. *Sleep '86.* Stuttgart/New York: Gustav Fischer Verlag.

Irene Tobler

FLOWER CLOCK

Carolus Linnaeus (1707–1778), a renowned Swedish naturalist of the eighteenth century, is still honored in the history of science because he devised the first logical system for classifying the plant world. Among the many observations Linnaeus made about plants were that they regularly open and close their flowers each day and that different species of plants have characteristic times of day at which these activities occur. In Uppsala, where Linnaeus lived, he noted that rough hawkbit flowers opened by 4 A.M., dandelions by 5 A.M., and both closed by 8 A.M. White water lilies opened around 7 A.M. and closed by 5 P.M., while the ice plant's flowers "slept" until 11 A.M. and were closed again by 3 P.M. In his monumental book on plants, *Philosophia Botanica* (1751), he listed the flower opening and closing times of dozens of plants and suggested that a fairly accurate "flower clock" could be constructed by planting the appropriate plants in a circular garden. Whether or not Linnaeus actually planted such a garden is unknown, but attempts to do so in the nineteenth century apparently failed because many of the plants Linnaeus listed do not flower at the same season. Even those that flower throughout the summer open and close at different times of day across the season in the temperate zones of the earth. This is because the times of sunrise and sunset, which synchronize this internal rhythm of plants, vary considerably from month to month (see BIOLOGICAL RHYTHMS; DE MAIRAN, JEAN JACQUES D'ORTOUS). Obviously, a flower clock would not be feasible in the cold months of the year, except perhaps in a greenhouse.

Despite the drawbacks, it must be remembered that most people of Linnaeus's era had no personal timepieces, and depended on a town square clock to know the time. Town clocks had become reasonably accurate during the 200 years since their invention, but required considerable attention from master craftsmen to be even kept running. Had they been practical, flower clocks would have been a much cheaper alternative, and if planted strategically, would have been useful to those who worked or traveled out of earshot of the town clock's chimes.

(See also ALARM CLOCKS.)

REFERENCES

Fraser JT. 1987. *Time, the familiar stranger.* Amherst: University of Massachusetts Press.

Kerner AvM. 1895. *The natural history of plants,* vol II, Oliver FW, trans. and ed. London: Blackie & Son.

Daniel R. Wagner

FLYING IN DREAMS

Many ordinary activities in dreams can be interpreted literally; for example, dreaming of driving a car does not necessarily stand for something else. Dreams of flying under one's own power, however, invite symbolic interpretation. Freud considers flying to be a symbol of sexual longing; other psychologists regard dream flying as an expression of freedom (see ADLER'S DREAM THEORY; FREUD'S DREAM THEORY; JUNG'S DREAM THEORY; PHENOMENOLOGY OF DREAMS). Flying can convey a dreamer's feeling of being "on top of the world" at the time of the dream. On the other hand, it can also reflect a struggle to "rise above" a problem or restriction. The emotional tone of a flying dream is thus important for interpretation; elation or anxiety in the dream may indicate how the dreamer really feels about the waking situation. Even the height to which the dreamer flies can be seen as relevant symbolic information. Thus, anxiety in a dream about flying higher may suggest that the dreamer does not feel "up" to an actual challenge in the waking world.

One researcher examining dream content from 250 nights of laboratory dreams in young adults—art students, farmers, medical students—found that flying dreams occurred infrequently. Only one of the 635 dream reports included flying (Snyder, 1970). When they do occur, dreams of flying are often remembered vividly. Although flying in dreams can be frightening, most people find it a fun and sometimes thrilling event. It can also serve to help "induce" a lucid dream (see LUCID DREAMING).

Certain researchers have recently suggested a physiological cause rather than a purely psychological explanation for dream flying. Although the sleeping body is quiescent and sensory input to the sleeping brain is restricted, animal studies have shown that the brainstem's motor system is activated during dreaming sleep, leading to neuronal discharge in related systems higher in the cortex. Many scientists agree that in humans these signals for body actions are normally incorporated into the dream story and the sleeper cannot run, jump, or move around the room because of the simultaneous suppression of motor effector systems in REM sleep (see REM SLEEP PHYSIOLOGY). McCarley (1989) notes that the vestibular system, which functions in wakefulness to sense the body's movement and position in space, is highly activated during dreaming sleep, and the dreaming brain may interpret such sensations as flying. Similarly, psychologist Harry Hunt speculates that conflicting signals arise because the real body lies inert but the "dream body" moves about when the brain is in REM sleep. This difference may destabilize balance perception and lead to the dream experience of strange body distortions, nightmares, or lucid dreams (Hunt, 1989).

(See also CONTENT OF DREAMS.)

REFERENCES

Faraday A. 1974. *The dream game*. New York: Harper & Row.

Gackenback J, Bosveld J. 1989. *Control your dreams*. New York: Harper & Row.

Hunt HT. 1989. *The multiplicity of dreams: Memory, imagination, and consciousness*. New Haven, CT: Yale University Press.

McCarley RW. 1989. The biology of dreaming sleep. In Kryger MH, Roth T, Dement WC, eds. *Principles and practice of sleep medicine,* pp 173–182. Philadelphia: WB Saunders.

Snyder F. 1970. The phenomenology of dreaming. In Madow L, Snow L, eds. *The psychodynamic implications of the physiological studies on dreams,* pp 124–150. Springfield, IL: CC Thomas.

Krista Hennager

FOLK AND OTHER NATURAL REMEDIES FOR SLEEPLESSNESS

Awakening refreshed from a deep and restful sleep is one of the hallmarks and rewards of good emotional and physical health. There is nothing more precious than a good night's sleep, and every culture from earliest recorded history to the present has its own favorite nostrum for problems affecting this universal need. Some remedies are bizarre, from putting one's feet in the refrigerator for ten minutes to rubbing garlic on the soles of the feet or sleeping with a cut raw onion under the pillow. Other treatments seem to come from a mother's instinctive common sense: a warm relaxing bath, a glass of warm milk with honey, a cup of herbal tea. A favorite Japanese formula is two tablespoons of honey followed by a glass of hot water and lemon juice taken one hour before retiring. Other beverages reputed to have sleep-inducing qualities are warm grapefruit juice, elderberry juice, and goat's milk.

Bad Foods and Good Foods

Nutritionally speaking, certain foods and drinks act as stimulants and keep one awake; others have a more relaxing, sedative effect. The first step an insomniac might take would be to reduce or eliminate caffeine-containing stimulants like COFFEE, TEA, COLA DRINKS, and CHOCOLATE (see CAFFEINE). Other foods and substances that might keep one awake by increasing the heart rate are sweets and refined carbohydrates, excess salt, alcohol, tobacco, and MSG or other chemical additives.

Foods high in the amino acid tyramine (a precursor of norepinephrine, a brain chemical stimulant) eaten before bed may cause sleeplessness in certain people. Tyramine-rich foods include cheese, sauerkraut, wine, bacon, ham, sausage, eggplant, spinach, and tomatoes. Many people have reported that overeating in general, especially fatty foods, close to bedtime may also inhibit sleep.

On the other hand, a light snack containing the amino acid tryptophan (a precursor to serotonin, the brain's own sedative and relaxant) may help one to fall asleep more quickly (see L-TRYPTOPHAN). Milk is a major food source of tryptophan, as are turkey, yoghurt, and bananas. A small bowl of cereal with milk, a few whole-grain crackers with nut butter, or a plain baked potato eaten thirty minutes before bed may activate this sleeping aid. Warm milk flavored with either honey, nutmeg, or a few threads of saffron may also do the trick (the flavoring is not chemically necessary). Children seem to be more responsive to prebedtime foods than most adults. Interestingly, people have also reported that skipping lunch causes a restless sleep.

A controlled scientific study has proven the effectiveness of at least one prebedtime drink: Horlick's hot malted milk. Those who drank Horlick's slept longer and had fewer wakeful periods during the night than those who did not. Sleeping improved even more with the repeated use of this product, and it was especially effective for those ages forty-two to sixty-six (Regestein and Rechs, 1980, p. 176).

The magic of milk as a sedative may be due not only to tryptophan but to calcium as well. If muscle tension is keeping someone awake, nutritionists often recommend a supplement of 1,000 mg of both calcium and magnesium taken at bedtime.

Herbal Remedies

The use of plants for healing goes back to the dawn of humanity. Nature's safest and—many feel—most effective sleep inducers, herbal formulas for sleep have been handed down from generation to generation. Herbs have rewarded their users with deep, relaxing sleep long before barbiturate drugs came on the scene at the beginning of the twentieth century. Unlike certain modern sleep medications, herbs produce no unpleasant side effects when used properly: they are nonaddictive.

Valerian root is probably the most widely used herbal sedative and sleep aid in both Europe and the United States. It may be prepared as a tincture (one dropperful in a little water); freeze-dried in capsule form (take two at bedtime); or as an herbal tea (steep one teaspoon in boiling water for ten minutes). The only complaint on record about valerian is that it smells of "old socks."

Hops, a close botanical relative of marijuana, is another favorite of herbalists. It can be used by itself as a tea or along with valerian root (one-half teaspoon of each steeped in a cup of boiling water). A variety of people since the Middle Ages, from English kings to American pioneers, have used hops flowers sewn into a small pillow to induce sleep. Hops should be avoided by persons who are depressed, as it may worsen depression. Tea made from lady's slipper, on the other hand, is a mood elevator *and* a sleep inducer.

Other popular herbal sleep teas include chamomile, passion flower, catnip, scullcap, lime flowers, and cowslip flowers and various combinations of these. Favorite mixtures combine equal amounts of chamomile, lime flower, and red clover or passion flower, hops, and valerian. Other herbs with relaxant qualities—many familiar from the kitchen—are anise, balm, cayenne pepper, dill, heather, marjoram, peppermint, rosemary, gotu kola, poppyseed, lemon verbena, and California poppy (a nonaddictive cousin of the opium poppy). Jamaican dogwood in equal combination with hops and valerian is recommended especially when sleeplessness is due to pain.

Hydrotherapy, Aromatherapy, Massage

Hydrotherapy or "water healing" is also one of the oldest and among the cheapest and safest natural therapies for many common ailments including insomnia. There may be nothing more soothing and relaxing than immersion in a deep tub of warm water. A tepid bath with a temperature of 92°F to 97°F (33°C to 36°C) is best. A hotter bath may stimulate, rather than relax. Scientific evidence is now accumulating that suggests that moderate body warming has a specific enhancing effect on deep, slow-wave sleep (see SLOW-WAVE SLEEP). If time is short or hot water is scarce, try a hot foot bath.

Ancient Egyptian hieroglyphics show that aromatherapy is among the most ancient of the healing arts. In aromatherapy, essential oils extracted from the roots, bark, leaves, or seeds of plants are massaged into the skin, added to the bath water, or simply inhaled in steam. For sleeplessness, six drops of chamomile or lavender oil or five drops of orange blossom oil may be added to a warm bath. To use dried herbs, one practice is to steep a handful or two of valerian root, lime blossom, and/or chamomile in 2 pints of boiling water for ten minutes, strain, and add the water to a warm bath. If one then sips a cup of tea made from the same mixture and takes several deep breaths while relaxing in the warm tub, she or he will be receiving hydrotherapy, aromatherapy, and herbalism simultaneously!

When sleeplessness is due to muscle tension or anxiety, massage or the healing touch of another person can relax both body and mind. A simple stroking or kneading of the neck and shoulder area will loosen the tight muscles that may cause discomfort and inhibit sleep. A warm bath beforehand plus the use of a relaxing massage oil of lavender or chamomile may enhance the effectiveness of a simple massage. When a full body massage is not possible, a simple foot massage or reflexology may yield the same beneficial results.

BIBLIOGRAPHY

Balch JF, Balch PA. 1990. *Prescription for nutritional healing*. Garden City Park, N.Y.: Avery.

Carroll D. 1980. *The complete book of natural medicines*. New York: Summit Books.

Hoffman D. 1988. *The holistic herbal*. 2nd ed. Longmead, England: Element Books.

Regestein R, Rechs J. 1980. *Sound sleep*. New York: Simon & Schuster.

Stanway A, Grossman R. 1987. *The natural family doctor*. New York: Simon & Schuster.

Trattler R. 1985. *Better health through natural healing*. New York: McGraw-Hill.

Weil A. 1990. *Natural health, natural medicine*. Boston: Houghton Mifflin.

Wilen J, Wilen L. 1986. *More chicken soup & other folk remedies*. New York: Fawcett Columbine.

Phyllis Herman

FOOD

See Chocolate; Eating Disorders; Metabolism; Nutrition and Sleep; Postprandial

FORENSICS

See Violence

FRAGMENTATION

Sleep fragmentation is a general term used to describe the degree to which a period of sleep is interrupted by awakenings or arousals. While the sleep scoring guidelines established by Rechtschaffen and Kales in 1968 provide clear rules for the identification of stages of sleep in normal young adults, the guidelines did not anticipate scoring difficulties in individuals with severely fragmented sleep. Patients with sleep AP-NEA, PERIODIC LEG MOVEMENTS, fibrositis, or ARTHRITIS or in environments with significant intrusion (e.g., intensive care units) may be disturbed as often as once each minute by events that can cause awakening or AROUSAL. In patients with severe SLEEPINESS, the sleep electroencephalogram (EEG) changes commonly associated with sleep fragmentation include the periodic, brief appearance of higher-frequency EEG rhythms (usually a 3- to 5-second burst of ALPHA RHYTHM or theta frequencies) often associated with a physiological event such as a leg jerk or termination of an apnea. The brief appearance of the higher-frequency EEG rhythm, which may also be accompanied by increased muscle tone, body movement, or increased heart rate, is rapidly followed by slow rolling eye movements or other signs of stage 1 sleep (see STAGES OF SLEEP). Stage 1 characteristics are rapidly followed by SLEEP SPINDLES or other clear signs of stage 2 sleep, but a 30-second transition to well-defined sleep is frequently interrupted by another physiological event that produces a new arousal and a new attempt to resume sleep. Patients with sleep apnea or periodic leg movements, for example, have events that repeat at 15- to 60-second intervals regardless of the severity of their disease. Overall indices of average numbers of events per night actually reflect the proportion of the night that is characterized by the appearance of the periodic physiological phenomena rather than the average interval between events. As a result, interest in the consequences of these disordered sleep processes has served as an impetus for investigators to define several aspects of sleep continuity.

Identification of patients with frequently disturbed sleep as overwhelmingly sleepy resulted in initial hypotheses that the fragmentation of sleep somehow interrupts the restorative function that results in most individuals feeling awake and alert after a night of NORMAL SLEEP (see FATIGUE-RECOVERY MODEL; NONRESTORATIVE SLEEP; THEORIES OF SLEEP FUNCTION). Initial studies documented that, in groups of patients with sleep disorders causing fragmentation as defined above, there was a positive correlation between the amount of nocturnal sleep disturbance and the degree of residual sleepiness on the day that followed. Other patients, who have sleep disorders characterized by fewer but longer-lasting awakenings, commonly report INSOMNIA without significant daytime sleepiness. It is known that reduction in total sleep time will result in the development of daytime sleepiness and PERFORMANCE lapses (see DEPRIVATION). However, the sleepiness that develops in patients with severely fragmented sleep is independent of the total number of minutes of sleep obtained.

In several empirical studies with both animals and normal human participants, experimental arousals have been systematically performed in an attempt to understand the relationship between periodic sleep disturbance and the restorative function of sleep. It has been shown that brief arousals during sleep in normal young adults reduce daytime alertness. The extent of the reduction in daytime alertness depends upon the frequency of the arousals, the type of arousal, and the age of the subject. When periodic arousals occur at intervals greater than 20 minutes, no effects on daytime function are seen. Increasing loss of daytime function is found when the period of sleep between arousals is reduced from 20 minutes to 1 minute. When arousals are very frequent (i.e., once per minute), performance and alertness on the following day are approximately at the level seen in subjects who have been totally sleep deprived. Any manipulation resulting in frequent changes in ongoing EEG results in daytime deficits, whereas no deficits are seen in a condition of frequent, passively produced leg movements that do not result in EEG arousals. Older subjects are less sensitive to sleep fragmentation than are young adults. Results from several studies indicate that effects are dependent upon the rate of sleep fragmentation and not upon associated changes in the amount of REM SLEEP or SLOW-WAVE SLEEP. The fact that daytime residual effects following frequent sleep disruption are of a magnitude similar to that seen after total sleep loss suggests that, when the sleep process is disturbed at a rate of once per minute or more, the very brief periods of sleep are of insufficient duration for a basic restorative process to occur.

Human studies indicate that when 1- to 20-minute periods of sleep are allowed, sleep is partially restorative. These studies imply that a specific process time—greater than 1 minute and less than 20 minutes—without EEG disturbance is required for sleep restoration. This process time has been referred to as the *basic sleep unit*. The relationship between sleep continuity and sleep restoration also suggests that sensory thresholds are greatly increased during sleep (see DEPTH OF SLEEP; SENSORY PROCESSING AND SENSATION DURING SLEEP) as a means of preserving sleep continuity and thus sleep restoration. Specific biochemical or physiological processes that operate in the 1- to 20-minute range and may therefore be associated with the sleep restorative process have not been identified, although it is known that frequently fragmented sleep results in significantly elevated overall body METABOLISM. The rate of fragmentation required to produce significant daytime residual effects is so high that few individuals without sleep apnea or severe periodic leg movements experience sufficient natural sleep fragmentation to suffer negative daytime consequences.

REFERENCES

Bonnet MH. 1986. Performance and sleepiness as a function of frequency and placement of sleep disruption. *Psychophysiology* 23(3):263–271.

————. 1989. The effect of sleep fragmentation on sleep and performance in younger and older people. *Neurobiol Aging* 10:21–25.

Bonnet MH, Berry RB, Arand DL. 1991. Metabolism during normal sleep, fragmented sleep, and recovery sleep. *J of Appl Physiol* 71:1112–1118.

Carskadon MA, Brown ED, Dement WC. 1982. Sleep fragmentation in the elderly: Relationship to daytime sleep tendency. *Neurobiol Aging* 3:321–327.

Rechtschaffen A, Kales A, eds. 1968. *A manual of standardized terminology, techniques and scoring system for sleep stages of human subjects.* Los Angeles: UCLA Brain Information Service/Brain Research Institute.

Stepanski E, Lamphere J, Badia P, Zorick F, Roth T. 1984. Sleep fragmentation and daytime sleepiness. *Sleep* 7(1):18–26.

Michael H. Bonnet

FREE RUNNING

CIRCADIAN RHYTHMS persist in the absence of external time cues. For example, a mouse kept in total darkness and constant ambient temperature and given free access to food and water wakes and sleeps with about a 23-hour periodicity. The same mouse in the wild, however, would adhere to a strictly 24-hour schedule, because it could entrain (see ENTRAINMENT) to environmental cues (called ZEITGEBERS) with 24-hour periodicity. Some properties of circadian rhythms (such as the period of the rhythm in the above example) change depending on whether zeitgebers are present in the organism's environment. Rhythms occurring in the absence of all zeitgebers are referred to as *free running*. An organism exhibiting a free running circadian rhythm is said to be *in free run*.

What features of rhythms differ between entrained and free-running conditions? The period of the rhythm (also called *tau*) can change markedly when an organism is moved from a light–dark cycle into free-running conditions. The mold *Neurospora crassa,* for example, will make its spores every 24 hours when it is grown in a cycle of 12 hours light and 12 hours dark. In free-running conditions, the tau for spore formation shortens to 21.5 hours. In other cases, a rhythm may completely disappear in constant conditions. Rats that have been surgically altered to remove the part of the brain believed to contain the circadian clock (SUPRACHIASMATIC NUCLEUS OF THE HYPOTHALAMUS) continue to wake and sleep with a 24-hour period in a standard light–dark cycle, but show no rhythms at all when placed in total darkness. In this instance, the rhythm observed in the light–dark conditions is not considered a circadian rhythm, and the effect of the zeitgeber in producing a rhythm is called a *masking* effect. Other rhythm features that can change between entrained and free-running conditions include the phase at which particular events occur in the circadian cycle, and decoupling of the periods of several free-running rhythms (see INTERNAL DESYNCHRONIZATION; TEMPORAL ISOLATION).

Free-running circadian rhythms have been noted since the eighteenth-century work of Jean Jacques d'Ortous DE MAIRAN. However, the detailed study of the free-running circadian clock really began only in the latter half of the twentieth century. These studies, which established the extreme precision and persistence of free-running circadian rhythms in a variety of creatures from unicellular organisms to humans, provided the crucial evidence suppporting the hypothesis that circadian rhythms are timed by oscillators *internal* to the organism. Elucidating the mechanisms by which organisms can keep time in free-running conditions remains a major area of research.

Today, free-running rhythms are used to study the phase response characteristics of the circadian clock. By pulsing an animal in temporal isolation with light or other zeitgebers at times in the circadian cycle relative to the free-running rhythm and measuring the resulting phase of the rhythm one can determine a "resetting curve" for the circadian clock. Such curves are very useful for comparing rhythms between and within species. Additionally, by measuring the phase response curves produced by drugs that selectively perturb specific cellular functions (such as RNA transcription or protein synthesis) researchers can gain insight into the molecular mechanisms underlying circadian timekeeping. (See also PHASE RESPONSE CURVE.)

Russell N. Van Gelder

FREUD'S DREAM THEORY

It is generally unrecognized that Sigmund Freud's contribution to the scientific understanding of dreams derived from a radical reorientation to the dream experience. During the nineteenth century, before publication of *The Interpretation of Dreams,* the presence of dreaming was considered by the scientific community as a manifestation of mental activity during sleep. The state of sleep was given prominence as a factor accounting for the seeming lack of organization and meaning to the dream experience. Thus, the assumed relatively nonpsychological sleep state set the scientific stage for viewing the nature of the dream. Freud radically shifted the context. He recognized—as myth, folklore, and common sense had long understood—that dreams were also linked with the psychology of waking life. This shift in orientation has proved essential for our modern view of dreams and dreaming. Dreams are no longer dismissed as senseless notes hit at random on a piano keyboard by an untrained player. Dreams are now recognized as psychologically significant and meaningful expressions of the life of the dreamer, albeit expressed in disguised and concealed forms. (For a contrasting view, see ACTIVATION–SYNTHESIS HYPOTHESIS.)

Contemporary Dream Research

During the past quarter-century, there has been increasing scientific interest in the process of dreaming. A regular sleep–wakefulness cycle has been discovered, and if experimental subjects are awakened during periods of rapid eye movements (REM periods), they will frequently report dreams. In a typical night, four or five dreams occur during REM periods, accompanied by other signs of physiological activation, such as increased respiratory rate, heart rate, and penile and clitoral erection. Dreams usually last for the duration of the eye movements, from about 10 to 25 minutes. Although dreaming usually occurs in such regular cycles, dreaming may occur at other times during sleep, as well as during hypnagogic (falling asleep) or hypnopompic (waking up) states, when REMs are not present.

The above findings are discoveries made since the monumental work of Freud reported in *The Interpretation of Dreams,* and although of great interest to the study of the mind–body problem, these findings as yet bear only a peripheral relationship to the central concerns of the psychology of dream formation, the meaning of dream content, the dream as an approach to a deeper understanding of emotional life, and the use of the dream in psychoanalytic treatment.

Rudiments of the Dream

In his initial psychological work, Freud was led to the dream via his interest in neurotic symptoms. In his attempt to understand the meaning of symptoms, he asked his patients to associate freely, and in doing so they began to report dreams. He then treated the dream much like a symptom, amenable to the formation of associational links and susceptible to interpretation. Freud asked patients to report freely what came to mind in response to specific elements of the dream. The method of free association required the curtailment of the mind's tendency to judge, evaluate, and criticize, and thus block the natural flow of association.

This method, which is also the method used by the patient in revealing his thoughts and feelings in psychoanalytic psychotherapy, led Freud to clarify the meaning of the dream. The dream as reported is called the *manifest dream* and is the dream as consciously perceived and subsequently remembered. Freud discovered that behind the manifest dream could be uncovered a number of *latent* thoughts, and these thoughts were transformed by a process of dream work into the manifest dream. When the manifest dream was analyzed by the method of free association, the dream representation could be understood as an attempt at the fulfillment of wishes of which the dreamer was not consciously aware.

On the surface, such a proposition seemed even more radical than the view that the seemingly senseless and chaotic dream is an understandable part of psychological life; however, Freud presented evidence to support such a proposition. To support the *wish-fulfillment* theory, for example, one can point to the small number of dreams that are clearly wish-fulfilling even in their manifest content. Explorers deprived of food and drink dream of huge banquets and luscious, clear, thirst-quenching mountain streams. Also, some children's dreams are manifestly wish-fulfilling. A medical student who must report to the hospital early in the morning to make rounds dreams of lying in a hospital bed, and continues to sleep, comforted in the thought that she is already in the hospital. Such a dream is called a *dream of convenience*. The wish fulfilled is the universal desire to continue to sleep.

Such easily decipherable dreams are the exception, however; most dreams do not readily present wishes as fulfilled in the manifest content. Instead, the manifest dream is the end product of a process of disguise and distortion. To account for the masking of the wish, it is necessary to understand that the difficulty the dreamer experiences in recognizing his or her wishes is explained by the fact that the wishes that underlie the dream are unacceptable to the dreamer's *ego*. The wishes are objectionable on moral grounds or unacceptable because they lower self-esteem or produce anxiety, guilt, shame, disgust, or embarrassment. Thus, the wishes are unconscious, and the thoughts and feelings connected with such wishes are subjected to a *censorship* that interferes with ready access to conscious awareness. Many dreams that occur during a night's sleep are forgotten and fade away with awakening. The dream censorship also affects the retention of dream content. Thus, one may forget a dream because of the presence of a repressive force. Other similar defensive forces use a variety of psychological techniques to distort the representations of clear wish fulfillment. As an example of distortion, an unconscious hostile wish directed toward a loved one on the previous day may be presented in a dream by the dreamer's attempt to rescue the loved one from a dangerous and painful situation invented by the dream representation.

Psychoanalysis is interested in the varied sources involved in the formation of a dream. If we simply examine the dream on a manifest level, the dream is made of a large number of elements. The images of the dream may consist of previously experienced real events, waking thoughts, feelings, and ideas. Body sensations, memories from the previous day, or memories of experiences from the distant and even infantile past may find a place in the manifest dream. The immediate source for the dream is some psychological remnant, such as a longing, worry, or concern—some incomplete task from the previous day that has not been resolved and put to rest. In *The Interpretation of Dreams*, Freud offers several examples of such *day residues* that serve as precipitants to the imagery of the dream. Freud had a dream of turning over a colored picture of a plant in a monograph he had written. The imme-

diate source of this dream was the sight of a new book about the plant, which he had seen the previous day. The dream was also instigated by a conversation Freud had on the previous day with a man on a topic related to the book he saw. The second instigator, the conversation, was much more emotionally meaningful to Freud than the sight of the book in the window. It is common for dreams to use indifferent recent memories to conceal other situations that stir emotion and conflict. It is also common for the thoughts about the current life of the dreams to evoke related memories from the past with which the immediate experiences resonate.

The Dream Work

The latent dream thoughts, stirred by the day residues, seek some form of expression. The vehicle for this expression, the means by which the latent dream thoughts are transformed into manifest dream content, is known as the *dream work*. Before embarking on a description of dream work, one should point out that the latent dream thoughts, when they are revealed through dream interpretation, follow the ordinary laws of logic and everyday speech. Latent dream thoughts are understandable as forms of expression in the optative mood; that is, "if only it were true that . . . ," "given such and such a condition, I would wish that . . . ," and other such ordinary means of expressing a desire.

The dream work is the vehicle and language available to the dreamer for expressing thought. The language resembles a rebus or pictographic puzzle more than a written language, in which words bear a clear symbolic relation to a referent. The mechanisms of dream work: *condensation, displacement, plastic representation,* and *secondary revision* (also known in older psychoanalytic literature as secondary elaboration). The first three mechanisms are archaic, prelogical modes of thinking. The last, secondary revision, is a component of rational, logical thought.

Condensation refers to the tendency to combine a number of latent dream thoughts into a more succinct element. Thus, in Freud's well-known dream of Irma's injection, which he discussed at length in the second chapter of *The Interpretation of Dreams,* the figure of Irma in the manifest content stands for at least seven women including herself. Thus, a number of latent thoughts about women are condensed into a single manifest element. Displacement is a mechanism that allows the dreamer to shift the emotional intensity from one dream thought to another. Freud maintained that there is never any doubt about the psychological value of the latent dream thoughts. We know their value on the basis of our direct judgment, our shared humanity, empathy, and introspection. In the formation of the dream, however, the accent is shifted, the psychologically important is treated casually, and the seemingly innocuous in the manifest content may stand for the emotionally intense. Displacement is facilitated by the dream censorship, resistance, and defensive needs to conceal conflicted thoughts from the dreamer's ego. Freud was fond of illustrating the concept of dream displacement by the tale of a town in which a tailor had committed a crime punishable by execution. As the town had only one tailor but had three butchers, it was decided to execute a butcher instead.

The contents of the latent dream thoughts are also revealed through the processes used in constructing the dream. As primary process mechanisms are inadequate to express relations between dream thoughts, they may be expressed in the formal means available to the dreamer. Thus, a close connection between two events or people may be expressed by their occurrence simultaneity in time or by juxtaposing figures side-by-side in the manifest dream. Furthermore, causal relation in latent thought may be represented by a short dream sequence that introduces another dream. A contradiction may be expressed by a reversal. Various qualities about the dreamer's perception of the dream may represent components of the latent dream thoughts. Thus, the sensory quality of the dream may stand for ideas about clarity or vagueness, which are components of the latent dream thoughts. For example, a patient has a "vague" dream that expresses his view of the psychotherapist's interpretation of the previous day; it, too, was vague.

The dream work may also make use of a universal tendency to depict a psychologically important person, body part, or experience by a repertoire of common *symbols*. A father or the analyst may be represented by a king or president, a penis by a knife, a vagina by a cave, birth by water. These symbols, however, are traps for the unwary. In the absence of confirming associa-

tions, the psychotherapist will not be taken in by the facile glibness such symbols offer, but will explore their meaning via associations from the patient.

The third mechanism of the dream work is the capacity to form plastic representations of the dream thoughts. The dreamer tends to form visual images rather than to express formal relations among thoughts in conceptual terms. Occasionally, the images are in other sensory modalities besides the visual; auditory, kinesthetic, and olfactory are also used. Some dreams may lack all sensory qualities and be present only as thoughts, isolated ideas, feeling states, or single words.

The fourth factor responsible for the work of constructing a dream is secondary revision. This mechanism strives to make the confusion and seeming chaos of dream images and thoughts coherent and intelligible. The organized narrative and storylike quality of the dream is attributable to this factor. Occasionally, the dreamer will fit the dream contents to an available daydream from waking life, much as a Renaissance painter may choose to express personal infantile wishes for maternal care by making use of conventional Nativity iconography.

The dream work is the manner by which a dream is created; dream analysis and interpretation are the techniques by which the meaning is revealed.

Harry Trosman

FUNCTIONS OF DREAMS

The functions of dreams constitute their psychologic purpose—the answer to the question, "What good are they?" Many functions have been proposed but only a few have any scientific support. The most famous of these are the functions offered by Freud in his landmark book *The Interpretation of Dreams* (1955). The one that became best known was his proposal that dreams act as a safety valve for the expression of forbidden impulses. Dreams, according to Freud, allow us to gratify in fantasy our sexual and aggressive impulses that are not permitted to us in waking behavior. In this way they drain off the possibility of our getting into trouble. Another dream function Freud proposed was that dreams protect our sleep. While we pay attention to the dream we do not heed other stimuli that might rob us of our rest.

Later, Freud (1920) added a third function that helps account for bad dreams. These, he said, are attempts to master events we could not cope with when they occurred. By repeating them in dreams, we attempt to bring under control the anxiety we felt at the time of some real-life upsetting event. In this way, dreams are a kind of internal coping mechanism. It is this last function that has been taken up by some more modern writers and researchers who see the purpose of dreams as a way to work on emotional problems, both personal and interpersonal (French & Fromm, 1964; Erikson, 1954; Jones, 1970). One test of this proposal was carried out by Breger, Hunter, and Lane (1971), who studied the dreams of people before and after surgery. The patients dreamed of surgery and its possible consequences beforehand, but did not after it was over. Dreams seemed to help them cope with the anxiety that surgery brings. (See also FREUD'S DREAM THEORY.)

Alfred Adler (1936) proposed that dreaming was a kind of thinking ahead to prepare the feelings we need in order to act courageously the next day to work out our life plan. If not for our dreams, we might remain lazily in bed. The purpose of dreams is to stir up our feelings, Adler said. (See also ADLER'S DREAM THEORY.)

Kramer and Roth (1973) carried out research to test whether dreams in fact change our feelings from night to morning. They argued that, if feelings change, the content of what we dream should be related in some way. They found that a reduction in the amount of unhappiness from before sleep to the morning was related to the number of characters included in the intervening dreams. The more people we dreamed about, the less unhappy we are when we wake up.

Another point of view on the functions of dreams was developed by Carl Jung (1974), who theorized that dreams compensate for personality distortions in the waking state. Dreams help us to keep our psychologic balance by reminding us of important parts of our personality we do not adequately express in waking life; they regulate inner harmony. When we are out of harmony, they give evidence of what needs to be corrected. This theory suggests that persons with good balance in waking will have dreams that are like their waking thoughts, but persons who suppress important feelings like anger or sex or power

drives, will have dreams that express these feelings. The hen-pecked husband who dreams of breaking free of his wife would be an example. Although there has not been a good test of this theory as yet, Jung opened up the thinking about dreams by challenging Freud's belief that all dreams relate to early childhood wishes. (See also JUNG'S DREAM THEORY.)

Other views on the function of dreams make use of modern computer models and speak of the information-processing function of dreams (Dewan, 1970). This view has been elaborated by Breger (1967) in a way that links this thinking to Freud's insights into the importance of the early emotional elements stored in memory. Thus, such early memories continue to be available throughout our life in dreams. Dreams make use of the early memories, not as they were originally experienced, but reconstructed and linked to the present day's experience by way of the emotional significance of this experience to us. This explains why you might dream of a house you once lived in, a long dead relative, or a schoolmate mixed in with present-day images. The particular memory bits that come back in our dreams are not accidental; they are emotionally related to some presleep events that trigger their retrieval in sleep. Any emotion can do it—not just the pleasure of expressing repressed wishes. According to Breger, the purpose of this dream system is to relate our present "hot" issues to older solutions of similar emotion-provoking problems from the past. These blends of old and new memories are displayed in our dreams. This thinking suggests that experiencing some emotional event, such as a divorce, will invoke in dreams memories of earlier loss experiences, such as the death of a friend or parent. These dreams will illustrate earlier solutions to problems with the same feelings.

Quite a different function of dreams has been suggested to account for why we remember so few of them. Evans and Newman (1964) proposed that dreams serve as a filter of the day's experiences, reviewing and rejecting the redundant or unimportant information unworthy of being stored permanently in memory. Dreams display these odd bits, and this is why they are difficult both to remember and to understand. This suggestion was more recently revived by Crick and Mitchison (1983), who summarized their hypothesis as "we dream in order to forget," that is, dreams represent a reverse learning process.

Their idea is that the brain needs some way to eliminate information it does not need to keep and the dream was evolved to do this. This raises an important question: Who decides? Often in waking we throw something out only to find out we need it later. Is it likely that dreams can make such important decisions about what should be preserved in memory?

Whatever the function of dreams, one way to go about discovering what this might be is to eliminate them experimentally and see what happens. Such experiments have been done in many ways by many people with mixed results.

In the first place it is hard to do. Humans struggle to maintain their dreams. When they are awakened at the beginning of each REM sleep period, some subjects begin to dream again more quickly (Dement, 1960; Cartwright and Monroe, 1968; Cartwright, Monroe, and Palmer, 1967), and some begin to experience dreams in other sleep states. Whether this happens depends on what state the experimenter allows to occupy the subjects' time instead of dreaming. If the subjects are allowed to express fantasy at the time they are awakened, they don't seem to be as affected by the dream loss as when they are forced instead to do mathematical problems.

Moreover, it is not only the type of task taking the place of dreaming that produces varied effects, but also the nature of the people involved. After REM deprivation of a few nights, some people become a little more free to express their impulses the next day. At worst, some experience transitory episodes of paranoid thinking and impulses to act out (Dement, 1960). At best there are reports that a few become more creative in their waking writing and painting, less conventional and more expressive. Some people have strict controls on their fantasy behaviors; they are practical all day and only indulge in creative imagery in dreams. These persons seem to be more affected by dream loss than those who are in better touch with their feelings and fantasies in waking. The latter show less effect from dream deprivation (see also DEPRIVATION, SELECTIVE).

One group clearly appears to profit from dream deprivation: those who are chronically depressed. Vogel et al. (1980) demonstrated that many patients who experience low mood, low sex drive, less interest in other people and in food, and take no pleasure in things that used to delight them can show a reversal of these symptoms after 3 weeks of REM sleep deprivation.

Dreams of depressed people have the characteristic of being more self-blaming (Beck and Ward, 1961). When these dreams are experimentally suppressed, patients become more outgoing, energetic, and engaged with others; their mood becomes less unhappy. If Freud is right that dreams are a safety-valve to allow the safe expression of infantile wishes, they do not seem to carry out this function in the depressed. The dreams of depressed patients do not give them much pleasure.

Once we understand the function of dreams more fully, we will be in a better position to make repairs to the system when it seems not to be working well. Current research on this question is being done in persons who are depressed while going through divorce (Cartwright, 1991). It appears that those who include the missing spouse in their dreams and deal overtly with the divorce are more likely to get over their depression and make a better waking adjustment than those who do not. Dreams appear to carry forward emotional work in some people under some circumstances. Much work is still needed to improve our understanding of the dream function or functions, as well as their malfunctioning.

REFERENCES

Adler A. 1936. On the interpretation of dreams. *Int J Individual-Psychology* 1:3–16.

Beck A, Ward C. 1961. Dreams of depressed patients: Characteristic themes in manifest content. *Arch Gen Psychiatry* 5:462–467.

Breger L. 1967. Function of dreams. *J Abnormal Psych Monograph* 72(5), whole no. 641.

Breger L, Hunter I, Lane R. 1971. The effects of stress on dreams. *Psychol Issues* 7:Monograph 27.

Cartwright R. 1991. Dreams that work: The relation of dream incorporation to adaptation to stressful events. *Dreaming* 1:3–9.

Cartwright R., Monroe L. 1968. The relation of dreaming and REM sleep: The effects of REM deprivation under two conditions. *J Pers Soc Psychol* 10:69–74.

Cartwright R, Monroe L, Palmer C. 1967. Individual differences in response of REM deprivation. *Arch Gen Psychiatry* 16:297–303.

Crick F, Mitchison G. 1983. The function of dream sleep. *Nature* 304:111–114.

Dement W. 1960. The effect of dream deprivation. *Science* 131:1705.

Dewan E. 1970. The programing (P) hypothesis for

REMs. In E. Hartmann E, ed. *Sleep and dreaming,* pp 295–307. Boston: Little, Brown.

Erikson E. 1954. The dream specimen of psychoanalysis. *J Am Psychoanal Assoc* 2:5–55.

Evans C, Newman E. 1964. Dreaming: An analogy from computers. *New Sci* 419:577–579.

French T, Fromm E. 1964. *Dream interpretation.* New York: Basic Books.

Freud S. 1953. Beyond the pleasure principle (1920). In *Standard Edition of the Complete Works of Sigmund Freud,* 18, pp 7–64. London: Hogarth Press.

————. 1955. *The interpretation of dreams.* New York: Basic Books.

Jones R. 1970. *The new psychology of dreaming.* New York: Grune and Stratton.

Jung C. *Dreams.* 1974. Princeton, N.J.: Princeton University Press.

Kramer M, Roth T. 1973. The mood regulating function of sleep. In Koella W, ed. *Sleep,* pp 563–761. Basel: S. Karger.

Vogel G, Vogel F, McAbee R, Thurmond A. 1980. Improvement of depression by REM sleep deprivation. *Arch Gen Psychiatry* 37:247–253.

Rosalind D. Cartwright

FUNCTIONS OF SLEEP

Before the functions of sleep are discussed, it is best to indicate how we are using the term *function,* since it has many meanings. We are concerned with function in the sense of that for which a phenomenon exists, that is, its purpose. In short, why do we sleep?

When we try to answer such questions, we typically seek the effect or effects accomplished. For example, the purpose of a chair is to sit upon it; the purpose of the heart is to pump blood. We should, however, notice several aspects of this approach. First, a thing, organ, or activity may have a range of effects that vary from vital to trivial to unfortunate. A nose permits access to oxygen and a sensitivity to odors. It also furnishes a place for glasses and may enhance or spoil attractiveness. The sexual act is vital for reproduction, but it may also serve in mate bonding or as a pleasure. Also, a purpose may be simply a link in a complex chain of events. For example, the pumping of the heart is one vital aspect of the cardiovascular system, and the carburetor is one aspect of the gasoline engine. Frequently, various ways are available to accomplish the same effect.

Thus, a functional analysis must ask as specifically as possible about the particular and unique functions a phenomenon efficiently performs to accomplish necessary effects. We can tighten this analysis by asking, If the system failed to function, would it make a difference? In our particular case, we want to ask, What effects does sleep efficiently accomplish; further, if it did not accomplish these effects, would it make a difference?

The search for the purpose of sleep has a long history. One of the earliest answers was that given by Aristotle, who observed: "Every creature is endowed by nature with the power to move, but cannot move itself always and continuously, rest [sleep] is necessary and beneficial . . ." (1931, p. 454). Aristotle specifically described sleep as "an inhibition of function . . . imposed on sense perception" during which "the nutrient part does its own work better" (1931, p. 455). Simply, we become tired during wakefulness and recover during sleep.

More than 2,000 years later, in 1965, one of the great pioneers in sleep research, W. R. Hess, reiterated this position in more modern language: "Physical and mental fatigue automatically makes itself felt [as] a signal that performance . . . is no longer up to external demands. . . . The effects of involuntary rest during sleep . . . can be none other than that restorative processes have been in play . . ." (p. 5).

This dominant position holds that the purpose of sleep is to restore the organism's capacity to be awake. This has been labeled the *restorative* model (see also FATIGUE-RECOVERY MODEL).

Some variations on this model have been proposed. Claparede, early in this century, focused on the preventive role of sleep rather than its restorative function (Webb, 1983). He asserted that we sleep in order to prevent ourselves from becoming exhausted. Similarly, the Russian physiologist Pavlov conceived of sleep as an evoked "cortical inhibition" that protected the organism from excessive and conflictual stimulation (although he did not deny the restorative aspect).

In more recent times, an alternative or additional role of sleep has been proposed by Zepelin and Rechtschaffen (1974), who noted that the total sleep amounts of different animals range from 3 or 4 to as many as 18 of every 24 hours. These amounts show a strong relationship to body weight; smaller animals tend to sleep more than larger animals. Smaller animals also have higher rates of metabolism, which are related to higher energy-level requirements. This relationship suggests that higher sleep amounts may serve the purpose of energy conservation.

In the 1970s, a distinct alternative to the restorative model emerged, called the *adaptive* model (Meddis, 1977; Webb, 1974, 1975). A review of sleep patterns of animals indicated that—rather than being dangerous—sleep was adaptively related to the foraging, predatory relations, and physiological capacities of each species. For example, grazing animals tended to sleep for only a few hours in short episodes, which reflected grazing herd behavior and predator pressures. Hunting animals, such as large felines, on the other hand, showed variable highly flexible sleep patterns. Small burrowing animals with high predator pressures had higher total sleep. These data led to the proposal that sleep in each species was an evolved adaptive form of behavior serving the purpose of enhancing survival. From this perspective, the purpose of sleep was to aid the survival of the animal in relationship to environmental pressures.

Separately, the restorative and the adaptive concepts each fit some of the facts of sleep very well. The restorative model accounts for the results of sleep deprivation; not getting sleep makes us sleepy, and getting sleep helps us to recover. On the other hand, the adaptive model neatly handles the wide range of animal sleep and recognizes the crucial role of the timing of sleep.

Both theories have their limitations. A reasonable restorative model predicts that a linear increase in sleepiness and length of recovery sleep will occur as some direct function of length of wakefulness. However, sleepiness does not increase linearly. Many animals require 20 hours to recover from 4 hours of wakefulness, while others require 4 hours of sleep in relation to 20 hours' wakefulness. Moreover, the restorative model cannot be fitted to the problems we see in humans as a result of SHIFTWORK and JET LAG. On the other hand, the adaptive theories tend to ignore the importance of sleep deprivation and apparent recovery effects.

Both theories also had real difficulties in defining underlying mechanisms. The restorative models, in spite of intensive searches, have not been supported by any evidence of a physiological substance or condition that shows a systematic increase (or decrease) in waking and a reversal in sleep. The adaptive model initially leaned heavily on the concept of "instincts"; however, the evidence of sleep as a biological rhythm has tended to furnish a reasonable mechanism for the adaptive model (see BIOLOGICAL RHYTHMS).

In the 1980s, the two positions, restorative and adaptive, were sensibly combined in a two-factor model (Borbely, 1982; Daan, Beersma, and Borbely, 1984). In this model, sleep has a need/restorative component (restorative) and a biological-rhythm timing component (adaptive). This model has since been extended into a three-factor model, which also emphasizes the behavioral control of sleep (Webb, 1988).

Let us now return to our initial question. What is the purpose (or purposes) of sleep? We have interpreted this question to mean, What does sleep efficiently accomplish and, if it did not, would it make a difference?

Our review of attempts to answer this question indicates that there is certainly a need to stop being awake. If we continue awake, we become sleepier and sleepier and less and less capable of performing efficiently; if this wakeful period is extended, the organism will die. This limitation on wakefulness is species-specific; that is, different species have different limitations on wakefulness time (see DEPRIVATION, TOTAL).

We do not know the physiological or neurophysiological basis of this vital need for sleep. The preponderance of evidence indicates that this need is simply a function of waking time. Activities within a given time interval tend to have little effect on the length of wakefulness; indeed, decreased activity tends to increase the probability of sleep onset.

This need or demand for sleep that accumulates with prolonged wakefulness is offset by the well-defined process of sleep. While we can describe the process, again we do not know the physiological or neurophysiological nature of the recovery. The amount of time associated with recovery is also species-specific and appears to be primarily related to length of wake time per se.

Research on the effects of sleep loss (see DEPRIVATION) and our common-sense evidence attest to the necessity of sleep for maintenance of wakeful functioning. There is also evidence that this function is efficiently accomplished. Earlier notions held that sleep was a dangerous condition that provided restoration at risk of the organism's state of vulnerability. Quite to the contrary, biological rhythm research has established that sleep is an endogenously timed event. The adaptive theory of sleep function maintains that the timing of sleep within each day occurs at a phase most appropriate for the survival of a particular species. Indeed, this position asserts that sleep may serve the additional purpose of effectively relating the organism's behavior to its environment with respect to foraging, predator pressure, and physiological limitations.

Moreover, the sleep process itself is directed toward efficiently maintaining itself. Thus, the arousal threshold to external stimulation is markedly increased to reduce the probability of awakening (see DEPTH OF SLEEP). The sleep period tends to be self maintaining, such that in the absence of danger or interference, sleep resumes after awakenings.

The extension of the two-factor model (restoration and timing) to include a behavioral component points to an additional efficiency of the sleep system. With the inclusion of this component, the model permits sleep a necessary flexibility within broad limits. Thus, in relation to environmental and psychological demands, wakefulness may be extended, the placement of sleep may be modified, and sleep may be terminated. Within limits, therefore, the organism can extend waking time for pleasure or protection, can undertake shift work or adjust to jet travel, can respond to dangers from within sleep, and can answer an alarm to get to work.

Why do we sleep? Sleep is a natural endowment that terminates extended wakefulness and, with its occurrence, permits a return to effective wakefulness. This process is accomplished with maximum efficiency; it requires no learning or effort; it is regularly timed; and this timing may serve additional functions in aid of survival. Sleep is flexible, within limits, to permit adjustments to environmental demands.

REFERENCES

Aristotle. 1931. *The works of Aristotle,* Ross WD, ed. Oxford: Clarendon Press.

Borbely AA. 1982. A two process model of sleep regulation. *Human Neurobiol* 1:195–204.

Daan S, Beersma SGD, Borbely AA. 1984. Timing of human sleep: Recovery process gated by a circadian pacemaker. *Am J Physiol* 246:R161–178.

Hess WR. 1965. Sleep as phenomenon of the integral organism. In Akert K, Bally C, Schade JP, eds. *Sleep mechanisms.* New York: Elsevier.

Meddis R. 1977. *The sleep instinct.* London: Routledge & Kegan Paul.

Webb WB. 1974. Sleep as an adaptive response. *Percept Motor Skills* 38:1023–1027.

_____. 1975. The adaptive functions of sleep. In Levin P, Koella WP, eds. *Sleep 1974,* pp 13–19. Basel: Karger.

_____. 1983. Theories in modern sleep research. In Mayes A, ed. *Sleep mechanisms and functions.* London: Van Nostrand Reinhold.

_____. 1988. An objective behavioral model of sleep. *Sleep* 11:488–496.

Zepelin H, Rechtschaffen A. 1974. Mammalian sleep, longevity, and energy metabolism. *Brain Behavior Evol* 10:425–470.

Wilse B. Webb

G

GALVANIC SKIN RESPONSE

Galvanic skin response (GSR) is a classic method for measuring the electrical activity of the skin. Electrical activity of the skin varies as a function of the degree of sweating. Sweating, in turn, is controlled by the sympathetic branch of the autonomic nervous system (ANS) (see AUTONOMIC NERVOUS SYSTEM; SYMPATHETIC NERVOUS SYSTEM). Autonomic control of sweating is unusual in that this is the only part of the ANS where the neurotransmitter at the end of the pathway is acetylcholine and not noradrenaline. Stimulation of ANS results in increased sweating in the eccrine glands of the skin.

Although well known, the term *galvanic skin response* is no longer in common use because it has been defined in a variety of ways. In current usage, the measure is more frequently called a skin resistance response (SRR) or a skin conductance response (SCR). Originally, GSR referred to the technique whereby a small electrical current is passed through the skin between two electrodes. The amount of sweat present determines the level of resistance or conductance of the electrical current between the electrodes. GSR equipment determines the level of the response in millivolts and other electrical measurement units. Increased GSR is defined as corresponding to decreased resistance or increased conductance, which accompanies an increase in sweating.

Galvanic skin response studies in sleep have shown a reliable pattern of increasing responses during NREM sleep, with the maximum number of responses occurring in stage 4 sleep (Johnson and Lubin, 1966). Galvanic skin response is reported to be essentially absent during REM sleep, occurring only during phasic bursts of rapid eye movements (Broughton, Poire, and Tassinari, 1965). The high frequency of GSRs during deep NREM sleep has been described as "GSR storm" and may be associated with night sweats that occur primarily during deep NREM sleep (McDonald et al., 1976; see also NIGHT SWEATS). Several early reports also suggested that a higher level of GSR activity during sleep was related to increased presleep levels of arousal, emotion, or anxiety (see ELECTRODERMAL ACTIVITY).

REFERENCES

Broughton RJ, Poire R, Tassinari CA. 1965. The electrodermogram (Tachanoff effect) during sleep. *Electroencephalogr Clin Neurophysiol* 18: 691–708.

Johnson LC, Lubin A. 1966. Spontaneous electrodermal activity during waking and sleeping. *Psychophysiology* 3(1):8–17.

McDonald DG, Shallenberger HD, Keosko RK, Kinney BG. 1976. Studies of spontaneous electrodermal responses in sleep. *Psychophysiology* 13:128–134.

Prokasy WF, Raskin DC. 1973. *Electrodermal activity in psychological research.* New York: Academic.

Mark R. Pressman

GAMMA-AMINOBUTYRIC ACID (GABA)

See Benzodiazepines; Chemistry of Sleep: Amines and Other Transmitters

260

GARDNER, RANDY

Randy Gardner is considered to be one of the folk heroes of modern sleep research. In a field in which most research subjects remain anonymous, Randy Gardner is well known for staying awake for 264 hours—11 straight days without sleep. This experiment began as the 17-year-old high-school student's research project for the 1964 Greater San Diego Science Fair; however, his vigil was of considerable interest to sleep researchers and provided important data about prolonged sleep loss in the human being.

Randy Gardner started his vigil at 6 A.M. on December 28, 1963, and stayed awake without the use of any drugs or caffeinated beverages until a few minutes after 6 A.M. on January 8, 1964. He broke the previous world's record for continuous wakefulness. Randy was observed at all times by at least one of two high-school friends who acted as his co-investigators, helped him to remain awake, and collected temperature and other data from him every 6 hours. When sleep researchers became aware of Randy's success in staying awake, they immediately made plans to study him. William C. Dement and George Gulevich came from Stanford to San Diego to join Laverne C. Johnson at the Navy's Neuropsychiatric Research Unit at Naval Hospital to perform awake and sleep electroencephalographic, autonomic, and psychological studies.

Randy found that it was most difficult to stay awake during the very early morning hours. He experienced overwhelming fatigue at times and gave up watching television on the second day because his eyes burned and it was difficult for him to focus his gaze. As the vigil progressed, he became irritable, developed memory lapses, and was nauseated. At 3 A.M. on the fourth day without sleep, Randy responded to a street sign as though it were a person. Later, he imagined himself to be a famous football player. On the fourth and fifth days, Randy began to have microsleeps, in which dreamlike thoughts occurred and during which he was unresponsive to the environment for very brief periods. His speech became noticeably slurred on the seventh day. He also developed ptosis (drooping of the eyelids), finger tremor, and hyperactive reflexes. It was also found that Randy's electroencephalogram (EEG) no longer showed alpha activity near the end of his vigil. Although Randy experienced considerable changes in mood, ability to concentrate, and mild hallucinations and delusions, he did not become psychotic as a result of this long period of sleeplessness, as some people feared that he would. (See also SLEEPINESS.)

Of considerable interest to sleep researchers was the nature of Randy's recovery sleep. The first three recovery sleep periods, as well as follow-up sleep at 1 week, 6 weeks, and 7 months, were recorded in the sleep laboratory of the Neuropsychiatric Research Unit. Randy wore electroencephalographic and other recording electrodes so that precise measurements of his sleep, waking, and other physiological functions could be made. In the first recovery sleep recorded on January 8, 1964, Randy went to bed at 6 A.M. and took 2 minutes to fall asleep. He slept for 14 hours, 40 minutes and arose from bed at approximately 8:45 P.M. After this first recovery sleep, Randy's fatigue, irritability, and neurological symptoms generally disappeared. In addition, alpha activity reappeared in his waking EEG. He then stayed awake nearly 23 hours to go to bed at a more regular bedtime—8 P.M. on January 9—and slept for 10 hours, 25 minutes. On the third recovery night, his bedtime was 9 P.M., and he slept for 9 hours, 3 minutes. On all three recovery nights, both his percentage of slow-wave sleep and REM sleep were substantially elevated. One week later, Randy's total sleep time and sleep stage percentages had returned to normal levels.

At the time of Randy's vigil, sleep researchers knew very little about the effects of severe sleep deprivation, and many believed that psychosis would be the result. Randy's experience showed that it was possible for a healthy individual to go without sleep for long periods of time without becoming psychotic. In addition, the data collected from Randy showed that there were many psychological, behavioral, and physiological changes associated with prolonged sleep loss, but that these changes were readily reversible by recovery sleep.

Randy Gardner is married, lives in the San Diego area, is still interested in sleep research, and reports that he sleeps very well.

(See also DEPRIVATION.)

REFERENCES

Gulevich G, Dement W, Johnson L. 1966. Psychiatric and EEG observations on a case of prolonged (264

hours) wakefulness. *Arch Gen Psychiatry* 15:
29–35.

Johnson LC, Slye ES, Dement W. 1965. Electroencephalographic and autonomic activity during and after prolonged sleep deprivation. *Psychosom Med* 27:415–423.

Ross JJ. 1965. Neurological findings after prolonged sleep deprivation. *Arch Neurol* 12:399–403.

Cheryl L. Spinweber

GASTROESOPHAGEAL REFLUX

See Heartburn

GENETICS OF SLEEP

Although specific genes that influence sleep have not yet been identified, it is clear that sleep patterns are heritable. Species-specific sleep patterns have been documented in birds and mammals and are relatively stable characteristics both across species and among individuals within a species. Although environmental factors can have significant acute effects on sleep, there is little evidence that they induce permanent changes in sleep requirements or patterns.

Heritability of sleep patterns has been studied most extensively using inbred strains of rodents. Strain-specific differences in total sleep, total REM SLEEP, and circadian parameters of sleep have been documented in rats and mice. Results of cross-breeding studies by Friedmann (1974) showed that amount of REM sleep, amount of SLOW-WAVE SLEEP, and CIRCADIAN RHYTHMS could be inherited independently, suggesting that they are controlled by different sets of genes. Attempts to determine the genetic mechanisms for inheritance of specific traits have shown that total daily sleep, slow-wave sleep, REM sleep, and circadian rhythms were transmitted additively; that is, each parental strain influenced the sleep characteristics in the offspring, with some parental strains increasing and others decreasing the amounts of the particular sleep characteristics. In some cases, dominant transmission of a given sleep characteristic has also been observed; that is, the offspring's sleep behavior closely resembled that in one of the parent strains. No sex-linked factors have been identified for any sleep parameters in the rodent studies.

It has also been possible to breed rodents selectively for specific sleep characteristics. The Flinders Sensitive Line of rats, which were bred to have increased numbers of receptors in the brain for the neurotransmitter acetylcholine (see CHEMISTRY OF SLEEP), show elevated REM sleep percentage of total sleep, reduced REM latency, and reduced REM–NREM cycle length. A single-gene, spontaneous mutation has been identified that leads to shortening of the circadian period in hamsters; the trait is inherited in a dominant manner (Ralph et al., 1990). Finally, inbred lines of mice have been established that exhibit short or long sleep times in response to ethanol and other hypnotic agents.

Association of normal sleep behaviors with particular chromosomal expression has also been best studied in rodents. Valatx (1984) has shown that the sleep pattern of an albino strain of mice is expressed in association with the transmission of albinism in breeding studies with nonalbino strains. The specific gene for albinism alone does not appear to control sleep, however, since black mice with a spontaneous mutation for albinism did not exhibit the sleep pattern of the albino strain. The association of sleep patterns with the genes coding for transplantation antigens (the histocompatibility complex) has also been studied in mice. The results suggest that amounts of slow-wave sleep and REM sleep may be related to histocompatibility genes, but that genes in other chromosomes also must affect slow-wave and REM sleep patterns.

Heritability of sleep patterns is evident in human studies as well. According to large-scale studies by Partinen et al. (1983) and Heath et al. (1990) of self-reported sleep behavior in adult twins, sleep patterns, including bedtime, length of sleep, and sleep quality, show greater concordance in identical (monozygotic) than in fraternal (dizygotic) twins. In addition, a study by Webb and Campbell (1983) of polysomnographically recorded sleep in young adult twin pairs showed significant correlation of sleep efficiency, total sleep time, and REM amount in monozygotic but *not* dizygotic twins. Although twin studies suggest that there is a heritable component of sleep behavior, it is also apparent that acute effects of environment on sleep are stronger than genetic factors.

Sleep disturbance is also strongly correlated with psychiatric disorders, which themselves appear to be regulated significantly by genetic factors. In at least one of the twin studies described above, genetic influences on sleep were distinguished from influences affecting psychiatric symptoms; however, other evidence has suggested that sleep patterns and susceptibility to psychiatric illness may be linked (Giles et al., 1989; Sitaram et al., 1987). Two sleep parameters that have been studied in depressed individuals and their immediate families are REM latency (which is often reduced in depression) and the triggering of REM sleep with drugs that affect acetylcholine receptors in the brain, referred to as the *cholinergic REM induction test*. REM latencies tended to be similar in family members with major DEPRESSION. Similarly, depressed individuals and their relatives with major depression showed more rapid onset of REM sleep in response to the cholinergic REM sleep induction test. It is not yet clear whether reduced REM latency and/or cholinergic sensitivity were the result of prior episodes of affective illness. Recent work has shown that rates of reduced REM latency were increased in nondepressed relatives of depressed patients with short REM latency, suggesting that genes involved in the genesis of depression might also affect sleep independently.

Further evidence for genetic control of sleep is seen in the increased incidence of sleep disorders in some families. NARCOLEPSY, a disorder of REM sleep, is strongly associated in humans with the expression of the histocompatibility genes *DR2/DQw6*. Although narcolepsy in dogs (see CANINE NARCOLEPSY) does not appear to be linked to histocompatibility genes, it is heritable in a dominant fashion. Other sleep disorders that have been reported to be heritable include idiopathic HYPERSOMNIA, sleep drunkenness, isolated familial CATAPLEXY, SLEEP PARALYSIS, SLEEP WALKING, SLEEP TERRORS, BEDWETTING, and sleep APNEA. Neither the specific genes nor the mode of transmission for any sleep disorder has yet been identified, although the data for most of the disorders are consistent with a model of autosomal dominant transmission with incomplete penetrance; that is, the disorder may be inherited from one parent, but inheritance of the genes does not necessarily mean that the individual will develop the disorder.

It is clear that sleep is a complex behavior, probably regulated by somewhat independent groups of genes responsible for specific aspects of sleep. It is likely that most sleep characteristics are affected by multiple genes. The ultimate identification of the genes controlling sleep will be intimately related to the discovery of the purpose of sleep: the evolutionary pressures shaping sleep must have selected genes both within and across species that would best subserve the ultimate functions of sleep.

(See also FUNCTIONS OF SLEEP; HERITABILITY OF SLEEP AND SLEEP DISORDERS; HUMAN LEUKOCYTE ANTIGEN.)

REFERENCES

Friedmann JK. 1974. A diallele analysis of the genetic underpinnings of mouse sleep. *Physiol Behav* 12:169–175.

Giles DE, Roffwarg HP, Kupfer DJ, Rush AJ, Biggs MM, Etzel BA. 1989. Secular trend in unipolar depression: A hypothesis. *J Affect Disorders* 16:71–75.

Heath AC, Kendler KS, Eaves LJ, Martin NG. 1990. Evidence for genetic influences on sleep disturbance and sleep pattern in twins. *Sleep* 13(4):318–335.

Partinen M, Kaprio J, Koskenvuo M, Putkonen P, Langinvainio H. 1983. Genetic and environmental determination of human sleep. *Sleep* 6(3): 179–185.

Ralph MR, Foster RG, Davis FC, Menaker M. 1990. Transplanted suprachiasmatic nucleus determines circadian period. *Science* 247:975–978.

Sitaram N, Dube S, Keshavan M, Davies A, Reynal P. 1987. The association of supersensitive cholinergic REM-induction and affective illness within pedigrees. *J Psychiatr Res* 21(4):487–497.

Valatx J-L. 1984. Genetics as a model for studying the sleep-waking cycle. In Borbély A, Valatx J-L, eds. *Experimental brain research, Supplementum 8,* pp 135–145. New York: Springer-Verlag.

Webb WB, Campbell SS. 1983. Relationships in sleep characteristics of identical and fraternal twins. *Arch Gen Psychiatry* 40:1093–1095.

Ruth M. Benca

GLUTAMATE

See Chemistry of Sleep: Amines and Other Transmitters; REM Sleep Mechanisms and Neuroanatomy

GONADOTROPIC HORMONES

The gonadotropic hormones, luteinizing hormone (LH) and follicle-stimulating hormone (FSH), are a dynamic pair of hormones secreted from the anterior PITUITARY GLAND. Their role is to stimulate the gonads (ovaries in females and testes in males) and induce ovulation and testosterone and sperm production. LH is secreted in a pulsatile fashion. FSH pulses have been more difficult to detect. The importance of these LH pulses is alluded to by the relationship between LH secretion and sleep. (See also ENDOCRINOLOGY.)

For example, one of the very first changes that takes place in the body during the onset of puberty is an augmentation of both the amplitude and frequency of LH pulses released during sleep. Daytime LH secretion is similar to the prepubertal level until later in puberty when it approaches the adult pattern (Kapen et al., 1974). This increase in LH secretion during sleep occurs even before there are physical signs of PUBERTY.

A second connection between sleep and LH secretion has been demonstrated in menstruating women (see MENSTRUAL CYCLE). The pulsatile release of LH varies in women depending on the phase of the menstrual cycle. The early follicular phase (EFP) occurs at the time of menstrual bleeding. During this phase, there is a sleep-related slowing in the pulsatile release of LH (Kapen et al., 1976). The clinical significance of this phenomenon is uncertain, but loss of this slowing of LH secretion may play a role in the infertility seen in night shift workers (see SHIFTWORK).

Investigators have attempted to explain the mechanisms by which sleep influences the secretion of LH. Several different substances and hormones have been implicated. For example, serotonin, a neurotransmitter involved in the maintenance of SLOW-WAVE SLEEP (see CHEMISTRY OF SLEEP: AMINES AND OTHER TRANSMITTERS), has been shown to inhibit LH secretion in a variety of mammals; however, when the drug methysergide, which is a serotonin blocker, is administered to women in the EFP of the menstrual cycle, the sleep-related slowing of LH secretion still occurs (Kapen, Vagenakis, and Braverman, 1980). On the other hand, when naloxone, an opioid receptor blocker is given, the frequency of LH pulses increases to waking level (Rossmanith and Yen, 1987). These results suggests that naturally occurring opioids, which are morphinelike substances, are at least in part responsible for the relationship between sleep and LH secretion observed in women.

The secretion of the hormones PROLACTIN and MELATONIN (which are released from the pituitary gland and PINEAL GLAND, respectively) is augmented during sleep. Independently, these two hormones have been shown to inhibit the release of LH. It is therefore reasonable to infer that they may somehow be involved in the sleep-related decrease in LH secretion. The picture may actually be more complex. Perhaps changes in the level of the neurotransmitter dopamine (which normally inhibits the release of prolactin) are responsible for changes in LH secretion during sleep (Kapen et al., 1976).

Overall, the relationship between the secretion of LH and sleep is a complex one. LH secretion appears to be augmented during sleep in pubertal males and diminished during sleep in females during the EFP of the menstrual cycle. Both of these characteristic phenomena are probably important in the biological function of the reproductive organs. Various neurotransmitters and hormones have been implicated as mediators of this relationship, but there is still much to be discovered about their precise roles and mechanisms.

REFERENCES

Griffin JE, Wilson JD. 1985. Disorders of the testes and male reproductive tract. In Wilson JD, Foster DW, eds. *Williams textbook of endocrinology,* 7th ed, p 273. Philadelphia: Saunders.

Kapen S, Boyar RM, Finkelstein JW, Hellman L, Weitzman ED. 1974. Effect of sleep–wake cycle reversal on luteinizing hormone secretory pattern in puberty. *J Clin Endocrinol Metab* 39:293.

Kapen S, Boyar R, Hellman L, Weitzman ED. 1976. The relationship of luteinizing hormone secretion to sleep in women during the early follicular phase: Effects of sleep reversal and a prolonged three-hour sleep–wake schedule. *J Clin Endocrinol Metab* 42:1031.

Kapen S, Vagenakis A, Braverman L. 1980. Failure of a serotonergic receptor-blocking drug to change the twenty-four-hour luteinizing hormone secretory pattern in women. *J Clin Endocrinol Metab* 51:302.

Rossmanith WG, Yen SSC. 1987. Sleep-associated decrease in luteinizing hormone pulse frequency during the early follicular phase of the menstrual cycle: Evidence for an opioidergic mechanism. *J Clin Endocrinol Metab* 65:715.

Linda S. Jaffe

GRADUAL SLEEP REDUCTION

In a number of studies the total sleep time of human subjects has been reduced by small increments over the span of several weeks in order to measure the effects of this restriction on variables such as time spent in specific sleep stages, SLEEPINESS, PERFORMANCE during the day, and daytime mood. The general hypothesis underlying these studies was that gradual reduction of sleep time might allow shortening of sleep time without the adverse consequences of acute sleep DEPRIVATION.

The first study of this type was reported in 1973 by Johnson and MacLeod. Two men and one woman reduced their total nightly sleep time by 30 minutes every 2 weeks for 5 months, starting at 7.5 hours. One male subject stopped reduction at 4.5 hours, and the other two decreased sleep time to 4 hours and maintained this sleep time for 3 weeks. In this study, no changes were found in the performance tests, sleep–wake diary, or mood tests of these subjects, compared with the tests before the study began, until the 4-to 5-hour level was reached. The length of time spent in SLOW-WAVE SLEEP dropped somewhat between the baseline sleep time and the 5.5-hour mark and then increased again almost to baseline levels when only 4 hours of sleep time was allowed. This finding is similar to the results from acute sleep deprivation studies, in which subjects spend significantly more time in slow-wave sleep than any other stage of sleep during recovery sleep after severe deprivation. REM sleep time steadily declined throughout the study, suggesting to some scientists that slow-wave sleep is preserved at the expense of REM sleep. The subjects were asked to keep sleep-wake records for the following eight months after the study. Even 8 months after the study, two subjects slept for 5 and 6 hours, 2.5 and 1.5 hours less than their baseline sleep time. (See also STAGES OF SLEEP; DEPRIVATION, TOTAL: PHYSIOLOGICAL EFFECTS.)

Another study, performed by Friedman and colleagues in 1977, evaluated four couples who wanted to reduce their sleep time. Three couples reported baseline sleep of 8 hours, and one couple reported baseline sleep of 6.5 hours. These subjects reduced their total nightly sleep by 30 minutes every 2 weeks, then every 3 to 4 weeks as the reductions became more difficult. The couples were asked to stop the program when they thought they could not reduce their sleep time further and to stay within 30 minutes of that time for 3 months. Performance tests did not show a decline in waking vigilance, but subjects began complaining of difficulty keeping the schedule at the 6 to 6.5-hour level. They had trouble waking up in the morning and staying awake in the daytime. As before, REM sleep time decreased and slow-wave sleep increased as a percentage of total sleep time throughout the study. Here, stage 2 sleep was also shown to be reduced, particularly in the sleep cycles near the end of sleep. Below 5.5 hours of sleep, subjects were shown to fall asleep more quickly. As in the earlier study, the 8-hour sleepers continued to sleep 1 to 2.5 hours less than that for at least the next year; the 6.5-hour sleepers, however, went back to sleeping 6.5 hours per night.

One criticism of both of these studies was that no control subjects were included. The conclusion that there was no decrement in performance should be evaluated relative to other subjects performing the tests repeatedly without sleep deprivation. In 1985, Horne and Wilkinson reported an experiment in which six subjects gradually decreased their sleep time by 1 to 2 hours, and compared these subjects with six control subjects who continued to sleep normally. The experimental subjects did not differ from the control subjects on performance or sleepiness tests except briefly at the 1.5- and 2-hour reduction points. As in the other studies, subjects maintained reduced sleep times after the study for at least 3 months. Together these studies suggest that it may be possible to achieve some reduction gradually in total sleep time without the adverse impact on daytime function associated with acute partial sleep deprivation (see DEPRIVATION, PARTIAL).

One potential explanation for these results has been offered by Horne (1989). He proposes that human sleep consists of two components, core sleep and optional sleep, and that optional sleep, consisting of stages 1 and 2 and REM sleep, can be eliminated without significant impact on daytime function. An alternate view suggests that these last hours of sleep of the night are important, but that their impact is too subtle to be measured with the performance tests used by earlier researchers. The MULTIPLE SLEEP LATENCY TEST (MSLT), a standardized electroencephalographic measure of alertness, can detect the effect of very small reductions in sleep time. The MSLT has not yet been used to evaluate daytime function in subjects undergoing gradual sleep reduction, but this and other test results are necessary before the sleep at the end of the night may be dismissed as optional.

REFERENCES

Friedman J, Globus G, Huntley A, Mullaney D, Naitoh P, Johnson L. 1977. Performance and mood during and after gradual sleep reduction. *Psychophysiology* 14:245–250.

Horne J. 1989. *Why we sleep: The functions of sleep in humans and other mammals.* New York: Oxford University Press.

Horne JA, Wilkinson S. 1985. Chronic sleep reduction: Daytime vigilance performance and EEG measures of sleepiness, with particular reference to 'practice' effects. *Psychophysiology* 22:69–78.

Johnson L, MacLeod WL. 1973. Sleep and awake behavior during gradual sleep reduction. *Percept Motor Skills* 36:87–97.

Laura Walhof

GROWTH HORMONE

Growth hormone, a peptide hormone secreted by the anterior pituitary gland, has been of long-standing interest to sleep researchers because of the close association of its secretory pattern with sleep. Although its best-known function is to stimulate the growth of long bones, cartilage, and soft tissues, growth hormone plays an important role in metabolic regulation (Mendelson, 1987). Growth hormone is found in the brain, and there have been reports that it may induce some kinds of behavioral effects after injections into animals. In mice, for instance, it enhances isolation-induced aggression. Injection of growth hormone into animals and humans increases REM sleep.

The release of growth hormone from the pituitary gland is determined by the summation of effects of two hypothalamic agents, somatostatin (which inhibits release) and growth hormone–releasing hormone (Daughaday, 1985). After release, its main physiological effects may result from stimulation of the liver and possibly kidney to secrete compounds known as *somatomedins*. Repeated injections of growth hormone result in decreased secretion during sleep long after the exogenous hormone itself has left the blood, suggesting that the nervous system responds to elevations in somatomedins or some related compounds by decreasing growth hormone secretion. The results of growth hormone secretion include enhancement of protein synthesis and increases in concentration of blood glucose. Insulin administration results in secretion of growth hormone. It has been shown that this response is due specifically to the lowering of blood sugar rather than to the insulin per se, since tumors that cause hypoglycemia without secretion of insulin cause elevations of growth hormone. Oral ingestion of glucose decreases growth hormone; fasting increases it.

Illnesses result from either oversecretion or undersecretion of growth hormone (Spilotis et al., 1984). Acromegaly, characterized by hyperplasia of the jaw, nose, fingers, and toes, results from oversecretion. (The enlarged jaw found in acromegaly may affect function of the upper airway and can be an unusual contributing factor in some cases of obstructive sleep APNEA.) Short stature can result from undersecretion caused either by decreased amounts of hormone or by subtle alterations in the hormone so that, although it is present in normal amounts, its biological function is impaired. Treatment with synthetic growth hormone is now available. Children who suffer long-standing emotional deprivation or stress may also have decreased growth hormone and subsequent impaired growth, which returns to normal after they are placed in a happier environment.

Sleep-related elevation of growth hormone in adults was first recognized in the 1960s. At first this elevation was thought to be a response to relatively low blood glucose levels during sleep. In 1968, however, investigators at Washington University, who drew blood samples for hormone analysis while sleep electroencephalograms (EEGs) were recorded, found that approximately 90 minutes after sleep onset, a large burst of growth hormone secretion occurs that constitutes almost three-fourths of a person's 24-hour secretion (Takahashi, Kipnis, and Daughaday, 1968). The timing of this secretion tended to be associated with SLOW-WAVE SLEEP; over 40 percent of the peaks of secretion occurred during slow-wave sleep, even though slow-wave sleep constituted only 15 percent of sleep. When patients were purposely awakened by the investigators and then returned to sleep, new peaks of secretion occurred roughly 90 minutes after the new sleep onsets. Subsequent studies have indicated that newborn infants have little difference in blood levels of growth hormone between waking and sleep, but that after the third month, elevation of growth hormone and "quiet sleep" begin to appear. In adolescence, both sleep-related and daytime secretion of growth hormone increase. In adults, growth hormone secretion is somewhat less than in adolescents, and in old age it declines, possibly in association with the age-related decrease in slow-wave sleep. (See also AGING AND SLEEP; INFANCY, NORMAL SLEEP PATTERNS IN; PUBERTY.)

The exact association of growth hormone to slow-wave sleep remains a subject of controversy. It is clear that they can be dissociated in certain special situations. The BENZODIAZEPINES potently decrease slow-wave sleep, and one study has shown that reduction of slow-wave sleep by flurazepam does not result in alterations in sleep-related growth hormone secretion (Rubin et al., 1973). Conversely, some anticholinergic drugs can greatly decrease growth hormone secretion without altering sleep (see CHEMISTRY OF SLEEP: ACETYLCHOLINE). The possible association of growth hormone with circadian rhythmic processes also remains uncertain. Early studies showed that under conditions of 12-hour sleep–wake reversal, growth hormone (in contrast to CORTISOL) secretion immediately changed its pattern to be associated with the new sleep time, implying an absence of circadian effects. Later studies indicating abnormal secretion during JET LAG have raised the possibility that body clocks do affect growth hormone release. This view has also been strengthened by the observation that monkey pituitary glands kept alive in vitro may show rhythmic release of growth hormone.

Traditionally, growth hormone secretion has been studied by observing its release during the daytime in response to injections of insulin or arginine or, alternatively, by following blood levels during the night after bedtime administration of drugs. Such studies have suggested that the effects of drugs on growth hormone secretion during daytime tests may be very different from, even opposite to, the effects during sleep. For example, the medicine methysergide, which blocks serotonin receptors and is used in the treatment of migraine headaches, decreases growth hormone response to insulin but actually increases secretion during sleep. Such observations emphasize the many important differences in a variety of physiological processes during waking and sleep.

There has also been interest in alterations in growth hormone secretion in psychiatric illnesses and particularly in DEPRESSION. Depressed adults may have decreased daytime release of growth hormone in response to insulin or amphetamine, as well as decreased sleep-related secretion. Interestingly, children with endogenous and nonendogenous depression may have elevated sleep-related secretion. Sleep-related secretion is decreased in schizophrenia (see PSYCHOPATHOLOGY, NONDEPRESSION) and ALCOHOLISM, both of which are characterized by decreased slow-wave sleep. In one study, "dry" alcoholics were given a drink; during the subsequent sleep, slow-wave sleep returned to normal but regular growth hormone secretion failed to occur. Abnormal growth hormone secretion during sleep and in response to arginine also occurs in sleep APNEA and NARCOLEPSY.

REFERENCES

Daughaday WH. 1985. The anterior pituitary. In Wilson JD, Foster DW, eds. *Williams textbook of endocrinology,* pp 568–613. Philadelphia: Saunders.

Mendelson WB. 1987. *Human sleep: Research and clinical care.* New York: Plenum.

Rubin RT, Gouin PR, Arenander AT, Poland RE. 1973. Human growth hormone release following prolonged flurazepam administration. *Res Commun Chem Pathol Pharmacol* 6:331–334.

Spilotis BE, August GP, Hung W, Sonis W, Mendelson WB, Bercu BB. 1984. Growth hormone neurosecretory dysfunction. *JAMA* 251:2223–2251.

Takahashi Y, Kipnis DM, Daughaday WH. 1968. Growth hormone secretion during sleep. *Clin Invest* 47:2079–2090.

Wallace B. Mendelson

H

HALLUCINATIONS

Hallucination refers to the apparent perception of sensory stimuli that are not physically present. The hallucination may be experienced in any of the sense modalities, although auditory and visual hallucinations are the most common. Hallucinations have many origins and may reflect normal physiological processes as well as abnormal processes. The most universal experience of a hallucinatory event is a dream. When individuals dream they see, or less commonly hear, things that are not physically present. These hallucinatory dream experiences most commonly occur during REM sleep (see REM SLEEP, PHYSIOLOGY OF; ACTIVATION–SYNTHESIS HYPOTHESIS).

Dream experiences may also occur during other stages of sleep (see HYPNAGOGIC REVERIE). Variations in sleep processes can also produce dreamlike hallucinations in the waking state. For example, it is not uncommon for individuals who undergo total sleep deprivation to experience visual hallucinations during wakefulness (see DEPRIVATION, TOTAL; BEHAVIORAL EFFECTS). This experience resolves when the sleep deprivation is resolved. These hallucinations are thought by some to reflect REM sleep processes escaping into wakefulness.

NARCOLEPSY, a disorder of REM sleep, has as one of its symptoms the experience of visual hallucinations at sleep onset. These hallucinations have been referred to as HYPNAGOGIC HALLUCINATIONS. Patients with narcolepsy often fall asleep by going directly into REM sleep. The presence of sleep-onset REM periods has been offered as the explanation for the hallucinations narcoleptics experience as they are falling asleep (see also REM LATENCY).

Mental illness, especially schizophrenia, has been associated with reports of hallucinations. This observation has led some individuals to speculate that sleep loss is somehow related to mental illness, whereas sleep per se maintains mental health. Research on the relation of sleep and schizophrenia has failed to confirm this speculation (see PSYCHOPATHOLOGY, NONDEPRESSION). First, people who are sleep deprived for very long periods of time (200 hours) do not show any signs of mental illness with the exception of hallucinations. Also, whereas hallucinations related to sleep and sleep loss are primarily visual in nature, the hallucinations of schizophrenics tend to be auditory. Finally, with recovery sleep, hallucinations related to sleep deprivation cease, whereas extending sleep in schizophrenics has no effect on the frequency of hallucinations.

Thomas Roth

HEADACHES, NOCTURNAL

Sleep may be either the balm or the bane of headache sufferers. All the primary headache conditions share two features. The first is their propensity to occur periodically—during the year, month, sleep–wake, or REM–NREM portion of the sleep cycle. For those headaches related to sleep, it is not known whether the sleep–wake cycle per se is the trigger or whether some other cyclic phenomena such as hormonal variations associated with the sleep–wake cycle are involved. The second feature is that despite their severe, frightening, or incapacitating nature, headaches are almost never the symptom of any serious underlying neurological condition. Extensive and expensive neurological evaluation is infrequently warranted. Headaches are also rarely due to significant psychological or psychiatric causes. Most can be controlled to varying degrees by medication.

Headaches occurring during sleep may be divided into two major categories: primary (headaches interrupting sleep) and secondary (headaches resulting from some other phenomenon occurring during sleep).

Primary Sleep Headaches

Migraine

The most common headache associated with sleep is the migraine. The term *migraine* is derived from *hemicrania,* meaning pain affecting only one side of the head. This one-sided headache is the "classic" migraine. In fact, however, the majority of migraine sufferers experience a diffuse, generalized headache, termed the "common" migraine. Migraine affects at least 10 percent of the population, with women affected three times as frequently as men. Women may experience more headaches around the time of menstruation (see MENSTRUAL CYCLE). There is a strong genetic component—the majority of migraineurs have additional affected family members. Migraines often begin in childhood or adolescence and sometimes disappear with increasing age, after menopause in women and late middle age in men.

The classic migraine may be heralded by an *aura,* most commonly visual (the sensation of flashing lights, zigzag lines, or loss of a portion of the visual field). Other auras include numbness or tingling of parts of the body (often the hand and corner of the mouth region), confusion, or rarely, weakness of an extremity or double vision. The nature of both the classic and common migraine is one of periodic, severe, incapacitating pain, often associated with other symptoms such as light and sound sensitivity, nausea, or vomiting. The headache often lasts the better part of 24 hours. The typical refuge for a migraineur during an attack is in bed in a dark quiet room, with provisions made for the nausea/vomiting that may occur. The drug methysergide, which blocks

serotonin receptors, is used in the treatment of migraines.

The relationship between migraine headaches and sleep is variable. The majority of sufferers find that, even after medication that attenuates the pain, sleep (termed "recovery sleep") is desirable or mandatory to terminate an attack completely. Some find that their migraines may be triggered by either insufficient or unusually long sleep periods (hence the term "weekend" or "holiday/vacation" migraines).

Another group of migraineurs finds that their spells often or always begin during sleep, resulting in a rude and painful awakening to a full-blown attack. Sleep studies performed on those suffering from nocturnal migraine have shown that, in some, the headaches arise during or close to a period of REM sleep. There is also an association between migraine headaches and disorders of arousal, such as SLEEP TERRORS and SLEEPWALKING in children. The significance of this relationship is not known.

Cluster Headaches

Another type of headache, often confused with migraine, is the cluster headache. Unlike migraine, it affects men nine times as frequently as women, is not familial in nature, is not preceded by an aura, and is generally brief (often less than 30 minutes in duration). The headaches occur in clusters (hence the name), often daily or nightly for a period of time, then disappear as mysteriously as they came—sometimes for months, or even years, at a time. They are more prevalent in the spring and fall. Some victims can predict with great accuracy when the next cluster will appear. In some, during a period of cluster, even very small amounts of alcohol (particularly red wine) will inevitably trigger a headache.

The cluster headache often begins with a burning sensation around one eye, then rapidly progresses to an excruciating pain confined to the region of the eye, often associated with redness, tearing, pupillary dilation, and drooping of the eyelid of the affected eye. The pain is often incapacitating, driving the victim to distraction. Suicide threats are occasionally made during a spell.

Cluster headaches are more apt to occur during sleep than are migraines, often developing toward the last portion of the sleep period. They occur 2.5 times as frequently from the sleep period as from wakefulness. Sleep studies indicate that cluster headaches are often REM sleep-locked. This concept is supported by the fact that the peak frequency of cluster headaches coincides with the time of maximal REM tendency (4 to 10 A.M.).

Chronic Paroxysmal Hemicrania

A rare variant of the cluster headache is "chronic paroxysmal hemicrania," which unlike conventional cluster headache, most frequently affects young women. This headache may be sleep period-related, often occurring multiple times (up to twenty or so) per 24 hours. It, too, tends to be associated with REM sleep.

Hypnic Headache Syndrome

A recently described condition affecting elderly individuals is the hypnic headache syndrome. This condition is characterized by regular awakenings from sleep, often at a consistent time. The headaches are diffuse, last less than an hour, and may be accompanied by nausea but no other symptoms suggestive of cluster headache. They may occur multiple times nightly. No sleep studies have been performed on this condition.

Secondary Sleep Headaches

Sleep-Disordered Breathing

Rarely, headaches during the sleep period may be a manifestation of an underlying sleep-related respiratory disturbance. They have been reported in association with obstructive sleep APNEA. They may also be seen in other conditions associated with hypoventilation during sleep—particularly in patients with neuromuscular weakness (as in some forms of muscular dystrophy) whose compromised respiratory function becomes exaggerated by the sleeping state—particularly during REM sleep. These headaches are probably caused by dilation of the extracerebral blood vessels induced by a reduction of the blood oxygen and/or elevation of the blood carbon dioxide levels resulting from inadequate respiration during sleep. Subtle sleep-breathing irregularities may trigger some of the varieties of primary sleep headaches in susceptible individuals.

REFERENCES

Dalessio DJ, ed. 1980. *Wolff's headache and other head pain.* New York: Oxford University Press.
Saper JR. 1983. *Headache disorders. Current concepts and treatment strategies.* Boston: John Wright.

Mark W. Mahowald

HEADBANGING

See Rhythmic Movement Disorder

HEAD INJURY

The incidence of head injury in the United States is staggering. Approximately 400,000 individuals per year require hospitalization for treatment and/or observation of head injuries; of this number, approximately 45 percent, or 180,000, are persons with severe or moderately severe closed-head injuries. Seventy percent of all head-injured persons are aged less than 34 years. The national financial burden associated with head injuries has been estimated at $4 billion annually (Frankowski, Annegers, and Whitman, 1985).

The effects of a head injury are devastating to the person as well as to his or her family. The hours spent in a critical care unit are often recalled by family members as a blurred nightmare. Once the comatose closed-head–injured person reaches a stable period and life support systems are no longer required, the patient is usually transferred out of the critical care unit and into a short-term care unit of a hospital to begin a long course of treatment. Ultimately, the patient continues treatment in a rehabilitation facility.

When removed from the critical list in a stabilized condition, the head-injured person appears to be asleep but cannot usually be aroused from the coma state. In certain cases, vigorous and/or noxious (painful) stimulation will produce arousal (see COMA). By placing electrodes in a standardized array on the scalp to measure brain waves, as well as electrodes to measure eye movements, muscle tension of the chin, and heart rate, it is possible to identify the brain state or sleep stage experienced by a person in a coma or semicomatose state (see POLYSOMNOGRAPHY).

As far back as the 1930s, electroencephalographers observed that the brain waves of the comatose head-injured person differed from those described for normal persons. Interest in sleep research in the 1950s and 1960s stimulated renewed efforts to identify the types of sleep in head injury and coma. Normally, sleep is divided into REM sleep and the four stages of NREM sleep based upon the distinctive polysomnographic patterns of each stage (see STAGES OF SLEEP; REM SLEEP, DISCOVERY OF). Criteria for analyzing and scoring these electrophysiologic measurements were established for normal persons in 1968 (Rechtschaffen and Kales); however, different guidelines and criteria were needed for brain-injured persons. Subsequently published reports of scientists in the United States (Chatrian, White, and Daly, 1963), Italy (Bergamasco et al., 1968; Bergamasco, Bergamini, and Doriguzzl, 1968; Bricolo et al., 1968; Bricolo and Turella, 1973), and Austria (Rumpl et al., 1979; 1983) found that various electroencephalographic (EEG) waveforms usually seen in sleeping patients were present in comatose patients, although often with an unusual pattern or distribution. In 1986, Parsons performed forty-four long-term studies on twenty-two severe–head-injured persons and formulated guidelines that could be used to evaluate and specify the sleep of persons in coma following head injury (Table 1). These guidelines are based upon hypnogram charts of sleep stages derived from analyzing the EEG records and comparing them with those of normal subjects. For this comparison, the head-injured patients were grouped according to the severity of their injury and level of consciousness or unconsciousness at the time of sleep evaluation with use of the Glasgow Coma Scale (GCS) (Table 2), which ranges from a score of 3 (deep coma) to 15 (awake).

When the head-injured person is in deep coma (GCS 4 to 6), the EEG is dominated by very high amplitude and slow waveforms commonly referred to as delta and theta, respectively. These waveforms fluctuate in a monotonous, rhythmic manner known as delta coma and theta coma. When these EEG waveforms are analyzed using Parsons's criteria and condensed into a hypnogram, the overnight sleep pattern appears as illustrated in Figure 1.

As the head-injured person begins to emerge

Table 1. Parsons's Criteria: EEG Sleep Stages in Closed-Head Injury

REM = rapid eye movement sleep
REM_v = rapid eye movement sleep associated with variants
$A-1_a$ = fluctuation between wake and drowsiness
1_b = light sleep with a predominance of small spindles
2_a = light sleep with spindles
2_b = light sleep without spindles; diphasic
2_{bv} = light sleep without spindles; monophasic
2_{bt} = light sleep without spindles; predominantly small amplitude theta
3 = delta sleep without spindles
3_s = delta sleep with spindles
4 = delta sleep without spindles
4_s = delta sleep with spindles

from coma, EEG waveforms change, indicating a lighter and altered stage of sleep. Unlike stage 2 sleep in normal subjects, this lighter stage of sleep is very fragmented. The only part of normal stage 2 sleep that appears intact is the theta waveforms and what appears to be a remnant of K-complexes (see K-COMPLEX). Sleep spindles (12 to 14 hertz), usually associated with stage 2 sleep, are not found in this light sleep (see SLEEP SPINDLES). The predominant theta waveforms in the patient's EEG record meet criteria for theta coma; sleep spindles appear later, after a definite improvement in the head-injured person's level of consciousness as indicated by an increase in the GCS score.

By the time the head-injured person's neurologic status improves to a GCS level of 7, 8, or 9, the EEG waveforms indicative of light NREM sleep occur, although REM sleep is still lacking. Sleep spindles at this level of coma define two stages: spindles associated with a K-complex (stage 2_a) and predominance of sleep spindles (stage 1_b). Based on neurophysiologic evidence, the reappearance of sleep spindles usually indicates a reestablishment of functional anatomic links between the cerebral cortex and aggregates of pacemaker cells located deep in the brain—for example, in the thalamus (see THALAMUS). Thus, the sleep spindles are a sign of healing.

Sleep spindles in light sleep gradually increase in amplitude and definition as the brain contin-

Table 2.   Glasgow Coma Scale (GCS): Changes in level of consciousness are monitored by giving the patient's best single response in each of the three categories and expressing responsiveness as the total score.

Category	Response	Score
Eyes		
	Open	
	Spontaneously	4
	To verbal command	3
	To pain	2
	No response	1
Best motor response		
	To verbal command	
	Obeys	6
	To painful stimulus*	
	Localizes pain	5
	Flexion: withdrawal	4
	Flexion: abnormal	
	(decorticate rigidity)	3
	Extension	
	(decerebrate rigidity)	3
	No response	1
Best verbal response†		
	Oriented and converses	5
	Disoriented and converses	4
	Inappropriate words	3
	Incomprehensible sounds	2
	No response	1
Total score		3 (deep coma) to 15 (awake)

Apply knuckles to sternum; observe arms. †Arouse patient with painful stimulus if necessary.

ues to reorganize and reestablish connections with thalamic pacemaker cells, as well as other collections of neurons in the brainstem, specifically the pons and medulla (see MEDULLA; PONS). Figure 2 depicts a series of four EEGs from the same patient recorded between the 19th and 53rd day of coma, when GCS scores ranged from 5 to 9. At this point, the sleep record includes stages 4, 3, 2_b (or 2_{bv}), 2_a, and 1_b; however, no signs of wakefulness or REM sleep are yet apparent in the EEG.

The next waveforms to reappear in the course of recovery are those associated with a form of wakefulness. By this time, the head-injured person's eyes begin to open and can follow the movement of family members about the room. The patient may lie quietly with eyes closed or begin rolling back and forth in bed for extended periods of time. The EEG waveforms during this period tend to show alphalike activity (8 to 13 hertz), a pattern typical of normal subjects in the awake state with eyes closed but mentally free-associating (see ALPHA RHYTHM). Parsons has termed this stage A-1_a to signify fluctuation between wakefulness (stage A) and drowsiness (stage 1_a). The hypnogram at this stage of recovery (e.g., a patient with GCS score between 10 and 12) shows EEG patterns including delta, theta, light NREM sleep, and wakefulness.

The last aspect of normal-appearing sleep to occur during recovery from head injury is indicators of an altered form of REM sleep. The sawtooth waves of REM sleep appear but have a reduced amplitude and are mixed with spindles (see SAWTOOTH WAVES). Curiously, even with the presence of the EEG waveforms typical of REM sleep, the eye movements under the closed eyelids greatly diminish. Finally, fully integrated REM sleep reappears when the GCS score reaches 13, 14, or 15 and the hypnogram indicates that

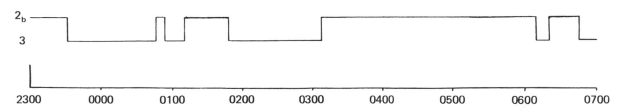

Figure 1. Overnight hypnogram of head-injured patient in deep coma (GCS 4), showing fluctuation between delta coma and theta coma (see Table 1 for Parsons's criteria).

all stages of sleep and wakefulness have returned (Figure 3). The resequencing of stages also suggests that the normal nocturnal architecture of sleep is beginning to reestablish itself (see CYCLE OF SLEEP ACROSS THE NIGHT). At this point, the outlook on recovery from the head injury appears somewhat optimistic; that is, sleep measurements demonstrate progressive improvement in the brain, and some functional recovery is likely. One should keep in mind, however, that the time required to reach this point may have been as long as three months. When the patient reaches this period of recovery, a more normal pattern of

sleep begins to reform, with better definition of sleep stages, less fragmentation, and improved organization, as illustrated in Figure 4.

Almost all injuries, including head injury, are preventable. About 35 percent to 50 percent of head injuries are associated with the use of alcohol or other mind-altering drugs, especially among those aged 15 to 30 years. Younger persons (aged 5 to 14 years) tend to experience head injuries because they fail to wear protective helmets or take foolish risks associated with "childish dares." Children aged 6 months to 5 years who suffer head injuries that are not the result of

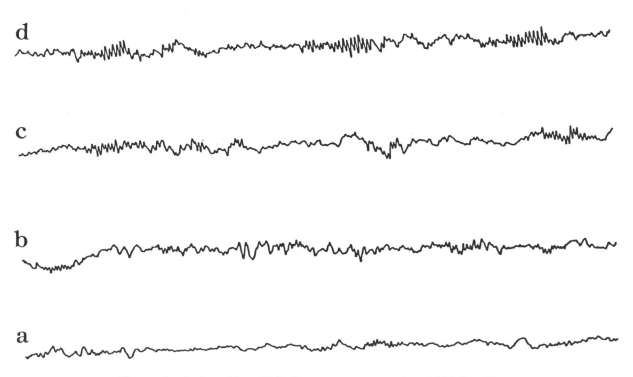

Figure 2. Series of four EEGs from a comatose patient (GCS 5 to 9) recorded (a) 19, (b) 27, (c) 43, and (d) 55 days after head injury, showing progressive changes in spindle morphology during light sleep.

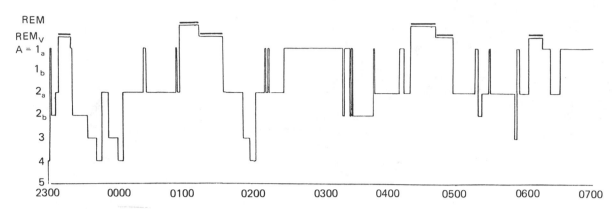

Figure 3. Overnight hypnogram of head-injured patient (GCS 13), showing return of all stages of sleep and wakefulness with persistent fragmentation.

a car or bicycle accident may be victims of child abuse.

In summary, alterations of the sleep–wake cycle associated with severe to moderately severe head injury are brought about by a functional dissociation among the cerebral cortex, the thalamus, and the lower brainstem (see NREM SLEEP MECHANISMS; REM SLEEP MECHANISMS AND NEUROANATOMY). Over time, and assuming that only minimal complications (i.e., pneumonia and brain swelling) occur secondary to the comatose state, neuronal recovery will occur and be manifested by neuron sprouting within and between regions of the brain as well as by pre- and postsynaptic reattachment of axon terminals. Recovery of normal sleep stages is a marker for general brain recovery. Nevertheless, the time required to recover from a brain injury is frequently several months to several years. Even then, the head-injured person may never be able to achieve a preinjury level of physical and mental ability. Children and young adults need to consider seriously these alternatives before riding bicycles without helmets and driving motorcycles and cars under the influence of alcohol or mind-altering drugs.

REFERENCES

Bergamasco B, Bergamini L, Doriguzzl T. 1968. Clinical value of the sleep electroencephalographic patterns in post-traumatic coma. *Acta Neurol Scand* 44:495–511.

Bergamasco B, Bergamini L, Doriguzzl T, Fabiani D. 1968. EEG sleep patterns as a prognostic criterion in post-traumatic coma. *Electroencephalogr Clin Neurophysiol* 24:374–377.

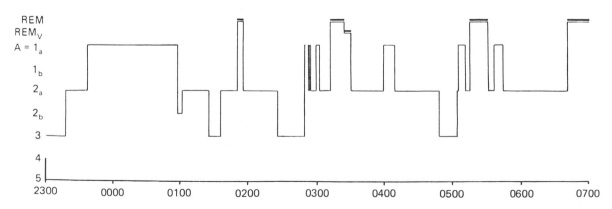

Figure 4. Overnight hypnogram of head-injured patient (GCS = 15), showing increasingly normal pattern of sleep/wake stage organization and less fragmentation.

Bricolo A, Gentilomo A, Rosadini G, Rossi GF. 1968. Long-lasting post-traumatic unconsciousness. A study based on nocturnal EEG and polygraphic recording. *Acta Neurol Scand* 44:512–532.

Bricolo A, Turella G. 1973. Electroencephalographic patterns of acute traumatic coma: Diagnostic and prognostic value. *J Neurosurg Sci* 17:278–285.

Chatrian GE, White LE, Daly D. 1963. Electroencephalographic patterns resembling those of sleep in certain comatose states after injuries to the head. *Electroencephalogr Clin Neurophysiol* 15:272–280.

Frankowski RF, Annegers JF, Whitman S. 1985. Epidemiological and descriptive studies Part I. In Becker DP, Povlishock JT, eds. *Central nervous system trauma status report*, pp 33–51. Bethesda, Md.: NINCDS of NIH.

Parsons LC. 1986. *Traumatic coma*. Final report submitted to Division of Nursing, Bureau of Health Professions, HHS Grant NU00772.

Rechtschaffen A, Kales A. 1968. *A manual of standardized terminology, techniques, and scoring system for sleep stages of human subjects*. Washington, D.C.: Public Health Service, U.S. Government Printing Office.

Rumpl E, Lorenzi E, Hackl JM, Gerstenbrand F, Hengl W. 1979. The EEG at different stages of acute secondary traumatic midbrain and bulbar brain syndromes. *Electroencephalogr Clin Neurophysiol* 46:487–497.

Rumpl E, Prugger M, Bauer G, Gerstenbrand F, Hackl JM, Pallua A. 1983. Incidence and prognostic value of spindles in post-traumatic coma. *Electroencephalogr Clin Neurophysiol* 56:420–429.

L. Claire Parsons

HEARTBURN

Heartburn is a common symptom among the general population in the United States and is generally described as a "burning" sensation directly beneath the breast bone, or sternum. It is caused by the retrograde flow of acidic gastric contents into the esophagus. This physiologic event may occur during waking or during sleep and frequently occurs without the individual experiencing any concomitant symptom. Although daytime gastroesophageal reflux (GER) and associated heartburn are usually benign, when GER occurs during sleep, there is considerable risk of more serious complications.

Nocturnal GER is an infrequent occurrence in normal individuals. It is usually provoked by late evening meals, which tend to leave a large volume of acid in the stomach at the time the individual retires for the night. The large gastric volume and the recumbent position will predispose to GER. Nocturnal GER appears to be considerably more common in individuals with gastroesophageal reflux disease. The latter term generally applies to individuals with significant daytime symptoms (i.e., heartburn or regurgitation several times per week) and inflammation of the lining of the esophagus.

In patients with significant heartburn suggestive of gastroesophageal reflux disease, the actual reflux of gastric contents into the esophagus can be continuously monitored by placing a pH probe into the esophagus (via nasal intubation). This allows the clinician or the medical researcher to identify the timing of reflux events, the duration of reflux events, whether events tend to occur during sleeping or waking, and the timing of reflux with regard to meals and other physical activities. It also provides unique information concerning the relationship between symptoms experienced by the patient and the reflux events. These studies are conducted on an ambulatory basis with patients conducting their normal daily activities. Other studies can be conducted in the sleep laboratory, where more precise information can be obtained concerning reflux events and their relationship to specific stages of sleep, and how acidification of the distal esophagus alters the state of consciousness. These investigations collectively have led to a number of interesting findings that relate to the occurrence of GER during waking and sleeping, the pattern of acid clearance (acid neutralization) during waking and sleep, and the relationship between these phenomena and development of gastroesophageal reflux disease and its attendant complications (i.e., severe inflammation of the esophagus) or aspiration of the refluxed gastric contents. These studies have revealed that GER occurs most commonly in the daytime after meals. In individuals with a more severe condition, this may continue for several hours after the meal. In some individuals, nocturnal GER is identified to occur with acid exposure time in the esophagus nearly equivalent to that noted in the daytime. Many investigators feel that it is these individuals who develop the most severe problems with gastroesophageal reflux disease.

Nocturnal reflux appears to be primarily associated with brief arousals from sleep, but these events are clearly not exclusively related to arousal responses. The neutralization and clearance of acid from the esophagus has been shown to take considerably longer when reflux occurs during sleep. The length of time necessary for acid clearance from acidification of the esophagus during sleep appears to be directly related to the degree of sustained waking obtained by the patient after the reflux event. That is, reflux events that are associated with a brief arousal and an immediate return to sleep take considerably longer to neutralize than those events that are associated with an arousal and subsequent period of time primarily associated with wakefulness. It is uncertain why patients develop problematic nocturnal GER.

Gastroesophageal reflux can also be the source of multiple awakenings from sleep with the resultant complaint of insomnia occurring during sleep. In an obvious state of depressed consciousness, GER places a patient at increased risk to aspirate the refluxed gastric contents. This is especially true in patients with depressed consciousness resulting from traumatic head injuries or other serious medical illnesses. There are physiological data that demonstrate a variety of autonomic reflexes associated with acidification of the esophagus. That is, there is a reflex constriction of the small air passages in the lung in response to acid in the esophagus. This has been linked to triggering of wheezing in patients with asthma, particularly those who experience nocturnal asthma. There are data to support the fact that in many patients nocturnal wheezing may often be secondary to sleep-related GER.

Both daytime and nocturnal GER are most effectively treated by antacids, which neutralize refluxed contents into the esophagus or by prescription drugs that suppress acid secretion. By effectively reducing the amount of gastric acid in the stomach, there is a concomitant reduction in the frequency of GER. The availability of 24-hour monitoring either on an ambulatory basis or in a sleep laboratory allows the clinician much greater insight and flexibility into an effective diagnosis and treatment for gastroesophageal reflux disease.

REFERENCES

Johnson LF, DeMeester TR. 1974. Twenty-four hour pH monitoring of the distal esophagus. *Am J Gastroenterol* 62:325–332.

Mansfield LE, Stein MR. 1978. Gastroesophageal reflux and asthma: A possible reflex mechanism. *Ann Allergy* 41:224–226.

Nebel OT, Fornes MF, Castell DO. 1976. Symptomatic gastroesophageal reflux: Incidence and precipitating factors. *Am J Dig Dis* 21:953–956.

Orr WC, Johnson LF, Robinson MG. 1984. The effect of sleep on swallowing, esophageal peristalsis, and acid clearance. *Gastroenterology* 86:814–819.

Orringer MB. 1979. Respiratory symptoms and esophageal reflux. *Chest* 76:618–619.

William C. Orr

HEART REGULATION DURING SLEEP

Control of the heart undergoes dramatic changes as an individual passes from waking to different states of sleep. These changes are not necessarily associated with rest or restoration, particularly in individuals who are enduring certain types of cardiac or respiratory disease; for these individuals, sleep imposes severe stress on the heart and blood vessels.

Several aspects of cardiac control are of interest during sleep. Heart rate in humans slows in the transition from waking to NREM sleep and usually increases after the individual passes from NREM to REM sleep. Heart rate, however, is only one aspect of cardiac functioning in which important physiological changes take place from waking to sleep. The moment-to-moment changes from one heartbeat to the next are an important indicator of cardiac functioning, as are changes in blood pressure during different types of sleep and blood flow through the vessels that supply the heart muscles.

The most marked sleep effect on heart activity in the human is the nature of changes from one heartbeat to the next. Heart rate is seldom unvarying in normal humans; indeed, a fixed, unvarying heart rate is usually indicative of severe disease. Heart rate normally accelerates on inspiration and slows on expiration; this coupling of heart rate with breathing (called respiratory sinus arrhythmia) results from reflexive interactions between the respiratory and cardiac systems. One can experience these momentary rate changes by listening to his or her heartbeat while sitting quietly and breathing very regularly. As breathing in quiet NREM sleep is very regular, and each breath is rather deep in that state, the highly regular acceleration and slowing of heart rate associated with respiration are accentuated during the quiet sleep state. On the other hand, changes in heart rate from movement or other sources is greatly diminished during quiet NREM sleep. Thus, heart rate is usually slow during quiet sleep, and the rate increases and decreases rhythmically with each breath.

During REM sleep, heart rate usually increases, but again, the most remarkable changes are those that occur from one beat to the next; during REM sleep, heart rate occasionally accelerates for sustained periods and then slows; the range of heart rate changes is much more pronounced than in quiet NREM sleep. The changes in rate typically accompany twitches and movements that also occur during REM sleep.

The distribution of blood flow to various organs can change markedly during sleep. Of particular interest is the nature of blood flow to the heart muscles through the vessels supplying this pumping organ; these vessels are called *coronary arteries*. Adequate blood flow to the heart is essential for maintaining healthy cardiac action. REM sleep is characterized by a peculiar phenomenon: Enormous surges in coronary blood flow occur episodically, and these surges occur without the heart rate changes that would normally accompany such a flow increase during waking. Disturbed changes in blood flow to the heart may underlie nocturnal angina (heart-related pain occurring at night).

The coupling of breathing and heart rate that leads to the normal acceleration and deceleration of heart rate with respiration can be greatly exaggerated during particular breathing disorders that occur during sleep. In some patients, airflow through the oral cavity and pharynx becomes sufficiently obstructed during sleep to block air movement. This disturbance is called obstructive sleep APNEA (*apnea* means "no breath"). When the upper airway is obstructed, negative pressure is generated in the thorax by diaphragmatic descent, venous blood returns to the heart with each attempt to inspire, and the heart reflexively slows very dramatically. Blood pressure markedly increases with each attempted breath, and patients may be at increased risk for STROKE.

Arterial blood pressure drops slightly from waking to quiet NREM sleep (although that finding is species specific) but can vary markedly during REM sleep. In addition to increased varia-

tion during REM sleep, animal studies suggest that a redistribution of blood flow occurs, such that flow to the peripheral limbs is diminished with increased constriction of the vessels, and flow to the vessels supplying the major organs of the gut is increased.

REFERENCES

Orem J, Barnes CD. 1980. *Physiology in sleep.* New York: Academic Press.
Verrier R. 1988. Behavioral state and cardiac arrhythmias. In Lydic R, Biebuyck J, eds. *Clinical physiology of sleep,* pp 31–51. Bethesda, Md.: American Physiological Society.

Ronald M. Harper

HERITABILITY OF SLEEP AND SLEEP DISORDERS

Family studies often help to elucidate the mechanisms of various physiological processes and disease states. Family members are studied to determine their degree of similarity regarding the property or condition under study, patterns of inheritance are identified, and inferences are made regarding the nature of the genes responsible for given traits. In the case of a disorder, the influences of specific environmental and host-specific risk factors on the expression of the disorder are also sought, allowing more specific determinations of disease mechanisms and elucidation of interactions between genetic and environmental factors. Hundreds of conditions—including color blindness, muscular dystrophy, cancer, heart disease, asthma, schizophrenia, and alcoholism—have been studied with such approaches; these studies often have resulted in advances in disease treatment and prevention strategies.

Studies of the familial determinants of sleep and various sleep disorders are likely to increase our understanding of normal and pathophysiological processes that influence sleep. A strong genetic component has been identified for sleeping pattern (i.e., habitual bedtime, sleep duration, and daytime napping) (Heath et al., 1990). Thus, inheritance appears to influence significantly those factors that regulate sleep–wake cycles. However, the specific genes responsible for such regulatory processes have not yet been identified.

Disorders of sleep are also significantly influenced by inherited factors. Insomnia and other sleep disturbances characterized by poor sleep quality and disturbed sleep are in large part determined by genetic factors (see INSOMNIA; FATAL FAMILIAL INSOMNIA). One study indicates that inherited factors explain approximately 30 percent to 40 percent of the variability in these traits (Heath et al., 1990). Genetic factors appear to be especially important for those problems in initiating and maintaining sleep that are associated with mood disorders, such as depression and anxiety. This relationship may be surprising in light of commonly held notions that mood disorders are a result of situational stresses, and it highlights the need to appreciate the biological bases of mood-associated sleep disorders (see NONDEPRESSION).

NARCOLEPSY may occur in 10 percent to 50 percent of the first-degree relatives (i.e., parents, brothers, sisters, and children) of patients with this disorder compared with an overall population prevalence of 0.1% (Guilleminault, 1989). Furthermore, virtually all patients with narcolepsy share an identical genetic marker, known as human leukocyte antigen (HLA-DR2). This HLA-disease association is the strongest such association known; however, the inheritance of a specific gene does not seem to be sufficient itself for the development of narcolepsy. In fact, among identical twins—siblings with identical genes—narcolepsy is often observed in only one member of the twinship. Thus, in this disorder, an inherited predisposition may be a necessary prerequisite for disease development; however, environmental and developmental influences may significantly influence the likelihood that any given "genetically predisposed" individual will develop narcolepsy.

Disruptive snoring, a symptom associated with partial obstruction of airflow in the upper airway during sleep, is most commonly reported among middle-aged and older men and in children with enlarged adenoids and tonsils. However, inherited factors also appear to influence the likelihood that any given person will snore loudly; relatives of loud snorers are two to four times more likely to be loud snorers themselves than are persons who are unrelated to loud snorers (Redline and Tishler, 1993). Familial similarities in snoring may relate to similarities in the size and shape of upper airway structures or in body size among relatives. As a result of such clustering of snoring among family members, some people who have lived in households with multiple loud snorers perceive disruptive snoring to be commonplace and often may underestimate the severity of their own loud snoring. For example, one young, recently married man who always had been a loud snorer encouraged his wife to sleep in a separate bedroom to minimize disruption of her sleep from his loud snoring—his parents had practiced this bedtime behavior, which he considered to be "normal." (See also SNORING.)

Sleep apnea, characterized by repetitive episodes wherein breathing stops during sleep and the subject gasps or struggles for breath, often occurs in association with disabling daytime sleepiness; this condition also clusters within families. Clustering of sleep apnea has been observed among parents and their children and among siblings. Figure 1 demonstrates one family with multiple affected relatives, including the brother and one son of the *proband* (first identified patient). Additionally, in this family, two members had sudden infant death syndrome (SIDS) or near-miss SIDS, suggesting that in certain instances sleep apnea and SIDS may share a common basis. The degree to which inheritance increases one's risk of developing sleep apnea is currently under active investigation. (See also APNEA; SUDDEN INFANT DEATH SYNDROME.)

No single predisposing factor for sleep apnea among family members has yet been identified. Some family members with sleep apnea are similarly obese; in others, there are similarities in jaw structure. But in many such families, the familial basis for sleep apnea remains elusive, although it may be related to abnormalities in lung function and the control of breathing among affected family members. Allergy, which has a clear familial basis, may also predispose to sleep apnea by causing nasal congestion and increased airway resistance (see ALLERGIES). Tobacco consumption and evening alcohol use, habits influenced in part by genetic factors, may also alter the properties of the upper airway and increase a given subject's risk of developing sleep apnea (see SMOKING AND SLEEP; ALCOHOL). It is very likely that the development of sleep apnea may be influenced by several factors (e.g., a small airway size and an abnormality in breathing regulation) that may interact to produce a critical level of "susceptibility."

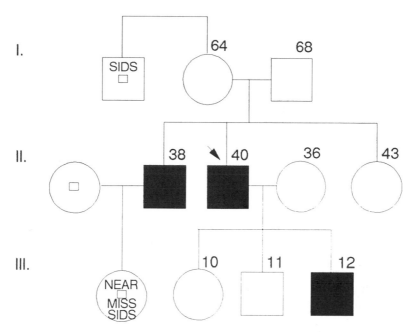

Figure 1. Pedigree analysis (a family tree). The index case (*arrow*) was identified after coming to a sleep disorders clinic with symptoms of loud snoring and sleepiness. Subsequent members of his family were studied as part of a research study. His brother and 11-year-old son were observed also to have significant sleep apnea. Additionally, the index case's uncle and niece were reported as having SIDS and near-miss SIDS, respectively. Females are depicted with circles, males with squares. Age of each subject is provided above each figure. Subjects with sleep apnea are depicted by shaded figures.

In summary, there appear to be strong inherited bases for factors that govern normal and abnormal sleep–wake cycles and familial factors that influence the propensity for snoring and sleep apnea. Further elucidation of the nature of the genes responsible for these physiological and pathophysiological processes will be important for future efforts at designing better treatment strategies.

REFERENCES

Guilleminault C. 1989. Narcolepsy syndrome. In Kryger MH, Roth T, Dement WC, eds. *Principles and practice of sleep medicine,* pp 338–346. Philadelphia: Saunders.

Heath AC, Kendler KS, Eaves LJ, Martin N. 1990. Evidence for genetic influences on sleep disturbance and sleep pattern in twins. *Sleep* 13:318–335.

Redline S, Tishler PV. 1993. Familial influences on sleep apnea. In Saunders NA, Sullivan CE, eds. *Sleep and breathing.* 2d ed. New York: Marcel Dekker.

Susan Redline

HIBERNATION

The word *hibernation* derives from the Latin *hibernare,* meaning "to pass the winter." Any animal that spends the winter in a resting or dormant state can, in general usage, be described as hibernating. Physiologists, however, make a distinction between the continuous winter dormancy of *ectotherms* (animals that cannot use metabolic heat production to sustain a temperature differential between their bodies and the environment) and the recurring bouts of seasonal torpor used by *endotherms* (animals that can maintain a high and constant body temperature by means of metabolic heat production). In strict usage, hibernation is recurring, regulated, multiday episodes of reduced metabolism and body temperature—an adaptation used by some species of endotherms to survive seasonal cold and food scarcity (see THERMOREGULATION).

Many species of mammals hibernate, but only one species of bird, the poorwill, is a confirmed hibernator. The mammalian hibernators are scattered among a number of families that also include species that do not hibernate. This pattern suggests that hibernation is a suite of physiologic and behavioral adaptations that have evolved independently a number of times. In all cases, however, hibernation occurs seasonally in antiphase with the reproductive season.

Animals prepare for hibernation by fattening, caching food, and usually preparing a hibernaculum—a nest in which the animal hibernates. During the hibernation season, the animal cycles through bouts of torpor punctuated by spontaneous arousals to periods of *euthermia* (normal body temperature) that may last a few hours to a day or more. Initial bouts in hibernation season may be short, a few hours to a day, and then lengthen to reach a maximal duration of a week or more. Toward the end of the hibernation season, bouts again shorten until a final arousal marks the end of hibernation and the onset of the reproductive season.

Physiologically, a bout of hibernation is characterized by a cessation of cold-induced heat production so that metabolic rate decreases to basal levels (Figure 1). Body temperature then begins to decrease as heat loss exceeds heat production. As body temperature decreases, so does metabolic rate, until the animal comes into a new thermal equilibrium usually within a degree of environmental temperature. Metabolic rate in deep hibernation may be one-thirtieth to one-fiftieth of the basal metabolic rate. Arousals are marked by dramatic increases in metabolic heat production that return body temperature to normal levels. If these complex physiologic adaptations evolved independently a number of times, they probably arose from preadaptations common to all endotherms. Those preadaptations were most likely physiologic adjustments associated with NREM sleep.

During NREM sleep, body temperature is regulated at a slightly lower level than during wakefulness. Hypothalamic regulation of body temperature is severely inhibited during REM sleep. Electroencephalo-, electrooculo-, and electromyographic recordings of ground squirrels entering hibernation show that they enter hibernation

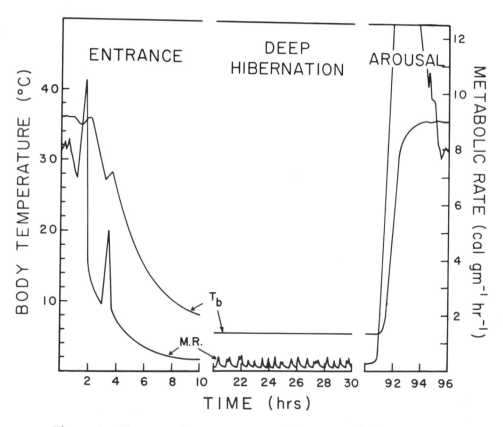

Figure 1. Changes in body temperature (T$_b$) and metabolic rate (M.R.) during a bout of hibernation.

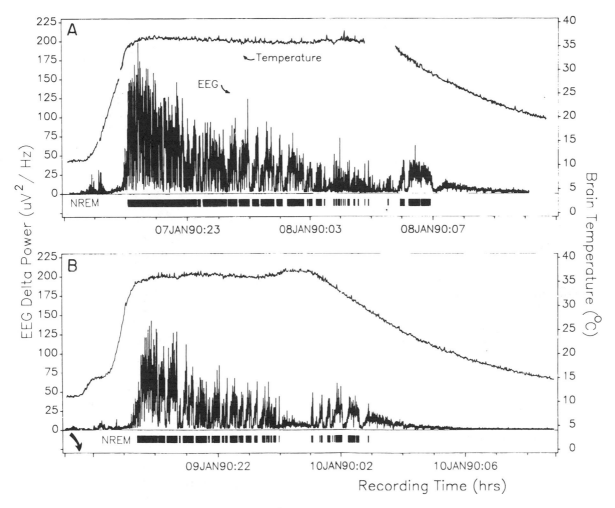

Figure 2. Recordings of brain temperature and electroencephalographic delta power during hibernation, euthermia, and reentry into hibernation obtained from one ground squirrel after a long bout (A, 4.25 days) and a short bout (B, 1.5 days) of hibernation.

mostly through NREM sleep, with the occurrence of REM sleep decreasing to virtually zero by the time body temperature reaches 25°C. Manipulations of hypothalamic temperature, the major feedback signal in the regulation of body temperature, show that the set point for metabolic heat production gradually declines as the animal enters hibernation. The evolutionary hypothesis drawn from these various findings is that, in species exposed to seasonal cold and food scarcity, hibernation could have evolved by a natural selection that favors a decrease in regulated body temperature during NREM sleep because of the resulting energy conservation.

Biologic rhythms play important roles in hibernation. Many species of hibernators have been shown to have circannual rhythms of hiberna-

tion, reproduction, fattening, and food storage. Under constant environmental conditions in the laboratory the seasonal changes in the physiology and behavior of these animals continues to cycle with an endogenous periodicity of usually less than 1 year. Hibernators have normal CIRCADIAN RHYTHMS when they are euthermic. Their circadian clocks continue to run during hibernation with a temperature-compensated free-running periodicity. In other words, their circadian clocks can still accurately tell time even at the reduced temperatures experienced during hibernation. The circadian system appears to time the arousals from multiday bouts of torpor.

If a bout of hibernation is a multiday period of mostly NREM sleep, what causes this condition of HYPERSOMNIA? Does a bout of hibernation end when the animal is sleep satiated? Currently, it is not known what causes the extreme hypersomnia of hibernators, but the animal arousing from a bout of hibernation is not sleep satiated and, in fact, appears to be sleep deprived. The high spectral power of the electroencephalogram (EEG) in the delta band characteristic of deep NREM sleep is most pronounced immediately after arousal from a bout of hibernation, and the longer the preceding hibernation bout, the greater is the EEG delta power on arousal (Figure 2). The animal is mostly asleep during the euthermic period between bouts, and the EEG delta power during this time decreases until just before the entrance into the next bout. At the time of entrance, there is a relatively small increase in EEG delta power. The conclusion is that hibernators achieve great savings of metabolic energy by an exaggerated lowering of body temperature during NREM sleep and by a hypersomnia that increases the amount of NREM sleep. The low body temperature during a bout of hibernation, however, seems to inhibit the restorative properties of NREM sleep as reflected by EEG delta power (an index of the intensity of NREM sleep). It is conceivable that the characteristic periodic arousals from hibernation are driven by sleep need. Hibernators are thus proving to be a valuable model for sleep research.

REFERENCES

Krilowicz BL, Glotzbach SF, Heller HC. 1988. Neuronal activity during sleep and complete bouts of hibernation. *Am J Physiol* 255:R1008–R1019.

Lyman CP, Willis JS, Malan A, Wang LCH. 1982. *Hibernation and torpor in mammals and birds.* New York: Academic Press.

Trachsel L, Edgar DM, Heller HC. 1991. Are ground squirrels sleep deprived during hibernation? *Am J Physiol* 260:R1123–R1129.

H. Craig Heller

HIPPOCAMPAL THETA

During REM sleep, the hippocampus generates a remarkably regular rhythm of electrical activity.

This rhythm has a frequency of about 7 cycles per second and is referred to as hippocampal theta activity, or rhythmic slow activity. In rodents, theta activity is easily observed because it dominates the cortical ELECTROENCEPHALOGRAM (EEG) (see Figure 1) and is used to define REM sleep. In cats, its detection requires deep electrodes. In primates, the hippocampal theta rhythm has been very difficult to detect at all.

Neuroanatomical Basis

Theta activity arises when the firing patterns of individual nerve cells in the hippocampus are synchronized such that their synaptic potentials add together. Populations of neurons giving rise to theta activity are located in three distinct regions of the hippocampus: the entorhinal cortex, the dentate gyrus, and CA1. Synchronization of these neurons depends on input from the medial septal nucleus, although it is not certain whether the input itself must be rhythmic or whether septal input merely activates a rhythm intrinsic to the hippocampus. The ultimate trigger probably involves cells of the pontine reticular formation, where stimulation can induce a coordinated response involving not only hippocampal theta but also cortical desynchrony and muscle ATONIA, which together define the state of REM sleep (see REM SLEEP, PHYSIOLOGY OF).

Pharmacology

Drugs such as atropine that block cholinergic input from the septum only partly suppress theta activity. Theta activity normally occurs throughout REM sleep, during both tonic muscle suppression (atonia) and phasic muscle twitches. Atropine suppresses only the subset of theta activity that occurs during atonia. Thus, there are two different types of theta activity: one atropine-sensitive and associated with atonia, the other atropine-resistant and associated with phasic motor activation. The second form of theta activity may depend on serotonergic input from the raphe nucleus.

REM SLEEP

ECoG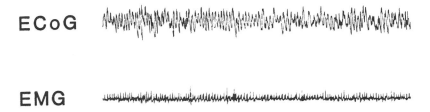

EMG

THETA-DOMINATED WAKE

ECoG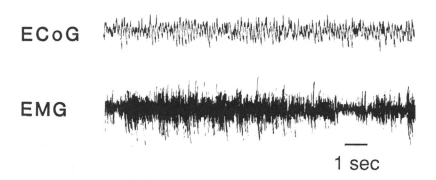

EMG

1 sec

Figure 1. Recordings of an electrocorticogram (ECoG) and electromyogram (EMG) from a mouse during REM sleep (above) and during active wakefulness (below). Both records illustrate hippocampal theta activity at 7 cycles per second.

Waking Theta Activity

Hippocampal theta activity also occurs prominently during active wakefulness. In rodents, the presence of theta activity in the EEG makes REM sleep and active wakefulness difficult to distinguish by EEG criteria alone (see Figure 1). Both atropine-sensitive and atropine-resistant forms of theta activity occur during wakefulness, just as during REM sleep. Atropine-sensitive theta occurs during alert immobility, whereas atropine-resistant theta occurs during certain motor behaviors such as head movement, rearing, walk-

ing, and running. More stereotypical behaviors, such as feeding or grooming, are not associated with theta activity.

It might seem peculiar that hippocampal theta activity is associated with behaviors as different as REM sleep and running. But REM sleep and active wakefulness are closely related in a physiologic sense. In addition to the presence of hippocampal theta, both behavioral states are characterized by rapid eye movements, PGO spikes (see PGO WAVES), high brain temperature, and high neuronal activity in the pontine reticular formation. Furthermore, cats that have lost motor inhibition during REM sleep as a result of pontine lesions exhibit such behaviors as head movement, orienting, walking, and even "attack" or "rage" behavior during REM sleep. Such observations have given rise to the popular description that REM sleep represents an "active brain in a paralyzed body" (see ANIMAL'S DREAMS).

Function

The functional significance of hippocampal theta activity is unclear. Hippocampal damage often results in learning and memory impairments. Lesions of the septum, which suppress hippocampal theta activity without damaging the hippocampus, can produce similar impairments, suggesting a possible role for theta activity in learning. In addition, electrical stimulation of the hippocampus most effectively induces long-term synaptic changes when delivered at frequencies in the theta range, especially when in phase with endogenous theta activity. On the basis of such findings, Winson (1990) has suggested that hippocampal theta activity is instrumental for storage of memories during wakefulness, and for strengthening or reprocessing of those memories during REM sleep. Nevertheless, it remains possible that theta activity is merely an easily observable but incidental reflection of a more fundamental process of arousal, attention, or learning (see LEARNING; MEMORY).

REFERENCES

Robinson TE. 1980. Hippocampal rhythmic slow activity (RSA; theta): A critical analysis of selected studies and discussion of possible species differences. *Brain Res Rev* 2:69–101.

Siegel JM. 1989. Brainstem mechanisms generating REM sleep. In Kryger MH, Roth T, Dement WC, eds. *Principles and practice of sleep medicine*, pp. 104–120. Philadelphia: W.B. Saunders.

Stewart M, Fox SE. 1990. Do septal neurons pace the hippocampal theta rhythm? *Trends Neurosci* 13(5):163–168.

Winson J. 1990. The meaning of dreams. *Sci Am* 263(5):86–96.

David K. Welsh

HISTAMINE

See Antihistamines; Chemistry of Sleep: Amines and Other Transmitters

HIV

See AIDS and Sleep

HOMEOTHERMY

See Thermoregulation

HUMAN LEUKOCYTE ANTIGEN

The major histocompatibility complex (MHC) refers to a group of genes found on the short arm on chromosome 6. The products of these genes (the specific protein or polypeptide molecules, frequently enzymes, which depend on the presence of a gene) are present on cell surfaces, expressed as antigens (substances capable of inducing a specific immune response and of reacting with the products of that response), or circulate in the blood. Cells bearing MHC antigens play a major role in self recognition by the immune system and determine if there will be rejection of a transplant or tissue graft. Much of our knowledge of MHC, immunity, and transplantation comes from the analogous H-2 gene complex in mice. In humans, because products of MHC genes are expressed on cell surfaces, including leukocytes (white blood cells or corpuscles), this system is sometimes referred to as the human leukocyte antigen (HLA) system.

Three classes of gene product (called classes I, II, and III) are encoded within a small region of the MHC consisting of three closely linked areas or loci (HLA-A,-B,-C) and one, more remote region (HLA-D region) (Figure 1). By nature of their different molecular structures and biological functions, HLA antigens are divided into two categories: (1) class I (HLA-A,-B,-C) and (2) class II (HLA-D,-DR,-DQ,-DP) (Figure 2). Class I molecules, glycoproteins, are found on all cell

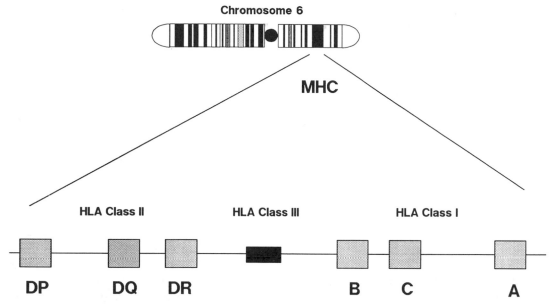

Figure 1. Location of major histocompatibility complex (MHC) on the short arm of chromosome 6. The relative relationship of the HLA genes is outlined. The genes for class III proteins of the complement system are between the HLA-A, -B, -C region and the HLA-D region.

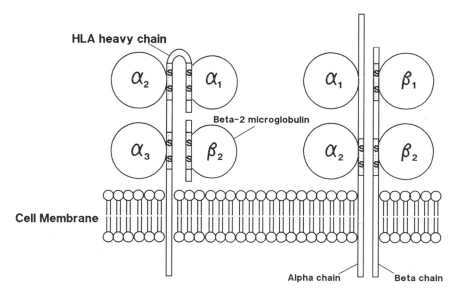

Figure 2. MHC class I molecules consist of two polypeptide chains held together noncovalently. The polypeptide heavy chain is glycosylated (has sugar/carbohydrate molecules attached) and has three regions designated α_1, α_2, and α_3. It traverses the cell membrane while the smaller protein chain (known as and β_2-microglobulin) remains entirely outside of the cell. MHC class II molecules consist of two glycosylated polypeptide chains both of which extend through the cell membrane. Areas of disulfide bonds are indicated by an "S" within a stippled box.

types except red blood cells and trophoblasts (embryonic cells that have not yet differentiated). Some cells (striated muscle and liver cells) express their class I molecules only during times of inflammation. Class I molecules are composed of two polypeptide chains. Class II molecules, also glycoproteins, are restricted to certain cells involved with the immune response (e.g., B lymphocytes, some monocytes, activated T lymphocytes).

Class III molecules are components of the complement system, a series of enzymes made in the liver and involved in immune response. These molecules are not expressed on cell surfaces but can bind to cell surfaces as part of the immune response. Class I and II molecules are involved with the presentation of antigens or peptides from intracellular protein breakdown to T lymphocytes and other cells involved in the immune response. Because HLA antigens represent a portion of a person's genetic makeup and because certain conditions appear to have a hereditary basis, it is not surprising that many diseases are positively associated with certain HLA antigens. The highest association to date is with HLA-DRw15 (previously called HLA-DR2) and narcolepsy, a disorder of excessive daytime sleepiness (see NARCOLEPSY). In this disorder, more than 98 percent of white, Caucasian narcoleptics express DRw15. In other sleep disorders, such as idiopathic central nervous system hypersomnolence, the B27, Cw2, and DR5 antigens are present five to eight times more commonly than in controls. Certain HLA-associated diseases have an autoimmune or inflammatory nature, but there is no evidence in narcolepsy or other sleep disorders for autoimmune dysfunction; however, B lymphocytes of HLA-DRw15,-DQw6 narcoleptics show altered binding to muramyl peptides (see SLEEP-PROMOTING SUBSTANCES), and this suggests that the effect of the DRw15 gene (or another closely linked gene) is to modify the presentation and/or metabolism of neurotransmitters important for sleep (see also CANINE NARCOLEPSY).

REFERENCES

Carpenter CB, David J. 1991. Histocompatibility antigens and immune response genes. *Sci Am* (Med) 6:1–10.
Silverman DH, Sayegh MH, Alvarez CE, Johnson TS, et al. 1990. HLA class II restricted binding of muramyl peptides to B lymphocytes of normal and narcoleptic subjects. *Hum Immunol* 27:145–154.

Charles F. P. George

HYPERNYCHTHEMERAL SYNDROME

Imagine that you went to bed at the same time every night, but it took an extra hour each night to go to sleep. After a week or so, if you continued to get up at the same time every morning despite the increasing lack of sleep, you would have a night with no sleep at all. You would also be very sleepy in the daytime. If you had the opportunity, you might just sleep through the morning. But what if this process continued so that sleep onset continued to delay by an hour or so each day—as if your sleep were traveling west around the world while you were stuck at home? If you decided to keep up with your sleep's westward travel by only going to bed when you became sleepy, you would go to bed later each day and also get up about an hour later. After about 3 weeks, you would again sleep at your usual home time zone hours. But if this process continued, you would sleep "at home" or close to it (in time) only for a few nights each month. You would have to choose between getting enough sleep and getting to school, work, movies, or parties on time on most days of the month. If you tried to follow a regular schedule for bedtime and getting up, you would again find yourself lying awake for more and more hours each night.

The sleep disorder just described is known as the non-24-hour sleep–wake syndrome or the *hypernychthemeral syndrome,* the latter meaning "more than a day and night," that is, more than 24 hours. Although this condition is uncommon, many cases are reported in the medical studies on sleep. In this condition, sleep onset and wake times occur about every 25 hours, and occasional noncircadian (longer than 27 hours) sleep–wake cycles occur from time to time, some lasting more than 40 hours. This is similar to the sleep–wake behavior of people who have participated in human time-isolation experiments, which have been conducted in caves and special laboratories since about 1960. The experiments have revealed that when humans have no access to clocks, television, radio or the light–dark cycle outside, they usually decide to go to sleep and get up about every 25 hours. In some cases, much longer sleep–wake cycle lengths, up to 52 hours, have occurred, a phenomenon called INTERNAL DESYNCHRONIZATION. Patients with the non-24 hour syndrome behave similarly in their sleeping behavior, but while they are living in the "normal" world and not in a laboratory or cave. Their body clocks apparently ignore the everyday social and environmental (light) time cues that serve to synchronize most of us to the 24-hour rotation of the earth. Over long periods of time, the non-24-hour patient may alternate between being symptomatic and asymptomatic, depending on the relative synchrony between the internal (25-hour) biological rhythm and the 24-hour world (see FREE-RUNNING; ZEITGEBERS).

This condition has been observed most often in blind individuals (see BLINDNESS: EFFECTS ON SLEEP PATTERNS AND CIRCADIAN RHYTHMS), but a few patients with intact vision have been described as well. Many of these individuals abandon trying to synchronize their sleep to conventional hours. Others persistently attempt to sleep and get up at conventional social times. Their persistence is rewarded with progressively less sleep and secondary daytime sleepiness that interferes with daytime functioning. The prevalence of the syndrome in the blind population is unknown, but one survey of blind individuals (Miles and Wilson, 1977) showed a high incidence of sleep–wake complaints, and 40 percent had recognized a cyclic pattern to their symptoms. One sighted patient was later discovered to have a large tumor of his PITUITARY GLAND involving the optic chiasm, the part of the visual system where some of the nerve fibers from each eye cross to the other side of the brain. The chiasm is also where some nerve fibers enter the SUPRACHIAS-MATIC ("above the chiasm") NUCLEUS OF THE HYPO-THALAMUS, which is now generally accepted as the site of the body clock in mammals. Light signals traveling through this pathway are thought to be one of the major ways that the body clock is reset each morning. The absence of the daily light time cue in blind individuals probably underlies their difficulty in synchronizing their sleep to the 24-hour environment.

Some blind individuals with this problem may respond to strict 24-hour social scheduling of their lives, but there has been no clear demonstration that this is true. Avoidant or schizoidal personality characteristics may underlie the syndrome in some of the few sighted individuals who have had it. Vitamin B_{12} in pill form helped alleviate the condition in three reported cases, and bright light (sunlight) exposure in the morning was added in one (sighted) patient to help move the patient's sleep back into the nighttime hours. Obviously, light would not be useful in blind patients with this sleep disorder (see LIGHT THERAPY).

REFERENCES

Miles LE, Wilson MA. 1977. High incidence of cyclic sleep-wake disorders in the blind. *Sleep Res* 6:192.
Wagner DR. 1990. Circadian rhythm sleep disorders. In Thorpy MJ, ed. *Handbook of sleep disorders,* pp 493–527. New York: Marcel Dekker.

Daniel R. Wagner

HYPERSOMNIA

Hypersomnia literally means "sleeping too long." In the field of sleep medicine, however, *hypersomnia* is used interchangeably with *excessive daytime sleepiness* (see SLEEPINESS). These terms are used to refer to patients who complain of sleeping too much, being sleepy during the day, or being unable to stay awake during the day. The prevalence of excessive sleepiness or hypersomnia has been reported to be between 3.8 and 5.0 percent of the population in studies from several different countries. The exact rate found depends on the nature of the questions used to elicit the complaint. It is generally thought that the actual prevalence rate is higher than reported because individuals who are chronically sleepy often perceive themselves as being normal. Several studies have shown that there exists a group of patients who are objectively sleepy, yet deny hypersomnolence or excessive sleepiness.

There is no question that excessive sleepiness is associated with morbidity (see LONGEVITY). Patients with disorders of daytime sleepiness have been reported to have higher rates of automobile accidents, unemployment, and neuropsychological deficits as well as social and personality problems. Most if not all of these impairments are reversed when the condition causing the sleepiness is treated.

The sleep clinician has two major responsibilities in evaluating patients with excessive sleepiness: to determine the cause of the sleepiness and to determine the severity of the sleepiness. The primary tools used to make these determinations are nocturnal POLYSOMNOGRAPHY and the MULTIPLE SLEEP LATENCY TEST (MSLT). On the MSLT, patients with severe excessive sleepiness fall asleep within 5 minutes when they are put in a sleep-conducive environment several times in the course of the day. In other studies, 24-hour AMBULATORY MONITORING has been used to evaluate these patients. The assumption is that patients with hypersomnia will sleep longer, nap more frequently, and have more microsleeps (see MICROSLEEP) than the general population.

Four principal causes of sleepiness have been identified in patients. First, the patient may be sleepy because of drug use. Many drugs (e.g., TRANQUILIZERS, ANTIHISTAMINES) make people sleepy. Similarly, withdrawal from STIMULANTS (e.g., CAFFEINE, COCAINE, OVER-THE-COUNTER STIMULANTS) also can cause sleepiness. CIRCADIAN RHYTHM DISORDERS cause sleepiness; it is not uncommon for shiftworkers, or people experiencing JET LAG, to fall asleep at inappropriate times. Third, sleep DEPRIVATION or sleep FRAGMENTATION makes patients sleepy. Sleep APNEA causes patients to awaken frequently to resume breathing, hence fragmenting their sleep—this is the most common cause of sleepiness seen in medical practice. Sleep fragmentation can also be caused by periodic leg movements or other nocturnal PARASOMNIAS (see EPILEPSY, REM SLEEP BEHAVIOR DISORDER, PERIODIC LEG MOVEMENTS). Finally, sleepiness can result from disorders of the CENTRAL NERVOUS SYSTEM (CNS). The two most common CNS disorders causing sleepiness are NARCOLEPSY and idiopathic hypersomnia syndrome. The former syndrome has its onset most commonly during the second decade of life. Hypersomnolence may be related to an infectious agent such as Epstein–Barr virus, ECHO virus, or hepatitis. In other instances, hypersomnia develops following a bout of infectious MONONUCLEOSIS, atypical pneumonia, hepatitis, or aseptic meningitis. It is very similar to the hypersomnia seen secondary to ENCEPHALITIS or to hydrocephalus. In many cases of idiopathic hypersomnia, however, no causal relationship can be found. A subgroup of patients with isolated hypersomnia may have a specific HUMAN LEUKOCYTE ANTIGEN (HLA) typing, but this finding has not yet been replicated. A familial element may also exist in certain cases. The different known causes of daytime sleepiness must be considered and ruled out before a diagnosis of idiopathic hypersomnia can be made; such assessments are most effectively performed at SLEEP DISORDERS CENTERS.

Therapeutic approaches to hypersomnia or excessive sleepiness range from treating the underlying condition to using stimulants to manage the daytime sleepiness symptomatically. In the case of sleep apnea, treatments are directed at reversing the respiratory abnormalities and preventing sleep fragmentation. In other cases of sleep fragmentation, medications are used to prevent frequent arousals during the night. Finally, idiopathic hypersomnia and narcolepsy are treated with stimulant medications.

Christian Guilleminault
Thomas Roth

HYPNAGOGIC HALLUCINATIONS

Hallucinations occurring at the interface between wakefulness and sleep are referred to as *hypnagogic* when they occur at the onset of sleep and *hypnopompic* when they occur at the end of sleep. The hallucinations have a dreamlike quality, but they differ from dreams because of the lack of full participation of the subject and the absence of a theme or story. Hallucinations of this type constitute one of the four classical symptoms of NARCOLEPSY and can also occur in persons without narcolepsy. During the hallucinations, the subject is not fully asleep and often remains aware of being in bed or lying down.

The hallucinations almost always include visual imagery, and auditory components are also common; tactile and olfactory elements are less frequent but can occur. The visual images may be simple forms such as floating circles or lights or may be complex hallucinations of landscapes or animals. Auditory hallucinations also may be simple repetitive sounds or complex musical themes. One patient reported, "I hear a scratched record which plays the same sentence over and over" (Ribstein, 1975). Multiple sensory modalities may be involved as in a patient who felt the fur of animals and heard their chirping sounds as they ran over his body (Daniels, 1934). There may be a sensation of weightlessness, falling, or loss of balance. Body parts may be transformed or there may be a hallucination of movement associated with sleep paralysis: "I move quickly to get up and turn out the light, but then I realize that I have not moved at all and that, in fact, I am unable to move" (Ribstein, 1975).

Images from the previous few hours or days may be revisualized, and sometimes hallucinations recur night after night. The experiences may be pleasant and relaxing, or they may be terrifying. Sometimes the hallucinations are so vivid and realistic that the subject may have difficulty believing they are not real and may take actions to escape from the images or to block them from sight by closing windows or barricading doors.

Hallucinations are divided into "release" hallucinations, implying the release of visual systems from a normal inhibitory mechanism, and "irritative" hallucinations, implying an irritative process such as epilepsy that activates visual systems in an abnormal fashion. Studies of hypnagogic hallucinations in persons with narcolepsy have demonstrated that they often occur just as the subject is passing from wakefulness to REM sleep or vice versa. It seems likely that the hallucinations represent an intrusion of REM sleep imagery into consciousness during the transition from one state to the other and thus are an example of release hallucinations that occur as a result of defective inhibition during wakefulness of the systems responsible for REM sleep imagery.

REFERENCES

Daniels LE. 1934. Narcolepsy. *Medicine* 13:1–122.
Ribstein M. 1975. Hypnagogic hallucinations. In Guilleminault C, Dement WC, Passouant P, eds. *Narcolepsy*, pp 145–160. New York: Spectrum.

Michael Aldrich

HYPNAGOGIC REVERIE

The hypnagogic (hypnogogic) state is the transitional state from wakefulness to sleep. It is sometimes called the sleep-onset state. Subjectively the state is an orderly sequence of stages from awake but drowsy through drifting off to sleep to light sleep. The subjective sequence is paralleled by a sequence of brain wave patterns, with either rapid or slow eye movements. This parallel brain wave sequence ranges from a continuous alpha pattern with rapid eye movements (REM) through an alpha pattern with slow eye movements (SEM) through stage 1 sleep to early stage 2 sleep (see SLEEP ONSET; STAGES OF SLEEP).

Individuals differ in the correspondence between the subjective stages and brain wave stages of sleep onset. In healthy humans who are good sleepers, sleep onset usually occupies about 5 to 10 minutes. Arousals made from the hypnagogic state almost always produce reports of prearousal mental activity. In one study (Foulkes and Vogel, 1965), percentages of arousals with mental content from sleep onset stages were as follows: alpha REM, 96 percent; alpha SEM, 98 percent; stage 1, 98 percent; stage 2, 90 percent. In contrast, 83 percent of REM sleep arousals resulted in recalled content. The length of the mental content report as measured by word count was the same in hypnagogic reports and REM sleep reports.

Hypnagogic mental activity is not simply meaningless flashes of light or an isolated image. Rather, the content is usually a meaningful and dramatic visual sequence that forms a story or part of a story. At the beginning of sleep onset, the subject is aware that he or she is in the laboratory and has some control over the course of mental activity. Later in sleep onset, subjects lose control over their mental activity and become unaware of their location. Finally, subjects begin to dream; that is, they believe that what is going through their minds is really happening in the external world. Individuals differ in the match between this sequence of mental changes and the sequence of brain wave changes. Nevertheless, the hypnagogic dreams are like REM sleep dreams. Specifically, hypnagogic and REM sleep dreams are indistinguishable in terms of bizarreness and in terms of aggressive, sexual, and pleasurable content. The significance of this finding is that REM sleep is not, as originally thought, the only state during which frequent dreaming occurs. Dream investigators and dream theories must take into account both REM sleep and hypnagogic dreaming.

REFERENCES

Foulkes D, Vogel G. 1965. Mental activity of sleep onset. *J Abnorm Psychol* 70:231–234.

Vogel G. 1991. Sleep onset mentation. In Arkin AM, Antrobus JS, Ellman SJ, eds. *The mind in sleep: Psychology and psychophysiology,* 2nd ed. pp. 125–142. New York: Wiley.

Gerald W. Vogel

HYPNIC JERKS

Hypnic jerks are sudden, spontaneous jerks of part or all of the body (usually the legs) that occur during the drowsy period or during light sleep. Usually they occur infrequently; a few, scattered hypnic jerks are part of normal sleep, and especially sleep onset and REM sleep. In cases of greater frequency they are often a source of anxiety and complaint. They are occasionally accompanied by hallucinations. Polygraphic recordings of the subject will demonstrate leg movement with artifacts that can obscure the entire recording. Hypnic jerks occurring during stage 1 NREM sleep have been associated in reports with a poorly formed K-COMPLEX (a specific EEG wave which frequently occurs in response to a discrete stimulus or momentary activation of the sleeper); however, the jerks may be seen during clear alpha EEG frequencies or during persistent wakefulness. They are periodic; they may be brief (20 to 100 milliseconds) and involve upper, lower, or combined extremity movement, or may last longer (> 1 second) and involve other muscle groups. Hypnic jerks are more likely to occur when sleep has been disrupted or curtailed.

Hypnic jerks can be violent, and it is in these cases that consultation is usually sought. Reassurance about the benignity of the phenomenon allows the subjects to withstand the events, even if jerks recur frequently. Hypnic jerks are nonepileptic. They are also distinct from periodic leg movements, which are bursts of anterior tibialis muscle activity with a duration between onset and resolution of 0.5 to 5 seconds. Repetition occurs within 90 seconds of the previous burst.

Restless legs syndrome may be associated with leg movements at sleep onset and during sleep. This urge to move the legs is associated with an unpleasant but not painful sensation. "Painful legs and moving toes syndrome" is a syndrome characterized by pain in one or both feet, with or without a sensation of burning, and involuntary movements of the toes. These movements are irregular and unrelated to the sleep–wake cycle. These disorders are distinct from hypnic jerks.

REFERENCES

Broughton R. 1986. Pathological fragmentary myoclonus, intensified hypnic jerks and hypnagogic foot tremor: Three unusual sleep-related movement disorders. In Koella P, Obal F, Schulz H, Visser P, eds. *Sleep 86,* pp 240–243. New York: Fischer Verlag.

Gastaut H, Broughton RA. 1965. A clinical and polygraphic study of episodic phenomena during sleep. *Recent Adv Biol Psych* 7:197–221.

Oswald I. 1959. Sudden bodily jerks on falling asleep. *Brain* 82:92–103.

Christian Guilleminault

HYPNIC MYOCLONIA

See Hypnic Jerks

HYPNOSIS AND DREAMING

People have long wondered about the similarities between hypnosis and sleep, and it is interesting to note that the term *hypnosis* itself is derived from the Greek word for sleep. Nevertheless, even though the two conditions are similar in the sense that both can be regarded as altered states of consciousness, they are not the same. During hypnotic trance, for example, the electroencephalographic (brain wave) patterns are those of waking, not of sleep.

It is possible, however, to influence nocturnal dream content by means of hypnotic suggestions. Actually, dream content can be influenced in many ways, but the strongest method so far discovered has been the use of posthypnotic suggestion (Tart, 1988); that is, the dream content is suggested to the subject in a hypnotic trance prior to sleep. This method has demonstrated powerful effects, especially with persons of high hypnotic suggestibility (see CONTENT OF DREAMS).

During the first quarter of the twentieth century, several pioneering psychoanalysts began exploring posthypnotically suggested dreams in patients undergoing psychoanalytic therapy (see Rapaport, 1951). These clinicians reported that patients dreamed about suggested topics, primarily sexual ones, in the manner that had been predicted from psychoanalytic theory. Specifically, the suggested material was (symbolically) transformed in ways that were consistent with Freudian theories of dream formation (Rapaport, 1951, pp. 249–253) (see FREUD'S DREAM THEORY).

The first study to investigate hypnotically suggested dreams with modern sleep laboratory techniques was carried out by Stoyva (1965). Subjects were selected for high hypnotic susceptibility and then, during a 20-minute trance period immediately before sleep, were given simple suggestions such as, "You will dream in every dream tonight of climbing a tree," or "You will dream in every dream tonight of rowing a boat." Awakenings from REM sleep periods showed the following:

1. Subjects dreamed about the suggested topic not only in the first REM sleep period of the night, but often in later REM periods as well.

2. About 50 percent of these highly hypnotizable individuals reported dreams in accordance with the suggested topic in nearly every REM sleep period (from 70 percent to 100 percent of awakenings).

3. These successive reports resembled variations on a theme. In each dream, the influence of the suggested topic was clearly visible, but the topic did not appear as a lump of obviously "foreign" material. Rather, it was smoothly and naturally woven into the content of the dream: The suggested material was contextually related to the nonsuggested part of the dream.

4. The influence of the suggested topic was also apparent in roughly one half the reports from NREM awakenings, although, as in other studies of the NREM awakenings, the overall incidence of recall was much less than in REM sleep. The fact that dreams in accordance with the suggestion were also reported from NREM sleep showed that subjects do not sharply discriminate between REM and NREM mental activity. At least in the subjects' experience, there was no absolute distinction between the two.

5. These posthypnotically induced dreams, however, did not support the Freudian theory of dream formation, in the sense that there were dramatic transformations or the topic was disguised and appeared in symbolic form. On the contrary, the presence of the suggested topic was fairly obvious from the manifest dream content. Tart (1988), who studied this particular issue more extensively, drew the same conclusion. Even when he used fairly unpleasant suggestions, which might have been expected to produce a greater degree of distortion, the hypnotically influenced dream content was fairly obvious. Thus, Tart's findings did not support the psychoanalytic view of dream formation.

6. Subjects who regularly dreamed about the suggested topic showed a significant reduction in REM sleep time on those nights when they had been given a hypnotic dream suggestion but were not awakened (Stoyva, 1965). The scientific reason for this curious reduction in REM sleep time is not known, but it may be part of a more general stress reaction, since it is now known that various stress and anxiety situations act to decrease REM sleep time.

The foregoing observations about posthypnotic dream content have been confirmed and expanded by Tart (1988) and others. Additional findings described by Tart include (1) the observation that suggested dreams occurring during the hypnotic trance period itself are not the same physiologically as those occurring during REM sleep; and (2) the observation that highly hypnotizable subjects are capable of incorporating a great many parts or elements of a suggested story into their subsequent dreams.

A methodological question has occasionally been raised as to whether posthypnotically suggested dreams are genuine dreams or simply a *fabrication* of the subject made up to please the experimenter. Perhaps these "dreams" are actually put together as the subject surfaces into wakefulness. According to this hypothesis, a long period of waking up should result in a longer dream report, since there is more time for the fabrication process to take place. A later study by Stoyva, however, showed the opposite effect: Rapid awakenings yields longer dream reports, whereas gradual awakenings produced short dream accounts (Stoyva and Budzynski, 1968). This result is consistent with the idea that the subjects were recalling genuine REM sleep dream experiences, rather than simply generating material during the awakening process.

It seems probable that the suggested dream will see further use in exploring hypotheses about hypnosis, imagery, and the process of dreaming.

REFERENCES

Rapaport D, ed. 1951. *Organization and pathology of thought*. New York: Columbia University Press. See especially papers by Schrötter, Nachmansohn, and Roffenstein.

Stoyva J. 1965. Posthypnotically suggested dreams and the sleep cycle. *Arch Gen Psychiatry* 12: 287–294.

Stoyva J, Budzynski T. 1968. The nocturnal hypnotic dream: Fact or fabrication? (Abstract) *Psychophysiology* 5:218.

Tart C. 1988. From spontaneous event to lucidity: A review of attempts to consciously control nocturnal dreaming. In Gackenbach J, LaBerge S, eds. *Conscious mind, sleeping brain,* pp. 67–103. New York: Plenum Press.

Johann Stoyva

HYPNOTICS

See Antihistamines; Barbiturates; Benzodiazepines; Chemistry of Sleep: L-tryptophan; Over-the-Counter Sleeping Pills; Sleeping Pills

HYPNOTOXIN THEORY OF SLEEP

See Chemistry of Sleep: Sleep Factors; Early Sleep Theories

HYPOPNEA

See Apnea

HYPOTHALAMUS

Interest in the hypothalamic regulation of sleep and waking dates to the early part of this century. In 1918, von Economo published observations on the victims of an ENCEPHALITIS epidemic in Austria. In those cases where excessive sleep was present, inflammatory lesions were found in posterior portions of the hypothalamus. Where insomnia was a prominent symptom, anterior hypothalamic disease was frequently observed. Based on these clinical–anatomic correlations, his hypothesis of a waking mechanism in the posterior hypothalamus and a sleep system in the anterior hypothalamus remains valid today.

Although small—only about 5 millimeters in front-to-back length in the rat—the hypothalamus possesses enormous anatomic, chemical, and functional complexity. It lies at the very base of the brain, directly over the pituitary gland and surrounding the fluid-filled third cerebral ventricle. The hypothalamus can be divided into smaller groups of neurons, called nuclei. The locations of the major cell groups in and around the hypothalamus of the rat are shown in Figure 1.

The hypothalamus can be divided into three zones: periventricular, medial, and lateral. The periventricular zone surrounds the third ventricle. The ventricles are a series of fluid-filled cavities that act as an auxiliary circulatory system for the brain. Most periventricular cell groups regulate the secretion of hormones from the pituitary gland. Some cells send long axons that travel to the pituitary gland and secrete hormones directly into the blood stream. Others secrete hormone-releasing factors, which travel to the pituitary gland in a specialized circulatory system connecting the hypothalamus and pituitary and, in turn, stimulate hormone release into the general circulation. One periventricular cell group, the SUPRACHIASMATIC NUCLEUS OF THE HYPOTHALAMUS, controls the timing of all the body's 24-hour, or circadian, rhythms (see CIRCADIAN RHYTHMS).

The medial zone consists of several large (by hypothalamic standards) cell groups, such as the preoptic, anterior, ventromedial, and dorso-

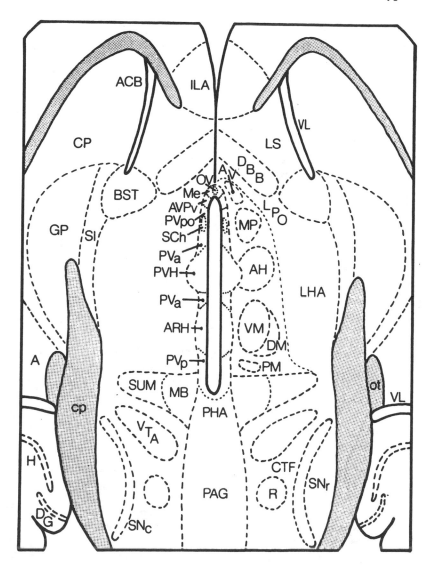

Figure 1. A drawing of the major cell groups in and around the hypothalamus of the rat brain, representing a horizontal cross-section with the front of the brain toward the top of the diagram. The hypothalamic tissue surrounds the third cerebral ventricle, which is shown as the thin elliptical structure in the exact center of the figure. A, amygdala; ACB, nucleus accumbens; AH, anterior hypothalamic nucleus; ARH, arcuate nucleus; AV, anteroventral preoptic nucleus; AVPv, anteroventral periventricular nucleus; BST, bed nucleus of stria terminalis; CP, caudoputamen; CTF, central tegmental field; DBB, nucleus of the diagonal bands; DG, dentate gyrus; DM, dorsomedial nucleus; GP, globus pallidus; H, hippocampus; ILA, infralimbic area; LHA, lateral hypothalamic area; LPO, lateral preoptic area; LS, lateral septal nucleus; MB, mammillary body; Me, median preoptic nucleus; MP, medial preoptic nucleus; OV, vascular organ of the lamina terminalis; PAG, periaqueductal gray; PHA, posterior hypothalamic area; PM, premammilary nucleus; PVa, anterior periventricular nucleus; PVp, posterior periventricular nucleus; PVpo, preoptic periventricular nucleus; PVH, periventricular nucleus; R, red nucleus; SCh, suprachiasmatic nucleus; SI, substantia innominata; SN_{c,r}, compact and reticular parts of the substantia nigra; SUM, supramammillary nucleus; VL, lateral ventricle; VM, ventromedial nucleus; VTA, ventral tegmental area; cp, cerebral peduncle; ot, optic tract. *Reproduced from Swanson, 1987, with permission.*

medial nuclei. These nuclei are involved in the regulation of physiologic functions, including blood pressure, heart rate, respiration, and body temperature. They also influence such important behaviors as feeding, drinking, sexual, and maternal behavior. In combination with the periventricular zone, the nuclei of the medial zone are of paramount importance in maintaining the constancy of the body's internal environment, a process named *homeostasis* by physiologist Walter B. Cannon. Nuclei of the medial zone also have extensive connections with structures of the limbic system, including the hippocampus and amygdala, among others. The limbic system is involved in the generation of emotions. Limbic system influences on the hypothalamus are thought to underlie the ability of emotional states to exert profound effects on the body's physiology.

The lateral zone of the hypothalamus is morphologically very different from the periventricular or medial zones. It contains many nerve fiber systems, both those ascending from the brainstem and those descending to the brainstem from the forebrain. Scattered among these fibers are the neurons of the lateral zone. Lateral cell groups participate in the control of feeding and in the perception of reward, or pleasure. Lateral cell groups that send axons directly to the neocortex have been identified, and some of these may participate in the control of cortical activation. The rostral lateral zone merges with the magnocellular BASAL FOREBRAIN, a region involved in both the control of arousal and NREM sleep.

Elucidation of hypothalamic mechanisms will be a key to understanding the neurobiology of sleep. Virtually all hypothalamic-regulated functions vary with sleep–waking state. State-dependent changes in blood pressure, hormone release, body temperature, etc., must involve changes in hypothalamic function. In fact, this relationship has been documented for the control of body temperature (see THERMOREGULATION). In addition, the hypothalamus itself is an organ of sleep–wake control. The suprachiasmatic nucleus regulates the timing of waking and sleep. The anterior hypothalamic nuclei exert NREM sleep–promoting actions that appear to be closely associated with the regulation of body temperature. The posterior hypothalamus is important for the maintenance of wakefulness. Contemporary evidence suggests that reciprocal interactions between anterior and posterior cell groups are involved in the generation of sleep–waking cycles, just as von Economo had hypothesized almost 70 years ago.

REFERENCES

Cannon WB. 1932. *The wisdom of the body.* New York: Norton.

Kupferman I. 1985. Hypothalamus and limbic system I: Peptidergic neurons, homeostasis and emotional behavior. In Kandel ER, Schwartz JH, eds. *Principles of Neural Science.* pp 611–625. New York: Elsevier.

Swanson LW. 1987. The hypothalamus. In Bjorkland A, Hokfelt T, Swanson LW, eds. *Handbook of chemical neuroanatomy,* Vol 5: *Integrated systems of the CNS,* pp 1–124. New York: Elsevier.

von Economo C. 1930. Sleep as a problem of localization. *J Nerv Ment Dis* 71:249–259.

Ronald Szymusiak

HYPOXIA

See Altitude; Apnea; Pressurization; Respiration Control in Sleep

I

ILLNESS

See Medical Illness and Sleep

IMAGERY IN DREAMS

See Content of Dreams; Hypnagogic Reverie

IMMUNE FUNCTION

Relationships between sleep and the immune system are suggested by the increased fatigue and sleep that often accompany infectious illnesses. In addition, it has long been suspected that sleep is important for optimal functioning of the immune system and therefore loss of sleep may result in increased susceptibility to infection. (See also INFECTION.)

The immune system functions through lymphocytes, which are white blood cells with specific receptors on their surfaces that recognize and bind to foreign substances (antigens). Lymphocytes circulate between the lymphoid organs and the blood and tissues, where they recognize and bind to such antigens. Two general types of immune responses are known. One response is that of B-lymphocytes, which produce antibodies—proteins that bind to antigens. Cell-mediated responses are carried out by T-lymphocytes and include cytotoxic reactions (killing another cell) as well as recruitment of other inflammatory cells. Immune responses re-

quire the participation of several interacting cell types, including lymphocytes and antigen-presenting cells such as macrophages, which communicate to each other with specialized molecules called cytokines. In addition to their involvement in immune responses, cytokines have a number of other biological activities, including effects on the central nervous system (Plata-Salaman, 1991). Conversely, neurotransmitters and neuroendocrine systems are able to influence immune function, suggesting bidirectional communication between the immune and nervous systems.

Studies of effects of sleep on the immune system and vice versa have also provided evidence for immune–nervous system interactions. Several cytokines have sleep-promoting effects, most notably interleukin-1 (IL-1) (Borbely and Tobler 1989; Krueger et al., 1990). IL-1 is primarily produced by macrophages (antigen-presenting white blood cells) during an immune response, and its major function is to activate lymphocytes. Glial cells (nonneuronal support cells) in the central nervous system are also capable of synthesizing IL-1, and IL-1 receptors have been found in many areas of the brain, including the hypothalamus, hippocampus, and brainstem. Experimental administration of IL-1 into the central nervous system induces NREM sleep in rats, cats, rabbits, and primates. Furthermore, it has been postulated that the sleep-promoting effects of muramyl peptides derived from bacterial cell walls may be mediated by IL-1, since these peptides induce IL-1 production. (See CHEMISTRY OF SLEEP: PEPTIDES and SLEEP FACTORS.)

One possible mechanism by which IL-1 induces sleep is through its effects on temperature regulation. IL-1 increases heat production and decreases heat loss in rats by inducing prostaglandin release in the preoptic area of the hypothalamus. IL-1 has potent fever-producing effects in other mammalian species as well. Increased brain and/or body temperature is known to enhance NREM sleep. IL-1 may also act directly on neural systems controlling NREM sleep, since NREM is also increased by the co-administration of IL-1 and antipyretics (compounds that reduce fever) (Krueger et al., 1984; see also HYPOTHALAMUS).

A number of other macrophage and lymphocyte products also increase temperature and NREM sleep. Tumor necrosis factor (TNF), a mediator of inflammation released by macrophages in response to endotoxin (from cell walls of gram-negative bacteria), can increase body temperature by direct effects in the preoptic area of the hypothalamus as well as by stimulating IL-1 production. TNF administration also results in NREM sleep enhancement and REM sleep inhibition. Interferons (IFNs), antiviral proteins produced by lymphocytes and macrophages, can induce IL-1 production as well. Administration of IFN also increases fever and NREM sleep. (See also BODY TEMPERATURE; THERMOREGULATION.)

In addition to the effects of centrally or peripherally administered cytokines on sleep discussed above, induction of immune responses by pathogens also appears to cause increased NREM sleep and fever. For example, rabbits challenged with bacteria capable of stimulating the immune system showed significant increases in temperature and sleep (Toth and Krueger, 1988). Further evidence of a role for the immune system in regulating sleep is the observation that plasma levels of IL-1 and interleukin-2 (IL-2) increase during sleep in humans (Moldofsky et al., 1986).

In addition, lymphocyte proliferation in response to mitogens, nonspecific stimulators of lymphocyte cell division, increases during sleep. Although all these studies show relationships among sleep and components of immune responses, they do not prove specifically that immune function is facilitated by sleep; rather, the hypothesis that sleep may enhance immune function has been tested primarily by assessing the effects of sleep deprivation on immune function.

Results from such studies in humans have been equivocal. Short-term sleep deprivation accompanied by a stressor resulted in increased production of IFN and slightly decreased phagocytic activity by lymphocytes early in the sleep deprivation/stress period (Palmblad et al., 1976). In this study, it was not clear whether the changes resulted from the sleep loss, the stress, or both. In another study, sleep deprivation alone caused mitogen-induced lymphocyte proliferation to decrease significantly, although not below the normal range (Palmblad et al., 1979). No changes in the activity of granulocytes, nonspecific mediators of inflammation, were observed. In a more recent study, Moldofsky and colleagues (1989) showed that 40 hours of sleep DEPRIVATION caused alterations in subjects' circadian patterns of immune function, including increased nocturnal IL-1 and IL-2 activities, delayed nocturnal increases in response to only one of several mitogens, and a decrease in natural killer cell activity that persisted during recovery sleep.

More extensive immune system challenges have been performed in sleep-deprived rodents (Benca et al., 1989). Prolonged deprivation of total sleep or REM sleep in rats inevitably leads to death. Lymphocytes obtained from sleep-deprived rats that were near death were tested in vitro for their ability to respond to primary antigen challenges and mitogens. No significant reductions were observed in either antibody production or lymphocyte proliferation in response to a variety of antigens. Furthermore, animals receiving an in vivo injection of antigens shortly before expiring from sleep deprivation also failed to show suppression of antibody responses. In addition, sleep-deprived rats do not die from infectious diseases, which suggests that significant suppression of the immune system is not the primary mechanism of death.

Studies of the effects of short-term sleep deprivation on immune function in mice and rats showed, however, that secondary immune responses (i.e., antibodies produced following repeated administrations of antigen) were somewhat reduced (Brown et al., 1989a). No significant suppression of primary immune responses (i.e., following the first exposure to antigen) were observed. When either IL-1 or muramyl peptide was coadministered with the antigen, however, sleep deprivation resulted in significantly increased antibody production (Brown et al., 1989b). (Both IL-1 and muramyl peptide were shown to have immunosuppressive effects when administered to non-sleep-deprived animals.)

Overall, these results indicate that sleep-related fluctuations in immune function may occur and that sleep deprivation may perturb some immune parameters. It is not yet clear, however, that sleep deprivation results in clinically significant immunosuppression.

REFERENCES

Benca RM, Kushida CA, Everson CA, Kalski R, Bergmann BM, Rechtschaffen A. 1989. Sleep deprivation in the rat: VII. Immune function. *Sleep* 12:47–52.

Borbely AA, Tobler I. 1989. Endogenous sleep-promoting substances and sleep regulation. *Physiol Rev* 69:605–670.

Brown R, Pang G, Husband AJ, King MG. 1989a. Suppression of immunity to influenza virus infection in the respiratory tract following sleep disturbance. *Regional Immunol* 2:321–325.

Brown R, Price RJ, King MG, Husband AJ. 1989b. Interleukin-1 B and muramyl dipeptide can prevent decreased antibody response associated with sleep deprivation. *Brain Behav Immunity* 3:320–330.

Krueger JM, Opp MR, Toth LA, Johannsen L, Kapas L. 1990. Cytokines and sleep. In Ganten D, Pfaff D, eds. Behavioral aspects of neuroendocrinology. *Current Topics in Neuroendocrinology 10*, 243–261.

Krueger JM, Walter J, Dinarello CA, Wolff SM, Chedid L. 1984. Sleep-promoting effects of endogenous pyrogen (interleukin-1). *Am J Physiol* 246:R994–R999.

Moldofsky H, Lue FA, Eisen J, Keystone E, Gorczynski RM. 1986. The relationship of interleukin-1 and immune functions to sleep in humans. *Psychosom Med* 48:309–318.

Palmblad J, Cantell K, Strander H, Froberg J, Claes-Goran K, Levi L, Grantstrom M, Unger P. 1976. Stressor exposure and immunological response in man: Interferon-producing capacity and phagocytosis. *J Psychosomatic Res* 20:193–199.

Palmblad J, Petrini B, Wasserman J, Akerstedt T. 1979. Lymphocyte and granulocyte reactions during sleep deprivation. *Psychosom Med* 41:273–278.

Plata-Salaman CR. 1991. Immunoregulators in the nervous system. *Neurosci Biobehav Rev* 15:185–215.

Toth LA, Krueger JM. 1988. Alterations in sleep during *Staphylococcus aureus* infection in rabbits. *Infect Immun* 56:1785–1791.

Ruth M. Benca

INCORPORATION INTO DREAMS

Dream incorporation refers to the appearance in a dream of some aspect of an external stimulus. In the narrowest sense, the external stimulus occurs during the dream and appears in some way in the dream. A typical example might be a ringing alarm clock that appears in a dream of a classroom situation as a ringing bell signifying the end of the class. The external stimulus appears but has been altered to fit the context of the dream. In a broader sense, dream incorporation studies have attempted to find the determinants of dream content by considering the effects of both presleep and sleep stimuli on dream content. In the broadest sense, incorporation studies might be considered to include the possible "incorporation" of waking personality styles in dream content. For example, does the good man dream of what the evil man does, as the ancient Greeks believed?

Modern sleep laboratory studies indicate that the sources of specific dream content are unclear. Presleep stimuli have no substantial effect on dream content. Thus, REM and NREM dream reports are only slightly affected by an evening of physical exercise, challenging mental work, or relaxation (Hauri, 1970). Compared with presleep emotionally neutral films, presleep violent films do not evoke more violent REM or NREM dreams in adults, preadolescents, or children (Foulkes and Rechtschaffen, 1964; Foulkes et al., 1967). In fact, only about 5 percent of REM reports show incorporation of the filmed presleep violence. Presleep pornographic films are not followed by obviously sexual REM dreams (Cartwright et al., 1969). Thirst induced by 24-hour fluid restriction is followed by isolated references to drink rather than persistent themes of thirst, and the isolated references occur in only one third of REM reports (Dement and Wolpert, 1958).

Just as with presleep stimuli, stimuli presented during sleep have minimal effect on dream content. Such events are usually not incorporated into dreams. For example, stimulus objects in front of eyes taped open during sleep are not incorporated into REM dreams (Rechtschaffen and Foulkes, 1965). Tones, light flashes, cold water stimuli, and wrist shocks during REM sleep are incorporated into only 9 percent, 24 percent, 47 percent, and 20 percent of dream reports, respectively (Dement and Wolpert, 1956). In virtually all instances of incorporation, the stimulus was represented in the dream report as a momentary event that fit into the ongoing dream narrative, not as a determinant of the dream's theme. (See also INSTANTANEOUS DREAMING.)

Like external stimuli before and during sleep, physiological events during sleep have no substantial relationship to dream content. In the male, for example, 95 percent of REM sleep periods are accompanied by ERECTIONS, but the frequency of manifest sexuality of REM dreams is very low (Hall and Van de Castle, 1966).

During REM sleep, some physiological events are tonic or continuous (e.g., relatively low-voltage, mixed-frequency ELECTROENCEPHALOGRAM) and others are phasic, that is, brief and intermittent (e.g., PGO spikes, rapid eye movements, bursts of electroencephalographic SAWTOOTH WAVES; see also PHASIC ACTIVITY IN REM SLEEP). It has been hypothesized that mental activity during phasic REM sleep would be more perceptual, intense, bizarre, or distorted than mentation during tonic REM sleep. For practical purposes, however, the findings show that tonic and phasic REM reports are not significantly different in these qualities (Pivik, 1991). Similarly, mental activity during phasic events of NREM sleep (e.g., the K-COMPLEX) is not different from that reported during "tonic" NREM sleep. Hence, dream content is remarkably independent of external psychological and physical stimuli both before and during sleep and equally independent of currently measurable physiological processes during sleep. Therefore, the sources of dream content, that is, its themes and its specific elements, remain a mystery.

Certain formal characteristics of dreams, however, are modestly related to waking personality. Imaginativeness in REM sleep dreams correlates positively with imaginativeness in stories reported in a psychological test called the Thematic Aperception Test (TAT) (Foulkes and Rechtschaffen, 1964). For dream reports from both NREM and REM sleep, length, vividness, emotionality, and distortion each correlate positively with psychopathology scores on the MMPI, a personality test. Evidently, emotional activation or tone during sleep parallels emotional activation or tone during wakefulness. Following a stressful presleep film, individual differences in waking anxiety correlate positively with individual differences in anxiety shown in REM sleep dream reports (Goodenough et al., 1975). Over the menstrual cycle of normal women, changes in waking mood correlate positively with mood changes in REM reports. Depressed patients have a depressive tone in their REM reports; schizophrenic patients have disorganized, incoherent REM reports. These findings do not support the complementarity hypothesis about the relationship of waking mentation to sleep mentation, which states that dreams form a complement to waking life by reflecting characteristics that are hidden or suppressed during waking life. The good person does not dream of what the evil person does. Rather, the findings support a continuity hypothesis—that dreams "continue" certain formal characteristics of waking mental life. (See also PERSONALITY AND DREAM RECALL.)

REFERENCES

Cartwright RD, Berniche N, Borowitz G, Kling G. 1969. Effect of an erotic movie on sleep and dreams of young men. *Arch Gen Psychiatry* 20:263–271.

Dement W, Wolpert EA. 1956. The relation of eye movements, body motility, and external stimuli to dream content. *J Exp Psychol* 55:543–553.

Foulkes D. 1966. *The psychology of sleep*, Chap. 8. New York: Charles Scribner's Sons.

Foulkes D, Pivik T, Steadman HS, Spear PS, Symonds JD. 1967. Dreams of the male child. An EEG study. *J Abnorm Psychol* 72:457–467.

Foulkes D, Rechtschaffen A. 1964. Presleep determinants of dream content: Effects of two films. *Percept Motor Skills* 19:983–1005.

Goodenough DA, Witkins HA, Koulach D, Cohen H. 1975. The effects of stress films on dream content and on respiration and eye movement during rapid eye movement sleep. *Psychophysiology* 15:313–320.

Hall CS, Van de Castle RL. 1966. *The content analysis of dreams*. New York: Appleton.

Hauri P. 1970. Evening activity, sleep mentation, and subjective sleep quality. *J Abnorm Psychol* 76:270–275.

Pivik RT. 1991. Tonic states and phasic events in relation to sleep mentation. In Ellman SJ, Antrobus JS, eds. *The mind in sleep*, pp 214–247. New York: Wiley.

Rechtschaffen A, Foulkes D. 1965. Effect of visual stimuli on dream content. *Percept Motor Skills* 20:1148–1160.

Gerald W. Vogel

INCUBATION OF DREAMS

See Interpretation of Dreams

INCUBUS ATTACKS

The term *incubus* has been used indiscriminately and promiscuously over the years. Current usage most often (erroneously) refers to the night terror (sleep terror, *pavor nocturnus*). *Incubus* is derived from the Latin *incubare,* and originally referred to "an evil spirit supposed to lie upon persons in their sleep and especially to have sexual intercourse with women by night." It is synonymous with the terms *nightmare,* as originally defined, and *succubus,* which refers to "a demon assuming female form to have sexual intercourse with men in their sleep" (*Webster's Third New International Dictionary,* 1970).

Experientially, all refer to the combination of (1) dreaming occurring during the onset of sleep, (2) a sense of impending doom, and (3) a perception of total-body paralysis. Physiologically, all three terms represent the appearance of two elements (dreaming and total-body paralysis) of REM sleep occurring during the transition from wakefulness to sleep. These events differ from conventional dreams and dream anxiety attacks in that they occur at sleep onset, there is some perception of wakefulness, and they are associated with the perception of paralysis (Mahowald and Ettinger, 1990). This phenomenon occurs frequently in those suffering from the sleep disorder narcolepsy, but may appear in perfectly normal individuals, particularly in the setting of sleep deprivation. Reassurance of its benign and normal nature is sufficient treatment.

(See also HYPNAGOGIC HALLUCINATIONS; SLEEP PARALYSIS.)

REFERENCES

Mahowald MW, Ettinger MG. 1990. Things that go bump in the night: The parasomnias revisited. *J Clin Neurophysiol* 7:119–143.

Mark W. Mahowald

INDIVIDUAL DIFFERENCES

There are two aspects of individual differences in sleep: the presence of differences between individuals and the consistency with which these differences are maintained by individuals. With regard to human sleep, the differences among total sleep time, the timing of sleep, and measures of sleep architecture are considered first.

Total Sleep Time

Analyses of the differences in amounts of sleep per night have been reported on for two large samples. Self-reports about "average sleep per night" were obtained from over one million Americans (Kripke, Simons, and Garfinkel, 1979). In another study 30,000 people in eleven countries were asked to report total sleep for the preceding night (Webb, 1987). The data from these studies are given in Table 1.

Table 1   Percentage Distribution of Sleep Amounts from Two Studies

	Minutes of Sleep						
	Less than 300	300–359	360–419	420–479	480–539	540–599	600 or More
Kripke, Simons, and Garfinkel (1979)	1	2	12	35	44	6	1
Webb (1985)	2	6	19	33	26	9	5

The discrepancies in Table 1 point to the difficulties encountered in measuring individual differences. The "piling up" of numbers in the Kripke, Simons, and Garfinkel analysis probably reflects a self-reporting bias of an easy and conventional guess by subjects at what their sleep "should be." The time-budget reports of subjects in the Webb study contain more extreme sleep amounts and reflect the fact that a one-day sampling of sleep is more likely to measure unusual periods of longer- or shorter-sleep circumstances than an average of a number of nights of individuals. The generally lower values in the Webb study likely reflect using only workday sleep estimates (see CULTURAL ASPECTS OF SLEEP).

Figure 1 is an idealized estimate of individual differences in sleep length among young adults. The distribution is based on many self-report surveys and sleep diaries maintained over periods of time. This idealized distribution assumes that amounts of sleep, like many biologically based traits, are normally distributed and that the average sleep length, which has been confirmed often, is 7½ hours. The estimated standard deviation of 1 hour fits many studies and approximates the often reported ranges of normal sleep. This figure indicates that about 68 percent of young adults have an average sleep length of between 6½ and 8½ hours, and an equal number have higher or lower sleep lengths. About 1 in 100 averages more than 10 hours or less than 5 hours.

Total sleep time in infants is, of course, greater and more widely distributed. Parmalee, Schultz, and Disbrow (1961) found an average of 16.5

hours of total sleep for the neonate (range 10.8 to 21 hours; standard deviation 1.6 hours). A slight rise in total sleep time as well as a broader distribution of sleep may occur in late life as compared to middle age. For example, in the Kripke, Simons, and Garfinkel study, 27 percent of 90-year-old persons reported approximately 10 or more hours of sleep, and 5 percent reported less than 5 hours. This contrasts with about 1.5 percent and 2.5 percent in these ranges in 30-year-old persons.

The Timing of Sleep

In one study of college students, the standard deviation of sleep onset times was about 1½ hours. This means that, on the average, sleep onset times varied by as much as 3 hours from night to night for 68 percent of these students. There are apparent systematic individual differences in the onset of sleep time (see EARLY BIRDS AND NIGHT OWLS; MORNINGNESS/EVENINGNESS) and the ease of going to sleep (see INSOMNIA). The presence of differences in sleep patterning is also seen in napping tendencies. Because napping is heavily influenced by work–rest schedules (see SHIFTWORK) and cultural factors (see CULTURAL ASPECTS OF SLEEP), the extent of these differences is best seen in infants and children. Ragins and Schachter (1971) found that 8 percent of 2-year-olds did not nap, whereas 27 percent had naps of 2 hours or longer. Another study reported that

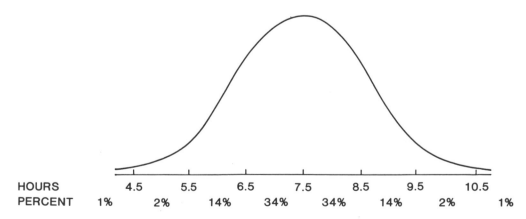

HOURS		4.5	5.5	6.5	7.5	8.5	9.5	10.5	
PERCENT	1%	2%	14%	34%	34%	14%	2%	1%

Figure 1. A theoretical distribution of total sleep. *Reproduced with permission from Webb, 1992.*

the number of children not napping rose from 8 percent (2 years) to 12 percent (3 years), 36 percent (4 years), and 95 percent (5 years). These differences reflect differences in both developmental rate and the strength of napping tendencies.

Sleep Structure

Sleep structure measures also show a wide range of individual differences and age-related changes in these differences. Table 2 presents the means and standard deviations from a set of standardized measures of female sleep stages (data from Williams, Karacan, and Hursh, 1974).

Measures typically extend three standard deviations above and below the mean or average score. These data indicate that, in young females (who do not differ significantly from young males), there are a wide range of individual differences in sleep structure measures. Stage 2 scores extend from about 34 percent to 70 percent, REM scores from about 15 percent to about 35 percent, and awake time during sleep from 0 to about 2.5 percent. These ranges increase in older persons, particularly in amount of time awake.

Traits Versus States

A crucial question is the extent to which these are consistent differences between individuals, like, say, height or skin color, or transient tendencies, such as moods or opinions. The former we label *traits* and the later we label *states*. The answer is dependent on the consistency of differences that is found in repeated measures across time and situations. If the measures of

Table 2   Means and Standard Deviations of Percentage of Sleep Stages

	20–29 years		60–70 years	
	Mean	SD	Mean	SD
Stage 2	52%	6.0	55%	8.5
REM	25%	3.5	21%	4.0
Awake	1%	0.5	9%	8.5

differences are highly correlated, that is, if individuals are ranked with consistency across measurements, then they represent consistent individual differences. As with most variables that involve behavioral tendencies, some sleep measures reflect traitlike tendencies whereas others do not.

Our best measures of total sleep amounts are sleep logs or diaries kept over several weeks. These data show that sleep onset times and wakeup times (and, consequently, total sleep time) vary from night to night and on weekends. There is, however, a consistency of sleep amount when averaged weekly sleep amounts are correlated. A study of a set of 6-week sleep diaries found that weekly averages were highly correlated (.85) with the 6-week average of these logs (Mullington, Speilman, and Wells, 1987). This indicates that, although sleep varies somewhat each night, there are strong tendencies for individuals to maintain consistent "long" or "short" sleep amounts.

There are few data on the consistency of timing of sleep. Sleep onset times vary widely. As noted, among college students, the standard deviation of sleep onset times is about an hour and a half. Night-to-night sleep latencies in normal subjects show little correlation; however, it is clear that there are consistent tendencies in maintaining "lark" and "owl" patterns of sleep (see EARLY BIRDS AND NIGHT OWLS) and insomnias may show consistency (see INSOMNIA). Some consistencies are noted in napping (see NAPPING).

In regard to sleep structures, the measures of the stages of sleep show both consistency and inconsistency. For example, the consistency of REM sleep from night to night is quite low; however, the amount of slow-wave sleep is much more consistent. Slow-wave sleep is correlated about .60 from night to night.

In general we may conclude that, like the dimensions of most biological systems, the dimensions of sleep show a wide range of individual differences. Total sleep amount, although somewhat variable from night to night and responsive to situational demands, shows evidence of being an individual trait. The timing of sleep is more variable and responsive to extrinsic variables, although systematic individual patterns may be maintained. The structure of sleep as measured by sleep stages shows a wide range of individual differences with both state and traitlike variability in relation to different stages.

REFERENCES

Kripke DF, Simons RN, Garfinkel L, Hammond EC. 1979. Short and long sleep and sleeping pills: Is increased mortality associated? *Arch Gen Psychiatry* 36:103–116.

Mullington J, Speilman A, Wells R. 1987. Subjective estimation of nocturnal sleep length and stability of sleep patterns: A 42 night sleep log study. *Sleep Res* 16:342.

Parmalee AH, Schultz HR, Disbrow MA. 1961. Sleep patterns in the newborn. *J Pediatr* 65:575–582.

Ragins N, Schachter J. 1971. A study of sleep behavior in two-year-old children. *J Am Acad Child Psychiatry* 10:463–480

Webb WB. 1985. Sleep in industrialized settings in the northern hemisphere. *Psychol Rep* 57: 591–598.

———. 1992. *Sleep, the gentle tyrant.* Bolton, Mass.: Anker.

Williams R, Karacan I, Hursh C. 1974. *Electroencephalography (EEG) of human sleep and clinical applications.* New York: Wiley.

Wilse B. Webb

INFANCY, NORMAL SLEEP PATTERNS IN

Sleep in infants is dramatically different from sleep in adults. It is even quite different from sleep in children or adolescents. Infant sleep patterns begin to develop in the uterus, before birth. A fetus of 6 or 7 months' gestation experiences REM sleep, with NREM sleep beginning shortly afterward. By the end of the eighth month of gestation, sleep patterns are well established.

Instead of using the terms REM and NREM sleep, as in older children and adults, researchers classify the sleep in a newborn infant as either *active* or *quiet*. During active sleep, which is the developmental precursor of REM sleep in adults, infants, though asleep, are quite active. They move their arms or legs, cry or whimper, and have their eyes partly open. Their breathing is irregular and their eyes dart back and forth under their eyelids. During quiet sleep, which is equal to NREM sleep in adults, infants are behaviorally quiescent. Their breathing is regular and they lie very still; however, they may have an occasional startle or jerk and make sucking movements.

Another difference between sleep of infants and sleep of adults is how their sleep patterns are organized. Infants have polyphasic sleep periods; that is, they have many sleep periods throughout the day. Adults, by contrast, typically have only one sleep period lasting about 8 hours. A newborn infant typically sleeps for 3 or 4 hours and wakens to be fed, which results in about seven sleeping and waking cycles per day. Also, sleep in the newborn is equally spaced throughout the day, with no clear differentiation between daylight hours and nighttime hours. This pattern may be cause for dismay for the child's parents. As infants get older, however, their sleep begins to consolidate and they also sleep a bit less (Figure 1). For example, typical newborns sleep 17 to 18 hours a day; by 1 month of age, infants sleep 16 to 17 hours on average; and by 3 or 4 months a baby sleeps about 15 hours a day. At this age, sleep has consolidated into about four or five sleep periods, with two-thirds of total sleep time occurring at night. Thus, 3- to 4-month-old babies already show a diurnal pattern of daytime wakefulness and nighttime sleep, which continues to develop into fewer daytime sleep periods and progressively longer sleep at night by 6 months. Whereas newborn infants sleep almost three-quarters of the time, 6-month-olds sleep only about half of the time, approximately 13 hours per day. At this age, the longest sustained daily sleep period is about 7 hours, with many children waking for brief periods but able to put themselves back to sleep. Thus, parents who assume their 6-month-old sleeps continuously 10 to 12 hours may be mistaken; their child may actually wake briefly several times without disturbing anyone. By 24 months of age, toddlers sleep about 12 hours per day, and most children continue to take one or two naps during the day. By 4 years of age, children sleep about 10 to 12 hours per day, consisting of a long nighttime sleep and perhaps one daytime nap (see CHILDHOOD, SLEEP DURING).

An important feature to consider when evaluating infant sleep patterns is night waking. At 1 month of age, about two thirds of babies wake more than once per night. By 6 months of age, most infants have "settled." That is, they sleep through most of the night. Only about 15 percent of infants wake more than once a night, although this percentages increases for babies between 6 and 9 months of age. However, age is not the only factor affecting night wakings. Boys, and infants who are breast-fed (as discussed below), are also more likely to wake during the night.

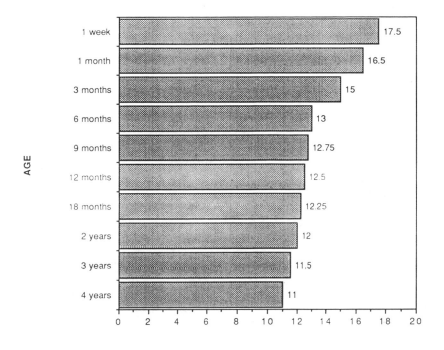

Figure 1. Typical sleep patterns of infants.

Napping is another important aspect of the sleep of infants and young children. As an infant ages, the amount of nap time decreases. By four months of age, most children take either two or three naps per day; by 6 months, nearly 90 percent of all children take only two naps per day; and by 15 months, almost half of all children take just one nap per day. In addition, the timing of the nap affects the type of sleep that occurs. Early naps, occurring midmorning, have more active sleep, and afternoon naps have more quiet sleep. Thus, naps at different times of day are actually different. What's more, naps are very beneficial. Children who nap often have longer attention spans and are less fussy than their nonnapping counterparts. Some parents, concerned about their child's nighttime sleeping habits, try to encourage more sleep at night by depriving their child of a nap. This is not always effective and may in fact be detrimental, as children need naps. Also, evidence shows that keeping children up during the day does not necessarily help them sleep more at night (Weissbluth, 1987).

Not only is the organization of infants' sleep different from that of adults, so is its type and structure. For example, about 50 percent of the sleep of newborns is active sleep, but for adults

REM constitutes only about 20 percent to 25 percent of the time spent sleeping. As in adults, active sleep is cyclical, but infants' cycles are sixty minutes long rather than the 90-minute cycle of adults. Also, infants may immediately have active sleep upon falling asleep, which is unusual for adults to experience. Quiet sleep in infants is also different from NREM sleep in adults. First, newborn infants do not have the characteristic stage 1, 2, 3, and 4 sleep experienced by older children and adults. Also, quiet sleep accounts for a smaller proportion of total sleep time. Quiet sleep accounts for 50 percent of total sleep time in infants, but almost 75 percent of adult sleep is spent in NREM. These particular differences between infants' and adults' sleep patterns quickly dissipate, however, and by 3 months of age, the sleep stages of infants begin to resemble those of adults. For example, by 3 or 4 months, mature stage 2 SLEEP SPINDLE activity occurs and the spontaneous K-COMPLEX, another sleep EEG pattern, develops at 6 months. Other changes include a decrease in REM sleep and an increase in NREM sleep, so that, by 6 months of age, REM sleep accounts for 30 percent and NREM for 70 percent of total sleep time, more like adult sleep. Finally, the transition to sleep shifts from the newborn pattern—wake to active to quiet sleep—to the mature pattern—wake to NREM to REM sleep.

Several methods are used to assess infants' sleep. In early studies, sleep was measured with behavioral observation. Infants were watched as they slept, and determinations were made about their state of sleep or wakefulness based on observations of movements, breathing patterns, and eye movements. Others have incorporated the use of video recordings into behavioral observation, with a method called *time-lapse video somnography* (Anders and Sostek, 1976). The video tapes can be accurately scored for quiet sleep, active sleep, and wakefulness. Another method is the use of polysomnography in the laboratory (see POLYSOMNOGRAPHY); infants stay overnight at a sleep laboratory and numerous physiological measures are continuously recorded. This method has several disadvantages, including concerns about how much infants' sleep in a lab setting resembles sleep at home and the expenses associated with this method. More sophisticated and less cumbersome methods to study sleep in infants have recently been developed. One such method is a pressure-sensitive crib pad, which records infants' respiration and body movements. From these measures active sleep, quiet sleep, and wakefulness can be determined. Another method is the actigraph, an instrument that infants wear on their leg to keep track of their movements and measure the duration, stages, and quality of sleep.

Many factors may affect infant sleep patterns. For example, there are documented differences between infants who are breast-fed versus those who are bottle fed. Breast-fed babies wake more often during the night than bottle-fed babies. One study found that 52 percent of breast-fed infants and only 20 percent of bottle-fed infants woke during the night, and at 12 months of age or older, nearly two thirds of the breast-fed group continued to wake at night (Carey, 1975). No evidence shows that these multiple awakenings have negative consequences for the infant. Also, many people believe that eating solid foods affects infants' sleep; however, this is not true. Infants who eat solid foods do not sleep any better than those who do not eat solid foods (Macknin, Van der Brug-Medendorp, and Maier, 1989). Sleeping results from maturation, not changes in diet.

Finally, it is also important to understand that every infant displays a unique sleeping pattern. The information presented here provides broad generalizations drawn from the behavior of hundreds of infants; however, each infant will define his or her own unique sleeping pattern. Certain newborns sleep through the night immediately, whereas the sleep of others does not consolidate for several months. In all ways, the sleep patterns of infants are as different and varied as those seen in adults. (See INFANCY, SLEEP DISORDERS IN, for problems related to sleep in infancy.)

REFERENCES

Anders TF, Sostek AM. 1976. The use of time-lapse video recording of sleep-wake behavior in human infants. *Psychophysiology* 13:155–158.
Carey WB. 1975. Breastfeeding and night waking. *J Pediatr* 87:327.
Ferber R. 1985. *Solve your child's sleep problems.* New York: Simon & Schuster.
Macknin ML, Van der Brug-Medendorp S, Maier MC. 1989. Infant sleep and bedtime cereal. *Am J Dis Children* 143:1066–1068.
Weissbluth M. 1987. *Healthy sleep habits, happy child.* New York: Fawcett Colombian.

Jodi A. Mindell

INFANCY, SLEEP DISORDERS IN

Parents commonly complain of sleep problems in their infants, and several studies have reported that as many as one out of every three or four infants has some type of sleep disorder. The most common of these disturbances is sleeplessness, either difficulty falling asleep or problems with waking up during the night.

Before discussing sleep disorders, it is helpful first to understand the normal sleep patterns of infants (see also INFANCY, NORMAL SLEEP PATTERNS IN). Most babies by 6 weeks of age begin to show a clear day–night sleep pattern. By 6 to 9 months of age, most infants have "settled"; that is, they sleep from at least midnight to 5:00 A.M. (Moore and Ucko, 1957); however, it is important to note that infants continue to wake regularly, for brief periods, throughout the night. Many infants can fall back asleep on their own after these regular partial wakings, and these infants are called "selfsoothers." Most parents of a self-soother never even know their baby was awake several times during the night.

On the other hand, infants known as "signalers" cannot return to sleep on their own after waking during the night. They cry when they awaken and often need their parents to intervene in some manner so they can fall back to sleep. This type of sleep problem is usually referred to as night wakings. By 6 months of age, about 15 percent of infants—and their parents—suffer from night wakings more than once per night (Moore and Ucko, 1957). For unknown reasons, this problem becomes even more prevalent (up to 40 percent) in babies between the ages of 6 and 9 months (Guilleminault and Anders, 1976).

Signalers who wake often during the night usually get caught in a cyclical pattern. Many of these babies appear to form negative sleep associations (Ferber, 1985). These infants often fall asleep while being breastfed or while drinking a bottle, or they may fall asleep being rocked or having their back rubbed while lying in the crib. Some infants may even fall asleep in the living room with the television on. When these infants wake during the night they cannot return to sleep until the conditions they have learned to associate with sleep, such as being fed or rocked, are reinstated. Signaling continues because the infant has not learned how to fall back to sleep on his or her own. Parents also continue to respond to their baby during the night because the baby so quickly returns to sleep on being picked up, rocked, or fed. Once this pattern becomes established, it often persists, as both parents and infants are caught in a cycle that perpetuates the night waking problem (see NIGHT WAKING IN INFANCY).

Another struggle for many parents is getting their baby to fall asleep at bedtime. This is often related to the same negative sleep associations mentioned above. The instant the parent stops rocking or feeding the baby, the baby wakes again. Often, babies will resist falling asleep, apparently conditioned to realize that the minute they do, their parents will stop whatever behavior they are doing and place them in their crib.

Environmental factors, including hunger, light, noise, and the lack of a regular sleep–wake schedule, contribute to infants' sleep difficulties. In addition, infants who sleep in their parents' bed are observed to wake more often during the night than those who sleep alone. Breastfed babies are also more likely to wake during the night in comparison with bottle-fed babies: in one study, 52 percent of the breast-fed babies and only 20 percent of the bottle-fed babies woke during the night (Carey, 1975). A disrupting event, such as a family vacation or a move, also frequently results in sleep problems for infants.

Inherent temperamental and medical factors may also cause particular infants to be more susceptible to sleep problems. First, certain babies have more difficulty learning to fall asleep, are more easily aroused from sleep, and are more sensitive to changes in routines that affect their sleeping patterns. Second, medical conditions, especially those involving pain, can cause sleep problems in infants. Chronic *otitis media,* otherwise known as chronic ear infections, can lead to prolonged night wakings even after successful treatment of the infection (Ferber, 1985). This condition is often overlooked by parents and pediatricians, as it is difficult to determine whether the child is still in pain or is having difficulty returning to sleep without parental intervention. Another condition, milk intolerance, may lead to frequent night wakings; infants with this condition may also take longer to fall asleep at bedtime and sleep fewer hours (see MILK ALLERGY AND INFANT SLEEP).

The most common cause of sleep disturbances in babies from birth to 3 months, however, is a condition known as COLIC. Colic is excessive crying in an otherwise healthy infant that can result in an inability to sleep. The cause of colic is unclear and may be different for individual babies; there is also no known cure, which can be frustrating for the parents and the pediatrician. Doctors may suggest changing the infant's and nursing mother's diets or prescribe sedatives or rhythmic movement for the infant, such as riding in a moving car or being placed in a moving swing. All in all, the most common approach is simply the wait-it-out method. Unfortunately, even after the colic has resolved, sleep disruption may continue.

What can be done to help infants and their parents with disorders involving sleeplessness? Changes in sleep routines and changes in parents' behavior can be quite successful. Establishing a set bedtime with a bedtime routine and maintaining a regular daytime nap schedule are both effective in alleviating many infants' sleep problems (Milan et al. 1981). The elimination of negative sleep associations (such as feeding or being rocked to sleep) is also important. Babies should be put to bed while awake in an environment that will be the same throughout the night. Studies have shown that infants who fall asleep while in their cribs are much less likely to wake and signal during the night than infants put in their cribs already asleep (Anders, 1978). In short, parents need to establish bedtime rules and to teach their infants how to fall asleep without parental involvement. It is important to recognize and treat infant sleep disorders rather than to ignore the problem, as many who experience sleep difficulties early in life continue to experience them as they age (Richman, 1981; Zuckerman, Stevenson, and Bailey, 1987). (For a contrasting view, see COSLEEPING.)

Furthermore, sleep disturbances in infancy are not only problematic for the baby but also are stressful for the family, as parents may become sleep-deprived themselves. Many parents begin to feel depressed and anxious and have difficulties being productive at home or at work. Many couples also begin to argue about the best way to handle their infants' sleeping behavior and the causes of the problem. Therefore, sleep disorders such as night waking, sleep onset struggles, and colic should not be taken lightly but treated as health issues that have consequences for the entire family.

REFERENCES

Anders TF. 1978. Home-recorded sleep in 2- and 9-month-old infants. *J Acad Child Psychiatry* 17:421–432.

Carey WB. 1975. Breast feeding and night waking. *J Pediatr* 87:327.

Ferber R. 1985. *Solve your child's sleep problems.* New York: Simon and Schuster.

Guilleminault C, ed. 1987. *Sleep and its disorders in children.* New York: Raven.

Guilleminault C, Anders TF. 1976. Sleep disorders in children. *Adv Pediatr* 22:151–175.

Kryger MH, Roth T, Dement W, eds. 1989. *Principles and practice of sleep medicine.* Philadelphia: Saunders.

Milan MA, Mitchell ZP, Berger MI, Pierson DF. 1981. Positive routines: A rapid alternative to extinction for elimination of bedtime tantrum behavior. *Child Behav Ther* 3:13–25.

Moore T, Ucko LE. 1957. Night waking in early infancy. *Arch Dis Child* 32:333–342.

Richman N. 1981. Sleep problems in young children. *Arch Dis Child* 56:491–493.

Zuckerman B, Stevenson J, Bailey V. 1987. Sleep problems in early childhood: Continuities, predictive factors, and behavioral correlates. *Pediatrics* 80:664–671.

Jodi A. Mindell

INFECTION

Many people experience fatigue and a desire for more sleep than usual when suffering from an infectious disease. In fact, some diseases, such as African sleeping sickness and mononucleosis, are particularly noted for this symptom. Like fever, sleep may represent a major physiological response of the body to infectious disease. Although the role of fever in infectious disease has been studied extensively, the role of sleep has received much less attention, perhaps because sleep is more difficult to measure. Most physicians, however, recognize that sleep probably is important for recovery from infectious disease, because they frequently recommend that their patients get plenty of rest. Many people also believe that insufficient rest can make them more likely to get a cold or "the flu."

Historically, the study of sleep has been associated with studies of infectious disease. About 50 years ago, for example, the study of brain lesions induced by viral infections led von Economo to describe sleep as an active process that was mediated by specific brain regions, a view that is still widely held by sleep researchers. Until recently, however, the precise relationship between sleep and infectious disease has received little systematic scientific study. Evidence has now confirmed the common presumption that sleep is in some way linked to the body's response to infectious disease. In fact, it now seems likely that the biological systems involved in the regulation of immune responses, sleep, and body temperature are very closely interrelated.

Experiments that studied animals with bacterial or fungal infections found that changes occur in both slow-wave sleep ("deep" sleep, or nondreaming sleep) and REM sleep ("dream" sleep) after exposure to an infectious organism. Slow-wave sleep increases for up to a day after the infection, but then decreases to levels that are actually less than normal. In contrast, REM sleep is suppressed for 2 or more days. Other aspects of sleep remain relatively unchanged. For example, sleep still occurs in discrete episodes from which animals can be easily awakened, and the circadian ("light–dark" cycle) organization of sleep persists. The time of occurrence of these sleep effects does not correspond closely to the time course of other signs of infectious disease, such as fever and changes in white blood cell counts. The amount of increased sleep and the time course with which it appears do, however, vary depending on the type of infectious organism and the route by which the microbe entered the body. In addition, the severity of the disease and the state of the immune system of the animal also influence the type of sleep changes that develop after exposure to infectious organisms. For example, drugs that enhance or suppress immune function also alter the pattern of sleep that occurs during infection.

In contrast to bacterial and fungal infections, sleep has not yet been systematically evaluated during a viral infection; however, abundant indirect evidence suggests that sleep might be altered during viral disease. Experimental animals injected intravenously with a noninfective strain of influenza virus show increased sleep for several hours after the injection. Moreover, viral infections have been linked to such diseases as CHRONIC FATIGUE SYNDROME and fibrositis (see ARTHRITIS AND OTHER MUSCULOSKELETAL DISORDERS), which are characterized in part by problems with sleep and have also been implicated as a contributing factor in SUDDEN INFANT DEATH SYNDROME (crib death). Recent observations have shown that people who are infected with the human immunodeficiency virus (HIV) but are still in good health have an excess of slow-wave sleep. Sleep deprivation, on the other hand, has been reported to increase the susceptibility of experimental animals to viral disease.

In addition to live infectious organisms, even killed microbes or purified microbial components can enhance sleep. In fact, macrophages, which are cells that phagocytize or "eat" infectious organisms as part of the body's defense mechanisms, can digest bacteria to produce sleep-inducing substances. Microbial components also stimulate the body to produce and release substances that mediate the immune response. A specific group of these compounds is known as the cytokines. Cytokines are of funda-

mental importance in the regulation of immune responses and probably also help to mediate other physiological and behavioral effects of infectious disease, such as fever and an increased desire to sleep.

Sleep could serve an adaptive role in combating infectious disease. It is possible, for example, that sleep, which is associated with a decreased metabolic rate and reduced muscular activity, permits an animal to conserve metabolic energy, particularly during fever when overall energy requirements are high. Currently, however, the survival advantage of enhanced sleep during infectious disease remains a topic for conjecture.

The changes in sleep that occur during infectious disease are likely to result from the activation of normal sleep regulatory mechanisms. As has often been demonstrated in other fields of physiology, investigation of the impact of disease on sleep together with further study of sleep in normal animals is likely to enhance our understanding of how sleep is regulated and how sleep benefits the animal. (See also AIDS AND SLEEP.)

REFERENCES

Toth LA, Krueger JM. 1988. Alteration of sleep in rabbits by *Staphylococcus aureus* infection. *Infect Immunity* 56:1785–1791.

———. 1989. Effects of microbial challenge on sleep in rabbits. *FASEB J* 3:2062–2066.

———. 1990. Infectious disease, cytokines and sleep. In Mancia M, Marini G, eds. *The diencephalon and sleep,* pp 331–341. New York: Raven Press.

Linda A. Toth

INFRADIAN RHYTHMS

See Biological Rhythms

INSECTS, SLEEPLIKE STATES IN

Most insects have a preferred time of day for activity, which is usually very short and often occurs at the transitions of dawn and dusk, and prolonged periods of inactivity. This daily rest–activity rhythm is endogenous (driven by an internal timekeeping mechanism), because it is not merely a reflection of the light–dark changes of the environment. The rhythm is still present when the animals are observed under conditions where the environment does not provide time cues. The question remains whether the prolonged periods of behavioral inactivity resemble sleep as it is defined for mammals. Application of the behavior criteria for sleep has shown that for some insect species, this inactivity bears close resemblance to sleep. In addition, physiological measures (e.g., muscle activity and neuronal activity) have provided more information about the resting state in bees.

Preferred sleeping sites and specific sleep postures have been described in several insects. Moths, for example, show five body postures with typical antennae and wing positions (Andersen, 1968). Touching the moths' wings does not elicit a response in the posture where the antennae are folded under the wings. The researchers concluded that this posture represented "deep sleep." In cockroaches, a distinct position of the body, head, and antennae is associated with an elevated arousal threshold to a vibration stimulus. Similarly, the reaction of "resting" mosquitoes to touch stimulation depends on their body position.

The forager bee is the insect that has been most extensively studied to identify electrophysiological signs of behavioral sleep (Kaiser and Steiner-Kaiser, 1983; Kaiser, 1988). The signs of rest, which occur mainly during the late hours of the night, include immobility, characteristic postures of body, head, and antennae, decreased body temperature, reduced neck muscle tone, increased arousal threshold (i.e., decreased response to stimulation), and decreased sensitivity of visual nerve cells to air puffs. As the bees change their body position from the upright state, with the abdomen and head off the ground to a position where the body rests on the ground, the head and antennae are inclined, and neck muscle tone is lowered, the arousal threshold to an external stimulus increases, suggesting that the latter posture characterizes a sleeplike state in these bees.

The nightly motor activity of the rhinoceros beetle decreases in proportion to the quantity of injected uridine, an active component of "sleep-promoting substance" (SPS), which has been extracted and purified from the brainstems of sleep-deprived rats. The control injection of saline (salt water) has no effect (Inoué et al., 1986) on the beetles. Similarly, an increase of nocturnal sleep has been found in rats after injection of uridine. This finding in the rhinoceros beetle may indicate a biochemical similarity of insect inactivity to mammalian sleep.

Sleep deprivation in mammals is followed by compensatory sleep during recovery, and this experimental technique has been used to investigate whether disturbances of rest are similarly compensated in insects. For example, cockroaches that were disturbed for 3 hours at the end of their resting period showed a decrease in active behavior in the subsequent recovery period (Tobler, 1983). On the other hand, preliminary data on rest deprivation in honey bees indicate that in some individuals an increase in resting behavior occurs during recovery, whereas in others, a prolonged activation is elicited. Thus, it is premature to conclude that rest disturbances are followed by compensatory mechanisms in insects.

In conclusion, behavioral inactivity in several insects is not a uniform state. Substates of rest can be discriminated on the basis of body posture, arousal level, and neuronal activity. Thus, there are phases of inactivity that in some aspects resemble sleep in vertebrates.

REFERENCES

Andersen FS. 1968. Sleep in moths and its dependence on the frequency of stimulation in *Anagasta kuehniella*. *Opusc Entomol* 33:15–24.

Inoué S, Honda K, Okano Y, Komoda Y. 1986. Behavior modulating effects of uridine in the rhinoceros beetle. *Zool Sci* 3:727–729.

Kaiser W. 1988. Busy bees need rest, too. Behavioral and electromyographical sleep signs in honeybees. *J Comp Physiol A* 163:565–584.

Kaiser W, Steiner-Kaiser J. 1983. Neuronal correlates of sleep, wakefulness and arousal in a diurnal insect. *Nature* 301:707–709.

Tobler I. 1983. Effect of forced locomotion on the rest–activity cycle of the cockroach. *Behav Brain Res* 8:351–360.

Irene Tobler

INSOMNIA

Insomnia is a subjective report of having difficulty falling asleep or staying asleep. Insomnia is a frequent medical complaint and is easily the most common type of sleep problem. Seventeen percent of the adult population of the United States is estimated to experience serious insomnia each year (Mellinger, Balter, and Uhlenhuth, 1985). Everyone is vulnerable to difficulty sleeping at least one or two nights per year.

Patterns of Insomnia

The characteristics of insomnia vary considerably among individuals. One primary factor used to classify types of insomnia is the duration of the problem. *Transient* insomnia lasts up to 1 week, *short-term* insomnia lasts weeks to months, and *chronic* insomnia is insomnia lasting greater than 3 months. Because occasional episodes of transient and short-term insomnia occur normally, it is chronic insomnia that is most often a focus of treatment in a sleep center. Most of the information presented below has come from research with patients experiencing chronic insomnia.

Insomnia may be experienced in many different patterns. Some individuals are unable to fall asleep initially, and others fall asleep quickly but wake up in the middle of the night or early morning and are unable to return to sleep. Still another pattern is numerous brief awakenings throughout the night. In the recent past, insomniacs were categorized solely on the basis of the time of night that difficulty sleeping occurred. The categories consisted of "sleep-onset," "sleep maintenance," and "terminal" insomnia to denote difficulty sleeping at the beginning, middle, or end of the night. People with severe insomnia often have both difficulty falling asleep initially and awakenings during the night. In addition to differences in sleep patterns, people with insomnia also vary greatly as to the specific cause and severity of the consequences of their sleep disturbance.

Daytime Effects of Insomnia

A common component of complaints of insomnia is that sleep is either too short or too light to produce a refreshed feeling the next day. Daytime symptoms that patients frequently attribute to poor sleep are fatigue, difficulty concentrating, depression, and irritability (Stepanski et al., 1989). As a result of these cognitive and mood changes people feel that their ability to do their job, relate to their families, and perform other responsibilities is negatively affected. This is true even after one night of insomnia. It is usually these daytime consequences of insomnia that are most upsetting to those unable to sleep. An individual who loses sleep at night but has no deficits during the day is unlikely to seek treatment. For this reason, the severity of an insomnia complaint is determined as much by the level of daytime impairment as by the frequency of the sleeplessness itself.

In contrast to the pervasiveness of these subjective reports of daytime impairment, no consistent decrements in objective measures of cognitive or motor skills have been found. Further, insomniacs as a group have not been found to be sleepier than normal sleepers during the day when objective tests are used.

Objective mood and personality tests nearly always find differences between insomniacs and normal sleepers. Insomniacs have higher levels of depression, tension, and anxiety. It is unclear from the research whether these personality differences are a cause or a consequence of sleep disturbance.

Causes of Insomnia

Insomnia is not a disorder in itself, but is usually a symptom of some other disorder. Therefore, a thorough understanding of the various causes of insomnia is necessary before a careful evaluation can be performed. Historically, insomnia was often perceived to be related to psychological or psychiatric problems. Although it is true that many people with severe DEPRESSION or anxiety disorders have disrupted sleep, most patients with insomnia do not have a psychiatric disorder. Sleep experts have come to view insomnia as a symptom common to many different disorders or causes.

The monitoring of physiological activity during sleep, in conjunction with the development of standard criteria for categorizing the sleep ELECTROENCEPHALOGRAM (EEG) into distinct stages, led to more objective analysis of sleep. This increased ability to analyze sleep objectively allowed for greater specificity in making diagnoses of sleep problems. Sleep recordings of patients complaining of insomnia generally find reduced total sleep time and an increased percentage of light sleep (Zorick et al., 1981). At times a specific cause for the sleep disturbance is evident in the recording, as in the case of stopped breathing episodes (sleep APNEA) or abnormal muscle activity (PERIODIC LEG MOVEMENTS/restless legs syndrome).

The American Sleep Disorders Association (ASDA) has developed a diagnostic system that is used to classify types of insomnia (American Sleep Disorders Association, 1990). Most diagnoses denote the immediate cause of the insomnia. Although there are many diagnoses, most of these fall within five general categories: insomnia secondary to (1) medical disorders, (2) psychiatric disorders, (3) behavioral factors, (4) CIRCADIAN RHYTHM DISORDERS, and (5) primary sleep pathology.

Medical Disorders

Insomnia can be caused by many different medical conditions. Obviously, any condition producing pain, such as arthritis, can lead to difficulty sleeping. Patients with pulmonary disease often have disturbed sleep, as they may become hypoxemic during sleep or experience difficulty breathing on lying down (George and Kryger, 1987). Also, many NEUROLOGIC DISORDERS such as PARKINSON'S DISEASE are associated with disrupted sleep. An additional factor that elicits insomnia with these conditions is the adverse effects on sleep caused by many medications used to treat medical conditions. (See also DRUGS FOR MEDICAL DISORDERS; FATAL FAMILIAL INSOMNIA; MEDICAL ILLNESS AND SLEEP.)

Psychiatric Disorders

DEPRESSION, when severe, leads to either insomnia or hypersomnia in nearly 100 percent of affected patients. An overwhelming majority of these patients, particularly if they are over 30 years old, have insomnia as a prominent symptom of their depression. Specific abnormalities of the sleep cycle have been described in patients with endogeneous depression (Reynolds and Kupfer, 1987).

Anxiety disorders, especially obsessive–compulsive disorder, have been cited as causes of sleep-onset insomnia. Some patients with PANIC DISORDER may suffer attacks during sleep, leading to abrupt awakenings and difficulty returning to sleep. (See also AFFECTIVE DISORDERS OTHER THAN MAJOR DEPRESSION.)

Behavioral Factors

Behavioral insomnia occurs when an individual engages in routine habits (or behaviors) that promote disrupted sleep. Insomnia can result when a person uses his or her bed for watching TV, eating meals, studying, or doing other "wake" activities. Other behavioral causes of insomnia include use of caffeine late in the day, daytime naps, working right before bedtime, and leaving the TV or radio on through the night. The precise mechanism by which these behaviors interfere with sleep is not clear. Theories have suggested that insomnia results from certain behavioral patterns because of physiological arousal, cognitive arousal, or negative conditioning. These theories have some support from research studies, but none of them has proven to be definitive. The ambiguity in this area may result because all of of these explanations may be true, but only for certain a subgroup of insomniacs. Also, two or more of these factors may all operate within a given individual, but in different degrees.

Circadian Rhythm Disorders

The CIRCADIAN RHYTHM refers to the 24-hour cycle that regulates the sleep–wake cycle. Patients experience great difficulty falling asleep if they have a kind of circadian rhythm disorder called a *phase delay syndrome*. This means that the biological clock is set later (delayed) compared with the environmental schedule for sleep. For example, a college student accustomed to sleeping from 2 to 10 A.M. may get a summer job and need to arise at 6 A.M. If the student tried to lie down at 10 P.M. to get 8 hours of sleep by 6 A.M., he will likely lie awake until close to 2 A.M., the time that the biological clock says he should fall asleep. The student will experience sleep-onset insomnia until his circadian rhythm for sleep adjusts to his summer schedule. (See also DELAYED SLEEP PHASE SYNDROME.)

A similar type of problem occurs when people work rotating shifts (see SHIFTWORK). In general, people sleep better when on a consistent schedule 7 days a week. Widely varying sleep schedules (e.g., arising at 7 A.M. some days and at noon other days) will lead to poor-quality sleep.

Primary Sleep Pathology

Periodic leg movements and sleep apnea are conditions that arise in sleep and can awaken a patient repeatedly during the night. Leg twitches are associated with certain medical conditions (e.g., anemia, uremia, neuropathy) and in some cases occur with no clear cause. The significance of these movements is controversial, as many people with no sleep complaints have also been found to have twitches. A related disorder, restless legs syndrome, occurs in older patients and is characterized by a tingling sensation in the legs that is relieved by movement of the affected limb. Breathing abnormalities, such as apnea, most often lead to a complaint of daytime sleepiness, but do cause insomnia in some instances.

Subjective Insomnia

One of the first findings of physiological monitoring in insomniacs was that these patients uniformly exaggerate the severity of their sleep problem. It is common for individuals with insomnia to overestimate the time it takes to fall asleep and to underestimate their total amount of sleep. In extreme cases, some patients complain of severe insomnia even after a night of 7 to 8 hours sleep with no apparent abnormalities. In fact, 9.2 percent of patients who are evaluated at sleep centers for a complaint of insomnia are found to have normal sleep (Coleman et al., 1982). The reason that these patients believe they are wide awake even though their EEG shows sleep is unknown. Some experts believe that the sleep of these patients is flawed by some defect not detected by EEG recordings of sleep.

Effects of Aging

A 1-month-old infant sleeps for 15½ hours each day. Insomnia, in the sense of lying in bed quietly during the night wide awake, is rare in children. If given a regular schedule and safe sleep environment, children will sleep well; however, refusing to go to bed or leaving the bed once placed there are common problems for 2- to 3-year-olds. This is a normal expression of issues inherent to this developmental stage, and is analogous to a child refusing to eat certain foods or comply with other parental demands. This type of sleep problem responds very well to appropriate behavior modification. (See also INFANCY, NORMAL SLEEP IN; INFANCY, SLEEP DISORDERS IN.)

It is well documented that sleep worsens as people grow older. Total sleep time and amount of deep sleep decrease steadily across the life span. It was previously believed that individuals needed less sleep as they aged, and this belief was used to explain lower sleep times in elderly people. Careful research has shown that decreased sleep time or sleep quality in the elderly is accompanied by increased daytime sleepiness. It appears that older sleepers suffer the same consequences of lessened or fragmented sleep as do younger sleepers. Therefore, it can be inferred that sleep *need* is the same, but sleep *ability* becomes impaired with age. As a person ages, her sleep becomes lighter, she awakens more often, and she feels less rested in the morning. This is often compensated for by staying in bed longer or by taking daytime naps. As expected, the prevalence of insomnia is increased in older populations. Primary sleep pathologies, such as restless legs syndrome and sleep apnea, occur more frequently in older individuals.

Treatment of Insomnia

The treatment for insomnia is aimed at the primary cause of the sleep disturbance. In many instances, the treatment is for a primary medical or psychiatric disorder that, when successful, also leads to improved sleep. Treatments specifically developed for insomnia fall into two modalities: behavioral and pharmacological.

Behavioral Treatment

Behavioral treatments are those that require changes in schedule, habits, life-style, or level of relaxation to improve sleep. The most commonly employed behavioral program is to enforce rules for good SLEEP HYGIENE. These rules represent the minimal conditions needed for improvement of a disrupted sleep pattern, and are usually combined with other behavioral or pharmacological treatments. Sleep hygiene treatment entails instructing patients to avoid a wide range of habits known to interfere with normal sleep. Maintaining a comfortable sleep environment with adequate regulation of noise and temperature, limiting use of caffeine and alcohol, and avoiding afternoon naps are examples of sleep hygiene rules.

A number of other behavioral treatments have been developed (Bootzin and Nicassio, 1978). Each is based on one of several theories. Progressive muscle relaxation, electromyogram BIOFEEDBACK, and self-hypnosis are treatments whose goals are to give the patient the ability to decrease tension and promote relaxation prior to bedtime. These treatments evolved from the belief that physiological hyperarousal at bedtime is responsible for insomnia.

STIMULUS CONTROL is a treatment based on the theory that insomnia results from negative conditioning to the bedroom or sleep environment. This treatment attempts to undo this conditioning by teaching the patient to associate the bedroom only with relaxation and sleep.

Cognitive refocusing, guided imagery, and meditation techniques have been used for insomnia as a way of calming the mind. These treatments are a response to the possibility that cognitive, rather than physiological, arousal is responsible for insomnia.

A chief drawback of any behavioral treatment is that the patient must be very motivated to make difficult changes in their customary habits and life-style. Also, this approach requires a great amount of time on the part of the sleep specialist or therapist.

(See also BEHAVIORAL MODIFICATION; FOLK AND OTHER NATURAL REMEDIES FOR SLEEPLESSNESS; RELAXATION THERAPY; SLEEP RESTRICTION THERAPY.)

Pharmacological Treatment

Pharmacological treatment has been much more extensively studied than has behavioral treatment. This approach most commonly consists of using sedating drugs 30 to 60 minutes before bedtime. The drowsiness produced by these drugs can shorten the time it takes to fall asleep, and decrease the amount of time spent awake during the night (Nicholson, 1989).

Many medications used to promote sleep are members of the class of drugs called BENZODIAZEPINES. These compounds are generally safe when taken at appropriate dosages, but some patients may experience side effects such as morning grogginess. The possibility that tolerance to the hypnotic (sleep-inducing) effects of these drugs develops with steady use is controversial, but chronic use is not often recommended. For this reason, this treatment approach is most useful for episodes of transient or short-term insomnia. Insomnia in these instances is often related to acute situational factors that may not be easily addressed by behavioral treatments. For patients with chronic insomnia, use of medication may be helpful at times but is usually not the treatment of choice. "Rebound insomnia" can result when a short-acting hypnotic medication is abruptly discontinued. *Rebound* refers to a worsening of sleep to levels even worse than that experienced at the pretreatment phase. This phenomenon only occurs in certain individuals and is usually limited to one night.

(See also BARBITURATES; CHEMISTRY OF SLEEP; L-TRYPTOPHAN; SLEEPING PILLS.)

REFERENCES

American Sleep Disorders Association. 1990. *The international classification of sleep disorders.* Rochester, Minn.: ASDA.

Bootzin RR, Nicassio PM. 1978. Behavioral treatments for insomnia. In Hersen M, Eissler R, Miller P, eds. *Progress in behavior modification,* vol 6, pp 1–45. New York: Academic Press.

Coleman R, Roffwarg H, Kennedy S, Guilleminault C, Cinque J, Cohn M, Karacan I, Kupfer D, Lemmi H, Miles L, Orr W, Phillips E, Roth T, Sassin J, Schmidt H, Weitzman E, Dement W. 1982. Sleep–wake disorders based upon a polysomnographic diagnosis: A national cooperative study. *JAMA* 247:997–1003.

George CF, Kryger MH. 1987. Sleep in restrictive lung disease. *Sleep* 10:409–418.

Mellinger GD, Balter MB, Uhlenhuth EH. 1985. Insomnia and its treatment. Prevalence and correlates. *Arch Gen Psychiatry* 42:225–232.

Nicholson AN. 1989. Hypnotics: Clinical pharmacology and therapeutics. In Kryger MH, Roth T, Dement WC, eds. *Principles and practice of sleep medicine,* pp 219–228. Philadelphia: Saunders.

Reynolds C, Kupfer D. 1987. Sleep research in affective illness: State of the art circa 1987. *Sleep* 10:199–215.

Stepanski E, Koshorek G, Zorick F, Glinn M, Roehrs T, Roth T. 1989. Differences in individuals who do or do not seek treatment for chronic insomnia. *Psychosomatics* 30:421–427.

Zorick FJ, Roth T, Hartze KM, Piccione PM, Stepanski EJ. 1981. Evaluation and diagnosis of persistent insomnia. *Am J Psychiatry* 138(6):769–773.

Edward J. Stepanski

INSPIRATION

See Creativity in Dreams

INSTANTANEOUS DREAMING

The length of REM sleep episodes varies across the night in a fairly consistent fashion—shorter REM episodes occur earlier in the night and longer episodes follow later in the night. Ordinarily, the longest REM episode is at most thirty to forty minutes, occurring toward the end of the night (see CYCLES OF SLEEP ACROSS THE NIGHT). Dream stories are often shorter than the entire REM episode, which may be fragmented into segments, each associated with a different dream story. Dreams lasting fifteen to twenty minutes, however, are probably not unusual.

A common nineteenth-century notion held that dreams were generated instantaneously; in other words, a complex, lengthy dream story was elaborated as a split-second response to some outside stimulus. A famous story that helped to foster this notion is the "French revolution" dream of Alfred Maury, a nineteenth-century French dream researcher. Freud (1961) describes this dream in *The Interpretation of Dreams.*

> He [Maury] was ill and lying in his room in bed, with his mother sitting beside him, and dreamt that it was during the Reign of Terror. After witnessing a number of frightful scenes of murder, he was finally himself brought before the revolutionary tribunal. There he saw Robespierre, Marat, Fouquier-Tinville and the rest of the grim heroes of those terrible days. He was questioned by them, and, after a number of incidents which were not retained in his memory, was condemned, and led to the place of execution surrounded by an immense mob. He climbed on to the scaffold and was bound to the plank by the executioner. It was tipped up. The blade of the guillotine fell. He felt his head being separated from his body, woke up in extreme anxiety—and found that the top of the bed had fallen down and had struck his cervical vertebrae

just in the way in which the blade of the guillotine would actually have struck them.

From dream experiences similar to this, Freud (1961) drew the conclusion that "an apparently superabundant quantity of material" was compressed into "the short period elapsing between his perceiving the rousing stimulus and his waking." In other words, the entire dream experience was interpreted as virtually instantaneous.

Are dreams really instantaneous responses to unusual stimuli, as the Maury dream suggests? In an early study of REM sleep, Dement and Kleitman (1957) examined the length of the dream after assuming that dreaming depended on the presence of REM sleep (see REM SLEEP). These investigators simply correlated the number of words in the dream reports to the length of the REM episode. They found a significant positive correlation in each subject. This preliminary observation, at a minimum, suggests that REM episode length is somehow related to dream story length.

Dement and Wolpert (1958) then evaluated several additional features of REM sleep and dreaming. One of their experiments involved applying stimuli to sleepers during REM sleep to see whether the event would be incorporated into dreams (see INCORPORATION INTO DREAMS). They used three different stimuli: a loud tone, a bright flash of light, and a spray of cold water. The water was incorporated far more often than the other stimuli. The length of the dream was measured as the interval between incorporation of the stimulus and the time the volunteer woke up from REM sleep to a loud door bell tone. The following samples are excerpts from this study.

> The S [subject] was sleeping on his stomach. His back was uncovered. An eye-movement period started and after it had persisted for 10 min., cold water was sprayed on his back. Exactly 30 sec. later he was awakened. The first part of the dream involved a rather complex description of acting in a play. Then, "I was walking behind the leading lady, when she suddenly collapsed and water was dripping on her. I ran over to her and felt water dripping on my back and head. The roof was leaking. I was very puzzled why she fell down and decided some plaster must have fallen on her. I looked up and there was a hole in the roof. I dragged her over to the side of the stage and began pulling the curtains. Just then I woke up."
>
> [This] example is included because of its special interest. It was obtained fortuitously. The S was

standing by a record player in his dream listening to some music, intending to leave for home. "The doorbell rang and she asked me if I would answer it. I hesitated for a moment and, as I started to go, it rang again." In this instance E's [the experimenter's] finger accidentally slipped off the awakening bell, and hence it was rung twice to rouse S. About 3 or 4 sec. elapsed between the two rings.

After evaluating these and many other examples, Dement and Wolpert (1958) concluded that their findings and those of others "tend to support the hypothesis that dream events and real events proceed at about the same rate." Subsequent studies have not altered this conclusion.

REFERENCES

Dement WC, Kleitman N. 1957. Cyclic variations in EEG during sleep and their relation to eye movements, body motility, and dreaming. *Electroencephalogr Clin Neurophysiol* 9:673–690.

Dement WC, Wolpert EA. 1958. The relation of eye movements, body motility, and external stimuli to dream content. *J Exp Psychol* 55(6):543–553.

Freud S. 1961. *The interpretation of dreams.* New York: Science Editions.

Mary A. Carskadon

INSTINCT

Whether one calls sleep an instinct depends on the definition of the term *instinct*. Most biologists agree to the following technical definition: a pattern of behavior that is elicited by a pattern of stimuli (internal or external) without a background of learning. In addition, instincts typically end in an adaptive, stereotyped consumatory (fulfilling) response and are universal within species. This definition describes many mating, maternal, migratory, and foraging behaviors in many species. Problems arise when the term *instinct* is extended to mean any kind of species-typical behavior that on the surface seems to be "innate" or "natural," such as aggression, curiosity, display, acquisitiveness, and playfulness. In the 1920s, an extreme position was promulgated, with a resultant listing of thousands of "instincts" proposed to explain behavior.

The central problem typically involves the extent to which the behavior in question depends on or is modifiable by learning. The difficulty is compounded by the apparent presence of technically defined instincts in lower organisms that may be less apparent in higher organisms.

In regard to sleep, it is clear that species-specific patterns of sleep are typical. For example, grazing animals such as cattle, sheep, and deer sleep in short bouts for about 4 hours per 24 hours. Primates, like humans and monkeys, sleep for long periods of about 8 hours per 24 hours. Many rodents sleep in brief episodes, mostly during the daylight hours, totaling as much as 12 hours per 24 hours. Other animals, such as the opposum and sloth, sleep as much as 18 hours per 24 hours. Furthermore, such patterns are evidently not learned, as they are essentially identical across generations, emerge in a developmental sequence, and may be maintained even when an animal is raised in isolation or in widely different surrounds. Thus, in the broad sense of an innate and species-specific behavior, sleep can be called an instinct.

Limitations of a pure instinctive notion, however, should be noted. Even in lower animals, for example, there is little evidence that sleep is tightly tied to "eliciting" cues, as is the case for classical instinctive mating or maternal behaviors. Further, within limits, sleep is responsive to learning or environmental influences. For example, diurnal animals may become nocturnal under heavy daytime predatory pressures, and total sleep amounts may be influenced by such behavioral controls as confinement. In humans, sleep patterns may be culturally influenced (see CULTURAL INFLUENCES). Nevertheless, the innate and adaptive nature of animal sleep patterns has led some authors to speculate about sleep as an instinctive behavior (Meddis, 1977, Webb, 1974).

(See also EVOLUTION OF SLEEP.)

REFERENCES

Meddis R. 1977. *The sleep instinct.* London: Routledge & Kegan Paul.

Webb WB. 1974. The adaptive functions of sleep. *Percept Motor Skills* 38:1023–1027.

Wilse B. Webb

INTERNAL ALARM CLOCK

A long-standing belief in a human capacity to measure the passage of time while asleep is based on the reputed ability of some individuals to awaken themselves at or very near preselected, nonhabitual times without reliance on external cues. This belief has been sustained by recurrent anecdotal accounts of such feats and by several scientific reports; but contemporary sleep research has cast serious doubt on it.

Skepticism about this concept is in order because, prior to the modern era of sleep research, seemingly supportive investigations of timed self-awakenings typically relied on self-observations without objective confirmation of reportedly accurate outcomes by independent observers (for example, Brush 1930; Omwake and Loranz, 1933). As a rule, such investigations also failed to distinguish between truly accurate single awakenings and what amounts to inaccurate performance when a sleeper awakes prematurely, consults a clock, and then manages to awake near the target time on a second or third attempt.

Modern investigations based on closely monitored electrophysiological recordings have shown that self-awakenings, whether single or multiple and whether accurately timed or not, occur with disproportionately high frequency from REM sleep and at points of likely transitions to REM sleep (Lavie, Oksenberg, and Zomer, 1979; Zepelin, 1986). This finding holds true for both experienced self-awakeners and unpracticed novices. A similar distribution has been found for unintentional, spontaneous awakenings in humans (Hono et al., 1990) and other mammals (Snyder, 1966).

The activated condition of the brain during REM sleep increases the likelihood of awakening and apparently also facilitates recall of the sleeper's intention to awake. As indicated by the self-awakening ability of unpracticed individuals, no special gift or training is required. Although sleepers typically do not know when their REM periods will occur, occasional coincidence of target times and REM periods is ensured by the cyclical recurrence of REM across the night. Such coincidence gives the impression of astonishing accuracy. Awakenings even 15 to 20 minutes away from target time reinforce this impression.

Supporting this explanation are contemporary findings that self-described accurate self-awakeners perform very inconsistently when studied in the laboratory (Lavie, Oksenberg, and Zomer, 1979; Zepelin, 1986). There has yet to be a witnessed demonstration of accurate self-awakenings at a variety of target times during sleep by any individual. Without such demonstrations, coincidence is the only plausible explanation of accuracy. Should the need for an alarm clock arise when one is available, however, the REM cycle can be recommended as a built-in substitute of limited reliability.

REFERENCES

Brush, EN. 1930. Observations on the temporal judgment during sleep. *Am J Psychol* 42:408–411.

Hono T, Matsunaka K, Hiroshige Y, Miyata Y. 1990. Behaviorally signaled awakenings during a nocturnal sleep in humans: The special preference to REM sleep and their coupling with NREM/REM cycle. *Psychologia* 33:21–28.

Lavie P, Oksenberg A, Zomer J. 1979. "It's time, you must wake up now." *Percept Motor Skills* 49:447–450.

Omwake KT, Loranz M. 1933. Study of ability to wake at a specified time. *J Appl Psychol* 17:468–474.

Snyder F. 1966. Toward an evolutionary theory of dreaming. *Am J Psychiatry* 123:121–134.

Zepelin H. 1986. REM sleep and the timing of self-awakenings. *Bull Psychon Soc* 24:254–256.

Harold Zepelin

INTERNAL DESYNCHRONIZATION

Internal desynchronization is the loss of synchrony between two CIRCADIAN RHYTHMS. It has been observed in many, though not all, human TEMPORAL ISOLATION experiments, in which subjects spend weeks in underground bunkers or special apartments, shielded from time cues such as sunrise and sunset, newspapers, television, radio, telephone, and the like. Researchers monitor a host of biological variables, including temperature, activity, urinary output, and blood levels of certain hormones and other substances.

Synchronization or *synchrony* means that there is a 1:1 relation between two rhythms and that the two rhythms maintain the same phase relation to each other. A marker event or particular phase in one rhythm (e.g., sleep onset in the sleep–wake rhythm) may be characterized by its timing with respect to the other rhythm (e.g., timing of sleep onset with respect to temperature minimum).

In a typical free run, a subject initially shows a synchronization between the temperature rhythm and the sleep–wake rhythm. Sleep onsets tend to occur at the same time of each temperature cycle, usually close to the minimum temperature, and not at other times during the temperature cycle. After several temperature cycles, the sleep onsets of many subjects would occur not just near the temperature minimum, but at a variety of times throughout the temperature cycle.

The temperature cycle can be imagined as a clock with 0 at twelve o'clock, 0.25 at three o'clock, 0.5 at six o'clock, 0.75 at nine o'clock, and other decimal fractions between 0 and 1 at any given position on the clock face. For example, five o'clock would be 5/12 or 0.4167. These fractions are called *phases* of the temperature cycle. By convention, phase 0 is assigned to the temperature minimum.

Around the edge of the temperature clock, a dot is placed every time there is a sleep onset. When the temperature and sleep–wake rhythms are in synchrony, the dots cluster near the same phase. When the temperature and sleep–wake rhythms are in desynchrony, dots occur at a variety of phases throughout the cycle. For example, a typical sequence of sleep-onset times during synchrony in a free run might be 0.85, 0.9, 0, 0.95, 0.05, 0. This might be followed by a run of desynchrony such as 0, 0.4, 0.7, 0.3, 0.6, 0.2.

Sometimes an individual might show a pattern such as two temperature cycles for one sleep onset, with a very long wake length. In some published data sets, sleep onsets in such cases occur at the same phase. Although this would seem to be an example of synchrony, the traditional name for such a pattern is *apparent internal desynchronization,* highlighting the fact that there is not a 1:1 relation between temperature and sleep–wake rhythms. Another term, *real internal desynchronization,* refers to the irregular pattern of sleep onsets at a variety of temperature phases.

Although the relation between temperature and activity during some free runs is often cited as an example of desynchronization, any two rhythms may show such a relation.

It is believed that some people suffering from JET LAG experience temporary internal desynchronization of temperature and activity rhythms.

(See also CIRCADIAN RHYTHMS.)

REFERENCE

Wever RA. 1979. *The circadian system of man.* New York: Springer-Verlag.

Kevin A. O'Connor

INTERNS

See Deprivation, Partial

INTERPRETATION OF DREAMS

The interpretation of dreams refers to a process of discovering the connection between the dream and the emotional life of the dreamer. The way we should go about interpreting dreams has been a matter of concern and debate all through our recorded history. Existence of this problem for at least the last 2,000 years is demonstrated by the records of dream guide books dating from as long ago as 500 B.C. Clay tablets with information on interpreting dreams were very common during that period. To dream of flying meant impending disaster. To drink water in a dream meant a long life, but to drink wine foretold a short one (Van de Castle, 1971). Some people still look for the meaning of their dreams in such dream "dictionaries." These may be fun, rather like fortune cookies, but they are not to be taken seriously.

The early Egyptians had the ancient equivalent of our modern sleep laboratories in their temples. People came to sleep there to find the answer to questions of importance to them. They would "incubate" dreams by praying or fasting beforehand. Dream interpreters, known as the Learned Men of the Magic Library, had offices in these temples and offered to decode the dream answer sent by the gods (Wallis-Budge, 1899).

Artemidorus, an Italian physician writing in about A.D. 150, had a rather more sophisticated view of what the interpreter needed to know before pronouncing what a dream was about. He stressed the importance of having more than one dream, preferably a sequence of dreams to work with, as well as some knowledge of the dreamer and his or her present circumstances (White, 1975).

The answer to the question, "What do dreams mean," and even "Do they mean anything at all," has been sought by many philosophers, physicians, poets and priests and continues to be asked today with only somewhat better methods to help in the hunt. The difficulty comes about because of three facts: (1) Dreaming is a plentiful but uniquely private mental experience; (2) it is common to us all throughout our life span, yet occurs spontaneously, outside our will; (3) dreaming occurs in a form quite different from our waking thoughts, so that it appears to us as strange. In other words, dreams are common but unique, our own but outside our control, and created by us but not understandable. What should we do with this experience? Being creatures of enormous curiosity, we try hard to find meaning in all our experience, and so we have invented many different ways to understand the meanings of our dreams.

The modern era of dream interpretation begins in 1900 with the publication of Sigmund Freud's major work "The Interpretation of Dreams" (1966). Freud gave us two keys to finding the meaning in our dreams. The first was his distinction between the obvious or manifest content of the dream (the dream story) and its hidden purpose or latent content. The important part is the latent content, which requires a skilled person to understand. The second key to the meaning of dreams came from Freud's idea of their function. He believed that dreams express unfulfilled wishes left over from early childhood—hidden away in our unconscious mind but still active. They are banished from our waking awareness because they are unacceptable in polite society. Even in sleep they must only show themselves in disguised form. To understand dreams we must use an indirect route. Freud's method was to train the patient to let his or her mind float freely. To help this along it was important that the person lay on a couch with the dream interpreter behind and out of sight. The patient's job was to say whatever came into his or her mind and not to follow the logical connections between the dream imagery and waking life. Presumably, these free as-

sociations would get at the underlying pattern of emotional connections between the dream and the past. These emotions are expressed in the dream through various tricks such as condensation (where one object or person perhaps represents several emotionally important streams of thought that are condensed into one image).

To interpret a dream correctly according to Freud, one needs to understand his theory of the mind—particularly the role of the unconscious—and to use the method of free association. This technique circumvents the barriers between our conscious and unconscious minds, barriers erected to keep the forbidden impulses "out of sight and out of mind." This approach proved to be too esoteric an idea and too slow a method to satisfy the more pragmatic-minded fast-track Americans.

Theories of the next generation of dream doctors differed greatly regarding how dreams are interpreted. Thomas French and Erika Fromm (1964), for example, saw the purpose of dreaming to be a search for solutions to current interpersonal problems. Their method, like that of Artemidorus, requires working with dreams in series rather than one at a time. Their emphasis is less on the dreamer's free association and more on the empathic intuition of the dream analyst. It is the analyst's job to fit together the dream's references to the past with the dreamer's present emotional situation.

These changes—from an emphasis on the past to looking for meaning in the dreamer's present, from the free association method, which was difficult to learn, to trusting to the listener's intuition—have culminated in new, typically American ways to approach dream interpretation, such as the group methods of Montague Ullman (Ullman and Zimmerman, 1979) and Gayle Delaney (1991).

Ullman and Delaney are professional therapists who have developed similar methods for understanding dreams. They believe that a dreamer can be helped to "see what the dream means" more clearly by being offered intuitions from other people not emotionally involved with the same problem as the dreamer. Dream groups using these methods meet in many communities.

Quite a different and more intellectual approach has evolved from the work of the French anthropologist Claude Lévi-Strauss (1981). It is a more formal structural analysis developed to understand the myths of primitive people, and

Kuper (1983) has applied it to dream interpretation. This method, too, goes back to Artemidorus's point that we need to work with a series of dreams if we are to discover their meaning. According to Kuper, dreams consist of a series of variations that obey a strict set of rules. The variations reflect a problem of the dreamer along sets of opposites like in-out, male-female, superior-inferior. These dimensions are the personal elements the dreamer uses to construct dream stories, all of which are attempts to deal with an emotional issue. To interpret the dream, one must identify the dimensions that will be used over and over, sometimes on one side and sometimes on the other. The elements are shifted about until the dreamer reaches some satisfying conclusion about the meaning of the dream.

Whether we take a theory-based approach to dream interpretation, an intuitive approach like Freud's, a group method like those of Ullman and Delaney, or a formal structural analysis approach, such as Kuper's, or some combination of these, the general consensus is that a dream's meaning lies in the current waking emotional life of the dreamer alongside what is in the memory bank of past experiences that are related to current problems.

REFERENCES

Delaney G. 1991. *Breakthrough dreaming*. New York: Bantam Books.

French T, Fromm E. 1964. *Dream interpretation*. New York: Basic Books.

Freud S. 1966. *The complete psychological works of Sigmund Freud* (Standard Edition). London: Hogarth Press.

Kuper A. 1983. The structure of dream sequences. *Cult Med Psychiatry* 7:153–175.

Lévi-Strauss C. 1981. *The naked man*. London: Jonathan Cape.

Ullman M, Zimmerman, N. 1979. *Working with dreams*. New York: Delacorte.

Van de Castle R. 1971. *The psychology of dreaming*, pp 1–46. New York: General Learning Press.

Wallis-Budge E. 1899. *Egyptian magic*. London: Paul, Trench & Truber.

White RJ. 1975. *The interpretation of dreams: Oneirocritica by Artemidorus*. Park Ridge, N.J.: Noyes.

Rosalind D. Cartwright

IRREGULAR SLEEP–WAKE CYCLE

A sleep disorder known as irregular sleep-wake pattern illustrates what happens when someone either ignores the environmental time cues that normally sychronize CIRCADIAN RHYTHMS or has a brain condition that reduces their ability to respond to such cues (see ZEITGEBER). The main feature of this condition is that sleep and waking no longer alternate in a predictable daily cycle. The total amount of sleep per 24 hours may be normal for age, but few if any individual sleep periods are of normal length. The likelihood that the person will be asleep at any particular time of day is relatively low.

If someone with this problem sees a doctor, it may be to complain about an inability to go to sleep or stay asleep at night (INSOMNIA); or they may be distressed by unpredictable and frequent daytime NAPPING. The complaint to the doctor may depend on who is doing the complaining. The patient whose higher mental functions are intact may emphasize the insomnia at night and regard the daytime napping as a necessary result of it. However, when this sleep pattern occurs in conjunction with brain damage, as it often does, the patient's family may ask that the physician prescribe SLEEPING PILLS or TRANQUILIZERS because their loved one wanders about the house at night and becomes agitated when asked to go back to bed. When such patients are hospitalized or placed in a nursing home, the night staff may report that sleeping pills do not work on them, while the patient's family complains that he or she is seldom awake when they come to visit in the daytime.

Unlike other syndromes of abnormal sleep timing (see DELAYED SLEEP PHASE SYNDROME; ADVANCED SLEEP PHASE SYNDROME; HYPERNYCHTHEMERAL SYNDROME; JET LAG; SHIFTWORK), a 1-or 2-week sleep–wake log or diary from an irregular pattern patient shows little or no regularity of sleep onsets or wake times. Instead, sleep occurs in three or more short, often broken episodes that are scattered across each 24 hours, with much day-to-day change in their timing. The pattern is actually somewhat similar to that of newborn infants, but sleep occupies a much lower fraction of the day than in infants.

The original cases of irregular sleep–wake pattern were described in mentally intact individuals who had stopped following a regular rest–

activity schedule, spent very large amounts of time in bed, and often did not eat on a regular basis (Hauri, 1977). The original loss of regularity of daily habits began during a prolonged period of bedrest resulting from a disabling illness or injury. Irregular sleep then persisted despite recovery from the original medical problem. Complaints of poor concentration and memory often accompany the nocturnal insomnia in such cases. Most efforts at medical treatment, including prescription sedatives and/or STIMULANTS, are unsuccessful in the long term. Drug dependence may ensue with long-term use of such medications, and prolonged use can contribute to DEPRESSION.

Irregular sleep is probably more common in patients with congenital, developmental, or degenerative brain problems (for example, in severe MENTAL RETARDATION or advanced ALZHEIMER'S DISEASE) than in mentally intact persons. Prolonged polygraphic recordings of sleep and wakefulness have been performed in a few patients with this problem and generally confirm the disrupted pattern and random timing of their sleep (Allen et al, 1987; Okawa, Takahashi, and Sasaki, 1986; Wagner, 1984). In brain-damaged patients, the irregular sleep–wake pattern may be a result of damage to the circadian timing system ("body clock") in the brain or to brain systems governing sleep and wakefulness, or both. In mentally intact patients, the syndrome probably results from lack of exposure to those social and environmental time cues that ordinarily synchronize our body clocks to the outside world. Such patients usually spend more than half of their daily lives in bed in futile attempts to get more sleep or "rest." They do not recognize that their excessive use of their beds causes the very unpredictability and disruption of sleep from which they are suffering.

These patients are exceedingly difficult for doctors to treat. Those who are mentally intact are often resistant to changing their poor sleep habits, suggesting that the pattern may serve some hidden psychological need, or that they have a concomitant depression. A regular daily sleep–wake and meal schedule combined with some kind of scheduled daily physical and social activities will help if they can be persuaded to follow such advice.

Mentally impaired patients are unable to understand what is wrong because of their brain damage. Nevertheless, a knowledgeable doctor can teach the patient's caretakers about the problem, and caretakers can try to establish a more reasonable daily schedule. Three or four regularly scheduled, short (e.g., 2-hour) "nap" periods, perhaps after each meal and another during the night, is a more sensible way of attempting to manage the sleep–wake schedules of these unfortunate patients. Trying to force sleep to occur only at night by the long-term administration of sleeping pills is very likely to lead only to significant drug toxicity (oversedation, agitation, falling) in these patients.

REFERENCES

Allen SR, Seiler WO, Stahelin HB, Spiegel R. 1987. Seventy-two hour polygraphic and behavioral recordings of wakefulness and sleep in a hospital geriatric unit: Comparison between demented and nondemented patients. *Sleep* 10(2):143–159.

Hauri P. 1977. *The sleep disorders.* Kalamazoo, Mich.: Upjohn.

Okawa M, Takahashi K, Sasaki H. 1986. Disturbance of circadian rhythms in severely brain-damaged patients correlated with CT findings. *J Neurol* 233:274–282.

Wagner DR. 1984. Sleep (in Alzheimer's disease). *Generations—J West Gerontol Soc* 9(2):31–37.

———. 1991. Circadian rhythm sleep disorders. In Thorpy MJ, ed. *Handbook of sleep disorders,* pp 493–527. New York: Marcel Dekker.

Daniel R. Wagner

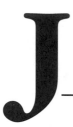

JACTATIO CAPITIS NOCTURNA

See Rhythmic Movement Disorder

JET LAG

The introduction of air travel in this century brought with it an unexpected side effect known as jet lag. Jet lag can occur when people cross several time zones, either east or west, but is not associated with travel north or south, in which the time zone is constant. The symptoms of jet lag can be produced by any situation that involves a change in the schedule of sleeping and waking. Since actual travel is not required, researchers can study the problem under controlled laboratory conditions. Jet lag researchers simulate jet lag in laboratory experiments using time-free apartments. These apartments have no windows, clocks, televisions, radios, or other sources of time cues. Any time zone shift can be achieved by manipulating sleep periods. The other major method of research on jet lag is to study actual travelers.

Potential Causes

The symptoms of jet lag probably result from several factors: (1) fatigue related to the travel itself; (2) a slow and uneven rate of adjustment of biologic rhythms to the new schedule; and (3) sleep loss. The biologic clock located in the brain uses environmental and social time cues to synchronize the biologic rhythms of an individual to the 24-hour day. These cues include, among others, the light–dark cycle, meals, bed and wake times, and social events. When a person crosses time zones, the clock needs to "reset," a process that takes about a day for each time zone crossed. Because the biologic clock tends to "run slow" in humans (see BIOLOGICAL RHYTHMS), it is thought to be easier to travel west, in the natural direction of the biologic clock (a delay), than it is to travel east (an advance). When the biologic clock has not yet adjusted, a person may be trying to sleep when the body is not quite ready, thus contributing to the poor sleep and daytime symptoms of sleepiness, irritability, and fatigue commonly reported with jet lag.

It is important to note that the change in schedule leads to jet lag. If a person stays on his or her home schedule even after traveling, jet lag may be avoided. When many time zones are crossed, however, trying to keep on home time may be extremely difficult.

Older men may cope less well with jet lag because they appear to have more problems sleeping at new times than younger men. Very little is known about women and jet lag because men have been much more frequently studied.

Symptoms

Many people report difficulties in sleeping, daytime sleepiness, and lack of alertness after traveling across time zones. The sleep problems can take many forms, but research has demonstrated shortened nighttime sleep periods, more time spent awake during the night, and changes in the sleep stage pattern, especially in deep sleep and dreaming (REM) sleep.

Many travelers also report irritability, difficulty concentrating, fatigue, and malaise. These mood changes may be due in part to problems with nighttime sleep on the new time schedule. Both laboratory and field studies have reported that subjects with jet lag perform less well on certain types of mental tasks. In addition, muscle strength, ability to sprint, and overall performance in sports may be decreased. Gastrointestinal problems are also frequently reported by travelers across time zones.

Treatments

Treatments are designed either (1) to shift the biologic clock to the new schedule faster than it would without treatment, or (2) to improve nighttime sleep in the hope that daytime symptoms will then improve as well. Some investigators recommend gradually adjusting to the new schedule before traveling, by about an hour a day, either by retiring and waking early (eastbound trips) or by retiring and waking late (westbound trips). These procedures are somewhat inconvenient and have not been rigorously tested. Alternatively, a traveler can maximize his or her exposure to the potential entraining cues at the destination. Resetting one's watch to the new local time, eating meals when the local people do, sleeping during the "new" night, and getting out of bed at the appropriate local time are important methods of using available temporal cues. In addition, people should go outside during daylight so that they are exposed to natural light. Using bright artificial light to alter the timing of biologic rhythms is currently an area of active investigation, but to date, the exact parameters of light exposure have not yet been determined.

Finally, laboratory studies of napping as a treatment for jet lag suggest that napping may increase a person's alertness after the nap, but this is a potentially problematic approach because the person may sleep less well that night and perpetuate the jet lag.

A jet lag treatment program has been proposed, combining the use of a special diet, exercise, and exposure to time cues at the destination. The diet component is performed before and during the days of travel and consists of alternating days of high-calorie and low-calorie consumption, eating high-protein breakfasts and lunches and high-carbohydrate dinners, and timing consumption of caffeine. This treatment program needs to be studied under controlled conditions before it can be recommended. Furthermore, because it must be implemented before traveling, it may be inconvenient or impractical for last-minute travelers.

Melatonin, a hormone produced by the pineal gland, has been used to treat jet lag on the assumption that it may speed adjustment of the circadian clock. Melatonin is not approved for this purpose, however, and more research is needed before this substance can be recommended.

Some studies have examined the use of sedative-hypnotics (sleeping pills) to treat jet lag. The results from several studies suggest that they can lengthen sleep during the destination night, but can worsen daytime symptoms, such as excessive sleepiness, if drugs with a long duration of action are used.

There are still many questions that need to be addressed by future research on jet lag, including the effects of age and gender, which have not been the focus of research to date. The best advice at this time is that travelers should maximize their exposure to the environmental and social time cues at their destination, avoid napping unless they need to be maximally alert immediately afterwards, and limit the use of hypnotics because of daytime sedation and side effects. Timed light exposure and melatonin administration may ultimately prove to be useful techniques as well.

Margaret L. Moline

JUNG'S DREAM THEORY

The dream theory of Carl G. Jung (1875–1961) is one of the most important and widely influential dream theories in modern depth psychology (that branch of psychology that studies the unconscious as its main object). Jung, a Swiss medical doctor, was at one time Freud's closest friend and leading student; however, Jung and Freud had a bitter falling out in 1914, in part because of their different theories of the nature and function of dreams (see FREUD'S DREAM THEORY).

In Jung's view, dreams are the direct, natural expression of the current condition of the dreamer's mental world. Jung rejected Freud's claim that dreams intentionally disguise their meanings; rather, Jung believed that the nature of dreams is to present "a spontaneous self-portrayal, in symbolic form, of the actual situation in the unconscious" (Jung, 1967, Vol. 8, par. 505). Jung claimed that dreams speak in a distinctive language of symbols, images, and metaphors, a language that is the unconscious mind's natural means of expression. We have trouble understanding dreams, Jung said, only because this symbolic language is so different from the language of our waking consciousness.

Dreams sometimes portray the dreamer's relation with the external world, that is, with the people, events, and activities of the dreamer's daily life. Jung called this the *objective* level of a dream's meaning. At other times, dreams portray the dreamer's inner world; the dream figures are personifications of thoughts and feelings within the dreamer's own psyche. This, Jung said, is the *subjective* level of a dream's meaning. Jung criticized Freud for acknowledging only the objective level; the true nature of dreams, Jung believed, is to portray both these levels of the dreamer's life.

Jung stated that dreams serve two functions. One function is to *compensate* for imbalances in the dreamer's psyche. Dreams bring forth unconscious contents that consciousness has either ignored, depreciated, or actively repressed. For example, if a person is overly intellectual, his or her dreams will work to balance this conscious excess by bringing forth images of the psyche's more emotion-oriented contents. According to Jung, when the dreamer recognizes and accepts these unconscious contents, greater psychological balance is achieved. The second function of dreams is to provide *prospective* images of the future. Jung agrees with Freud that dreams may look backward to past experiences, but he argues that dreams also look forward to anticipate what the dreamer's future developments may be. Jung did not mean that dreams predict the future, only that dreams can suggest what might happen, what possibilities the future might hold. Ultimately, Jung believed that dreams function to promote the most important developmental process of human life, namely, the uniting of consciousness and the unconscious in a healthy, harmonious state of wholeness. Jung calls this process *individuation*, the "complete actualization of the whole human being" (Jung, 1967, Vol. 16, par. 352).

One of the most distinctive features of Jung's theory of dreams is his claim that dreams express not just personal contents, but also collective or universal contents. Jung believed that dreams frequently contain *archetypes*, universal psychic images that underlie all human thought. (Common archetypal figures described by Jung are the wise old man, the great mother, the trickster, the divine child, and the shadow.) Archetypes reflect a natural wisdom deep within the human unconscious; archetypal images in dreams can provide the dreamer with special insights and guidance along the path toward individuation. Jung believed that the world's religious and mythological traditions contain a wealth of archetypal images, and he refers to these traditions in describing the nature and function of dreams.

Jung's dream theory has been criticized for being perilously close to mysticism and the occult. Jung insisted, however, that his theory of dreams is based on strictly empirical observations. He claimed to have interpreted over 80,000 dreams during his almost 60 years of clinical practice; Jung said his theory simply attempts to describe and classify the dream phenomena he had observed.

REFERENCES

Homans P. 1979. *Jung in context*. Chicago: University of Chicago Press. A study of Jung's relationship with Freud.

Jung CG. 1965. *Memories, dreams, reflections*. New York: Vintage. Jung's autobiography, filled with dream accounts; essential to understanding his life and theories.

———. 1967. *Man and his symbols*. New York: Dell. Jung's last work, an explanation of his psychology in nontechnical terms.

———. 1967. *The collected works of C.G. Jung*. Princeton, NJ: Princeton University Press, 1967. Jung discusses dreams throughout the 18 volumes of his writings. The key works on dreams are the following: General Aspects of Dream Psychology, Vol. 8; On the Nature of Dreams, Vol. 8; The Practical Use of Dream Analysis, Vol. 16; Individual Dream Symbolism in Relation to Alchemy, Vol. 12; Two Essays on Analytical Psychology, Vol. 7.

Samuels A. 1985. *Jung and the post-Jungians.* London: Routledge & Kegan Paul. Describes post-Jungian dream theories.

Kelly Bulkley

K
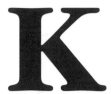

K-COMPLEX

One of the most striking features of the ELECTRO-ENCEPHALOGRAM (EEG) during sleep is the K-complex (Figure 1). This complex of waveforms, which is a defining characteristic of stage 2 sleep (see STAGES OF SLEEP), has an initial sharply contoured negative component that rises abruptly out of the background EEG activity and may have an amplitude of several hundred microvolts. This component is followed immediately by a lower-amplitude positive slow wave that may have a superimposed sleep spindle. The complex, which has a voltage maximum over the vertex or less commonly over the midline frontal scalp, has a total duration of at least 0.5 second and sometimes more than 1 second. K-complexes are first apparent at about age 5 months and are most prominent in older children and in early adolescence. With advancing age, the complex declines in voltage.

The K-complex is an example of an *evoked response,* a term used to describe brain potentials that are elicited by stimulation. During stage 2 sleep, the K-complex can be easily elicited by auditory stimuli, such as the tap of a pencil, and by other forms of mild stimulation. It can also occur spontaneously, perhaps in response to internal stimuli.

REFERENCES

Erwin CW, Somerville ER, Radtke RA. 1984. A review of electroencephalographic features of normal sleep. *J Clin Neurophysiol* 1:253–274.

Niedermeyer E. 1987. Sleep and EEG. In Niedermeyer E, Lopes da Silva F, eds. *Electroencephalography: Basic principles, clinical applications and related fields,* 2nd ed, pp 119–133. Baltimore: Urban & Schwarzenberg.

Michael Aldrich

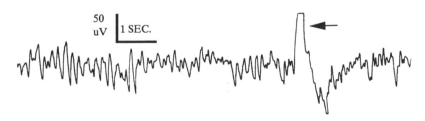

Figure 1. Electroencephalogram recording during stage 2 sleep from the left central scalp (C_3 electrode) using the right ear as a reference electrode. A K-complex is shown at the arrow. The peak of the initial negative phase is flattened because the excursion of the recording pen could not accommodate the entire amplitude of the wave. SEC., second; uV, microvolts.

KEKULÉ, FRIEDRICH AUGUST

See Creativity in Dreams; Problem Solving and Dreaming

KENNEDY, JOHN F.

See Short Sleepers in History and Legend

KLEINE-LEVIN SYNDROME

The association of behavioral disturbances with disordered eating and sleep has been known for centuries. Some of the earliest reports were in myths, plays, and even religious writings. So-called vegetative symptoms, including sleep and eating disturbances, are important diagnostic features of depression. In a 1942 survey of a small number of case reports of patients with episodic sleepiness, excessive eating, and psychological symptoms, this condition was named for Kleine and Levin to credit them for their earlier detailed descriptions of this illness.

Relatively uncommon, Kleine-Levin syndrome is a disorder of recurrent episodes of excessive drowsiness and associated behavior, mood, and thought abnormalities, each usually lasting days to weeks. The periodic symptoms may be substantially disabling but between recurrences the patients are usually normal. Typically, the symptoms recur without any definable precipitant at least once or twice per year. Symptomatic periods become less frequent with time. Eventually, recurrences stop and the patient remains symptom free.

When excessively drowsy, Kleine-Levin patients may sleep almost the entire day, awakening only to eat, urinate, or defecate. They are not incontinent. Despite their prolonged sleep the patients can be aroused from sleep but often remain lethargic. Curiously, a small proportion of patients with the behavioral features of Kleine-Levin have insomnia rather than excessive drowsiness. Symptoms that arise in epileptics during sleep—incontinence, biting of the tongue or lining of the mouth, falls from bed during sleep, or awakening with excessive aching in muscles—are absent.

During symptomatic periods overeating (and consequent weight gain) is often dramatic. Patients are observed to take in substantially more food than normal and, unable to defer eating, ingest any food available regardless of quality or preferences. Oddly, symptomatic Kleine-Levin patients do not complain of hunger, and when food is not present they do not crave it or attempt to find it.

Depression, anxiety, slow thinking, absentmindedness, inattention, memory disturbance, apathy, irritability, and aggression may occur during symptomatic periods. At these times, patients may have difficulty organizing or carrying out step-by-step plans. Effective study or other organized work may be precluded for the duration. Hallucinations may also occur.

Impulsiveness can be prominent during a recurrence. Otherwise uncharacteristic unrestrained sexual behavior may manifest. The patient may make provocative comments or actually initiate sexual contact with unfamiliar or otherwise inappropriate individuals. Masturbation may take place in an exhibitionistic setting. As with the excessive drowsiness and overeating, the disinhibition gives way to normal baseline behavior during remissions.

Kleine-Levin syndrome usually begins during adolescence. It is more frequent in males than females. In a minority of cases a flulike illness, head injury, or other event precedes the onset of symptoms. There is no evidence of familial occurrence.

Although the behavioral symptoms, drowsiness, and overeating suggest dysfunction of the HYPOTHALAMUS, high-resolution images of the brain generated by computerized tomographic scanning or magnetic resonance imaging show no characteristic structural abnormality. Postmortem examinations of the brains of two patients with histories suggestive but not typical of Kleine-Levin documented inflammatory reactions in the thalamus in one and similar abnormalities of the hypothalamus and portions of the temporal lobe in the other.

Reports of electroencephalographic recordings made during and between symptomatic episodes indicate a variety of nonspecific abnormalities. During episodes, slowing of brain wave frequencies was noted. More normal recordings were obtained between spells. Overnight simultaneous recordings of brain waves, eye movements, and muscle electrical activity documented some loss of slow-wave sleep and the early onset of REM sleep. In standardized tests consisting of multiple daytime naps, symptomatic Kleine-Levin patients were very sleepy and had sleep-onset stage REM sleep, a physiological feature of NARCOLEPSY and depression; however, a small number of other Kleine-Levin patients lacked HLA-DR2 and HLA-Dqw1 antigens, genetic markers that are an essentially constant feature of narcolepsy.

Like other, more common sleep disorders, Kleine-Levin is often misdiagnosed. Many patients may have only a few of the typical symptoms, and the intensity of those present may be mild. Patients, particularly those with the incomplete syndrome, may receive inappropriate and sometimes expensive or potentially harmful treatment. Excessive sleepiness, overeating, and asocial behavior do not engender empathy, further compounding the disability of Kleine-Levin patients. Even when the correct diagnosis is made the response to treatment is variable. Some patients respond to phenytoin (Dilantin), a commonly used anticonvulsant. Stimulant medi-cations may temporarily reduce the pervasive drowsiness during attacks. Lithium, a drug used most often to prevent recurrences of manic-depressive illness, has been effective in isolated cases.

REFERENCES

Billiard M. 1989. The Kleine-Levin syndrome. In Kryger M, Roth T, Dement WC, eds. *Principles and practice of sleep medicine,* chap 39, pp. 377–378. Philadelphia: Saunders.

Critchley M. 1962. Periodic hypersomnia and megaphagia in adolescent males. *Brain* 85:627–656.

Gallinek A. 1954. Syndrome of episodes of hypersomnia, bulimia, and abnormal mental states. *JAMA* 154:1081–1083.

Smolik P, Roth B. 1988. Kleine-Levin syndrome: Ethiopathogenesis and treatment. *Acta Univ Carol [Med Monogr] (Praha)* 128:5–94.

Michael P. Biber

L

LATERAL GENICULATE NUCLEUS

The lateral geniculate nucleus is the brain area relaying visual information from the eyes to the cerebral cortex. It is located in a brain region called the thalamus. It receives a direct projection from the eyes and thus is one of the two senses whose sensory messages do not pass through additional lower brainstem relays (the other sense is smell). The position of the lateral geniculate nucleus as the only link between the visual receptor apparatus and the cortex has made it a popular region in which to study sleep–wake influences on thalamic sensory processing. Like other thalamic relay nuclei during different states of arousal, lateral geniculate relay neurons are highly excitable during waking and pass to the cortex, almost unaltered, the visual messages received from the eyes. During NREM sleep, lateral geniculate neurons are inhibited and less responsive to visual stimuli. During REM sleep, however, lateral geniculate neurons are again highly excitable and are at least as active as during waking. Additionally, the separation of neurons into layers within the lateral geniculate nucleus permits large electrical waves to be recorded at this location during REM sleep. These waves are associated with an additional excitation of the lateral geniculate nucleus. The high level of activity in the lateral geniculate nucleus during REM sleep is relayed to visual cortex and may be the neuronal population underlying the prominence of visual imagery during dreaming. (See PGO WAVES; THALAMUS.)

REFERENCE

Steriade M. 1990. Thalamocortical systems: Inhibition at sleep onset and activation during dreaming sleep. In Mancia M, Marini G. eds. *The diencephalon and sleep*, pp. 231–247. New York: Raven.

Gerald A. Marks

L-DOPA

See Parkinson's Disease

LEARNING

Can factual information presented to an individual during sleep be stored and then remembered (retrieved) when awake? Asked differently, Can individuals learn while sleeping? Researchers usually focus on declarative knowledge when trying to provide an answer to the question. Declarative knowledge deals with explicit everyday remembering of facts such as names, numbers, and events. This type of knowledge can be easily communicated to others and is similar to what we learn in most classrooms. Before answering the question posed above we must distinguish between "learning during sleep" and "processing information during sleep." There is some confusion regarding the two phenomena.

We know that during sleep our brain continuously monitors the external environment and that we remain sensitive to changes in it. Thus, processing of information does occur in sleep in that we respond to sensory events and can retrieve, in sleep, material learned and stored in memory while awake (see PERCEPTION DURING SLEEP). But, can we form memories of having done so? Can we remember events that we experience during sleep?

Studies in which sleeping subjects respond to stimuli according to instructions they receive while awake indicate that short-term memory functions well in sleep and that memories established in waking can be accessed (Badia, 1990; see AMNESIA). However, the critical event for establishing learning in sleep—consolidation into long-term memory of events occurring in sleep—does not occur. This memory deficit in sleep closely resembles the memory (learning) deficit present in people with head (brain) injuries and also those with ALZHEIMER'S DISEASE. It is called anterograde amnesia. That is, old experiences can be retrieved from memory but new experiences cannot be stored in memory (learning does not occur).

There are both anecdotal and systematic accounts of amnesia (failing to learn) for events occurring during sleep. When the material to be remembered (learned) is factual (names, numbers, events, etc.) and sleep is objectively measured (polygraphically recorded brain wave activity), there is simply no evidence available that information presented in sleep is stored in memory and retained in waking. The latter conclusion regarding the absence of learning in sleep was drawn by Emmons and Simon (1956) and has been confirmed and strengthened by others (Aarons, 1976; Lehmann and Koukkou, 1974). For learning to occur or new memories to be formed regarding factual material, an individual must be awake; that is, the ELECTROENCEPHALOGRAM (brain waves) must show a waking pattern (e.g., alpha rhythm).

What about simpler forms of learning that do not involve factual knowledge? There is some evidence that classical conditioning and habituation of autonomic responses, such as heart rate and eye blink responses, can be learned during sleep. Thus the suggestion is that sleep may affect the brain areas involved in factual learning differently than the brain areas involved in simpler learning (Badia, 1990).

REFERENCES

Aarons L. 1976. Sleep assisted instruction. *Psychol Bull* 83:1–40.

Badia P. 1990. Memories in sleep: Old and new. In Bootzin BR, Kihlstrom JF, Schacter DL, eds. *Sleep and cognition*, pp 67–77. Washington, D.C.: American Psychological Association. This book is an excellent review of the cognition during sleep literature.

Emmons WH, Simon CW. 1956. The non-recall of material presented during sleep. *Am J Psychol* 6:76–81.

Harsh J, Badia P. 1990. Stimulus control and sleep. In Bootzin BR, Kilhstrom JF, Schacter DL, eds. *Sleep and cognition*, pp 58–66. Washington, D.C.: American Psychological Association.

Koukkou M, Lehmann D. 1968. EEG and memory storage in sleep experiments with humans. *Electroencephalogr Clin Neurophysiol* 25:455–462.

Lehmann D, Koukkou M. 1974. Computer analysis of EEG wakefulness–sleep patterns during learning of novel familiar sentences. *Electroencephalogr Clin Neurophysiol* 37:73–84.

Pietro Badia

LEG CRAMPS, NOCTURNAL

See Parasomnias

LEGENDARY SLEEPERS

See Long Sleepers in History and Legend; Short Sleepers in History and Legend

LIGHT

Early in the nineteenth century, it was discovered that the period or cycle length of daily BIOLOGICAL RHYTHMS, when monitored in constant darkness, is not exactly 24 hours (DeCandolle, 1832). Subsequent research has demonstrated that, of all the periodic changes of the external environment, the daily alternation between light and darkness is responsible for synchronizing these near-24-hour (or *circadian*) rhythms to the 24-hour day (see CIRCADIAN RHYTHMS).

At first, humans were thought to be an exception to this general rule. The human circadian system was thought to be more responsive to the influence of periodic social interaction than to the periodic environmental stimulus of the LIGHT–DARK CYCLE. More recent research, however, revealed that humans respond to light in much the same was as do plants, other MAMMALS (Czeisler et al., 1989), and insects (see INSECTS: SLEEPLIKE STATES IN). ENTRAINMENT to the 24-hour day can even be achieved with exposure to comparatively dim indoor room light during waking hours and to darkness during night sleep (Czeisler et al., 1981). Furthermore, properly timed exposure to bright light (comparable in intensity to outdoor light) and darkness can quickly (within one or two cycles) reset the human circadian pacemaker to any desired phase. Several factors determine how the circadian pacemaker responds to a light stimulus: the light's intensity, the light's wavelength (or color spectrum), the duration of light exposure, the phase of the circadian cycle at which light exposure occurs, and the number of consecutive daily light exposures.

The circadian phase dependence of the resetting response to light—first discovered in a species of blue-green algae (Hastings and Sweeney, 1958)—has since been verified in all other eukaryotic organisms (i.e., those made up of cells with true nuclei) studied, including humans (Czeisler et al., 1989). In fact, the PHASE–RESPONSE CURVE to light in humans is strikingly similar to that in other species. Thus, for example, light exposure that occurs later than usual (i.e., after our usual bedtime) *delays* the human circadian pacemaker to a later hour on subsequent cycles. Similarly, light exposure earlier than usual (i.e., before our usual rise time) *advances* the pacemaker to an earlier hour on subsequent cycles. Light exposure at the usual times (i.e., during the waking day) has much less of a resetting effect on the pacemaker, although daytime light exposure is important for entrainment of the pacemaker to the 24-hour day. As might be expected, bright light exposure at times when the pacemaker "expects" darkness has the most profound resetting effect on the pacemaker; in fact, repeated exposure to bright light at "night" reliably turns the biological night into day.

Nevertheless, the phase or timing of the pacemaker's oscillation is not the only rhythmic characteristic affected by light. Exposure to light also affects the amplitude or strength of the underlying oscillation (Winfree, 1987; Jewett, Kronauer, and Czeisler, 1991). Light exposure at an adverse phase, such as the biological night, diminishes the strength of the circadian oscillation; light exposure in synchrony with the rhythm, such as during the biological day, enhances the strength of the oscillation. These effects of light on the amplitude of the circadian oscillation interact with the phase-shifting response, since reducing the amplitude of the underlying oscillation increases its sensitivity to the resetting effects of light.

The circadian pacemaker's resetting response to light increases with the intensity of the light exposure. This intensity dependence, though well known in other species, has yet to be quantified in humans. Current evidence, however, suggests that there is a nonlinear relationship between the intensity of a light stimulus and the biological response that it elicits. In other words, a stimulus that is twice as bright will not elicit twice as great a response. To understand this quantitatively requires an understanding of the yardstick by which light intensity is measured. The *lux* is the metric unit used to quantify the intensity of visible light and represents the amount of visible light to which we are exposed by a single candle viewed from a distance of 1 meter. The lux is the metric counterpart of the British foot-candle. Light intensity in the latter case, however, is measured from a distance of 1 foot; hence, 1 foot-candle is roughly equivalent to about 10 lux. Although the precise relationship between such physical measures of light intensity (I) and measures of the biological effectiveness of light as a circadian phase-shifting agent (B) has yet to be determined, Richard Kronauer has hypothesized on the basis of available evidence that the formula $B=k(I)/3$ roughly approximates their nonlinear relationship (i.e., a ten-fold increase in light intensity increases the biological effectiveness of the stimulus by only a bit more than two-fold).

Although little is known about the influence of the color or wavelength of a light stimulus in humans, wavelength is well known to affect the resetting response to light in other species. For example, in organisms as diverse as algae and nocturnal rodents, red light is not effective in resetting the circadian pacemaker. The photoreceptive element mediating the circadian phase-shifting response has not yet been identified.

Recent studies in a strain of mice with a genetic defect that causes a nearly complete degeneration of the retina have yielded a very surprising result: The pacemaker's response to light is not at all diminished in those "blind" mice. Since removal of eyes does eliminate the resetting response, Foster and his colleagues at the University of Virginia suggest that the retina may contain a novel photoreceptive cell—other than the rods and cones—that may transduce "circadian photoreception," mediating entrainment of the circadian system to the light–dark cycle (Foster et al., 1991). A similar distinction is beginning to emerge from studies of blind human subjects. Studies of the visually impaired indicate that without light input, the circadian pacemaker of most totally blind subjects fails to remain synchronized to the 24-hour day, even if they maintain a rigid schedule of sleeping and waking at the same time every day (Klein et al., 1991). A recent case study of a blind subject whose pineal MELATONIN secretion could be acutely suppressed by exposure to bright light suggests, however, that the retinohypothalamic tract within the optic nerve may be spared in at least some otherwise "blind" patients, even if they lack conscious light perception (Martens et al., 1992). This tract may be sufficient to maintain photic entrainment to the 24-hour day, even in the absence of conscious vision (see BLINDNESS).

The magnitude of the resetting response generally increases with the duration of the light stimulus. For example, exposure to 8,000 lux of light for 7.5 minutes in the mosquito induces weak (Type I) circadian phase resetting, whereas exposure to the same light intensity for 2 hours induces strong (Type 0) resetting, yielding up to 12-hour phase shifts. There are limits to this process: Because of the cyclic nature of the underlying response curve, increasing the stimulus duration beyond about 12 hours reduces, rather than increases, the strength of the stimulus. Thus, the effect of a 16-hour light stimulus is approximately equivalent to that of an 8-hour stimulus. Furthermore, circadian light sensitivity changes with developmental stage in some species.

Kronauer (1987) has developed a mathematical model of the effect of light on the human circadian pacemaker that incorporates recent findings. This model makes it possible to predict the response of the pacemaker to any pattern of light exposure. The model has been used successfully to design light exposure patterns that come close to "stopping" the clock, so that the pacemaker oscillation has a very low amplitude (Jewett, Kronauer, and Czeisler, 1991). This finding indicates that the model accurately represents the effective strength of light on the pacemaker.

Practical application of these findings includes help for night shiftworkers who try to stay awake at night and sleep by day. Most of these workers are plagued by fatigue and lapses of attention at work and difficulty trying to sleep during the day. Properly-timed exposure to bright light during night SHIFTWORK can help them to adapt rapidly to a night work schedule, enabling them to be much more productive at night and to sleep more soundly during the day (Czeisler, Duffy, and Kronauer, 1990). In the future, these findings may also be used to help transmeridian travelers adjust to the rapid shifts in TIME ZONES encountered in jet travel (see JET LAG). In addition, patients with sleep scheduling disorders, such as DELAYED SLEEP PHASE SYNDROME (great difficulty falling asleep at night followed by great difficulty WAKING UP on time for school or work in the morning), may be treated effectively by bright light exposure in the early morning hours (see CIRCADIAN RHYTHM DISORDERS; LIGHT THERAPY).

REFERENCES

Czeisler CA, Duffy JF, Kronauer RE. 1990. Treatment of physiologic maladaptation to night work. (Letter to the editor.) *N Engl J Med* 323:918–919.

Czeisler CA, Kronauer RE, Allan JS, Duffy JF, Jewett ME, Brown EN, Ronda JM. 1989. Bright light induction of strong (Type 0) resetting of the human circadian pacemaker. *Science* 244:1328–1333.

Czeisler CA, Richardson GS, Zimmerman JC, Moore-Ede MC, Weitzman ED. 1981. Entrainment of human circadian rhythms by light-dark cycles: A reassessment. *Photochem Photobiol* 34:239–247.

DeCandolle AP. 1832. Du sommeil des feuilles. In: *Physiologie végétale, ou exposition des forces et des fonctions vitales des végétaux,* pp 854–862. Paris: Bechet Jeune.

Foster RG, Provencio I, Hudson D, Fiske S, De Grip W, Menaker M. 1991. Circadian photoreception in the retinally degenerate mouse (rd/rd). *J Comp Physiol A* 169:39–50.

Hastings JW, Sweeney BM. 1958. A persistent diurnal rhythm of luminescence in *Gonyaulax polyedra*. *Biol Bull* 115:440–458.

Jewett ME, Kronauer RE, Czeisler CA. 1991. Light-induced suppression of endogenous circadian amplitude in humans. *Nature* 350:59–62.

Klein T, Martens H, Seely EW, Czeisler CA. 1991. Chronic non-24-hour sleep/wake disorder: Circadian sleep regulation in a 63-year-old blind man. *Sleep Res* 20A:541.

Kronauer RE. 1987. A model for the effect of light on the human "deep" circadian pacemaker. *Sleep Res* 16:621.

Martens H, Klein T, Rizzo JF, Shanahan TL, Czeisler CA. 1992. Light-induced melatonin suppression in a blind man. *Soc Res Bio Rhythms Abstract* 58:52.

Sack RL, Lewy AJ, Blood ML, Keith LD, Nakagawa II. 1992. Circadian rhythm abnormalities in totally blind people: Incidence and clinical significance. *J Clin Endocrinol Metab* 75:127–134.

Winfree A. 1987. *The timing of biological clocks.* New York: Scientific American.

Charles A. Czeisler

LIGHT–DARK CYCLES

Light and dark cycles are dependent on the earth's rotation, which is close to a 24-hour cycle. The day and night length vary seasonally with the axial tilting of the earth and the revolution of the earth around the sun. The fluctuation of these daily cycles functions as a time cue (see ZEITGEBERS). Aside from behavioral and social time cues, light and dark cycles, particularly LIGHT, appear to be the primary exogenous factors that influence biological or CIRCADIAN RHYTHMS. These rhythms include such bodily functions as hormonal secretion, metabolic rate, sleep–wake cycles, and core body temperature. While light can entrain these circadian rhythms to the 24-hour light–dark cycle, these rhythms will persist even in the absence of these temporal prompts.

Light affects circadian rhythms at the level of the HYPOTHALAMUS in the brain, specifically at the SUPRACHIASMATIC NUCLEUS OF THE HYPOTHALAMUS, which is the origin of these biological rhythms. Neurological pathways link the retina of the eye to the suprachiasmatic nucleus. ENTRAINMENT of circadian rhythms by a light source does not require a lengthy exposure; on the contrary, short photoperiods (periods of light) of an hour or less

can synchronize biological rhythms to a 24-hour cycle. An example of the ability of bodily functions, notably sleep–wake cycles, to adapt to a change or shift in light–dark cycles is transmeridian travel. If one travels from America to Europe, which is a 6-hour time difference, one will experience a common phenomenon of tiredness and sluggishness known as JET LAG. After several days of exposure to this new schedule of light–dark cycles, the internal biological clock will be parallel with the external environment.

Amy E. Suessle

LIGHT THERAPY

Light therapy, a procedure for treating SEASONAL AFFECTIVE DISORDER (SAD) by exposing the depressed person to bright light, is also used to manipulate the human circadian timing system and treat certain types of INSOMNIA.

The use of light to treat mood disorders was described in past centuries (Wehr, 1989). Light therapy for SAD was rediscovered and popularized in the early 1980s by researchers in the United States at the National Institute of Mental Health (Rosenthal et al., 1984). In subsequent years, research groups throughout the world have begun to study SAD and its treatment with light therapy. Many studies have compared the effects of bright light exposure with effects of other procedures that were not thought to have an intrinsic effect (placebo treatments). Such studies are important since quite a few patients, especially those with relatively mild depression, improve after contacting a therapist or receiving something inactive, such as a sugar pill. In the case of SAD, many experts now believe that bright light treatment has been demonstrated to be more effective than inactive procedures (Terman et al., 1989; National Institute of Mental Health, 1990). Therefore, they have concluded that it is a valid treatment for SAD. However, it has not yet been proven how light therapy works (see CIRCADIAN RHYTHMS; LIGHT). It appears to help a majority of SAD patients, whether their depressions are extremely mild or quite severe, but light exposure does not improve mood in people who are not depressed (Kasper et al., 1989).

The first studies of light therapy for SAD used

full-spectrum light (light that includes all the wavelengths found in sunlight) and compared low illuminance levels, such as ordinary indoor room light, with much higher illuminance, such as found outdoors in the early morning on a clear day. It was shown that bright light was much more effective than dimmer indoor light. To receive such high-illuminance light indoors, special light fixtures are required. Several light therapy fixtures (light boxes) have been developed for home or office use. Most studies have tested fluorescent light bulbs, but incandescent lights have also been reported effective. It now seems that full-spectrum light is not required, but it is not yet known exactly which wavelengths are necessary (National Institute of Mental Health, 1990). Several new devices are being tested that may deliver light more conveniently.

Exposure of the eyes seems to be important for light therapy. Some bright light sources are dangerous to look at, however, because they can damage the eye. Many light boxes commercially available for use in SAD have been tested for safety, and these tests continue. Ophthalmological examinations (examinations of the health of the eye, not just tests of vision) are recommended for persons before they begin light therapy (Terman et al., 1990) and periodically over the years of continued treatment. Adverse effects of bright light exposure, including difficulty sleeping, excessive energy, headache, and nausea, have been transient and in many cases could be corrected by modifications of the treatment procedure. However, some medical conditions and drugs increase sensitivity to light and can increase the danger of adverse reactions. An international professional organization started in 1989, the Society for Light Treatment and Biological Rhythms in Wilsonville, Oregon, provides up-to-date information for both consumers and health-care providers.

As mentioned above, exposure to bright light has also been used in the treatment of disorders other than SAD (Anderson and Wirz-Justice, 1991). It is under evaluation for the treatment of nonseasonal depressions and of premenstrual dysphoria (often called PREMENSTRUAL SYNDROME). Certain sleep disorders of presumed circadian etiology have been treated, and light therapy has also been administered to alleviate difficulties related to the circadian timing system, such as JET LAG and SHIFT WORK maladaptation (see CIRCADIAN RHYTHMS; LIGHT). The term *phototherapy* has been used for many years to refer to a dermatological light-exposure treatment of newborn infants for jaundice. Although light therapy for SAD was also referred to in the 1980s as phototherapy, this terminology has been dropped to avoid confusion with the dermatological use of light. Light therapy has been used successfully to treat patients with CIRCADIAN RHYTHM DISORDERS, specifically DELAYED SLEEP PHASE SYNDROME, in which the phase-shifting capacity of light is thought to be the therapeutic mechanism (Rosenthal et al, 1990). Timed bright light exposure may also be useful to control the sleep disorders resulting from SHIFTWORK (Czeisler et al., 1990; Dawson and Campbell, 1991).

REFERENCES

Anderson JL, Wirz-Justice A. 1991. Biological rhythms in the pathophysiology and treatment of affective disorders. In Horton RW, Katona C, eds. *Biological aspects of affective disorders,* pp 224–269. London: Academic.

Czeisler CA, Johnson MP, Duffy JF, Brown EN, Ronda JS, Kronaver RE. 1990. Exposure to bright light and darkness to treat physiologic maladaptation to night work. *N Engl J Med* 322(18): 1253–1259.

Dawson D, Campbell SS. 1991. Timed exposure to bright light improves sleep and alertness during simulated night shifts. *Sleep* 14(6):511–516.

Hyman JW. 1990. *The light book.* Los Angeles, Tarcher.

Kasper S, Rogers SLB, Yancey A, Schulz PM, Skwerer RG, Rosenthal NE. 1989. Phototherapy in individuals with and without subsyndromal seasonal affective disorder. *Arch Gen Psychiatry* 46:837–844.

National Institute of Mental Health. 1990. Seasonal mood disorders: Consensus and controversy. *Psychopharmacol Bull* 26:465–530.

Rosenthal NC, Joseph-Vanderpool JR, Levendosky AA, Johnston SH, Allen R, Kelly KA, Souetre E, Schulty PM, Starz KE. 1990. Phase-shifting effects of bright morning light as treatment for delayed sleep phase syndrome. *Sleep* 13(4):354–361.

Rosenthal NE. 1989. *Seasons of the mind.* New York: Bantam.

Rosenthal NE, Sack DA, Gillin J, Lewy AJ, Goodwin FK, Davenport Y, Mueller PS, Newsome DA, Wehr TA. 1984. Seasonal affective disorder: A description of the syndrome and preliminary findings with light therapy. *Arch Gen Psychiatry* 41:72–80.

Smyth A. 1990. *SAD: Winter depression—Who gets*

it, what causes it and how to cure it. London: Unwin.

Terman M, Réme CE, Rafferty B, Gallin PF, Terman JS. 1990. Bright light therapy for winter depression: Potential ocular effects and theoretical implications. *Photochem Photobiol* 51:781–793.

Terman M, Terman JS, Quitkin FM, McGrath PJ, Stewart JW, Rafferty B. 1989. Light therapy for seasonal affective disorder: A review of efficacy. *Neuropsychopharmacology* 2:1–22.

Wehr TA. 1989. Seasonal affective disorders: A historical overview. In Rosenthal NE, Blehar MC, eds. *Seasonal affective disorders and phototherapy,* pp 11–32. New York: Guilford.

Janis Anderson

LITERATURE, SLEEP AND DREAMS IN

The literary world contains countless references to the topics of sleep and dreams. Subtle differences exist in the treatment of sleep and dreams in literature from author to author and society to society; this article focuses primarily upon Western literary traditions. A useful means of surveying these literary themes is to explore sleep and dreams separately, following their historical usage through the centuries to more contemporary manifestations.

Sleep in Literature

Sleep phenomena are prevalent in early Western myths, medieval and Renaissance fairy tales, and modern and contemporary fiction. Poets, playwrights, and storytellers have spun yarns regarding characters who sleep, can't sleep, cause others to sleep, or suffer from sleep disorders. Examples from the Judeo-Christian tradition include the story of the prophet Elijah, who is said to be asleep in the bosom of Abraham until the Antichrist appears. An example of New Testament narrative dealing with sleep is the story of Jesus on the eve of his crucifixion. He asks his disciples to spend the evening praying with him after the Last Supper, yet every one of them falls into a deep slumber. Perhaps the New Testament writers considered that the disciples' inability to remain awake represented a figurative abandon-

ment of Jesus and further distinguished him by illustrating his ability to overcome the mortal need for sleep.

Greek mythology includes many famous sleeping characters, such as the hero Endymion, with whom the moon falls in love. A kiss from the moon causes Endymion to sleep forever and thereby remain eternally youthful (Urdang and Ruffner, 1986). Hypnos, the god of sleep, also figures prominently in Greek myths.

The Arthurian legends of the medieval era are remarkable for several sleeping characters. King Arthur is said to be asleep by enchantment and will return to the world someday to regain the throne of England. Likewise, Merlin, the wizard who helped Arthur ascend to power, is said to be asleep rather than dead. It is likely that the Arthurian storytellers sought to show that England, like King Arthur and his counselor, was not dead but would someday rise again to glory and splendor.

Among the fairy tales that originated during the Middle Ages and the Renaissance, many deal with sleep and magic. Tales of the SANDMAN, who sprinkled magical, sleep-inducing sand in the eyes of children, are thought to be from this era, as are the popular fairy tales of Snow White and Sleeping Beauty. Snow White was poisoned by an apple that caused her to sleep until she was kissed by a prince; likewise, Sleeping Beauty was magically put to sleep for a hundred years until a prince's kiss woke her. The writers of these stories used sleep as a symbol to illustrate Snow White's and Sleeping Beauty's awakening to life as mature women. The two girls are not just physically asleep; their adult wisdom, intellect, and sexuality are symbolically asleep as well. (See also LONG SLEEPERS IN HISTORY AND LEGEND.)

One of the most famous English literary figures from the Elizabethan era, William Shakespeare, wove themes of sleep throughout his works. Perhaps the most memorable reference to sleep in the work of Shakespeare is the appearance of the sleepwalking Lady Macbeth in the tragedy *Macbeth.* The Scottish lord Macbeth kills the king of Scotland in order to become king himself; Lady Macbeth not only urges him to the hideous murder but helps him commit it. Later she suffers from NIGHTMARES and SLEEPWALKING, and eventually admits to the murder in her sleep. Shakespeare may have meant to suggest that these sleep disorders punished Lady Macbeth for her crime.

Writers of Shakespeare's and earlier times were both puzzled and awed by the sleep process.

Sleep was as compelling to their minds as it is to our own, but they did not have the scientific and physiological explanations that we have now. As this premodern literature illustrates, our predecessors often viewed sleep as a mystical or death-like occurrence. Modern writers have a more sophisticated understanding of sleep, and therefore tend to focus less upon the supernatural aspects of slumber and more upon the phenomenon itself.

Perhaps the most famous British novelist to write of a specific sleep disorder was Charles Dickens. In *The Pickwick Papers,* Dickens tells of a boy named Joe (sometimes referred to as "the fat boy") who continually falls asleep during the day. Joe's affliction came to be known as *Pickwickian syndrome.* This disorder is a close cousin of sleep APNEA.

An important modern work incorporating a sleep theme is Anton Chekhov's short story "Let Me Sleep" (Miles and Pitcher, 1982, pp. 191–196), which deals with the human need for sleep and the effects of sleep deprivation. The tale's main character is Varka, a nurse who has been chronically sleep deprived in caring for her master's newborn child. She spends the days hard at work with the household chores and the evenings fighting to stay awake so the master's child may sleep. As her weariness grows, she comes to feel that the baby is the cause of her misery. If it weren't for the child, Varka might get the sleep that she so desperately craves. With a smile upon her face, Varka smothers the baby and quickly lies down on the floor beside the cradle to sleep. Chekhov's tale, a chilling social message to pre-Communist Russia about the common worker's needs, is also a testament to the human craving for sleep. (See also DEPRIVATION; VIOLENCE)

Dreams in Literature

Dream motifs abound in the Western literary tradition. Literary works not only show a continuing fascination with dreaming throughout the ages, but also display shifts in peoples' beliefs about the nature and process of dreaming. The earliest Western writings tell us that the ancients believed dreams were caused by gods, devils, and the dead (see DREAM THEORIES OF THE ANCIENT WORLD). Dreams were thought to influence the actions of the living or to foreshadow events (Weidhorn,

1988; see also CULTURAL ASPECTS OF DREAMING; PSYCHIC DREAMS). This motif is found throughout the Homeric epics. In the *Iliad,* for example, Zeus deceives the Greek king Agamemnon by advising him in a dream to advance the warrior Achilles. In another Homeric tale, Odysseus's wife Penelope has a prophetic dream about an eagle killing twenty geese. Penelope's dream is interpreted to mean that her husband will return from his long years at sea to vanquish the suitors for her hand in marriage.

Plato and the Stoics opposed these common beliefs about prophetic dreams, suggesting that dreams were generated internally rather than by external powers of the supernatural. Thinkers such as Hippocrates elaborated upon the Platonic notion of dreaming and hypothesized that dreams were strictly physiological events. Hippocrates believed that the mind continued functioning, thus causing dreams, while the body was inoperative. This Platonic perspective shifted the notion of dreams from a mystical, external manifestation to a psychological or philosophical internal manifestation.

A final concept about dreams that coexisted with these other theories was best articulated by Herodotus, the fifth-century B.C. Greek historian who believed that dreams simply reflected and represented the waking thoughts and concerns of the dreamer. Herodotus's way of understanding dreams suggests that they can be seen as mirrors of reality.

By the Elizabethan period, the Herodotian view of dreaming became the more prevalent perspective, exemplified by the works of Shakespeare, which are loaded with dream motifs. *Macbeth,* mentioned earlier for its treatment of sleepwalking, is full of anxiety-related dreams fueled by guilt. Another of Shakespeare's plays involving particularly vivid dream sequences is *Richard III,* in which Clarence experiences an elaborate anxiety dream, and Richard is plagued by dreams of guilt that are prophetic in the classical tradition. The characters of *A Midsummer Night's Dream* undergo enchantments while sleeping that cause them to act against their accustomed natures and ultimately change their destinies; the play's title suggests that its action, and perhaps life itself, may be a dream. Other notable works of Shakespeare that employ dreaming as a dominant theme or plot device include *Romeo and Juliet, Henry IV, Measure for Measure,* and *The Tempest.*

Manfred Weidhorn (1988) suggests that the seventeenth-century materialist philosophies of Bacon, Locke, and Hobbes caused a decrease in literary dream motifs. These three empiricists were concerned primarily with the measurable universe and found little merit in reflecting upon or writing about subjective states; similar patterns of thought persisted in the rationalist Enlightenment of the 1700s. In the nineteenth century, the advent of the Romantic movement made room for subjective experience once again. This broadened realm of discourse permitted dreaming to return as a theme in literature.

Thus, in the 19th century, dissatisfaction with the current state of society led to a renewed fascination with dreaming or dreamlike states as providing routes to greater self-awareness and pathways to the unconscious. Specifically, many writers involved with the growing drug culture became interested in the dreamlike states produced by opium. Thomas De Quincey's *Confessions of an English Opium Eater,* Samuel Taylor Coleridge's "Kubla Khan," and Lewis Carroll's *Alice in Wonderland* are but a few examples of literature influenced by opium-induced dreams (see CREATIVITY IN DREAMS). As dreaming returned to literary vogue, vivid nightmares appeared in Tolstoy's *War and Peace* and *Anna Karenina* as well as Dostoevsky's *Crime and Punishment* and *The Brothers Karamazov.*

Modern literature has been greatly influenced by the psychological theorizing of Sigmund Freud. Freudian schools of thought increased the incorporation of dream motifs in fiction (see FREUD'S DREAM THEORY). With the increase in popular attention to dreaming, modern fiction writers not only utilized dreams to develop characters psychologically, but also began to attempt to capture the essence of dreaming in highly surrealist works. Examples include Thomas Mann's *The Magic Mountain,* August Strindberg's *A Dream Play* and *The Ghost Sonata,* Franz Kafka's *The Trial* and *The Castle,* and James Joyce's *Ulysses* and *Finnegan's Wake.* These works represent another profound step in the evolution of public and scholarly attitudes toward dreams—from thinking of them as supernatural phenomena or simple mirrors of reality to using them to reveal important aspects of personal identity. A survey of dreaming as reflected in literature not only displays our continued fascination with this nocturnal phenomenon, but also illustrates the way that each generation has thought about and explained dreaming.

REFERENCES

Miles P, Pitcher H, trans. 1982. *Chekhov: The early stories.* New York: Macmillan.

Urdang L, Ruffner FG Jr, eds. 1986. *Allusions—cultural, literary, biblical, and historical: A thematic dictionary.* Detroit.: Gale.

Weidhorn M. 1988. *The dictionary of literary themes and motifs,* vol. I, pp. 406–414. New York: Greenwood.

Thomas Wheatland

LONGEVITY

According to popular anecdotes, which may or may not be true, Thomas Edison and President John F. Kennedy needed only a few hours of sleep each day, whereas Einstein could sleep as much as twelve hours a day. Who can say if the achievements of Edison and Kennedy were greater than Einstein's, or if their genius was multiplied by the ability to work long hours?

On the other hand, Edison lived to age eighty-four and Kennedy to age forty-five, whereas Einstein lived to age seventy-six. Does cutting down on sleep cut down on life span? Nobody believes Kennedy's life was cut short by a sleep problem. Does more sleep cause longer life? This also may not be correct.

In 1959 and 1960, thousands of volunteers working for the American Cancer Society gave health questionnaires to about a million of their friends. Because the people who completed the questionnaires *were* friends, the volunteers were able to trace more than 98 percent of them six years later to determine if the subjects were still alive. This was an important study showing that cigarette smokers died younger than nonsmokers (Hammond, 1964). The study also showed that subjects who said that they usually slept *either* less than seven hours a night or more than eight hours were more likely to have died within the six years (Kripke et al., 1979). Both unusually short sleep and unusually long sleep predicted early mortality from several causes such as heart disease, stroke, and cancer.

Several similar studies have since repeated the finding that both unusually long sleep and unusually short sleep predict early death. These studies showed that a number of factors, including age, sex, exercise, diet, and cigarette smoking, do not explain the differences in longevity between seven- to eight-hour sleepers and those who sleep either less or more. Use of sleeping pills was not an explanation; although people who reported using sleeping pills died earlier, short sleepers who said they never used sleeping pills and never had insomnia also had higher mortality than people of similar age and sex who slept seven to eight hours.

Long sleepers, adults who usually slept nine or more hours, also had increased mortality. Indeed, as there were more long sleepers than short sleepers in the sample(s), especially among the elderly (who are most likely to die from any cause), most of the deaths associated with unusual sleep times were among elderly people reporting long sleep. Although the largest studies depended on questionnaires to determine sleep times, a recent study that measured sleep time in the homes of elderly persons confirmed that measured long and short sleep times predicted higher mortality (Kripke et al., 1991).

Up to now, research has not explained why long and short sleep are associated with early death. We are not certain that the sleep differences are the primary *cause* of the mortality with which they are associated. For example, it has not been proven that the six-hour sleeper who stays in bed an hour longer will consequently live longer. Similarly, it has not been shown that the nine-hour sleeper will live longer if the alarm clock is set an hour earlier. Nevertheless, until we learn more, sleeping about seven to eight hours seems to be a reasonable goal.

(See also DEATH.)

REFERENCES

Hammond EC. 1964. Some preliminary findings on physical complaints from a prospective study of 1,064,004 men and women. *Public Health* 54:11–24.

Kripke DF, Ancoli-Israel S, Fell RL, Mason WJ, Klauber MR, Kaplan O. 1991. Health risk of insomnia. In Peter JH, et al., eds. *Sleep and health risk*. Berlin/New York: Springer-Verlag.

Kripke DF, Simons RN, Garfinkel L, Hammond EC. 1979. Short and long sleep and sleeping pills: Is increased mortality associated?. *Arch Psychiatry* 36:103–116.

Daniel F. Kripke

LONG SLEEPERS IN HISTORY AND LEGEND

Among historical and legendary figures credited with unusual sleeping patterns, relatively few are supposed to have had longer-than-normal sleep periods. This comparative paucity of reports may be due to societal expectations of sleep patterns and a historical emphasis on minimizing sleep to increase the number of hours available for work and play (see DEPRIVATION). In view of such expectations, it is no surprise that Thomas Edison, inventor of the electric light bulb, regarded "excessive sleep" (8–10 hours) as a waste of time as well as a symptom of weakness and stupidity (see SHORT SLEEPERS IN HISTORY AND LEGEND). Nevertheless, patterns of longer sleep periods can serve to illustrate the importance of SLEEP HYGIENE and variations in human sleep need.

Charlemagne, emperor of the Holy Roman Empire from A.D. 800 to 814, slept 3 hours after his midday meal in addition to having a "regular" sleep at night—but he was also known to wake up four or five times during the night. This pattern of behavior might now be labeled INSOMNIA.

The story of Rip Van Winkle (Irving, 1849) features a well-known legendary figure who sleeps for 20 years as the result of a potent drink. Hunting in the Catskill mountains, Rip Van Winkle encounters an oddly dressed little man carrying a keg and helps him carry the keg to a valley filled with other oddly dressed little fellows playing ninepins. Rip serves the bowlers from the keg and then drinks himself into a stupor. When he awakens, he finds himself on a grassy knoll; his gun has rusted and his dog is gone. Walking with less agility than before, Rip makes his way back to his village only to discover that he has grown a beard a foot long, 20 years have passed, and his nagging wife is dead. Rip spends the rest of his life contentedly telling others of olden times before his great sleep. Although the point of the legend seems to be the connection between the alcohol and his slumber, this is not the usual effect of alcoholic drinks on sleep (see ALCOHOL).

It is widely (and incorrectly) believed that most elderly people require less sleep (see AGING AND SLEEP). The French mathematician Moivre, however, is reported to have slept 20 hours a day during old age, leaving only 4 hours for science and the rest of life's necessities (Hall, 1911).

Perhaps the outstanding legend of a long sleeper is that of Sleeping Beauty, from the tales of the brothers Grimm (Grimm, 1977). This young princess sleeps for a hundred years after pricking her finger on a spindle poisoned by an angry witch's spell. All the other inhabitants of the castle, people and animals, fall asleep as well. A prince finally breaks the spell by kissing Sleeping Beauty, and the two marry and live happily ever after. As in other fairy tales, this magically induced sleep may serve a metaphorical purpose, ushering Sleeping Beauty from girlhood into womanhood—or it may be that the storytellers recognized an increased sleep need in puberty (see ADOLESCENCE AND SLEEP).

Sleep researcher Peretz Lavie (1987) has cited documented reports from the late nineteenth century of 11- to 32-year-old females sleeping for periods ranging from 3–4 days to several months or, in one case, a year. Thus, this "sleeping beauty" phenomenon may have been a reality of the time when these legends originated; cases of this type, however, have not been documented in the twentieth century. Lavie speculates that this fact may be related to a general change in mental symptoms from the nineteenth to the twentieth century, ascribing the "sleeping beauty" phenomenon to hysterical symptomatology. The pattern is seen in Greek mythology as well: Psyche falls asleep when she opens Persephone's box, and later is awakened by Eros.

(See also INDIVIDUAL DIFFERENCES; LITERATURE, SLEEP AND DREAMS IN; SLEEP LENGTH.)

REFERENCES

Grimm J. 1977. The sleeping beauty. In *Grimm's tales for young and old: The complete stories.* Garden City, N.Y.: Doubleday.
Hall B. 1911. *The gift of sleep.* New York: Moffat Yard.
Irving W. 1849. *Rip Van Winkle.* New York: American Art Union.
Lavie P. 1987. The "sleeping beauty"—an extinguished syndrome of excessive sleepiness. *Sleep* 16:382.

Jenifer Wicks

LSD

See Drugs of Abuse

L-TRYPTOPHAN

L-Tryptophan (or tryptophan) is one of the essential amino acids (protein building blocks) found in a variety of foods. Tryptophan can be metabolically converted to a variety of chemicals, such as serotonin [5-hydroxytryptamine (5-HT)] and kynurenine, which in the brain may act as neurotransmitters (messengers between nerve cells) (Wurtman, 1982; see also CHEMISTRY OF SLEEP; AMINES AND OTHER TRANSMITTERS). Early work in cats suggested that serotonin is responsible for SLOW-WAVE SLEEP (SWS) and/or REM SLEEP (Jouvet, 1968). As a result, many studies have been undertaken with tryptophan in humans to assess its effect as an hypnotic or sleep-promoting substance. A number of studies showed no effect on SWS or REM sleep with low dosages (<5 grams), of L-tryptophan; others showed a modest increase in SWS and/or a decrease in REM sleep with intermediate dosages (5 to 9 grams); and high dosages (10 to 15 grams) may produce paradoxical results (decreased SWS and increased REM sleep). Differences in the populations studied (only healthy volunteers in some studies, varying proportions of severe INSOMNIA or other psychiatric illnesses in other studies) and varying times of tryptophan administration likely account for certain of the conflicting results. Nonetheless, it is generally agreed that tryptophan allows more rapid onset of sleep and lowers the sensitivity to external stimuli during sleep. Concomitant administration of food or other drugs may enhance or diminish the onset of action. As tryptophan must compete with other amino acids for transport into the brain, its administration in the fasting state may enhance brain tryptophan levels and potentiate its sleep-promoting effect.

In normal individuals, a dose-dependent increase in blood levels during fasting correlates with more rapid sleep onset (increased objective sleepiness as measured by the MULTIPLE SLEEP LATENCY TEST, or MSLT) (George et al., 1989). In 1989, L-tryptophan was linked to development of eosinophilic myalgia syndrome, a serious blood disorder. Contaminants in the preparation and not L-tryptophan itself are most likely responsible for this syndrome (Belongia et al., 1990).

REFERENCES

Belongia EA, Hedberg CW, Gleich GJ, White KE, et al. 1990. An investigation of the cause of the eosinophilia–myalgia syndrome associated with tryptophan use. *N Engl J Med* 323:351–365.

George CFP, Millar TW, Hanly PJ, Kryger MH. 1989. The effect of L-tryptophan on daytime sleep latency in normals: Correlation with blood levels. *Sleep* 12:345–353.

Jouvet A. 1968. Biogenic amines and the states of sleep. *Science* 163:32–41.

Spinweber CL, Ursin R, Hilbert RP, Hildebrand FL. 1983. L-Trytophan: Effects on daytime sleep latency and the waking EEG. *Electroencephalogr Clin Neurophysiol* 55:652–661.

Wurtman RJ. 1982. Nutrients that modify brain function. *Sci Am*, April 1982:55–59.

Charles F. P. George

LUCID DREAMING

As a rule, we are not aware, while we are dreaming, of the fact that we are dreaming. Our dreams seem so real to our sleeping minds that we regularly accord them the status of physical reality. Only when we awaken do we usually recognize our dreams as the exclusively mental experiences they are. Although this is how we generally experience dreams, there is a significant exception: Sometimes, while dreaming, we know full well that we are in fact dreaming. This clear-sighted state of mind is referred to as *lucid dreaming*.

Lucid dreamers report being in possession of all their cognitive faculties: They are able to reason clearly, to remember the conditions of waking life, and to act voluntarily within the dream upon reflection or in accordance with plans decided upon before sleep. At the same time, they remain soundly asleep, vividly experiencing a dream world that can seem astonishingly real. Lucid dreamers can exert a remarkable degree of control over what happens in dreams, doing things that would seem magical, if not impossible, in the physical world.

Many people have experienced at least occasional and brief instances of lucid dreaming. In one common experience, the dreamer realizes near the end of a nightmare that "it's only a dream" and awakens with relief a few seconds later. Dreamers who wake up to escape a nightmare, however, are probably only partially lucid. Fully lucid dreamers realize that the nightmare is as harmless as a horror film; therefore, they may choose to stay in the dream, to face and successfully overcome their nightmare fears. They may then wake up with boosted self-confidence and, perhaps, one less irrational fear. This approach appears promising as a method for overcoming nightmares.

Dreamers typically become lucid when they puzzle over some oddity in a dream and conclude that the explanation is that they are dreaming. Although for most people lucid dreaming is a rare experience, there is reason to believe that it is a learnable skill. Thus, certain people appear to be able to carry a specific intention into sleep, such as to wake by a certain time (see INTERNAL ALARM CLOCK) or to have lucid dreams. Several methods for inducing lucid dreams are based on this approach. Diligent practice with these techniques has reportedly allowed highly motivated individuals with good dream recall to become lucid whenever they wish (LaBerge, 1980).

Another approach to lucid dream induction uses biofeedback: Low-level sensory stimuli are presented to dreamers in REM sleep. If the stimuli become incorporated into dreams, the dreamers can use them as cues to recognize that they are dreaming. LaBerge and his colleagues at Stanford have tested a variety of cues, including tape recordings of the phrase "This is a dream!" Unfortunately, sound tends to wake sleepers. The most promising results so far have been obtained with flashing lights used as a cue.

Although accounts of lucid dreaming go back at least as far as Aristotle, for many years sleep researchers doubted that the dreaming brain was capable of such a high degree of mental functioning and consciousness. Studies by Howard

Roffwarg and William Dement had shown that the directions of eye movements recorded during REM sleep sometimes closely corresponded to the directions in which subjects reported they had been looking in their dreams. LaBerge reasoned that because lucid dreamers can act volitionally in dreams, they should be able to make prearranged eye movement signals marking the exact times they became lucid. With the eye-movement signaling method, LaBerge and his colleagues (1981) verified reports of lucid dreams from five subjects. All of the signals, and therefore lucid dreams, had occurred during uninterrupted REM sleep (Figure 1).

The signaling technique was independently developed by Keith Hearne and Alan Worsley in England, who also found that lucid dreaming occurred exclusively during REM sleep. Studies in several other sleep laboratories have obtained nearly identical results. The Stanford group has

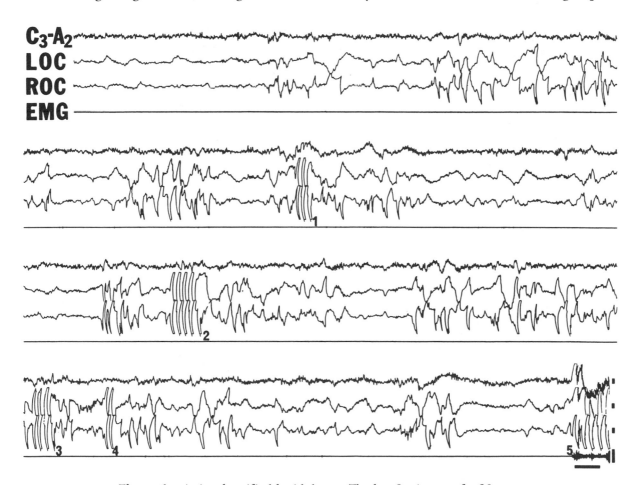

Figure 1. A signal-verified lucid dream. The last 8 minutes of a 30-minute REM period are shown. Upon awakening, the subject reported having made five eye movement signals (labeled 1–5 in figure). The first signal (1, two pairs of left–right eye movements, LRLR) marked the onset of lucidity. During the following 90 seconds the subject "flew about" exploring his dream world until he believed he had awakened, at which point he made the signal for awakening (2, LRLRLRLR). After another 90 seconds, the subject realized he was still dreaming and signaled (3) with three pairs of eye movements. Realizing that this was too many, he correctly signaled with two pairs (4). Finally, upon awakening 100 seconds later he signaled appropriately (5, LRLRLRLR). Abbreviations: C_3-A_2, electroencephalogram; LOC, ROC, electrical activity in left and right eye muscles, respectively; EMG, electromyogram. Scale bars at bottom right represent 50 microvolts and 5 seconds.

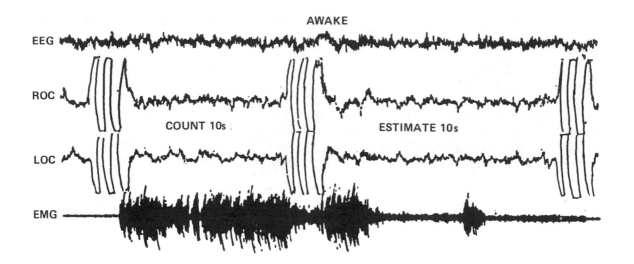

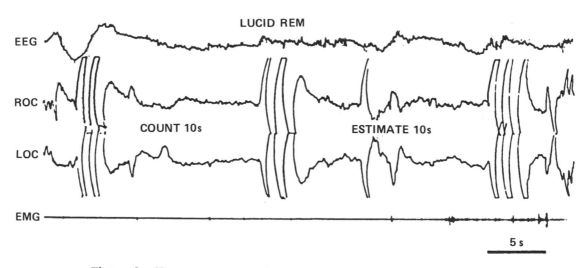

Figure 2. Time estimates during waking and REM lucid dreaming. While awake (top panel), the subject signaled with eye movements, estimated 10 seconds by counting, signaled again, estimated 10 seconds without counting, and signaled a third time. The lower panel shows the subject carrying out the same task in lucid REM sleep. The time estimates are very similar in both states.

further determined that lucid dreams tend to begin at moments of relatively high brain activity in REM sleep, most frequently during later REM periods of the night (LaBerge, Levitan, and Dement, 1986).

The fact that lucid dreamers can remember to perform predetermined actions and signal to the laboratory suggested to LaBerge a new approach to dream research: Lucid dreamers could carry out experiments marking the exact time of particular dream events, allowing precise correlations between the dreamer's reports and recorded physiology and enabling the methodical testing of hypotheses. The Stanford group has used this strategy in a series of studies demonstrating parallelism between dreamed actions and physiological responses.

A study of "dream time" revealed that time intervals estimated in lucid dreams are very close to actual clock time (Figure 2). A study of dreamed breathing showed a correspondence between dreamed and actual respiration (LaBerge and Dement, 1982). Other studies demonstrated that dreamed movements result in corresponding patterns of muscle twitching, and that dreamed sexual activity is associated with physiological responses very similar to those associated with actual sexual activity (LaBerge, Greenleaf, and Kedzierski, 1983).

LaBerge (1985) concludes from the results of these and related studies that dreamed experiences produce effects on the dreamer's brain (and, to a lesser extent, body) remarkably similar to the physiological effects produced by actual experiences of the corresponding events while awake. If it were not for the fact that most of our muscles are paralyzed during REM sleep, we would actually do what we dream we are doing. Perhaps this explains in part why we are so inclined to mistake our dreams for reality: To the perceptual systems of the brain, dreaming of perceiving or doing something may be equivalent to actually perceiving or doing it. (For alternative explanations, see ACTIVATION–SYNTHESIS HYPOTHESIS; PSYCHOPHYSIOLOGY OF DREAMING.)

REFERENCES

Gackenbach J, LaBerge S, eds. 1988. *Conscious mind, sleeping brain: Perspectives on lucid dreaming.* New York: Plenum.

LaBerge S. 1980. Lucid dreaming as a learnable skill: A case study. *Percept Motor Skills* 51:1039–1042.

———. 1985. *Lucid dreaming.* Los Angeles: Tarcher.

LaBerge S, Dement W. 1982. Voluntary control of respiration during REM sleep. *Sleep Res* 11:107.

LaBerge S, Greenleaf W, Kedzierski B. 1983. Physiological responses to dreamed sexual activity during lucid REM sleep. *Psychophysiology* 20:454–455.

LaBerge S, Levitan L, Dement W. 1986. Lucid dreaming: Physiological correlates of consciousness during REM sleep. *J Mind Behavior* 7:251–258.

LaBerge S, Nagel L, Dement W, Zarcone V. 1981. Lucid dreaming verified by volitional communication during REM sleep. *Percept Motor Skills* 52: 727–732.

LaBerge S, Rheingold H. 1990. *Exploring the world of lucid dreaming.* New York: Ballantine.

Roffwarg H, Dement W, Muzio J, Fisher C. 1962. Dream imagery: Relationship to rapid eye movements of sleep. *Arch Gen Psychiatry* 7:235–258.

Stephen LaBerge

LULLABY

Most lullabies are folk songs. By definition, a folk song is music that evolves from a culture as an expression of daily life. Therefore, folk music develops anonymously and, because it is passed aurally, frequently changes. The lullaby, another term for a cradle song, evolved naturally as parents used gentle sounds and steady motions to put their babies to sleep. The root of the word is "lull," meaning to calm or quiet with soothing sounds, rocking motions, or both. For this reason, lullabies are typically tranquil flowing melodies accompanied by a rhythmic pattern to represent the rocking of a cradle.

In many cultures, bedtime is a traditional time for song. Music was used to calm children down in the transition to bedtime, thus aiding the sleep process. Children, wanting to prolong bedtime, requested long songs; consequently, many verses were often added. Sometimes lullabies are personalized by substituting the child's name for the name in the song, thereby enhancing the intimacy of the moment.

Perhaps the most popular folk lullaby is "Rock-A-Bye-Baby." From the southern United States comes "All the Pretty Little Horses," the spiritual "By'm Bye," and the well-known "Hush, Little Baby," a multiversed song about offering gifts to encourage happy thoughts. Sir Harold Boulton's words inspired the beautiful, traditional melody for the famous Welsh lullaby "All Through the Night." The lullaby "Schlaf, Kindlein, Schlaf" ("Sleep, Baby, Sleep") originated in Germany. The French "La Poulette Grise" ("The Old Grey Hen"), in which the child's name may be used, describes a different-colored hen in each verse. When this piece is sung in English, the verses use a hen, a dog, and a fish to encourage the child to sleep. One Yiddish lullaby is even intended to be sung by babysitters, "Vigndig A Fremd Kind" ("Baby Sitter's Lullaby").

In addition to the folk lullabies, two well-known composed cradle songs may be found in many homes and many music boxes. The most famous is "Brahms' Lullaby," composed by

Johannes Brahms to the words written by Fritz Simrock, his publisher and friend.

> Lullaby and goodnight,
> With roses bedight,
> With lilies bespread
> Is baby's wee bed.
>
> Lay thee down now and rest,
> May thy slumber be blessed,
> Lay thee down now and rest,
> May thy slumber be blessed.

The other, less familiar composition is "Mozart's Lullaby," by Wolfgang Amadeus Mozart. It is a lilting melody resting over an expressive accompaniment.

The folk lullaby not only inspired vocal compositions such as those by Mozart and Brahms; it also evolved into an instrumental form called a berceuse. The berceuse, the French word for cradle song, was particularly popular in nineteenth- and twentieth-century piano literature, when descriptive titles were frequently used by composers. Its main features are an undulating theme set over a repeating bass figure. Two examples of well-known keyboard cradle songs are Frédéric Chopin's Berceuse in D-flat, Op. 57, and Gabriel Fauré's Op. 56, No. 1.

Just as there are lullabies to help children fall asleep, there is a category of morning songs to aid children and adults alike in waking up. Rather than the smooth, undulating rhythm of a lullaby, morning songs are bright and loud. The abundance of morning songs suggests that the difficulty of waking children up is universal. The folk song "Lazy Mary" typifies this parental challenge. (Often, other children's names are substituted for Mary.)

> Lazy Mary, will you get up,
> Lazy Mary, will you get up,
> Will you get up, will you get up?
> Will you get up today?
>
> No, no mother, I won't get up,
> No, no mother, I won't get up,
> I won't get up, I won't get up,
> I won't get up today.

REFERENCES

Sadie S, ed. 1988. *The Norton/Grove concise encyclopedia of music*. New York: Norton.

Winn M, ed. 1966. *The fireside book of children's songs*. New York: Simon and Schuster.

Pamela J. Bigler

M

MAMMALS

Mammals are distinguished from other vertebrates by the secretion of milk for nourishment of their young and by the possession of hair (or fur). Sleep is not among their uniquely distinguishing characteristics, for other creatures also sleep, but it is a prominent feature of mammalian existence, occurring in all species without exception and occupying a substantial portion of every 24-hour period. Mammals are the principal source of scientific knowledge about sleep, gained chiefly from humans, rats, and cats studied in laboratories and clinics, and also from about 100 other, less intensively studied species. This knowledge guides the exploration of sleep in the rest of the animal kingdom and dominates thinking about the regulation of sleep and its basic purpose.

Sleep in mammals, as in other animals, is recognizable as a state of sustained immobility or quiescence in a characteristic posture accompanied by reduced responsiveness to external stimuli. Immobility need not be absolute, for some mammals (e.g., dolphins, seals, whales) may float or swim as they sleep. Terrestrial mammals typically sleep lying down with eyes closed, but there are exceptions and striking postural variations. Cattle, for example, may sleep with eyes open. Horses and elephants can sleep while standing. Some species sleep lying on the belly, others lying on the side or back or haunches. Domestic cats and their wild relatives incorporate all the recumbent positions in their sleep repertoire. Bats and sloths, on the other hand, sleep while hanging by their feet, head down. In general, posture is a convenient behavioral sign of ongoing or impending sleep.

Where mammals sleep is determined by their physical characteristics and life styles, and sometimes also by an apparent desire for comfort. Whales and dolphins, for example, have no choice but to sleep under water, piercing the surface periodically to breathe. Seals can sleep in or out of water; so can the hippopotamus. Sea otters may sleep pleasurably floating on the surface. The great apes sleep in nests constructed in trees or on the ground. Baboons, who forage on land, retire to trees or cliffs for safety from predators. Monkeys sleep in trees, which are their homes, sometimes huddled together for warmth. In contrast, zebras and wildebeest sleep in the open in large groups or herds, protected by their closeness to others who remain awake and alert for predators. A more common precaution is sleeping under cover. Rodents and insectivores (e.g., moles, shrews) sleep in burrows or crevices, rabbits in hollows or thickets, and deer in dense undergrowth. Though seemingly free to sleep wherever they choose, big predators such as the lion, cheetah, and wolf frequently sleep in lairs or dens where they may safely leave their young.

Reduced responsiveness to external stimuli sets sleep apart from simple rest. A related behavioral criterion of sleep is the quick reversion to normal responsiveness (i.e., to wakefulness) in reaction to moderate stimulation. This distinguishes sleep from conditions that superficially resemble it but are not quickly reversible (such as fainting, ANESTHESIA, and COMA). Physiologically, sleep is distinguished from wakefulness most clearly by distinctive patterns of electrical activity in the brain registered in the electroencephalogram (EEG), which is recorded from the scalp in humans and from the surface of the brain in laboratory animals. Details of the EEG vary from one species to another, reflecting differences in brain structure, but similar EEG signs of sleep are recognizable in all. The critical signs are EEG activity at reduced frequency (slowing, fewer waves per second), greater synchronization (more regularity in the form of individual waves), and increased amplitude (greater elevation of the waves, representing higher voltage) (see ELECTROENCEPHALOGRAM; STAGES OF SLEEP.)

A precise moment where wakefulness ends and sleep begins cannot be pinpointed, but EEG recordings make it possible to judge SLEEP ONSET within a minute or so. This judgment, especially in human sleepers, is facilitated by the appearance of EEG spindling, a waveform that is the hallmark of mammalian sleep. In some species (e.g., cattle, the cat), however, the transition to sleep may be hard to judge because of long periods of drowsiness, signified by a mixture of wakeful activity and transient sleep signs in the EEG. Distinguishing between wakefulness and REM sleep may also be difficult because of the desynchronized, low-amplitude EEG activity in both, but other signs of REM (to be discussed shortly) set it apart. Of great interest is the unihemispheric sleep present some of the time in dolphins, porpoises, and whales. Synchronized EEG patterns of sleep in one hemisphere of the brain are accompanied by a desynchronized waking pattern in the other hemisphere. This adaptation ensures these aquatic mammals the ability to breathe.

The timing of sleep and wakefulness plays a significant part in defining each species' niche in the environment. Some mammals, like humans, sleep exclusively or mainly at night and are active during the day. Many species follow the opposite pattern. Some have two activity periods (dawn and dusk, or part of the day and part of the night), with their sleep also divided into two major periods. In relatively few species (the domestic cat is one), sleep periods are arhythmic (irregular). The day-to-day consistency of these timetables suggests that sleep and wakefulness are governed by environmental cues, such as the alternation of light and dark. In fact, however, as shown by its persistence in the absence of any time cues, the sleep–wakefulness cycle is an endogenous (built-in) circadian rhythm that becomes synchronized with the 24-hour patterning of events dictated by the rotation of the earth (see BIOLOGICAL RHYTHMS). Sleep's occurrence is independent of other bodily needs and environmental pressures. This distinguishes sleep from other dormant states that outwardly resemble it but are prompted by shortages of food or water or by low ambient temperature (see HIBERNATION; TORPOR; and ESTIVATION).

Characteristic of sleep in virtually all mammals are the cycles of alternating REM sleep and NREM sleep. Depending on the species, 70 percent or more of mammalian sleep is NREM (also referred to as quiet sleep), which is distinguished by high-amplitude slow waves with intermixed spindling. REM sleep occurs in periods of relatively short duration and is distinguished by EEG activity reminiscent of wakefulness and accompanied by REMs, loss of muscle tone, irregular breathing and heart rate, and twitching of the extremities. Because of these puzzling features, REM sleep is also known as active or PARADOXICAL SLEEP. Figure 1 shows differences between wakefulness and the sleep states as they appear in recordings from the cat. In some species, REM sleep can be recognized by postural signs related to loss of muscle tone, as Figure 2 indicates. Twitching is a telltale

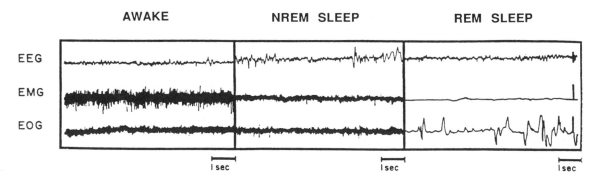

Figure 1. Wakefulness and sleep states as they appear in standard recordings from the cat. EEG, electroencephalogram; EMG, electromyogram (muscle tone); EOG, electrooculogram (eye movements).

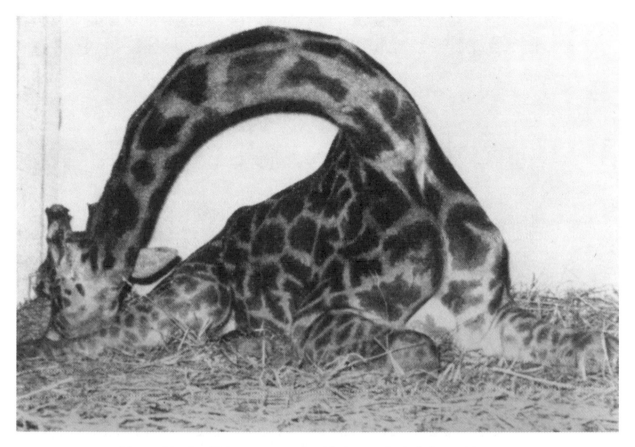

Figure 2. Giraffe in a zoo, presumably in paradoxical sleep. (*Reproduced, with permission, from Immelman K, Gebbing H. 1962. Schlaf bei Giraffiden.* Tierpsychologie *19:84–92. Copyright Verlag Paul Parey.*)

sign of REM sleep in human infants and in the dog and cat.

Figure 3 illustrates the alternation of REM and NREM sleep in three species. A NREM period and the successive REM period together constitute a sleep cycle, also known as the NREM–REM or REM–NREM cycle. Cycle duration, measured from the beginning of a NREM period to the end of the successive REM period (excluding intervening wakefulness) varies from one species to another. Human cycle length averages 90 minutes, the cat's, 25 minutes, and the rat's, 11 minutes. Measured in thirty or more mammalian species, cycle length is longest in species with large brains. An unsolved mystery, however, is the absence of REM sleep and a sleep cycle in the Australian echidna (spiny anteater), one of only three surviving egg-laying mammals (see ECHIDNA), and also reportedly in the dolphin and porpoise.

Another characteristic of mammalian sleep is its homeostatic regulation, which keeps the daily "supply" of sleep at a fairly constant level. Although individual requirements differ, each individual's sleep time normally varies within narrow limits. Part of the sleep lost one day tends to be regained the next; unusually prolonged sleep shortens subsequent sleep. This is similar to the self-regulation of other bodily conditions, such as body temperature and the water content of the blood. Working in concert, sleep homeostasis and the circadian sleep–wakefulness rhythm determine the placement and duration of sleep.

The sleep cycle itself also plays a part in this regulatory system, as is most apparent in humans, whose NREM sleep can be subdivided visually into four stages, as Figure 3 indicates. This subdivision is based partly on the variation of slow, high-amplitude EEG activity, which is at its

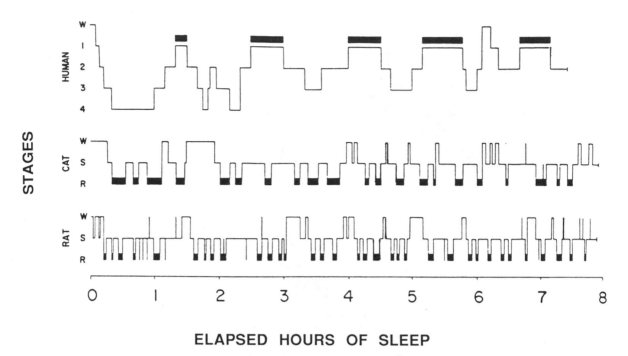

Figure 3. Sleep cycles in three species. W, wakefulness; S, NREM sleep; R, REM sleep. Black strips opposite "1" for humans represent REM sleep.

height in stage 4 and secondarily in stage 3, the two stages together being known as delta or SLOW-WAVE SLEEP. Concentrated early in the sleep period, when the pressure for sleep is presumably greatest, slow-wave sleep is also most sensitive to sleep loss. It increases dramatically in response to acute experimental sleep deprivation, taking priority over relatively small compensatory increases in other stages. This response includes an increase in the density and amplitude of slow waves, suggesting that homeostatic intensification of sleep makes it possible to fulfill sleep requirements without much extension of the sleep period. More subtle variation of EEG activity in almost all other species precludes subdivision of their NREM sleep into stages comparable to those in humans. Nevertheless, computerized, electronic analyses of EEG activity, especially in the rat, have disclosed a comparable distribution of high-amplitude, slow-wave activity during the sleep period and a similar propensity for its intensification in reaction to extended wakefulness.

Mammalian sleep patterns vary most importantly perhaps with respect to daily sleep quotas (amounts), which range widely (see Table 1). Such data are available for about 100 species but

are of uneven reliability because research settings have not always been ideal, and the number of animals studied for some species is very small. Extension and refinement of the data, however, will probably confirm the presently available picture. Overall, on the species level, total daily sleep time varies inversely with body size. Small animals, who generally are short-lived (e.g., rat, hamster, squirrel), tend to sleep more than large ones, who are long-lived (e.g., human, seal, horse, giraffe). Independent of body size, daily REM sleep quotas vary dramatically. Both at birth (when REM sleep time is at its peak) and in maturity (after a decline in REM sleep), altricial species, who are born helpless in large litters (e.g., dog, cat, hamster) have more REM sleep than precocial species, who are born fairly developed singly or in small litters (e.g., horse, giraffe, baboon). This pattern may explain the apparent absence of REM sleep in the highly precocial dolphin and porpoise, though not its absence in the echidna.

Relationships of sleep quotas to other variables may provide clues to the functions of sleep in general and specifically of REM sleep, but this remains controversial because the findings lend themselves to a variety of interpretations. For ex-

Table 1. Daily Sleep Quotas in a Sample of Mammalian Species

Species	Total Daily Sleep Time (hours)	Daily REM Sleep Time (hours)
Echidna	9.0	?
Opossum	18.0	5.0
Hedgehog	10.0	3.5
Mole	8.5	2.0
Bat	19.0	3.0
Baboon	9.5	1.0
Man	8.0	2.0
Armadillo	17.0	3.0
Rabbit	8.0	1.0
Hamster	14.0	3.0
Rat	13.0	2.5
Squirrel	16.0	3.0
Dolphin	10.0	?
Seal	6.0	1.5
Cat	12.5	3.0
Dog	10.0	3.0
Horse	3.0	0.5
Giraffe	2.0	0.5

Note. Total daily sleep time includes daily REM sleep time. Values are rounded to the half-hour and exclude prolonged drowsiness. Some values are averages for two or more members of the same genus. Question marks indicate reported absence of REM sleep.

ample, small mammals may have relatively high sleep quotas because they have little body fat for energy reserves; this could be taken as support for the theory that sleep is for energy conservation. An alternative explanation for the sleep quota–body size relationship is that big mammals sleep less because their food requirements necessitate more time awake for foraging. Other explanations may be couched in terms of prey–predator relationships, emphasizing the need for vigilance by large prey who lack hiding places and the ability of small prey to sleep where they hide. Left to be answered, however, is the critical question why sleep at all if it is dangerous or if foraging time is needed? By themselves, comparisons between mammalian species cannot give a conclusive answer (see THEORIES OF SLEEP FUNCTION).

(See also ANIMALS IN SLEEP RESEARCH; DOGS.)

REFERENCES

Borbely A. 1986. *Secrets of sleep.* New York: Basic Books.
Zepelin H. 1989. Mammalian sleep. In Kryger M, Roth T, Dement WC, eds. *Principles and practice of sleep medicine*, chap 4, pp 30–49. Philadelphia: Saunders.

Harold Zepelin

MANIA

See Affective Disorders Other Than Major Depression

MARIJUANA

Marijuana is the term used to refer to parts or extracts of the hemp plant, which has somatic and/or psychic effects in humans. Although a variety of compounds (cannabinoids) are synthesized by this plant, Δ^9-tetrahydrocannabinol (THC) is considered to be the principal active component mediating psychological and physiological effects in humans. The metabolism of THC occurs chiefly in the liver, with some breakdown taking place as well in the lungs and brain. These metabolic products are then sequestered in fatty tissues and slowly released. Marijuana may be ingested either through inhalation (smoking), orally, or intravenously. Behavioral and physiological effects occur within ½ hour and may persist for 3 to 5 hours.

Interest in the effects of this psychoactive compound on sleep developed from reports indicating marijuana-related sedation and hallucinatory-like behavior in lower animals, and sleepiness, hallucinations, and thought disruption in humans. Although aspects of sleep (e.g., amounts of REM sleep and eye movement activity during REM sleep) have been related to information processing, and marijuana has been shown to compromise cognitive functioning during wakefulness, sleep studies have focused on the physiological and not the cognitive effects of marijuana. Interpretation of the results of these studies has been complicated by variations in dose, route of administration, study design, and the extent to which subjects were experienced in psychoactive compound usage. Still, consistencies in results that emerge from these studies suggest reliable effects of both acute and chronic use of marijuana on sleep. Acute administration of the drug is reported to increase slow-wave sleep, decrease eye movements during REM sleep, and slightly reduce REM sleep with subsequent increases in REM sleep (REM rebound) following withdrawal.

Chronic exposure to marijuana also alters sleep patterns, and the most reliable observation is a decrease in slow-wave sleep that may extend beyond the drug administration period. Abrupt discontinuation of marijuana by chronic users is followed by sleep disturbances that take the form of difficulty falling asleep and increased awakenings. These latter observations are in agreement with previous research indicating that psychological, but not physical, dependence may develop with chronic use of this drug.

Despite increased concern and awareness of the potential negative effects on the fetus of pharmacological agents taken during pregnancy, very little is known about the effects of this compound on infants born to mothers who have been exposed to marijuana during pregnancy. Information is beginning to emerge on this topic, however, and early indications are that alterations in sleep patterns and motor activity are evident within hours of birth in infants born under such conditions. Among other observations, these infants were noted to have less quiet sleep, more mixed active sleep, fewer rapid eye movements, and more body movements (Scher et al., 1988). A complicating factor in the interpretation of these results is the fact that drug exposure occurred under noncontrolled, naturalistic conditions and it is likely that multiple pharmacological agents may have been involved. For example, marijuana is often used in combination with alcohol, and it has been determined that the physiological and behavioral effects of this combination are greater than those observed when either drug is taken alone.

Clearly, marijuana can modify physiological features of sleep; however, the implications of these effects for waking behavior remain to be clarified.

REFERENCES

Feinberg I, Jones R, Walker J, Cavness C, Floyd T. 1976. Effects of marijuana tetrahydrocannabinol on electroencephalographic sleep patterns. *Clin Pharmacol Ther* 19:782–794.

Halikas JA, Weller RA, Morse CL, Hoffmann RG. 1985. A longitudinal study of marijuana effects. In *Int J Addictions* 20:701–711.

Mendelson JH. 1987. Marijuana. In Meltzer HY, ed. *Psychopharmacology: The third generation of progress*, chap 168, pp 1565–1571. New York: Raven.

Pivik RT, Zarcone V, Dement WC, Hollister LE. 1972. Delta-9-tetrahydrocannabinol and synhexl: Effects on human sleep patterns. *Clin Pharmacol Ther* 13:426–435.

Scher MS, Richardson GA, Coble PA, Day NL, Stoffer DS. 1988. The effects of prenatal alcohol and marijuana exposure: Disturbances in neonatal sleep cycling and arousal. *Pediatr Res* 24:101–105.

R. T. Pivik

MATTRESS

A mattress is an article consisting of filling materials, covered with ticking and used for sleeping. The word is derived from the Arabic *matrah* meaning "to throw down." Early designs of the mattress were simple sacks filled with batts or layers of cotton felt. Ostermoor, a name associated with the cotton felt mattress, began manufacture in the United States in 1895 and met with much success. The felt mattress was very popular until the 1930s when it succumbed to the competition of the innerspring. Records indicate the first patent for an innerspring was issued in 1853, but this product was never marketed. Other patents were issued but the first commercially successful venture of the innerspring mattress did not occur until Marshall, a Canadian, took out patents on a pocketed coil design in 1900. Growth of the innerspring mattress in the United States accelerated in 1921 with the introduction of the burlap pocketed-type of unit for mattresses. In 1924 the innerspring mattress accounted for 5 percent of the industry production. Utilization of this type of mattress construction has grown to where innerspring accounted for approximately 80 percent of all mattresses produced in the United States in 1990.

Early innerspring mattresses used natural materials in the upholstery layers to achieve a level of comfort over the innerspring. These materials were generally sisal, jute, coir, or coconut fiber with additional layers of cotton felt. These early constructions were soft and yielding and lacked support. Techniques were developed to improve the firmness of the product through improvements in the innerspring and mechanical bonding of the upholstery layers. "Tufted" and single-needle or "scroll quilted" mattresses were the result of these efforts. The introduction of the multineedle quilted mattress in the late 1960s, along with the utilization of synthetic upholstery materials such as polyurethane foam and polyester fiber batting, resulted in the development of the innerspring mattress we are familiar with today. The combination of firm innersprings with thick upholstery layers affords today's user the option of mattresses with a wide range of comfort and support factors.

Although innerspring construction accounts for 80 percent of the mattresses produced in the United States, several other types of support systems are used in the manufacture of mattresses. They include foam (both latex and polyurethane), which accounts for approximately 5 percent of the total US market, flotation (waterbeds and airbeds) accounting for approximately 14 percent and fiber (futons, etc) for the remaining 1 percent of the US market.

Standard sizes of mattresses in the United States are twin 39 × 75 inches, full or double 52 × 75 inches, queen 60 × 80 inches, king 76 × 80 inches, and California or western king 72 × 84 inches. These sizes are modified in the international market to be consistent with metric standards.

The mattress industry is considered very mature, with recent innovations being the introduction of the waterbed in the late 1960s and, more recently, the popularity and use of the action bed or adjustable mattress. This latter development is consistent with the change in usage of the bedroom as primarily a sleep room to its utilization as an area for additional activity such as television viewing and reading.

The influence of the innerspring mattress on the European continent is not as strong as that on the domestic market. Latex foam mattresses are dominant in that market, with innerspring-type constructions lagging. The innerspring or "Western-style" mattress is gaining significant acceptance in Asian countries. The Asian traveler has been introduced to this type of mattress while staying at hotels in Western countries. Conversely, in recent years there has been an increase in popularity of the futon as a mattress in the USA, particularly in the West Coast states.

REFERENCES

Bedding Magazine/Buyers' Guide. 1972, pp 23–30. Available from ISPA (formerly NABM), 333 Commerce St, Alexandria, VA 22314.

Burgess A. 1982. *On going to bed*, pp 149–183. New York: Abbeville.

Dittrick M. 1980. *The bed book*, pp 5–20. New York: Harcourt, Brace, Jovanovich.

Robert Wagner

MATURATION

See Development; Ontogeny; Puberty

MAXILLOFACIAL SURGERY

Maxillofacial surgery is an effective treatment for obstructive sleep apnea syndrome and other breathing disorders during sleep that involve a narrow upper airway (see APNEA). It may be used not only in patients who have obvious skeletal malformations of the jaw but also in those with more subtle anatomical anomalies, which can be identified only by a thorough evaluation. The evaluation must always include several techniques to visualize the upper airway; for example, x-rays of the head (cephalometric x-rays), upper airway computed tomography (CT) scans, and upper airway visualization with an endoscope are commonly performed.

Several types of maxillofacial surgery are used to treat sleep apnea: uvulopalatopharyngoplasty (UPPP), tonsillectomy, adenoidectomy, septoplasty, and posterior tubinectomy, to name a few. Each of these surgical procedures involves removing tissue from the throat or upper airway (see UVULOPALATOPHARYNGOPLASTY; TONSILLITIS). The surgical procedure appropriate for each case is determined by the location of upper airway narrowings found in presurgical testing. Most cases can be classified as one of three types:

abnormal oropharynx (type I), abnormal oro-pharynx and hypopharynx (type II), or abnormal hypopharynx (type III). These types indicate levels of the throat where narrowing occurs (Figure 1).

Another type of maxillofacial surgery is performed when the surgeon considers that the airway can be enlarged best by pulling the large tongue (genioglossus) muscle forward. One way to accomplish this is by an operation that moves the upper (maxilla) and lower (mandible) jaws forward and therefore moves the tongue as well. In certain patients, this surgery corrects an obvious facial malformation and hence improves the way they look as well as improving their sleep disorder. A variation of this operation also repositions the hyoid bone under the jaw so that the tongue is moved forward. Several other approaches may be used, usually in combination with or following UPPP (Figure 2). In all, the goal is to provide a wider airway so that when the muscles relax during sleep, the airway space remains sufficiently large to prevent collapse with inhalation. These surgical procedures can be quite complex, lasting several hours and requiring difficult dissections of tissue. Certain patients will require a dental appliance to help correct changes in dental alignment that may occur as a result of surgery.

The difficulty of these surgical procedures is that they involve two different techniques that are rarely acquired by a single specialist: otorhinolaryngoplasty (ear, nose, throat) and oral surgery. Few medical teams have developed this combination, and younger specialists may wish to consider receiving this type of training. Positive results have been reported predominantly by one surgical group. This team has performed the largest postoperative study of maxillofacial patients, including 306 who were observed up to 4 years

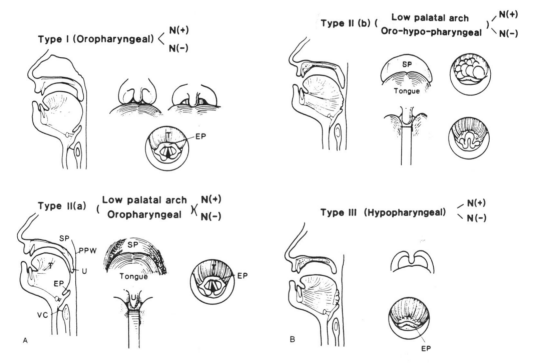

Figure 1. These drawings illustrate how surgeons classify the location of the airway obstruction in patients with upper airway sleep apnea syndrome. These classifications can be useful for determining the type of surgery that is likely to be most helpful. Type I is an obstruction high in the throat (oropharynx). Type IIa and Type IIb are lower in the throat (orohypopharyngeal). Type III is lower still, in the hypopharynx. Abbreviations: EP = epiglottis, T = tongue, SP = soft palate, PPW = posterior pharyngeal wall, VC = vocal chord, U = uvula. (*Reprinted with permission from Fairbanks et al., 1987.*)

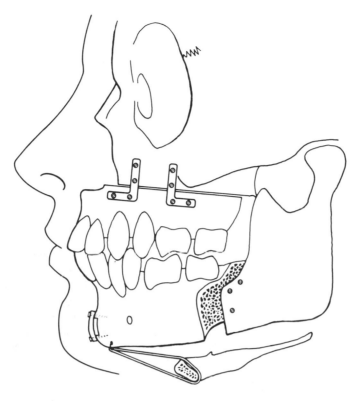

Figure 2. This diagram shows maxillofacial surgery that has moved the maxilla and mandible forward (stabilizing the maxilla) and moved the hyoid bone forward and up. The net result is an enlargement of the airway space in the upper throat. (*Reprinted with permission from Riley, Powell, and Guilleminault, 1990.*)

past surgery (Riley, Powell, and Guilleminault, 1990). Results of surgery cannot be determined for at least 6 months. Available data indicate an overall success rate of 76.5 percent at an average of 9.3 months with polysomnographic follow-up. The percentage of complications is low. Transient numbness of the cheek and chin area is seen in all subjects for 6 to 12 months. Immediate postsurgical bleeding requiring new general anesthesia was reported in 1 percent of subjects. Twelve percent of patients experience transient nasal reflux. From the available data, these results appear better overall than those of less specialized teams performing these procedures.

Surgical procedures represent one option for the treatment of sleep apnea. Other options include CONTINUOUS POSITIVE AIRWAY PRESSURE, medications, dental appliances, and so forth. The success rate of any treatment depends upon many factors, including the level of the airway obstruc-

tion, patient compliance with procedures over time, and surgical skill. Physicians treating sleep apnea take all of these factors into account when helping patients to decide which treatment may be best for them.

REFERENCES

Fairbanks DNF, Fujita S, Ikematsu T, Simmons FB, eds. 1987. *Snoring and obstructive sleep apnea.* New York: Raven.

Riley RW, Powell NB, Guilleminault C. 1990. Maxillofacial surgery and nasal CPAP: A comparison of treatment for obstructive sleep apnea syndrome. *Chest* 98:1421–1425.

Christian Guilleminault

MEASUREMENT OF SLEEP

[*The measurement of sleep can be accomplished using a wide variety of approaches, and the approach chosen depends upon a number of factors, including the type of organism to be studied, the age of the animal or person to be studied, and the reason for taking the measurement. At times, a very precise, fine-grained, second-by-second measurement is required; at other times, a grosser measure will suffice. Furthermore, for certain purposes in clinical and experimental sleep studies, the measurement of sleep is combined with measurements of other features of behavior or physiology.*

The most common technique for measuring sleep in humans is called POLYSOMNOGRAPHY *and is ordinarily performed at a sleep laboratory. The primary sleep-related measures in polysomnography are the* ELECTROENCEPHALOGRAM *(EEG),* ELECTROOCULOGRAM *(EOG), and* ELECTROMYOGRAM *(EMG). In humans, these recordings of electrical activity are taken from electrodes applied to the surface of the scalp and face; to identify the various stages of sleep in other animals, these recordings can be taken from electrodes placed directly in contact with brain tissue (EEG) or within the muscles (EMG). Other measures that can be taken concomitantly with the EEG, EOG, and EMG include the* ELECTROCARDIOGRAM *and measures of respiration, blood pressure,* NOCTURNAL PENILE TUMESCENCE, *and many other variables.*

An alternative means of measuring sleep in very young organisms, including human infants, is behavioral observation (see INFANCY, NORMAL SLEEP PATTERNS IN*). At times, such measures may even be more accurate than the EEG, because the immature level of central nervous system development in a very young organism makes state classification by EEG rather difficult. Observational techniques are often used for invertebrate species, such as* INSECTS. *Behavioral observation has proven particularly useful in evaluating the sleep of many types of* AMPHIBIANS, REPTILES, FISH, BIRDS, *and* MAMMALS *under natural conditions.*

Depending on the observer's needs and the available technology, sleep–wake behaviors can be coded directly and continuously, or observations can be made intermittently, as has been done in studies of nursing home residents.

SLEEP POSITIONS *and patterns have been documented by means of time-lapse photography, and similar techniques have been used with animals in a zoo. Time-lapse videotape has also been used quite effectively, particularly in the study of infant sleep.*

AMBULATORY MONITORING *is a general set of techniques that enable measurement outside of the laboratory setting; typically, a portable measuring device is attached to the person (or animal) whose sleep is being studied. For example, a compact but fully operational eight-channel polygraph—no bigger than a Walkman—can be carried around by a person wearing electrodes connected to the machine. Such a device can record EEG, EOG, and EMG, as well as many other physiological variables or behavioral events, on normal audio tape or in electronic memory.*

Finally, scientists have developed additional techniques called ACTIVITY-BASED MEASURES OF SLEEP. *In one such measure, actigraphy, the individual being studied wears a miniature motion detector on a wristband or belt or (in infants) on the ankle to track activity levels around the clock for up to several weeks at a time. Alternatively, a static charge–sensitive bed or a pressure-sensitive mattress can be used to measure the movements of a person in bed.*

The methods described here represent the most common approaches to the measurement of sleep, and each provides reliable and valid data with regard to sleeping and waking patterns.]

MEDICAL ILLNESS AND SLEEP

[*Since "getting a good night's sleep" is often cited as a characteristic of a healthy person, it is not surprising to find that sleep disturbances are often an aspect of medical illness.*

The quality of sleep itself is a major characteristic of some illnesses, such as NARCOLEPSY *and* CHRONIC FATIGUE SYNDROME. *The entry below focuses on four serious and widespread illnesses that also have a significant effect on sleep: cancer, rheumatoid arthritis, congestive obstructive pulmonary disease, and osteoarthritis. The entry opens with a consideration of two groups of chronic pain sufferers whose sleep patterns have been studied most often: those in intensive care units, and those suffering from psychogenic pain, as in DEPRESSION.*]

Pain

There are many causes of pain, as well as many degrees of severity. To some extent, as has been seen in osteoarthritis (see below), the degree of sleep disturbance is related to area of the body affected. Two major groups of patients have been studied—those with chronic pain as a result of a variety of medical illnesses and those in intensive care units either for surgical recovery or for recovery from myocardial infarctions (heart attacks). Generally speaking, patients with chronic pain have a decreased total sleep time, but not as much as patients with psychiatric illnesses such as depression and anxiety. Alpha intrusion is seen in the sleep ELECTROENCEPHALOGRAM (EEG) in as many as one-third of patients with chronic pain (Wittig et al., 1982). Patients with psychogenic pain, which is often caused by difficulty coping, frequently have depression and as a result have a decreased REM sleep latency (Blumer et al., 1982). Behavioral techniques, such as relaxation exercises and biofeedback, have been found useful in some patients with chronic pain in relieving the symptoms and the sleep disturbance (Morin, Kowatch, and Wade, 1989).

Of those individuals in the intensive care unit, at least 25 percent complain of difficulty sleeping (Jones et al., 1979). Many patients may attribute poor sleep to the inability to lie comfortably, but studies have indicated that staff activity, noise, pain, nursing interventions, lights, various apparatus used, and coldness are significant factors (Dlin et al., 1971). The "intensive care unit syndrome," in which there are a few hours or days of hallucinations and confusion after surgery, has been partially attributed to sleep loss (Johns et al., 1974). Patients with a variety of surgical procedures usually show an increase in stage 1 sleep, reduced REM and slow-wave sleep (SWS), with substantial reduction in the total sleep time in the first 2 days of recuperation (Aurell and Elmqvist, 1985). Patients with myocardial infarctions who are in an intensive care unit also have a reduction in total sleep time, increase in stage 1, increase in the number of arousals, and decline in

REM sleep. It has been reported, however, that SWS is normal in these patients with an increase in SWS with recuperation. Over several days, patients with myocardial infarction may continue to have a relative reduction in total sleep time and reductions in REM sleep parameters (Broughton and Baron, 1978).

(See also ALPHA–DELTA SLEEP; ARTHRITIS AND OTHER MUSCULOSKELETAL DISORDERS.)

REFERENCES

Aurell J, Elmqvist D. 1985. Sleep in the surgical intensive care unit: Continuous polygraphic recording of sleep in nine patients receiving postoperative care. *Br Med J* 290:1029–1032.

Blumer D, Zorick F, Heilbronn M, Roth T. 1982. Biological markers for depression in chronic pain. *J Nerv Ment Dis* 170(7):425–428.

Broughton R, Baron R. 1978. Sleep patterns in the intensive care unit and on the ward after acute myocardial infarction. *Electroencephalogr Clin Neurophysiol* 45:348–360.

Dlin BM, Rosen H, Dickstein K, Lyons JW, Fischer HK. 1971. The problems of sleep and rest in the intensive care unit. *Psychosomatics* 12(3):155–163.

Johns MW, Large AA, Masterson JP, Dudley HAF. 1974. Sleep and delirium after open heart surgery. *Br J Surg* 61:377–381.

Jones J, Hoggart B, Withey J, Donaghue K, Ellis BW. 1979. What the patients say: A study of reactions to an intensive care unit. *Intensive Care Med* 5:89–92.

Morin CM, Kowatch RA, Wade JB. 1989. Behavioral management of sleep disturbances secondary to chronic pain. *J Behav Ther Exp Psychiatry* 20(4):295–302.

Wittig RM, Zorick FJ, Blumer D, Heilbronn M, Roth T. 1982. Disturbed sleep in patients complaining of chronic pain. *J Nerv Ment Dis* 170(7):429–431.

Virgil Wooten

Cancer

Sleep disturbances associated with cancer have not been defined for every form of cancer; however, knowledge about the effects of specific kinds of cancer on sleep patterns is expected to grow. Brain cancers usually cause changes in sleep patterns because of the direct effect of brain tumors on the various areas governing sleep. In certain instances, brain wave patterns may become so distorted that sleep stages cannot be easily identified (Kanno, Hosaka, and Yagamuchi, 1977). In cancers affecting other parts of the body, there is usually a reduction in the amount of total sleep time (Beszterzey and Lipowski, 1977). The most important factor, in most instances, is not the presence of the cancer itself, but instead the anxiety and depression that often accompanies a diagnosis of cancer (Beszterczey and Lipowski, 1977; Lamb, 1982). Sleep disturbance does not appear to be any worse in those with cancer than in individuals with other medical problems (Kaye, Kaye, and Madow, 1983). The best approach to treating sleeping difficulties in individuals with cancer involves good psychological support and medications aimed to reduce anxiety, depression, and pain. Training in relaxation techniques can also be very beneficial (Cannici, Malcolm, and Peek, 1983).

REFERENCES

Beszterczey A, Lipowski ZJ. 1977. Insomnia in cancer patients. *Can Med Assoc J* 116:355.

Cannici J, Malcolm R, Peek LA. 1983. Treatment of insomnia in cancer patients using muscle relaxation training. *J Behav Ther Exp Psychiatry* 14(3): 251–256.

Kanno O, Hosaka H, Yagamuchi T. 1977. Dissociation of sleep stages between two hemispheres in a case with unilateral thalamic tumor. *Folia Psychiatr Neurol Jpn* 31(1):69–75.

Kaye J, Kaye K, Madow L. 1983. Sleep patterns in patients with cancer and patients with cardiac disease. *J Psychol* 114:107–113.

Lamb MA. 1982. The sleeping patterns of patients with malignant and nonmalignant diseases. *Cancer Nurs*, Oct., pp 389–396.

Virgil Wooten

Rheumatoid Arthritis

Rheumatoid arthritis is a systemic (affecting the whole body) disease characterized by the progressive destruction of the joints because of the body's immune system's attacking the tissues. Individuals with rheumatoid arthritis usually develop fatigue, weakness, loss of appetite, weight loss, joint stiffness, joint pain, muscle pain, and sleep disturbance.

There may be great variability among individuals as to how much the rheumatoid arthritis causes sleep disturbance. In many, there is no abnormality of sleep onset or of sleep stage distribution; however, there may be a marked increase in the number of arousals (Mahowald et al., 1989), an increase in the number of stage shifts (for example, shifting frequently from stage 2 to stage 1), increased stage 1, and reduction in the total sleep time (Moldofsky, Lue, and Smythe, 1983). Many patients with rheumatoid arthritis have alpha rhythm occurring in the sleep EEG (Mahowald et al., 1989; Moldofsky, Lue, and Smythe, 1983). The alpha brain wave pattern is usually seen with the eyes closed while awake and should not occur very often after sleep begins.

Few studies have been performed on patients with rheumatoid arthritis to determine the effectiveness of medications in improving sleep. Surveys indicate that benzodiazepine hypnotics (drugs related to diazepam) give a feeling of improvement in sleep and less nighttime pain; however, complaints of morning stiffness may not be altered or may actually be increased. The use of medications that reduce inflammation, like ASPIRIN, either alone or with sedative hypnotics appear to improve the impression of sleep quality as well as improving the morning stiffness, which is usually one of the more serious complaints (Bayley and Haslock, 1976). Tricyclic antidepressants, such as amitriptyline, may also help reduce the pain and improve the sleep quality. Antidepressants have many uses and are very helpful in reducing pain regardless of whether the person treated is depressed.

(See also ARTHRITIS AND OTHER MUSCULOSKELETAL DISORDERS; SLEEPING PILLS.)

REFERENCES

Bayley TRL, Haslock I. 1976. Night medication in rheumatoid arthritis. *J R Coll Gen Pract* 26:591–594.

Mahowald MW, Mahowald ML, Bundlie SR, Ytterberg S. 1989. Sleep fragmentation in rheumatoid arthritis. *Arthritis & Rheumatism* 32(8):974–983.

Moldofsky H, Lue FA, Smythe HA. 1983. Alpha EEG sleep and morning symptoms in rheumatoid arthritis. *J Rheumatol* 10:373–379.

Virgil Wooten

Chronic Obstructive Pulmonary Disease

Chronic obstructive pulmonary disease (COPD) is a term that usually implies a combination of chronic bronchitis and emphysema and is most frequently caused by tobacco smoking. Emphysema is the term that is most often used by the general public to describe this condition. Emphysema per se refers to enlargement of the air spaces in the lungs caused by destruction of the tissues. Chronic bronchitis is caused by prolonged irritation of the tracheobronchial tree, which results from excessive mucus secretion. The combination of emphysema and chronic bronchitis results in "trapping" of air in the lungs. As a result of airways obstruction, breathing is difficult and wheezing is often heard, especially upon breathing out. Because of impaired breathing, the oxygen level in the blood is often lowered, while the carbon dioxide level increases. During sleep the reduced oxygen and elevated carbon dioxide levels may markedly worsen, particularly during REM sleep.

Individuals with COPD have reduced total sleep time, increased stage shifts and arousals, and decreased slow-wave and REM sleep. When hypoxemia occurs, it is usually much worse in REM sleep. Administering extra oxygen may help normalize the oxygen level during sleep in individuals with milder COPD; however, in individuals with moderate or severe COPD with high blood carbon dioxide levels, the addition of oxygen may actually reduce the effort to breath. The result is extremely high carbon dioxide levels that in turn can lower the pH (or increase the acid concentration in the blood), thereby endangering the afflicted individual's life. Even if the oxygen level is improved during sleep, it does not appear to improve sleep quality.

Milder cases of COPD may benefit from bronchodilator drugs such as theophylline and albuterol, which relax and open the air passages in the lungs. Sometimes these agents contribute to sleep disturbance because of their stimulant properties. Some sedatives can be used as necessary to help individuals with milder COPD; however, in patients with advanced COPD, these drugs may make breathing during sleep worse. Alcohol should be avoided in individuals with COPD, as it has been shown that alcohol can sometimes cause marked worsening of breathing.

REFERENCES

Flenley DC. 1989. Chronic obstructive pulmonary disease. In Kryger MH, Roth T, Dement WC, eds. *Principles and practice of sleep medicine,* pp 601–610. Philadelphia: Saunders.
Wooten V. 1989. Medical causes of insomnia: Chronic obstructive pulmonary disease. In Kryger MH, Roth T, Dement WC, eds. *Principles and practice of sleep medicine,* pp 457–458. Philadelphia: Saunders.

Virgil Wooten

Osteoarthritis

Osteoarthritis, also known as degenerative joint disease, is caused by chronic wear (trauma) of the joints. Although most individuals who live long enough sustain trauma over a number of years and develop osteoarthritis, the problem may be accelerated by exercises or occupations that are known to result in damage to the joints.

Studies of individuals with severe osteoarthritis of the hip and/or knee show increases in stage 1 sleep and less stage 2 sleep than in normal individuals (Leigh et al., 1980). It has been suggested that in patients with osteoarthritis affecting the hands or other joints that are not aggravated by sleeping positions, there is little sleep disturbance (Moldofsky, 1989); however, in individuals whose sleeping position may aggravate the affected joints, such as in cervical (neck) spine disease, there may well be an increase in sleep disturbance.

REFERENCES

Leigh TJ, Hindmarch I, Bird HA, Wright V. 1980. Comparison of sleep in osteoarthritic patients and age and sex matched healthy controls. *Ann Rheum Dis* 47:40–42.

356   Medications

Moldofsky, H. 1989. Sleep influences on regional and diffuse pain syndromes associated with osteoarthritis. *Semin Arthritis & Rheum* 18(4):18–21.

Virgil Wooten

MEDICATIONS

See Amphetamines; Antidepressants; Antihistamines; Aspirin; Barbiturates; Benzodiazepines; Drugs for Medical Disorders; Monoamine Oxidase Inhibitors; Narcotics; Over-the-Counter Sleeping Pills; Over-the-Counter Stimulants; Pharmacology; Sleeping Pills; Stimulants

MEDITATION AND SLEEP

People used to regard meditation as a kind of thinking or even prayer. Within the past twenty-five years meditation has become associated with specific practices brought to the West from places like India, Thailand, and Japan. There are many different kinds of meditation practices. Some are either physical or mental; some are both. Many people have heard of the popular "name brand" techniques like Transcendental Meditation (TM), Insight Meditation, Zen, Kung Fu, Tai-Chi-Kwan, Kundalini Yoga, Iyengar Yoga, and Integral Yoga. Yet, there is unity in this diversity: Meditative disciplines have a common goal. The classic definition of yoga is "the control of the thought waves in the mind" (Prabhananda and Isherwood, 1969). Curiously, this idea of "thought waves" predates our understanding of brain waves by at least 2,500 years! Yet, no matter how ancient the technique, the control of thought waves may seem very desirable with the stress of modern life. Indeed, according to a Hindu proverb, "If you conquer the mind, you have conquered the world." Like the need for sleep, perhaps the need for meditation is timeless.

Traditional teachers (often referred to as *gurus*) and the ancient texts that guide them often claim that meditative practices give extraordinary control of mind and body. For example, some teachers claim that practice of their

techniques can give the ability to control breathing, heartbeat, and blood flow. Other gurus claim to teach practices that lead to levitation, clairvoyance, and telepathy.

Within the past few decades, scientific interest has moved toward objectively documenting the effects of various meditation practices. Still, as a new area of investigation, meditation research needs to clarify three basic questions: First, do all the various meditation practices produce the same effects? Second, what differences are there between novices and long-term meditators? Finally, are the subjects who volunteer for meditation research people who are naturally disposed toward meditative practices?

In spite of these important missing pieces, many benefits of meditation have been confirmed. Some effects, such as inducing the relaxation response and aiding the reversal of coronary artery disease, have been documented in well-controlled studies. Much of the experimental research on the effects of meditation has applied the same technology and methods developed to study sleep, hypnotic trance, and relaxation.

What are the similarities and differences between meditation and sleep? Most researchers agree that the physiological characteristics of meditation (such as specific brain wave patterns) are very similar to the characteristics of relaxation training and hypnosis (Delmonte, 1984). Meditators also look very sleepy. At least one electroencephalographic study found that some meditators spent almost 60 percent of their meditation time in scorable stage 1, stage 2, and delta sleep (Delmonte, 1984). Most meditating subjects show increased and slowed alpha electroencephalographic activity; a forward spread of alpha, theta trains; and slow eye movements. These features are all consistent with stage 1 sleep (see STAGES OF SLEEP).

In spite of these physiological similarities to sleep, meditation is more than training in drowsiness. When comparing meditators to resting or untrained subjects, many studies on perception have shown that meditators are actually quite alert. In studies that compare meditators with untrained subjects, *during meditation,* meditators can (1) sense and report more with their eyes (Brown, Forte, and Dysart, 1984) and ears (Ikemi, 1988), (2) relax more quickly when subjected to stressful sounds (Delmonte, 1984), and (3) make fewer mistakes on tasks requiring physical speed and thought (Ikemi, 1988).

Research has also shown that meditation provides a great variety of mental benefits. Some of these benefits are reduced anxiety and depression, increased self-regulation of chronic pain, improved psychotherapy, decreased neuroticism, and emotional release (Murphy and Donovan, 1988). The HYPNAGOGIC REVERIE that can occur during meditation has also been associated with increased potential for creative problem solving.

These findings suggest that meditation may be regarded as deliberately held state of consciousness that appears to have psychological, if not physiological, characteristics that distinguish it from the ordinary, unconscious drowsiness of stage 1 sleep.

How does practicing meditation affect sleep? Given the physiological similarities between meditation and sleep, one might wonder if regular periods of meditation reduce the amount of sleep needed or improve the quality of sleep. There is not much support for the idea that meditators require less total sleep or can do without sleep. Some of the studies show that meditation may generate more efficient dream (or REM) sleep. Meditators seem to require less time in REM sleep and, when deprived of REM, tend to return sooner to their predeprivation levels of REM sleep (Miskiman, 1974).

As meditation can reduce ANXIETY and DEPRESSION, and as anxiety and depression may be factors contributing to INSOMNIA, meditation also may help with insomnia. Research on meditation and insomnia has been mixed but has yielded some supportive findings. Meditation, like progressive relaxation training, can significantly reduce the amount of time a person remains awake after sleep onset (see RELAXATION THERAPY). Curiously, subjects' expectations affect how their insomnia will be helped. In one study subjects learned meditation–relaxation and controls were given a supposed placebo (Carr-Kaffashan and Woolfolk, 1979). All were told not to expect any improvements for four weeks. The subjects who practiced meditation–relaxation reported improvements during the first three weeks. Yet by the fourth week *all* subjects reported the same significant improvement. It seems that it was equally helpful to tell everyone they would sleep better, four weeks into *whichever* technique they were using.

In another study three techniques were compared for their ability to reduce insomnia (Schoicket, Bertelson, and Lacks, 1988): (1) provision of information about the "do's and don'ts" of behaviors before bedtime (called *sleep hygiene information*); (2) training in associating the bed and bedroom with sleepiness rather than with wakeful behaviors like reading, eating, and watching TV (this is called *stimulus control therapy*); (3) clinically standardized meditation (CSM) (Carrington, 1979). After the experiment, all three subject groups reported comparable improvements in wake time after sleep onset, number of awakenings, and duration of awakenings. Surprisingly, significantly more of the subjects given the SLEEP HYGIENE instructions rated their treatment *less favorably* and considered themselves still insomniac.

What accounts for this difference in self-perception when all subjects reported the same amount of symptom improvement? Meditation and stimulus control therapy require active and regular practice. Perhaps the subjects who used these techniques felt more improvement because action may be psychologically more powerful than information alone.

In summary, science has yet to prove that meditation generates a state of consciousness that is distinct from either wakefulness or sleep. Most of the physiological evidence supports the idea/notion/concept that meditation and stage 1 sleep are more similar than different; however, even if the meditation state resembles sleep, practicing meditation does not substitute for sleep. Among the many reported benefits of practice, meditators appear more alert during meditation than during ordinary wakefulness. Like sleep, meditation is an exciting and promising area of body–mind research.

REFERENCES

Brown D, Forte M, Dysart M. 1984. Visual sensitivity and mindfulness meditation. *Perceptual Motor Skills* 59:775–784.

Carrington P. 1979. *Clinically standardized meditation: Instructor's manual.* Kendall Park, NJ: Pace Educational Systems.

Carr-Kaffashan L, Woolfolk R. 1979. Active and placebo effects in treatment of moderate and severe insomnia. *J Consult Clin Psychol* 46:1072–1080.

Delmonte MM. 1984. Electrocortical activity and related phenomena associated with meditation practice: A literature review. *Int J Neurosci* 24:

217–231. Contains concise and thorough summaries of physiological studies and an excellent bibliography.

Ikemi A. 1988. Psychophysiological effects of self-regulation method: EEG frequency analysis and contingent negative variations. *Psychother Psychosom* 49:230–239.

Miskiman DE. 1974. Long-term effects of transcendental meditation on compensatory paradoxical sleep. In Orme-Johnson DW, ed. *Scientific research on transcendental meditation: Collected papers,* vol 1. Los Angeles: MIU Press.

Murphy M, Donovan S. 1988. *The physical and psychological effects of meditation.* San Rafael, CA: Esalen Institute. A comprehensive bibliography.

Prabhananda S, Isherwood C. 1969. *How to know god.* New York: Mentor Books, New American Library. This is a most concise translation and commentary of the Raja Yoga Sutras—the 2,500-year-old "blueprint" or "roadmap" of the purposes and practices of the many yoga systems of meditative discipline.

Schoicket S, Bertelson A, Lacks P. 1988. Is sleep hygiene a sufficient treatment for sleep-maintenance insomnia? *Behav Ther* 19:183–190.

Lakshyan Schanzer

MEDULLA

The medulla is the brainstem region located just above the spinal cord and just below the PONS (see Figure 1; see also Figure 1 in REM SLEEP MECHANISMS). The medulla alone contains mechanisms sufficient to keep us breathing, keep our hearts beating and regulated, and produce arousal in response to intense stimuli. The medulla is not sufficient to generate REM sleep; however, it does contain neurons contributing to the control of both REM and NREM sleep (see NREM SLEEP MECHANISMS; REM SLEEP MECHANISMS AND NEUROANATOMY).

A key neuronal group for NREM sleep control is located in the lateral medulla. Stimulation of the region adjacent to the nucleus solitarius can induce sleep, as can stimulation of the receptors in the carotid body (adjoining the carotid artery) monitoring blood pressure. The carotid body receptors connect with the region of the nucleus solitarius. The more medial portions of the medulla are critical for the suppression of muscle tone that occurs in REM sleep (see ATONIA). The nuclei involved in muscle tone suppression in-

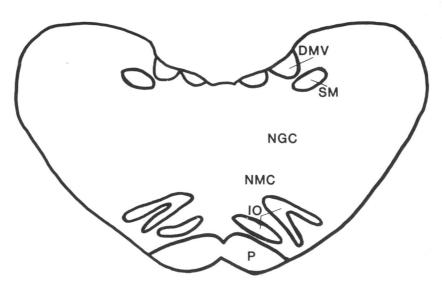

Figure 1. A cross-section of the medulla. DMV = dorsal motor nucleus of the vagus nerve, which controls certain visceral motor functions such as the heart and intestines; IO = inferior olive, a motor nucleus that works with the cerebellum; NGC = nucleus gigantocellularis; NMC = nucleus magnocellularis; P = pyramidal tract, which conveys motor information to the spinal cord; SM = medial nucleus of the solitary tract, which receives sensory signals from visceral areas and the circulatory system.

clude portions of the nucleus gigantocellularis (named for its large neurons) and, beneath this, the nucleus magnocellularis containing somewhat smaller cells. Closer to the spinal cord (just behind the nucleus gigantocellularis and magnocellularis) is a cell group called the nucleus paramedianus, also involved in the suppression of muscle tone in REM sleep. The medial medulla also contributes to the regulation of arousal through projections going forward through the brainstem to arousal-related regions of the PONS, MIDBRAIN, and THALAMUS. Therefore, this region can coordinate motor activity with level of arousal.

REFERENCE

Siegel JM. 1989. Brainstem mechanisms generating REM sleep. In Kryger MH, Roth T, Dement WC, eds. *Principles and practice of sleep medicine,* pp 104–121. Philadelphia: Saunders.

Jerome Siegel

MELATONIN

Over three decades ago, Lerner et al. (1958) set out to isolate the factor present in the PINEAL GLAND that lightened amphibian skin. From an extract of 250,000 beef pineals, he and his colleagues were able to identify the major bioactive indolamine, melatonin or 5-methoxy-*N*-acetyltryptamine, produced by the pineal gland. The physiological function of melatonin remains to be defined; however, the melatonin rhythm can be used as a marker of the circadian timing system (see CIRCADIAN RHYTHMS). Melatonin has also been reported to have hypnotic properties, leading some to suggest that melatonin, which is released at night, may be an endogenous sleep-inducing factor.

Melatonin production is highest during the nighttime hours in both diurnal (day-active) and nocturnal (night-active) animals. The biosynthetic pathway for melatonin is stimulated by sympathetic innervation of the pineal gland. The amino acid L-TRYPTOPHAN is converted into serotonin within the pinealocyte. *N*-acetyltransferase, the rate-limiting enzyme in the pathway,

then acts on serotonin to produce melatonin. Unlike hormones controlled by the hypothalamic–pituitary axis, the release of melatonin from the pineal gland does not appear to be pulsatile in nature (see CHEMISTRY OF SLEEP; NEUROENDOCRINE HORMONES; PINEAL GLAND).

The pineal gland is the primary location of melatonin production, although the retina is also accepted as a secondary source of the hormone. High-affinity melatonin binding sites have been identified in the pineal gland, the SUPRACHIASMATIC NUCLEUS OF THE HYPOTHALAMUS, the retina, and the PITUITARY GLAND. Melatonin, which is highly lipid soluble, has been detected in blood, cerebrospinal fluid, and saliva. 6-Hydroxymelatonin, the major metabolite of melatonin following conjugation in the liver, can be measured in the urine. (See also ENDOCRINOLOGY.)

The 24-hour melatonin pattern in humans is characterized by a gradual rise that, on average, begins around 10 P.M. Melatonin levels continue to climb thereafter, reaching peak values by approximately 3 A.M., and then fall to low daytime levels, which are often undetectable, by 8 A.M. The endogenous melatonin rhythm is stable and reproducible from night to night within an individual when observed under CONSTANT ROUTINE conditions; however, large unexplained differences in the amplitude of melatonin production occur among individuals.

The endogenous circadian melatonin rhythm persists both in constant darkness and in blind individuals (see BLINDNESS) with a near-24-hour period. Melatonin production can be suppressed by bright light exposure. Light detected by the retina is relayed to the pineal gland via a circuitous pathway. The signal is first transmitted along the retinohypothalamic tracts to the suprachiasmatic nuclei (SCN). Efferent fibers from the SCN then travel down the interomediolateral cell columns of the thoracic spinal cord to the superior cervical ganglia, from which the pineal's afferent sympathetic innervation originates.

Release of melatonin from the pineal gland is highly dependent on the light–dark cycle. Timed exposure to bright light and darkness that resets the circadian system shifts the timing of both endogenous body temperature and melatonin rhythms by equivalent amounts, suggesting that both rhythms are controlled by a common circadian pacemaker.

The amplitude of melatonin production has been shown to decrease with advancing age. Furthermore, this decline appears to be independent of the age-related calcification of the pineal gland. Young children have high levels of circulating melatonin that decrease significantly around the time of puberty. This observation has prompted the investigation of a possible involvement of melatonin in reproductive function.

Many species of seasonally breeding animals reproduce during a specific time of the year to increase the chances of survival for their offspring. As light inhibits the secretion of melatonin, many seasonal breeders use the interaction between their endogenous melatonin rhythm and the evoked effect of light on melatonin secretion to measure day length effectively. For example, as day length increases in the spring, a longer light period effectively inhibits melatonin production, causing the duration of the melatonin peak to narrow. The narrow melatonin peak signals the hamster that it is time to reproduce. Likewise, during the shorter days of winter, the duration of the melatonin peak widens to indicate an undesirable breeding season, and the testes of the male hamster regress. Administration of exogenous melatonin to these animals in patterns designed to mimic spring environmental lighting conditions can stimulate reproductive development.

Melatonin has also been administered to humans, and the primary effect of the agent is increased sleepiness. Melatonin administration has been reported to alleviate some of the symptoms of JET LAG that often accompany travel across time zones (see SLEEP PATTERNS AND CIRCADIAN RHYTHMS). Melatonin has also been employed to stabilize sleep onset in a blind individual who had previously experienced disturbed sleep (see BLINDNESS; EFFECTS ON SLEEP PATTERNS AND CIRCADIAN RHYTHMS). Disrupted sleep in the blind can be the result of a loss of synchronization of the circadian pacemaker by the light–dark cycle. If melatonin proves to be an effective treatment for this circadian rhythm sleep disorder, it may be one of the first clinically viable pharmacological agents shown to reset the human circadian pacemaker.

In conclusion, melatonin appears to be involved in the translation of light–dark information into a hormonal message. In some animals, melatonin is involved in reproductive function, but evidence of reproductive effects in humans is still speculative. In fact, it is unclear at this point what biological effect melatonin has in humans. Melatonin is certainly regulated by the circadian timing system, and the sensitivity of melatonin to the light–dark cycle makes it a potential modulator of circadian function.

REFERENCES

Arendt J. 1988. Melatonin. *Clin Endocrinol* 29: 205–229.

Cassone VM. 1990. Effects of melatonin on vertebrate circadian systems. *Trends Neurosci* 13:457–464.

Lerner AB, Case JD, Takahashi Y, Lee TH, Mori W. 1958. Isolation of melatonin, the pineal gland factor that lightens melanocytes. *J Am Chem Soc* 80:2587.

McIntyre IM, Norman TR, Burrows GD, Armstrong SM. 1989. Human melatonin suppression by light is intensity dependent. *J Pineal Res* 6:149–156.

Shanahan TL, Czeisler CA. 1991. Light exposure induces equivalent phase shifts of the endogenous circadian rhythms of circulating plasma melatonin and core body temperature in men. *J Clin Endocrinol Metab* 73:227–235.

Theresa L. Shanahan

MEMORY

[*This entry discusses the effect of sleep on memory for events during sleep. For a theory suggesting that sleep is implicated in memory formation for events during wakefulness, see* HIPPOCAMPAL THETA.]

Events occurring during sleep are not remembered, as a number of experiences and evidence attest. It is not uncommon for an individual to awaken during the night, perform a brief activity, immediately go back to sleep, and have no memory of the awakening in the morning. On the average, people recall dreams about once every couple of days, although modern sleep research has shown that people dream during REM sleep, which occurs four to six times each night (Webb and Kersey, 1967). In fact, when people are awakened during REM sleep, they can recall dreams 80 percent of the time (Goodenough, 1978). Sleep LEARNING has in the past been heralded in the popular press as a breakthrough and the boon of every student. Nevertheless, there is no scientific evidence for sleep learning. One classic study showed that among all the items presented throughout the night, only those items presented while the ELECTROENCEPHALOGRAM (EEG) indicated wakefulness were remembered; those presented while the EEG indicated sleep were not remembered (Simon and Emmons, 1956). Thus, both common experience and scientific evidence attests to the fact that sleep is amnesic (see AMNESIA).

The question then arises, What aspect of memory is inhibited during sleep? One can use a very simplistic model of memory and hypothesize three possibilities. First, memory is impaired because there is a failure of stimulus registration during sleep. Second, memory is not possible because the consolidation of information from short-term to long-term memory is inhibited. Finally, long-term memory may be somehow impaired during sleep.

The failure of stimulus registration during sleep is an unlikely explanation for sleep-associated amnesia. Research has shown that although auditory thresholds are elevated during sleep compared to wakefulness, stimuli can be perceived (Williams, Morlock, and Morlock, 1966). Stimuli presented during sleep evoke responses that subjects have learned during prior wakefulness. Further, people can discriminate between stimuli during sleep by responding differentially to them (Wilson and Zung, 1966). Thus, for example, most mothers of newborn babies will attest to their ability to hear their babies' smallest whimpers, whereas the roar of a truck does not awaken them (see PERCEPTION DURING SLEEP; SENSORY PROCESSING AND SENSATION DURING SLEEP).

Long-term memory deficiencies also fail to explain sleep-associated amnesia. Early research on this issue indicated that long-term memory for material presented during wakefulness is better if sleep intervenes before recall than if a comparable period of waking has occurred (Jenkins and Dallenbach, 1924). More recent research has confirmed these findings, showing recall is best after periods of NREM sleep, worst after periods of wakefulness, and intermediate after REM sleep (Yaroush, Sullivan, and Ekstrand, 1971). The explanation for these findings is disputed, but it is clear that sleep does not disturb long-term memory.

The most likely explanation for sleep-associated AMNESIA is the failure of consolidation of short-term information into long-term memory. In other words, the stimulus information is registered during sleep, but it is not converted to a long-term memory trace. Several lines of evidence support the hypothesis that sleep-associated amnesia is due to failure of memory consolidation.

Studies on dream recall show that recall of dreams collected from REM sleep is greatly dependent on the proximity of the awakening to the REM sleep period (Dement and Kleitman, 1957). Dream recall is highly probable if the awakening is done during REM sleep, but delaying the awakening by several minutes after the transition from REM sleep to NREM sleep greatly reduces recall rate. Furthermore, the morning recall of a nighttime REM sleep dream report depends on the length of the nighttime awakening after the dream report has been made (Baekeland and Lasky, 1968). Thus, the longer one remains awake, the greater the likelihood that a nighttime dream report will be remembered in the morning.

Studies on sleep and memory also support the memory consolidation hypothesis. Memory for stimuli presented during wakefulness decreases as the given stimulus is closer to sleep onset. One study in which words were presented continuously to subjects lying in bed showed that those words presented within 5 minutes of sleep onset could not be recalled, whereas words presented earlier were easily recalled (Guilleminault and Dement, 1977). In another study, subjects were awakened several times during the night and given verbal stimuli to recall in the morning (Goodenough et al., 1971). If subjects spontaneously remained awake for a long period of time after the material was presented, they were able to recall the material in the morning. These findings suggest that some period of wakefulness is necessary for memory consolidation to take place. More recent studies suggest that certain types of memory (implicit as opposed to explicit) may be better preserved (see COGNITION).

Finally, studies of the amnesia associated with SLEEPING PILLS suggest that it is the hastened sleep onset produced by the drugs that disrupts memory consolidation and thus produces amnesia. A typical study involves giving various sleeping pills (including a variety of BENZODIAZEPINES and BARBITURATES), presenting stimuli for recall, obtaining immediate recall, permitting sleep to occur, and then obtaining delayed recall. In the majority of such studies, it was noted that amnesia is usually associated with a sleep onset latency of less than 8 minutes; normal recall occurs if sleep latency is longer than 10 minutes. In one study directly testing this observation, subjects who had received sleeping pills were made to remain awake for 15 minutes after the material to be remembered was presented. In this study, the sleeping pills had no amnesic effect (Roehrs et al., 1983). Thus, various areas of research indicate that sleep, or the process of sleep onset, inhibits the consolidation of memory.

Speculation regarding the neurobiology of the sleep-associated amnesia is also possible. Although a complete and satisfactory neurobiology of memory is not available, several of the critical brain structures are known. For example, animal research and studies of patients with memory problems indicate that the HIPPOCAMPUS is one area of the brain that is important for memory (Squire, 1987). As with memory, many aspects of the neurobiology of sleep also are unclear. Nevertheless, basic animal research indicates that one of the sleep-associated neural pathways leads to the hippocampus (Jones, 1989). Furthermore, the neurotransmitter in this pathway is gamma-aminobutyric acid (GABA), an inhibitory transmitter system. Incidentally, the benzodiazepines—common sleeping pills—are known to facilitate GABA transmission. Thus, certain of the mechanisms generating sleep may also inhibit the activation of memory systems in the hippocampus.

REFERENCES

Baekeland F, Lasky R. 1968. The morning recall of rapid eye movement period reports given earlier in the night. *J Nerv Ment Dis* 147:570–579.

Dement WC, Kleitman N. 1957. The relation of eye movements during sleep to dream activity: An objective method for the study of dreaming. *J Exper Psych* 53:339–346.

Goodenough DR. 1978. Dream recall: History and current status of the field. In Arkin AM, Antrobus JS, Ellman SJ, eds. *The mind in sleep: psychology and psychophysiology,* pp 113–140. Hillsdale, NJ: Erlbaum.

Goodenough DR, Sapan J, Cohen H, Portnoff G, Shapior A. 1971. Some experiments concerning the effects of sleep on memory. *Psychophysiology* 8:749–762.

Guilleminault C, Dement WC. 1977. Amnesia and disorders of excessive daytime sleepiness. In Drucker-Colin RR, McGaugh JL, eds. *Neurobiology of sleep and memory,* pp 439–456. London: Academic Press.

Jenkins JG, Dallenbach KM. 1924. Obliviscence during sleeping and waking. *Am J Psych* 35:605–612.

Jones BE. 1989. Basic mechanisms of sleep-wake state. In Kryger MH, Roth T, Dement WC, eds. *Principles and practice of sleep medicine,* pp 121–138. Philadelphia: Saunders.

Roehrs T, Zorick F, Sicklesteel J., Wittig R, Hartse K, Roth T. 1983. Effects of hypnotics on memory. *J Clin Psychopharmacol* 3:310–313.

Simon CW, Emmons WH. 1956. Responses to material presented during various levels of sleep. *J Exper Psych* 51:89–97.

Squire LR. 1987. *Memory and brain.* New York: Oxford University Press.

Webb WB, Kersey J. 1967. Recall of dreams and the probability of stage 1-REM sleep. *Percept Motor Skills* 24:627–630.

Williams HL, Morlock HC, Morlock JV. 1966. Instrumental behavior during sleep. *Psychophysiology* 2:208–216.

Wilson WP, Zung WWK. 1966. Attention, discrimination, and arousal during sleep. *Arch Gen Psychiatry* 15:523–528.

Yaroush R, Sullivan JJ, Ekstrand BR. 1971. Effect of sleep on memory: II. Differential effect of the first and second half of the night. *J Exper Psych* 88: 361–366.

Timothy A. Roehrs

MENOPAUSE

It is well known that sleep patterns (the components of sleep and their interrelationships) change gradually with age. Women and men in their forties and fifties wake more frequently during the night than they did in their earlier years. For women, however, these nighttime awakenings and other sleep problems occur with increased frequency in the years surrounding menopause. The most common sleep-related problems that menopausal women complain of are trouble falling asleep, waking frequently at night, and feeling unusually tired during the day. Laboratory investigations confirm that menopausal women take longer to fall asleep, experience more nighttime awakenings, and have somewhat less REM SLEEP than do younger women. While some of these effects are attributable to the aging process (see AGING AND SLEEP), the response to hormone replacement (see below) suggests that the menopause is the most important factor (see GONADOTROPIC HORMONES).

Strictly speaking, *menopause* is defined as the occurrence of the last menstrual period. More generally, however, the term is used to describe a broader time period. During puberty, menstrual cycles are gradually established (see MENSTRUAL CYCLE); similarly, as menopause approaches, the reverse process occurs, and menstrual cycles tend to become increasingly irregular before they finally stop. This transition period is sometimes called the *perimenopause,* and it may last for several years. Also, like PUBERTY, menopause is a time of adjustment to a new balance of sex hormones. Thus, during the perimenopause, and after menopause as well, women may experience physical and psychological changes that are correlated with changes in hormone levels.

A primary sign of menopause is the hot flash. A hot flash (also called hot flush, night sweat, or vasomotor flush) is a sensation of heat often accompanied by sweating, rapid heart rate, and a feeling of anxiety, which lasts, on average, about 5 minutes. About 75 percent of women will have hot flashes as they enter menopause. For some women, hot flashes occur once a week, or once a month; others (perhaps 10–15 percent of those with hot flashes) may have them hourly, everyday for several years. Women with severe hot flashes may be awakened repeatedly during the night. Often, their clothes and sheets are so wet from the sweating during the hot flash, they have to get up to change their clothes and bedding. Hot flash sufferers often sleep with windows open, even in the winter, and are constantly throwing the blankets off and on, disrupting not only their own sleep, but that of any sleep partner. Lack of sleep resulting from hot flashes can lead to fatigue, irritability, or mood shifts. Before the phenomenon was taken seriously, women were frequently told that hot flashes were "all in their head." Hot flashes are now recognized as a well-defined physiological phenomenon.

Hot flashes have now been measured in the laboratory, where increases in skin temperature, heart rate, skin blood flow, and sweating have been recorded. Surprisingly, despite the sensation of heat during a hot flash, internal body temperature never increases above normal. Although we do not know what triggers each hot flash episode, hot flashes are related to the level of estrogen (the primary female sex hormone) in the body, and

are most likely the result of a disturbance in the body's temperature-regulating system.

Laboratory studies using objective physiological measures have shown that when women who have hot flashes wake up during the night, the awakenings are primarily caused by hot flashes (Figure 1). These women also take longer to fall asleep (sleep onset latency), and the time to their first REM sleep episode is longer (REM LATENCY). When these women are treated with estrogen for their hot flashes, they have fewer hot flashes, awaken less often during the night, and have a shorter REM latency. There are certainly additional reasons for INSOMNIA and FATIGUE in menopausal women, but hot flashes seem to be responsible for most of the sleep-related problems in the years immediately surrounding menopause. Although much more research remains to be done on the hormonal relationships among menopause, sleep, and hot flashes, estrogen surely plays a key role.

The amount of estrogen in women's bodies declines in the years leading up to menopause. Because estrogen's effects are widespread, influencing a wide range of physical and psychological functions, many of the symptoms of which menopausal women complain are related to their reduced level of estrogen.

It is well known that DEPRESSION and other psychiatric problems can adversely affect sleep. The sleep problems that menopausal women report can be made even worse by depression. The specific relationship of estrogen to depressive illness has not been fully determined, and leaves a number of questions unanswered. Does a decline in estrogen increase depression and therefore increase sleep problems, or does it increase chronic sleep problems and therefore lead to depression? Either way, the quality of sleep is disturbed.

Researchers are also investigating the relationship between estrogen and sleep-related respiratory problems that affect the quality of sleep. There is evidence that before menopause, sex hormones may protect women from sleep-disordered breathing episodes. These disturbances occur primarily in men through middle age. After menopause, the incidence of such disturbances in women approaches that of men. Apneas and hypopneas tend to be reduced in menopausal women who are treated with estrogen and progesterone (see APNEA). Lowered estrogen level in menopausal women can also influence respiratory patterns by another means. After

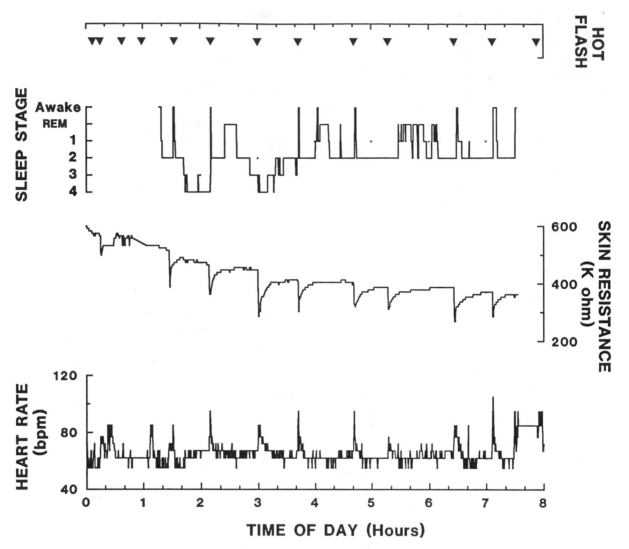

Figure 1. Pattern of hot flashes, sleep stages, skin resistance, and heart rate for an 8-hour period. The triangles indicate hot flashes. REM sleep and stages 1 through 4 of NREM sleep are indicated; absolute clock time is on the abscissa. This subject went to bed shortly after 1:00 A.M. and awoke at about 7:30 A.M. *(Modified from Kronenberg, 1990.)*

menopause, many women find that they gain weight. Significant weight gain can also cause sleep-related respiratory disturbances.

Other hormones such as prolactin, growth hormone, and gonadotropins are of importance to the regulation of sleep. Their role in the maintenance of proper sleep function may be adversely affected by the decrease in estrogen levels.

The biology of sleep is extremely complex, as is the biology of menopause. Study of the interrelationships between sleep and menopause is in its infancy, with serious investigations having begun only in the late 1970s. Simplistic explanations for the root of menopausal sleep problems are confounded by a number of interrelated processes: changes in age, general health, hormones, psychological state, and temperature regulation. Whether changes in sleep patterns proceed normally or become the source of problems depends on relationships among these variables. Investigators have just begun to scratch the surface of this complex phenomenon.

REFERENCES

Fry JM. 1987. Sleep disorders. *Med Clin North Am* 71:95–110.

Kronenberg F. 1990. Menopausal hot flashes: Epidemiology and physiology. *Ann NY Acad Sci* 592: 52–86.

Ravnikar VA, Schiff I, Regestein QR. 1983. Menopause and sleep. In Buchsbaum HJ, ed. *The Menopause,* pp 161–171. New York: Springer-Verlag.

Schiff I, Regestein QR, Schinfeld J, Ryan KJ. 1980. Interactions of oestrogens and hours of sleep on cortisol, FSH, LH and prolactin in hypogonadal women. *Maturitas* 2:179–183.

Fredi Kronenberg

MENSTRUAL CYCLE

The normal human menstrual cycle is characterized by constantly changing levels of hypothalamic, pituitary, and ovarian hormones. The reproductive cycle is dependent on secretion of gonadotropin-releasing hormone (GnRH or LHRH) from the HYPOTHALAMUS, which stimulates the pituitary to secrete luteinizing hormone (LH) and follicle-stimulating hormone (FSH). LH and FSH, in turn, are responsible for stimulation of sex steroid production from the ovary (see GONADOTROPIC HORMONES). From the time of menses, when sex steroid levels are low, estrogen increases progressively across the follicular phase with development of the follicle, until ovulation occurs at midcycle. After ovulation, the follicle is transformed into a corpus luteum, which produces both progesterone and estrogen. The corpus luteum has a finite life span, and with its regression, progesterone and estrogen levels decline and menses occur, signaling the end of the second half of the cycle, the luteal phase.

It has been hypothesized that the varying levels of sex steroids across the menstrual cycle may affect patterns of sleep and dreaming. Marked changes in the architecture of sleep from childhood to adulthood, and again during the menopause, may be mediated by sex steroids. The central nervous system effects of estrogen and progesterone are not limited to the reproductive hormonal axis. For example, estrogen plays a major role in menopausal symptomatology in women (see MENOPAUSE). Furthermore, progesterone exerts a thermogenic effect, which is responsible for the rise in basal body temperature that can be used clinically as a sign of ovulation. Progesterone also acts as a mild respiratory stimulant in the luteal phase of the menstrual cycle and has been shown to have anesthetic properties in pharmacological doses. In addition, there are several case reports of menstruation-linked hypersomnia in women that respond to treatment with estrogens that inhibit ovulation and progesterone production (Billiard, Guilleminault, and Dement, 1975). In rats, motor activity increases and REM sleep decreases during proestrus and estrus when sex steroid levels are high; the opposite effects are seen with waning hormone levels in diestrus (for review, see Parry et al., 1989).

Effect of the Menstrual Cycle on Sleep

Few studies in humans address the impact of the menstrual cycle on sleep parameters, and results have not been consistent. Most investigators have divided their observations into four cycle phases: (1) early follicular or menstrual, (2) late follicular or ovulatory, (3) early to midluteal, and (4) late luteal or premenstrual. One study that employed self-reported assessments of sleep described an increase in the total duration of sleep and greater sleep disturbance in women in the premenstrual phase of the cycle in comparison with other cycle stages (Patkai, Johannson, and Post, 1974). A higher incidence of intermittent awakenings was also observed premenstrually in another study that used ELECTROENCEPHALOGRAM (EEG) monitoring (Parry et al., 1989; see also PREMENSTRUAL SYNDROME). The increase in sleep duration premenstrually has not been confirmed in other studies. An increase in REM sleep in the premenstrual phase was reported in a widely quoted study of a mixed group of normal women and psychiatric patients (Hartmann, 1966). Although these results have not been confirmed in other studies of normal women (for review, see Lee et al., 1990; Parry et al., 1989), one study did report a decrease in REM latency in the luteal phase (Lee et al., 1990).

A number of methodological problems bear significantly on this literature: (1) Because of the intensive and repetitive nature of the monitoring required, few normal women have been studied. (2) Not all studies have confirmed cycle phase using hormonal measurements. (3) Not all studies have used EEG monitoring in a carefully controlled setting. (4) Not all studies have carefully excluded patients with premenstrual affective disorder. This last point is particularly important. Although the diagnosis of premenstrual affective disorder is still controversial, it may have a profound effect on the architecture of sleep (see PREMENSTRUAL SYNDROME). Inclusion of such patients in a normal sample might overshadow the more subtle hormonally associated changes occurring in normal menstrual cycles.

Effect of Sleep on Reproductive Hormones

The effect of sleep on the pattern of secretion of the pituitary gonadotropin hormones, LH and FSH, has also been studied. LH is secreted episodically in pulses that reflect the pulsatile secretion of its stimulatory hormone, GnRH (Crowley et al., 1985). In childhood, gonadotropin levels are low. With the onset of puberty, LH and FSH are secreted only during sleep in both sexes; during later stages of puberty and in adulthood gonadotropins are secreted throughout the day and night (Boyar et al., 1972). The frequency of secretion of LH pulses and, by implication, of hypothalamic GnRH pulses is not different between daytime and nighttime over the majority of the menstrual cycle. In the early follicular phase, however, there is ample evidence of a decrease in LH pulse frequency and in some cases a striking suspension of LH secretion (Filicori et al., 1986; Soules et al., 1985). Further studies have shown that these changes in LH secretion are related to sleep, although the sleep stage associated with the decrease in LH secretion has not yet been determined. This pattern of LH secretion is characteristic of ovulatory cycles, suggesting that progesterone may be involved in its genesis. It is possible that the slowing of GnRH stimulation of LH and FSH during sleep in the early follicular phase is important for the preferential increase in FSH that is critical for normal follicular recruitment at this stage of the cycle; however, these hypotheses have yet to be investigated.

Evidence that the circadian timing system may also influence normal menstrual cycles has been reviewed by Czeisler, Rogacz, and Duffy (1990). Studies of rotating shift workers and flight attendants subjected to transmeridian travel indicate that a high proportion of these women have menstrual cycle irregularities.

Conclusion

There is ample evidence that sleep influences hypothalamic GnRH and pituitary gonadotropin secretion in normal women. It is possible that the adverse effects of disrupted sleep/work schedules on menstrual cyclicity function through this mechanism. The evidence for an effect of reproductive hormones on sleep and dreaming is less clear-cut in normal women, although women with premenstrual syndrome exhibit changes in the pattern of sleep in comparison with normal women. Further well-controlled investigations of this area are required.

Effect of the Menstrual Cycle on Dreams

The effect of the menstrual cycle on dream recall and content has also been studied and reviewed by Severino, Bucci, and Creelman (1989). Again the number of studies and the number of normal subjects studied are small, cycle stage was not confirmed by hormonal measurements in any of the studies reported, and a variety of different measurement tools were used. One study noted that dream recall was highest in the periovulatory phase. A second study found no change in content recall across the cycle, but an increase in contentless dreams with a decrease in dreamless episodes. Yet a third study found no change in recall of contentless or content dreams across the menstrual cycle. Intellectual style may influence the pattern of changes in dream recall across the cycle and account for the variability in study results. In studies of the effect of the cycle on dream interpretation, an increase in manifestly sexual dreams during menses was found in two studies, whereas a third study found no change in dream content across the menstrual cycle. Using a psycholinguistic approach in preliminary studies, Severino, Bucci, and Creelman have suggested that the ability to access and communicate nonverbal images is facilitated in the follicular phase and diminished in the luteal phase.

REFERENCES

Billiard M, Guilleminault C, Dement WC. 1975. A menstruation-linked periodic hypersomnia. Kleine-Levin syndrome or new clinical entity? *Neurology* 25:436–443.

Boyar R, Finkelstein J, Roffwarg H, Kapen S, Wietzman E, Hellman L. 1972. Synchronization of augmented luteinizing hormone secretion with sleep during puberty. *N Engl J Med* 287:582–586.

Crowley WF Jr, Filicori M, Spratt DI, Santoro NF. 1985. The physiology of gonadotropin-releasing hormone (GnRH) secretion in men and women. *Recent Prog Horm Res* 41:473–531.

Czeisler CA, Rogacz S, Duffy JF. 1990. Reproductive function in women: Circadian interaction. In Naftolin F, Gutmann JN, DeCherney AH, Sarrel PM, eds. *Ovarian secretions and cardiovascular and neurological function,* pp 239–247. New York: Raven.

Filicori M, Santoro N, Merriam GR, Crowley WF Jr. 1986. Characterization of the physiological pattern of episodic gonadotropin secretion throughout the human menstrual cycle. *J Clin Endocrinol Metab* 62:1136–1144.

Hartmann E. 1966. Dreaming sleep (the D-state) and the menstrual cycle. *J Nerv Ment Dis* 143:406–416.

Lee KA, Shaver JF, Giblin EC, Woods NF. 1990. Sleep patterns related to menstrual cycle phase and premenstrual affective symptoms. *Sleep* 13:403–409.

Parry BL, Mendelson WB, Duncan WC, Sack DA, Wehr TA. 1989. Longitudinal sleep EEG, temperature, and activity measurements across the menstrual cycle in patients with premenstrual depression and in age-matched controls. *Psychiatr Res* 30: 285–303.

Patkai P, Johannson G, Post B. 1974. Mood, alertness and sympathetic-adrenal medullary activity during the menstrual cycle. *Psychosomat Med* 36: 503–512.

Severino SK, Bucci W, Creelman ML. 1989. Cyclic changes in emotional information processing in sleep and dreams. *J Am Acad Psychoanalysis* 17:555–577.

Soules MR, Steiner RA, Cohen NL, Bremner WJ, Clifton DK. 1985. Nocturnal slowing of pulsatile luteinizing hormone secretion in women during the follicular phase of the menstrual cycle. *J Clin Endocrinol Metab* 61:43–49.

Janet E. Hall

MENTAL RETARDATION

Mental retardation is characterized by a faulty development of intelligence that results in an inability to learn and difficulty interacting with the environment. Mental retardation can result from hereditary disorders, abnormalities of embryonic development, other prenatal problems or birth injuries, acquired childhood diseases, and environmental deprivation. Unknown causes account for many cases, particularly cases of mild mental retardation. Since brain dysfunction is the underlying defect in all children with mental retardation, it is not surprising that sleep, which requires the coordinated effort of multiple areas of the central nervous system, is often disturbed. In addition, specific disorders such as Down syndrome are especially linked with certain sleep problems.

One of the first developmental goals of the infant is to establish an organized, daily sleep–wake rhythm. By 4 months of age infants already sleep mostly at night with adultlike cycles of well-defined NREM and REM sleep (see ONTOGENY; INFANCY, NORMAL SLEEP PATTERNS IN). Infants with brain abnormalities may not develop this sleep–wake rhythm. Parents may then complain that the child suffers from INSOMNIA, reversal of day and night, or excessive sleeping. Severely brain damaged and blind children may have FREE-RUNNING rhythms of sleeping and waking that do not relate to a regular daily schedule. The expected electroencephalographic features of sleep reflect the disturbance of brain function by demonstrating absent or excessive SLEEP SPINDLE activity or indistinguishable SLEEP STAGES. Such disturbed sleep organization can be associated with NONRESTORATIVE SLEEP or with clinical seizures.

The treatment of schedule disorders in mentally retarded children is often quite difficult; however, it is important to remember that treatable sleep disorders such as obstructive apnea, SLEEP TERRORS, epilepsy, and developmental insomnia can also occur in brain-damaged individuals. Although there have been no comparative studies, the incidence of sleep problems from inappropriate sleep-onset associations, excessive fluids, or inconsistent parenting is probably even higher in retarded children whose parents are overwhelmed or who overly sympathize with their child's problems (see INFANCY, SLEEP DISORDERS IN). EPILEPSY is a common condition associated with mental retardation. Seizures can disrupt sleep, and even abnormal brain waves without clinical seizures can disturb sleep continuity and may lead to daytime SLEEPINESS. Sedating anticonvulsant medication used to treat seizures can also disrupt sleep–wake rhythms. On the other hand, poor sleep can produce excessive daytime sleepiness which causes irritability, impairs ability to participate in school or therapeutic programs, and even directly exacerbates seizures.

DOWN SYNDROME (trisomy 21) is one of the most common causes of hereditary mental retardation. In addition to the characteristic mongoloid facial features and frequently associated congenital heart lesions, there is an increased risk for sleep disorders. Obstructive sleep apnea is found in one half to two thirds of children and adults with Down syndrome. APNEA is caused by crowding of the upper airway from the abnormally developed bony and soft tissue structures, a large tongue, floppy muscles, and obesity. It has been suggested that obstructive apnea in these youngsters may contribute to pulmonary hypertension out of proportion to any coexistent heart disease. Fortunately, tonsillectomy and adenoidectomy can often improve the problem by clearing the airway.

Prader-Willi syndrome is another genetic syndrome associated with mental retardation in which sleep disorders are common. This syndrome is usually associated with deletion of the long arm of chromosome 15. Typical facial features include narrowly set eyes with antimongoloid slant (the outside of the eye slanting downward), downturned mouth, and high arched palate with a crowded posterior throat region (pharynx) leading to obstructive apnea. Marked hypotonia (low muscle tone) and hypogonadism (small genitalia) are additional features of this syndrome. Early failure to thrive is replaced in the second year of life by dramatic increase in appetite and massive weight gain. Sleep disturbances include obstructive apnea and the obesity–hypoventilation (Pickwickian) syndrome, which produce excessive somnolence. Some of the psychomotor retardation and poor learning in these children can be improved by weight loss and tonsillectomy. The intellectual improvement is perhaps secondary to improving the sleep disorder.

Sleep problems are extremely common in certain congenital metabolic disorders. Phenylke-tonuria was once the most common metabolic cause of mental retardation. This syndrome has been almost eliminated by universal screening of newborns followed by effective dietary treatment initiated in the first months of life. Untreated children have disturbed sleep from seizures as well as the direct effects on brain norepinephrine and serotonin, both critical in the control of sleep (see CHEMISTRY OF SLEEP: AMINES AND OTHER TRANSMITTERS). Rett syndrome is a recently recognized and still incompletely understood mental retardation syndrome seen only in girls. Typical findings include autistic behavior, progressive microcephaly, seizures, and peculiar hand wringing movements, which are the disorder's most distinctive feature. The majority of children with Rett syndrome have frequent night arousals and periodic hyperventilation during the waking state.

There has been little careful research in retarded children on the relationship between night sleep and daytime function. While it is true that all children perform suboptimally if sleep is too short or otherwise disturbed, the mentally retarded individual is already functioning less efficiently than normal. Furthermore, visual and hearing deficits, epilepsy, motor disabilities (e.g., cerebral palsy), ATTENTION DEFICIT HYPERACTIVITY DISORDER, and emotional problems are all more common in the retarded population. Each of these additional handicaps can also impair daytime function. Therefore, scrupulous attention to sleep is important to provide the retarded child with the best chance to maximize his or her limited abilities. Enforcement of a strict sleep schedule, restriction of the child to the bed at night, avoidance of sedating medications, optimal seizure management, and reasonable nap opportunities during the day can go a long way to improving learning. When stimulant medications such as methylphenidate (Ritalin) are used for educational purposes, careful attention to level and dosage schedule is essential to avoid toxicity or sleep-onset insomnia.

REFERENCES

Marcus C, Keens TG, Bautista DB, et al. 1991. Obstructive sleep apnea in children with Down syndrome. *Pediatrics* 88:132–139.
Okawa M, Sasaki H. 1987. Sleep disorders in men-

tally retarded and brain-impaired children. In Guilleminault C, ed. *Sleep and its disorders in children,* pp 269–290. New York: Raven.

Shibagaki M, Kiyono S, Takeuchi T. 1986. Nocturnal sleep in infants with congenital cerebral malformation. *Clin Electroencephalogr* 17:92–104.

Lawrence W. Brown

METABOLIC CONTROL OF REM SLEEP

The ULTRADIAN RHYTHM of REM sleep, which represents the duration of the intervals between two successive REM sleep episodes, correlates with both brain size and general metabolic activity. Thus, in mice this interval is about 10 minutes, whereas it is 24 minutes in the cat, 90 minutes in humans, and around 120 minutes in the elephant. These data suggest that in some direct or indirect way REM sleep is related with metabolism or energetic mechanism (see PHYLOGENY).

The relationships between energetic mechanisms and REM sleep could be summarized as follows (see references in Giuditta, 1984, and Siesjö, 1978). The cells of the brain (the neurons and glia) need some fuel (energy) to perform their various tasks. The brain chiefly utilizes glucose, which is taken from the blood by special "wagons," which transport it to glia cells (astrocytes). Therein it is metabolized into pyruvate—the main fuel of neurons. In the neurons, the pyruvate may be processed along two different metabolic pathways according to the availability of oxygen. Thus, pyruvate is either metabolized into lactate without oxygen by the enzyme lactate dehydrogenase or metabolized by the so-called oxidative pathway (the Krebs cycle) into carbon dioxide and water. This oxidative metabolism necessitates another enzyme, the pyruvate dehydrogenase complex, which transforms pyruvate into acetylcoenzyme A. In sum, the brain either can work without oxygen (the anaerobic lactate pathway) or needs oxygen (the Krebs cycle). When does the brain utilize one pathway and when the other? Are these pathways selectively used during either waking or sleep?

The waking brain must sometimes perform in situations of emergency during which there might be a decrease of oxygen availability. It is also well known that arousal increases in such conditions. In fact, most of the "waking systems,"

like the monoaminergic systems, contain lactate dehydrogenase so that waking can operate in anaerobic conditions (like muscles during extended effort). This anaerobic metabolism does not only occur in emergency situation but also during attention at the cortical level, as has been demonstrated by Fox et al. (1988) with the imaging techniques of positron emission tomography. In human subjects during visual attention, the occipital cortex utilizes more glucose (50 percent increase) but no more oxygen (5 percent increase) than during relaxed waking; thus, the pyruvate has to be metabolized into the lactate pathway.

During SLOW-WAVE SLEEP (SWS), there is a decreased utilization of both glucose and oxygen. As a result, there is a decrease in the metabolism of the brain and of the body. The temperature of the brain decreases because of the decrease of general metabolism and also because of the inhibition of the sympathetic system, which leads to vasodilation (increase of heat loss). Therefore, at the energetic level, slow-wave sleep performs two main functions: It decreases brain metabolism (and brain temperature); and at the same time, it enables the glucose that is not utilized to be stored as glycogen in glial cells (glycogenesis).

Thus, after a sufficient duration of SWS (which represents the ultradian rhythm of REM sleep), there appears to be a positive balance between the increase of energetic fuel (glycogen) and the decrease of energy utilization. This positive balance would be "weighed" by some still unknown mechanism and would permit REM sleep to occur and utilize aerobically the energy that has been stored in the glia cells.

Much indirect evidence suggests that REM sleep utilizes at least as much energy as during waking and that this energy has to be utilized according to the oxidative pathway (see REM SLEEP PHYSIOLOGY). As shown by the C^{14}-deoxyglucose technique, glucose utilization is increased during REM sleep at a level much higher than during SWS and even higher than during waking in some parts of the brain. This increase is correlated with an increase in brain circulation. Although there has not yet been any simultaneous measurement of oxygen utilization during REM sleep (in relation with glucose or pyruvate utilization), the following indirect evidence suggests the importance of oxidative metabolism: REM sleep is indeed decreased or selectively suppressed during hypoxic or ischemic hypoxia (conditions of low blood oxygen), whereas SWS or waking may be enhanced. The decrease in REM sleep during hyperthermia (high body temperature) might also be related to a negative balance between increased energy utilization and relative decreased oxygen availability. On the contrary, Jouvet, Buda, and Sastre (1989) observe a dramatic increase (up to 90 percent) of REM sleep in experimental ectothermic pontile preparations, which do not regulate central temperature during hypothermia and hyperoxia. This result may be explained by a positive balance between decreased energy utilization (resulting from the hypothermia) and an increased oxygen availability (see TEMPERATURE EFFECTS ON SLEEP). It is also possible that the REM sleep–suppressing effect of some psychotropic drugs may be obtained through their inhibitory effect on the pyruvate dehydrogenase complex.

Finally, why does REM sleep necessitate the aerobic metabolism of pyruvate? A possible answer is provided by some of its mechanisms. Converging lines of indirect evidence indicate that REM sleep depends on cholinergic mechanisms. Now, acetylcholine is the central neurotransmitter that depends most strongly on oxidative metabolism. For this reason, lower oxygen availability could decrease or suppress cholinergic metabolism (see CHEMISTRY OF SLEEP; ACETYLCHOLINE).

The importance of pyruvate dehydrogenase may also explain why most of the neurons involved in the cholinergic "executive mechanisms" of REM sleep are particularly rich in this oxidative enzyme. It is possible that some alterations of this enzyme may explain the suppression of REM sleep in some human degenerative diseases.

REFERENCES

Fox PT, Raichle ME, Mintun MA, Dence C. 1988. Nonoxidative glucose consumption during focal physiologic neural activity. *Science* 241:462–464.

Giuditta A. 1984. The neurochemical approach to the study of sleep. In Lajthe A, ed. *Handbook of neurochemistry,* 2nd ed., pp 443–476. New York: Plenum.

Jouvet M, Buda C, Sastre JP. 1989. Hypothermia induces a quasi-permanent paradoxical sleep state in pontine cats. In Malan A, Canguilhem B, eds. *Living in the cold,* pp 487–497. London: John Libbey Eurotext.

Siesjö BK. 1978. *Brain energy metabolism.* New York: Wiley.

Michel Jouvet

METABOLISM

Energy metabolism is the use of chemical energy obtained from food to drive the processes necessary for life (Blaxter, 1989). The energy in food is in three forms: carbohydrates (sugars), lipids (fats), and proteins. By oxidizing ("burning") these compounds, animals supply the energy to synthesize body constituents (e.g., muscles, bones, hormones) and to power activities such as movement, thinking, and digestion. Because energy utilization is the most fundamental process of life, it is not surprising that metabolism has effects on and is affected by almost every other physiological process, including sleep.

Although the metabolic process is continuous (and stops completely only at death), it is not constant. The rate of energy utilization [metabolic rate (MR)] varies considerably and is influenced by many factors. Therefore, to compare MR measurements, the conditions under which they are recorded must be specified. The basal metabolic rate (BMR) is the minimum MR required for maintenance of the animal. In humans, BMR is measured in a relaxed but awake subject, 10 to 12 hours after the last meal and at a comfortable environmental temperature, typically in bed after morning awakening. The conditions required to measure BMR indicate several of the important modifiers of MR. Physical activity can have a dramatic effect on MR. Intense exercise can increase it by ten times or more. Another factor affecting MR is the digestive process; consuming a meal increases MR. Finally, endotherms (mammals and birds) require energy to produce the heat necessary to maintain a relatively high and stable body temperature. Below the critical environmental temperature (see THERMOREGULATION), metabolic heat production increases as environmental temperature decreases to maintain a constant body temperature.

As with many biological processes, MR fluctuates on a daily (circadian) basis. The lowest MR occurs during the sleep portion of the rest–activity cycle, which is during the night in day-active (diurnal) animals, such as humans. Following relatively high daytime levels, MR decreases during the first half of the sleep period, and begins a gradual rise 1 to 2 hours before morning awakening. The decline in MR ranges from approximately 8 percent to 20 percent below BMR.

On the basis of electrophysiological criteria, human sleep has been divided into four stages of NREM sleep and REM sleep (see STAGES OF SLEEP). Although a few studies reported no changes in MR among these sleep stages (White, Weil, and Zwillich, 1985), most have found differences. The most consistent finding is that MR is lowest during slow-wave sleep (SWS; NREM stages 3 and 4) (Shapiro et al., 1984) and highest in REM sleep (Palca, Walker, and Berger, 1986).

In nonhuman endotherms, sleep is usually divided into only two states, NREM and REM sleep. Although in humans MR appears to be lowest in SWS, in rats it is highest in waking, decreases and plateaus in NREM, and decreases further in REM sleep (Schmidek, Zachariassen, and Hammel, 1983). This species difference may be explained by the activation of the brain during REM sleep, which because of the relatively large brains of humans, constitutes a much higher proportion of the total MR (20 percent). In rats, decreased energy expenditure associated with the dramatic and progressive reduction of muscle tone from waking to NREM to REM sleep may overwhelm small increases in brain metabolism during REM sleep. Birds also consistently show lower MRs during the major sleep period. Unfortunately, REM periods last only a few seconds, and reliable MR measurements cannot be obtained for such a short interval. Therefore, comparisons of MR cannot be made between NREM and REM sleep in birds (see BIRDS).

The daily rhythm of MR is synchronized with the rhythm of sleep and waking, but to what extent does the MR rhythm depend on sleep? A portion of the daily MR rhythm results from rhythmic changes in processes that modify MR, such as activity, feeding, and body temperature. Additionally, there are physiological changes directly associated with sleep that decrease MR and body temperature. Thus in humans, the nighttime decline in MR can be divided into two approximately equal components. One is a gradual decline in MR that occurs independently of sleep; the other is a more rapid decline that is always associated with sleep onset regardless of

when in the night sleep begins (Fraser et al., 1989). Sleep-dependent reductions in MR and body temperature can be markedly accentuated in small mammals and birds during periods of fasting, when they enter torpor on a daily basis to conserve their declining bodily energy reserves (Phillips and Berger, 1991) and during multiday bouts of torpor in seasonal hibernators (Berger and Phillips, 1988) (see ESTIVATION; HIBERNATION; TORPOR).

REFERENCES

Berger RJ, Phillips NH. 1988. Regulation of energy metabolism and body temperature during sleep and circadian torpor. In Lydic R, Biebuyck JF, eds. *Clinical physiology of sleep*, pp 171–189. American Bethesda, MD: American Physiological Society.

Blaxter K. 1989. *Energy metabolism in animals and man*. Cambridge: Cambridge University Press.

Fraser G, Trinder J, Colrain IM, Montgomery I. 1989. Effect of sleep and circadian cycle on sleep period energy expenditure. *J Appl Physiol* 66:830–836.

Palca JW, Walker JM, Berger RJ. 1986. Thermoregulation, metabolism, and stages of sleep in cold-exposed men. *J Appl Physiol* 61:940–947.

Phillips NH, Berger RJ. 1991. Regulation of body temperature, metabolic rate, and sleep in fasting pigeons diurnally infused with glucose or saline. *J Comp Physiol* B161:311–318.

Schmidek WR, Zachariassen KE, Hammel HT. 1983. Total calorimetric measurements in the rat: Influences of the sleep–wakefulness cycle and of the environmental temperature. *Brain Res* 288: 261–271.

Shapiro CM, Goll CC, Cohen GR, Oswald I. 1984. Heat production during sleep. *J Appl Physiol* 56:671–677.

White DP, Weil JV, Zwillich CW. 1985. Metabolic rate and breathing during sleep. *J Appl Physiol* 59: 384–391.

Nathan H. Phillips

MICROGRAVITY AND SPACE FLIGHT

Many people spend a lifetime searching for the perfect bed or mattress—the one they can rely on to provide a "good night's sleep" all night, every night. Gravity makes comfort critical when sleep is the goal. In space you have no need for the perfect mattress. You never sleep lying down, or for that matter standing up, because there is no "up" or "down." What could be more comfortable than sleeping while floating weightlessly? Soft mattresses, heavy blankets, and lumpy pillows no longer matter. Although you may want to anchor yourself to something solid and wrap up in the "feel" of a blanket or sleeping bag, you could close your eyes expecting to experience the best sleep ever.

In fact, few of those who have slept in space have slept that well. In the early years of the U.S. space program, astronauts aboard the Gemini and Apollo spacecraft sometimes experienced dramatic sleep loss necessitating changes in the mission schedule. It was difficult to determine whether this sleep deprivation was due to equipment problems (e.g., confinement, noise, failed air conditioning), emotional stress, or microgravity. Such sleep disruption was documented in the first electroencephalographic studies of sleep in space on Gemini VII in 1965, but no ELECTROENCEPHALOGRAM (EEG) abnormalities were found during the 55 hours of recording at the beginning of the 14-day mission. Other astronauts and cosmonauts appear to sleep well in space but differently than they usually sleep on earth. Understanding why this is so first requires some knowledge about the different types of space missions and how they vary with regard to factors known to affect sleep.

The most common missions are relatively short Earth-orbital missions lasting several days. NASA Space Shuttle missions are a good example (see SPACE SHUTTLE SLEEPING ARRANGEMENTS). One prominent factor here is the space motion sickness that many astronauts experience during the first few days of flight. Although recently developed medications can provide substantial relief, astronauts experience wide individual differences in the duration and severity of such symptoms and in their detrimental impact on the ability to sleep. Regardless, most individuals adjust within 4 or 5 days. A second disruptive factor is the sudden change in the LIGHT–DARK CYCLE from 24 hours to approximately 90 to 120 minutes (depending on the orbit altitude), with 30 percent to 40 percent of this period in relative darkness from the earth's shadow. This dramatic change in day length removes a critical environmental cue, or ZEITGEBER, for synchronizing the timing of the body's numerous circadian rhythms (see CIRCADIAN RHYTHM DISORDERS). It is well known that sleep is detrimentally affected when these rhythms be-

come desynchronized. To counter this factor, both the U.S. and Russian space agencies make it a practice to adhere to "home" time (i.e., Houston or Moscow) in scheduling daily activities throughout the mission.

A third factor common to these missions, as well as others, is a shift in the usual distribution of body fluids. Contrary to our experience on Earth, gravity is no longer present to exert downward pressure. As a result, there is an increase in fluid concentration in the upper extremities including the head. This shift has well-known effects on cardiovascular function and might be expected to affect the brain's ability to sleep; however, most evidence suggests that the impact is minimal. Such evidence comes from laboratory studies on Earth in which volunteers mimic the effects of weightlessness by spending a week or more remaining in bed with their head 6 degrees lower than their feet. This procedure enables scientists to isolate the effects of the fluid shift on sleep from other factors common to spaceflight. Sleep is generally no different from normal in such head-down positions.

Of course, the results of such studies are limited by the extent of bedrest and may not predict the combined effects of microgravity and weak circadian zeitgebers during long-term space missions, that is, those lasting several weeks to a year. The Russian space program has had much more experience of this type. During the past decade numerous cosmonauts have lived aboard the Salyut or Mir space stations for up to a year or more; however, the only in-depth studies of sleep occurred during the U.S. Skylab missions of the 1970s. Polysomnographic monitoring was carried out on one astronaut per mission on specified nights during missions lasting 28, 59, or 84 days. Although the findings support the general conclusion that sleep was both normal and adequate, they also emphasize the importance of individual differences and the subtlety of altered sleep during and after spaceflight. The 84-day subject exhibited wide variations in total sleep time and increases in awake time while trying to sleep, yet another awakened less often in flight than on Earth. Consistent sleep changes also occurred immediately after returning to Earth. In general, the percentage of SLOW-WAVE SLEEP (stages 3 and 4) decreased, and the percentage of REM sleep increased. At the time, some experts suspected the latter might indicate a basic alteration in the sleep–wake mechanism of the central nervous system, but no further evidence has been forthcoming. One important sidelight to the Skylab studies is the astronauts' subjective report that they were less able to tolerate poor sleep when performing the next day as compared with their experiences on Earth. This may be the reason both Russian and U.S. space programs have observed substantial reliance on sleeping pills by some individuals during flight.

Russian knowledge about sleep during such missions is limited to subjective and observational data. They provide the only clues as to how sleep is affected in the long-term missions common to orbiting space stations. Cosmonauts on some of the longer Salyut-7 missions experienced a steady increase in the need for sleep after about the fourth month in space. Although cosmonauts have used drugs to counter sleep problems (once with serious emotional side effects), the space agency has cautioned against their prolonged use. Instead, they have made serious efforts to further reinforce the stability of the terrestrial circadian rhythm by exposing cosmonauts to appropriately timed sensory zeitgebers and by insisting on rigid adherence to scheduled sleep times.

Part of this renewed emphasis on circadian factors comes from the fact that both nations have witnessed the most severe sleep problems during missions that require a shift in the crew's usual sleep–wake cycle. Part of this result is due to mission requirements that often preclude simultaneous sleep by all crewmembers. Thus, part of the crew is always on duty, and some must sleep at times out of synchrony with the terrestrial circadian system. Sometimes the whole crew undergoes a circadian shift. This first occurred during the initial Apollo flights (7 and 8) and resulted in a pilot falling asleep during his watch and some real-time changes in the flight plan. During the Soyuz program, cosmonauts were put on a schedule with migrating days requiring a 30-minute daily advance or delay of their sleep–wake cycle. The result was increased sleep loss and fatigue coupled with unacceptable reductions in work capacity. Although mission duties and reentry trajectory requirements sometimes necessitate shifts in the crew's daily sleep–wake cycle, the potential impact on sleep and its outcome, that is, performance, are now part of any mission planning activity.

There is one other type of space mission for which we have no data on sleep but in which sleep could play a critical role. Interplanetary missions will last at least a couple of years and will require large crews living under highly constrained conditions far removed from Earth. Constant sunlight will be the norm, rather than the ultrashort "days" of orbital missions. Under such conditions, the Earth's 24-hour cycle may not be the most advantageous for crews. Perhaps a day length nearer the body clock's natural period of about 25 hours would be better. There are also related issues about sleeping on another planet and adjusting to its night. Unfortunately the answers to these and other questions relevant to interplanetary missions will be very difficult, if not impossible, to obtain on Earth.

REFERENCES

Bluth BJ, Helppie M. 1986. *Soviet space stations as analogs,* 2nd ed. NASA Grant NAGU-659. Washington, D.C.: NASA.

Frost JD, Shumate WH, Salamy JG, Booher CR. 1976. Sleep monitoring: The second manned Skylab mission. *Aviat Space Environ Med* 47:372–382.

Graeber RC. Sleep in space. In Roussel B, Jouvet M, eds. *Proceedings, 27th DRG Seminar: Sleep and its implications for the military,* pp 59–69. Lyon: NATO Defence Research Group.

Litsov AN, Bulyko, VI. 1983. Principles of organization of rational schedules for crew work and rest during a long-term spaceflight. *Kosmich Biol Aviakosmich Med* 17:9–12.

Santy PA, Kapanka H, Davis JR, Stewart DF. 1988. Analysis of sleep on Shuttle missions. *Aviat Space Environ Med* 59:1094–1097.

R. Curtis Graeber

MICROSLEEP

A microsleep episode is a very brief, usually somewhat unexpected episode of sleep that occurs in the midst of ongoing wakeful activity. Microsleeps are common in individuals undergoing sleep DEPRIVATION and in specific sleep disorders that cause people to be excessively sleepy in the daytime. Microsleep episodes as short as several seconds can be identified, principally through close inspection of the electroencephalogram (see ELECTROENCEPHALOGRAPHY). Figure 1 shows an example of a microsleep in a person who has been sleep deprived for two consecutive nights

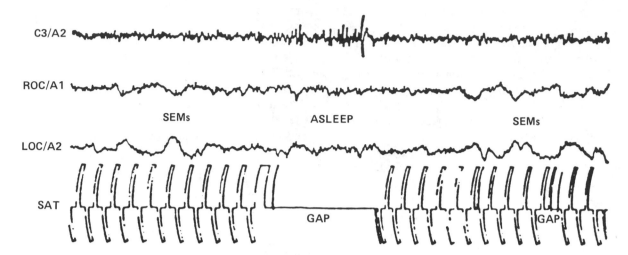

Figure 1. *Microsleep after sleep deprivation.* The top channel is the central electroencephalogram (EEG), the second and third channels are electrooculograms from right and left eyes, and the bottom channel shows performance on the serial alternation task (switch tapping). Note the transition from EEG alpha rhythm, slow eye movements, and correct switch tapping on the left to microsleep and performance gap in the center. (*Reprinted with permission from Carskadon MA, Dement WC. 1979. Effects of total sleep loss on sleep tendency. Percept Motor Skills 48:495–506. Copyright Perceptual and Motor Skills, 1979.*)

and is attempting to perform a simple behavioral task—tapping two switches alternately with the index and middle finger of the dominant hand. Note that slow rolling eye movements occur before the actual change in the electroencephalographic pattern, and these slow eye movements continue during the microsleep episode (see STAGES OF SLEEP; STAGE 1). Such slow eye movements may account for the blurred or double vision that is a common complaint of excessively sleepy people.

Microsleep events have been used by researchers to account for other problems that occur in individuals with disorders of excessive SLEEPINESS and in people who are sleep deprived. For example, researchers in Sweden have recorded brain waves continuously for twenty-four hours in train drivers who work the overnight shift. These investigators found that drivers operating trains in the middle of the night showed signs of microsleeps (Torsvall and Åkerstedt, 1983). Such microsleeps may interfere with performance and may account for an increased accident rate in overnight shift workers (see SHIFTWORK; TRUCKERS). Experiences of "nodding off" at work or in school are probably microsleep episodes that would be visible on an electroencephalogram.

REFERENCE

Torsvall L, Åkerstedt T. 1983. Sleepiness during day and night work: A field study of train drivers. *Sleep Res* 12:376.

Mary A. Carskadon

MIDBRAIN

The midbrain, also called the mesencephalon, constitutes the rostral (nearest the top of the head) third of the brainstem (Figure 1). It contains three parts. The tectum is located dorsally (nearest the back), the tegmentum is in the middle, and the crus cerebri make up the ventral (nearest the throat) portion. The tectum includes the inferior colliculi, important for processing auditory information and, rostrally, the superior colliculi, important for the interaction between visual information and eye movements. The crus cerebri are composed largely of fiber tracts connecting the motor cortex to the spinal cord for controlling voluntary movements. The midbrain tegmentum contains two of the three motor

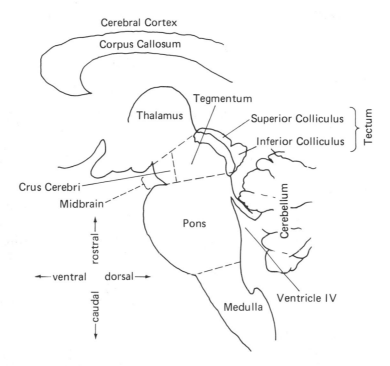

Figure 1. The midbrain.

nuclei that control eye movements during waking and REM sleep. (A nucleus is a grouping of similar neurons. There are many nuclei throughout the brain.) Located in the dorsolateral area of the tegmentum and of special relevance to sleep physiology are two nuclei composed of a majority of neurons that employ acetylcholine as their neurotransmitter. They are the lateral dorsal tegmental nucleus (which extends into the PONS) and the pedunculopontine tegmental nucleus. Finally, in the midline region of the midbrain tegmentum is another nucleus important to the control of sleep and waking, the dorsal raphe nucleus. Over 50 percent of the neurons in the dorsal raphe nucleus employ serotonin as their neurotransmitter.

(See also CHEMISTRY OF SLEEP; REM SLEEP MECHANISMS AND NEUROANATOMY.)

REFERENCE

Carpenter MB, Sutin J. 1982. *Human neuroanatomy*, 8th ed. Baltimore: Williams and Wilkins.

Robert W. Greene

MIDDLE EAR MUSCLE ACTIVITY

Middle ear muscle activity (MEMA) refers to the contractile action of the two smallest skeletal muscles of the body: the stapedius and tensor tympani, which reside within the middle-ear cavities on each side of the head. These muscles attach to a chain of tiny, interfaceted bones that span the middle-ear cavity.

External sound waves actuate proportional mechanical vibrations in the eardrum (tympanic membrane). The vibrations are transmitted by the ossicular chain across the middle-ear space to the neural elements of the inner ear. When the middle-ear muscles contract, they pull on the chain, rendering it more taut. Consequently, sound wave–induced vibrations of the ossicles are "damped" before entering the inner ear. In effect, therefore, activation of the middle-ear muscles reduces perceived sound volume.

Discrete, albeit indirect, electrophysiological monitoring of MEMA is made possible by MEMA's effect upon the position of the eardrum in space. The eardrum moves during MEMA because the ossicular chain, at its lateral end, adheres to the inner surface of the eardrum. The eardrum position shifts when MEMA stretches the chain. If the external ear canal is physically sealed, even a very minute eardrum displacement produces a measurable alteration in air pressure within the canal. For purposes of MEMA recording, the canal is plugged by a custom-fitted, airtight earmold (Figure 1). A tiny, air pressure-sensitive transducer protrudes into the canal through the earmold to register an air-pressure change and convert it to an electrical signal (Figure 2).

Inasmuch as MEMA is rapidly evoked by the first portion of a loud sound burst, usually exceeding 85 decibels, MEMA's principal function is thought to be protection of the auditory system against overwhelming acoustic excitation. It is now known, however, that the middle ear muscles also discharge *during sleep in the absence of external stimulation.* This occurs in cats and presumably other mammals, as well as in human beings (Dewson, Dement, and Simmons, 1965; Pessah and Roffwarg, 1972). Such "spontaneous MEMA" during sleep is observed almost exclusively in connection with REM sleep. Individuals differ considerably in the quantity of spontaneous MEMA that they produce during REM sleep; 2.5 to 3.5 bursts per minute is about average, but some individuals display as few as 0.7 and others as many as 6.5 bursts per minute (Pessah and Roffwarg, 1972).

Though appearances of MEMA during sleep would not logically be expected in the absence of loud acoustic stimulation, such seemingly unprovoked activity in the course of REM sleep has parallels in other motor systems. MEMA is only one of a number of muscle and autonomic phenomena exhibited during REM sleep that mirror the intrinsic, brainstem-initiated, phasic discharges characterizing this activated state (Pessah and Roffwarg, 1972). The brain activity responsible for MEMA, as well as for the eye movements of REM sleep and other motor discharges, is called ponto-geniculo-occipital (PGO) activity because it appears to ascend from the PONS through the LATERAL GENICULATE NUCLEUS to the occipital region of the cerebral cortex. The middle-ear muscles are innervated by the fifth and seventh cranial motor nerves in the pons, which are activated by the eighth nerve, responding to loud sound experienced in waking. During REM sleep (of course in a sound-free environment), however, either the fifth- or the seventh-nerve nuclei, or both, exhibit phasic activity (PGO WAVES) just before each burst of spontaneous MEMA (Roffwarg et al., 1979). (See also PHASIC ACTIVITY IN REM SLEEP.)

Given that PGO waves are recorded simultaneously in auditory cortex at the times they appear during REM sleep in motor fifth- and seventh-nerve nuclei, it was not surprising to find that

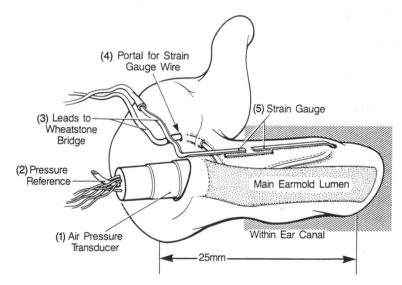

Figure 1. Illustration of the earmold used to close the external ear canal, showing the air-pressure transducer situated within the mold's main lumen. The tip of the transducer probe in the ear canal can register slight pressure shifts resulting from MEMA-provoked eardrum displacements. Note the strain gauge on the surface of the earmold. Its purpose is to monitor jaw-movement artifact that can mimic MEMA.

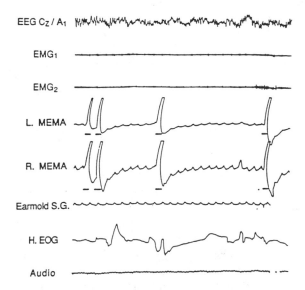

EEG Cz / A₁

EMG₁

EMG₂

L. MEMA

R. MEMA

Earmold S.G.

H. EOG

Audio

Figure 2. Electrophysiological recording in REM sleep. Spontaneous middle ear muscle contractions are indicated by phasic deflections (underlined) in the air-pressure recordings taken from the sealed external ear canals (L. and R. MEMA channels). The H. EOG channel shows phasic eye movements, some of which occur together with and some independent of the MEMA bursts. The oscillating background waves in the MEMA tracings do not indicate MEMA; they derive from pulsations of small arteries near the external canal. No activity is observed on the external strain-gauge channel, indicating the absence of MEMA artifact generated by jaw movement in this tracing. Abbreviations: EEG, electroencephalogram of midline central lead (Cz) referred to left mastoid (A₁); EMG₁, electromyogram of chin/masseter leads; EMG₂, anterior neck EMG at level of larynx; L. MEMA and R. MEMA, left and right middle ear muscle activity; Earmold S.G., strain gauge on external surface of earmold; H. EOG, horizontal electrooculogram; Audio, audio recording from bedroom to ensure that no actual sound impinges upon the sleeping subject.

episodes of MEMA during human REM sleep correspond in time and duration to instances of vivid auditory sensations in the ongoing dream. Significantly, MEMA in REM sleep coincides only with dreamed *loud sound,* not with the other, lower-volume dreamed sound experiences. Further, the close coupling of MEMA and auditory sensation during REM sleep parallels the intimate relationship seen between the direction and timing of the REM sleep rapid eye movements and the visual imagery of the dream. This reminds us, once again, that the singular neurophysiology of REM sleep is able to reproduce the very same type of sensori-

motor correspondence in REM-stage dreaming that obtains in the waking state. Finally, analyses of EEG specimens coinciding with MEMA and eye movements in REM sleep have demonstrated small but definite PGO-like waves, which are usually lost within the EEG background.

(See also EYE MOVEMENTS AND DREAMING; PSYCHOPHYSIOLOGY OF DREAMING; REM SLEEP MECHANISMS AND NEUROANATOMY.)

REFERENCES

Dewson JH III, Dement WC, Simmons FB. 1965. Middle ear muscle activity in cats during sleep. *Exp Neurol* 12:1–8.

Pessah MA, Roffwarg HP. 1972. Spontaneous middle ear muscle activity in man: A rapid eye movement sleep phenomenon. *Science* 178:773–776.

Roffwarg HP, Adrien J, Marks G, Farber J. 1979. Central and peripheral REM-sleep activity in the auditory system of the cat. *Sleep Res* 8:35.

Howard P. Roffwarg

MILK ALLERGY AND INFANT SLEEP

Of the many potential psychological, social, and physiological causes for sleep problems in childhood, several factors have been clearly identified and are commonly considered in assessing and treating children who suffer from sleep problems. Nevertheless, there is still a sense that the vulnerability of some children to sleep disturbance is not always understood and therefore cannot be treated appropriately.

One factor that has recently been associated with sleep problems in children is milk allergy, or the physical intolerance to cow's milk products. Cow's milk is the most common allergen (substance that causes allergy) in infants' food. The allergy may manifest itself in such symptoms as wheezing, eczema, diarrhea, and vomiting. Sleep problems that have been associated with ingestion of milk in children are increased night waking, prolonged sleep latency, and reduced sleep duration (Kahn et al., 1985, 1988, 1989).

The role of milk allergy in childhood sleep disturbances has been investigated by Dr. André Kahn and his colleagues (Kahn et al., 1985,

1988, 1989) in Belgium. They found that in nearly 10 percent of children under 5 years of age referred to treatment for chronic night waking, the problem could be traced to milk allergy. This relationship was established by the disappearance of sleep problems when these children were kept on a diet free of cow's milk products. The sleep problems reappeared when cow's milk products were reintroduced (Kahn et al., 1989).

These studies indicate that food intolerance should be considered as a possible contributing factor in sleep problems in young children. (See INFANCY, SLEEP DISORDERS IN; NIGHT WAKING IN INFANCY.)

REFERENCES

Kahn A, François G, Sottiaux M, et al. 1988. Sleep characteristics in milk-intolerant infants. *Sleep* 10:116–121.

Kahn A, Mozin MJ, Casimir G, Montauk L, Blum D. 1985. Insomnia and cow's milk allergy in infants. *Pediatrics* 76:880–884.

Kahn A, Mozin MJ, Rebuffat E, Sottiaux M, Muller MF. 1989. Milk intolerance in children with persistent sleeplessness: A prospective double-blind cross-over evaluation. *Pediatrics* 84:595–603.

Avi Sadeh

MIND–BODY RELATIONSHIPS

See Psychophysiology of Dreaming

MINNESOTA MULTIPHASIC PERSONALITY INVENTORY

The Minnesota Multiphasic Personality Inventory (MMPI) is a personality test commonly used in sleep disorder centers for psychological evaluation of both patients and research subjects. The MMPI was developed during the 1940s by Starke Hathaway and Jovian McKinley. It is composed of 566 statements that are answered true or false depending on whether the individual taking the test believes the statement is a true description of himself or herself. Scores for ten clinical scales and three validity scales constitute the basic profile that is derived from this test. The clinical scales are hypochondriasis, DEPRESSION, hysteria, psychopathic deviance, masculinity/femininity, paranoia, psychasthenia (ANXIETY), schizophrenia, mania, and social introversion.

Several innovations in the design of the MMPI made it different from any personality test that had been previously constructed. First, the validity of the scales of the MMPI was determined empirically. "Validity" means that a test really measures what it claims to measure. For example, just because an author states that his or her new test measures depression does not prove it to be true. Obviously, validity is of prime importance in the development of a useful test. To validate the MMPI, groups of patients already diagnosed with a certain disorder answered over 1,000 test questions. Their responses were compared with responses from normal subjects, and those questions that they answered differently were formed into a scale. The scale was "cross-validated" by having another sample of patients and sample of normal subjects take the test to see if the response sets could differentiate the two groups.

A second innovation of the MMPI is that it contains validity scales that check the honesty of the person taking the test. One problem that limits the accuracy of all self-report tests is that subjects may lie, exaggerate, or even answer randomly without the knowledge of the test administrator. As there is no way to guarantee that a person will be truthful while responding to the test items, the makers of the MMPI decided to measure how often the subject distorted his or her responses and use this in the interpretation of the test. Certain items on the MMPI are specifically included to measure the extent to which an individual may be consciously or unconsciously trying to manipulate the test outcome.

Use of psychometric tests can be helpful for sleep experts because psychological disturbances can be related to sleep problems in certain people. Therefore, patients seen in a sleep disorder center are often given the MMPI to screen for depression or anxiety. Although a diagnosis of depression is based on the clinical impression of the patient, the MMPI can provide a helpful "second opinion." The MMPI profile may also be helpful in predicting the patient's response to treatment. In research studies, the MMPI may be used to classify patients into different groups based on their personality characteristics. Again, because certain psychological factors can influence sleep, it is important for researchers to document the presence or absence of any psychological abnormalities within the subjects.

The MMPI has recently been revised, and the MMPI-2 is now being used as well. The MMPI-2 has been updated by changing some test items and providing new validation studies, but is essentially the same test as the original MMPI. Psychometric assessment is an important task for clinicians and researchers in sleep disorders centers, and the MMPI is the most widely used test in this assessment.

REFERENCES

Dahlstrom WG, Welsh GS, Dahlstrom L. 1972. *An MMPI handbook, vol 1: Clinical interpretation.* Minneapolis: University of Minnesota Press.
———. 1975. *An MMPI Handbook, vol. 2: Research applications.* Minneapolis: University of Minnesota Press.
Graham JR. 1987. *The MMPI: A practical guide,* 2nd ed. New York: Oxford University.
Zorick F, Kribbs N, Roehrs T, Roth T. 1984. Polysomnographic and MMPI characteristics of patients with insomnia. *Psychopharmacology* 2S–10S.

Edward J. Stepanski

MONOAMINE OXIDASE INHIBITORS

Monoamine oxidase (MAO) is an enzyme that is naturally present in the cells of the liver and other tissues and is responsible for metabolizing various substances in the body. Certain diseases are thought to result from inadequate amounts of some of these substances. In 1951, iproniazid, a drug that inhibits the activity of MAO, was tried in the treatment of tuberculosis. It was quickly noted that iproniazid elevated the mood of the patients. The inhibition of MAO is thought to cause an increase in the availability of specific neurotransmitters (e.g., dopamine, norepinephrine) within the nervous system, thereby alleviating depression.

As the mood-elevating property of MAO-inhibiting drugs (MAOIs) was recognized, they were increasingly applied in the psychiatric treatment of depressed patients. The first MAOIs used in this way included phenelzine and isocarboxazid. Tranylcypromine and phenelzine are the most frequently used MAOIs today. MAOIs are also used to treat some anxiety disorders.

MAOIs can have many side effects, some of them dangerous. For this reason, they are now used less frequently than other antidepressant medications, and in some cases only when other methods for treating depression have failed. MAOIs have complex and sometimes severe interactions with other drugs and some foods, including chocolate, cheese, and red wine. Common side effects of MAOIs include fainting, tremors, weight gain, dizziness, headache, blurred vision, dry mouth, skin rash, insomnia, and fatigue or sleepiness during the day.

Monoamine Oxidase and Sleep

Severe sleep disruption is a frequent side effect during use of MAOIs and shortly afterward. Patients often complain of insomnia characterized by interrupted, restless sleep and frequent awakenings. They also often experience sleepiness during the day. This sleep disruption and sleepiness can occur even as the depression improves.

Specific changes in the sleep of patients who are taking MAOIs are seen when their sleep is recorded in the sleep laboratory. Figure 1 shows what sleep looks like across the night for a normal, healthy adult. Notice the normal cycling of various sleep stages, including REM SLEEP, the stage in which we do most of our dreaming. Compare this histogram with Figure 2, which shows the disrupted sleep of a person who is taking an MAOI medication. Note the frequent awakenings, significantly delayed first REM sleep period, and decreased overall amount of REM sleep in comparison with the sleep of the healthy person. REM sleep is suppressed with MAOI treatment. The consequences of chronic REM suppression are not fully known, but it is an effect shared by many drugs successfully used in the treatment of depression, and may be fundamental to the beneficial actions of these drugs.

Furthermore, MAOIs result in an increased level of motor activity during sleep, leading to a pattern of REM sleep without the usual decrease in muscle tone and sometimes to increased occurrence of leg jerks (see PERIODIC LEG MOVE-

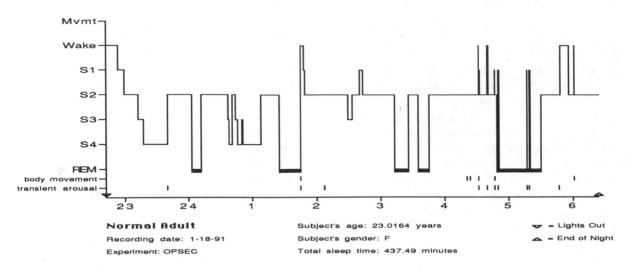

Figure 1. Idealized sleep histogram for a normal adult.

MENTS). These leg movements often result in brief awakenings during sleep and can contribute to the sleepiness experienced during the day by people who take MAOI medication.

Treatment of the sleep disruption associated with MAOI medications sometimes involves an alteration in the dose or type of MAOI or a switch to a different class of antidepressant medication. In the case of periodic leg movements, addition of another type of medication is often recommended.

After MAOI medication is stopped, another type of disruption can occur, characterized by a REBOUND of REM sleep following its suppression. This REM rebound can result in upsetting night-

mares for the patient. Luckily, the nightmares usually go away as the patient adjusts to the absence of the drug.

(See also ANTIDEPRESSANTS; DEPRESSION.)

REFERENCES

Graedon J. 1977. *The people's pharmacy: A guide to prescription drugs, home remedies, and over-the-counter medications.* New York: Avon.

Simon GI, Silverman HM. 1990. *The pill book.* New York: Bantam.

Cynthia M. Dorsey

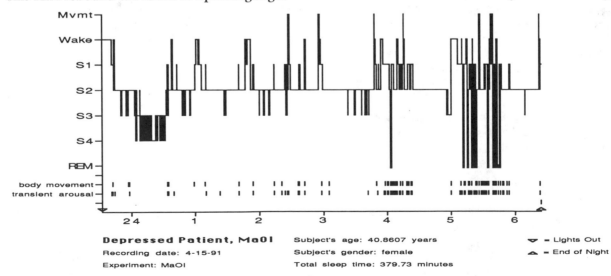

Figure 2. Sleep histogram based on actual data for a patient who was taking MAOI medication.

MONOAMINES

See Chemistry of Sleep: Amines and Other Transmitters

MONONUCLEOSIS

Infectious mononucleosis is an acute and generally benign infectious disease. It occurs most commonly in teenagers and young adults and is caused by the Epstein–Barr virus. Its clinical picture consists of fever, sore throat (pharyngitis), and swollen lymph glands (lymphadenopathies). Frequently, the spleen is enlarged, and a rash is found on the trunk and extremities in 10 to 20 percent of affected subjects at onset of the illness. The infection is marked by changes in the blood, including an increase in relative and absolute numbers of lymphocytes and monocytes, with abnormal lymphocytes. The concentration of characteristic abnormal antibodies is increased and remains elevated well after the disappearance of clinical symptoms. Results of liver function tests may also be abnormal.

Infectious mononucleosis may be associated with any of several neurological complications, such as ENCEPHALITIS, aseptic meningitis, and Guillain–Barré syndrome (also called Landry–Guillain–Barré syndrome). The latter syndrome consists of several neurological symptoms that develop during the midphase of the infection. Paresthesias (tingling, numbness) are reported, and pain may be present, particularly with skeletal muscle pressure. Flaccid paralysis, at times severe, is associated with reduced muscle tone and reflexes. In rare instances, the respiratory muscles and cranial nerves are involved in the neurological syndrome.

The paralyses seen with Guillain–Barré syndrome and the neurological complications of infectious mononucleosis are usually completely reversible. Some individuals, however, develop a persistent tiredness with no obvious neurological complications during the recovery phase of infectious mononucleosis, Guillain–Barré syndrome, aseptic meningitis, or mild encephalitis. These patients complain of a need for more nocturnal sleep and a persistent daytime fatigue. In the earliest phases of recovery, napping and increased nocturnal sleep are used to reduce the daytime tiredness, but the sleepiness persists. The naps occur on a daily basis, and they are long (1 to 2 hours) and nonrefreshing. This daytime sleepiness is isolated: There is no SNORING, breathing disorder, CATAPLEXY, or SLEEP PARALYSIS—thus no sleep APNEA or NARCOLEPSY. The toxic and other medical causes of daytime SLEEPINESS are also absent. A Multiple Sleep Latency Test clearly documents excessive sleepiness, with mean sleep latency scores varying from 1 or 2 to 7 or 8 minutes.

Treatment of excessive sleepiness in these patients is often difficult. As mentioned above, subjects respond poorly to naps. Nonspecific stimulant medications are the only drugs that may be of help. AMPHETAMINES must often be used together with scheduled naps. The sleepiness is fairly stable over time, and there is little likelihood of spontaneous improvement. In many cases, sleepiness is severe and responds poorly to stimulant medications, thus resulting in a chronic, lifelong disability. The lack of good treatment for daytime sleepiness has resulted in difficulty obtaining long-term gainful employment, leading to significant socioeconomic disruption for some patients.

Christian Guilleminault

MOOD DISTURBANCE

See Affective Disorders Other Than Major Depression; Depression

MORNINGNESS/EVENINGNESS

Early to bed, early to rise,
Makes a man healthy, wealthy and wise.

This maxim characterizes nicely the value that society places on being "up with the dawn" like a morning lark. Unfortunately, for many people such a goal is largely unattainable, and for various reasons (which we discuss below) these people are much more like the "night owl." Scientifically, the division of humanity into different circadian "types" has been referred to as *morningness/eveningness,* with morning types

(M-types) being more like the lark and evening types (E-types) more like the owl. (See also EARLY BIRDS AND NIGHT OWLS.)

Questionnaires to distinguish between M-types and E-types originated in Sweden in the late 1960s with the work of Oquist and Patkai who showed that scores from such pencil-and-paper tests could relate (at the extremes) to time-of-day differences in various physiological and psychological measures. Patkai (1971), for example, showed that the adrenaline rhythm peaked earlier in the day in M-types than in E-types.

The best known English-language morningness test was developed by Horne and Östberg in 1976. They built on the earlier Swedish work and tested the questionnaire on a group of British undergraduates, showing differences in the circadian temperature rhythm between extreme M-types and extreme E-types. Importantly, though, no rigorous psychometric testing was done on the instrument. Despite the absence of standardization, Horne and Östberg's test has become the instrument of choice, cited in more than fifty recent studies. This is unfortunate, because other morningness instruments are possibly better. Recently, Smith, Reilly, and Midkiff (1978) have published an excellent, easy-to-administer instrument that incorporates the best features of several earlier tests and shows promise as being an attractive new tool.

There are three different ways one can be E-type rather than M-type. The first is simply through choice. Those who prefer late-night television shows and indulge that preference will emerge on morningness tests as E-type even if there is no *biological* basis for the classification. Should circumstances change (e.g., the birth of a child or the lengthening of a morning commute) the move to a more M-type orientation is usually accomplished in a week or so with no long-term detrimental consequences.

More difficult to change is an E-type pattern that results from *biological* effects. The human circadian system (biological clock; see CIRCADIAN RHYTHMS) naturally runs slow, typically by about 1 hour per day. Thus, to retain a 24-hour periodicity there has to be a certain pressure, squeezing the rhythms, as it were, into a 24-hour day. The presence of this pressure leads to the two other mechanisms by which one can become an E-type. The first is if the "natural" period happens to be rather long (e.g., 25.5 hours), increasing the natural tendency to stay up late. The second is

if the time cues or ZEITGEBERS are weak (e.g., through the absence of daylight exposure and/or a chaotic routine), providing insufficient pressure to keep the rhythmic mechanisms running at 24 hours. In either case, all that can be done to change to a more M-type orientation is to enhance and strengthen the zeitgebers. This may not be easy, however, and will need to be ever-present; otherwise the individual will quickly revert to being an E-type.

Summarizing a number of different studies, Kerkhof (1985) concluded that "on average M-types go to bed/fall asleep 88 minutes earlier and awaken/arise 72 minutes earlier than E-types." Similarly, circadian (approximately 24-hour) rhythms in adrenalin and body temperature typically differ by less than 2 hours, even when extreme M-type and E-type groups are studied. Differences between the groups in subjective activation and performance can, however, be much more profound, and conflicts between M-types and E-types can arise when they try to live together. As people age they tend to become more M-type, perhaps because of the shortening of their natural free-running period. Although being an M-type is an asset for a dayworker, for a shift worker it is usually a liability. Hildebrandt and Stratmann (1979) have shown that morningness score is a reliable predictor of SHIFTWORK intolerance.

The division of the world into M-types and E-types is a valid one, though many lie "in between." There are both social and biological origins for these "circadian-type" differences.

REFERENCES

Hildebrandt G, Stratmann I. 1979. Circadian system response to night work in relation to the individual circadian phase position. *Int Arch Occup Environ Health* 43:73–83.

Horne JA, Östberg O. 1976. A self-assessment questionnaire to determine morningness–eveningness in human circadian rhythms. *Int J Chronobiol* 4:97–110.

Kerkhof GA. 1985. Inter-individual differences in the human circadian system: A review. *Biol Psychol* 20:83–112.

Patkai P. 1971. Interindividual differences in diurnal variations in alertness, performance, and adrenaline excretion. *Acta Physiol Scand* 81:35–46.

Smith CS, Reilly C, Midkiff K. 1978. Evaluations of three circadian rhythm questionnaires with suggestions for an improved measure of morningness. *J Appl Psychol* 74:728–738.

Timothy H. Monk

MOTOR CONTROL

Hidden beneath the calm exterior of sleeping humans and other mammals, dynamic forces are hard at work. These forces are responsible for both the suppression of muscle (i.e., motor) activity and the excitation of muscle activity that occur during sleep. Investigators have spent a considerable amount of time unraveling the ways in which these opposing forces work, especially during REM sleep, when inhibitory as well as excitatory forces reach their highest levels of activity.

When we fall asleep, we first enter into the state of NREM sleep (see CYCLES OF SLEEP ACROSS THE NIGHT; NREM SLEEP MECHANISMS). Our eyes drift slowly back and forth, and every once in a while we shift our sleep position. Because there is only a very low level of muscle activity during NREM sleep, there is apparently very little need for motor inhibition.

The second state of sleep, which follows NREM sleep, is called REM SLEEP. It is also called active sleep and for a very good reason—during REM sleep certain areas of the brain become incredibly active, resulting in storms of neuronal activity. This activity commences as soon as REM sleep begins, when inhibitory motor commands are sent by the brain to motoneurons, the nerve cells that control our muscles. These inhibitory commands result in the release of a chemical, named glycine, onto the surface of motoneurons. Glycine makes motoneurons more electrically polarized. This change in polarization prevents motoneurons from discharging; thus, they become extraordinarily inexcitable. This results in a kind of muscle paralysis, also called ATONIA, that is a primary characteristic of REM sleep.

Not only are these motor inhibitory forces maintained for the duration of REM sleep, but they actually increase during the rapid eye movement periods of REM sleep. (See REM SLEEP MECHA-NISMS AND NEUROANATOMY.) It is therefore surprising, when one considers the enormous amount of inhibition that is present during REM sleep, that the eyes and limbs are able to make any movements at all. The reason that they can move is that at the same time that inhibition is being increased, strikingly potent motor excitatory forces also come into play. These excitatory forces have the potential for inducing movements that could awaken us or allow us physically to act out our dreams. These movements do not occur, because inhibition generally reigns supreme, although excitation, from time to time, may momentarily become predominant. When the bastions of motoneuron inhibition are breached by excitatory forces, motoneurons are able to discharge, especially during periods of rapid eye movements; the interaction of the excitatory and inhibitory forces produce muscle contractions and subsequent movements unlike those that occur during any other state. It is like applying pressure to the brakes of a car and at the same time to the accelerator. When motoneurons are simultaneously driven by opposing inhibitory and excitatory motor forces, the resulting muscle movements are abrupt—they are twitchy, jerky, and without apparent purpose.

When these normal patterns of motor control go awry, pathological behaviors occur during sleep as well as during wakefulness; they can become so severe that individuals are prevented from sleeping or functioning in an effective manner while they are awake. One of the most dramatic of these abnormal behaviors is REM sleep behavior disorder, which may cause individuals to act out their dreams, even though they are asleep! (See REM SLEEP BEHAVIOR DISORDER.) CATAPLEXY is another common sleep disorder. Surprisingly, the problems of cataplexy are expressed during wakefulness. Known as "waking paralysis," cataplexy is generally considered to be the result of the inappropriate triggering during wakefulness of the motor inhibition that is normally present only during REM sleep. As a result, the unfortunate individual becomes paralyzed—although still conscious—for anywhere from several seconds to many minutes. Individuals have experienced cataplectic attacks while driving, flying a plane, scuba diving, and procreating, as well as during many other activities. Thus, a malfunction in the sleep motor inhibitory system can cause a loss of muscle paralysis during sleep (resulting in REM behavior disorder) as well as the inappropriate presence of muscle paralysis during wakefulness (resulting in cataplexy).

Other muscle-related sleep disorders include (1) sleep APNEA, which involves the cessation of breathing during sleep; (2) SUDDEN INFANT DEATH SYNDROME (SIDS), which is thought to involve the inactivation or lack of proper functioning of respiratory muscle activity during sleep; and (3) somnambulism, better known as SLEEPWALKING. There are also a variety of motor disorders that are not part of the sleep states, but that are influenced by them, such as the intense motor "fits" of epilepsy and the tremors of Parkinson's disease.

Learning how our muscles are so finely controlled during sleep by the interaction of motor inhibitory drives and motor excitatory drives will shed light on the manner in which the brain controls the thousands of patterns of motor activity that are unique and essential in sustaining our lives while we are asleep as well as while we are awake.

Understanding why we are normally paralyzed during sleep from our facial muscles to those tiny muscles that wiggle our toes, and why we sometimes have some rather strange movements while we sleep, will help us to develop cures for many of the sleep and sleep-related motor disorders that affect millions of individuals. But fortunately for the majority of us, most of the time our motor systems function correctly, and we rest securely and pleasantly, tucked safely away each night beneath the blanket of motor inhibition that covers us all while we sleep.

(See also HYPNIC JERKS; PERIODIC LEG MOVEMENTS.)

REFERENCES

Chase MH. 1983. Synaptic mechanisms and circuitry involved in motoneuron control during sleep. In Bradley RJ, ed. *International review of neurobiology*, vol 24, pp 213–258. New York: Academic.

Chase MH, Morales FR. 1989. The control of motoneurons during sleep. In Kryger MH, Roth T, Dement WC, eds. *Principles and practice of sleep medicine*, pp 74–85. Philadelphia: Saunders.

———. 1990. The atonia and myoclonia of active (REM) sleep. *Annu Rev Psychol* 41:557–584.

Michael H. Chase
Francisco R. Morales

MOUNTAIN SICKNESS

See Altitude

MOVIES, DREAMS IN

In the opening scene of the 1983 movie *Risky Business*, Tom Cruise dreams that he is looking around for some people when he hears water running. Upon investigating, he finds a beautiful girl taking a shower. She asks him to wash her back, but when he goes closer she disappears in the steam. Then Cruise suddenly wakes up to find himself in a room of students taking the college boards. He's three hours late and has two minutes to take the whole test.

Unfortunately, we have all experienced dreams very similar to the one presented. But, in one critical respect, our dreams are different from film dreams. Unlike our own dreams, whose meanings and possible purposes may often be unknown and unclear, every film dream is created with one singular objective—to further the film's story.

In *The Sure Thing* (1985), for example, the main character, Gib, travels across the country for a date with his ideal woman, the Sure Thing. Through a series of misadventures he winds up traveling with Alison, who is definitely not Gib's idea of the perfect woman. One night, Gib dreams about his date with the Sure Thing, but when she turns her face to him, she is Alison. Gib wakes with the realization that the woman he really wants is Alison. In this case, the film dream functions dramatically because it makes the audience, as well as Gib, aware of Gib's feelings for Alison, furthering the storyline as their adventures become more emotionally complicated.

Film dreams are often used to increase the audience's emotional involvement in a film's characters and their situations. Charlie Chaplin's character in his silent film *The Gold Rush* (1925) dreams that he is being kissed by the woman he loves. Simultaneously, the film shows that the woman is actually out dancing with other men. The irony of the reality versus the desire expressed in the dream heightens the emotional tension by showing Chaplin's love interest to be unattainable for him.

Highly emotional film dreams are often found in "scary" movies such as *Aliens* (1986). Although the lead character, Ripley, may seem cool and calm when she is awake, her nightmares are meant to demonstrate that she is emotionally trapped in a web of fear. In another example, John Landis uses the film dream in *An American Werewolf in London* (1981) to show a character, David, haunted in his dreams by a truth he refuses to admit when he is awake. Such frightening film dreams dramatize the characters' internalized terrors while heightening the films' emotional intensity.

Films also use dreams to rationalize the existence of a fantasy world. By saying or implying that everything unrealistic in the film is actually just part of a dream, filmmakers encourage their audiences to accept the film's underlying premise—perhaps to forget that they are watching a dream sequence and not a segment of real life. *The Wizard of Oz* (1939) is almost entirely a film dream. Although we never see Dorothy fall asleep, the fact that the Land of Oz is in color, unlike her "real" black and white world, hints early on that the movie is basically a film dream. In one respect, *The Wizard of Oz* mimics real dream behavior by incorporating day residue in the form of people from Dorothy's life—the farm hands, the nasty neighbor, the traveling salesman—into characters in her dream—the Scarecrow, the Tin Man, the Lion, the Wicked Witch of the West, and the Wizard. In general, however, if a film puts most of its actions in a *dream world,* that dream world functions almost identically to the film's portrayal of normal life.

Films may capitalize on another aspect of dreaming that makes dreams so "dreamlike," when the dreamer does or experiences bizarre things and strange associations. For example, the main character in *Brazil* (1985), Sam Lowry, has dreams in which he suddenly moves from one locale to another and people change into other people. Another type of film dream depicts the premonition dream. This type of dream is used as a dramatic device, known as foreshadowing, in which tension is heightened by giving the audience a glimpse of the future. In the beginning of *La Bamba* (1987), Richie Valens dreams of a plane crash that foreshadows his demise.

Filmmakers characteristically follow certain widely accepted conventions when depicting the dream experience. When the purpose is to reveal to the audience the innermost feelings of a character, a film dream is usually derived from events within the film's context, and the dream employs a straightforward structure to make all of its "hidden" meanings obvious. Alfred Hitchcock's celebrated film dream in *Spellbound* (1945) used animations by Salvador Dalí to portray the dream of Gregory Peck's character. The surrealistic style of this dream sequence is characterized by stark "optical illusion"-style backgrounds, where objects and distances become elongated while the dreamer is thrust from one peril to another, highlighting rather than hiding his anxieties. Similarly, Hitchcock employed spiraling animation in his film *Vertigo* (1958) when the character of John Scott, who suffers from vertigo, dreams that he is falling from a great height—this scene was later parodied by Mel Brooks in *High Anxiety* (1978). In these examples, the events and symbols of the film dream make explicit the inner fears of the dreamer. Unlike these film dreams, however, real dreams' meanings are rarely so obvious and therefore much more difficult to interpret.

With the exception of infants and young children, most everyone in modern society recognizes that what occurs in one's dreams is isolated from the real world and does not affect waking physical reality. Thus, no matter what one dreams at night, the next day things are relatively similar to the day before; the line between the real world and the dream world cannot be crossed. This dichotomy holds true for most films, except for those in which dramatic license is taken with both dream and film. Movies such as the series of *A Nightmare on Elm Street* (1984, 1985, 1987, 1988, 1989, 1991) and *Dreamscape* (1984) exploit the inner fear that some outside force can take control of our dreams. Freddy Kruger, the demonic ghost haunting Elm Street, attacks by first entering his victims' dreams and then taking them back to *his* reality. Once in Freddy's nightmarish world, the dreamers are trapped and this causes them to die in their cinematic real life. *Dreamscape* portrays people with certain psychic powers who enter another person's dream and manipulate it from within, for better or worse.

A film dream is a particularly versatile device that filmmakers use to tell a dramatic story. People respond emotionally to dreams; as dreamers themselves, audiences can empathize with a film character's dream experiences when they recognize similarities both to their own dreams and to their feelings about their dreams. Even though dreams in "reel" life are not exactly the same as dreams in "real" life, there is a resonance between film dreams and one's own dreams that makes the cinematic portrayal of dreams one of the filmmaker's most powerful dramatic tools. (See also ART, SLEEP AND DREAMS IN WESTERN; LITERATURE, SLEEP AND DREAMS IN; POPULAR MUSIC, SLEEP AND DREAMS IN.)

REFERENCES

Dement WC. 1972/1974/1976. *Some must watch while some must sleep: Exploring the world of sleep.* New York: Norton.

Koulack D. 1991. *To catch a dream: Explorations of dreaming.* Albany: State University of New York Press.

Susan Franzblau
John Franzblau

MULTIPLE SLEEP LATENCY TEST

The Multiple Sleep Latency Test (MSLT) has been used in human studies since the 1970s to measure the brain's tendency to fall asleep. The MSLT was devised by experimenters at Stanford University to obtain an objective measure of daytime sleepiness (Carskadon and Dement, 1977). Until this test, introspection was the method most commonly used to assess sleepiness in patients with severe daytime sleepiness or in experimental subjects undergoing sleep restriction or sleep DEPRIVATION; that is, individuals were simply asked, "How sleepy are you?" This question can be asked simply or with a high degree of sophistication; nevertheless, the responses of perceived sleepiness are clearly subjective and often imprecise. (See also STANFORD SLEEPINESS SCALE.)

The MSLT grew out of an experiment called the ninety-minute day, in which sleep was evaluated in people sleeping thirty out of every ninety

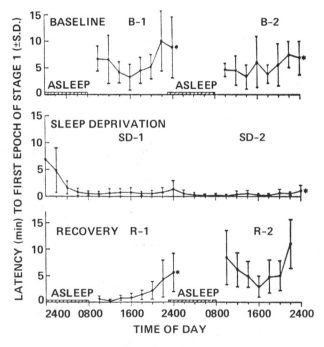

Figure 1. *The MSLT shows sleepiness as speed of falling asleep during the day.* Results (means and standard deviations) of sleep latency tests in college students after two nights of normal sleep (B-1, B-2), two nights of sleep deprivation (SD-1, SD-2), and two nights of recovery sleep (R-1, R-2). Note how short the sleep latencies were throughout the days following sleep loss, not returning to baseline pattern until R-2. (*Reprinted with permission from Carskadon MA, Dement WC. 1979. Effects of total sleep loss on sleep tendency.* Percept Motor Skills 48:495–506. Copyright *Perceptual and Motor Skills, 1979.*)

Table 1. The Multiple Sleep Latency Test (MSLT): A Standardized Method for Measuring Physiological Sleepiness in Humans

- Physiological sleepiness = speed of falling asleep (sleep latency) under standard test conditions
- Measuring tool = polygraph, recording activity of brain (electroencephalogram), eyes (electrooculogram), and muscle (electromyogram)
- Schedule = at least four short naps across the day, 2 hours between each nap, no sleep in between
- Nap conditions = lying comfortably in bed in a dark, quiet room
- Faster speed of falling asleep (shorter sleep latency) = higher level of physiological sleepiness
- Slower speed of falling asleep (longer sleep latency) = lower level of physiological sleepiness

minutes. The length of time it took people to fall asleep in this experiment showed a consistent pattern of variation across each twenty-four hours. The investigators thought that measuring the speed of falling asleep repeatedly in an everyday setting would give an objective value for daytime sleepiness; to test this possibility, speed of falling asleep (sleep latency) was measured with polysomnography in college students before, during, and after two nights without sleep. These sleep latency measures were compared with their subjective sleepiness ratings (Carskadon and Dement, 1979). The results showed clearly that speed of falling asleep varied as a function of prior sleep loss, with a return to baseline levels after recovery sleep (Figure 1). Subsequent studies have confirmed the MSLT's usefulness as a tool for quantifying daytime sleepiness (see SLEEPINESS).

The MSLT is also used in the clinical evaluation of excessively sleepy patients to determine their level of sleepiness and whether they may have NARCOLEPSY (Richardson et al., 1978). When administered under standard conditions (Table 1), the MSLT involves four to six opportunities to fall asleep. Normal adults always fall asleep by going from wakefulness to NREM sleep and only much later to REM sleep. Patients with narcolepsy, however, often go directly from wakefulness to REM

sleep. Such abnormal transitions can be properly evaluated with the MSLT: Patients who show this abnormal EEG pattern at the start of two or more naps are thought to have narcolepsy (Mitler et al., 1979).

REFERENCES

Carskadon MA, Dement WC. 1977. Sleepiness and sleep state on a 90-minute schedule. *Psychophysics* 14:127–133.

———. 1979. Effects of total sleep loss on sleep tendency. *Percept Motor Skills* 48:495–506.

Mitler MM, van den Hoed J, Carskadon MA, Richardson GS, Park R, Guilleminault C, and Dement WC. 1979. REM sleep episodes during the multiple sleep latency test in narcoleptic patients. *Electroencephalogr Clin Neurophysiol* 46:479–481.

Richardson GS, Carskadon MA, Flagg W, van den Hoed J, Dement WC, and Mitler MM. 1978. Excessive daytime sleepiness in man: Multiple sleep latency measurement in narcoleptic and control subjects. *Electroencephalogr Clin Neurophysiol* 45:621–627.

Mary A. Carskadon

MURDER

See Violence

MYTHS ABOUT DREAMING

Just as society has perpetuated myths about sleep, so too are there myths about dreams. Perhaps these myths have evolved because dreams are a source of wonderment. Whatever the reason, dreams are not yet fully understood, but we do know that at least some common myths are false.

Some people never dream. All people experience an average of three to six REM sleep periods each night, and as dreaming occurs in nearly every REM period, it seems highly likely that everyone dreams each night. Yet not everyone remembers dreams. According to research studies, however, even individuals who claim they do not dream remember dream content if awakened from REM sleep.

It is possible to teach oneself to remember one's dreams more clearly by thinking back, upon awakening, on one's thoughts of the night, rather than by concentrating on what one will do that day, as most people do (see RECALL OF DREAMS).

Dreams occur only in black and white. Or, conversely, *everyone dreams in color.* Another variation is the myth that *men are more likely to dream in black and white and women to dream in color.* The truth is that despite those who claim to dream only in black and white, laboratory studies show that everyone dreams in color. Colors in the first REM period are pale but become more vivid and varied by the last REM period. Because our memory for color is generally unreliable and because we tend to notice color only when it is unusual or significant, some of us simply do not remember the colors (see COLOR IN DREAMS).

Two people sleeping together can have the same dream. Although it seems extremely unlikely that two individuals can have the exact same dream (just as two individuals interpret the same environment differently when awake), it is possible for two people to have similar dream *content.* Two people sleeping together are likely to have shared similar presleep experiences that influence dream content; in fact, any two people (very close friends or siblings, for example) who have had a similar experience may have similar dreams (see TELEPATHY AND DREAMING).

If you sleep with a piece of wedding cake under your pillow, you will dream of the person you are to marry. Or *if you sleep with a piece of wedding cake under your pillow, you will soon find true love.* Although some people believe that dreams can predict the future (the Bible tells how Jacob's son Joseph interpreted dreams of others to foretell the future), it is generally accepted that dreams are a compilation of thoughts and memories and not of what will actually happen in the future. As an individual who sleeps with a piece of wedding cake under the pillow may have attended a wedding recently, the probability of dreaming about marriage or romance is increased (see PSYCHIC DREAMS).

If you dream that you are falling and hit the ground, you die. Or more broadly, *if you die in your dream from any cause, you die in your sleep.* Those who would know the truth of these statements are not able to communicate it to us, but one sleep researcher reports that he did die in one of his dreams and is still alive to relate the story.

You will never harm yourself within the story of a dream. In our dreams, as in our waking lives, we have self-protective mechanisms; thus we tend to wake up before a trigger is pulled or before being thrown in the ocean in our dreams. Just as in our waking lives, however, these mechanisms may not always function.

Some people dream only in the printed word, as if they are reading. Certain people dream with less imagery than others, giving the impression that they are only reading a newspaper or listening to the radio, but in fact all sighted people dream with some degree of visual imagery. As individuals vary on the degree to which they attend to visual information in their waking lives, they do in their dreaming lives as well (see CHARACTERISTICS OF DREAMS).

Eating spicy food in the evening causes nightmares. Nightmares can be caused by medications such as beta blockers and L-dopa and by traumatic experiences such as a near drowning and a narrow escape from a fire, but not by spicy foods. Spicy foods can, however, cause indigestion, which in turn may disturb sleep. Nightmares are actually common in many people (see HEARTBURN; NIGHTMARES; POSTTRAUMATIC NIGHTMARES).

A similar myth is that *eating chili makes you dream more.* Events during the day may appear in dreams—hence, eating chili may cause one to dream about chili or about food in general—but consuming certain foods does not affect the length of the dream or induce nightmares. Consuming excessive alcohol, though, is known to increase the intensity of dreams late in the sleep period and the fact that alcohol is frequently consumed with spicy foods, such as pizza, may have given rise to this myth (see ALCOHOL).

Blind people cannot dream. The dreams of people blind from birth reflect their waking world; they have imaginations and thoughts as do people who can see, but their dreams lack visual imagery. Children who become blind before the age of five or seven lose the ability to have visual imagery in their dreams, but those who become blind after this critical age retain visual imagery for an extended period, sometimes for life (see BLINDNESS: DREAMS OF THE BLIND; DEAFNESS AND DREAMING).

You cannot dream about something that you have never seen or someplace that you have never been. Many, if not all, of us have dreamed about things we have never seen and may not even exist. Generally, these images are a compilation of people or things with which we are familiar (see PICTORIAL REPRESENTATION; SYMBOLISM IN DREAMS).

You can have "reruns" of dreams. It is possible to dream about a situation or place more than once, especially one that is familiar. Although there have been no reports of recurring normal dreams, experts do not discount the possibility that such dreams could recur. Posttraumatic stress (generally stress that involves an unexpected incident) may cause recurring nightmares (see RECURRING DREAMS).

Other myths with no scientific basis include the following:

1. When sleeping dogs twitch, they arc dreaming of chasing rabbits (see ANIMALS' DREAMS).
2. If you dream that someone is dead or has died, it means that someone is pregnant.
3. Dreaming of pigs brings good luck.
4. Telling your dreams before breakfast makes them come true.
5. Your will have a nightmare if you sleep in the moonlight (see ENVIRONMENT; INCORPORATION INTO DREAMS).

REFERENCES

Anch MA, Browman CB, Mitler MM, Walsh JK. 1988. *Sleep: A scientific perspective.* Englewood Cliffs, NJ: Prentice-Hall.

Cartwright D. 1977. *Night life: Explorations in dreaming.* Englewood Cliffs, NJ: Prentice-Hall.

Cartwright RD. 1989. Dreams and their meaning. In Kryger MH, Roth T, Dement WC. *Principles and practices of sleep medicine.* Philadelphia: Saunders.

Foulkes, D. 1985. *Dreaming: A cognitive psychological analysis.* Hillside, NJ: Erlbaum.

James K. Walsh
Christin L. Engelhardt

MYTHS ABOUT SLEEP

Myths about sleep abound and vary from one culture to another. Given that sound sleep is such an important part of a healthy life, however, it is important for myths to be eradicated. No one knows the exact origin of these myths (some of which have more than one version), but they have been perpetuated by many.

It is dangerous to awaken a sleepwalker. In fact, it can be dangerous *not* to awaken a sleepwalker. Sleepwalkers have been known to fall down stairs and to walk through glass doors. They will not have a heart attack or go insane on being awakened, as some believe. It may be difficult to wake a sleepwalker; gently guiding the sleeper back to bed may be an easier course of action than trying to wake him or her. A related myth is that a sleepwalker who falls while sleepwalking will not be injured as she or he would be while awake because the muscles are more relaxed; however, sleepwalkers are capable of seriously hurting themselves (see SLEEPWALKING; REM SLEEP BEHAVIOR DISORDER).

You can learn a person's secrets when he or she talks in his or her sleep. Each sleeptalker is different; some only mumble incoherently whereas others speak in clear sentences. It is rare for a sleeper to respond to questions or instructions, but some do respond.

Generally, people are most likely to talk during stages 1 and 2 of NREM sleep, although it is possible to do so during REM sleep when words may be more meaningful and relate to an ongoing dream. Speech during stage 1 or 2 sleep is generally short and meaningless, such as "yeah" and "of course." It is true that more women than men talk in their sleep, and sleeptalkers can be of any age. Talking in one's sleep is not medically significant (see SLEEPTALKING). Coherent "sleep conversations" may often occur when the individual has awakened but is very sleepy, and then returns quickly to sleep. The fast return to sleep affects memory of the conversation and thus perpetuates the myth the person was sleeptalking.

A warm room, a big lunch, or a boring situation will make you sleepy. Although such statements have been made for so long that they are often accepted as fact, they are actually false. A warm room or a heavy meal or an uninteresting lecture will only reveal a person's sleepiness but will not cause it. A well-rested person will not feel very sleepy, no matter what the environment or circumstances. One sign of sleep deprivation is frequently getting sleepy or falling asleep unintentionally while in sedentary positions: watching television, reading, or sitting at a desk (see SLEEPINESS).

People sleep in 20-minute or 2-hour or 3-hour cycles; if you awaken before completing a cycle, you will feel tired. We do sleep in cycles of approximately 90 to 100 minutes, but the cycles change as the night goes on. We begin in a brief period of stage 1 and then move into stage 2 and delta sleep. After this, our first REM SLEEP stage, the shortest one of the night, begins. This cycle recurs, with the amount of delta sleep decreasing and the amount of REM sleep increasing throughout the night (see CYCLES OF SLEEP ACROSS THE NIGHT).

How one feels when one awakens is not related to the completion of a cycle but to the total number of hours slept and the time of day and the stage from which one awakens. Thus, although some believe, for example, that sleeping eight hours is not as beneficial as sleeping six or nine hours, it is important to obtain a sufficient amount of sleep each night, generally from seven to nine hours, but each individual's needs vary (see INDIVIDUAL DIFFERENCES; NEED FOR SLEEP; SLEEP LENGTH; TIMING OF SLEEP AND WAKEFULNESS).

Alcohol helps you to sleep better. It is true that alcohol helps one to fall asleep quickly, but alcohol actually decreases the quality and quantity of sleep. People who have trouble sleeping are often advised to avoid alcohol (see ALCOHOL).

Warm milk induces sleep. Warm milk may make one feel sleepy because of its soothing effect. Moreover, there is an ingredient in milk, cheese, beans, nuts, turkey, and other foods that may promote sleep (see FOLK AND OTHER NATURAL REMEDIES FOR SLEEPLESSNESS). It is an amino acid, L-tryptophan. A single glass of milk at bedtime, however, is unlikely to provide enough L-tryptophan to induce sleep then, nor is it likely to be converted rapidly enough into a neuro-chemical involved in sleep. More likely, regular consumption of L-tryptophan in the diet is necessary (see L-TRYPTOPHAN).

You change body positions every seven minutes regularly. The average person has significant body movements twenty-five to thirty times during the night, generally when changing from one sleep stage to another or during a brief awakening. Most large movements cluster near the start or end of REM periods, not every seven minutes. Slight movements and muscle twitches are much more frequent.

During REM sleep, one is virtually paralyzed and does not move, other than eye movements and occasional twitches. Persons with REM be-havior disorder (see REM SLEEP BEHAVIOR DISORDER) are an exception to this rule: they appear to act out their dreams, at times harming themselves or their bed partners (see VIOLENCE).

You can get by on ten-minute "power naps" every couple of hours or so. Although our society seems to believe that sleep is dispensable, sleep deprivation can have severe consequences. Numerous accidents have been attributed to an individual's falling asleep or to decreased alertness resulting directly from sleep deprivation. "Power naps," no matter what length, are not a substitute for a regular schedule of adequate sleep. It is true, however, that naps taken by sleep-deprived individuals or by night workers at the appropriate time in their circadian rhythm are likely to improve their alertness, at least temporarily.

A related myth is that you can teach yourself to need less sleep. Although one can voluntarily reduce the usual amount of sleep obtained at night, it is likely that mood and performance will suffer (see GRADUAL SLEEP REDUCTION; NAPPING; SLEEP RESTRICTION, THERAPEUTIC).

Older people need less sleep. Many people find it difficult to sleep as they age and may have heard that their need for sleep has decreased. In actuality, to feel refreshed and alert for the day's activities, older people need as much sleep as they did in earlier years, generally seven to eight hours each night. It is true that as people age, the quality of their sleep decreases. Sleep may be more fragmented and lighter and more easily disrupted by noises (see AGING AND SLEEP; ONTOGENY).

Putting a sleeping person's hand in water causes urination. Although this is a well-known trick among guests at grade school sleepovers, there is no evidence that it works. It is true that water imagery is common in dreams of people who have enuresis (see BEDWETTING).

Snoring is a sign of sound sleep. Loud snoring can actually be a sign of a disorder called sleep apnea (see APNEA). Not all snorers have sleep apnea (as many as 1 in 10 adults snores but only 1 in 100 has sleep apnea), but almost all who have sleep apnea snore and snore loudly. Some snore so loudly that the hearing of the snorer and the bed partner is damaged (see SNORING).

It's bad to sleep on your stomach. There are many different sleep positions; different people prefer different positions. There is no scientific evidence that sleep is better or worse in any one position. Some people with sleep apnea are advised not to sleep on their backs, and those with certain neurological disorders are told to avoid certain positions. As long as one does not have a medical condition that necessitates a particular position and is comfortable, any position is fine. One exception to this rule is that severely intoxicated individuals have died sleeping on their back, unconscious, after choking on what they regurgitated (see SLEEP POSITIONS).

The hours of sleep one obtains before midnight are twice as valuable as those obtained after midnight. It is true that stage 3 and 4 NREM sleep (slow-wave sleep), considered by many to be the deepest stages, occurs predominantly in the first half of the night (see SLOW-WAVE SLEEP). The occurrence of slow-wave sleep is not dependent on the time of day or night but on the time when sleep is initiated; depending on bedtime, slow-wave sleep will occur just as readily after midnight as before. Optimal sleep is best obtained by maintaining regular sleep times, whether or not this time includes the hours before midnight.

You can learn while you sleep. Although many students may wish this were not a myth, one must be awake to store new material in memory. Studies have shown that material heard while lying in bed may be recalled the next day, but only if that material was presented while the person was actually awake. Because brief awakenings at night are not always perceived accurately, a person may believe he or she learned this information during sleep, but lessons on a tape that plays while one sleeps are absorbed into memory only if one is not physiologically sleeping (see LEARNING; MEMORY; SLEEP LEARNING).

You cannot make up for lost sleep. If a person obtains inadequate sleep and is sleepy as a result, the sleepiness can be reversed by sleep. From this perspective, one can make up for lost sleep. Interestingly, if you lose four hours of sleep by sleeping from 11:00 P.M. to 3:00 A.M. (instead of from 11:00 P.M. to 7:00 A.M.), you do not need to sleep an additional four hours the next night to restore alertness. Increasing sleep time by two hours may be sufficient. Thus it appears we do not make up sleep on a minute-to-minute basis (see DEPRIVATION, PARTIAL; DEPRIVATION, TOTAL: BEHAVIORAL EFFECTS; DEPRIVATION, TOTAL: PHYSIOLOGICAL EFFECTS; SLEEP EXTENSION).

Resting is as beneficial as sleeping. Although resting as opposed to activity may leave you less fatigued, physical inactivity does not replace the crucial processes of sleep that result in an alert and energetic person. During sleep the brain produces the biochemical and physiological changes that are apparently necessary for restoration. The capacity to produce such changes is not found in the brain during wakefulness (see FUNCTIONS OF SLEEP; NONRESTORATIVE SLEEP; REST).

The brain is "turned off" during sleep. In fact, nothing could be farther from the truth. Some areas of the brain are more active during sleep than during wakefulness. Although scientists have not completely determined all of the brain's activities during sleep, it is clear that sleep is actively controlled by the brain. Studies show that animals deprived of sleep die within a few weeks and that sleep deprivation in humans leads to poorer mood, as well as decreased motor and mental ability (see BRAIN MECHANISMS; REM SLEEP MECHANISMS AND NEUROANATOMY).

If you can't get a full night of sleep, it is better to get no sleep at all. Although it is ideal to get a full night of sleep each night, occasions will arise when this is not possible. In such a situation, one should still attempt to obtain as much sleep as possible. It is true that one may feel exhausted on waking after an insufficient amount of sleep. Thus, not sleeping at all, especially when one has much adrenalin, may seem like a better option; however, studies show that complete sleep deprivation leads to greater performance deficits than sleep restricted to a few hours.

REFERENCES

Anch AM, Browman B, Mitler MM, Walsh JK. 1988. *Sleep: A scientific perspective.* Englewood Cliffs, NJ: Prentice-Hall.
Kryger M, Roth T, Dement WC. 1989. *Principles and practice of sleep medicine.* Philadelphia: Saunders.
Lamberg, L. 1984. *The AMA guide to better sleep.* New York: Random House.
Mendelson WB. 1987. *Human sleep: Research and clinical care.* New York: Plenum.

James K. Walsh
Christin L. Engelhardt

N

NAPPING

In the broadest sense *napping* refers to any period of sleep that is of shorter duration than the typical habitual sleep taken by an individual or characteristic of a species. Thus a nap is most often considered to be any sleep that is less than approximately 4 hours in duration in humans. Studies have shown that most naps last between 20 minutes and 2 hours. Another criterion often used to define a nap is the time of day it is taken. Most often, naps are taken sometime during daylight hours by humans and other species that have their longest sleep periods at night. Although daytime napping is discouraged in some cultures, much scientific evidence now supports the view that napping is a normal part of the human sleep–wake cycle. Thus, there is a biologically based tendency to fall asleep in midafternoon, just as there is a tendency to fall asleep at night. Moreover, if sleep the night before is reduced or disturbed for any reason, a nap the subsequent afternoon is not only more likely to occur, but it can also help relieve sleepiness and enhance alertness. How often naps are taken, when naps occur, and the factors that influence the benefits and consequences of naps vary as a function of biological and behavioral factors.

Factors Affecting Napping Behavior

Age

Just as the amount of nocturnal sleep humans obtain changes across the life span, so does the amount of daytime napping. Newborn infants nap many times each day, showing the polycyclic sleep–wake pattern characteristic throughout the life span of such animals as cats and rabbits. As a human baby's circadian system develops, daytime naps decrease in frequency. By 2 years of age most babies take one daytime nap, usually in the afternoon. By 5 years of age the majority of children do not give in to the tendency to nap in the afternoon, unless they have not obtained adequate sleep at night. Daytime nap tendency decreases further from ages 6 to 15 years, and then begins to increase again. The majority of teenagers and young adults nap at least once a week. Although this increased napping tendency is part of their biologically driven sleep–wake cycle, it is also a result of many teenagers and young adults obtaining too little sleep at night. Increased freedom and control over sleep–wake cycles in adolescence and young adulthood, as well as the demands of school, extracurricular, social, and work activity, contribute to the loss of nocturnal sleep and the increased need for daytime naps at these ages (*see* ADOLESCENCE AND SLEEP; INFANCY, NORMAL SLEEP PATTERNS IN).

Throughout adulthood, especially from ages 30 to 60, the tendency to feel sleepy in midday and the ability to nap at that time appear to be relatively stable. Whether or not an adult takes a daytime nap depends greatly on the work–rest cycle of the person, the control the person has over his or her time, and the culture to which the person belongs. In some countries, the life-style of most adults includes timeout for a brief daytime nap. These SIESTA cultures include the countries China, Greece, Nigeria, and Mexico. Other countries, especially those that have undergone major industrialization, do not allow for siesta. Exam-

392

ples of these countries are Japan, Russia, Germany, and the United States. This distinction between siesta cultures and nonsiesta cultures signifies only whether the culture endorses daytime napping, not whether the tendency to nap is present. In all cultures in which sleep tendency and behavior have been carefully studied, the tendency for a daytime nap, typically in midafternoon, is present. Within a nonsiesta culture this tendency gives way to napping among those adults who have the opportunity to nap at midday. Thus, in a nonsiesta country such as the United States, daytime napping is quite common among adults who have work–rest schedules that are flexible enough to permit a daytime nap. These include college students, homemakers, shift workers, and some executives. Conversely, among adults who must work during the time of midday nap tendency, napping behavior is relatively rare.

As humans enter the later decades of life (ages 60 to 90), daytime napping appears to increase in frequency: more of the elderly nap, and they nap more often. It is not yet certain whether this reflects a change in the biological regulation of sleep and sleepiness as we age, or the freedom to take naps because of retirement, or some combination of these factors. (See also AGING AND SLEEP.)

Nap Time

One of the most striking scientific findings about napping is that humans have a biological predisposition to nap at a certain period of the day. That is, the tendencies to feel sleepy and to make mistakes because of sleepiness are increased at midday, which is when the tendency to fall asleep rapidly, as reflected in the MULTIPLE SLEEP LATENCY TEST, is increased. Napping has a very high likelihood of occurring at this time. The nap zone occurs between 12:00 noon and 5:00 P.M. for children and adults who do not have sleep disorders and who normally sleep at night. The precise hour of the nap tendency within this zone appears to depend on the person's habitual nocturnal sleep time. For those who go to bed relatively early at night and awaken early in the morning, such as children and the elderly, the nap zone is typically 12:00 P.M. to 3:00 P.M. For young adults and those who tend to delay their nocturnal sleep until later at night (e.g., after midnight), the nap zone is typically 2:00 P.M. to 5:00 P.M. Thus, the period of the day when there

is an increased tendency to nap occurs approximately 12 hours after the midnocturnal sleep time of an individual. This temporal relationship and other data supporting the view that naps are biologically driven have prompted some scientists to suggest that there is a 12-hour rhythm of sleepiness underlying nocturnal and daytime nap sleep tendencies.

Sleep Need

Although the tendency to nap appears to reflect a biological timing process in the brain, napping behavior is most likely to occur in the preferred daytime nap zone when the amount of sleep obtained by a person is reduced relative to the biological sleep need of that individual. Thus, a new-born baby will nap as a result of an endogenous sleep need that is programmed into the brain to ensure the baby obtains adequate sleep. As we age and gain more control over our sleep behavior, we may elect to reduce the amount of sleep we obtain at night below our basal sleep need, thereby increasing our daytime sleepiness, especially during the midafternoon nap zone. For example, a 10-year-old child who does not ordinarily take daytime naps may suddenly find sleepiness to be overwhelming in midafternoon after he stayed awake until 3:00 A.M. one night with friends during a "sleepover." Similarly, studies of college students showed napping behavior was most prevalent when nocturnal sleep had been reduced. Napping behavior that occurs primarily in association with reduced nocturnal sleep is referred to as compensatory or replacement napping: the person is thought to be compensating for or replacing the lost nocturnal sleep. In nonsiesta cultures, compensatory napping is the most common reason for naps taken by healthy adults with busy life-styles.

Sleep Disorders

Just as napping can occur in response to life-style reductions of nocturnal sleep, it can also occur as a function of medical and psychological disruptions of nocturnal sleep (see MEDICAL ILLNESS AND SLEEP). For example, chronic pain and discomfort can disrupt nighttime sleep and increase the tendency for daytime napping. Among persons who suffer from disorders of excessive sleepiness (DOES), such as NARCOLEPSY and sleep APNEA, daytime napping can be frequent and involuntary, meaning that the person cannot stop falling asleep for brief naps. In such cases, the naps often occur throughout the day, not just during the nap zone, and they may or may not be refreshing. Many persons with narcolepsy find brief daytime naps to be helpful, whereas persons with untreated sleep apnea derive no benefit from frequent naps. Similarly, there are patients who nap during the day, but find that they cannot fall asleep or remain asleep at night. In all such cases napping can be a sign or symptom of a sleep disorder or disturbance of the sleep–wake cycle. For this reason, doctors who diagnose and treat sleep disorders often discourage napping by patients. For otherwise healthy persons, however, napping is normal and can be quite beneficial.

Napping and Human Functioning

Naps are often alleged to be refreshing disproportionate to their length, and there are apocryphal tales of great persons who reputedly survived for long periods solely on nap sleep (e.g., Leonardo da Vinci, Napoleon Bonaparte, Thomas Edison, Winston Churchill). Although no one has ever been documented to live solely by napping, research has shown that naps can have very important benefits, depending on the sleep need and work–rest schedule of the person. They can also have some unwanted consequences (*see* SHORT SLEEPERS IN HISTORY AND LEGEND).

Consequences of Napping

Daytime naps taken by otherwise healthy persons generally have more benefits than negative consequences. There are only two potentially serious negative effects of napping. The first is called sleep inertia, which refers to the feelings of grogginess and difficulty thinking that accompany awakening from some daytime naps. Typically SLEEP INERTIA lasts only a few minutes, giving way to feelings of alertness. Therefore, sleep inertia from napping poses a problem only for persons who must be able to perform quickly on abrupt awakening from a nap. Examples of these circumstances might include a medical doctor who is on call or a fighter pilot. The other potentially negative effect of napping is that if the nap is too long, it can interfere with the subsequent night of sleep. This does not appear to be nearly as serious

a problem as was once assumed by sleep specialists. For a midafternoon nap to adversely affect the ability to sleep that night, the nap must be at least 2 hours long. Studies of healthy adult nappers reveal that afternoon naps rarely last this long, with the average duration being around 70 minutes.

Benefits of Napping

Most naps enhance the alertness and reduce the sleepiness of the napper. If the napper does not have a significant sleep debt and naps to relieve mild daytime sleepiness, then the effects of the nap are generally an enhancement of subjective alertness. If the nap is taken after the napper has accumulated a substantial sleep debt, the benefits of the nap may or may not be an improvement of subjective alertness, but the nap will almost always improve performance. Thus, when sleepiness has accumulated to the point where performance is adversely affected, such as when a forest ranger remains awake 26 hours to fight a fire, a nap can greatly improve performance on a wide range of tasks including the ability to attend and respond quickly, to remember what was said or read, and to think clearly. The napper may still feel tired by virtue of only getting an hour or two of sleep during a day or two of wakefulness, but after the nap, no matter when it is taken, performance will typically improve dramatically. The duration that performance will remain improved can vary from 3 to 18 hours, depending on how much sleep was obtained, the magnitude of the sleep debt remaining, and the type and amount of work being carried out.

Prophylactic Napping

One of the more useful and surprising scientific discoveries about napping is that "prophylactic napping" is not only possible, but quite often it is very helpful for persons who must work for prolonged hours (Dinges et al., 1987). Prophylactic napping refers to the practice of taking a nap in advance of a period of work that will either last an abnormally long time, occur at night when sleepiness is naturally greater, or both. Prophylactic napping has also been called *preparatory napping, preplanned napping*, and *power napping*; the last term is not descriptively accurate, but it has been used by laypersons who attribute performance-enhancing effects to napping.

In its simplest form prophylactic napping refers to taking a nap to prevent sleepiness from increasing to a level that impairs performance capability. Prophylactic napping not only has been shown to enhance human performance in laboratory studies; recently it has also been shown to enhance vigilance functioning and physiological alertness in airline pilots flying long flights over many time zones. The remarkable aspect of prophylactic napping is that the benefits of the nap, even a nap of only 25 minutes, can be evident in performance for many hours afterward, including during periods when sleepiness would ordinarily be quite intense. The results of studies on prophylactic or preplanned napping were unexpected because a prophylactic nap taken in advance of prolonged work appears to yield greater benefits than naps taken after sleep pressure has built up from prolonged wakefulness, despite the fact that the earlier prophylactic nap contains less consolidated sleep. It appears that the prophylactic nap reduces the potential for later sleepiness. For this reason preplanned napping is now viewed as a viable countermeasure to performance impairment accompanying many modern sustained work scenarios.

Nap Sleep Structure and Napping Cycles

The type and occurrence of sleep stages during naps are like those of nocturnal and longer periods of sleep. Thus, there is no sleep stage or pattern that is unique to naps, and the same chronological factors that regulate nocturnal sleep also regulate nap sleep stages. Naps taken during the midafternoon nap zone typically contain little or no REM sleep, as they last less than 90 minutes and occur at a time of day when REM sleep requires about 90 minutes of prior sleep.

Napping has been used scientifically to study the factors that regulate and affect sleep stages and timing. Many unusual sleep experiments have been done using naps, such as having people live on a 90-minute day (i.e., 30 minutes to sleep and 60 minutes to stay awake). These studies have yielded very important insights into how sleep tendency and stages vary as a function of prior wakefulness and time of day. Napping has also proven to be a very practical tool, as it is used by sleep disorder specialists and sleep scientists to study daytime sleep tendency in the Multiple Sleep Latency Test and variants of it.

Napping, once considered irrelevant to understanding the secrets of sleep, has proven to be a remarkably important process for identifying and preventing sleepiness.

REFERENCES

Dinges DF, Broughton RJ, eds. 1989. *Sleep and alertness: Chronobiological, behavioral and medical aspects of napping.* New York: Raven Press. Contains an exhaustive bibliography of napping in animals and humans.
Dinges DF, Orne MT, Whitehouse WG, Orne EC. 1987. Temporal placement of a nap for alertness: Contributions of circadian phase and prior wakefulness. *Sleep* 10:313–329. Evidence of benefits of prophylactic napping.

David F. Dinges

NARCOLEPSY

Narcolepsy is a sleep disorder characterized, in its fullest expression, by excessive daytime SLEEPINESS, CATAPLEXY, SLEEP PARALYSIS, and HYPNAGOGIC HALLUCINATIONS. These symptoms are known as the *narcolepsy tetrad.* The term *narcolepsy,* which means sleep seizure, was introduced in 1880 by Gélineau; however, it was not until 1957 that Yoss and Daly operationalized the criteria for the diagnosis of the disorder. They required the presence of one or more symptoms of the tetrad. At first, the diagnosis rested on the clinical history and no laboratory tests were available for confirmation of narcolepsy. Nevertheless, several events have enabled achievement of laboratory confirmation on patients in whom the diagnosis is suspected. Primarily, Vogel (1960) using polysomnographic techniques showed that patients with narcolepsy frequently enter REM sleep from wakefulness. These events have been called *sleep-onset REM periods* (SOREMPs). Documenting the occurrence of SOREMPs has become an essential part of the laboratory confirmation of narcolepsy. More recently, a significantly high association, greater than 90 percent, between the class II human leukocyte antigen (HLA)-DR2 and narcolepsy has been reported in these patients.

Studies on the prevalence of the disorder show that narcolepsy is found in about 0.06 percent of the population; however, some populations show extreme variation. For example, in Japan the prevalence is as high as 0.16 percent, in contrast with Israel where the condition is extremely rare (1 in 500,000). In the United States, it is estimated that at least 250,000 people have narcolepsy. This means that narcolepsy is more frequent in the U.S. population than other well-known neurological disorders (e.g., myasthenia gravis, amyotrophic lateral sclerosis, Huntington's chorea, and multiple sclerosis).

Clinical Manifestations

The peak age of onset for narcolepsy is in adolescence and young adulthood (15 to 35 years). Some studies suggest that males are affected somewhat more often than females. Usually, excessive daytime sleepiness is the initial symptom. This is manifested by unwanted episodes of sleep that recur several times a day (SLEEP ATTACKS). Occasionally, a patient may report feeling sleepy throughout the day without ever feeling fully alert. Although most of the unwanted sleep episodes occur during sedentary situations, when sleepiness is more likely to be manifested (e.g., attending a boring lecture, play, concert, or movie), they can also be experienced during monotonous activities. Depending upon the activity, the unwanted sleep episode is potentially dangerous, for example, if it occurs while driving. Infrequently, sleep attacks may occur in more active situations such as eating or during a conversation. Relief from this extreme sleepiness can be obtained by a brief nap. People afflicted with this symptom frequently report feeling refreshed after a 10- to 20-minute nap. Moreover, some patients with narcolepsy may nap for more than an hour.

Cataplexy is reported by 70 percent to 80 percent of narcoleptic patients. These episodes are recognized as characteristic and unique to this disorder, and many consider cataplexy essential for the diagnosis of narcolepsy. The episodes consist of sudden muscular weakness (loss of muscular tone or ATONIA) that is triggered by emotional stimuli. The latter can be any affect-laden situation such as anger, laughter, surprise, sexual encounters, and sporting events. During episodes of cataplexy, patients are conscious, their memory is not impaired, and the oculomotor and respiratory muscles remain intact. Cataplectic episodes are usually short (less than a minute); they may involve all skeletal muscle groups or be localized to the knees, face, eyelids, or lower or upper extremities (partial episodes). The frequency of the episodes shows wide interpersonal variation from very occasional (less than once a year) to several attacks in a single day. Although some patients learn to recognize the warning signs of cataplexy and have time to sit or lie down, others do not recognize them and thus may injure themselves.

Hypnagogic hallucinations are vivid perceptual experiences occurring at sleep onset and they may be concomitant with sleep paralysis. They are reported by 50 percent to 70 percent of the patients. The hallucinations are most often visual and auditory but may also be tactile or kinetic. Patients commonly report experiencing being caught in a fire, the telephone ringing, being about to be attacked, or flying through the air. They usually experience these episodes as real and may be confused when awakened from them.

Sleep paralysis consists of a temporary loss of muscle tone that occurs in the transition between wakefulness and sleep (hypnagogic) or on awakening (hypnopompic). It is reported by 40 percent to 65 percent of the patients. Because of the inability to move or speak, these episodes are frequently reported as very frightening experiences. The episodes last several minutes and patients with these symptoms report an inability to overcome the paralysis unless touched or called by another person.

The full narcoleptic tetrad is seen in 20 percent to 30 percent of all patients. In addition, other symptoms have also been frequently reported by patients with narcolepsy. These include disturbed nocturnal sleep, automatic behaviors and memory problems, and visual symptoms. The majority of patients report frequent awakenings during sleep (70 percent to 85 percent) and some complain of vivid dreams. Although the etiology of the awakenings may be periodic leg movements during sleep, the majority of patients suffer from awakenings of unknown cause.

Automatic behaviors occur during monotonous or repetitive activities and involve a semipurposeful activity for which the patient has no memory. These episodes may be responsible for poor performance at work and memory lapses during which patients may put away things in unusual places, utter words out of context, or drive a car far from their intended destination. The visual symptoms include ptosis, blurred vision, and diplopia.

The symptoms associated with narcolepsy represent a challenge to the patient. The initial symptoms may follow abrupt changes of the sleep–wake schedule or life stressors (e.g., death of a relative or a divorce). Although the severity of the symptoms may fluctuate over time, for most patients this is a chronic disease. The pervasive effects of narcolepsy are reflected on work, education, driving, recreation, personality, and interpersonal relationships. Symptoms of depression are not infrequent, and marital and family problems are reported by the majority of the patients.

The etiology of the disorder remains unclear. Although the occurrence of narcolepsy in families has been recognized, cases with no genetic predisposition are also found. Monozygotic twins may be concordant or discordant for narcolepsy, which suggests that genetic factors may be necessary but not sufficient to manifest the disease (multifactorial model of heritability). Other studies have found that first-degree relatives of people with narcolepsy are at or about eight times greater risk of having some disorder of excessive sleepiness than are individuals in the general population.

The finding of a greater than 90 percent frequency (98 percent to 100 percent when only patients with cataplexy are considered) of an HLA-DR2 haplotype in patients with narcolepsy is remarkable. This association is significantly greater in narcolepsy when compared with that found in normals or in other conditions with HLA associations. Despite this strong association, the exact location of the narcolepsy-susceptibility gene has not been determined. The existence of well-documented cases of classic narcolepsy in patients who do not have the HLA-DR2 haplotype has prompted suggestions that the gene may be outside the HLA-DR subregion on the short arm of chromosome 6 [see HUMAN LEUKOCYTE ANTIGEN (HLA)].

Pathological studies on brains donated by nar-coleptic patients are just emerging. Preliminary results have not found clear histopathological abnormalities using light microscopy. Furthermore, no definite quantitative analysis of neurotransmitter receptors is yet available. Based on studies of CANINE NARCOLEPSY, changes in muscarinic-M2 and dopamine-D2 receptor density in several areas of the brains of narcolepsy patients are expected. These results concur with neurochemical studies, indicating reduced dopamine levels in dogs and in cerebrospinal fluid from patients with narcolepsy. The neurochemical studies also support cholinergic involvement in narcolepsy, in particular as it relates to REM sleep.

Polysomnographic studies have contributed to a better understanding of the pathophysiology of the disorder. In particular, SOREMPs have been shown to be characteristic of narcolepsy. Relevant to this finding is the preservation of the 90-minute NREM/REM cycle in narcoleptics and the comparable percentage of REM sleep during nocturnal recordings between patients and normal controls; however, some narcoleptics have very disturbed sleep secondary to idiopathic arousals and awakenings and increased stage 1 NREM sleep (see STAGES OF SLEEP). Ambulatory 24-hour sleep–wake monitoring has shown that no differences exist in the total sleep time between narcoleptic patients and normal controls. In addition, these recordings have documented that most sleep attacks last 1 to 10 minutes, some with SOREMPs. A few episodes may last less than 30 seconds and these have been called *micro-sleep episodes*. In fact, studies using performance testing have documented that microsleep episodes were responsible for poor performance. Microsleep episodes are also believed to be the causal factor responsible for the automatic behaviors reported by some patients in their activities of daily living. The polysomnographic data available to date indicate that patients with narcolepsy have difficulty maintaining a given neural state, whether sleep or wake. Thus, these patients tend to fall asleep during their waking hours and to wake up more frequently during their sleeping period.

The neurophysiological basis of cataplexy has also been studied. Measurement of the H-reflex during a cataplectic episode has shown it to be decreased or absent as happens normally during REM sleep. The conclusion from this finding is that the motor inhibition of REM sleep intrudes into the wake state during a cataplectic episode.

A similar dissociative process of REM sleep occurs in sleep paralysis. Hypnagogic hallucinations are thought to be REM sleep mentation (dreaming) that intrudes into wakefulness. Thus, cataplexy and the auxiliary symptoms (hypnagogic hallucinations and sleep paralysis) represent the intrusion into wakefulness of various physiological components of REM sleep.

Polysomnographic Features

The polysomnographic evaluation (nocturnal clinical POLYSOMNOGRAPHY [CPSG] followed by a MULTIPLE SLEEP LATENCY TEST [MSLT]) is the most valuable laboratory test for evaluating patients with excessive daytime sleepiness. Before polysomnographic evaluation, patients with suspected narcolepsy undergo a thorough clinical evaluation, including questions about the patient's sleep schedule on weekdays and weekends, scheduled naps, and involuntary sleep episodes. This will provide a clinical assessment of the severity of excessive daytime sleepiness (EDS). The patient is also questioned about the occurrence of cataplexy and the other auxiliary symptoms, automatic behavior, and disturbed nocturnal sleep. Questions also address other possible causal factors of symptomatic EDS like a history of loud and interrupted snoring (frequently encountered in patients with sleep apnea), psychiatric symptomatology, unusual movements during sleep, and use of prescribed and nonprescribed medications. An assessment of alcohol and illicit use of drugs is important, given the potential confounding effects they may have on the evaluation. A physical examination is performed, and any suggestions of a medical or neurological condition are followed up with the appropriate testing. When the clinical assessment is completed, the CPSG and MSLT are scheduled.

Before the polysomnographic evaluation is done, the patient is withdrawn from any medications with central nervous system (CNS) effects and follows a regular sleep schedule. The polysomnographic evaluation provides an objective assessment of the patient's sleep. It enables an accurate differential diagnosis, objectively quantifies the severity of the patient's sleepiness, and documents the presence of SOREMPs. Specifically, the polysomnographic diagnosis of narcolepsy requires a pathological level of sleepiness (mean MSLT ≤ 5 minutes), two or more SOREMPs, and the absence of other potential causes of EDS (e.g., sleep apnea, insufficient sleep, effects of medication). Other disorders in which a single SOREMP may be seen are virtually ruled out (e.g., alcohol or drug withdrawal, depression and other psychiatric conditions, circadian sleep disturbances, and obstructive sleep apnea syndrome) by the high degree of specificity derived from the MSLT and SOREMP criteria. An HLA-DR2-positive haplotype is considered supportive of the diagnosis, although this haplotype is found in 20 percent to 30 percent of the general population. Furthermore, a diagnosis of narcolepsy in patients negative for this haplotype may lead one to question the accuracy of the diagnosis, except in African-Americans, in whom the association of narcolepsy with the HLA-DQw1 antigen is stronger than for the HLA-DR2 haplotype.

Treatment

The treatment of narcolepsy is mainly symptomatic. Treatment needs to be individualized depending on the patient's clinical presentation and the severity of the auxiliary symptoms. If the polysomnographic evaluation shows significant sleep APNEA, it needs to be treated first, since normalization of sleep-disordered breathing may ameliorate the severity of daytime sleepiness and allow a more accurate evaluation of the other symptoms associated with narcolepsy. In general, the sleepiness associated with narcolepsy is treated with CNS stimulants (methylphenidate and pemoline being the most widely used). These medications are thought to enhance the synaptic availability of norepinephrine. When cataplexy and the auxiliary symptoms of narcolepsy are present, their treatment usually includes tricyclic ANTIDEPRESSANTS because of their REM-suppressing effects. Other novel treatments can be found in medical textbooks. Among these, γ-hydroxybutyrate has been used successfully in the treatment of both EDS and cataplexy (see also STIMULANTS).

Another important aspect of the treatment of narcolepsy is patient education. An understanding of sleep physiology and the effects of a regular sleep schedule and prophylactic naps is likely to benefit patients afflicted with this disorder.

The deleterious effects of ALCOHOL on sleep should be known by the patients, and a thorough review of the symptoms associated with narcolepsy will likely alleviate some of the confusion experienced by both patients and their families. A lack of understanding of these issues is likely to result in poor adjustment to the disorder and underachievement. This, in turn, may lead to psychological impairment which needs to be recognized and treated if necessary. Self-help groups such as the American Narcolepsy Association and the Narcolepsy Network have been helpful to many patients. In summary, the treatment of narcolepsy needs to include appropriate medical management and ample discussion of the impact of the disease on life-style, work, family, and family planning. Inclusion of these aspects in the care of narcolepsy patients will likely assist them in adapting to the limitations of the disease, thus improving their chances to lead productive and enjoyable lives.

REFERENCES

Aldrich MS. 1990. Narcolepsy. *N Engl J Med* 323: 389–394.

Amira SA, Johnson TS, Logowitz NB. 1985. Diagnosis of narcolepsy using the Multiple Sleep Latency Test: Analysis of current laboratory criteria. *Sleep* 8:325–331.

Billiard M, Besset A, Cadilhac J. 1983. The clinical and polygraphic development of narcolepsy. In Guilleminault C, Lugaresi E, eds. *Sleep/wake disorders: Natural history, epidemiology and long-term evolution*, pp 171–185. New York: Raven Press.

Broughton RJ. 1989. Sleep attacks, naps, and sleepiness in medical sleep disorders. In Dinges DF, Broughton RJ, eds. *Sleep and alertness*, pp 267–298. New York: Raven Press.

Broughton RJ. 1990. Narcolepsy. In Thorpy MJ, ed. *Handbook of sleep disorders*, pp 197–216. New York: Marcel Dekker.

Gélineau J. 1880. De la Narcolepsie. *Gaz Hop (Paris)* 53:535–637.

Guilleminault C. 1989. Narcolepsy syndrome. In Kryger MH, Roth T, Dement WC, eds. *Principles and practice of sleep medicine*. Philadelphia: WB Saunders.

Guilleminault C, Dement WC, Passovant P, eds. 1976. *Narcolepsy*. New York: Spectrum.

Honda Y, Juji T, eds. 1988. *HLA in narcolepsy*. Heidelberg: Springer-Verlag.

Kleitman N. 1963. *Sleep and wakefulness*. Chicago: University of Chicago Press.

Neely S, Rosenberg R, Spire JP, et al. 1987. HLA antigens in narcolepsy. *Neurology* 37:1858–1860.

Rechtschaffen A, Wolpert EA, Dement WC, et al. 1963. Nocturnal sleep of narcoleptics. *Electroencephalogr Clin Neurophysiol* 15:599–609.

Richardson G, Carskadon M, Flagg W, et al. 1978. Excessive daytime sleepiness in man: Multiple sleep measurement in narcolepsy and control subjects. *Electroencephalogr Clin Neurophysiol* 45: 621–637.

Rosenthal L, Merlotti L, Young D, et al. 1990. Subjective and polysomnographic characteristics of patients diagnosed with narcolepsy. *Gen Hosp Psychiatry* 12:191–197.

Rosenthal L, Roehrs TA, Hayashi H, et al. 1991. HLA-DR2 in narcolepsy with sleep-onset REM periods but no cataplexy. *Biol Psychiatry* 30:830–836.

Thorpy MJ (Chairman, Diagnostic Classification Steering Committee of the American Sleep Disorders Association). 1990. *The international classification of sleep disorders: Diagnostic and coding manual*. Lawrence, Kans.: Allen Press.

Vogel G. 1960. Studies in psychophysiology of dreams. III. The dream of narcolepsy. *Arch Gen Psychiatry* 3:421–428.

Yoss RE, Daly DD. 1957. Criteria for the diagnosis of the narcoleptic syndrome. *Mayo Clin Proc* 32: 320–328.

Leon D. Rosenthal

NARCOTICS

Narcotics are a class of drugs used to relieve pain and induce sleep. Morphine, codeine, and heroin are among the most well-known narcotics. They are classified as *opiates* because of their relationship to opium, a drug obtained from the juice of the opium poppy, *Papaver somniferum*. Opium has been used for various medical and recreational purposes. The ancient Greeks and Romans were aware of its pharmacological action as well as its sleep-inducing effects, but opium's addictive properties were first recognized in nineteenth-century England. Approximately twenty distinct opiate alkaloids are obtained from crude preparation of opium, including morphine, heroin (diacetylmorphine), codeine, hydromorphine, meperidine, and propoxyphene. Compounds such as naloxone, naltrexone, and nalorphine may be used to counteract the effects of opiates.

Opiate administration produces pain relief, changes in mood, sedation, and modification of digestive functions. These effects are largely the result of the drugs' interaction with specific *receptor* sites for opiates in the brain. Receptors are large glycoprotein molecules, spanning the thickness of a cell membrane, whose structure allows them very specifically to bind to certain compounds such as neurotransmitters or neuromodulators (see CHEMISTRY OF SLEEP). After the discovery of the brain's opiate receptors, the existence of an internal (endogenous) opiate factor was proposed. In 1974, the enkephalins—endogenous pentapeptides with opiatelike action—were identified. The enkephalins and another class of endogenous opiates called endorphins are involved in neural transmission in several neurobiological functions, including pain modulation.

One of the main effects of this group of drugs on the CENTRAL NERVOUS SYSTEM is sedation; indeed, morphine is named for Morpheus, the Greek god of dreams. Studies of sleep following acute administration of opiates have shown, however, that morphine produces an increase in wakefulness during the sleep period as well as an increase in the lighter stages of NREM sleep, whereas deep sleep (SLOW-WAVE SLEEP stages 3–4) is reduced, as is REM SLEEP. With chronic administration of morphine, adaptation or tolerance to the awakening effects develops, but REM sleep and slow-wave sleep remain reduced. The same findings have been reported for methadone, a synthetic opiate compound.

Endogenous opiates (enkephalins and endorphins) are thought to function as neurotransmitters or neuromodulators (see CHEMISTRY OF SLEEP: PEPTIDES). For that reason, the role of these substances in sleep mechanisms has been explored on the basis of the following premises: First, certain of them are known to have a sedative effect; second, all the endogenous peptides appear to be involved in sensory modulation and analgesia, which could be important in the onset of sleep; and third, endorphin concentration shows a circadian (approximately 24-hour) rhythm in brain tissue and cerebrospinal fluid in rats. Blocking the endogenous opiates' action with naloxone (a selective antagonist) is an experimental technique used to evaluate the possible role of these factors in sleep. Thus far, the main finding with this pharmacological manipulation has been an increase in REM LATENCY, that is, the time between the beginning of sleep and the first minute of REM sleep. It seems unlikely that endogenous opiates play a direct role in the regulation of sleep, but more work is needed before any firm conclusion can be drawn.

REFERENCES

Jaffe JH, Martin WR. 1985. Opiate analgesics and antagonists. In Gilman AG, Goodman LS, Rall TW, Murad F, eds. *The pharmacological basis of therapeutics,* pp 491–531. New York: Macmillan.

Kay DC, Eisenstein RB, Jasinski DR. 1969. Morphine effects on human REM state, waking state and NREM sleep. *Psychopharmacologia* 14:404–416.

Simon EJ, Hiller JM. 1989. Opiate peptides and opiate receptors. In Siegel G, Agranoff B, Albers RW, Molinoff P, eds. *Basic neurochemistry,* 4th ed, pp 271–285. New York: Raven.

Sitaram N, Gillin JC. 1982. The effect of naloxone on normal human sleep. *Brain Res* 244:387–392.

Rafael J. Salin-Pascual

NEED FOR SLEEP

[*The need for sleep is an individual function that varies across species and among individuals. Sleep need changes with age and maturational status as well (see* ADOLESCENCE; AGING AND SLEEP; CHILDHOOD, SLEEP DURING; INFANCY, NORMAL SLEEP PATTERNS IN; NORMAL SLEEP; ONTOGENY). *Questions about the* GENETICS OF SLEEP *have been illuminated by comparisons within and between species, which point to a biological source of sleep need. The* HERITABILITY OF SLEEP AND SLEEP DISORDERS *has also been demonstrated by studies in humans and in dogs with* CANINE NARCOLEPSY.

Another line of evidence based upon behavioral phenomena suggests that need for sleep may be related to personality factors (see PERSONALITY AND SLEEP*), though the direction of this relationship is unclear. Thus, one might ask, "Do people with type A personality have short sleep, or do short sleepers have type A personalities?" Many anecdotes and stories have de-*

scribed LONG SLEEPERS and SHORT SLEEPERS IN HISTORY AND LEGEND. Certainly, INDIVIDUAL DIFFERENCES in SLEEP LENGTH and in the TIMING OF SLEEP AND WAKEFULNESS occur, and it is not surprising that certain individuals with ultrashort or ultralong sleep needs do occur from time to time.

Across the human lifespan, if one considers the "typical" amount of sleep to be an indicator of the need for sleep, infancy is the time at which sleep need is highest. Children also have a higher sleep need than adults, and this sleep need may be manifested by the DEPTH OF SLEEP as well as by its length (see CHILDHOOD, SLEEP DURING). Across adolescence, the need for sleep does not seem to decline as had once been thought; in fact, adolescents appear to undergo an increase in sleep need during the pubertal years (see ADOLESCENCE AND SLEEP; PUBERTY).

The need for sleep is highlighted by the effects of sleep DEPRIVATION, either TOTAL or PARTIAL. Experiments in which rodents have been sleep deprived for many, many days have shown that without sleep, animals do not survive. In humans, sleep deprivation experiments show marked deterioration of behavioral functioning, including high levels of SLEEPINESS. Survival in sleep-deprived humans can be endangered through consequent behavioral problems that may impact on PUBLIC SAFETY IN THE WORKPLACE or PUBLIC SAFETY IN TRANSPORTATION.]

NEUROANATOMY

[As understanding of sleep state control progresses, researchers have been able to identify the locations and anatomical connections of the neurons controlling and being controlled by sleep. While the entire brain is involved in sleep generation, particular brain regions have been shown to be critical for various aspects of REM sleep, NREM sleep, and waking. These regions are discussed in the entries on REM SLEEP MECHANISMS AND NEUROANATOMY; NREM SLEEP MECHANISMS; BASAL FOREBRAIN; MEDULLA; PONS; MIDBRAIN; THALAMUS; LATERAL GENICULATE NUCLEUS; HYPOTHALAMUS; and SUPRACHIASMATIC NUCLEUS OF THE HYPOTHALAMUS. See THALAMUS for a figure depicting the midline of the human brain and indicating some of the brain regions implicated in sleep control. BRAIN MAPPING techniques have shown localized changes in brain activity with sleep. BRAIN TUMORS have effects on sleep and waking states that depend on the anatomical location of the tumors. Increasing knowledge about the brain chemistry of sleep (see CHEMISTRY OF SLEEP) allows scientists to determine the neurotransmitters in regions implicated in sleep control.]

NEUROENDOCRINE HORMONES

Neuroendocrinology has traditionally been defined as the study of the interaction between the central nervous system (CNS) and the endocrine system. Neuroendocrine hormones are the subset of hormones within the endocrine system that are directly under CNS control. It should be noted that the distinction between neurohormones and the rest of endocrinology is arbitrary; all hormonal systems are at least indirectly influenced by the CNS and thus, in a sense, all are neuroendocrine hormones (see ENDOCRINOLOGY). Nonetheless, when we consider the hormonal systems that are intimately controlled by the brain and, more specifically, hormonal systems with prominent modulation by sleep–wake state changes in the brain, a relatively well-defined subset of neuroendocrine hormones can be identified. By this definition, the neuroendocrine hormones consist of the secretory products of the anterior and posterior PITUITARY GLAND and the principal secretory product of the PINEAL GLAND, MELATONIN.

Secretory Products of the Anterior Pituitary Gland

The anterior pituitary gland secretes several neuroendocrine hormones that have diverse and extensive effects throughout the rest of the endocrine system. These hormones share a common functional organization; they are synthesized and released in response to specific stimulating factors released by the HYPOTHALAMUS that reach the anterior pituitary gland through a system of small blood vessels in the pituitary stalk. These hormones also share a general structure; they are all peptides (proteins) and, as such, each one consists of a unique sequence of amino acids.

In humans, secretion of the anterior pituitary hormones is prominently influenced by sleep–wake state, but the nature of the effect—inhibition or stimulation—varies from hormone to hormone and can vary with age and sex as well. Table 1 summarizes the anterior pituitary hormones and the known effect of sleep on their secretion.

Secretory Products of the Posterior Pituitary Gland

The posterior pituitary gland also secretes peptide hormones, but its functional organization is different from that of the anterior pituitary gland. The hormones of the posterior pituitary gland, oxytocin and vasopressin, are synthesized in the hypothalamus and then travel to the posterior pituitary gland via long axons of the hypothalamic neurons themselves. No intermediary secretory factors are involved as they are with the anterior pituitary hormones. Oxytocin is important in the production of milk in nursing mothers, and vasopressin controls the rate at which urine is produced. Although the secretion of these two hormones appears to vary with time of day (see CIRCADIAN RHYTHMS), it has not been possible to demonstrate a direct effect of sleep state on their secretory rate.

Melatonin and the Pineal Gland

Melatonin is secreted from the pineal gland under the control of the SUPRACHIASMATIC NUCLEUS OF THE HYPOTHALAMUS. Melatonin differs from the other neuroendocrine hormones in that it is a much smaller molecule, consisting of a single modified amino acid rather than a complete peptide. Although it has a prominent circadian rhythm, there is currently no evidence for a direct effect of sleep–wake state on its secretion or vice versa.

Table I. Neuroendocrine Hormones of the Anterior Pituitary

Name	Function	Effect of sleep
Adrenocorticotropic hormone	Stimulates the adrenal gland to release CORTISOL, a hormone with important effects on metabolism of carbohydrate, fat, and protein	Inhibition
GROWTH HORMONE	Stimulates skeletal and muscle growth	Stimulation (particularly by SLOW-WAVE SLEEP)
THYROID-STIMULATING HORMONE	Stimulates the thyroid gland to release thyroxine, a hormone with important effects on metabolic rate	Inhibition
PROLACTIN	Women: stimulates milk production in the breast; men: no known function	Stimulation
Luteinizing hormone and follicle-stimulating hormone (gonadotropic hormones)	Control production of sex steroid hormones and sperm/eggs by gonads	Puberty: stimulation; adult women: inhibition during the follicular phase of the menstrual cycle; adult men: no apparent effect

Other Neuroendocrine Hormones

In addition to the well-studied examples already mentioned, other putative neuroendocrine hormones have been described to varying degrees. For example, atrial natriuretic factor, a hormone released by the heart to control plasma salt concentration, has been found in the hypothalamus as well. Other peptides have been found in the anterior and posterior pituitary. While it may ultimately be shown that these are also neuroendocrine hormones, the evidence for this functional role is not yet available (*see* CHEMISTRY OF SLEEP: PEPTIDES).

REFERENCES

Martin JB, Reichlin S. 1987. *Clinical neuroendocrinology.* Philadelphia: Davis.

Mendelson WB. 1987. *Human sleep: Research and clinical care.* New York: Plenum.

Weitzman ED, Boyar RM, Kapen S, Hellman L. 1975. The relationship of sleep and sleep stages to neuroendocrine secretion and biological rhythms in man. *Recent Prog Horm Res* 31:399–446.

Gary S. Richardson

NEUROLOGIC DISORDERS

[*Neurologic disorders are typically divided into two large groups: those involving the* CENTRAL NERVOUS SYSTEM *(the brain and spinal cord) and those affecting the peripheral nervous system (the peripheral nerves and the connections between nerve and muscle). Within each group are extensive subclassifications and literally hundreds of specific diseases. Reviewing the relationship between each of these and sleep is not feasible; instead, the examination of a few specific diseases will illustrate the changes in sleep and wakefulness seen in patients with these disorders.*

Patients with NARCOLEPSY *are extremely sleepy, and most also suffer from* CATAPLEXY, *the abnormal occurrence of* REM SLEEP *paralysis during wakefulness, as well as* HYPNAGOGIC HALLUCINATIONS *and* SLEEP PARALYSIS; MICROSLEEP *epi-sodes probably contribute to other behavioral manifestations of narcolepsy such as* MEMORY lapses. *In* REM SLEEP BEHAVIOR DISORDER, *the* ATONIA *of REM sleep fails and motor activity occurs during REM sleep. Research using animal models for both of these disorders has provided important information about underlying mechanisms (see* ANIMALS IN SLEEP RESEARCH; CANINE NARCOLEPSY; REM SLEEP, PHYSIOLOGY OF). *In* PARKINSON'S DISEASE, *the discomfort associated with the disorder is clearly an important part of patients' sleep problems, but abnormalities of dopamine-dependent neuronal activity may also play a direct role in the sleep disruption. (See also* CHEMISTRY OF SLEEP: AMINES AND OTHER TRANSMITTERS.)

Disruption of sleep and of the normal sleep-wake cycle is a common feature in neurologic disorders of all kinds. Until more is known about the anatomy and physiology of sleep, identifying the link between damage to a specific part of the brain and a specific sleep disruption is not possible. For example, certain patients with HEAD INJURY *often have sleep disruption, but other patients with seemingly equivalent injuries may have no apparent sleep problems. In other cases, the link may be fairly nonspecific. For example, patients with certain headache syndromes often complain of difficulty sleeping, presumably as a consequence of the discomfort, while other headache syndromes are characterized by onset preferentially during sleep (see* HEADACHES, NOCTURNAL) *—this suggests an important relationship between sleep-related changes in neuronal activity and blood flow and the genesis of headache.*]

NEUROMODULATORS

See Chemistry of Sleep: Peptides; Chemistry of Sleep: Sleep Factors

NEUROPHYSIOLOGY

See NREM Sleep Mechanisms; REM Sleep Mechanisms and Neuroanatomy

NEUROTRANSMITTERS

See Chemistry of Sleep; NREM/REM Mechanisms; Pharmacology; Sleeping Pills

NICOTINE

Nicotine is an alkaloid (a family of organic bases found in plants) that is found mainly in tobacco. It is a water-soluble base and smells like tobacco when exposed to air. Nicotine is readily absorbed through the respiratory tract, the mucous membrane lining the mouth, and the skin. The absorption of nicotine from the lungs during cigarette smoking is almost as efficient as intravenous administration. Nicotine contained in cigarette smoke reaches the brain in 8 seconds. The half-life of nicotine following inhalation is about 1 hour, which may explain the periodic need to smoke. Nicotine is present in the breast milk of mothers who smoke, and this may adversely affect the nursing infant.

Nicotine produces arousal, increases alertness, and may facilitate memory. There is also an accompanying feeling of relaxation and reduced anxiety. Nicotine decreases appetite and irritability and stimulates the release of norepinephrine and epinephrine, which increase heart rate and blood pressure. Some of these factors may be reinforcing and this might explain why tobacco is used; however, nicotine is not as powerful a reinforcer as AMPHETAMINE or COCAINE.

Nicotine exerts its action via specific nicotine receptors, which are located on the terminals of nerves controlling skeletal muscles, on the autonomic ganglia, and in the central nervous system. The nicotinic receptor is a protein made up of five subunits. Two of the subunits are identical and are called alpha; the other three are called beta, gamma, and delta. Research on the nicotinic receptor has been facilitated by the discovery that large numbers of these receptors are found in the electricity-producing organs of the electric eel, *Electrophorus electricus,* and the ray, *Torpedo californica.* For instance, in the ray as many as 10,000 receptors are packed in a square micrometer. The venom from the deadly Formosan snake, *Bungarus multicinctus,* binds irreversibly with the nicotinic receptor, and the scientific use of this venom has contributed sig-

nificantly to our understanding of the nicotinic receptor. In the disease myasthenia gravis, the nicotinic receptor degenerates, and, as a result, muscles cannot contract. Individuals with this disease typically have droopy eyelids and reduced tone in other muscles.

In the brain, nicotinic receptors are found in the cerebral cortex, substantia nigra (an area in the midbrain), THALAMUS, neostriatum, and hippocampus (the neostriatum and hippocampus are parts of the forebrain). It is not known which brain area is associated with the addicting features of nicotine. The thalamic and cortical receptors are likely to be involved in the arousing effects that nicotine has on the ELECTROENCEPHALOGRAM. Smoking increases alpha and beta electroencephalographic activity, both of which are indicators of arousal. Smokers (consuming about one pack per day) typically have difficulty falling asleep. Nevertheless, chronic smoking does not adversely affect expression of the various sleep stages, including REM sleep. During abstinence from smoking, sleep onset occurs faster, and there is increased stage 4 sleep and REM sleep. Even though sleep recordings indicate that there is an improvement in sleep, smokers who have quit smoking initially complain of sleepiness because of the loss of the activating effects of nicotine during wakefulness.

In animals, nicotine significantly increases REM sleep. It has also been determined in animals that the nicotinic receptors in the lateral geniculate nucleus might be involved in triggering the ponto-geniculo-occipital (PGO) waves, which occur just before and during REM sleep (see LATERAL GENICULATE NUCLEUS; PGO waves). The lateral geniculate nucleus relays visual information into the cortex. The presence of these waves in this nucleus signifies the activation of visual pathways during REM sleep, which may denote the mental imagery occurring during dreams.

Nicotine withdrawal produces a well-characterized cluster of symptoms following cessation of smoking. These symptoms include irritability, restlessness, feeling sleepy, difficulty concentrating, dizziness, coughing, constipation, mouth sores, tightness in the chest, anxiety, difficulty concentrating, increased appetite and the ensuing weight gain, and decreased heart rate. These symptoms begin about 24 hours after the individual stops smoking, and they peak within the next 1 to 2 days. A gradual decline in severity of the symptoms is followed by a resurgence of the symptoms by about the tenth day of abstinence. Another peak is noted around the end of the third week. Heavy smokers (consuming about two packs per day) experience greater withdrawal symptoms. Smokers who receive nicotine-containing chewing gum experience fewer withdrawal symptoms; however, the individual should be weaned off the gum by the fifth week when the gum has no further effect on withdrawal symptoms.

REFERENCES

Cummings KM, Giovino G, Jaen CR, Emrich LJ. 1985. Reports of smoking withdrawal symptoms over a 21 day period of abstinence. *Addict Behav* 10: 373–381.

Gross J, Stitzer ML. 1989. Nicotine replacement: Ten-week effects on tobacco withdrawal symptoms. *Psychopharmacology* 98:334–341.

Soldatos CR, Kales JD, Scharf MB, Bixler EO, Kales A. 1980. Cigarette smoking associated with sleep difficulty. *Science* 207:551–553.

Priyattam J. Shiromani

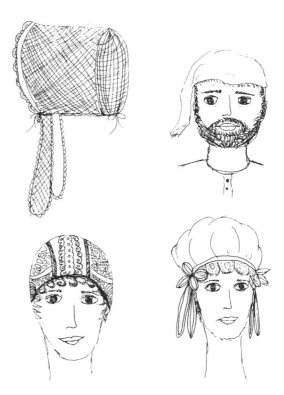

Figure 1. Clockwise from upper left: American woman's nightcap, ca. 1785; man's nightcap, ca. 1790; boudoir cap, ca. 1865; slumber helmet, ca. 1922. *Illustration by Katherine M. Sharkey.*

NIGHTCAPS

Throughout different historical periods, both men and women have gone to bed with their heads covered. This practice originated for a variety of reasons, including social mores and cosmetic purposes. For instance, during the 1700s, it was the custom among European men and women to wear elaborate wigs and hairpieces during the day. As a result, many had shaved heads or closely cropped hair that they covered with a cap to keep warm at night. Traditionally, men's nightcaps were pointed at the top and relatively plain. Women's nightcaps often tied at the chin and were adorned with a variety of ribbons and bows. In most cases, the nightcaps were washable and most people owned more than one. During the eighteenth and nineteenth centuries, women in America and Europe had special nightcaps for bridal and mourning wear. When Indian clothing began to exert a strong influence on European fashions during the early 1800s, both men and women wore turbans to bed (see PAJAMAS AND NIGHTWEAR). In the 1920s, the most chic ladies had their hair styled short with curls all over their heads. In an effort to keep her coiffure intact overnight, a "flapper" would don a close-fitting, richly decorated "slumber helmet" to protect her hairdo.

To some people, a "nightcap" is an alcoholic drink taken before bed. Although ingesting alcohol might relax a person temporarily, it is known that alcohol disrupts sleep and that drinking large quantities of alcohol before bedtime is not conducive to restful sleep (see ALCOHOL).

REFERENCES

Earle AM. 1903. *Two centuries of costume in America.* New York: Macmillan.

Holliday RC. 1933. *Unmentionables: From figleaves to scanties.* New York: Ray Long & Richard R. Smith.

Jackson S. 1978. *Costumes for the stage.* New York: EP Dutton.

Payne B. 1965. *History of costume—From the ancient Egyptians to the twentieth century.* New York: Harper & Row.

Yarwood D. 1978. *The encyclopedia of world costume.* New York: Charles Scribner's Sons.

Katherine M. Sharkey

NIGHTMARES

The term *nightmare* is used by the general public in at least three senses. Some use the term to mean "a frightening dream"; some use it to mean simply "waking up frightened at night," whether or not there is any dream; and finally, the term has sometimes been used to refer to the fearful "demon" or "creature" that supposedly produces the awakening as in "the nightmare in my closet." Sleep laboratory research of the last 25 years has greatly clarified the situation, although not much scientific light has been shed on the third sense of nightmare: the closet generally turns out to be empty.

Nightmares Versus Night Terrors

When someone who describes having nightmares is studied in the sleep laboratory, one of the following two situations is almost inevitably found when an episode occurs during that night. In the more common type, there is an awakening during the second half of sleep, from a long REM period usually at least 15 minutes in length. Physiologically, the REM period may show more eye movements than usual and perhaps a small increase in pulse and respiratory rate, but nothing very unusual. The subject lies quietly in bed; does not move or get up; and when he or she awakens, a long frightening dream is reported. This dream is commonly a detailed vivid dream that becomes more frightening as it goes on and ends at the most terrifying point, when the dreamer is being hurt, attacked, killed, or something of the kind. This sort of nightmare event is clearly a dream, and like most dreams it is reported from a REM period.

The other sort of event, less common, usually occurs within the first 2 hours after sleep onset. It involves an unusual kind of arousal from sleep. The sleeper is usually in stage 3 or 4 NREM sleep and wakes up over a period of 15 to 30 seconds during which the pulse and respiratory rate may double, and there is a great deal of activity, which may include screaming, sitting up, or even sleepwalking. The subject wakes up terrified, but either remembers nothing or remembers a single image such as "something was crushing me." The experience is *not* described as a dream.

This second sort of experience, sometimes loosely called nightmare, is now designated as a night terror or sleep terror (see SLEEP TERRORS). The first sort of episode is what we refer to as the *nightmare*. It is sometimes called a *REM-nightmare*, because it occurs in REM sleep, and sometimes a *dream anxiety attack*. Night terrors and nightmares are very different phenomena. They are experienced differently: The nightmare is a dream; the night terror is not. As we have seen, they are different in terms of physiology. And generally, they are experienced by different people (see below).

Most, though not all, nightmare experiences fall into these two groups. Occasionally someone has a nightmare at sleep onset during the transition from waking to NREM sleep. And posttraumatic nightmares (see POSTTRAUMATIC STRESS DISORDER) are unusual in that although they appear to be dreams, they occur in NREM sleep as well as in REM sleep.

Definition and Content of Nightmares

Thus, as the term is currently used, a nightmare is a frightening dream during REM sleep from which the dreamer awakens. It is almost always a long, vivid, detailed dream. This is the best definition available at present, although logically it is not entirely precise. For instance, if someone describes a particular nightmare that seems to wake him or her up a couple of times during the night, and then says on another occasion he or she remembers having had the same nightmare but it did not awaken him or her, the definition requires one to say the last event was not a nightmare. Commonsense suggests it was the same thing, but perhaps a bit less severe.

Although the nightmare can be differentiated from the night terror, the nightmare cannot be differentiated from a dream. The nightmare is a specific sort of dream.

The content of a nightmare may include any

number of actions or events frightening to the dreamer. Occasionally the material may not sound frightening to an impartial observer, for example, "a long shadow that felt ominous." However, the most common content involves the dreamer being chased, threatened, hurt, or attacked in some way; simply being chased is the most common nightmare theme. In childhood, the perpetrator who chases or hurts the dreamer is often a wild animal or a monster; in adults it is more frequently a threatening man, a group of people, or a gang.

In almost all cases, the dreamer is the victim—the person being chased or attacked. It is relatively rare for the dreamer to commit violence or simply to watch a violent dangerous scene. One major exception occurs in the case of parents, usually mothers, of young children; the victim in the nightmare is frequently the dreamer's child rather than the dreamer herself: "I dreamt that someone broke into the house and was attacking my child." A pregnant woman will often have a nightmare that something bad is happening to her developing fetus—that she will give birth to a deformed child. Apart from these situations, we are usually concerned with ourselves and our own safety and not for that of others in our nightmares.

Who Has Nightmares?

Almost everyone has nightmares. At least in childhood—especially during the ages 3 to 6 years—nightmares are very frequent. There is some disagreement as to what percentage of children report nightmares. The percentage is lower for instance when one speaks of children whose nightmares are reported to their pediatricians, but much higher when one speaks directly to children or to sensitive parents. It is likely that almost all children aged 3 to 6 years experience at least a few nightmares. Nightmares become less frequent with age; however, they are by no means rare. Studies suggest that the average college student experiences four to eight nightmares per year, and the average adult aged 25 years or older may have one or two per year.

A small percentage of adults—less than 5 percent—report frequent nightmares (generally defined as one or more per week over long periods). Who are these people who report hav-

ing nightmares regularly or all the time? Recent studies have compared groups of frequent nightmare sufferers with various control groups. The nightmare group could not be described as simply sicker (more mentally ill) or even as more anxious, nor did most of them describe especially traumatic childhoods.

What did characterize the nightmare sufferers and separate them from the control groups was a number of characteristics that can be summarized as their having "thin boundaries" in many senses. First, they were unusually open. They told the interviewers far more about their lives than is usual in such interviews. They were interpersonally open in terms of getting into relationships very quickly. They seemed unprotected or undefended; everything "got to them." They were easily hurt and would remember for a long time the suffering of an animal for instance. Many of them described themselves as having been sensitive in several respects for their whole lives: sensitive to bright lights or loud sounds, sensitive emotionally, and also empathic to the feelings of others. Mostly, they tended to have been artistic and creative in some way since childhood. Most of these people with nightmares had jobs relating somehow to the arts or crafts, rather than ordinary blue collar or white collar positions. They also had thin boundaries between fantasy and reality, often describing fantasies or daydreams so real and vivid as to be difficult to distinguish from waking reality. Likewise, they described in-between states when they were not certain whether they were awake or asleep and dreaming. They would describe waking up after a dream but not being really sure they were awake for one-half hour or more. Most of them also had thin boundaries in such senses as sexual identification: They were very willing to recognize both masculine and feminine aspects of themselves, and they could easily imagine themselves as a member of the opposite sex. Some of them even described vivid daydreams, as well as night dreams in which they were someone of the opposite sex or in which they were animals.

In general, the best way to describe frequent nightmare sufferers psychologically seemed to be that they had thin boundaries in many senses; and in fact this was confirmed by findings on the Rorschach test. On this well-known inkblot test, the subjects with nightmares saw a great many more permeable, gauzy, amorphous, or torn things than did control subjects.

When Do Nightmares Occur? What Causes Nightmares?

Whether people ordinarily have frequent or infrequent nightmares, they report more nightmares and worse nightmares at times of change and stress. Almost any kind of stress appears sometimes to produce an increase in nightmare frequency and nightmare intensity; this is especially true of stresses such as the loss of an important person, the loss of a relationship, or a major change of occupation. Periods of great anxiety, such as the beginning of a psychotic episode, are also often associated with nightmares. It is likely that each of us has specific stressful situations that may be nightmare producing for us, though perhaps not for others. These appear to be situations that remind us of our childhood vulnerability, when we were all small and to a great degree helpless (and when most of us did in fact have nightmares).

Overall, then, there is no single cause of nightmares. It appears that a certain type of personality ("thin boundaries") may be predisposed to nightmares; stressful situations definitely increase nightmares; extremely stressful occurrences known as trauma can definitely produce nightmares (see POSTTRAUMATIC NIGHTMARES); also, certain neurologic conditions and some medications produce a sudden onset of nightmares in people who have not previously had them. Research data do not support older views that suffocation under blankets causes nightmares, nor the view that spicy foods frequently produce nightmares ("the pepperoni pizza theory"; see MYTHS ABOUT DREAMING).

Interpretation

Nightmares, like all other dreams, come from the mind of the dreamer and in some way refer to the dreamer's memories, problems, wishes, and fears. Thus, nightmares like any other dreams can be "interpreted" in the sense that connections with one's life can be examined and a better understanding of oneself obtained. Although one cannot generalize because everyone is different, associations to the content of the nightmare often lead to something in the adult's life that reminds him or her of a childhood experience and childhood helplessness. (*See also* INTERPRETATION OF DREAMS.)

Treatment

Nightmares should not be considered an illness that in itself requires treatment. In groups of people who experienced frequent nightmares, it was found that only about one-half actually wanted treatment and wanted to reduce the nightmares; many felt the nightmares were somehow a part of them and were perhaps useful; in fact, writers, painters, and other artists often use their nightmares in their work. When nightmares are very disturbing and treatment is desired, a number of treatments can be helpful. Psychotherapy of one kind or another is the most frequent treatment. There are also behavioral techniques, and techniques involving imagery and hypnosis can reduce nightmares. In serious cases, a number of medications can be useful. A person with frequent disturbing nightmares, however, first needs a detailed evaluation. The nightmares themselves may not require treatment, but at times they may be part of another condition, such as a neurologic illness, a psychosis, or post-traumatic stress disorder, which definitely requires treatment.

REFERENCES

Hartmann E. 1984. *The nightmare.* New York: Basic Books.
———. 1987. Who has nightmares? *Arch Gen Psychiatry* 44:49–56.
———. 1991. Boundaries in the mind. New York: Basic Books.

Ernest Hartmann

NIGHT OWLS

See Early Birds and Night Owls; Morningness/Eveningness

NIGHT SWEATS

> Amidst painful oppression of the stomach, the whole body was suffused with a fetid perspiration. . . .

This description portrays how the English described sweating that occurred in persons suffering from what was termed plague or "sweating sickness" during the sixteenth century.

Sweating, in and of itself, is considered a second line of defense and is called on only when the variations in the initial vasomotor system are insufficient to prevent a rise in core body temperature. Sweating is recognized as an active heat-dissipating mechanism. Local sweating has been described in waking humans as a function of both internal and mean skin temperatures, as well as local skin temperature. Psychogenic sweating is sweating that is brought on by an emotional/psychological cause, for example, anxiety, fear, and excitement.

Night sweats (sleep hyperhidrosis) are characterized by excessive sweating that occurs during sleep. Individuals with nights sweats may or may not have a similar problem during the day. This condition can be lifelong or limited to a short duration. Night sweats are categorized as acute (1 month or less), subacute (1 to 6 months), or chronic (6 months or longer).

Night sweats can cause a person to wake from sleep, usually because of the dampened nightwear or, in more severe cases, drenched bed sheets.

During the last two decades, the causes of fluctuations in body temperatures and subsequent episodes of sweating during daytime naps and during the night have been studied extensively. During afternoon naps, an increase in sweating and vasodilation has been observed.

There have been several explanations for the changes in sweat rate throughout the night. At neutral to warm ambient temperature, the sweat rate of humans increases at the onset of slow-wave sleep (SWS), but is severely depressed during REM sleep. The increase in sweat rate in association with the deepening of electroencephalographic sleep stage during daytime sleep may be attributed to the release of hypothalamic activity from cortical inhibition. During night sleep, reduction of the activity of the hypothalamus and reduction of metabolic heat rate production occur as sleep deepens, causing a gradual decrease in sweat rate. The subsiding trend of sweat rate as sleep progresses has been found to be independent of sleep depth. Little is known about the associated changes occurring in the central thermoregulatory system.

Nocturnal sleep is associated with a lowering of body temperature in normal individuals. In humans, the skin temperature increases in the first hour of sleep. The association of sweating with sleep suggests that reduction in body temperature during the night may in fact be a regulated response. (See THERMOREGULATION for further information).

Studies have revealed that although, in general, psychogenic sweating is absent during sleep it may appear during REM sleep. In this case psychogenic sweating is thought to be associated with dreams accompanied by emotional excitement, as well as a manifestation of the arousal response during sleep. In such studies, sweating only appeared during REM sleep *with dream recall*.

Night sweats are due most often to a chronic or febrile disorder but, in some patients, may indicate an underlying autonomic disease. They are most commonly seen in early adulthood, but can occur at any age. Night sweats may occur as the primary or secondary symptom of several clinical disorders. The most common include diabetes insipidus; hypoglycemia (associated with diabetes mellitus); hyperthyroidism, nocturnal hot flushes (or flashes) of menopause; infectious diseases and viral syndromes such as tuberculosis, AIDS, influenza, and chronic fatigue syndrome (also referred to as chronic Epstein-Barr virus); Hodgkin's disease; and obstructive sleep apnea (from anecdotal reports and observations in over 60 percent of patients with this disorder, though no controlled studies have been performed; the sweating is presumably associated with autonomic disturbance).

Night sweats have also been reported in the following medical conditions: nocturnal esophageal reflux, pheochromocytoma, hypothalamic lesions, epilepsy, cerebral and brainstem strokes, cerebral palsy, chronic paroxysmal hemicrania, spinal cord infarction, HEAD INJURY, typhus, brucellosis, plague, and familial dysautonomia. Night sweats can occur in pregnancy and can also be caused by antipyretic (temperature-lowering) medications.

REFERENCES

Davison WC. 1960. Sweating sickness. *Am J Dis Child* 100:934.

Diagnostic Classification Steering Committee, Thorpy MJ, Chairman. 1990. pp 293–295. *ICSD— The international classification of sleep disorders: Diagnostic and coding manual.* Rochester, MN: American Sleep Disorders Association.

Geschickter EH, Andrews PA, Bullard RW. 1966. Nocturnal body temperature regulation in man: A rationale for sweating in sleep. *J Appl Physiol* 21(2):623–630.

Gobbi PG, Pieresca C, Ricciardi L, Vacchi S, Bertoloni D, Rossi A, Grignani G, Rutigliano L, Ascari E. 1990. Night sweats in Hodgkin's disease: A manifestation of preceding minor febrile pulses. *Cancer* 65:2074–2077.

Henane R, Buguet A, Roussel B, Bittel J. 1977. Variations in evaporation and body temperatures during sleep in man. *J Appl Physiol* 42(1):50–55.

Ogata K, Sasaki T. 1963. On the causes of diurnal body temperature rhythm in man. *Jpn J Physiol* 13:84–96.

Ogawa T, Satoh T, Takagi K. 1967. Sweating during night sleep. *Jpn J Physiol* 17:135–148.

Quinton PM. 1983. Sweating and its disorders. *Annu Rev Med* 34:429–452.

Reynolds WA. 1989. Are night sweats a sign of esophageal reflux? *J Clin Gastroenterol* 2(5):590–591.

Sagot JC, Amoros C, Candas V, Libert JP. 1987. Sweating responses and body temperatures during nocturnal sleep in humans. *Am J Physiol* 252: R462–R470.

Silbert PL. 1989. Diabetes mellitus, AIDS and night sweats. *Lancet,* November 25, p 1285.

Suzan E. Norman

NIGHT TERRORS

See Parasomnias; Sleep Terrors

NIGHT WAKING IN INFANCY

Night waking is usually defined as full arousal from sleep with awareness and responsiveness to the environment. These characteristics are essential to distinguish normal night waking from other nocturnal phenomena such as NIGHTMARES or SLEEP TERRORS.

Night wakings may result from internal stimuli (that is, sensations originating in the body or brain) or external stimuli from the environment. Internal stimuli include sensations such as hunger, thirst, pain, and bladder pressure (the need to urinate). External stimuli include temperature, noise, aversive smells, and so forth. Everyone is familiar with some of these experiences leading to an occasional night waking. In infancy, however, night wakings are very common and frequent. Surveys on infant sleep show that night waking is a very prevalent problem, reported by 20 to 30 percent of parents of young children (Richman, 1987). One of the crucial aspects of night waking in infancy is that it becomes a very disruptive factor in family life: Very often parents are the primary "victims," whereas the child seems to suffer no adverse effects.

There are different ways to understand why night wakings are frequent in early childhood. Newborn babies' sleep is very different from that in older children or adults, divided into a few, relatively short (4- to 5-hour) periods distributed throughout day and night. The shift to a more consolidated, prolonged major sleep episode during the nighttime is a gradual process that most babies achieve within their first year of life (see INFANCY, NORMAL SLEEP PATTERNS IN). In many cases, however, these changes are not accomplished easily, and the infant continues to wake up several times during the night, posing a serious problem to his exhausted parents.

In addition to the general developmental aspect of night wakings, there are a few special physiological causes. COLIC, for instance, is a condition that may cause great distress to babies and disrupt their sleep in their early months of life. Allergies (see MILK ALLERGY AND INFANT SLEEP), teething, ear infection, and even common colds or stuffed noses increase the likelihood of night wakings. In the emotional domain, night wakings have been associated with fears and ANXIETY. The most common anxiety in early childhood is that of separation. Going to sleep in the dark, usually separated from the parents and, in many cases, alone without siblings sharing the room, may be experienced as very frightening by a young child whose sense of security greatly depends upon the parents. It is not unusual to see infants wake up often during the night and check for their parents' presence (see CO-SLEEPING). Another way to view night waking is as a learned response associated with specific reinforcing behaviors, such as breast feeding, drinking, rocking, and soothing (Ferber, 1985). It has been shown that infants who fall asleep with such reinforcers tend to wake up more often, and once they wake up they tend to demand the same reinforcer, therefore requiring parental involvement in order to go back to sleep (Adair et al., 1991).

Night waking, however, does not necessarily entail parental intervention. In fact, studies of infant sleep using objective methods such as home video recordings or activity monitors revealed that many infants wake up during the night and resume their sleep without help; thus, parents often remain unaware of the fact that their infants do wake up (Anders, 1978; Sadeh et al., 1991). Although night wakings tend to decrease over time, the problem may persist for a long time and cause much distress to the child and the family (Zuckerman, Stevenson, and Baily, 1987). Studies have shown that counseling for parents regarding their bedtime interactions with the child can effectively reduce night waking in most babies (see INFANCY, SLEEP DISORDERS IN). Nevertheless, research has also shown that infants who tend to be night wakers share some vulnerability or set of characteristics that may be temperamental or physiological in nature (Carey, 1974).

REFERENCES

Adair R, Bauchner H, Philipp B, Levenson S, Zuckerman B. 1991. Night waking during infancy: Role of parental presence at bedtime. *Pediatrics* 87(4):500–504.

Anders T. 1978. Home recorded sleep in two and nine month old infants. *J Acad Child Psychiatry* 17: 421–432.

Carey WB. 1974. Night waking and temperament in infancy. *J Pediatrics* 84:756–758.

Ferber R. 1985. *Solve your child's sleep problems.* New York: Simon & Schuster.

Richman N. 1987. Surveys of sleep disorders in children in the general population. In Guilleminault C, ed, *Sleep and its disorders in children.* New York: Raven Press.

Sadeh A, Lavie P, Scher A, Tirosh E, Epstein R. 1991. Actigraphic home-monitoring of sleep-disturbed and control infants and young children: A new method for pediatric assessment of sleep-wake patterns. *Pediatrics* 87(4):494–499.

Zuckerman B, Stevenson J, Baily V. 1987. Sleep problems in early childhood: Continuities, predictive factors, and behavioral correlates. *Pediatrics* 80: 664–671.

Avi Sadeh

NOCTURNAL EMISSION

See Sexual Activation

NOCTURNAL PENILE TUMESCENCE

Nocturnal penile tumescence (NPT) is the cyclic, repetitive pattern of sleep-related ERECTIONS that occur in virtually all men who are sexually potent. The sleep erection cycle was first observed by Ohlmeyer in 1936; however, the close association between REM sleep and nocturnal erections was not systematically documented until 1965. Working independently, research groups led by Charles Fisher and Ismet Karacan confirmed the previous speculation that sleep-related erections occurred predominantly during REM sleep. Figure 1 illustrates the relationship between sleep stages and penile circumference increase in a normal male volunteer subject.

Typically, sleep erections are recorded using mercury-filled strain gauges placed around the penis. During an erection, penile circumference increases, causing the column of mercury to become longer and thinner, thus increasing the electrical resistance. This change is transduced to voltage and recorded polygraphically, usually in conjunction with brain electroencephalographic (EEG) activity, eye movements, muscle activity, and breathing. The standard measures, therefore, are based on changes in the girth, not the length, of the penis.

As with other physiological events, sleep-related tumescence can be quantified in terms of frequency, magnitude, and duration. The architecture of a tumescence episode is characterized by the durations of the three phases of erectile activity: the ascending phase (T-up), the plateau at maximum tumescence (T-max), and detumescence (T-down). Further quantification can index the coordination of erections with REM

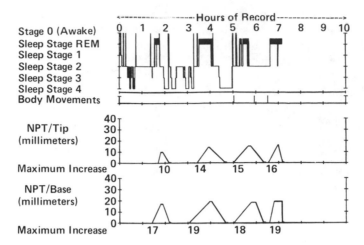

Figure 1.   Sleep stages and sleep-related erections recorded from the penile base (NPT/BASE) and the coronal sulcus (NPT/TIP). This figure illustrates a normal erectile pattern recorded from a 43-year-old, sexually potent Caucasian man who voluntarily participated in a research project.

sleep, the number of minutes of simultaneous REM sleep and tumescences, and the penile rigidity. Rigidity is measured by awakening the individual during a representative erection and applying a force to the tip of the penis until the shaft bends (or until some predetermined maximum is reached, e.g., 1,000 grams). This measure of axial rigidity is sometimes called buckling resistance.

Sleep-related erectile activity may decline slightly with advancing age; however, in the absence of significant neurogenic or vasculogenic diseases, the nocturnal tumescence cycle persists into old age. Established and replicated normative data are available; consequently, the recording of nocturnal penile tumescence is considered by many the "gold standard" for indexing erectile capacity. (For further discussion of the relationship between sleep-related erections and sexual potency, see SEXUAL ACTIVATION; SEX AND SLEEP; ERECTIONS; ERECTILE DYSFUNCTION.)

REFERENCES

Karacan I. 1982. Evaluation of nocturnal penile tumescence and impotence. In Guilleminault C, ed. *Sleeping and waking disorders: Indications and techniques.* Menlo Park, Calif.: Addison-Wesley.
Ware JC. 1989. Monitoring erections during sleep. In Kryger M, Roth T, Dement WC, eds. *Principles and practice of sleep medicine,* chap 75, pp 689–695. Philadelphia: WB Saunders.

Max Hirshkowitz

NOISE

Noise, defined most simply as unwanted sound, has been described as the most ubiquitous pollutant of the industrial world. Although noise predates civilization (people dwelling in the vicinity of large waterfalls may lose some hearing ability), it is in cities such as ancient Rome that noise first became a social problem requiring ordinances to control it, especially at night. In present-day industrial societies, noise originates from diverse sources ranging from highways, airports, and industrial plants to sleeping environments such as hospitals and apartment buildings. These sources commonly continue to generate noise at night and are likely to interfere with sleep.

Surveys show that about 7 percent of the residents of modern cities report sleeping difficulty that they attribute primarily to nighttime traffic noise. In the environs of airports, 60 percent of the residents may complain. Even when they are not sleeping or attempting to sleep, people expect not to be disturbed at night, and current governmental standards of noise measurement therefore more heavily weight noise occurring from 10:00 P.M. to 7:00 A.M.

Laboratory experiments have quantified the effects on sleep of road traffic, jet aircraft booms, and other kinds of noise. Noise may cause delay of sleep onset, awakenings from sleep, changes in sleep stages, delayed return to sleep, or premature awakening in the morning.

Two major effects on sleep have usually been reported: awakenings and shifts of sleep stage from deeper levels of sleep (stages 3 and 4) to lighter ones (stages 1 and 2). Whether such effects occur depends not only on the loudness of noise but also its pattern. Intermittent noises have greater effects than continuous ones, and the peak noise level more strongly determines how sleep is disturbed than do background levels.

Because sleep disturbances short of full awakening may occur, sleep disturbances related to noise may be even more common than surveys indicate. Both the overt disturbances of sleep and the subtle ones of which the sleeper is not aware may contribute to impaired performance on tasks the next day, impaired memory, and irritability.

Associated with changes in sleep are increases in heart rate and blood flow, as well as changes in sweating, breathing, and body movement. Such effects of noise may be greater during sleep than wakefulness, even when the noise is less intense.

Noise disturbs sleep by activating a specialized system of brain cells and fibers (the reticular activating system) that sample sounds and smells and interrupt sleep when meaningful events are detected. The system stops responding to repeated stimuli, which are unlikely to signify events requiring the sleeper to respond (habituation). Environmental noise has been found to lose its ability to disturb sleep over about 7 nights. Unfortunately, not all types of noise lose their effects on sleep; cannon shots originating from military bases, for example, do not. Furthermore, the complaints of long-time residents of noisy environments show that common traffic noise does not always lose its ability to disturb sleep. Thus, double glazing of apartment windows has improved both the sleep and the next-day performance ability of long-term residents. Changes in heart rate also do not necessarily habituate, and it is conceivable that such persistent effects of noise of which the sleeper is usually unaware could eventually impair health.

The same surveys that demonstrate the wide-spread effects of noise on sleep also show that large fractions of populations living or working in noisy environments report sleeping "very or extremely well." The worst effects of noise are therefore confined to certain groups or individuals. Elderly people, for example, are more susceptible to the effects of noise, even though the elderly are less likely to complain. Children are not immune to the effects of noise in the environs of schools, and noise may even affect the unborn fetuses of women living near airports. Also at risk are patients in noisy hospitals, as well as shift-workers, who must sleep in the daytime when traffic and industrial noises are maximal. Sensitivity to noise is also a trait of certain individuals, including those with INSOMNIA.

In conclusion, noise affects sleep in ways that are both apparent to the sleeper (delay in falling asleep, interruptions of sleep) and invisible (shifts toward lighter sleep and changes in heart rate, circulation, and breathing during sleep). There may be immediate effects on alertness, performance, and mood the next day as well as long-term effects on health. Combating the effects of noise requires not only regulation of noise sources but also the construction of quiet working and living environments and detection of individuals (including those with sleep disorders) who are susceptible to the effects of noise.

REFERENCES

Kryter KD. 1985. *The effects of noise on man,* 2nd ed. Orlando, Fla: Academic Press. The major general reference work in the field of noise.

Pollak CP. 1991. The effects of noise on sleep. In Fay T, ed. *Noise and health,* pp 41–60. New York: New York Academy of Medicine. Includes 101 references.

Charles P. Pollak

NONRESTORATIVE SLEEP

One of the theories about the function of sleep is that sleep permits the body and mind to recover from the wear and tear of wakefulness. The alternative, that sleep may be nonrestorative, is derived from the experience of awakening from sleep feeling physically and mentally unrefreshed. This experience may occur from time to time in healthy people or may be persistent in those with chronic sleep difficulties and ill health.

Nonrestorative sleep is usually light or restless as opposed to deep, quiet, undisturbed, and restful. With such light sleep, there may be awareness of any slight noise, many thoughts, or considerable dreaming. Such sleep is undesirable because, on awakening, there is an unpleasant sensation of physical exhaustion, often accompanied by generalized aching or stiffness, an inability to concentrate or think clearly, and an irritable or depressed mood. There may also be a sense of sleepiness, but usually not an irresistible urge to sleep. The poor quality of sleep is unrelated to its duration or its timing during a particular 24-hour period. Thus, unrefreshing sleep may follow a 15-minute afternoon nap or an overnight 8-hour sleep. By contrast, a normal daytime nap or overnight sleep of similar duration is typically quite restful. On arising from such sleeps, the person feels free of any discomfort and is energetic, alert, and in a good mood.

Nonrestorative sleep is usually experienced in a sleep-disturbing environment: The bed is uncomfortable and sleep is disrupted by noise, excessive heat, or cold. Consumption of stimulating substances (e.g., coffee, tea, chocolate, colas, nicotine), alcoholic beverages, or drugs that disturb sleep may result in feeling unrefreshed and miserable in the morning. Poor quality of sleep may occur with primary sleep disorders, such as sleep APNEA and periodic involuntary limb movements. Fever, as the result of bacterial or viral illnesses, is typically accompanied by unrefreshing sleep. Nonrestorative sleep can also occur with painful injuries or diseases and during periods of emotional distress as a result of worry or depression. Nonrestorative sleep is a feature of fibromyalgia (Wolfe et al., 1990) and CHRONIC FATIGUE SYNDROME (Moldofsky, 1990). With such chronic illnesses, people typically report light or restless sleep. They are vigilant even while asleep and rarely feel refreshed on awakening in the morning. The generalized aching, chronic fatigue, and unrefreshing sleep of patients with fibromyalgia may follow a motor vehicle accident or a physically noninjurious, but frightening industrial accident. Sometimes fibromyalgia, like chronic fatigue syndrome, follows a febrile illness (Moldofsky, 1990).

The electrophysiology of nonrestorative sleep in patients with fibromyalgia or chronic fatigue syndrome is characterized by an alpha rhythm (7.5 to 11 Hz) electroencephalographic (EEG) sleep anomaly during NREM sleep. Alpha rhythm normally occurs during quiet wakefulness and disappears with onset to EEG sleep. (see ALPHA RHYTHM). External stimulations that are used experimentally to induce arousals during sleep are accompanied by the alpha frequency. Initially, the term *alpha–delta sleep* was used to characterize a mixture of the faster alpha activity with the slower delta frequency (0.5 to 2.0 cycles per second) of slow-wave (stages 3 and 4) sleep that was found in some ill patients who described symptoms of malaise and fatigue. The alpha frequency is not confined to slow-wave sleep, however, but may also occur during stage 2, as well as stages 3 and 4 of NREM sleep (see ALPHA–DELTA SLEEP). The terms *alpha EEG NREM sleep* and *alpha EEG sleep* are more precise.

This EEG sleep anomaly occurs in 15 percent of healthy women and their female family members, and it is thought to indicate reduced depth of sleep. In patients with fibromyalgia, approximately 60 percent of NREM sleep is occupied by alpha EEG sleep. This atypical sleep EEG pattern and nonrestorative sleep symptoms have been artificially induced by noise disruption of stage 4 sleep in healthy sedentary people. Similarly, the disturbed restless sleep that accompanies the inflamed painful joints, morning stiffness, and fatigue of rheumatoid arthritis shows this alpha EEG anomaly. Assessment of daytime sleepiness with a series of 20-minute naps at 2-hour intervals (*see* MULTIPLE SLEEP LATENCY TEST) does not show an early onset to EEG sleep in patients with fibromyalgia or chronic fatigue syndrome.

Nonrestorative sleep symptoms that result from environmental disturbances and primary sleep disorders, such as sleep apnea and periodic limb movements, respond to interventions that ameliorate the identified sleep problem. In some patients with fibromyalgia, the drugs amitriptyline and cyclobenzaprine improve the unrefreshing sleep, as well as the pain, fatigue, and mood symptoms.

REFERENCES

Moldofsky H. 1990. The contribution of sleep–wake physiology to fibromyalgia. In Fricton JR, Awad E, eds. *Advances in pain research and therapy,* Vol. 17, pp. 227–240. New York: Raven Press.

Wolfe F, Smythe HA, Yunus MB, Bennett R, Bombardier C, Goldenberg D, et al. 1990.

Harvey Moldofsky

NON-24-HOUR SLEEP SCHEDULE

See Hypernychthemeral Syndrome

NORADRENALINE

See Chemistry of Sleep: Amines and Other Transmitters; Stimulants

NORMAL SLEEP

Describing "normal" sleep is difficult because sleep is a very dynamic and complex behavior. For example, normal sleep in infants is very different from normal sleep in children, adults, or elderly individuals (see INFANCY, NORMAL SLEEP PATTERNS IN; AGING AND SLEEP). Nevertheless, there are certain commonalities that may be used as a model for a normal night of human sleep.

Sensory processing is reduced during sleep, as is cognitive activity (*see* COGNITION; SENSORY PROCESSING AND SENSATION DURING SLEEP); and yet, the state of sleep is fairly easily reversed. Thus, sensory input of sufficient intensity will wake a sleeping person. One might therefore define sleep as a reversible behavioral state of reduced response to and reduced interaction with the environment. Humans evolved to sleep in the night, and the typical human sleeps while lying down with closed eyes. Different species may sleep in daylight and have quite varied specific postures for sleeping. In humans, sleep can occasionally occur while sitting or even standing. (For an electrophysiological description of normal sleep, see STAGES OF SLEEP; REM SLEEP; POLYSOMNOGRAPHY.)

Figure 1 illustrates the pattern of a normal night of sleep for a healthy 17-year-old who sleeps on a regular schedule. This figure is called a sleep hypnogram and illustrates stages of NREM sleep and REM sleep (vertical axis) as they occur over time (horizontal axis). When a teenager falls asleep, several moments of NREM stage 1 sleep occur, followed by a transition to stage 2 sleep, which may last for 5 to 15 minutes. Stage 3 sleep will appear briefly thereafter, to be followed by a relatively long episode of very deep stage 4 sleep, which may last for 20 to 40 minutes. At some point, the brain signals a change in the sleep pattern, and if we were watching our sleeping teen-

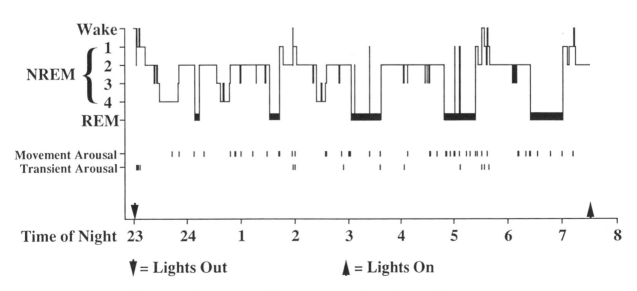

Figure 1. Hypnogram of normal night's sleep in a healthy teenager.

ager, we would see a number of body movements and a change on the ELECTROENCEPHALOGRAM to stage 2 sleep. This stage 2 sleep may last for 10 to 15 minutes, and then the night's first episode of REM sleep appears. The first REM sleep episode of the night is quite short and NREM sleep quickly follows, usually cycling through all four stages before returning to REM sleep about 90 minutes later. The second episode of REM sleep may last for 5 to 10 minutes. This NREM–REM sleep cycle continues with an alternating pattern until waking in the morning (see CYCLES OF SLEEP ACROSS THE NIGHT).

A number of generalizations about sleep can be made to describe this overnight pattern. First, normal individuals more than 1 year of age begin sleep with NREM sleep, and REM sleep normally appears 100 minutes or so later. Second, the deepest phases of NREM sleep (stages 3 and 4) tend to occur primarily during the first third of the night. Third, REM sleep episodes occur periodically through the night at about 90-minute intervals. Fourth, the length of REM sleep episodes increases across the night; thus, over half of REM sleep tends to occur in the last third of the night. Finally, body movements occur normally during sleep and often signal the transitions between NREM and REM sleep. Thus, it is not "normal" for people to lie in one position all night long (see SLEEP POSITIONS).

REFERENCE

Carskadon MA, Dement WC. 1989. Normal human sleep: An overview. In Kryger MH, Roth T, Dement WC, eds. *Principles and practice of sleep disorders medicine*, pp 3–13. Philadelphia: W.B. Saunders.

Mary A. Carskadon

NREM SLEEP MECHANISMS

Falling asleep involves changes in the activity and excitability of much of the central and peripheral nervous systems, resulting in the outward manifestations of sleep with which we are familiar. During transitions from wakefulness to NREM sleep (that portion of sleep during which high-amplitude synchronous brain waves are present), heart rate and respiration become slower and more regular and muscles relax. Body temperature decreases in an orderly fashion, as if the thermostat has been turned down. Throughout the brain, groups of cells involved in the control of waking behaviors dramatically slow their rate of discharge. Brain cells that convey information from the body's sense organs to the cerebral cortex begin to fire in a series of rapid bursts followed by long pauses, effectively impeding the flow of sensory information to the brain and allowing the sleeping animal to ignore minor disturbances in its environment. This rhythmic bursting in large groups of neurons gives rise to high-amplitude synchronous waves in the ELECTROENCEPHALOGRAM (EEG), which characterize NREM sleep in all mammals and birds.

Transitions from waking to sleep typically occur over the course of a few minutes. Therefore, brain mechanisms that control sleep onset must be capable of orchestrating changes in the activity of many different portions of the nervous system over a relatively short period of time (*see also* SLEEP ONSET). How is this accomplished, and what brain systems are involved? As might be expected for so complicated and important a task, there are multiple sleep-regulating systems, just as there are multiple systems involved in the control of wakefulness and waking behaviors.

Sleep: An Active or Passive Process?

First, what is the evidence that any part of the brain actively induces sleep? Not long ago, scientists believed that such a mechanism was not necessary. Sleep was thought to be a passive phenomenon of the nervous system. When animals seek out a quiet, warm, dark place to rest, decreased sensory stimulation was believed to cause declines in arousing impulses being conveyed from the brainstem to the cortex, leading to sleep. In the 1930s, physiologist Frederic Bremer studied EEG patterns in cats after the production of experimental brain lesions (see Moruzzi, 1972). The type of lesions Bremer made were transections, in which, under anesthesia, a cut was placed through a cross-section of the nervous system, completely disconnecting the parts of the brain above the cut from those below. When the most caudal part of the brainstem (the medulla) was separated from the spinal cord (Figure 1, A), the EEG recorded from the surface of the cerebral cortex still showed alternating periods of waking activity and synchronized, or sleeplike activity. When the cut was placed at the front of the midbrain (Figure 1, B), however, only the high-amplitude slow waves characteristic of sleep were seen on the EEG. Because several sensory nerves were located between the two transection sites, Bremer concluded that the lack of a waking EEG in cats with high brainstem transections resulted from the lack of sensory input to the isolated forebrain, thus supporting the passive sleep-control theory.

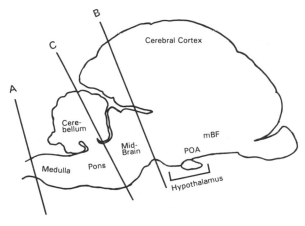

Figure 1. Drawing of a sagittal section (a cut down the middle of the brain along its entire front to back length) of a cat brain showing levels of transection. At level **A**, the rear-most part of the brainstem, the medulla, is separated from the spinal cord. (Bremer called this experimental preparation *encephale isolé*—detached head.) Following transections at this level, the EEG recorded from the surface of the cerebral cortex shows alternating periods of waking- and sleeplike activity. After a transection at level **B**, the EEG initially exhibits only high-amplitude synchronous waves of deep sleep. Within a few days after surgery, however, alternating periods of EEG waking and EEG sleep can be observed. (Bremer called this preparation *cerveau isolé*—detached brain.) With a transection a few millimeters behind **B**, in the middle of the pons (**C**), episodes of EEG waking quickly return, and cats eventually develop EEG insomnia. Important brainstem NREM sleep mechanisms appear to be located in the ventral medulla and pons. Important forebrain NREM sleep mechanisms are located within the preoptic and anterior hypothalamic nuclei (POA) of the medial hypothalamus, and in the magnocellular basal forebrain (mBF), which is located lateral to the POA.

The idea of sleep as a passive process has intuitive appeal as well, because it is easier to fall asleep in quiet or boring situations than in interesting ones.

Although sensory stimulation can prevent sleep, it is also true that the urge to sleep after sleep deprivation can be so powerful that wakefulness cannot be easily maintained even in normally arousing situations (e.g., while driving an automobile). Today, most sleep researchers believe that sleep is an active process. Evidence that led to this change in thinking came from studies of cats with brainstem transections—the same preparations used by Bremer to reach the opposite conclusion! In the early 1960s, neuroscientist Jaime Villablanca (1965) placed transections at the front of the midbrain, much as Bremer had done. Villablanca succeeded in keeping the cats alive and healthy for several days, largely because of refinements in surgical techniques. He discovered that, within a few days after surgery, episodes of EEG activation reappeared! These episodes persisted when cats were briefly isolated in a dark room, where stimulation of the two senses with inputs into the forebrain, vision and smell, would be minimized. Thus, the forebrain isolated from the brainstem and from sensory input is capable of generating EEG waking as well as EEG sleep.

Lower Brainstem NREM Sleep Mechanisms

Also in the early 1960s, a group of Italian investigators, including neurophysiologist Giuseppe Moruzzi, studied cats with transections at the middle of the PONS (Figure 1, C). This transection was just a few millimeters behind those of Villablanca and Bremer, and the forebrain of the midpontine cats had no additional sensory input (see Moruzzi, 1972). Yet the EEG patterns of this preparation were dramatically different: (1) Waking EEG patterns could be recorded within a few hours after surgery. (2) Within a few days, a profound INSOMNIA developed, in which EEG waking was present during 80 percent to 90 percent of the time (normally cats are awake for about 40 percent to 50 percent of the time). This finding pointed to several important conclusions about the organization of brainstem sleep and arousal mechanisms. First, it again demonstrated the independence of forebrain activation from the level of sensory input.

Second, it offered further proof that important arousal mechanisms were located in the midbrain, between the front of the brainstem and the mid-pontine area. In earlier studies, Moruzzi and Magoun had shown that electrical stimulation of this midbrain area in cats always evoked an abrupt change of a sleeping EEG pattern to one of intense wakefulness. This area became known as the midbrain reticular activating system (MRAS). Third, Moruzzi's finding suggested that behind the midpontine cut lay important sleep mechanisms, which when disconnected from the midbrain arousal systems, resulted in excessive EEG waking (*see also* AROUSAL).

Lower brainstem sleep-promoting mechanisms are localized to certain portions of the medulla and pons. In truth, many details regarding which cell types are most important and how they function to control sleep are not well understood, but some facts are known. For example, electrical stimulation of the ventral medulla can elicit a sleeplike EEG pattern in the forebrain (Magnes, Moruzzi, and Pomeiano, 1961) and inhibit cells within the MRAS (Mancia, Mariotti, and Spreafico, 1974). Some medullary cell groups exhibit increases in activity during sleep as compared with waking, suggesting an active role in generating and maintaining sleep (Eguchi and Satoh, 1980). These lower brainstem areas also have descending effects that inhibit spinal cord areas that control muscle activity (Lai and Siegel, 1988). Of course, reductions in muscle activity are an important behavioral component of normal NREM sleep. Electrical stimulation of these areas also causes reductions in blood pressure, heart rate, and body temperature (Chai et al., 1988), all physiological changes that normally accompany sleep. Future research will attempt to learn more about lower brainstem cells involved in promoting sleep. What kind of chemicals do these cells release at sleep onset, and where in the brain and spinal cord do they release them? Perhaps most important, what chemicals or stimuli excite sleep-promoting cell types in the lower brainstem during the transitions from wakefulness to sleep?

Forebrain NREM Sleep Mechanisms

The isolated forebrain of cats transected at the rostral midbrain level still exhibit periods of both EEG sleep and EEG waking. What forebrain areas are responsible for these periods of EEG sleep? Two prominently implicated brain regions are (1) the medial preoptic and anterior nucleus of the HYPOTHALAMUS, and (2) the adjacent magnocellular BASAL FOREBRAIN. The hypothalamus is a small bit of tissue, located in the middle of the base of the brain, just above the pituitary gland. Although small, it is a very important and complicated brain area, playing a regulatory role in many critical behavioral and autonomic functions. The hypothalamus comprises several even smaller groups of brain cells, called NUCLEI. The preoptic and anterior (POA) nuclei are located at the very front of the hypothalamus. These two nuclei participate in the control of thirst and body fluid regulation, the control of reproductive hormone release and sexual behavior, and the regulation of body temperature. These nuclei also participate in the regulation of sleep (see McGinty and Szymusiak, 1990). Localized damage of the POA nuclei causes long-lasting insomnia. Brain cells that increase discharge during sleep as compared with waking are found here in comparative abundance. Direct injection into the POA nuclei of very tiny quantities of benzodiazepine, a drug widely used in human sleeping pills, promotes sleep in rats (Mendelson et al., 1989).

Within the POA, brain cells that participate in the control of sleep are very closely related to those that control body temperature. The POA nuclei contain high concentrations of thermosensitive neurons, that is, brain cells whose discharge rate increases in response to either increases (warm sensitive) or decreases (cold sensitive) in local temperature (Boulant and Dean, 1986). In mammals, local warming or cooling of this area evokes appropriate whole-body thermoregulatory responses, for example, panting and shivering (*see also* THERMOREGULATION). Local warming of the POA nuclei also evokes reductions in muscle tone, relaxed body postures, and NREM sleep (Roberts and Robinson, 1969). NREM sleep is restored in animals made insomniac after POA nuclei damage by exposing them to abnormally high environmental temperatures (Szymusiak, Danowski, and McGinty, 1991). These findings suggest that activation of warmth-sensitive neurons of the POA nuclei is one event that can induce sleep. This pattern is consistent with the active decrease in body temperature that always accompanies

NREM sleep and the common experience of the sleep-enhancing effects of a hot bath or warm room.

Located just lateral to the POA nuclei is a brain region known as the *magnocellular basal forebrain* (mBF), so named because it contains groups of exceptionally large neurons located at the base of the brain. Electrical stimulation of portions of the mBF can evoke enhanced EEG synchrony and NREM sleep in cats (Sterman and Clemente, 1962). Conversely, localized lesions within this area can suppress sleep. Activity of one subgroup of mBF neurons is selective for NREM sleep (Szymusiak and McGinty, 1986). These cells are silent during waking, particularly when animals are alert. They begin to fire action potentials about 10 to 20 seconds before the initial occurrence of EEG slow wave activity during transitions from waking to sleep and reach peak discharge rates during deep stable NREM sleep. This property of increased activation before sleep onset is consistent with the possibility that such cells are involved in sleep induction.

The mBF, however, is not a "sleep center." Evidence suggests that mechanisms that regulate arousal and EEG activation co-exist with those that promote sleep. For example, one group of mBF neurons contains the chemical transmitter acetylcholine. Damage to these cell groups can cause an excess of EEG slow waves, even during waking (Stewart, MacFabe, and Vanderwolf, 1984). Activity of acetylcholine-containing neurons is greatest during activated waking states. Local interactions among mBF waking-active and sleep-active cell types may contribute to the regulation of the sleep–wake cycle (*see also* CHEMISTRY OF SLEEP: ACETYLCHOLINE).

Unanswered Questions

While some brain regions and cell types involved in NREM sleep regulation have been identified, many questions remain unanswered. For instance, how are responses integrated among the various forebrain and brainstem regions described above, to result in the coordinated, widespread changes in central and peripheral nervous system activation that characterize sleep? Do circulating sleep factors act on any or all of these sleep-promoting cell groups? Through what pathways do hypothalamic thermosensitive neurons influence sleep and arousal mechanisms? How does the clock within the brain (see CIRCADIAN RHYTHMS; SUPRACHIASMATIC NUCLEUS OF THE HYPOTHALAMUS) influence NREM sleep-regulating mechanisms such that sleepiness occurs at appropriate times during the day? These questions, and others, are sure to keep the next generation of sleep researchers busy.

REFERENCES

Boulant J, Dean JB. 1986. Temperature receptors in the central nervous system. *Ann Rev Physiol* 48:639–654.

Chai CY, Lin F, Lin, AMY, Pan CM, Lee, EHY, Kuo JS. 1988. Existence of a powerful inhibitory mechanism in the medial region of the caudal medulla— With special reference to the paramedian reticular nucleus. *Brain Res Bull* 20:515–528.

Eguchi K, Satoh T. 1980. Characterization of the neurons in the region of the solitary tract nucleus during sleep. *Physiol Behav* 24:99–111.

Lai YY, Siegel JM. 1988. Medullary regions mediating atonia. *J Neurosci* 8:4790–4796.

McGinty D, Szymusiak R. 1990. Keeping cool: A hypothesis about the mechanisms and functions of slow wave sleep. *Trends Neurosci* 13:480–487.

Magnes J, Moruzzi G, Pomeiano O. 1961. Synchronization of the EEG produced by low-frequency electrical stimulation of the region of the solitary tract. *Arch Ital Biol* 99:33–67.

Mancia M, Mariotti M, Spreafico R. 1974. Caudorostral brain stem reciprocal influences in the cat. *Brain Res* 80:41–51.

Mendelson WB, Martin JV, Perlis M, Wagner R. 1989. Enhancement of sleep by microinjection of triazolam into the medial preoptic area. *Neuropsychopharmacology* 2:61–66.

Moruzzi G. 1972. The sleep-waking cycle. *Ergeb Physiol* 64:1–165.

Roberts WW, Robinson TCL. 1969. Relaxation and sleep induced by warming of the preoptic region and anterior hypothalamus in cats. *Exp Neurol* 25:282–294.

Sterman MB, Clemente CD. 1962. Forebrain inhibitory mechanisms: Sleep patterns induced by basal forebrain stimulation in the behaving cat. *Exp Neurol* 6:103–117.

Stewart DJ, MacFabe DF, and Vanderwolf CH. 1984. Cholinergic activation of the electro-corticogram:

Role of the substantia innominata and effects of atropine and quinuclidinyl benzilate. *Brain Res* 322:219–232.

Szymusiak R, Danowski J, McGinty D. 1991. Exposure to heat restores sleep in cats with preoptic/anterior hypothalamic cell loss. *Brain Res* 541:134–138.

Szymusiak R, McGinty D. 1986. Sleep-related neuronal discharge in the basal forebrain of cats. *Brain Res* 370:82–92.

Villablanca J. 1965. The electrocorticogram in the chronic *cerveau isole* cat. *Electroencephalogr Clin Neurophysiol* 19:576–586.

Ronald Szymusiak

NUDITY IN DREAMS

The interpretation of nudity in dreams has changed dramatically through the years. At the turn of the century, when Freudian psychology was in its heyday, nudity in dreams was thought to represent an exhibitionistic wish (Freud, 1961; see also FREUD'S DREAM THEORY). Post-Freudian psychoanalysts often considered nudity to represent feelings of guilt or inferiority (Ward, Beck, and Rascoe, 1961) or a response to indifferent treatment by the dreamer's parents (Myers, 1989). Many current analysts believe that nudity in dreams should be interpreted not with generalizations, but on a case-by-case basis.

Although interpretative trends have changed, the incidence of nudity in dreams shows some consistency among survey studies. In 1958, Griffith and his collaborators surveyed several hundred Japanese and American college students about their dreams (Griffith, Miyago, and Tago, 1958). They found that 43 percent of the American students and 18 percent of the Japanese students reported having dreams in which they were nude. The investigators postulated that this cross-cultural difference was the result of Western civilization's relative emphasis on the nude in the fine arts. In 1961, Ward and his colleagues questioned several hundred psychiatric patients concerning the content of their dreams, and found that 21 percent of the patients reported dreams that involved being naked or scantily clothed (Ward, Beck, and Rascoe, 1961). (For both of these studies, sexual experiences in dreams were not considered in the same category as nudity, but were examined separately.) Although the percentage of American college students dreaming of being nude was higher than that of American psychiatric patients, this may be a result of the different survey techniques used in the studies. It seems most noteworthy that both studies found nudity to occur quite commonly in the reported dreaming histories of these very different populations.

A laboratory study, however, provides a different perspective on nudity as a theme or occurrence in dream stories. Snyder (1970) examined 635 dream reports from 250 nights of REM sleep awakenings in young adults, looking for categories of so-called typical dreams, including that of "being naked with embarrassment." Only 10 reports—approximately 1.6 percent—contained nudity involving the dreamer or another character in the dream story, with no accompanying description of feeling embarrassed. The popular conception of nudity as a common phenomenon in dreams may be due to nakedness being unusual or salient for the dreamer, and therefore more likely to be remembered over time than the ordinary state of being clothed. Thus, should an investigator inquire, "Have you *ever* had a dream in which you or someone else appeared naked?" (as in the surveys mentioned above), the percentage of positive responses might be expected to be higher than that found in Snyder's sample of one-night laboratory dreams.

REFERENCES

Freud S. 1961. *The interpretation of dreams*. New York: Science Editions.

Griffith RM, Miyago O, Tago A. 1958. The universality of typical dreams: Japanese vs. Americans. *Am Anthropol* 60:1173–1179.

Myers WA. The traumatic element in the typical dream of feeling embarrassed at being naked. *J Am Psychoanal Assoc* 37(1):117–130.

Snyder F. The phenomenology of dreaming. In Madow L, Snow L, eds. *The psychodynamic implications of the physiological studies on dreams*, pp 124–150. Springfield, Ill.: Charles C Thomas.

Ward CH, Beck AT, Rascoe E. 1967. Typical dreams: Incidence among psychiatric patients. *Arch Gen Psychiatry* 5:606–615.

Cecília Vieira

NUTRITION AND SLEEP

Food intake and nutrition have long been thought to have important effects on sleep in lower animals and humans. Hippocrates (500 B.C.), the father of medicine, observed that certain foods could induce SLEEPINESS in people. Aristotle later wrote in his essay on sleep and wakefulness (*De somno et vigilia*) that sleep in animals "arises . . . from the process of nutrition." These commonly held assumptions regarding the relationships between food intake, nutrition, and sleep are reflected in many classical works. For example, in *Henry IV,* Shakespeare described POSTPRANDIAL (i.e., postmeal) sleepiness in the gluttonous Falstaff, who was found "unbuttoning . . . after supper and sleeping upon benches after noon." Children's fables also allude to POSTPRANDIAL sleepiness, as portrayed in the tale of Goldilocks, who fell fast asleep after eating a meal of porridge.

Several investigators have attempted to document the relationship between food intake and sleep in laboratory animals. In the 1920s, Curt Richter was among the first to report that rats display a distinct pattern of activity before and after feeding. He described a behavioral sequence that is characterized by a gradual crescendo of activity prior to the onset of a meal, feeding, grooming, and then a long period of rest or sleep. These observations have been supported by the more recent finding that food intake often is followed by electroencephalographic evidence of sleep. Specifically, it has been shown that larger meals are associated with longer episodes of SLOW-WAVE SLEEP (SWS) and REM SLEEP during the dark (active) phase of the rats' sleep–wake cycle and that, under certain conditions, this association also is present in the light (dormant) phase of the cycle.

When the nutritional status of an animal is altered by increasing its food intake over an extended period, total sleep time increases dramatically. The administration of a highly palatable diet to laboratory rats over 10 days has been shown to result in a 60 percent increase in the daily production of SWS, and a 30 percent increase in the daily production of REM sleep. SWS rises during both the light and dark phases of the cycle, whereas REM sleep seems to rise mostly during the light phase. These effects are due to an increase in the duration, but not the number, of sleep episodes. On the other hand, animals that are maintained on restricted diets or prevented from feeding show dramatic reductions in total sleep time. After only 4 days of food deprivation, there can be as much as a 60 percent reduction in SWS and a 75 percent reduction in REM sleep.

It is not known why animals sleep after feeding. Animals may stay awake to hunt or forage for food, and may take the opportunity to sleep after feeding, when the demand to search for food is low. In fact, some scientists believe that starving animals remain awake primarily to continue their search for food. This may be because, even though rest or sleep can conserve some energy, the failure to consume food ultimately leads to death. The relationship between feeding and sleep may be modulated in other ways. It is known that some animals sleep or enter HIBERNATION when the availability of food is low. In these cases, the energy saved may be greater than the value of the small amounts of food that may be obtained, making the risk of searching for food (and expending too much energy) too high.

Much less is known about food intake, nutrition, and sleep in humans. One survey has shown that 23 percent of young adults report feeling sleepy often or always after meals and that 45 percent report feeling sleepy after big meals. Only 12 percent of the 435 subjects questioned in this study said that they never experienced bouts of SLEEPINESS after eating. Ratings of sleepiness tend to be greatest between 90 and 120 minutes after the end of a meal, and do not appear to be different from normal either before or after this period. Postprandial sleepiness may affect performance, as scores on tests that measure attention, reaction time, and other mental abilities have been found to be worse after meals.

Will a late snack help you to sleep at night? It probably is true that a glass of milk or a light snack before bed can help to lengthen sleep or decrease wakefulness during the sleep period. This may be, in part, because a snack can help to ward off hunger pangs. Large meals or large volumes of liquid taken before bedtime may actually disturb sleep, and can lead to an increased number of arousals from sleep. Many people describe awakenings, bad dreams, or the need to use the restroom after they've eaten or drunk too much before going to bed.

Not everyone agrees that food intake has an effect on sleep. One group has shown that subjects do not fall asleep when given the opportunity to take afternoon naps following a lunch meal. Another group of investigators divided subjects' daily caloric intake into twenty-four parts, and then administered meals of equal caloric value at 1-hour intervals over the course of one study day (Carskadon et al., 1985). They found that, even when the effects of food were thus controlled, subjects still tended to fall asleep faster during the middle of the day! This finding suggests that the circadian (daily) rhythm of sleep and wakefulness is independent of food intake. It does not, however, rule out the possibility that food intake has effects on sleep that occur in addition to its circadian rhythm. (See also CIRCADIAN RHYTHMS.)

Postprandial sleepiness tends to be most common after meals that are high in carbohydrate and not those that are protein rich or composed of blends of proteins, carbohydrates, and fats. This has led some to suggest that the amino acid tryptophan, which is abundant in carbohydrate foods, is responsible for postprandial sleepiness. Tryptophan promotes the synthesis of brain serotonin, a chemical neurotransmitter that has been thought to play an important role in the production of sleep; however, it is still unclear whether the tryptophan that is derived from dietary sources is sufficient to promote sleep in animals and humans. Alternative explanations have been proposed. It has been suggested that the rise and subsequent fall of glucose after a meal may result in a state of relative hypoglycemia, which is associated with extreme fatigue. This is unlikely, though, as postprandial glucose rarely falls below premeal levels. Two other hypotheses are now being actively investigated. Certain hormones (such as cholecystokinin, bombesin, somatostatin, and insulin) that are released during food intake may be involved in transmitting signals from the gut to the brain. Alternatively, the rise in heat production that follows food intake, which is the result of food metabolism, may be involved in promoting sleep. As the diversity of the research described here shows, scientists have only just begun to describe the complex mechanisms that link food intake, nutrition, and sleep.

REFERENCES

Carskadon MA, Dement WC. 1985. Midafternoon decline in MSLT scores on a constant routine. *Sleep Res* 14:292.

Christie MJ, McBrearty EM. 1979. Psychophysiological investigations of post lunch state in male and female subjects. *Ergonomics* 22:307–323.

Danguir J, Nicolaidis S. 1985. Feeding, metabolism, and sleep: Peripheral and central mechanism of their interaction. In McGinty DJ, et al., eds. *Brain mechanisms of sleep,* pp 321–340. New York: Raven Press.

Gary K. Zammit
Sigurd H. Ackerman

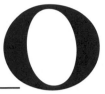

OBESITY

See Apnea; Eating Disorders

OBSTRUCTIVE APNEA

See Apnea

ONDINE'S CURSE

Ondine's Curse refers to a rare respiratory disorder that markedly worsens during sleep. This term has its roots in mythology and was first used by Severinghaus and Mitchell (1962) to describe the diminished respiratory drive of three patients who had undergone brainstem surgery.

The story of Ondine's curse originates in a German legend of a water nymph who obtained a soul by marrying a mortal man, recorded in the writings of Paracelsus (1493–1541), who applied the name Undine (from the Latin *unda* for wave) to describe this spirit of the water (Sugar, 1978). Throughout the ages, several authors have retold the story of Undine. The playwright Jean Giraudoux (1882–1944) inspired the naming of Ondine's Curse through his own interpretation, in which Ondine is a water nymph jilted by her mortal husband, the knight Hans. Although Ondine pleads for the life of Hans, the King of the Ondines demands his death since he has broken a pact that mandates death for an unfaithful husband. Thus, Hans is punished with the loss of all his automatic functions, including breathing: "... all the things my body once did by itself, it does now only by special order. . . . A single moment of inattention, and I forget to breathe. He died, they will say, because it was a nuisance to breathe. . . ." This disorder is named to acknowledge the mode of Hans's death—the loss of automatic breathing.

In medical terms, Ondine's Curse is a rare hypoventilation syndrome of unknown etiology that occurs in the absence of any identifiable abnormalities of the lungs, respiratory muscles, or central nervous system. The site of pathology is believed to be the respiratory centers of the brainstem, where input from central and peripheral chemoreceptors is integrated, because the normal ventilatory responses to carbon dioxide and oxygen are absent or diminished in these patients. Thus, the essential characteristic of the disorder is hypoventilation—that is, abnormally slow or shallow respiration causing an inadequate amount of air to enter the lungs. This abnormal breathing leads to chronically high levels of carbon dioxide (hypercapnia) and low levels of oxygen (hypoxemia) in the blood, both of which can be temporarily corrected by voluntarily increasing the breathing rate. Patients, therefore, show only a slight abnormality during wakefulness as they consciously continue to breathe, but their condition rapidly and markedly worsens at sleep onset because of the loss of voluntary breathing. Certain researchers report that the degree of hypoventilation does not vary significantly across the sleep stages (Coccagna et al., 1984); others have found that ventilatory performance worsens during NREM sleep, especially in infants (Fleming et al., 1980; Cornwell et al.,

1981). Central and peripheral respiratory pauses (see APNEA) may occur during sleep, but they are usually sporadic and not the sole cause of the reduced respiration. Patients with this syndrome typically develop symptoms including lethargy, fatigue, somnolence, disturbed sleep, and morning headache. Ondine's Curse is usually a progressive disease that eventually causes other serious medical problems (such as pulmonary hypertension and right heart failure) and ultimately causes death.

REFERENCES

Andersen, Hans Christian. 1961. *Fairy tales.* Kingsland LW, trans. Oxford: Oxford University Press.

Coccagna C, Cirignotta F, Zucconi M, Gerardi R, Medori R, Lugaresi E. 1984. A polygraphic study of one case of primary alveolar hypoventilation (Ondine's Curse). *Bull Eur Physiopathol Respir* 20:157–161.

Cornwell AC, Pollack MA, Kravath RE, Llena J, Nathenson G, Weitzman ED. 1981. Sleep apnea studies in an infant with congenital primary hypoventilation ("Ondine's Curse"). *Int J Neurosci* 15:155–162.

De la Motte-Fouqué FHK. 1909. *Undine.* Adapted from the German by WL Courtney. London: Heinemann; New York: Doubleday Page.

Fleming PJ, Cade B, Bryan MH, Bryan AC. 1980. Congenital central hypoventilation and sleep state. *Pediatrics* 66:425–428.

Giraudoux J. 1958. Ondine. In *Jean Giraudoux. Four plays, adapted, and with an introduction by Maurice Valency,* vol. 1. New York: Hill & Wang.

Phillipson EA. 1991. Disorders of ventilation. In Wilson JD, Braunwald E, Isselbacher KJ, Petersdorf RG, Martin JB, Fauci AS, Root RK, eds. *Harrison's principles of internal medicine,* pp 1116–1129. New York: McGraw-Hill.

Rodin AE, Key JD. 1989. *Medicine, literature & eponyms: An encyclopedia of medical eponyms derived from literary characters.* Melbourne, Florida: Krieger.

Severinghaus JW, Mitchell RA. 1962. Ondine's Curse—Failure of respiratory center automaticity while awake. *Clin Res* 10:122.

Sugar O. 1978. In search of Ondine's curse. *JAMA* 240:236–237.

Stephen S. Davis

ONTOGENY

Ontogeny is the biological development of an individual organism over time, as distinguished from PHYLOGENY, the evolution of a group of organisms such as a species, family, or order. The development of sleep from the fetal period to old age is similar in most warm-blooded vertebrates. Differences among animals in sleep–wake state distribution at birth are largely a function of differences in central nervous system maturity, with precocial animals such as the guinea pig showing more mature sleep–wake patterns than altricial animals such as the rabbit, rat, and human (see MAMMALS). (*Precocial* refers to animals that are quite mature when born; *altricial,* to animals that are immature at birth.) In general, three states of consciousness may be discerned by at least the time of birth in mammals: wakefulness, active sleep, and quiet sleep. The states of active and quiet sleep are assumed to be the immature precursors of REM and NREM sleep, respectively.

During the earliest period of an animal's life, sleep occupies a higher percentage of the 24-hour period than at later ages, and active sleep accounts for a higher percentage of the time asleep. For example, human infants at birth sleep approximately 17 to 18 of the 24 hours, and active sleep occupies over 50 percent of sleep time. The newborn infant's sleep occurs in episodes of 3 to 4 hours each, interspersed with brief periods of wakefulness. Sleep is more or less equally distributed over the day and night hours, although by 3 months of age it becomes clear that more sleep already occurs during the nighttime hours. Infants go directly from wakefulness to active sleep, a pattern that is gradually replaced during the first years of life by the adult pattern of entry into sleep through NREM sleep stages.

During the first year of life, many other changes in the nature of sleep bring the human infant's state organization closer to that of the adult. Thus, by about 4 months of age, four stages of NREM sleep may be distinguished in electroencephalogram (EEG) recordings. The number of sleep–wake cycles per day decreases with age. The short periods of sleep and wakefulness during infancy become consolidated into longer periods, until at about 4 to 5 years of age, the sleep period is monophasic, that is, once per 24-hour day (see INFANCY, NORMAL SLEEP PATTERNS IN).

Over the course of human development, total

sleep time decreases and the percentage of active or REM sleep decreases, while the majority of sleep time becomes NREM sleep. By age 4, the duration of sleep drops to about 10 to 12 hours and then to about 9 to 10 hours by age 10. By adolescence, the total duration of sleep has dropped to 7 to 9 hours. REM sleep decreases to 25 percent to 30 percent in childhood and to about 20 percent after puberty. With advancing age, the amount of SLOW-WAVE SLEEP is also gradually reduced, with an increased number of awakenings during the night (see ADOLESCENCE AND SLEEP; AGING AND SLEEP).

The very large amount of active or REM sleep seen in very young animals has intrigued researchers for a number of years. In 1966, Roffwarg, Muzio, and Dement hypothesized that one of the primary functions of REM (active) sleep in early development is to provide internal stimulation to the central nervous system at a time when the young organism's capabilities of receiving stimulation from the external environment are quite limited. The dramatic decrease in active sleep that occurs during the first months of life and the concomitant increase in alertness during this period were cited as support for this hypothesis. Although this hypothesis is appealing, REM sleep must also have other functions, as it persists as a portion of sleep time throughout life (see FUNCTIONS OF SLEEP; REM SLEEP, FUNCTION OF). Other researchers have studied the development and maturation of sleep patterns with the goal of relating the many changes that occur in the central nervous system during maturation to the changes in the way sleep and wakefulness are organized and expressed over the life span (see also CYCLES OF SLEEP ACROSS THE NIGHT).

REFERENCES

Anders TF, Keener M. 1985. Developmental course of nighttime sleep–wake patterns in full-term and premature infants during the first year of life, I. *Sleep* 8(3):173–192.
Hoppenbrouwers T, Hodgman J, Arakawa K, Geidel SA, Sterman MB. 1988. Sleep and waking states in infancy: Normative studies. *Sleep* 11(4):387–401.
Jouvet, Mounier D, Astic L, Lacote D. 1970. Ontogenesis of the states of sleep in rat, cat, and guinea pig during the first postnatal month. *Dev Psychobiol* 2:216–239.
Roffwarg HP, Muzio JN, Dement WC. 1966. Ontogenetic development of the human sleep–dream cycle. *Science* 152:604–619.
Williams R, Karacan I, Hursch C. 1974. *Electroencephalography (EEG) of human sleep: Clinical applications.* New York: Wiley.

Christine Acebo

ORGASM

See Female Sexual Response; Sex and Sleep

OUTER SPACE

See Microgravity and Space Flight; Space Shuttle Sleeping Arrangements

OVER-THE-COUNTER SLEEPING PILLS

Over-the-counter (OTC) SLEEPING PILLS (hypnotic medications) are the most widely used agents for inducing sleep. They are easily accessible to the public, since they can be purchased without a prescription. As a result, this class of medications is consumed in greater quantities than are prescription sleeping pills. In fact, according to a survey of U.S. adults by the Gallup organization ("Sleep in America," 1991), 40 percent of people with INSOMNIA report they self-medicate for their sleep problem with OTC sleeping pills, ALCOHOL, or both. In contrast, only 21 percent of adults with insomnia reported having taken prescription medications for sleep. These statistics confirm that OTC hypnotics enjoy widespread use by the adult population. Unfortunately, these medications are seldom used under the supervision of a physician, and their effectiveness has not yet been established in carefully controlled clinical trials.

Historically, scopolamine, bromides, and a variety of ANTIHISTAMINES were the active ingredients in OTC hypnotic preparations. In 1975, however, an advisory panel to the U.S. Food and Drug Administration (FDA) recommended that only certain antihistamines be allowed as nonprescription OTC hypnotics on grounds of safety and efficacy, and this recommendation was subsequently given the force of FDA regulation. Currently, diphenhydramine and doxylamine are the most popular antihistamines used in OTC hypnotic preparations. These antihistamines are known as H_1 blockers or H_1 antagonists because they block a population of histamine receptors called the H_1 receptors; interactions of histamine with these receptors affect capillary permeability and vascular and bronchial smooth muscle. Most H_1 antagonists also have central-nervous-system effects. They are known to diminish alertness, to slow reaction times, and to have sedative properties.

Abnormal release of histamine is encountered in allergic and hypersensitivity reactions, which are the primary indications for their use. Thus, sedation is technically a side effect of these medications. Furthermore, no systematic information is available about the range of doses needed to improve sleep. It is not known whether the sedating properties of the antihistamines continue after several days or weeks of continued use (i.e., whether tolerance develops).

Finally, the elimination half-life of these drugs needs to be considered, that is, how long they remain active. In particular, what may happen if they are taken at the wrong time (e.g., before driving or operating heavy machinery) or if the drug has a long half-life (e.g., doxylamine, with a half-life of 9 hours)? In the latter case, people might wake up with a hangover and be left with impaired cognitive abilities for several hours. Antihistamines also have anticholinergic side effects (dry mouth, dilated pupils, acceleration of the heart rate, difficulty urinating, and behavioral changes). These anticholinergic effects may be a particular problem for elderly people, a segment of the population frequently afflicted with insomnia. These characteristics of OTC hypnotics contrast sharply with the results of the safety and efficacy studies done on most FDA-approved prescription hypnotics.

REFERENCES

Mendelson WB. 1980. *The use and misuse of sleeping pills: A clinical guide*. New York: Plenum.

Physicians' desk reference for nonprescription drugs, 12th ed. 1991. Oradell, N.J.: Medical Economics Company.
Sleep in America: A national survey of U.S. adults. 1991. Princeton, N.J.: The Gallup Organization.

Leon D. Rosenthal

OVER-THE-COUNTER STIMULANTS

Over-the-counter (OTC) STIMULANTS are widely used as decongestants and as anorectic (appetite-suppressing) agents as well as for their stimulant properties. In some instances, they have been represented as AMPHETAMINES for sale to those attempting to buy this drug illegally. The most widely used OTC stimulants are phenylpropanolamine, pseudoephedrine, ephedrine, and CAFFEINE, which is the only compound approved by the FDA to be sold as a nonprescription stimulant.

Caffeine is a methylxanthine that is rapidly absorbed following oral administration and has a short half-life (about 3 hours). Its prevalence in foods and beverages makes it readily accessible if not unavoidable. COFFEE is regularly used by many people to wake up in the morning, to enhance concentration during the day, and to stay awake at night. Caffeine is present in coffee, TEA, COLAS, and CHOCOLATE. It may also be present in OTC cold medications, and it is marketed as a stimulant in tablets of 100 to 200 milligrams. Caffeine is a potent releaser of epinephrine from the adrenal glands and also causes stimulation of the central nervous system (CNS): It sensitizes postsynaptic dopamine receptors and perhaps adrenergic receptors, and is believed to antagonize CNS receptors for adenosine (see CHEMISTRY OF SLEEP).

The CNS effects of caffeine have been shown in laboratory tests of sleep latency (see MULTIPLE SLEEP LATENCY TEST). Ingestion of caffeine after 7:00 P.M. leads to reports of INSOMNIA in 53 percent of people who consume small amounts of coffee and 22 percent of people who usually drink large quantities of it. The consumption of more than 1,000 milligrams of coffee per day, called caffeinism, may result in symptoms that mimic anxiety disorders. In fact, intravenous administration of caffeine can cause panic attacks in people with preexisting panic disorder. Clinical and laboratory evidence indicates that tolerance to the CNS effects develops rapidly.

Phenylpropanolamine and pseudoephedrine are frequently used as nasal decongestants and in OTC cold remedies. When used as nasal decongestants, they may be administered orally or topically. When included in cold remedies, they are also intended for relief of nasal congestion; these products also include an analgesic and sometimes caffeine (for its stimulating properties) or an antihistamine (for sedating properties, in preparations for nocturnal use). Phenylpropanolamine and pseudoephedrine constrict blood vessels through their sympathomimetic effects (i.e., stimulation of the SYMPATHETIC NERVOUS SYSTEM). When this effect occurs in the nose tissue, it results in decrease of nasal discharge. Taken orally, these drugs may also cause heart palpitations (cardiac arrhythmias) and transient high blood pressure. Because they stimulate the CNS, these products may also cause nervousness and insomnia. Phenylpropanolamine is also encountered as the active ingredient in OTC appetite-suppressant products. Although the exact mechanism of its anorectic action is not understood, it is thought to derive from stimulation of the CNS, which may also increase metabolism.

Ephedrine, like phenylpropanolamine and pseudoephedrine, produces stimulation of the CNS, constriction of blood vessels, and heart palpitations. Ephedrine and pseudoephedrine are optical isomers, but ephedrine has greater beta-adrenergic properties, which cause widening of the bronchial tubes. Thus, this drug is found in OTC products for relief and control of bronchial asthma attacks.

Data on the efficacy of these drugs are limited, in particular when they are used over prolonged periods of time. Finally, they are frequently used free of any medical supervision and thus may bring about undesirable side effects or worsening of preexisting medical conditions.

Leon D. Rosenthal

OVERSLEEPING

A common question among many young people is, "Why do I feel so terrible when I sleep too much?" In 1969, sleep researcher Gordon Globus began to study what he called an "oversleeping syndrome" with a survey of fifty-one young adults. By asking these volunteers to indicate how they felt when they slept more than 10 hours a night, Globus identified two separate oversleeping syndromes: One was associated with feeling "worn out" (fatigued and so forth) and the other with feeling "just great" (refreshed and so forth) after a long night of sleep. Interestingly, these very different descriptions were reported in approximately equal numbers (Globus, 1969). Also in 1969, John Taub and Ralph Berger coined the term *Rip Van Winkle effect* for feeling bad after an extended night of sleep. Although no actual sleep recordings were made during this study of young adults, subjects instructed to sleep between 10:00 P.M. and 9:00 A.M. showed slight performance test difficulties when compared with subjects instructed to sleep between 1:00 A.M. and 9:00 A.M. (Taub and Berger, 1969). In a second study, Taub and his colleagues (1971) instructed all subjects to spend the same extended period in bed at night, only varying the portion of that time they were allowed to sleep, and obtained similar results: Performance was worse in those volunteers on the longer sleep schedule than on the shorter one.

Many of us who have slept too little, however, know that performance deficits can be produced by circumstances other than sleep extension, nor would we say that oversleeping necessarily leads to such a negative outcome. A series of sleep and performance evaluations by Taub and others demonstrated consistently that when young adult volunteers slept either more *or* less than their usual amount, their performance the next day was adversely affected. By contrast, Herscovitch and Broughton (1981) found that oversleeping when recovering from partial sleep deprivation actually led to improved performance after the long nights of sleep, and Carskadon and Dement's (1982) subjects showed similar positive results from oversleeping after a single night of sleep restriction.

Thus, investigations of oversleeping ever since Globus' original finding indicate that two distinct results of a long night's sleep may occur; furthermore, it may be possible to predict whether a person will feel "worn out" or "just great" based on the amount of sleep obtained before the oversleeping episode. The data suggest that people feel worse afterward if they had plenty of sleep just before oversleeping; conversely, people who have had too little sleep may be expected to feel "just great" after a night of oversleeping to recover.

In 1985, Carskadon and colleagues performed a study to test these hypotheses. Nine young male volunteers experienced a set of four sleep conditions over the course of four weeks and were evaluated repeatedly with the Multiple Sleep Latency Test (see MULTIPLE SLEEP LATENCY TEST), performance tests, and mood and sleepiness scales. Each sleep condition lasted four nights: the first three were either a baseline schedule of sleeping from 11:00 P.M. to 7:30 A.M. or a restricted schedule of sleeping from 1:00 A.M. to 7:30 A.M. On the fourth night, time in bed was elongated from 11:00 P.M. to 10:00 A.M., but sleeping was then permitted only from 11:00 P.M. to 7:30 A.M. or oversleeping was permitted for the entire time in bed. Surprisingly, all subjects reported feeling better and also demonstrated less sleepiness on the MSLT after the oversleeping nights, whether they occurred after restricted sleep or nonrestricted baseline sleep. With or without a prior sleep debt, the subjects' alertness was either unchanged or improved after acute oversleeping. Furthermore, actually sleeping more proved to be better for subjectively reported mood and objectively measured alertness than simply lying in bed awake for the extra hours. Only one of the many measures taken showed results as originally predicted; on the Stanford Sleepiness Scale (see STANFORD SLEEPINESS SCALE), subjects reported feeling worse after oversleeping when they were *not* previously sleep-deprived and feeling more alert after oversleeping when they *were* previously sleep-deprived. Nevertheless, the preponderance of other evidence indicated that long sleep led to a better sense of well-being in these experimental subjects (Carskadon et al., 1986).

Why, then, do people often feel worse when they oversleep in their ordinary lives and environments? Several explanations may account for this experience. (1) People generally expect to feel better after getting a longer night of sleep: their expectations may predict greater improvement than they actually obtain, in which case they could be disappointed and feel worse. (2) The specific type of sleep obtained in an oversleeping episode may differ from normal sleep patterns, and that may have some impact on how an individual feels. There is a bit of evidence that this possibility has some physiological basis: scientists in Roger Broughton's laboratory have found that when people sleep approximately twelve hours or longer, their electroencephalogram shows a reappearance of the very deep, slow-wave sleep stages (Gagnon, De Koninck, and Broughton, 1985). When people wake up from slow-wave sleep, they often feel worse or more "groggy" than when waking up from REM sleep or stage 2 sleep (see SLOW-WAVE SLEEP; REM SLEEP; STAGES OF SLEEP). (3) Many individuals obtain an occasional long night of sleep because of unusual circumstances such as being ill (see MEDICAL ILLNESS AND SLEEP), having had a great deal of ALCOHOL, and so forth; each of these circumstances in and of itself could lead a person to feel worse on awakening. (4) People typically oversleep by going to bed late and waking much later than usual: this raises the possibility that they wake up during the "midday dip" (see NAPPING; SLEEPINESS) which could then result in feeling worse or more tired than usual.

The most common pattern of oversleeping, particularly for individuals living in Western societies, is on the weekend (see SLEEP EXTENSION). It appears that many people establish a routine in which they consistently restrict sleep on week nights, often because of work or school commitments, and then lengthen sleep on the weekend. Whether this extension of sleep on weekends is sufficient for recovery from weekly sleep restriction, however, has not yet been established (see DEPRIVATION; FATIGUE–RECOVERY MODEL).

REFERENCES

Carskadon MA, Dement WC. 1982. Nocturnal determinants of daytime sleepiness. *Sleep* 5:S73–S81.

Carskadon MA, Mancuso J, Keenan S, Littell W, Dement WC. 1986. Sleepiness following oversleeping. *Sleep Res* 15:70.

Gagnon P, De Koninck J, Broughton R. 1985. Reappearance of electroencephalogram slow waves in extended sleep with delayed bedtime. *Sleep* 8:118–128.

Globus GG. 1969. A syndrome associated with sleeping late. *Psychosom Med* 31:528–535.

Herscovitch J, Broughton R. 1981. Sensitivity of the Stanford Sleepiness Scale to the effects of cumulative partial sleep deprivation and recovery oversleeping. *Sleep* 4:83–92.

Taub JM, Berger RJ. 1969. Extended sleep and performance: The Rip Van Winkle effect. *Psychon Sci* 16:204–205.

Taub JM, Globus GG, Phoebus E, Drury R. 1971. Extended sleep and performance. *Nature* 233: 142–143.

Kate B. Herman
Mary A. Carskadon

OWLS

See Birds; Early Birds and Night Owls

OXYGEN

See Apnea; Continuous Positive Airway Pressure

P

PAIN

The word *pain* is derived from *poena* (Latin) and *poine* (Greek), which mean "penalty." *Pain* is sometimes used in that sense, as in the legalistic phrase "on pain of death." More generally, pain is an unpleasant sensory experience usually caused by bodily injury or illness, but it also occurs in the absence of identifiable pathology. Intuitively, it is obvious that pain interferes with sleep. Pain is a common cause of *insomnia* (Kleitman, 1963), and difficulty with sleeping contributes to suffering and emotional distress in people who live daily with pain.

The degree of pain experienced is related to the extent of trauma or injury. A pinch of a finger hurts, whereas slamming a car door on it could be excruciatingly painful. The actual degree of pain experienced at the time of injury varies widely. For example, soldiers in battle or civilians injured in accidents sometimes report no pain until many hours later (Melzack and Wall, 1988).

Control over the transmission of pain is exerted at different levels in the central nervous system (brain and spinal cord), and specific nerve pathways from the brain to the spinal cord modulate pain sensations, but how and when these mechanisms are naturally activated is largely unknown. Bodily injury leads to increased sensitivity and spontaneous activity in areas of the central nervous system involved in the processing of both *noxious* (painful) and nonnoxious stimuli. Pain can even be triggered by light touch or slight movement and may spread to unrelated areas of the body where no injury exists. Pain persists long after removal of the noxious stimulus, a phenomenon called *sensitization*, which is gener-

ally transient but may persist long after injured tissue has healed. It is thus not surprising that insomnia is a common complaint of people who experience pain, but complete lack of sleep is unusual.

Sleep reduces responsiveness to environmental stimuli and blocks, to some degree, the transmission of and conscious awareness of bodily sensations; however, stimuli of sufficient strength inevitably will awaken a sleeper. For example, direct stimulation of nerves that transmit pain sensations produces arousal in sleeping animals, even during the recovery sleep that follows sleep deprivation.

The activity of nerve cells that respond to pain is unchanged from wakefulness to NREM sleep and to the portion of REM sleep without eye movements. These cells are, however, inhibited during the bursts of eye movements in REM sleep. Thus, transmission of pain signals in the nervous system is inhibited only during the eye movements of REM sleep and is largely unchanged during most stages of sleep.

Given the increased sensitivity and spontaneous activity of the nervous system associated with pain, and given that the sensory transmission of pain is largely unchanged during sleep, it is surprising that patients in pain sleep at all. In some poorly understood way, the response to pain signals must be reduced during most of sleep, just as responses to other signals are reduced. Nevertheless, pain does have well-recognized disturbing effects on sleep. Patients with and without a physical basis for their pain take a longer time to fall asleep, spend more time awake, and have less slow-wave sleep and more frequent arousals than either normal subjects or insomniacs (Moldofsky,

1989). They may also have an additional sleep disturbance characterized on the electroencephalogram (EEG) by the presence of alpha frequency waveforms, indicating arousal, during NREM sleep stages. This EEG arousal pattern, called alpha-NREM sleep, has been associated with more frequent reports of increased pain, tenderness, weakness, and fatigue upon waking up from sleep. In addition to sleep disturbances from pain, chronic pain patients may have disrupted sleep from a variety of sources, such as periodic leg movements, depressed mood, and psychological distress. Not all patients with chronic pain complain of disturbed sleep, but those who do report more pain. Thus, important consequences of lost and disrupted sleep in patients with chronic pain are increases in pain, fatigue, and sleepiness.

Increased sensitivity to pain and sleepiness are the most common symptoms of sleep loss (Kleitman, 1963). The selective deprivation of stage 4 sleep in normal subjects and of REM sleep in chronic pain patients increases pain sensitivity and complaints of pain and tenderness. REM sleep deprivation in animals also heightens pain sensitivity. The physiological basis for these changes in pain sensitivity with sleep loss is unknown.

(See also ALPHA–DELTA SLEEP; CHRONIC FATIGUE SYNDROME; NONRESTORATIVE SLEEP.)

REFERENCES

Kleitman N. 1963. *Sleep and wakefulness.* Chicago: University of Chicago Press.
Melzack R, Wall PD. 1988. *The challenge of pain,* rev. ed. New York: Basic Books.
Moldofsky H. 1989. Sleep influences on regional and diffuse pain syndromes associated with osteoarthritis. *Semin Arth Rheumatism* 18(suppl. 2):18–21.

Carol A. Landis

PAJAMAS AND NIGHTWEAR

The earliest written reference to clothing worn specifically for sleep is attributed to Isidor, Bishop of Seville, who reported that upper-class gentlemen began wearing nightshirts to sleep during the Byzantine period in the seventh century (Holliday, 1933). Unfortunately, documentation of the sleepwear of ancient times is scarce and that which exists is unsubstantial because, until very recently, it was thought blasphemous to discuss what ladies and gentlemen wore in the boudoir. Many early references to nightgowns and night clothes actually describe formal evening wear rather than garments worn especially for sleep. Poetry from the middle ages (A.D. 1100–A.D. 1300) refers quite often to an undergarment for women variously called a kirtle, smock, sherte, camise, or chemise. This was a cotton or linen dress, often trimmed with lace or ruffles; similar to the slips worn by modern women, this undergarment may have been the first definitively feminine item of sleepwear (see Figure 1).

Nevertheless, clothing historians report that before the Dark Ages (before the seventh century), people probably slept in the same underclothes that they wore during the day or went to bed wearing nothing at all. It is believed that during Greek and Roman times (1000 B.C.–A.D. 450), it was usual to wear the same underwear during the day and to bed at night. In addition, many medieval paintings portray women and men from a range of social classes sleeping in the nude. This practice continues to this day in parts of the world where climate does not necessitate warm nightclothes; in one survey from the 1960s, 70 percent of American men and 30 per-

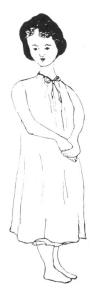

Figure 1. Early chemise, ca. 1500. *Illustration by Semra Aytur.*

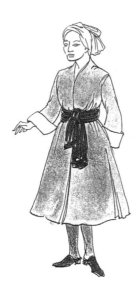

Figure 2.   Indian silk gown, ca. 1750. *Reproduced with permission from Yarwood, 1978. Copyright 1978 Doreen Yarwood.*

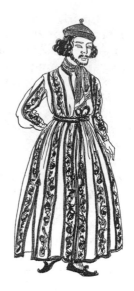

Figure 3.   Asian-influenced silk dressing gown, ca. 1840. *Reproduced with permission from Yarwood, 1978. Copyright 1978 Doreen Yarwood.*

cent of American women reported that they went to bed wearing nothing at all (Dunkell, 1977). A more recent probe into the habits of the American public found that 40 percent of Americans sleep in the buff (Sinrod and Poretz, 1991).

The word *pajamas* derives from the Hindi word *paejama,* a combination of the Persian *pai,* meaning leg or foot, and the Middle Persian *jamah,* meaning garment or clothing (*Webster's II, 1984*). Pajamas originated in ancient India as loose-fitting cotton trousers worn in bed by both men and women. They became a part of Western culture by 1610, when a Frenchman named Francis Pyrard wrote that Portuguese people wore cotton trousers to bed. Pajamas became known in England during the seventeenth century when they were coupled with a baggy shirt and were referred to as Turkish trousers or Moghul breeches. At the end of the nineteenth century, the pajama suit became popular in Europe for lounging as well as sleeping.

Nightwear inspired by India and the Orient also spread to the American Colonies. Well-to-do men and women donned loose-fitting often elaborately decorated robes, called nightgowns, Indian gowns, Indian robes, dressing gowns, night rails, or banyans (see Figure 2). Americans also adapted the traditional Japanese and Chinese kimono, which was usually made of richly embroidered silk and was sometimes quilted into a fancy robe (see Figure 3). However, some sources re-

port that these elaborate garments were not for sleeping, but were worn only when a wealthy person was going to be seen by others while relaxing at home. Colonial men and women of all social classes probably wore more simple night dresses or night shirts to sleep (see Figure 4).

The "roaring twenties" marked the beginning of the pajamas rage in the United States. Women were enamored of lounging pajamas and men often coupled their pajama sets with elaborate smoking jackets. During this time, manufacturers

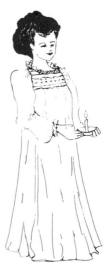

Figure 4.   North American sleepwear, ca. 1790. *Illustration by Semra Aytur.*

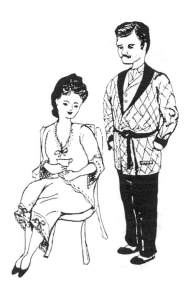

Figure 5. Woman's pajamas and dressing jacket, man's silk smoking jacket, ca. 1921. *Illustration by Semra Aytur.*

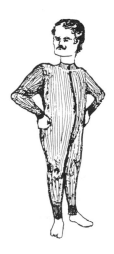

Figure 6. Man's union suit, ca. 1890. *Illustration by Semra Aytur.*

began fashioning pajamas with flared legs and short coats out of expensive silk or crepe de Chine; it was common for women to sport this fancy pajama ensemble in public, especially to the beach (see Figure 5). Pajamas soon became popular sleeping apparel not only for the fashion conscious, but also for the average American family, and the expensive pajama fabrics of the 1920s were replaced by cottons and flannels. A typical American sleeping costume of the nineteenth and twentieth centuries was the union suit, probably best known today as Dr. Denton's, although it was manufactured by a number of clothiers (see Figure 6). Resembling what is now commonly called long underwear, the union suit was a one-piece garment with long sleeves, long legs, and a high neck. Although the union suit was promoted as hygienic and "sensible" sleeping attire, its inherent appeal was most likely the warmth it provided to sleepers before the predominance of central heating and electric blankets. America's love for pajamas became a part of popular culture when the *Pajama Game,* a musical love story set in the Sleep Tite Pajama Factory, opened on Broadway in 1954. The show was based on the book 7 ½ *Cents,* written by Richard Bissell, who grew up working in his family's pajama factory in Dubuque, Iowa.

Throughout history, children were often dressed as though they were miniature adults and wore the same styles of nightwear as their elders.

Infants were sometimes put to bed dressed in swaddling clothes, a large piece of cloth that was wrapped and pinned around the baby's body and arms, forming a bundle. Another popular style of children's sleepwear is the one-piece pajama suit with a zipper up the front and "feet" sewn into the legs (see Figure 7). In the 1940s and 1950s, American manufacturers began styling children's pajamas from printed fabrics featuring toys, animals, and other tiny pictures. A major change in American children's nightwear occurred in 1975, when the Consumer Product Safety Commission began to enforce a regulation that all fabrics used to manufacture children's pajamas must meet stringent nonflammability criteria. In addition, the commission mandates that only garments that are tested and authorized by their researchers may be sold, advertised, or promoted as children's sleepwear.

Certain researchers suggest that the type of nightclothing a person wears could affect initiation or maintenance of sleep. One of the physiological characteristics of sleep is a decrease in body temperature, and nightwear that is too warm or heavy can interfere with the body's natural thermoregulatory processes (see THERMOREGULATION; TEMPERATURE EFFECTS ON SLEEP). To get a good night's sleep, experts recommend sleepwear that is roomy and comfortable and fashioned from a "breathable" fabric such as cotton, silk, or a cotton/polyester blend (Lamberg, 1989). (See also BEDS; CULTURAL ASPECTS OF SLEEP; NIGHTCAPS; PILLOWS.)

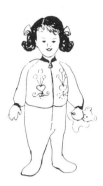

Figure 7.   Girl's one-piece pajama suit with "feet," ca. 1980. *Illustration by Semra Aytur.*

REFERENCES

Abbott G, Bissell R. 1954. *The pajama game.* New York: Random House.

Code of Federal Regulations. 1991. Vol 16, part 1616, pp 478–577. Washington, D.C.: U.S. Office of the Federal Register.

Dunkell S. 1977. *Sleep positions: The language of the body.* New York: Morrow.

Earle AM. 1903. *Two centuries of costume in America.* New York: Macmillan.

Holliday RC. 1933. *Unmentionables: From figleaves to scanties.* New York: Ray Long.

Jackson S. 1978. *Costumes for the stage.* New York: Dutton.

Lamberg L. 1989. Hot nights, cool clothes—the lightest, airiest, best-for-your-body sleepwear. *Health* 21:72–75.

Payne B. 1965. *History of costume—from the ancient Egyptians to the twentieth century.* New York: Harper and Row.

Sinrod B, Poretz M. *Do you do it with the lights on?* New York: Fawcett Columbine, 1991.

Webster's II new Riverside university dictionary. 1984. Boston: Houghton Mifflin.

Yarwood D. 1978. *The encyclopedia of world costume.* New York: Charles Scribner's Sons.

Katherine M. Sharkey

PANIC DISORDER

Panic disorders belong to the family of ANXIETY disorders. The essential feature of this psychiatric disorder is recurrent panic attacks, that is, discreet periods of intense fear that last for minutes, occasionally for hours, without the patient being in actual danger.

Panic attacks are characterized by at least four of the following thirteen symptoms: fear of dying, fear of going crazy or losing control, feeling that things are unreal or that oneself is unreal, shortness of breath or smothering sensation, chest pain, dizziness or faintness, palpitation or increased heart rate, trembling or shaking, sweating, choking, nausea, numbness or tingling in fingers and toes, and hot flashes or chills. Panic attacks are normal if one is in real danger (e.g., narrowly escaping a car accident). In patients who suffer from panic disorder, however, such panic attacks occur initially "out of the blue" (i.e., without any provocation whatsoever). Later, these panic attacks may occur more frequently in certain situations such as in elevators, shops, or crowds. Patients with panic attacks then often withdraw from situations where they fear that they may have panic attacks without possibility of escaping. In severe cases they may become confined to their own homes (agoraphobia) for fear that they might have a panic attack in public and make fools of themselves.

The causes of panic attacks are a matter of intense debate. Surprisingly, only a minority of scientists feel that panic disorder is a purely psychiatric disease. Most researchers believe that there is some abnormal, organic brain mechanism that triggers these panic attacks, be it some abnormal brain chemical, an anatomical abnormality, or another dysfunction. It is believed that initially this biological abnormality is the only reason for having panic attacks "out of the blue" and that patients later learn to fear the panics and to avoid places where having such an attack might be embarrassing.

In a minority of patients, panic attacks can also occur at night during sleep. If they do happen during sleep, they typically occur just as the sleeper moves from stage 2 into stage 3 sleep (see STAGES OF SLEEP), although panic attacks occurring during REM sleep have also been reported. At the beginning of the attack, there is increased body movement, the heart may speed up, and somewhat later the patient may wake up and report having a panic attack, or the patient may sleep through the attack and not remember it. The occurrence of these panic attacks during nondreaming sleep is interpreted by some as favoring a biological theory of panic disorder. Surprisingly, patients who suffer from panic attacks in general sleep relatively well, except when they are having an attack. They do show more body movement throughout sleep, but the length of sleep and the percentages of individual sleep stages are not disturbed.

Panic attacks need to be differentiated from dream anxiety attacks (NIGHTMARES) that occur later at night. In dream anxiety attacks, the dreamer typically remembers a long, nightmarish story; in panic attacks, very little or no content is remembered. Nocturnal panic attacks also need to be differentiated from SLEEP TERRORS, which occur during stage 4 sleep. Sleep terrors are much more stereotypic (sometimes starting with a blood-curdling scream). Patients return to sleep quite easily after a sleep terror, but they have great difficulties returning to sleep after a nocturnal panic attack. In the morning, sleep terrors are usually forgotten, whereas panic attacks are not.

Typically, nocturnal panic attacks occur only in patients who also have spontaneous daytime panic attacks. In a few rare cases, however, only nocturnal panic attacks are found.

Panic disorders are typically treated both with medication and with behavioral therapy that is designed to help patients deal with the fears and dreads of the panic attack. Sleep panic attacks are treated with the same medications, although somewhat higher doses may be needed to abolish nocturnal panic attacks than are needed to deal with daytime panic attacks.

REFERENCES

American Psychiatric Association. 1987. *Diagnostic and Statistical Manual of Mental Disorders, 3rd ed*, pp 235–254. Washington, D.C.: American Psychiatric Association.
Hauri PJ, Friedman M, Ravaris CL. 1989. Sleep in patients with spontaneous panic attacks. *Sleep* 12:323–337.
Uhde TW, Roy-Byrne P, Gillin JC, Mendelson WB, Boulenger JP, Vittore BJ, Post RM. 1984. The sleep of patients with panic disorder: A preliminary report. *Psychiatry Res* 12:251–259.

Peter Hauri

PARADOXICAL SLEEP

Also called active sleep or REM SLEEP, this stage of sleep is "paradoxical" in that, although muscle tone and general body posture indicate behavioral quiescence, heart rate, respiration, and many brain neurons display irregular activity akin to that of an awake animal. Equally paradoxical are the myoclonic jerks and twitches that often occur in this stage, unlike the behavioral quiescence observed in the rest of sleep. Paradoxical sleep and REM sleep are used as synonyms, although strictly speaking, the term *REM sleep* may be applied correctly only to those animals that exhibit rapid eye movements during the phasic parts of paradoxical sleep. The term *paradoxical sleep* was first used by Michel Jouvet in 1959. (See also REM SLEEP PHYSIOLOGY; REM SLEEP FUNCTION; SLEEP STAGES.)

REFERENCES

Jouvet M, Michel F, Courjon J. 1959. Sur un stade d'activité électrique cérébral rapide au cours du sommeil physiologique. *CR Soc Biol (Paris)* 153:1024–1028.
Sakai K. 1988. Executive mechanisms of paradoxical sleep. *Arch Ital Biol* 126(4):259–274.

Gina Rochelle Poe

PARASOMNIAS

[*As described in the* International Classification of Sleep Disorders *published by the American Sleep Disorders Association (1990), parasomnias include* "clinical disorders that are not abnormalities of the processing responsible for sleep and awake states per se but rather are undesirable physical phenomena that occur predominately during sleep." *Parasomnias comprise four rather general categories, including so-called* AROUSAL *disorders, disorders of the sleep–wake transition, disorders associated with* REM SLEEP, *and a rather loosely defined category of* "other parasomnias."

Arousal disorder parasomnias include several common phenomena often seen in young children: confusional arousals, SLEEPWALKING, *and* SLEEP TERRORS. *These events seem to be manifestations of an inability to execute a normal arousal; thus, the child does not fully awaken. Many arousal parasomnias occur early in the night during the transition from the very deepest stages of NREM sleep: Instead of a smooth transition to normal sleep stages, a partial arousal with abnormal behavior occurs.*

Sleep–wake transition parasomnias differ from arousal parasomnias in that the events occur in the course of going to sleep or from a full awakening, as in RHYTHMIC MOVEMENT DISORDER, *which is fairly common in young children. "Sleep starts" or* HYPNIC JERKS *are common occurrences at the onset of sleep and generally are not thought to be of great clinical significance; neither is* SLEEPTALKING. *This category of parasomnia also includes nocturnal leg cramps, however, which may be much more disruptive to sleep.*

Parasomnias associated with REM SLEEP *are much more serious in their presentation and consequences.* NIGHTMARES *are the most common of these parasomnias.* SLEEP PARALYSIS *is also fairly common and benign for many people who occasionally experience REM sleep* ATONIA *while falling asleep or upon awakening. The normal association of REM sleep with* ERECTIONS *has made* NOCTURNAL PENILE TUMESCENCE *an excellent medical test for male impotence; sleep-related painful erection are a rare phenomenon classified as a REM sleep parasomnia. Another rare but serious phenomenon is REM sleep sinus arrest, which has been reported in a small number of otherwise healthy young adults whose hearts briefly stop beating for more than 2.5 seconds, sometimes more than 5 seconds, during a flurry of* PHASIC ACTIVITY IN REM SLEEP. *When discovered, this serious condition may be treated by implantation of a ventricular-inhibited cardiac pacemaker to prevent full cardiac arrest during sleep.* REM SLEEP BEHAVIOR DISORDER *is also very serious and perhaps the most spectacular of all sleep disorders, involving a full loss of normal REM sleep atonia and the consequent acting-out of dreams during REM sleep.*

*The fourth category of parasomnias includes a wide variety of phenomena, ranging from bruxism (*TOOTHGRINDING*) to enuresis (*BEDWETTING*), the sleep-related abnormal swallowing syndrome,* SUDDEN NOCTURNAL DEATH SYNDROME IN ASIAN POPULATIONS, *primary* SNORING, SUDDEN INFANT DEATH SYNDROME, *and a congenital central hypoventilation syndrome (*ONDINE'S CURSE*). Thus, the parasomnias include a host of remarkable conditions, some of which are entirely without consequence and others of which may be life-threatening.]*

PARASYMPATHETIC NERVOUS SYSTEM

The parasympathetic nervous system is one of the two major subdivisions of the autonomic nervous system. The autonomic or visceral nervous system is responsible for the control of the heart, blood vessels, intestines, smooth muscles, and glands. Parasympathetic activation slows heart rate, narrows the pupil, and facilitates digestive activity by stimulating secretion of saliva and gastric juice and by contracting the smooth muscles of the gastrointestinal tract. Excretion of intestinal and urinary wastes is facilitated by the relaxation of the sphincters of the bladder and rectum and the contraction of the muscles in the wall of the bladder, both parasympathetic activities. In general, the parasympathetic system facilitates activities concerned with conserving and restoring the body's energy stores. Parasympathetic activity is normally closely integrated with the usually reciprocal sympathetic activity to regulate bodily functions (see SYMPATHETIC NERVOUS SYSTEM).

The parasympathetic output pathway involves two types of neuron. The first, or preganglionic, neuron is situated in the brainstem and in the sacral (lowest) region of the spinal cord. Fibers from these neurons exit the central nervous system through the third, seventh, ninth, and tenth cranial nerves in the brainstem and with the motor output nerves (ventral roots) of the spinal cord. These fibers then travel to groups of nerve cells called terminal ganglia, which are located near or within the target organ. In the ganglia, the preganglionic fibers make synaptic connections with the postganglionic neurons. The postganglionic neuron sends its axon out of the terminal ganglia and innervates the visceral organ, such as heart, gut, or pupillary muscle. The neurotransmitter released by both the pre- and postganglionic parasympathetic neurons is acetylcholine.

Most parasympathetic activity increases in both NREM and REM sleep, relative to waking levels. In REM sleep, phasic decreases in parasympathetic activity may occur on a background of increased activation. (See AUTONOMIC NERVOUS SYSTEM.)

REFERENCES

Carpenter MB, Sutin J, eds. 1983. *Human neuro-anatomy*, pp. 209–231. Baltimore: Williams and Wilkins.

Diamond MC, Scheibel AB, Elson LM. 1985. *The human brain coloring book.* New York: Harper and Row.

McGinty DJ, Drucker-Colin R, Morrison A, Parmeggiani PL, eds. 1985. *Brain mechanisms of sleep.* New York: Raven.

Orem J, Barnes CB, eds. 1980. *Physiology in sleep.* New York: Academic.

Stephen Morairty

PARKINSON'S DISEASE

Parkinson's disease, first described by James Parkinson in 1817, is a movement disorder characterized by tremor, muscular rigidity, and slowness of movement (bradykinesia) that affects 1 percent of people over age 50. The tremor of Parkinson's disease, most pronounced in the hands and fingers, occurs at rest, varies greatly over time, and is of 4 to 7 cycles per second. The rigidity produces a stooped posture and significant difficulties with gait. Although the most obvious feature, tremor, nearly disappears with sleep, most patients with this disorder have impaired sleep continuity and abnormal sleep architecture. Neurochemistry, PAIN, DEPRESSION, and medication side effects probably all contribute to the sleep disturbance in this disorder.

Idiopathic Parkinson's disease has a peak incidence at about age 55, and men and women are equally vulnerable. The etiology is unknown, and there are no known genetic mechanisms. The characteristic neuropathology is degeneration of the pigmented nuclei of the brainstem, most importantly the substantia nigra. This collection of cells supplies the extrapyramidal motor system with its rich supply of dopamine, a neurotransmitter that is important for normal movement and has also been implicated in the regulation of sleep and wakefulness (see also CHEMISTRY OF SLEEP: AMINES AND OTHER TRANSMITTERS). It is thought that the clinical symptoms of Parkinson's are not apparent until at least 75 percent of these cells are gone. The treatment of Parkinson's disease, replacement of lost dopamine, follows logi-cally from this underlying pathophysiology. Since dopamine cannot cross the blood–brain barrier, however, it is given in the form of its precursor *l*-dopa, which is chemically transformed (decarboxylated) in the brain to dopamine.

The symptoms of Parkinson's disease can also be produced by a variety of medical illnesses and medications (it is then called secondary Parkinson's). Antipsychotic medications cause the most common form by blocking dopamine receptors and producing reversible Parkinsonian symptoms. An epidemic of encephalitis in 1917 also led to a form of secondary Parkinson's, depicted in the film *Awakenings* (1990). Finally, severe irreversible Parkinson's symptoms can occur in intravenous users of the synthetic narcotic MPTP, which produces degeneration of the substantia nigra.

Sleep in Parkinson's Disease

The observation that Parkinson's disease is associated with disturbed sleep was originally made by Parkinson himself. More recently, controlled studies of Parkinson's patients have begun to elucidate how the waking clinical features change with sleep and to identify the features responsible for Parkinsonian sleep disturbances. It is not surprising that sleep is disturbed, since abnormalities in serotonin, acetylcholine, and norepinephrine are all present, and these neurotransmitters are vital in the coordination of normal sleep states (see CHEMISTRY OF SLEEP: NEUROTRANSMITTERS).

Although Parkinson believed that the tremor was responsible for awakening patients, POLYSOMNOGRAPHY has demonstrated that the classic alternating tremor nearly disappears with the onset of sleep, but recurs during brief arousals or a lightening of sleep stage. This latter observation may account for patients' belief that the tremor awakened them. On the other hand, sustained muscle bursts, without the characteristic alternating pattern of tremor, may appear in NREM sleep but not REM sleep. Waking bradykinesia and rigidity are reflected during sleep in a reduced number of position changes during the night, and these long periods of immobility often end in awakenings.

Sleep architecture is disturbed in Parkinson's, and the degree of disturbance appears to be correlated with the severity of waking symptomatology. Consistent with patients' descriptions, polysomnography has documented an increased number of awakenings along with a higher stage 1 sleep percentage (see STAGES OF SLEEP). In advanced cases, patients spend roughly one third of the night awake. In one study, pain (from muscle cramps or spasms, joints, and nerve roots) correlated with patient complaints of poor sleep maintenance. In addition, Parkinson's patients have a reduction in SLOW-WAVE SLEEP and REM SLEEP, and SLEEP SPINDLE frequency is reduced to roughly 50 percent of normal.

In addition to these sleep disturbances, 50 percent of patients with Parkinson's have dysthymia or major DEPRESSION, which can independently produce sleep disturbances. A recent study documented significantly lower REM LATENCY in Parkinson's patients with these affective disorders than in nondepressed Parkinson's patients, a finding characteristic of idiopathic major depression. PERIODIC LEG MOVEMENTS of sleep and sleep APNEA, common sleep disorders in the elderly, are also present in Parkinson's patients, although it is controversial whether they have a higher frequency than in age-matched controls. One subgroup of Parkinsonian patients with associated autonomic disturbances (Shy–Drager syndrome) do have an excess of abnormal respiratory events during sleep.

Treatment of Parkinson's disease with *l*-dopa or other dopaminergic compounds can both alleviate and produce sleep disturbances. In some patients, these medications can improve nocturnal symptoms (e.g., increase mobility) and thus improve sleep consolidation. On the other hand, *l*-dopa has stimulant properties, increasing arousal and extending REM sleep latency, and at higher doses these effects may prevail. In addition, reports of NIGHTMARES and vivid dreams are common after *l*-dopa use. Finally, myoclonus, periodic or aperiodic, may result from chronic *l*-dopa administration. The titration of *l*-dopa in Parkinsonian patients requires careful attention to the timing and quality of evolving symptoms. Other medications, including alternate dopamine agonists and the monoamine oxidase B–selective inhibitor selegiline, may aid in modifying treatment-resistant and treatment-emergent symptoms.

Conclusions

The causes of sleep disturbances in Parkinson's are manifold. In fact, it would be surprising if

Parkinson's disease were not associated with sleep disturbances. The cellular regions responsible for sleep regulation are those destroyed by the illness; patients with Parkinson's are often in pain; nearly half have major depression or dysthymia; and the primary treatment, *l*-dopa, can produce sleep disruption, nightmares, and periodic limb movements in sleep.

REFERENCES

Aldrich MS. 1989. Parkinsonism. In Kryger MH, Roth T, Dement WC, eds. *Principles and practice of sleep medicine,* pp 351–357. Philadelphia: Saunders.
Nausieda PA. 1990. Sleep in Parkinson disease. In Thorpy MJ, ed. *Handbook of sleep disorders.* New York: Marcel Dekker.

John Winkelman

PASSING OUT

It is generally accepted that sustained wakefulness is maintained by structures in the base of the brain (brainstem), including the well-known so-called reticular activating system, that stimulate the cortex or outer shell of the brain in which control of the majority of the higher nervous functions is located. Such activation permits awareness of the environment, voluntary actions, and other such activities. (See also AROUSAL.)

Passing out refers to the loss of consciousness of self and the environment. It can result from any process that impedes the activity of either these brainstem centers or the cortex they activate. The mechanisms are many. In the sleep attacks seen in certain sleep disorders, such as NARCOLEPSY, the activating brainstem centers are actively inhibited by the brain's sleep-inducing centers, as occurs normally at sleep onset. As brain cells can metabolize only the sugar glucose, which requires oxygen, two other main causes of loss of consciousness are insufficient glucose, such as occurs in low blood sugar in some diabetics (hypoglycemic coma), and insufficient oxygen. The latter most commonly occurs when blood pressure falls to levels not allowing sufficient blood to get to the brain, as in fainting spells (syncope), and in a variety of conditions in which the blood oxygen falls to critically low levels (hypoxemia).

Loss of consciousness may also occur because the normal brain cell firing patterns are disrupted by the discharges of an epileptic seizure (see EPILEPSY). Finally, unconsciousness, typically of much slower onset and often leading to COMA, may occur from the presence of internal toxic substances suppressing brain metabolism arising from, for instance, liver or kidney disease, or from ingestion of toxins external to the body such as excessive ALCOHOL or methanol.

Roger J. Broughton

PEPTIDES

See Chemistry of Sleep; Neuroendocrine Hormones

PERCEPTION DURING SLEEP

"Perception" encompasses all those processes by which we make sense of information from the world around us. By studying "what registers" when someone is asleep, we can gain insights into the psychology of sleep and dreaming, because differences between waking and sleeping perceptual abilities set limits on the availability of information the brain can respond to and process during sleep.

We know from physiological studies that the brain is continuously yet differentially active during all states of sleep and wakefulness, so it should not be surprising that the manner in which it receives and works with information varies when wakefulness and sleep are compared. That is, our perception of external events is greatly altered as we sleep. Of all the senses, changes in sensitivity to auditory information have been studied most thoroughly. Early experiments looked at auditory arousal thresholds (AATs)—at how loud a tone was required to awaken someone from each sleep stage (i.e., perceptual thresholds during sleep). Rechtschaffen, Hauri, and Zeitlin (1966), using a series of tones of increasing loudness to detect awakening

thresholds, found that auditory sensitivity was equal in stage 2 and REM sleep, whereas louder tones were necessary to arouse someone from slow wave sleep (SWS). Generally, AATs decreased (people became more sensitive to sounds) as the night progressed, regardless of sleep stage. Bonnet and Moore (1982) reported that AATs increase by more than 30 decibels within the first minute of electroencephalograph (EEG)-defined sleep, reaching over 60 percent of their maximal sleep values within that time.

So far, we have established that people are less sensitive to external, auditory information during sleep and that sensitivity (threshold) varies depending on sleep stage and time of night. But is perception during sleep otherwise identical to that of wakefulness? Studies cited below will show that there are also important qualitative differences in perceptual processing during different stages of sleep.

Okuma et al. (1966), using both optic and auditory stimuli, found that responses were made to stimuli presented in all but stage 4 sleep, and added that the perception of the correct number of stimuli presented was more accurate in REM than in any other stage. The unresponsiveness of people in stage 4 sleep was dramatically demonstrated by Oswald (1962), who showed an EEG tracing of a person deep in stage 4 sleep who remained asleep and unresponsive despite having his eyelids pulled open in the presence of a strong light, being poked, and spoken to loudly.

The meaningfulness of stimuli has been shown to have a marked effect on AATs from sleep. Oswald, Taylor, and Treisman (1960) used names as stimuli and found that a greater number of fist-clench responses and K-COMPLEXES (high-voltage EEG spikes with a spindle tail) occurred in response to one's own name than to one's own name read backward or the names of others. Langford, Meddis, and Pearson (1974) predicted that personally significant stimuli would be processed more accurately during REM than during other sleep stages. Adapting Oswald's forward and backward own-name procedure, they confirmed the prediction that responses were faster in REM than in stage 2 sleep. Forward own-name responses were more effectively perceived than backward own-names in both stages. These scientific data confirm common experience; for example, mothers frequently report being able to awaken from sleep in response to their baby's cry, while being able to sleep undisrupted through louder stimuli like thunder and traffic noise, which they have learned to ignore.

That we can learn to respond to some stimuli while paying less attention to others has been confirmed in other sleep laboratory studies. Williams, Morlock, and Morlock (1966) examined the ability to make simple discriminative responses during sleep. They instructed subjects to turn off tones by pressing a switch taped to their hand. Then they presented these tones during sleep and recorded the switch-pressing responses. Switch presses were always most frequent in stage 1 and least frequent in stages 3 and 4. Response frequencies were intermediate in stage 2 and REM sleep. If subjects were threatened with punishment (very loud sounds and electric shock) for failures to respond, response frequencies were increased in all stages. These findings were confirmed and extended by Harsh et al. (1987), who used voluntary increases in depth of breathing as the response measure to the tones. They reported a very consistent response rate to tones presented during REM and stage 2 sleep. Again, these findings show that the perceptual gate, while never fully open during sleep, is opened more fully in some sleep stages than in others. This is shown indirectly; the sleepers clearly had to perceive and process the signals before being able to respond to them during sleep. Of course, it is only their responses that we can observe directly.

Perry et al. (1978) showed that more complex perceptions and processing of verbal material can occur sometimes in sleep. While people were in REM sleep they were given suggestions like "Whenever I say the word 'itch', your nose will feel itchy until you scratch your nose." Of the 251 test word presentations, 117 responses were made, 36 of which were appropriate to the suggestion. This study shows that perception of and responding to complex information is possible, although not highly probable, during REM sleep.

The question of what level of complexity of information can be perceived during sleep is best approached by brief reference to studies on sleep LEARNING. An interesting set of conflicting findings is reviewed by Eich (1990), who notes that if the question of learning is addressed in a laboratory where care has been taken to shield the potential learner from prior information about the topic to be presented during sleep, and if care is also taken to insure that recordings are played only after definite EEG signs of sleep are established, sleep learning will not take place. Such studies address the issue of the possibility of perceiving difficult concepts during sleep and appear to rule out complex learning during established sleep. Nevertheless, if the focus is on the practical issue of whether or not one can further consolidate learning begun in wakefulness by playing tapes all night long, the answer is more positive. It appears that there may be some benefit in listening to nightly presentations of information, but if learning does occur, it does not take place during sleep per se, but during quiet periods of drowsy wakefulness preceding, following, and interspersed with sleep. (See also MEMORY.)

Conclusions

Nature has provided us with a perceptual system that continues to operate at reduced efficiency during sleep. Sounds and lights can still alert us during sleep, particularly if they have clear meaning to us—meaning derived from lengthy personal associations such as our names or stimuli made meaningful by positive or negative reinforcement. Sound presented during REM is generally more likely to be received than that presented during stage 2 sleep, whereas sounds of all complexity are least likely to register during SWS. The passage of time is perceived reasonably accurately during sleep. But despite these sleep abilities, if your friend needs to know about perception during sleep for a test tomorrow, don't wait until he has fallen asleep to read these paragraphs to him for the first time.

REFERENCES

Bonnet MH, Moore SE. 1982. The threshold of sleep: Perception of sleep as a function of time asleep and auditory threshold. *Sleep* 5:267–276.

Eich E. 1990. Learning during sleep. In Bootzin RR, Kihlstrom JF, Schachter DL, eds. *Sleep and cognition,* pp 88–108. Washington, D.C.: American Psychological Association.

Harsh J, Badia P, O'Rourke D, Burton S, Revis C, Magee J. 1987. Factors related to behavioral control by stimuli presented during sleep. *Psychophysiology* 24:535–541.

Langford GW, Meddis R, Pearson AJD. 1974. Awakening latency from sleep for meaningful and non-meaningful stimuli. *Psychophysiology* 11:1–5.

Okuma T, Nakamura K, Hayashi A, Fujimori M. 1966. Psychophysiological study of the depth of sleep in normal human subjects. *Electroencephalogr Clin Neurophysiol* 21:140–147.

Oswald I. 1962. *Sleeping and waking: Physiology and psychology.* Amsterdam: Elsevier.

Oswald I, Taylor AM, Treisman M. 1960. Discriminative responses to stimulation during human sleep. *Brain* 83:440–453.

Perry CW, Evans FJ, O'Connell DN, Orne EC, Orne MT. 1978. Behavioral response to verbal stimuli administered and tested during REM sleep: A further investigation. *Waking Sleeping* 2:35–42.

Rechtschaffen A, Hauri P, Zeitlin M. 1966. Auditory awakening thresholds in REM and NREM sleep stages. *Percept Mot Skills* 22:927–942.

Williams HL, Morlock HC, Morlock JV. 1966. Instrumental behavior during sleep. *Psychophysiology* 2:208–216.

Robert D. Ogilvie

PERFORMANCE

[*Performance can be affected in a number of ways by sleep, lack of sleep, or the* BIOLOGICAL RHYTHMS *of behavior. Sleep itself has a marked impact on performance, which can be best be seen through the effects of sleep on* MEMORY *and* LEARNING. *For example, despite a fairly widespread belief that learning can take place during sleep, this phenomenon has not been convincingly documented (see* MYTHS ABOUT SLEEP). PERCEPTION *and* SENSORY PROCESSING AND SENSATION DURING SLEEP *in general are greatly impaired; this implies that performance of most cognitive functions in sleep is quite limited. On the other hand, sleep is not entirely devoid of sensory and cognitive processing (see* COGNITION).

DREAMS AND DREAMING *have been related to several aspects of human performance, though even in these instances the quantity and quality of performance is reduced. For example, anecdotal evidence suggests that* PROBLEM SOLVING *can occur either during dreaming or with the help of dreaming. Successful resolution of a problem through dreaming is a rare occurrence; however, certain people have demonstrated an ability to apply the* CREATIVITY IN DREAMING *to problematic issues in their waking lives.*

Diminution of one's performance capacity is a significant and potent consequence of sleep DEPRIVATION. *In many instances, this reduced ability to perform a variety of tasks or functions is related specifically to the* SLEEPINESS *that results from sleep deprivation. Performance deficits are a major hazard to* PUBLIC SAFETY IN THE WORKPLACE *and* PUBLIC SAFETY IN TRANSPORTATION. *Performance decay as a result of sleep loss has been noted in such diverse groups as astronauts, airline* PILOTS, *and* TRUCKERS *(see also* MICROGRAVITY AND SPACE FLIGHT; SPACE SHUTTLE SLEEPING ARRANGEMENTS). *A classic description of the effects of sleep deprivation on performance and behavior resulted from an experiment undertaken by a young man who went without sleep for 11 days as part of a high school science project (see* GARDNER, RANDY). *In* ADOLESCENCE, *sleep at night is commonly shortchanged, and many teenagers suffer daytime sleepiness and significant performance decrements as a consequence. Such decrements are even greater when students pull* ALL-NIGHTERS. *Problems with performance are also common in people with such sleep disorders as* INSOMNIA, NARCOLEPSY, *and sleep* APNEA, *or who otherwise have either intrinsic or environmental disruptions of sleep (see also* FRAGMENTATION).

CIRCADIAN RHYTHMS *exert a powerful influence on performance; many aspects of waking abilities fluctuate across the day depending on underlying physiological and behavioral rhythms, including the sleep–wake cycle (see also* BASIC REST–ACTIVITY CYCLE; MORNINGNESS/ EVENINGNESS; TIMING OF SLEEP AND WAKEFULNESS). *This rhythmic relationship becomes particularly apparent following a night of sleep deprivation: Performance is terribly impaired in the depths of the night and then becomes markedly better, though not up to par, during the daytime. This phenomenon is largely a function of the circadian rhythm of performance.*

Many ingested substances, including drugs, have a major effect on performance. For example, CAFFEINE *can improve performance in someone who has been sleep deprived and is sleepy;* ALCOHOL, *on the other hand, can further impair performance, particularly in someone who is sleepy (see also* OVER-THE-COUNTER SLEEPING PILLS; OVER-THE-COUNTER STIMULANTS*).*]

PERIODIC LEG MOVEMENTS

The syndrome of periodic leg movements in sleep (PLMS) is one of the most common yet unusual of all sleep disorders. PLMS, as the name suggests, are periodic movements of the legs, feet, and/or toes during sleep. The movements are generally slow, lasting 0.5 to 5 seconds. The most unusual aspect of PLMS is that they occur in a periodic manner. This means that the movements repeat themselves at certain intervals. The most common interval is generally every 20 to 40 seconds. In many cases the interval between movements is very specific. It is not unusual to find in a particular patient that the periodic leg movements are separated by an interval of, for example, exactly 30, 24.2, or 43 seconds (Figure 1). The specific interval is different for different patients. This periodic aspect of the movement is most puzzling because research has shown that few other systems in the body or brain have a similar frequency.

Patients who are eventually found to have PLMS usually come to the doctor's office complaining of INSOMNIA, excessive daytime SLEEPINESS, frequent awakenings from sleep, or unrefreshing sleep. These symptoms are common to many sleep disorders. For this reason, the syndrome of PLMS is one the most difficult disorders to diagnose by simply talking to the patient. Patients are often not aware of moving their legs during sleep and are unaware of why their sleep is so unrefreshing. Occasionally, a bedpartner may complain of being kicked during the night or of the bed shaking, but most often there is no direct evidence in the patient's medical history to point to PLMS as the cause of the sleep problem.

Periodic leg movements in sleep can be diagnosed only during a polysomnogram (PSG) or sleep study (see POLYSOMNOGRAPHY). The PSG measures a variety of physiological parameters simultaneously. As part of the PSG, surface electrodes are placed over the anterior tibialis muscle, which is on the outside of both calves on the lower leg. This muscle contracts when the foot extends (dorsiflexes) or when the leg moves. The electrode detects increased electrical

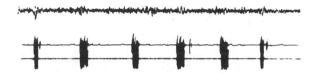

Figure 1.   Portion of polysomnographic recording showing repetitive movements of the legs (left and right legs from bottom to top) during sleep, and associated arousals in the electroencephalogram (topmost channel).

activity of the muscle, usually lasting 1.5 to 2.5 seconds. Four PLMS in a row with a typical interval of 20 to 40 seconds must occur for these movements to be called periodic. During the course of the night a PLMS index of 5 PLMS per hour of sleep must be detected (40 PLMS during 8 hours of sleep) for a clinical diagnosis of PLMS to be made.

One additional step must be taken to determine if these PLMS actually had an effect on sleep. Every time a periodic leg movement is noted in the PSG, the ELECTROENCEPHALOGRAM (EEG) (brain waves) occurring at the same time must be inspected to determine if the movement caused the patient to awaken. Often the EEG pattern will change for 1 to 30 seconds, and alpha waves, which are characteristic of drowsy wakefulness, or a K-COMPLEX, a sign of arousal, will appear. Occasionally, the patient may wake up for several minutes or longer and be completely unaware of what caused the awakening. It is the awakenings caused by the PLMS that are most important finding on the PSG, because they explain why the patient's sleep is fragmented and, thus, why the patient is so sleepy. PLMS that occur without disturbing sleep or causing awakenings may not be of importance. It is possible that hundreds of PLMS may occur during a recording without actually disturbing sleep. For this reason, a PLMS–arousal index (how many PLMS caused arousal or wakefulness per hour of sleep) is often computed and is very useful for determining just how severely sleep was fragmented (see FRAGMENTATION).

Periodic leg movements in sleep occur almost exclusively in NREM sleep and are absent in REM sleep. PLMS apparently are triggered somewhere in the brain, but what causes these puzzling movements and why they are periodic are not known.

Periodic leg movements in sleep are frequently associated with a waking disorder, restless legs syndrome, but not all patients with PLMS also have restless legs syndrome. On the other hand, most patients with restless legs syndrome do have PLMS. PLMS were originally called nocturnal myoclonus; however, this was changed because myoclonus suggests a very rapid movement of the muscles, and PLMS are relatively slow. Additionally, it was thought that the term *nocturnal myoclonus* might be confused with myoclonic or nocturnal epilepsy. PLMS are not thought to be a form of epilepsy. The brain waves that occur during the movements are usually normal.

The syndrome of PLMS is a common disorder that increases in frequency with age. It is rarely reported to affect children or adults below the age of 30 years. It has been reported to affect approximately 5 percent of people aged 30 to 50 years, 29 percent of those over age 50, and almost 44 percent of individuals older than 65. Both men and women may have PLMS, and it has also be reported to run in families.

Periodic leg movements in sleep can be provoked by or associated with many different medical disorders and medications. PLMS have been reported in patients with kidney failure and uremia as well as other medical disorders. Some depressant medications have been reported to provoke or dramatically increase the number and disruptiveness of PLMS. Additionally, withdrawal of drugs of the type used to treat PLMS may result in sudden increases in PLMS.

Periodic leg movements in sleep are treated exclusively with medications. Three general types of medications are used to treat PLMS. The most common treatment has been the use of the class of drugs called BENZODIAZEPINES, which include most prescription SLEEPING PILLS and antianxiety drugs. The benzodiazepine clonazepam is most frequently used to treat PLMS and restless legs syndrome; however, there is some controversy as to whether clonazepam works by actually reducing the number of PLMS or by mildly sedating the patient and therefore preventing PLMS from waking the patient. Additionally, clonazepam is a very long acting drug that remains in the body 20 to 96 hours after it is taken, possibly resulting in drug-induced grogginess during the daytime.

Recently, doctors have reported success using opiates. These include common drugs such as propoxyphene that are usually prescribed for pain. Additionally, several researchers have reported that drugs originally used for the treatment of abnormal movements of Parkinsonism patients significantly reduce the number of PLMS; however, these drugs, L-dopa and carbidopa/levadopa, have not yet come into common usage because of their potential side effects.

REFERENCES

Coleman R. 1982. Periodic movements in sleep (nocturnal myoclonus) and restless legs syndrome. In Guilleminault C, ed. *Sleeping and waking disorders: Indications and techniques,* pp 265–295. Menlo Park, Calif.: Addison-Wesley.
Montplasir J, Godbout R. 1989. Restless legs syndrome and periodic leg movements in sleep. In Kryger MH, Roth T, Dement WC, eds. *Principles and practice of sleep medicine.* pp 402–408. Philadelphia: Saunders.

Mark R. Pressman

PERIODIC MOVEMENTS IN SLEEP

See Periodic Leg Movements

PERSONALITY AND DREAM RECALL

Why do some people remember several dreams each night while others never recall a dream? This question is especially intriguing in view of sleep laboratory research demonstrating that all humans have three to five REM periods per night (SEE RAPID EYE MOVEMENT), and the vast majority of subjects awakened from a REM period or just after one will report a dream. Dreams are sometimes but less frequently reported from awakenings during NREM sleep and even during sleep onset. It appears then that most of us experience a number of dreams per night, but most of these are not recalled. Although there is not much difference between people in terms of amounts of REM sleep, there is a huge difference in the number of dreams spontaneously recalled. (See also RECALL OF DREAMS.)

Among the factors that make a difference are some purely physiological ones: Sound sleepers tend to recall fewer dreams than less sound sleepers, most likely because the latter are more likely to awaken during or just after a REM sleep period. Long sleepers (over 9 hours) recall more dreams than do short sleepers (under 6 hours), perhaps because the latter have less REM sleep and have fewer awakenings.

Personality factors also appear to be related to greater or lesser dream recall. Unfortunately, the results have not always been consistent and depend somewhat on variables such as whether the subject is simply asked once about dream recall, or is asked to keep a diary. However, a few points have emerged. Various studies have suggested that more dream recall may be related to high anxiety, low repression, field dependency, high tolerance for ambiguity, high "absorption," and high "creative interests." More recently, it has been demonstrated that there is a relationship between dream recall and having "thin boundaries." People with more dream recall demonstrate thin boundaries in a number of different psychological senses: They are open, trusting, sensitive, easily hurt; they tend to merge thoughts with feelings, fantasies with reality, and to experience vivid imagery and many in-between states such as reverie, dozing, or being "half asleep."

REFERENCES

Belicki K. 1986. Recalling dreams: An examination of daily variation and individual differences. In Gackenbach J, ed. *Sleep and dreams: A sourcebook,* pp 187–206. New York and London: Garland.
Hartmann E. 1990. Thin and thick boundaries: Personality, dreams, and imagination. In Kunzendorf R, ed. *Mental imagery.* New York: Plenum.
———. 1991. *Boundaries in the mind.* New York: Basic.

Ernest Hartmann

PERSONALITY AND SLEEP

One of the first comprehensive attempts to identify relationships between sleep and personality was carried out by Ernest Hartmann and his colleagues. Reflecting on the meaning of his data, Hartmann stated:

Assuming that our results are valid, it must be kept in mind that we have established only a correlation between the amount of sleep and certain personality or life-style characteristics. I consider the most likely explanation to be that certain life-styles or certain personalities require more sleep than others. However, it is possible that the inverse relationship might be true, that sleeping different lengths of time could produce personality changes.... (1973, pp 66–67)

In the years that have elapsed since these words were written, a fair number of studies have been carried out to identify possible relationships between sleep and personality traits. Almost all of these studies used correlational designs, and the quandary of interpretation posed by Hartmann's statement remains. That is, one cannot be sure whether certain personalities require more sleep or variations in sleep alter existing personality traits. Both alternatives have merit: personality may affect sleep habits, and amount of sleep may affect our personalities.

Hartmann's Research and Its Implications

Hartmann's original study forms the basis for much of the subsequent sleep and personality work. In the original study, a battery of psychological tests, interviews, and ratings of clinical behavior were used to measure the differences in personality between habitual short- and long-sleeping adults (Hartmann, Baekeland, and Zwilling, 1972). Drawing primarily on their clinical impressions, they described a fairly pronounced pattern of personality differences between these groups, and these findings were replicated in a subsequent study (Spinweber and Hartmann, 1976). Essentially, the short sleepers were seen as efficient, energetic, ambitious, but "preprogrammed" nonworriers who tended to "avoid problems by keeping busy and by denial which in some cases approaches hypomania" (Hartmann, Baekeland, and Zwilling, 1972, p. 467). On the other hand, long sleepers were described as less aggressive and more reflective individuals who were constantly "reprogramming" themselves.

These personality descriptions bear a striking similarity to those put forward by Friedman and Rosenman (1977) for individuals who are classified as exhibiting either the Type A or Type B behavior pattern. Thus, persons categorized as having a Type A personality are viewed as aggressive, impatient, hard-driving individuals who tend to engage in a greater number of activities than the fixed limitation of time allows. In doing this, the Type A person "more and more substitutes 'faster' for 'better' or 'different' in his way of thinking and doing. In other words, he indulges in stereotyped responses [and] substitutes repetitive urgency for creative energy" (p. 206). In contrast, Type B individuals are viewed as less aggressive, less likely to be in a struggle with time and/or with other individuals, and likely to be more reflective in their approach to problem solving. These differences in personality and/or life style are thought to have important implications for health: Type A persons seem to be at greater risk of stress-related disease because they are simultaneously more aroused and more engaged with life and its potential stressors, and when these stressors manifest themselves, they may be less able to cope by resolving problems.

Sleep and Type A/B Behavior

Several studies have linked type A/B behavior to sleep parameters. Research has documented an inverse relationship between level of Type A behavior and habitual sleep duration (Hicks et al., 1979), and a direct relationship between level of Type A behavior and the number of hours by which individuals have shortened their habitual sleep durations (Hicks et al., 1980). Thus, the person with stronger Type A personality characteristics is likely to sleep less and to have reduced the amount of time spent sleeping by a greater amount than a person with a weaker Type A personality. Logically, both these sets of data indicate that to meet life-style demands, the Type A person gives up sleep to gain more wakeful time for a greater number of activities.

On the other hand, the behaviors that are among the most salient aspects of the so-called Type A personality are influenced by sleep. For example, a number of *state* or *process* variables are altered by sleep and therefore have an effect on personality and/or life style. Such variables include arousal level, aggressiveness, problem solving-related abilities, and stress-management processes.

Sleep and Arousal Level

To explain the results of his monumental study demonstrating the psychoactive effects of REM sleep deprivation on people with endogenous depression (see DEPRESSION; DEPRIVATION, SELECTIVE; REM SLEEP), Gerald Vogel (1979) argued that REM sleep was a period during which drive energy accumulated during wakefulness was dissipated. Thus, reductions of REM sleep increase subsequent wakeful drive energy by reducing its discharge during REM sleep. Vogel also argued that loss of REM sleep activated a cluster of primary drive–linked motivational behaviors, such as eating and sexual activity. Although there is little evidence for the latter assertions, considerable evidence from a variety of research approaches indicates that REM sleep reductions produce an increased level of arousal in both humans and laboratory animals (see Ellman, Spielman, and Lipschutz-Brach, 1991, for review). Habits that alter REM sleep may therefore alter an individual's state and by that process have an influence on the expression of existing personality traits.

Sleep and Aggressiveness

It is a truism that sleep loss increases irritability and aggressiveness; however, the direct evidence for this widely held notion is sparse and difficult to interpret (Shaw et al., 1990). Positive evidence for this assertion comes from several studies. For example, laboratory animals deprived of REM sleep are less fearful of their environment and more likely to exhibit aggressive behaviors when coping with a stressor (Hicks and Moore, 1979; Hawkins et al., 1978). Another study examined coping styles of long and short sleepers immediately after the San Francisco Bay Area earthquake of October 17, 1989 (Hicks, Marical, and Conti, 1991). In responding to this substantial stressor, short sleepers were more likely to use confrontive (aggressive) coping than were longer sleepers. Such studies indicate that sleep habits may alter the way certain personality traits are manifested in behavior; reduced sleep appears to disinhibit certain forms of aggressiveness.

Sleep and Problem Solving

Studies designed to measure the relationships between sleep and human abilities report reliable relationships between amount of REM sleep and divergent thinking or general fluid intelligence. (*Fluid intelligence* is a label for a set of variables reflecting an individual's ability to deal with the environment on a day-to-day basis; it is contrasted with *crystallized intelligence,* a label for factors such as performance on tests of vocabulary, information, and arithmetic, thought to reflect level of acculturation.) Thus, for example, Feinberg, Koresko, and Heller (1967) reported that aged normal adults (mean age 77 years) showed significant correlations between amount of REM sleep (measured polygraphically) and measures of fluid intelligence. REM sleep was not related to *crystallized intelligence,* and SLOW-WAVE SLEEP was not correlated with either of these general factors of intelligence. In a related study, Glaubman and his colleagues (1978) found that divergent thinking was significantly lower after REM sleep deprivation than after NREM sleep deprivation. Two additional studies demonstrated that habitual short sleepers scored significantly lower than long sleepers on tests of divergent thinking and fluid intelligence (Hicks et al., 1978, 1980). The flexibility of intellectual functioning and especially the ability to solve problems may therefore be linked to the amount of REM sleep an individual normally experiences. Thus, if reductions in REM sleep promote stereotypical responding, the impact may be to alter the expresion of personality.

Sleep and Stress Management

Several studies suggest that sleep is related to stress management. For example, when subjects were selectively deprived of REM sleep, they were less able to cope with stress-induced anxiety than after selective NREM sleep deprivation (Greenberg, Pillard, and Pearlman, 1979). Another study showed that hospitalized patients dreamed about their upcoming surgery, but after successful operations such dreams were greatly reduced (Breger, Hunter, and Lane, 1972). Rosalind Cartwright, a noted psychologist in this field, has summarized the implications of such research:

> Dreaming is involved in reviewing, reorganizing, and rehearsing concepts of who we are and how we are doing in our own eyes. The system shows up best when we are under stress and threatened with a major life change that requires new responses. The system can be overloaded, which seems to happen in those with a biological vulnerability for REM sleep disruption. (1990, p. 188)

(See also INTERPRETATION OF DREAMS.)

In summary, data from several lines of investigation implicate sleep in stress management and suggest that sleep habits can alter coping processes. This relationship provides a way in which sleep may have an influence on the expression of personality traits.

REFERENCES

Breger L, Hunter I, Lane R. 1971. The effect of stress on dreams. *Psychological Issues Monograph,* 27 (7, suppl 3).

Cartwright R. 1990. A network model of dreams. In Bootzin RR, Kihlstrom JF, Schacter DL, eds. *Sleep and cognition,* pp 179–189. Washington, D.C.: American Psychological Association.

Ellman SJ, Spielman AJ, Lipschutz-Brach L. 1991. Update: REM deprivation. In Ellman SJ, Antrobus JS, eds. *The mind in sleep,* pp 369–376. New York: Wiley.

Feinberg I, Koresko RL, Heller N. 1967. EEG sleep patterns as a function of normal and pathological aging in man. *Psychiatric Res* 5:107–144.

Friedman M, Rosenman RH. 1977. The key cause: Type A behavior pattern. In Monat A, Lazarus RS, eds. *Stress and coping,* pp 203–216. New York: Columbia University Press.

Glaubman H, Orbach I, Aviram O, Frieder I, Frieman M, Pelled O, Glaubman R. 1978. REM deprivation and divergent thinking. *Psychophysiology* 15:75–79.

Greenberg, R, Pillard R, Pearlman C. 1972. The effect of dream (Stage REM) deprivation on adaptation to stress. *Psychosomatic Med* 34:257–262.

Hartmann E. 1973. *The functions of sleep.* New Haven: Yale University Press.

Hartmann E, Baekeland F, Zwilling GR. 1972. Psychological differences between long and short sleepers. *Arch Gen Psychiatry* 26:463–468.

Hawkins J, Hicks RA, Phillips N, Moore JD. 1978. Swimming rats and human depression. *Nature* 274:512.

Hicks RA, Allen JG, Armogida RE, Gilliland MA, Pellegrini RJ. 1980. Reductions in sleep duration and Type A behavior. *Bull Psychonomic Soc* 16:109–110.

Hicks RA, Guista M, Schretlen D, Pellegrini RJ. 1980. Habitual duration of sleep and divergent thinking. *Psychol Reports* 46:426.

Hicks RA, Marical CM, Conti PA. 1991. Coping with a major stressor: Differences between habitual short- and longer-sleepers. *Percept Motor Skills* 72:631–636.

Hicks RA, Moore J. 1979. REM sleep deprivation diminishes fear in rats. *Physiology Behavior* 22:689–692.

Hicks RA, Pellegrini RJ, Cavanaugh A, Sahatjian M, Sandham L. 1978. Fluid intelligence levels of short- and long-sleeping college students. *Psychol Reports* 43:1325–1326.

Hicks RA, Pellegrini RJ, Martin S, Garbesi L, Elliott D, Hawkins J. 1979. Type A behavior and normal habitual sleep duration. *Bull Psychonomic Soc* 14:185–186.

Shaw P, Puentes J, Reis C, Hicks RA. 1990. REM sleep deprivation fails to increase aggression in female rats. *Bull Psychonomic Soc* 28:448–450.

Spinweber CL, Hartmann E. 1976. Long and short sleepers: Male and female subjects' sleep, personality and biochemical measures. *Sleep Res* 5:112.

Vogel GA. 1979. A motivational function of REM sleep. In Drucker-Colin R, Shkurovich M, Sterman MB, eds. *The functions of sleep*, pp 233–250. New York: Academic.

Robert A. Hicks
Patricia Conti

PGO WAVES

PGO waves are electrical phenomena similar to the ELECTROENCEPHALOGRAM (EEG) that can be recorded from many locations within the brain. These waves occur both singly and as bursts of waves during REM sleep and only as single waves in NREM sleep 30 to 90 seconds before REM sleep begins. The name *PGO* derives from the three brain regions from which this activity was originally recorded—the pontine reticular formation, the lateral geniculate nucleus of the thalamus, and the occipital (visual) cortex—hence ponto-geniculo-occipital waves. PGO waves have since been recorded in many other brain structures, including several sensory and motor areas of the brainstem, cerebellum, all types of tha-

lamic relay nuclei, and cortical areas outside the occipital cortex. Because PGO waves are recorded from electrodes placed within the brain, they have been observed only in animals; however, PGO-like activity has been obtained in humans by using averaging techniques applied to the EEG recorded from scalp electrodes (see ELECTROENCEPHALOGRAPHY). The phasic, intermittent generation of PGO waves is probably a basic process of REM sleep in all mammals.

The electrical event resulting in a PGO wave is produced by simultaneous activity of many nerve cells in the vicinity of the recording electrode. The spatial distribution of these nerve cells is also important. The layered distribution of neurons in the lateral geniculate nucleus of the thalamus produces large-amplitude PGO waves, whereas PGO waves cannot be recorded from the midbrain reticular formation, yet bursts of activity in nerve cells located there occur in association with PGO waves recorded elsewhere. The underlying neural network(s) responsible for local PGO wave generation has a more widespread influence in brain than is indicated solely by the structures from which PGO waves can be recorded. The neuronal activity associated with PGO waves is most often excitation; however, certain nerve cell populations have recently been found to be initially inhibited during PGO waves.

Many behaviors that occur during REM sleep have the same phasic or periodic distribution in time as the PGO waves recorded in brain. Some of these behaviors include rapid eye movements, muscle twitches, muscle activity in the middle ear, and cardiorespiratory (heart and breathing) irregularities. Neuronal activity associated with PGO waves is probably responsible for these phasic behaviors. For example, PGO waves can be recorded from the brain cell groups containing motor neurons that control eye movements. Thus, the PGO wave-associated activity of these neurons is the proximal cause of the rapid eye movements during REM sleep. Phasic events, including the behaviors noted above, and the PGO waves and associated neuronal activity in brain, may be under the control of a single phasic event system. These phasic events, if not important to the function of REM sleep, are at least a prominent characteristic of it.

The neural networks constituting the REM sleep phasic event system are currently not well understood, nor are the cell populations responsible for the initiation and propagation of REM sleep phasic influence. Neurons that use the neurotransmitter serotonin are most certainly involved in restricting the temporal occurrence of PGO waves to REM sleep and the NREM sleep just preceding REM sleep onset. This relationship has been demonstrated by interfering with serotonergic synaptic transmission through a variety of methods, which results in the appearance of PGO waves throughout waking and NREM sleep. The inhibitory relationship between serotonin and PGO waves is consistent with the pattern of spontaneous activity of neurons that use serotonin as their transmitter: these neurons cease discharging at times when PGO waves normally occur.

The neurotransmitter acetylcholine, however, plays a positive role in PGO wave occurrence. Experimental manipulations that interfere with cholinergic synaptic transmission suppress PGO waves. Again, correspondence has been shown with the neurophysiology of a population of neurons in the brainstem that use acetylcholine as their neurotransmitter: These neurons discharge their greatest activity during waking and REM sleep. Located in the pons and midbrain and with widespread projections throughout the brain, this system has been referred to as the *mesopontine cholinergic system*. A small subset of these neurons are most active just preceding the occurrence of PGO waves recorded in the lateral geniculate nucleus. Additionally, many neurons in this subset of cholinergic nerve cells have connections with the lateral geniculate nucleus. Electrical stimulation of the region in which these cells containing acetylcholine reside results in a geniculate PGO wave; this induced wave is blocked when acetylcholine transmission is interfered with. These results indicate that the mesopontine cholinergic system is directly responsible for the appearance of PGO waves in the lateral geniculate nucleus. (See REM SLEEP MECHANISMS AND NEUROANATOMY.)

Although much of the neurophysiology and neurochemistry of the mesopontine PGO system has been identified, many questions remain unanswered. Is this system responsible for the propagation of phasic influences to structures other than the lateral geniculate nucleus? Does the phasic signal originate in the mesopontine system or is it generated elsewhere, such as in the reticular formation, and just relayed through the cholinergic system? Is there a single generator of phasic events or multiple linked generators? These questions are currently under investigation. A greater understanding of the neural mechanisms underlying REM sleep PGO waves and other phasic events may also increase our understanding of their functional significance.

At this time, however, the functional role played by phasic activity in REM sleep remains a complete mystery. Many hypotheses have been presented and a few have even garnered experimental support, none to the extent of being conclusive. The most prominent speculations are based on two characteristics of REM sleep phasic events. One is that they are present in neural networks that influence activity in widespread areas of the brain. The second is that they are triggered by processes internal to the organism but involve pathways that are subject to external (sensory) control during waking. As sensory input affects many functions of the brain, scientists have theorized that PGO wave activity is related to a resetting of drive or motivational states, facilitation of learning or memory consolidation, and influencing of the physical organization of the brain itself during development in early life. Furthermore, the stimulation of sensory pathways during REM sleep by phasic event mechanisms has lead to speculations that this activity is the basis of dreaming (see ACTIVATION–SYNTHESIS HYPOTHESIS). Just as higher cortical functions create sensory perceptions based on sensory stimuli, the stimulation associated with PGO wave activity may be the substrate of perceptions during sleep, which we call dreaming. (See also THALAMUS; LATERAL GENICULATE NUCLEUS; CHEMISTRY OF SLEEP.)

REFERENCES

Glenn LL. 1989. Brainstem and spinal control of lower limb motoneurons with special reference to phasic events and startle reflexes. In McGinty OJ, Drucker-Colin R, Morrison A, Parmeggiani PL, eds. *Brain mechanisms of sleep*, pp. 81–95. New York: Raven.

Steriade M. 1989. Brain electrical activity and sensory processing during waking and sleep states. In Kryger MH, Roth T, Dement WC, eds. *Principles and practice of sleep medicine*, pp. 86–103. Philadelphia: Saunders.

——— 1990. Thalamocortical systems: Inhibition at sleep onset and activation during dreaming sleep.

In Mancia M, Marin G, eds. *The diencephalon and sleep,* pp. 231–247. New York: Raven.

Gerald A. Marks

PHARMACOLOGY

[*Sleep is a fundamental function of the brain and relies upon a complex interplay of chemical actions (see* CHEMISTRY OF SLEEP*). Thus, many chemical compounds affect sleep—even those that are not prescribed or taken with the intent of changing sleep.* ALCOHOL, DRUGS OF ABUSE (MARIJUANA, COCAINE), *and* DRUGS FOR MEDICAL DISORDERS *can have a direct impact on sleep quantity or quality, as can such compounds as* ANTIHISTAMINES *and* ASPIRIN. *Foods and drinks that contain* CAFFEINE, *such as* COFFEE, TEA, COLA, *and* CHOCOLATE, *can affect sleep adversely through their stimulant effects. Other stimulants, such as* AMPHETAMINES *and* OVER-THE-COUNTER STIMULANTS, *may also have a negative effect on sleep.*

A number of compounds have been used specifically to enhance sleep. SLEEPING PILLS *include such drugs as the* BARBITURATES, BENZODIAZEPINES, OVER-THE-COUNTER SLEEPING PILLS, *and many* TRANQUILIZERS. *Although these compounds are intended to improve sleep, they may have the opposite effect when used over a prolonged time or otherwise taken inappropriately; when such medications are taken for many nights in a row and then abruptly stopped, the effects on sleep can be extremely disruptive.*

Drugs used to treat psychiatric conditions—such as ANTIDEPRESSANTS *(either tricyclics or* MONOAMINE OXIDASE INHIBITORS*)—also result in significant changes to sleep. These compounds, as do many others mentioned above, actually change the structure of* CYCLES OF SLEEP ACROSS THE NIGHT, *suppressing* REM SLEEP *significantly. Certain investigators have suggested that the mode of action on mood is related to the REM-suppressing action on sleep (see* DEPRIVATION, SELECTIVE: REM SLEEP*).*

In summary, almost all drugs that have any effect on the CENTRAL NERVOUS SYSTEM *will have an effect on sleep.*]

PHASE-RESPONSE CURVE

Since the discovery that our bodies are not controlled by *exactly* 24-hour clocks, but by *nearly* 24-hour clocks (see CIRCADIAN RHYTHMS), it has become clear that some mechanism exists that is responsible for synchronizing internal circadian rhythms to the 24-hour days of the external environment. Furthermore, it was early observed that effectiveness in setting this mechanism follows a circadian pattern itself and depends on the particular phase of the organism's circadian rhythm. For example, a time cue, or *zeitgeber,* may effectively entrain circadian rhythms during an animal's subjective night and not affect its circadian rhythms at all during that animal's subjective day (see ZEITGEBERS). A phase-response curve is the standard method for displaying the circadian pattern rhythm of a zeitgeber's effectiveness.

Deriving a Phase-Response Curve

The phase-response curve was developed in 1960 by Patricia DeCoursey, who used it to understand the effects of 10-minute light pulses on the circadian rhythms of flying squirrels that were kept in otherwise constant conditions so that their rhythms were FREE RUNNING—that is, maintaining the period of their internal clock unsynchronized to the external cycle. Figure 1 shows how the effects of these light-pulse zeitgebers applied at different phases of an animal's circadian rhythms constitute a phase-response curve. The animal in this example is free running with an internal period of 25 hours. A 60-minute LIGHT pulse is applied during different phases of its "subjective time." Light pulse A is administered in the middle of the animal's subjective day, when the animal is performing its daytime behavior and the brain is exposed to light as if in a natural setting. At this phase, the light pulse results in no adjustment in the phase of the animal's circadian rhythms.

Light pulse B is applied early in the animal's subjective night, when the animal is performing its nocturnal behavior. This pulse produces a delay in the phase of the circadian rhythms as if the animal's brain experiences the light when darkness was expected. When the light occurs early in the "dark phase," the free-running SUPRACHIASMATIC NUCLEUS (SCN) "interprets" the signal

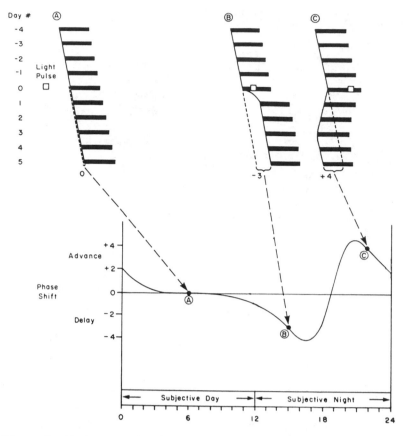

Figure 1.   Derivation of a phase-response curve. (A–C) Three experiments with an individual animal. Upper panel: the black bars represent the animal's subjective night. On days −4 to −1, the animal is free-running with a period of 25.0 hours. On day 0, a light pulse is given at midsubjective day (A), the beginning of the subjective night (B), and late in the subjective night (C). The light pulse in midsubjective day (A) has no effect, the light pulse at the beginning of the subjective night (B) delays the daily rhythms, and the light pulse late in the subjective night (C) advances the daily rhythms. Lower panel: direction and amount of phase shifts plotted against the time of light pulses. When light pulses are given at frequent intervals throughout subjective day and night, the waveform for the phase-response curve follows a solid line. *Modified and reprinted by permission from Moore-Ede, Sulzman, and Fuller, 1982, p. 86. Copyright © 1982 by the President and Fellows of Harvard College.*

to indicate that the internal clock is off-schedule and must be delayed so that light in the next cycle will occur only during the animal's subjective day. Because the light pulse occurred well into the subjective night, a fairly large (3-hour) phase delay was produced.

Light pulse C occurred later in the subjective night, before the anticipated beginning of the animal's "daytime" activities. This pulse produced an advance in the phase of the circadian rhythms.

In this case, the SCN experienced light earlier than expected. Consequently, the internal clock must shift to an earlier time so that the "morning light" will occur in the animal's subjective day, not its nighttime. Because the light pulse occurred well before the end of the subjective night, the phase advance produced by pulse C was fairly large (4 hours).

By giving light pulses at a number of phases to free-running animals, scientists can transform scattered data points into a smooth diagram called the phase-response curve (PRC). The lower panel of Figure 1 shows the PRC for which the time of the animal's subjective day is plotted along the horizontal axis, and the magnitude and direction of the phase shift produced are plotted along the vertical axis. As described above, light pulses during the animal's subjective day generally do not affect circadian rhythms (Pulse A), light pulses early in the animal's subjective night delay the circadian clock (Pulse B), and light pulses late in the animal's subjective night advance the circadian clock (Pulse C). In addition, larger phase shifts generally result from light pulses given closer to the middle of the night, because the SCN must make larger adjustments in order to adapt to the timing of the light. Phase shifts in the middle of the night are unpredictable, however, because the brain cannot always determine whether the light it sees is a late dusk or an early dawn. Consequently, a light pulse given in this unstable region may produce a large phase shift in either direction.

Types of Phase-Response Curves

Effects of light pulses are not the only data that can be plotted on a phase-response curve; the effects of any zeitgeber on the circadian rhythms of any organism can be similarly represented. For example, dark pulses given to an animal free-running in constant light can create phase shifts similar to those of light pulses, particularly in nocturnal species. The shape of the phase-response curve for dark pulses is somewhat different than for light pulses: Dark pulses administered during an animal's subjective night have no effect, dark pulses occurring early in the subjective day delay circadian rhythms, and dark pulses late in the subjective day advance circadian rhythms. The phase shifts induced by dark pulses are generally smaller than those produced by light pulses. In addition to dark and light pulses, phase-response curves have been generated for activity episodes as well as for administration of certain chemicals.

Uses of the Phase-Response Curves

With an appropriate phase-response curve, one can predict the effects of a zeitgeber adminis-

tered at any time of day. Such information is extremely useful when one wants to produce a phase shift voluntarily. For example, immediately after a 6-hour plane trip from New York to Rome, the environment has changed, but our internal clocks have not. By using the phase-response curve for light pulses in humans, it is possible to predict the best timing for bright light exposure in order to synchronize optimally to the new environment. Shift work is another area of application for the information imparted by phase-response curves (see JET LAG; LIGHT THERAPY; SHIFTWORK).

The phase-response curve also helps to explain our everyday adaptation to a 24-hour environment. Light has been shown to be perhaps the single most effective zeitgeber (see LIGHT; CIRCADIAN RHYTHMS; ZEITGEBER), and each day fine tunes our internal clocks to the external world. Every morning when we get up and see bright light, our circadian rhythms advance a little bit, and every evening when we see bright light our circadian rhythms delay a little bit. Dawn and dusk are thus continually pushing and pulling at our circadian rhythms, and the daily adjustments they (and other zeitgebers) make bring our not quite 24-hour clocks in line with the environment. Our circadian rhythms, when working correctly, should never stray too far from external rhythms imposed by our environment. When our internal rhythms are very different from external ones, our brains will encounter zeitgebers further from their anticipated times. These zeitgebers may then fall on the portion of the phase-response curve that leads to the largest phase shift, and a greater adjustment must be made to fit our internal clocks to the environment. The phase-response curve helps us understand how the circadian rhythms of organisms and their environment synchronize with each other.

REFERENCES

DeCoursey PJ. 1960. Daily light sensitivity rhythm in a rodent. *Science* 131:33–35.

Moore-Ede MC, Sulzman FM, Fuller CA. 1982. *The clocks that time us: Physiology of the circadian timing system.* Cambridge, Mass.: Harvard University Press.

Wever RA. 1979. *The circadian system of man: Results of experiments under temporal isolation.* New York: Springer-Verlag.

Max D. Stone

PHASE SHIFT

[*Specific reference points on a continuous cycle are called* phases *of the cycle. In the course of a 24-hour cycle, specific clock times such as noon can be thought of as phases of the day. Examples of phases of* CIRCADIAN RHYTHMS *include the maximum and minimum of the daily body temperature rhythm, the peak of* CORTISOL *secretion from the adrenal gland, or maximal* SLEEPINESS *in the circadian rhythm of sleep tendency. The entraining influence of* ZEITGEBERS *maintains the internal circadian clock and its dependent circadian rhythms in a fixed "phase relationship" to the external environment. That is, the specific phases of the internal rhythms occur at consistent times of day on successive cycles.*

When the timing of a zeitgeber changes, however, the timing of the phase of the circadian cycles changes as well, and a phase shift of the rhythms occurs. LIGHT *is the most important zeitgeber for all mammals, including humans. The* PHASE RESPONSE CURVE *demonstrates how light can induce a phase shift to produce* ENTRAINMENT *of the endogenous rhythm to the environmental light–dark cycle.*]

PHASIC ACTIVITY IN REM SLEEP

[REM SLEEP *includes both* tonic *and* phasic *phenomena. Tonic phenomena are those persisting throughout the REM sleep state and include the presence of a low-voltage* ELECTROENCEPHALOGRAM, *muscle* ATONIA, *reduced* SYMPATHETIC NERVOUS SYSTEM *activity, and penile* ERECTIONS. *Phasic phenomena, those occurring episodically during REM sleep, include rapid eye movements,* TWITCHES *of various muscles, transient increases in motor inhibition, and changes in activity of the* AUTONOMIC NERVOUS SYSTEM. *One phasic event that can be recorded within cer-*

tain regions of the brain is the occurrence of PGO WAVES *(see also* LATERAL GENICULATE NUCLEUS; REM SLEEP MECHANISMS AND NEUROANATOMY *). Phasic events gradually increase to a peak during the REM sleep episode and then decrease before REM sleep ends.*]

PHASIC INTEGRATED POTENTIALS

Phasic integrated potentials (PIPs) are indicators of muscle twitches that are too fast to be recorded by ordinary techniques on an ink-writing polygraph machine, because the pens on the machine cannot move fast enough to record the twitch. To circumvent this problem, the electrical output of the muscle is amplified and then integrated over time, thereby prolonging the signal so that it can be followed by the pens.

The recording of PIPs from eye muscles has been of particular interest, because research in cats has shown a good correspondence between twitches of the eye muscles and PGO spikes, which are bursts of electrical activity recorded from the PONS, LATERAL GENICULATE NUCLEUS, and occipital cortex of the brain (see PGO WAVES). These PGO spikes occur mostly during REM sleep, and they have been hypothesized to generate the bizarre images and abrupt shifts of content that sometimes occur in dreams. This theory has been difficult to test because we do not insert wires into the brains of humans to record their PGO spikes. Although many PGO spikes are undoubtedly reflected in eye movements, more PGO spikes are reflected in PIPs recorded from the skin over the eye muscles. Thus, the noninvasive recording of PIPs in humans can provide an opportunity to look more closely at the possible correspondence between PGO spikes and features of dream content.

One extensive study of four volunteers found that some subjects showed a modest association between PIPs recorded near the eye during REM sleep and distortions or discontinuities in the dreams reported on awakening from the REM sleep episode (Watson et al., 1978). In other subjects, there was no such association. Thus, the recording of PIPs and associated dream content has provided only very limited support for the idea that the strange twists and turns of dreams are caused by PGO spikes in the human brain.

REFERENCE

Watson RK, Bliwise DL, Friedman L, Wax D, Rechtschaffen A. 1978. Phasic EMG in human sleep. II. Periorbital potentials and REM mentation. *Sleep Res* 7:57.

Allan Rechtschaffen

PHOTOTHERAPY

See Light Therapy

PHYLOGENY

[Phylogeny *is the origin and evolution of a particular species or other grouping of living beings; it can be contrasted with* ONTOGENY, *the development of a single individual through time. A look at sleep and dreaming from a phylogenetic perspective raises several important issues.*

Alternation between resting and active phases is a virtually universal characteristic of animal behavior, whether or not the resting behavioral phase is specifically designated as sleep. *The strict definition of sleep in avian and mammalian species is based upon measurements of brain electrical activity, or* ELECTROENCEPHALOGRAPHY. *Behavioral criteria, on the other hand, are commonly used to describe sleep in other species and can also be applied to the description of sleep in mammals. The behavioral definition of sleep includes four required features:*

1. The animal assumes a species-specific stereotypic posture;

2. this posture is associated with behavioral quiescence;

3. the animal has an increased threshold for reacting to environmental stimuli; yet

4. the state is rapidly reversible with stimuli of moderate intensity.

These behavioral criteria define a state of sleep that is clearly distinct from wakefulness as well as from other biological or metabolic conditions such as HIBERNATION, ESTIVATION, TORPOR, *or* COMA. *(See also* ALTERED STATES OF CONSCIOUSNESS.) *The definition of sleep may also include a fifth component: that the state is regulated in some manner. Thus, if an animal is prevented from entering into or sustaining the resting phase for a period of time (i.e., is rest deprived), and is then permitted to behave normally, the resting phase will show a homeostatic rebound response to the previous deprivation. (See also* ANIMALS IN SLEEP RESEARCH.)

Although a firm electrophysiological description of sleep has been achieved for MAMMALS *and* BIRDS, *the distinction between sleep and wake is not always 100 percent clear-cut, even among these species. One of the most interesting adaptations in certain birds and aquatic mammals (such as dolphins and seals) is hemispheric sleep, in which one hemisphere of the brain shows the EEG pattern characteristic of sleep while the other hemisphere shows a waking EEG.*

Pet owners and sleep researchers alike have pondered the issue of ANIMALS' DREAMS. REM SLEEP, *highly associated with dreaming in humans, comprises only a tiny fraction of the sleep period in most birds; although it is present in virtually all mammals, REM sleep has not been found in two specific mammalian species, the* ECHIDNA *and the bottle-nosed dolphin. This finding has shaped scientists' understanding of the* EVOLUTION OF SLEEP, *an issue of debate that bears on sleep's phylogenetic diversity. Whether other species show either NREM or REM sleep is addressed in the entries on* FISH, INSECTS, AMPHIBIANS, *and* REPTILES. *(See also* DOGS; ENGLISH BULLDOGS AS AN ANIMAL MODEL OF SLEEP APNEA).]

PICKWICKIAN SYNDROME

See Apnea; Literature, Sleep and Dreams in

PICTORIAL REPRESENTATION

Although certain dreams have a vivid or lifelike story, others are unclear and confusing. It can be difficult to find meaning in a series of memories, childhood experiences, and seemingly insignificant mental images. Freud, however, offered a

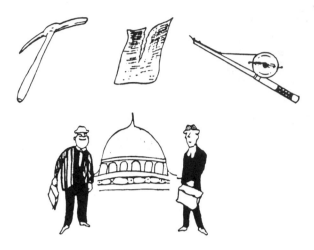

Figure 1. The process of pictorial representation in dream work. *Reprinted with permission from Van de Castle 1971.*

psychoanalytical explanation for this difficulty: that dreams express thoughts and emotions in a nonverbal language of sensory images for the very purpose of hiding their actual meaning from the consciousness of the dreamer. According to his "considerations of representability," various types of visual metaphors are the most effective—and often humorous—units of symbolic communication in dreams (Freud, 1965). Figure 1 demonstrates the pictorial representation of an abstract, verbal concept in the form of a rebus, or picture puzzle (Van de Castle, 1971).

Why is dream content disguised in this way? Freud theorized that people have many wishes that are too difficult for the conscious mind to entertain, in particular, sexual and aggressive drives, which he felt must be repressed during waking life. He suggested that this censorship process of the unconscious breaks down somewhat during sleep, but that sleep itself, as well as the dreamer, is protected from anxiety by "dream work," transforming unacceptable wishes or drives into symbolic picture language and releasing them as fantasy. Thus, Freud distinguished between latent dream content, which he considered the unconscious material underlying or motivating the dream, and manifest dream content, which he considered the images consciously remembered on awakening. Not all dream theorists make the distinction, but many see dreams as pictorial representations of the dreamer's wishes, conflicts, and problems, whether repressed or knowingly encountered in

waking life (see FREUD'S DREAM THEORY; INTERPRETATION OF DREAMS; SYMBOLISM IN DREAMS.)

REFERENCES

Freud S. 1965. *The interpretation of dreams.* New York: Avon Books.
Van de Castle RL. 1971. *The psychology of dreaming.* Morristown, NJ: General Learning Press, pp. 1–45.

Krista Hennager

PILLOWS

Pillows are used to cushion or support the head for sleep. Social customs and, especially, coiffures have influenced the types of pillows used in different cultures. Health considerations in selection of a pillow type have precedents in ancient and modern culture. Pillows are a very personal item and seem to influence an individual's ability to sleep well.

Not all pillows are soft. The oldest pillow may have been a round log. Wooden headrests were commonly used in ancient Egypt. The typical form had three parts: A crescent shape supported the neck, and this sat on a narrow pedestal that was attached to a flat base. Stone was also a common material, and alabaster and ivory headrests were used by the upper class.

Headrests made of wood are still used in Africa. There are a wide variety of shapes and artistic interpretations. Figure 1 shows a sculptural form, Figure 2 a geometric form. Sieber (1980) says Nuba tribesmen had a special reason to use a rigid headrest. Their goal was to sleep in one position so as not to rub and smudge their body paint and to keep the head from touching the ground, thus preserving their elaborate coiffures.

Rigid headrests have often been used when cultures employed elaborate hairdos. Tunis (1957) reports that in colonial North America, when the fanciful powdered hairdos of the time of George III of England were in fashion, women slept with their neck on a wooden block to protect their costly masterpieces. When the Japanese wore their hair in lacquered queues, the traditional pillow was called a *makura* (Figure 3). These

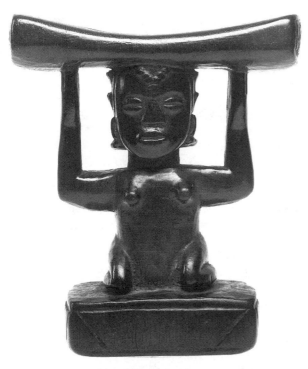

Figure 1. African headrest of carved wood from the Shakondi culture (height 14 centimeters). *Courtesy The Fowler Museum of Cultural History, UCLA.*

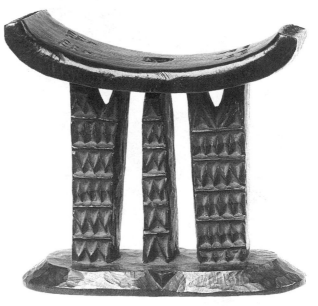

Figure 2. African headrest of carved wood from the Shona people of Zimbabwe (height 13 centimeters). *Courtesy The Fowler Museum of Cultural History, UCLA.*

were narrow wooden boxes with a flat or concave surface that were topped with a cylindrical pad filled with buckwheat husks. A pillow case of folded soft paper could be tied to the top of the pad. Morse (1961) noted the health benefit of having the neck elevated so that air can circulate around the head and keep it cool.

The Chinese, who often used rectangular ceramic pillows, also saw health benefits in keeping the head cool. Bushnell (1980) reports the Chinese thought that keeping the head cool during sleep preserved the eyesight. One type of porcelain pillow could be filled with ice in summer and hot water in winter. According to Kates (1948), besides porcelain, pillows in China were made of flexible strips of polished bamboo, lacquered leather, and finely woven rattan, hollow and stretched over a framework.

Pillows found in today's drugstore follow some of these ancient ideas. There is the Headache Ice-Pillo with a gel insert that can be frozen and placed inside a padded pillow with a neck cutout. The Wal-Pil-O claims to alleviate daytime pain with its design of a firm outside edge to sup-

port the neck and a softer inner cushion for the head. The satin pillowcase sold in beauty supply stores claims to preserve the hairdo. A cervical curve pillow supports the neck instead of cushioning the head. The Snore-No-More-Pillow claims to position the sleeper so that the airway will not be obstructed during sleep.

The stuffed bed pillow, however, is the favorite of this age. Although pillows have been stuffed with all sorts of things from cotton to kapok (from the silk floss tree), the most popular stuffings today are feathers, down, foam rubber, and polyester. The majority of pillows sold in the United States are filled with polyester fiber.

Pregnant women are sometimes advised to use two pillows, or one pillow between their knees as they sleep on their side. Eisenberg and colleagues (1988) promote this position because it prevents back sleeping that puts all the fetal weight on a major blood vessel, the inferior vena cava. Spock (1976) and Leach (1990) advise parents to use no pillow at all with newborns to avoid the possibility of suffocation. Allergic people may use polyester fiber-filled pillows or encase their pillows in plastic to avoid dust mites.

The pillow is a very personal item. Frequent travelers often bring their own pillow from

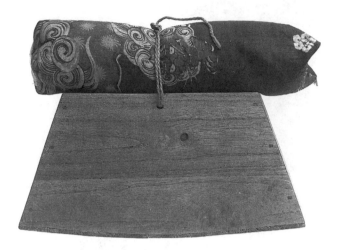

Figure 3. Japanese pillow or *makura* of wood with cushion stuffed with buckwheat husks (height 21 centimeters). *Courtesy The Fowler Museum of Cultural History, UCLA.*

home. Some sleep disorders clinics advise patients to bring along their personal pillow to better enable them to fall asleep in the sleep lab.

Without pillows, who could get a good night's sleep? And without pillows, where would the tooth fairy look for lost teeth?

REFERENCES

Bushnell S. 1980. *Oriental ceramic art,* p 94. New York: Crown.

Eisenberg A, Eisenberg Murkoff H, Eisenberg Hathaway S. 1988. *What to expect when you are expecting,* p 150. New York: Workman.

Kates N. 1948. *Chinese household furniture,* p 47. New York: Harper and Brothers.

Leach P. 1990. *Your baby and child, from birth to age five,* 2nd ed., p 491. New York: Knopf.

Morse ES. 1961. *Japanese homes and their surroundings,* pp 211–212. New York: Dover.

Sieber R. 1980. *African furniture and household objects,* pp 72, 105. Bloomington: Indiana University Press.

Spock B. 1976. *Baby and child care,* 4th ed., pp 57–58. New York: Elsevier–Dutton.

Treasures of Tutankhamen. 1976. Plate 29, pp 162–163. New York: Metropolitan Museum of Art.

Tunis E. 1957. *Colonial living,* p 145. Cleveland: World.

Wilkinson J. 1989. *The Ancient Egyptians,* pp 70–71. New York: Bonanza Books.

Diane J. Siegel

PILOTS

In a matter of hours, modern aircraft can transport people or cargo to virtually any destination in the world. The aviators responsible for the safe and efficient operation of these aircraft are the human pilots in the cockpit. Today, air transport operations encompass a broad range of flight environments, each with different demands for flight and duty schedules. Long-haul flying usually involves transoceanic or polar flights of 8 hours or longer (e.g., United States to Europe); short-haul operations involve shorter flight times (e.g., 1 to 5 hours). Overnight cargo operations involve working the "backside-of-the-clock," flying all night for morning delivery. Many corporations operate their own aircraft, and regional commuter airlines provide frequent flights that connect varied geographic locations. The flight length, number of takeoffs and landings, and time of day for operations can vary tremendously in these different flight environments. The aircraft also vary; the old Pan Am Clipper required five pilots, whereas today's planes usually operate with two or three pilots. Modern cockpits use computers and other advanced technology to automate many aspects of aircraft operation.

The operational requirements created by flight and duty scheduling have placed physiological demands on pilots that are frequently at odds with human biological processes. For example, long-haul flights can involve rapid, multiple time-zone changes and altered and extended duty schedules. These work requirements can affect pilots' sleep, circadian rhythms, and sleepiness. During layovers between flights, pilots will try to sleep at clock times not compatible with good sleep. Disturbed sleep on multiple layovers can result in the accumulation of a sleep debt. Pilots (and their internal circadian clocks) can be flown rapidly anywhere in world, but the clock does not adjust rapidly to a new environmental time (see CIRCADIAN RHYTHMS). The pilot's internal clock will thus be "out of phase" or desynchronized with the external world time. This can affect the quantity and quality of sleep, as well as waking performance and alertness. There is also a rhythm to sleepiness and pilots may be flying when physiologically their bodies are better suited to being asleep.

Since the early 1980s, the National Aeronautics and Space Administration's (NASA's) Ames Research Center has studied fatigue, sleep, and circadian rhythms in flight operations. In one study, the sleep of international longhaul pilots was examined in the sleep laboratory, and the results confirmed a common experience: Pilots showed more disturbed sleep and greater daytime sleepiness when flying east than when flying west (Graeber, 1986). This difference is a result of the natural tendency of the human circadian clock to lengthen our day. On a westward trip, adjusting to the new time zone involves staying up longer and lengthening the day, in synchrony with the clock. On the other hand, going east requires shortening the day, contrary to the circadian clock. (See TIME ZONES; JET LAG). Researchers have also found that 85 percent of longhaul pilots accumulate a sleep debt during a trip, and the deficit can range from 4 to 22 hours of sleep loss (Dinges et al., 1991). In another study of longhaul pilots, the duty periods averaged 10 hours and the layovers about 25 hours, typically involving two sleep periods during the layover (Gander et al., 1991). This study revealed a complex interplay between circadian factors and the accumulated sleep debt determining the length and quality of sleep during the layover sleep periods. In shorthaul operations, study results indicate that the time available on layovers can be insufficient for adequate sleep.

On the basis of these scientific findings, recommendations for pilots are designed to minimize the effects of sleep loss, circadian disruption, and fatigue. These recommendations include two basic approaches: preventive strategies and operational countermeasures. Preventive strategies are used before a duty period to minimize the effects during flight operations. Such strategies might include sleep scheduling, sleep hygiene, napping, and lifestyle changes. Operational countermeasures are used during flights to maintain performance and alertness. Examples include using physical activity, social interaction, and caffeine to offset fatigue and sleepiness. One possible operational countermeasure that is not currently sanctioned under federal regulations is preplanned cockpit rest. In a recent NASA study, long-haul pilots (one at a time) were allowed a 40-minute rest period during a low-workload, cruise portion of flight. Generally, the pilots were able to fall asleep quickly and to sleep efficiently for about 26 minutes. This nap was associated with better subsequent performance on a test of vigilance and sustained attention

and less physiological sleepiness compared with a group of pilots that were not allowed a rest period (Rosekind et al., 1992). (See also NAPPING.)

Today, air travel continues to be one of the safest modes of transportation. In the future, continuous 24-hour flight operations will become more complex (e.g., with automated aircraft and increased flight lengths). Continued research on the human factors associated with optimal pilot performance and alertness will help to maintain safe and efficient flight operations.

REFERENCES

Dinges DF, Connell LJ, Rosekind MR, Gillen KA, Kribbs NB, Graeber RC. 1991. Effects of cockpit naps and 24-hr layovers on sleep debt in long-haul transmeridian flight crews. *Sleep Res* 20:406.

Gander PH, Graeber RC, Connell LJ, Gregory KB. 1991. *Crew factors in flight operations. VIII. Factors influencing sleep timing and subjective sleep quality in commercial longhaul flight crews.* NASA Technical Memorandum. Moffett Field, CA: Ames Research Center.

Graeber RC, ed. 1986. Sleep and wakefulness in international air crews. *Aviat Space Environ Med* 57(Suppl 12):B1–B64.

Rosekind MR, Graeber RC, Dinges DF, Connell LJ, Rountree MS, Spinweber CL, Gillen KA. 1992. *Crew factors in flight operations. IX. Effects of preplanned cockpit rest on crew performance and alertness in long-haul operations.* NASA Technical Memorandum. Moffett Field, CA: Ames Research Center.

Mark R. Rosekind

PINEAL GLAND

The physiological function in humans of the pineal gland or epiphysis cerebri remains to be defined. The pineal gland received its name for its resemblance to a pine cone. Herophilos (325–280 B.C.), an Egyptian anatomist, was one of the first to describe this gland, which lies between the superior colliculi at the base of the brain. Early Greeks postulated that the pineal controlled the flow of thoughts forward to consciousness. René Descartes (1596–1650) later popularized the theory that the pineal gland was the "seat of the soul," which released "spirits" into blood vessels. The pineal gland does secrete a number of biologically active substances into the blood. The isolation by Lerner in 1958 of MELATONIN, the major hormone released by the pineal, has further stimulated investigation of this organ. Current work has focused on pineal involvement in the circadian timing system (see CIRCADIAN RHYTHMS) and reproductive function.

In lower vertebrates, the pineal gland functions as a photoreceptor; thus this light-sensitive organ is often referred to as the third eye. In certain species of birds, the pineal acts as a self-sustaining pacemaker capable of generating circadian rhythmicity, with pinealectomy leading to disorganization of circadian function. In higher vertebrates, the photoreceptive and pacemaker characteristics of the pineal are lost along with direct neural connections to the brain. Although its actual biological function remains unknown, the pineal gland is used by many radiologists as a landmark for the midline of the brain, as it normally undergoes calcification within the second decade of life. This calcified deposition, however, does not appear to be responsible for the age-related decline in the amplitude of the melatonin rhythm.

In mammals, pinealocytes secrete melatonin when stimulated by sympathetic neurons regulated by neural signals arising in part from the hypothalamic region (see HYPOTHALAMUS), an area thought to contain the circadian clock (see Figure 1). The circadian pacemaker, which receives light-dark information directly from the retina, times the daily rhythmic pattern of melatonin release by the pineal gland. The pineal is most active during darkness in both diurnal and nocturnal animals, and circulating melatonin reaches its lowest levels during the daytime hours. Although this rhythm persists in constant darkness, exposure to bright light or administration of a beta-adrenergic antagonist during the dark period leads to acute suppression of pineal melatonin secretion, demonstrating the sensitivity of the pineal gland to external photic and sympathetic signals.

The weight of the human pineal gland has also been observed to vary with the time of year. On average, the pineal gland weighs more during the winter months when there is less light to inhibit pineal activity than during the summer months when the day is longer. This annual variation in

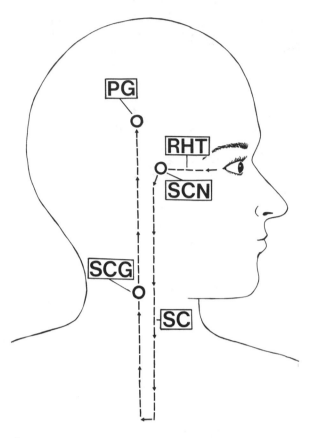

Figure 1. Light–dark information is transmitted to the pineal gland (PG) via a neural pathway that includes the retina, retinohypothalamic tract (RHT), suprachiasmatic nucleus (SCN), upper thoracic spinal cord (SC), and superior cervical ganglion (SCG). *Courtesy Elizabeth M. Shanahan.*

pineal activity, reflected by changes in the duration of the melatonin peak in some species, is hypothesized to serve as a signal for many seasonal breeding animals that selectively reproduce at specific times of the year (see ENDOCRINOLOGY). In humans, there is no direct evidence of similar effects of the pineal gland on reproductive function. However, pineal tumors have been reported in a number of patients diagnosed with precocious puberty.

Currently, the hypothesized function of the pineal gland, which lies outside of the blood-brain barrier in mammals, is the translation of photic information into hormonal messages. The length of the light-dark cycle is undoubtedly critical to the circadian timing system as well as for seasonal reproduction; thus the pineal gland may serve as a modulator in both of these processes.

REFERENCES

Arendt J. 1985. Mammalian pineal rhythms. In Reiter RJ, ed. *Pineal research reviews,* vol 3, pp 161–213. New York: Liss.

Binkley SA. 1981. Pineal biochemistry: Comparative aspects and circadian rhythms. In Reiter RJ, ed. *The pineal gland,* vol 1, pp 155–172. Boca Raton, Fla.: CRC Press.

Zrenner C. 1985. Theories of pineal function from classical antiquity to 1900: A history. In Reiter RJ, ed. *Pineal research reviews,* vol 3, pp 1–40. New York: Liss.

Theresa L. Shanahan

PITUITARY GLAND

The *pituitary gland* is a small endocrine gland located at the base of the brain immediately below the optic chiasm. It is connected via the slender pituitary stalk to the base of the hypothalamus, the center of the brain from which it receives its regulatory control (see HYPOTHALAMUS). Close connections to the CENTRAL NERVOUS SYSTEM allow the pituitary gland to serve as the "master gland," controlling the secretory function of a broad range of secondary endocrine glands (see ENDOCRINOLOGY).

Anatomy of the Pituitary Gland

Anatomically and functionally, the pituitary gland is divided into two parts. The anterior pituitary (also known as the adenohypophysis) secretes several neuropeptide hormones, including PROLACTIN, THYROID-STIMULATING HORMONE (TSH), GROWTH HORMONE (GH), adrenocorticotropic hormone (ACTH), luteinizing hormone (LH), and follicle-stimulating hormone (FSH) (see also GONADOTROPIC HORMONES). As their names imply, many of these hormones act by stimulating other endocrine glands (e.g., thyroid-stimulating hormone stimulates the thyroid gland) to release hormones. In turn, the anterior pituitary cells are regulated by specific stimulating proteins released by neurons in the hypothalamus into small vessels that supply the anterior pituitary via the pituitary stalk.

The posterior pituitary (neurohypophysis) secretes two important hormones, oxytocin and vasopressin (antidiuretic hormone). Organization of the posterior pituitary is different from that of the anterior pituitary. Neurons in the hypothalamus send axons down the pituitary stalk directly to the posterior pituitary, from which these hormones are secreted directly into the general blood circulation.

Effects of Sleep on Pituitary Gland Function

The close link between the pituitary gland and the hypothalamus provides the anatomic basis for the important influence of sleep–wake state on pituitary function. Secretion of all of the anterior pituitary hormones is altered by sleep in humans (see NEUROENDOCRINE HORMONES). Studies of pituitary function during sleep in animals are more limited, but most animal species do not appear to show prominent sleep-dependent modulation. One explanation for this difference may be the different organization of sleep itself; whereas humans commonly sleep uninterrupted for 8 or more hours, most animal species sleep in shorter segments, interrupting the sleep period with episodes of feeding and activity. Thus, many of the neuroendocrine changes seen during sleep in humans may represent adaptations to the special challenges to physiological regulation presented by an 8-hour period of fasting and water deprivation.

Effects of the Pituitary Gland on Sleep

The model outlined above suggests that the pituitary gland is important to normal sleep in humans, but studies of sleep after hypophysectomy (surgical removal of the pituitary gland) have not yet been done, and studies of humans with abnormal pituitary glands are complicated by the larger issues of endocrine abnormalities (e.g., hypothyroidism) that typically accompany pituitary tumors and other pituitary diseases (see THYROID DISEASE AND SLEEP). Systematic studies of the effects of hypophysectomy on sleep in animals are of limited relevance to the human, but they do support the notion that normal pituitary function is important to sleep. Additional studies must be performed before we can know the role of the sleep-dependent alterations in pituitary function in humans.

REFERENCES

DeGroot LJ, ed. 1989. *Endocrinology,* 2nd ed. Philadelphia: Saunders.

Martin JB, Reichlin S. 1987. *Clinical neuroendocrinology.* Philadelphia: Davis.

Valatx JL, Chouvet G, Jouvet M. 1975. Sleep-waking cFycle of the hypophysectomized rat. *Prog Brain Res* 42:115–120.

Gary S. Richardson

POLYSOMNOGRAPHY

The term polysomnography was coined by a group of sleep researchers in 1974 (Holland, Dement, and Raynal, 1974) and has Latin and Greek roots meaning "many sleep writings." Polysomnography is the generation of recordings during sleep, which serves as a central component of many sleep research studies and clinical evaluations. These recordings, known as polysomnograms, provide a continuous display of multiple aspects of the sleeping person's physiology.

A basic sleep recording displays the activity of three systems: brain activity is measured using electroencephalography (EEG) (see ELECTROENCEPHALOGRAPHY); eye movements are measured using electrooculography (EOG) (see ELECTROOCULOGRAPHY); and motor activity is measured using electromyography (EMG) (see ELECTROMYOGRAPHY). Information from these three systems is collected and used to differentiate stages of sleep (Rechtschaffen and Kales, 1968). In general, such evaluations are made through visual inspection of data written on a moving chart. A trained technologist determines sleep stages by examining 20-, 30-, or 60-second segments of the tracing. Modern technology is on the brink of automating this process with use of computerized algorithms that will assist human scorers with the analysis of hundreds of pages of sleep recordings. To date, however, no system has been able to automate these scoring judgments completely, although this is an area of rapid development in sleep research.

Polysomnography routinely includes several other physiological variables in addition to EEG, EOG, and EMG. Monitoring of heart rate (ELECTROCARDIOGRAM) [ECG]) and monitoring of breathing are typical. Many techniques have been used to evaluate breathing during sleep: temperature change of air flow near the nose and mouth associated with breathing, pressure changes inside the chest associated with effort of breathing, electromyography of intercostal muscles (muscles between the ribs), electromyography using small wires that are attached directly to the diaphragm muscle (the major muscle for breathing), sensors to measure percentage of carbon dioxide in air moving in and out of the nose and mouth, and many others. Another important measure is oxygen saturation, an indicator of the amount of oxygen bound to hemoglobin molecules in the blood. This measure can be made using an oximeter, which transmits a beam of light through a finger, toe, or ear, and measures the wavelength of light that passes through. This wavelength is converted by an equation to determine the percentage of oxygen in the blood. Measures of breathing during sleep are very important, particularly for the diagnosis of sleep apnea syndrome (see APNEA) and other sleep-related breathing disorders.

Virtually every physiological measurement that can be made in the waking state can also be made during sleep. For example, blood pressure can be measured continuously, either with an external cuff as one would during wakefulness, or with pressure monitors that are placed within a blood vessel. The latter is more invasive and used less frequently, but can be an important technique to be used with people who have significant sleep-related abnormalities. Body temperature can be measured with a probe that is positioned in the rectum or with a capsule that is swallowed. These devices monitor core body temperature, which is usually different from the temperature measured with a thermometer inserted into the mouth or placed under the arm. Another interesting physiological measure taken during sleep is the measurement of changes in the circumference of the penis associated with REM sleep. These measurements, used with other information, allow for the determination of a physiological versus psychological cause of erectile dysfunction (impotence) in males (see

ERECTILE DYSFUNCTION; ERECTIONS; NOCTURNAL PENILE TUMESCENCE; SEX AND SLEEP; SEXUAL ACTIVATION).

Polysomnography is also used to evaluate sleep in animals. Measurements taken in animals are often different from those in humans. For example, the EEG recorded during sleep in most animals is taken from electrodes that are placed deep within the brain to measure the electrical activity of specific groups of neurons. Such recordings can help to determine how various brain regions are involved in the control and regulation of sleep. Individual neurons can be monitored continuously during sleep in animals and their activity levels can be related to the polysomnographically observed sleep states (Zepelin, 1989). Such recordings have been valuable in distinguishing brain centers that are active during different phases of sleep. When these recordings are made in conjunction with measurements of brain chemical activity, the potential for unraveling the mechanisms that control sleep is increased. (See also ANIMALS IN SLEEP RESEARCH.)

Thus, polysomnography has become an essential tool for describing and understanding many physiological processes that take place during sleep in humans and other animals. Physicians have called polysomnography the physical examination of the sleeping patient. The clinical usefulness of polysomnography in understanding the sleeping patient has significantly advanced the field of sleep disorders medicine in the last two decades and remains the most important tool for scientists and physicians in understanding normal sleep and evaluating its disorders.

REFERENCES

Holland JV, Dement WC, Raynal DM. 1974. "Polysomnography": A response to a need for improved communication. Paper presented at the 14th annual meeting of the Association for the Psychophysiological Study of Sleep, Jackson Hole, Wyoming, June 1974.

Rechtschaffen A, Kales A, eds. 1968. *A manual of standardized terminology, techniques, and scoring system for sleep stages of human subjects.* Los Angeles: UCLA Brain Information Service/Brain Research Institute.

Zepelin H. 1989. Mammalian sleep. In Kryger MH, Roth T, Dement WC, eds. *Principles and practice of sleep medicine,* pp 30–49. Philadelphia: Saunders.

Sharon A. Keenan
Mary A. Carskadon

PONS

Although other regions are involved in REM sleep generation and control, the pons is clearly the brain region most critical for REM sleep control (see Figure 1; see also REM SLEEP MECHANISMS AND NEUROANATOMY). The pons is defined by a bulge at the bottom of the brainstem called the basilar pons, which contains the main connection between the brainstem and the cerebellum (a brain region that helps to control movement and posture). The brain substance within the midbrain, pons, and medulla is called *reticular formation,* meaning a net of neuronal cell bodies and axons (output fibers from neuronal cell bodies). Within the reticular formation of the pons are a number of clusters of neuronal cell bodies called *nuclei.*

Intense research interest in the pons has resulted in a very detailed naming scheme for its parts. The main pontine nuclei are called the nucleus reticularis pontis oralis (RPO; i.e., the pontine reticular region nearer the mouth) and the nucleus reticularis pontis caudalis (RPC; i.e., the pontine reticular region nearer the tail).

At the top of the pons is a pigmented region called the locus coeruleus ("blue place"). The locus coeruleus contains neurons that have the neurotransmitter norepinephrine, similar to adrenalin. Regions just below this area (the subcoeruleus) also contain norepinephrine. On the midline of the pons, as well as the midbrain and medulla, are the raphe (Greek for "seam") nuclei. These cells contain the neurotransmitter serotonin.

Just lateral to the locus coeruleus is the brachium conjunctivum. This is a major connection between the cerebellum and the rest of the brain. The areas around the brachium and medial to it contain concentrations of cells containing the transmitters acetylcholine and glutamate.

The interaction of these cell groups and transmitters, particularly norepinephrine, serotonin, acetylcholine, and glutamate, is believed to play

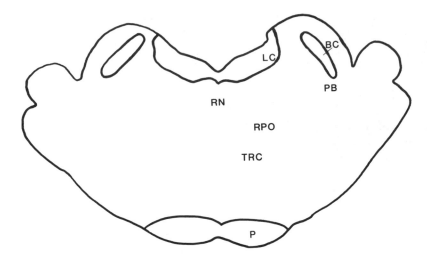

Figure 1. A cross section of the pons. BC, brachium conjunctivum; LC, locus coeruleus; P, pyramidal tract; PB, parabrachial nucleus; RPO, nucleus reticularis pontis oralis—just behind this level (towards the spinal cord) is the nucleus reticularis pontis caudalis; TRC, tegmental reticular nucleus, central division.

a major role in the generation of REM sleep and to control the level of arousal in waking (see REM SLEEP MECHANISMS AND NEUROANATOMY).

REFERENCE

Siegel JM. 1989. Brainstem mechanisms generating REM sleep. In Kryger MH, Roth T, Dement WC, eds. *Principles and practice of sleep medicine,* pp 104–121. Philadelphia: Saunders.

Jerome Siegel

POPULAR MUSIC, SLEEP AND DREAMS IN

Because of the rapid growth of the music industry during the latter half of this century, much of the music in existence today is considered "popular" for its availability to the masses via records, radio, television, nightclubs, concerts, and festivals. This vast collection of music contains elements of many different styles (blues, jazz, folk, rock), all of which influence one another and are shaped by the recording industry, radio, and audience demand. Popular musicians have written about love, about curfews, and about parental dismay over teenage activities. They have pon-

dered civil rights and social rebellion. Some have ventured into the controversial world of drugs, sex, and violence, whereas others have preferred to stay on the beach and dance. Nevertheless, all of these musicians are linked by the common experience of sleep and dreaming. Thus, it is not surprising that sleep and dreams are frequent themes in popular music, regardless of the artist, the style, or the era.

One of the most visible measures of success in the popular music industry today is the famed position of number 1 on Billboard's Top 40 Chart. The themes of sleep and dreaming have reached this pinnacle of the popular music world seven times. The first two number 1 "sleep hits" were by the Everly Brothers in 1957 and 1958. "Wake Up Little Susie" hit the top of the charts in 1957 despite the fact that it was banned by several radio stations for its "suggestive" lyrics concerning Susie and her boyfriend, who fell asleep at a drive-in movie and missed her curfew! Phil Everly considered their second hit, "All I Have to Do Is Dream," one of the most important songs the duo ever wrote. This sweet ballad conjures up a touching image of unrequited love. The next number 1 "sleep" song was an instrumental recording by Santo and Johnny on September 21, 1959. They spent two weeks at number 1 with the song "Sleepwalk." Bobby Lewis hit the top in 1961 with one of the most successful singles by a solo male singer in the entire rock era—"Tossin' and

Turnin'." This song aptly expressed the frustrations and trials of transient insomnia. Obviously, the public sympathized with Mr. Lewis, for the song remained at number 1 for seven weeks. That same year, on December 18, "The Lion Sleeps Tonight" by The Tokens reached the top spot, making 1961 rock music's most sleep-oriented year.

Two other sleep songs have reached number 1 since 1961, one in 1977 and the other in 1984. The first was "Dreams" by Fleetwood Mac, which stayed at number 1 for only a single week. The second was by the rock group Wham!, who topped the chart with the single "Wake Me Up Before You Go-Go." This song has an interesting origin; it was based on a late-night note a band member left his mother. While writing the note, the artist accidentally wrote, "up-up." He compensated for this slip at the end of the message, confusing his mother and making rock'n'roll history.

Although only seven songs containing sleep and dreaming references have made it to Billboard's top position, these themes have pervaded the rock era. During the late sixties and early seventies, Roger Daltry and The Who sang of noise pollution and insomnia in "Squeeze Box." The Beatles expressed similar sleep difficulties on their "white" album with the song "I'm So Tired"; by the end of the album, however, they had resolved their love-stricken insomnia in the lullaby "Good Night."

The 1980s brought different images of sleep and dreaming to the popular music scene. For instance, Pink Floyd moved far away from the Beatles' "sweet dreams" on their 1983 album, "The Final Cut." The lyrics of "The Gunner's Dream" describe a recurring dream of war that inspires fears of insanity in the dreamer. The power of dream imagery was also expressed on the 1987 album "The Joshua Tree" by the rock group U2 in their song "In God's Country": Sleep is likened to a drug, and a dream of a desert landscape represents both desolation and hope.

Sleep and dreaming as themes in popular music have not been exclusive to the rock genre. For example, blues musicians often sympathized with their rock counterparts by singing of insomnia-related loneliness and heartache, as in "No Nights by Myself" by Sonny Boy Williamson, who complained that he couldn't sleep at all without his sweetheart. Other bluesmen crooned of dreaming as an escape from their cruel reality. For instance, Johnny Shines describes his special dream of living in a rich man's paradise in "Living in the White-

house." Finally, blues artists often sang of the morning and waking from sleep to find an unpleasant reality. In "The End" by James Reed, the singer wakes to find his woman has left him: "Well, I woke up soon one morning;/I had the blues all 'round my bed./Yes, I woke up soon one morning;/I had the blues all 'round my bed./Well, I reached/for my baby,/and I got these/blues instead."

A more modern addition to the popular music genre—new age music—has attempted to go beyond this straightforward lyrical approach. By blending original compositions with a variety of natural sounds, new age musicians attempt to create a certain response in the mind of the listener. For example, several pieces have been developed specifically to promote sleep and relaxation, including "A Time to Dream" by Chazz and "Somona Surf" by Lou Judson. Both works use natural sounds, such as birdsong and the sound of the surf, to create a relaxing and quiet atmosphere in which to sleep and dream. Thus, new age music represents an attempt by artists to incorporate sleep and dreaming into their work through the listener's physiological and psychological responses to the music.

The prevalence of sleep and dreaming throughout the history of popular music in all of its many styles (rock, blues, folk) and the modern example of new age music with its own approach to these two themes indicate that sleep and dreaming will remain lasting themes in this popular art form.

BIBLIOGRAPHY

Birosik PJ. 1989. *The new age music guide: Profiles and recordings of 500 top new age musicians.* New York: Collier.

Bronson F. 1988. *The Billboard book of #1 hits.* New York: Billboard Productions.

Titon JT. 1988. *Downhome blues lyrics: An anthology from the post-World War II era.* Providence, RI: Jeff Todd Titon, Brown University.

John P. Spencer

POSTPRANDIAL

[Postprandial *is a term describing the period immediately after eating. It refers to a broad range of changes in physiological systems that occur in response to food intake. The digestive system activates and blood is diverted to the stomach, intestines, liver, and other digestive organs to facilitate absorption of the meal. These changes are mediated by the* SYMPATHETIC NERVOUS SYSTEM.

In addition to the changes in blood flow, the postprandial period involves important endocrine responses to feeding and to the subsequent absorption of nutrients. Insulin and other pancreatic hormones are released as the plasma concentration of glucose changes. Secretion of NEUROENDOCRINE HORMONES *(such as* GROWTH HORMONE *and adrenocorticotropic hormone) is also affected, as the body anticipates and responds to the altered availability of nutrients.*

People often associate the postprandial period with an increase in SLEEPINESS, *particularly after a large meal. It is commonly thought that such a decrease in alertness is caused by a reduction of blood flow to the brain as blood is diverted to the digestive tract; this simplistic explanation, however, is not correct. It is now known that sleepiness increases in the early afternoon even when no meal is consumed (see* MULTIPLE SLEEP LATENCY TEST*). Whether the physiological responses to feeding that characterize the postprandial period also contribute to increased sleepiness is not yet known.*]

POSTTRAUMATIC NIGHTMARES

Nightmares are dreams with intense feelings of fear or helplessness. Although nightmares may appear for no apparent reason, they are frequently the result of traumatic life events, such as war, terrorist attacks, work, or car accidents. The association of nightmares with traumatic events is so preponderant that posttraumatic nightmares are accepted as one of the diagnostic symptoms of posttraumatic stress disorder (PTSD) syndrome. Posttraumatic nightmares may appear at any age and continue many years after the trauma. Survivors of Nazi concentration camps and prisoners of war from World War II have been shown to suffer from nightmares more than 50 years after their traumatic experiences.

Sleep laboratory studies reveal that posttraumatic nightmares mainly occur during REM sleep, although some reports indicate they may also occur during NREM sleep, particularly during stage 2. The time elapsed from the trauma appears to be a critical factor regarding the vividness and emotionality of nightmares. Usually, the posttraumatic nightmare is initially an exact rerun of the actual traumatic events, later blending with persons and events from the victim's family and immediate environment. For instance, a sea-disaster survivor of an incident where half of the crew were drowned in the stormy "Bermuda triangle" had the following nightmare, recorded in the sleep laboratory 4 months after the event. He was trapped in his locked cabin unable to escape, while the water was rapidly rising. Just before waking up in great panic, he heard his sister calling for help from a nearby cabin. Although his sister had not been present during the incident, she was incorporated into the dream plot months later.

When dream content is highly emotional or frightening, there are extreme changes in respiration and heart rate and muscle twitches—indications of intense physiologic activation. Occasionally, this activation is so intense that sleep is momentarily interrupted. Such an interruption may fragment REM sleep every few minutes, a clinical condition know as "REM interruption insomnia." An interruption may be associated with vigorous behavior. In another survivor of the same drowning accident, REM periods were fragmented by multiple arousals, strong body movements, and vocalizations. On one of these occasions, the sailor woke up from REM sleep, jumped out of his bed, tore the electrodes from his head, and shouted, "The ship is sinking, the ship is sinking." After calming down, he reported that he had had a vivid nightmare in which the sea disaster had been reenacted.

The duration and intensity of the trauma may also influence the type of posttraumatic nightmare. Survivors of Nazi concentration camps described "rerun" nightmares that, almost every night, virtually brought to life the persecution experiences in the camps. In these terrifying dreams the survivors saw themselves being chased, running, hiding, or being beaten or humiliated. Some always managed to escape at the last moment; others had to wake up to abort the terror. After waking, frequently in panicky fear and screaming out loud, they would remain awake for a long time until they managed to calm themselves by repeatedly saying, "It's only a dream."

Can a trauma victim overcome posttraumatic nightmares? The treatment of posttraumatic nightmares cannot be separated from the treatment of the other posttraumatic symptoms. Freud believed that posttraumatic dreams, through the repeated reliving of the traumatic events during the dreams, represented attempts on the part of the ego to master the trauma, much the way repeated viewing of a horror film reduces anxiety and fear. Therefore, treatments of posttraumatic nightmares based on psychodynamic orientation repeatedly expose the victim to noises and pictures related to the trauma. Other treatments include psychotherapy and medications. Recent findings based on sleep laboratory studies indicate that suppression of dreaming altogether may be one of the ways for the trauma sufferer to combat posttraumatic nightmares. War-related traumatized patients and survivors of Nazi camps were found to have considerably lower recall of dreams when awakened from REM sleep than normal control subjects. We do not yet know why some traumatized victims can suppress their dreams while others cannot.

REFERENCES

Hartmann E. 1984. *The nightmare.* New York: Basic Books.

Hefez A, Metz L, Lavie P. 1987. Long-term effects of extreme situational stress on sleep and dreaming. *Am J Psychiatry* 144:344–347.

Lavie P, Kaminer H. 1991. Dreams that poison sleep: Dreaming in Holocaust survivors. *Dreaming.* 1:11–21.

Mack EM. 1974. *Nightmares and human conflict.* Boston: Houghton Mifflin.

Peretz Lavie

POSTTRAUMATIC STRESS DISORDER

See Posttraumatic Nightmares

PRECOGNITIVE DREAMS

See Psychic Dreams; Telepathy and Dreaming

PREGNANCY, SLEEP IN

Pregnancy is a state characterized by many dramatic changes in bodily functions and processes, including alterations in sleep patterns. From conception to delivery, pregnancy spans approximately 40 weeks, or 9 months. These 9 months are further divided into three periods of 3 months each, called trimesters. Each of the three trimesters is characterized by very specific alterations in the pregnant woman's physical and emotional functions, as well as specific changes in the growth and development of the unborn child. The first 3 months after delivery of the baby, often referred to as the fourth trimester or postpartum period, is also a time of dramatic change for the new mother, as the body's functions return to a nonpregnant state and the woman adapts to meeting the continuous care demands of the infant.

Women frequently identify disturbed sleep patterns and insufficient amounts of sleep, with subsequent feelings of tiredness and fatigue, as primary complaints and sources of distress during pregnancy and the early weeks after delivery. The dramatic changes in the body during this period of childbearing contribute to the sleep disturbances. Just as the bodily changes occur systematically and predictably in each of the trimesters, so do the changes in sleep.

The First Trimester

All of the major organ systems of the unborn child are developed and functional by the end of the first trimester. This period of very rapid growth is accomplished by an increase in the function of the mother's major organ systems and results in a high energy demand and expenditure for the pregnant woman. The most commonly reported changes during these first 3 months are feeling high levels of fatigue and tiredness and needing more sleep (see SLEEPINESS). In fact, total sleep time and nap-taking behaviors are increased during the first trimester, perhaps as a compensatory mechanism to alleviate feelings of fatigue and to restore energy reserves. In addition to elevated energy demands for the pregnant woman, nighttime interruptions in sleep may also contribute to the high levels of fatigue during the first trimester. At this time, the growing fetus places pressure on the pregnant woman's bladder, and sleep is often interrupted by the need to urinate frequently.

In general, the first trimester is characterized by high levels of fatigue, an increase in daytime napping, and an increase in total sleep time. These reports are primarily based on the subjective reports of pregnant women; very little sleep research has been done on women in the first trimester to document specific changes in their sleep patterns.

The Second Trimester

The middle 3 months of pregnancy are characterized by a normalization of sleep patterns and general feelings of well-being. Although energy demands remain high for nourishment of the unborn child, development does not progress as rapidly compared with the first trimester. It may also be that by the second trimester the maternal system has adapted to the higher energy demands. Nighttime disruptions in sleep from the need for frequent urination are infrequent because the uterus, the muscular organ that houses the growing fetus, moves from within the pelvic bone structure, where it pressed against the bladder, into the abdominal area, above the bladder.

The reports that sleep is improved and similar to prepregnancy sleep patterns are based primarily on subjective reports from pregnant women; once again, there is little research to document the reported changes in sleep during the second trimester.

The Third Trimester

During the last 3 months of pregnancy, women frequently complain of altered sleep patterns and poor sleep quality. The fetus again undergoes a dramatic growth increase that results in profound alterations in maternal respiratory function, digestion, bowel and bladder elimination, musculoskeletal system, and general level of comfort. All of these factors can contribute to the disturbed sleep patterns of late pregnancy. Reasons for disturbed sleep include backache, need for frequent urination, fetal movements, heartburn,

leg cramps, hip pain, and shortness of breath. Additionally, many women report having more vivid dreams with bizarre or unusual content (see PREGNANCY AND DREAMING).

Sleep research in women during the third trimester indicates that these women take longer to fall asleep, have more awake time during the night, have reduced amounts of slow-wave sleep (SWS), and have difficulty returning to sleep after nighttime awakenings as compared with nonpregnant women of the same age (Karacan et al., 1969; Petre-Quadens and De Lee, 1973). These alterations in sleep patterns during late pregnancy may result in a state of sleep deprivation for women as they near delivery.

The Fourth Trimester

After delivery, new mothers are responsible for the 24-hour care demands of the newborn. Because the sleeping, waking, and feeding behaviors of a newborn are unpredictable, the new mother's sleep continues to be disrupted. This can be even worse for mothers of twins. Additionally, pain from the labor and delivery process contributes to altered sleep patterns and frequent awakenings during the night.

When relieved of the responsibility for nighttime feeding of the newborn after delivery, new mothers take less time to fall asleep and have an increase in SWS (indicating a recovery from the SWS deprivation experienced in the final months of pregnancy) and a decrease in the amount of stage REM. However, new mothers still experience frequent awakenings, less total sleep time, and reduced sleep efficiency compared with nonchildbearing women of the same age. Some research results indicate that sleep patterns return to normal 2 weeks after delivery. Until the newborn sleeps through the night, however, maternal sleep continues to be disrupted by the need to feed and comfort the baby.

Conclusions

It has been said that the disturbed sleep during pregnancy, especially in the third trimester, prepares the woman for caring for the newborn during the fourth trimester. When a new mother's sleep patterns are severely disturbed, however, she may be at risk for developing postpartum depression or be predisposed to child abuse or neglect. Complaints of sleep disturbances by new mothers should be evaluated seriously to prevent adverse consequences to the mother and her newborn.

REFERENCES

Karacan I, Heine W, Agnew HW, Williams RL, Webb WB, Ross JJ. 1968. Characteristics of sleep patterns in late pregnancy and the postpartum periods. *Am J Obstet Gynecol* 101(5):879–882.

Karacan I, Williams RL, Hursch CJ, McCaulley M, Heine MW. 1969. Some implications of the sleep patterns of pregnancy for postpartum emotional disturbances. *Br J Psychiatry* 115:929–935.

Moorcroft WH. 1989. *Sleep, dreaming, and sleep disorders: An introduction.* Lanham, Md.: University Press of America.

Petre-Quadens O, De Lee C. 1972. Sleep cycle alterations during pregnancy, postpartum, and the menstrual cycle. In Ferin M, Halberg F, Richart RM, Vande Wiele RL, eds. *Biorhythms and human reproduction*, pp 331–351. New York: Wiley.

Schweiger MS. 1972. Sleep disturbance in pregnancy. *Am J Obstet Gynecol* 14:879–882.

Kathryn Lee

PREGNANCY AND DREAMING

Dream content changes during pregnancy, demonstrating how dreams appear to reflect what is currently important in a person's waking life, and, thereby, how dreams may be meaningful. During a woman's first pregnancy, dream content changes not only with the onset of conception, but also with the various stages of pregnancy (Stukane, 1985).

Early in the pregnancy (sometimes even before the conception is confirmed) the dreams focus on the woman herself and what is happening inside her body. Dreams about fertility and reproductive ability are much more frequent. Small animals (interpreted as representing the fetus) are more noticeable in dreams at this time. Sometimes the fetus is portrayed as dangerous or intrusive. Miscarriage (reflecting a normal fear and

concern) is another common topic. Dreams that appear to reflect ambivalence over the conception and the major changes in lifestyle that will follow the pregnancy may likewise occur.

During midpregnancy, the focus of the dreams changes. Images of being a bad mother and of things that could go wrong become more frequent and are thought to reflect the dreamer's concern about adequacy for motherhood. Also, relationships with others, especially the father of the baby, and the pregnant woman's self-comparison with her own mother become noticeable dream themes. Gradually, images of actual babies replace those of small animals. At times, the babies may be characterized as abnormal, reflecting a normal and common worry, whereas they appear very appealing at other times, especially later, as the pregnancy progresses. Near the end of midterm there may be frequent dreams of a wide range of disasters, focusing especially on unresolved issues including labor and delivery, careers, money matters, and marriage.

During the last 3 months of pregnancy, dream recall tends to increase because the woman awakens more frequently during the night (see PREGNANCY, SLEEP IN). Some themes, including abnormal or unusual babies as well as the relationship and comparison with the dreamer's mother, continue from midterm, but new themes also emerge in the dreams of the pregnant woman. There is a special focus on how her body is changing and how she perceives herself to be the focus of attention of others. As the due date approaches, the pregnant woman may dream of the birthing process. A recurrent dream character may be the attending gynecologist/obstetrician.

Subsequent pregnancies also influence dreams but with some differences (Stukane, 1985). The dreamer's mother is not as frequent a character. Dreams about how the new child will relate to the rest of the family and what effect the new baby will have on the dreamer's relationship with her family become more common.

The basis for these alterations in dreams during a woman's pregnancy may be either the many physiological changes that occur during pregnancy, the psychological changes that accompany pregnancy, or both. We cannot tell for certain, as both kinds of changes occur simultaneously. However, since the dreams of the father also shift during pregnancy (Siegel, 1983), the conclusion is less ambiguous; the alterations in the dreams of the father are unaccompanied by physiological changes and thus the dreams must be primarily psychologically based.

Early in the pregnancy the father dreams more of overtly sexual themes. Likewise, dreams about being "macho," being nurturing, and balancing these two roles are prevalent. During midpregnancy, the father continues to dream about nurturing, but themes of sex are replaced by comparison with his father, childhood family, and current family. At this time, he may additionally dream about being left out of the entire process. The last 3 months of pregnancy bring dreams that are less about the father's childhood family and more about his current family (especially the woman he impregnated). Images of what is happening to the mother's body and what the baby will be like are frequent. (A large percentage of the babies dreamt about by fathers are male.) As the due date approaches, the father may dream about the delivery process.

Thus, pregnancy affects the dreams of both the pregnant woman and the father. Following conception the dreams of both have a predominantly internal focus. By the end of pregnancy, both mother and father focus on the baby, the birth process, and their current family. In all, changes in dreams during pregnancy are a good illustration of how dreams reflect our current waking concerns and needs.

REFERENCES

Moorcroft WH. 1989. *Sleep, dreaming, and sleep disorders: An introduction.* Lanham, Md.: University Press of America.

Siegel A. 1983. Expectant fathers' dreams. *Dream Craft* 2:5–7.

Stukane E. 1985. *The dream worlds of pregnancy.* New York: Quill.

William H. Moorcroft

PREMATURE INFANTS

Infants who are born before the normal end of pregnancy (40 weeks) are called premature infants. These babies are typically born sometime after the 26th week of pregnancy and weigh between 1,000 grams (2.2 pounds) and 2,500 grams (5.5 pounds). As the premature baby is exposed to an environment that is very different from the mother's womb at a time when the brain is still very immature, many researchers have hypothesized that the subsequent development of the premature baby's brain is different from that of normal full-term infants. One of the ways to look for differences in brain development is to study the development of sleep and waking states in premature babies and to compare it with that of full-term infants at the same conceptional age. (Conceptional age is the sum of gestational age plus chronological age, where gestational age is the age in weeks from conception to birth, and chronological age is the age since birth). Another reason for studying the sleep of premature babies is an interest in describing what may be the very earliest forms of human sleep and waking behavior.

By the use of electroencephalographic (brain wave) measures along with measures of behavior, such as eye movements, body movements, and breathing regularity, recordings of sleep–wake patterns in premature babies during the preterm period (that is, prior to their formerly expected time of birth) have demonstrated that the states of active sleep, quiet sleep, and wakefulness may be identified as early as 28 weeks of conceptional age. At these very early ages, however, the states are not well differentiated, and there are times when it is not clear whether the baby is awake or asleep. These times are called the *indeterminate state*. Premature infants show greater amounts of active sleep and more indeterminate state than full-term infants. This finding was one factor supporting the ontogenetic hypothesis of REM sleep (see ONTOGENY; FUNCTIONS OF REM SLEEP). Over the course of the preterm period, the amount of active sleep eventually decreases and wakefulness increases. There is also a gradual increase in the overall organization of the sleep and waking states; by 40 weeks of conceptional age, the states resemble more closely the consistent recurring patterns of electroencephalographic and behavioral clusters that characterize the states seen in full-term infants (Curzi-Dascalova, Peirano, and Morel-Kahn, 1988; Dreyfus-Brisac, 1970; Holditch-Davis, 1990; Parmelee et al., 1968). Dreyfus-Brisac described the evolution of five distinct electroencephalographic patterns in premature infants. Beginning at 32 weeks of conceptional age, the predominant pattern is one of discontinuous bursts of nonspecific electrical activation; a definite tracé alternans pattern emerges by 34 weeks; a continuous slow-wave pattern provides a background to the tracé alternans by 36 weeks; and shortly thereafter, the typical high-voltage slow and low-voltage fast patterns of the neonate become evident. (See IN-FANCY, NORMAL SLEEP PATTERNS IN.)

When premature infants are compared with full-term infants at the same conceptional ages *after* term, subtle differences are seen in sleep–wake state expression. Thus, the premature infant in the first weeks after term may show state characteristics that are more mature than those of full-term infants in some ways—such as longer periods of quiet sleep or more time awake in the daytime—and less mature than those of full-term infants in other ways—such as more body movements during sleep or more frequent rapid eye movement episodes and changes between states (Dreyfus-Brisac, 1970; Parmelee et al., 1968).

In one long-term study, premature babies and full-term babies were observed using a time-lapse video recording procedure throughout the night over the first year of life. The results of this study indicated that premature and full-term infants showed the same general pattern of state development. That is, in both groups of infants, active sleep decreased and quiet sleep increased as they matured. Furthermore, the patterns of change generally occurred at the same rate in both groups. These results suggest that the general development of sleep states may be determined more by biological processes than by environmental influences. The researchers also found that, although both groups of infants spent the same amount of time awake during the night, parents of full-term infants took their babies out of their cribs when they woke up more often than did the parents of premature infants. The premature babies also spent a longer time awake after being put into their cribs to sleep (Anders and Keener, 1985). These observations suggest that there may be significant differences in either the way premature babies are able to initiate and maintain sleep, the way parents interact with their premature babies, or both.

One difficulty in describing the development of premature infants is the fact that not all premature infants are alike. Certain infants are relatively big and healthy, whereas others are very

small and sick and require long stays in the hospital with many invasive medical procedures just to keep them alive. Studies have demonstrated that although the overall pattern of state development is similar between healthy and sick premature babies, the rate of development may be somewhat slower and the organization of states may be different at various ages for the smaller and sicker premature babies (Holditch-Davis, 1990; Holmes et al., 1979). For this reason, several research groups have tried to discover ways to help the premature infant adapt and mature. Techniques intended to promote quieter and more consolidated sleep have included the use of waterbeds and "breathing" teddy bears to provide watery or rhythmic stimulation that may regularize respiration and soothe the infant (Korner, 1985; Thoman and Graham, 1986). (See also FETAL SLEEP–WAKE PATTERNS; ONTOGENY.)

REFERENCES

Anders TF, Keener M. 1985. Developmental course of nighttime sleep–wake patterns in full-term and premature infants during the first year of life: I. *Sleep* 8:173–192.

Curzi-Dascalova L, Peirano P, Morel-Kahn F. 1988. Development of sleep states in normal premature and full-term infants. *Dev Psychobiol* 21:431–444.

Dreyfus-Brisac C. 1970. Ontogenesis of sleep in human prematures after 32 weeks of conceptional age. *Dev Psychobiol* 3:91–121.

Holditch-Davis D. 1990. The development of sleeping and waking states in high-risk preterm infants. *Infant Behav Dev* 13:513–531.

Holmes GL, Logan WJ, Kirkpatrich BV, Meyers EC. 1979. Central nervous system maturation in the stressed premature. *Ann Neurol* 6:518–522.

Korner AF. 1985. Preventive intervention with high-risk newborns: Theoretical, conceptual, and methodological perspectives. In Osofsky JD, ed. *Handbook for infant development*, 2nd ed., pp 1006–1036. New York: Wiley-Interscience.

Parmelee AH Jr, Schulte FJ, Akiyama Y, Wenner WH, Schultz MA, Stern E. 1968. Maturation of EEG activity during sleep in premature infants. *Electroencephalogr Clin Neurophysiol* 24:319–329.

Thoman EB, Graham S. 1986. Self-regulation of stimulation by premature infants. *Pediatrics* 78: 855–860.

Christine Acebo

PREMENSTRUAL SYNDROME

Premenstrual syndrome (PMS) is a constellation of physical, behavioral, and emotional symptoms that affect up to 80 percent of women toward the end of each MENSTRUAL CYCLE. Up to 150 symptoms have been reported in association with PMS, including DEPRESSION, anxiety, confusion, irritability, breast tenderness, abdominal bloating, and sleep disturbances. Difficulty falling asleep (see INSOMNIA), sleeping too much, lethargy, fatigue, and unpleasant dreams are also commonly reported by women with PMS.

Few studies, all with small numbers of subjects, have focused specifically on the sleep disorders in these women. Those that do tend to fall into three categories: (1) surveys regarding the nature and frequency of occurrence of specific sleep complaints, (2) physiological studies of ELECTROENCEPHALOGRAM (EEG) and CIRCADIAN RHYTHMS abnormalities, and (3) investigations into the nature of dreams and emotional information processing across the menstrual cycle.

In one survey that specifically monitored sleep behavior, PMS patients reported a higher incidence of sleep disturbances than women in the general population, although premenstrual sleep difficulties are commonly observed in both groups. The most often reported sleep disorders in the women with PMS were frequent awakenings with higher mental activity during the night and, on rising, failure to wake at the expected time because of morning tiredness and unpleasant dreams. Increased daytime SLEEPINESS was also reported during the premenstrual and menstrual phases of the cycle. These symptoms appear to constitute an important component of the premenstrual syndrome, although the etiology of these disturbances remains poorly understood.

The few sleep EEG studies that have been done using subjects with PMS report conflicting results. One study demonstrated an increase in stage 2 sleep (see STAGES OF SLEEP) as a percentage of total sleep, and less REM SLEEP (percentage and minutes), in eight women with PMS compared with eight normal controls. Another study found that stage 1 sleep was elevated in the early to midcycle and premenstrually, whereas SLOW-WAVE SLEEP was increased in the midluteal phase. No reliable changes were observed in stage 2 or REM sleep. No significant fluctuations in EEG sleep parameters across the menstrual cycle were seen in nine PMS clinic patients in yet another study, although one investigation of women with severe premenstrual depression found shortened REM latencies and reduced slow-wave sleep, similar to the sleep abnormalities that have been described in major depression.

Other studies suggest the existence of a phase-advance disturbance of circadian rhythms in relation to the sleep–wake cycle in women with PMS. Evidence for this abnormality is found in studies that demonstrate the phase-advanced offset of melatonin secretion, symptom improvement with a phase advance of the sleep–wake cycle (i.e., late-night sleep deprivation) or a phase delay of circadian rhythms (evening bright-light treatment), and earlier minimum nocturnal temperatures. A similar phase advance of circadian rhythms in relation to the sleep–wake cycle has been observed in some patients with affective disorders, suggesting an element of commonality between these two disorders. (See also CIRCADIAN RHYTHM DISORDERS; DEPRESSION; IRREGULAR SLEEP-WAKE CYCLE; PHASE SHIFT.)

The results of investigations regarding dream recall and content across the menstrual cycle are also inconclusive and none has focused specifically on women with PMS. Methodological differences in the various studies, including the use of different subject populations and procedures for collecting dreams and even classification of menstrual cycle phases, may account for some of the confusion. Different investigators have variously reported no association of dream content with cycle phase, increased sexual and hostile dream content with menses, an increase in hostile themes during menses, and higher maternal scores in the luteal phase.

Most of these studies, though preliminary, suggest that sleep disturbances are a significant component of premenstrual syndrome. Whether these disturbances reflect exaggerations of "normal" changes in sleep patterns across the menstrual cycle or are an entity unto themselves, possibly reflecting the mood disturbance observed in women with PMS, has yet to be determined.

REFERENCES

Mauri M. 1990. Sleep and the reproductive cycle: A review. *Health Care Women Int* 11:409–421.

Parry BL, Mendelson WB, Duncan WC, Sack DA, Wehr TA. 1989. Longitudinal sleep EEG, temperature, and activity measurements across the menstrual cycle in patients with premenstrual depression and in age-matched controls. *Psychiatry Res* 30: 285–303.

Stephanie Jofe

PRESLEEP STIMULI

See Exercise; Incorporation into Dreams; Sex and Sleep; Sexual Activation

PRESSURIZATION

The twentieth century has seen a dramatic technological advance that has enabled humans to explore the environment at both high altitude and high pressure below the sea. This technological advance has forced us, however, to explore the limits of human physiological tolerance at these environmental extremes. This is exemplified by the human intolerance of the high G-forces experienced in fighter jet maneuvers.

Humans are subjected to high pressure or hyperbaric conditions in a variety of professions. Certainly scuba divers and submarine inhabitants are the obvious examples; however, other individuals such as tunnel diggers and water construction workers are also exposed to the effects of hyperbaria. In the future, the development of more advanced undersea exploration and perhaps underwater communities may again place individuals under the stress of high pressure.

High pressure has several adverse effects on the human. Ear and lung damage from rapid pressure changes during descent or ascent is well known. Other adverse effects related to gas mixtures under high pressure include oxygen, nitrogen, or helium toxicity. The "high-pressure nervous syndrome" (HPNS) characterized by nausea, vomiting, fatigue, and muscle twitching may be related to rapid descent and the amounts of nitrogen and carbon monoxide present in the body at high pressure. The Seadragon VI dive in 1987 evaluated the physiological effects of a 7-day dive at 31 atmospheres of pressure, equivalent to a 300-meter dive. The investigators noted changes in body temperature regulation and urine production and flow, and found evidence of cardiovascular deconditioning similar to that seen in those who are weightless or on bedrest. The long-term consequences of these physiological changes in those exposed to prolonged hyperbaria is unclear, but may impact work safety, efficiency, and capability.

In an attempt to define further the neurological syndromes seen with high-pressure exposure, several investigators have looked for electroencephalographic changes with diving. There have been observed electroencephalographic changes associated temporally with symptoms of the high-pressure nervous syndrome. Corriol, Chouteau, and Catier (1973) describe the development of prominent theta waves and a decrease in alpha activity on the ELECTROENCEPHALOGRAM (EEG) tracings of divers compressed to 31 atmospheres of pressure. These EEG changes were associated with symptoms of lethargy and fatigue, and both were reversed with increased time spent at depth or with decompression. Both symptoms and EEG changes were minimized with a slower compression rate, suggesting that a rapid compression rate may be an important factor in the development of the high-pressure nervous syndrome. In addition to the increased theta and decreased alpha activity in their divers, Shi and colleagues (1987) also described a prominent diffuse slowing of the EEG that increased with pressure. The long-term sequelae of these changes are unclear.

The effect of high pressure on sleep has not been extensively evaluated. One of the few studies examining this topic was reported by Serbanescu, Fructus, and Naquet in 1969. In this study, termed *Ludion II,* two trained divers lived in a caisson at 85 meters for 10 days with twice-daily excursions to 125 meters. EEG tracings were obtained before entering the caisson, before and during compression, during decompression, and after exiting the caisson. The waking EEG tracings did not vary; however, the sleep tracings during compression did show several interesting changes. Stage 2 sleep was described as more complex than before or after compression. There was an increase in the percentage of stage 2 sleep at the expense of stage 3 and 4 sleep. Additionally, there was an increase in the percentage of REM while under pressure. It is unknown whether these changes were due to the gas mixture, pressure, or both. The overall impact of the sleep tracing changes on the quality and quantity of sleep is also unclear.

Recently, Mohri (1990) evaluated the performance of divers exposed to 180 meters. Subjective complaints as well as objective sleep recordings were obtained. In contrast to the Ludion II findings, this study actually found a decrease in the percentage of REM sleep and an overall description of sleep quality as poor. It is unclear if this was due to higher pressure or other factors such as anxiety, temperature, or sleeping conditions.

Because the literature is limited in this area, it is difficult to know the full effect of high pressure on sleep quality or quantity. If sleep disorders do exist under these conditions, they many have an adverse impact on the duration and type of underwater exploration in the future. Certainly, more detailed and careful studies addressing the effect of pressure and gas mixture on sleep will be needed to answer these questions.

REFERENCES

Corriol J, Chouteau J, Catier J. 1973. Human simulated diving experiments at saturation under oxygen–helium exposures up to 500 meters: Electroencephalographic data. *Aerospace Med* 44(11):1270–1276.

Mohri M. 1990. Fatigue and performance of divers during a simulated, non-saturated oxygen–helium dive to 180 meters. *Nippon Eiseigaku Zasshi [Jpn J Hyg]* 45(2):619–626.

Nakayama H, Murai T, Hong SK. 1987. Seadragon VI: A 7-day saturation dive at 31 ATA. I. Objectives, design, and scope. *Undersea Biomed Res* 14(5): 377–385.

Serbanescu T, Fructus P, Naquet R. 1969. Study of the EEG of sleep under prolonged increase of pressure (the Operation Ludion II). *Electroencephalogr Clin Neurophysiol* 26:639.

Shi ZY, Zhao DM, Mei XH, Liu ZR, Sheng TM. 1987. The influence of simulated saturation diving on electroencephalogram of human at different depths. *Ann Physiol Anthropol* 6(3):123–132.

Smith E. 1984. The biological effects of high pressures: Underlying principles. *Philos Trans R Soc London Ser B*. 304(1118):5–16.

Thomas J. Meyer

PROBLEM SOLVING AND DREAMING

Dreams have been recognized as a source of solutions to problems almost since history has been recorded. Dreams have also been viewed as a source of creativity (see CREATIVITY IN DREAMS.) More recently, dreams have been seen as providing answers to emotional dilemmas.

Historical examples abound of the ideas that dreams have provided to inventors and artists. For example, Elias Howe had tried unsuccessfully for several years to invent a sewing machine. He dreamed one night that he had been captured by a tribe who, when he failed to perfect a sewing machine, began throwing spears at him. There were two unusual things about these spears: Each had a hole near its sharp end, and the spears would repeatedly partially penetrate the ground only to bounce up again. On awakening, Howe realized that his dream had given him two clues to completing the sewing machine: Move the hole for the thread to the sharp end of the needle, and have the needle repeatedly penetrate the cloth without completely going through.

Another example is James Watt's invention of the shot tower for the manufacture of shotgun pellets. Watt dreamed that he was in a storm in which it was raining hot lead. He dreamed this same dream three times before he realized its meaning: Allow drops of molten lead to fall through the air and thereby cool into the near-perfect spherical shapes ideal for shot.

Such insights from dreams are not limited to mechanical inventions; there are literary, artistic, scientific, and religious examples as well. Robert Louis Stevenson said that he had dreamed many of his story ideas, including the key characters in *Dr. Jekyll and Mr. Hyde*. Samuel Taylor Coleridge dictated the "Rime of the Ancient Mariner" just as it occurred in one of his dreams. (There is some question, though, of whether the dreams of Stevenson and Coleridge were natural or drug induced.) Mohammed stated that much of the *Koran* was dictated to him in his dreams. Tartini's violin sonata *The Devil's Trill* was written down by him just as he heard it in a dream. Friedrich August Kekulé, the famous chemist of the nineteenth century, dreamed that six snakes formed a ring by each biting and holding the tail of the snake in front of it. This ring shape, he realized on awakening, was the solution he had been seeking to the chemical nature of the benzene molecule.

Several elements common to these and many other examples give insight into the nature of and importance of dreams. First, the solutions were to problems that were areas of struggle in the person's waking life. In many cases, the person had been focusing on the quandary for days, weeks, or longer without success. Second, the problem and its solution were emotionally important to the dreamer. Struggling with the dilemma had resulted in frustration, and discovering the solution was very satisfying. Third, the solution was often presented in the dream as a metaphor rather than a direct, logical statement. The dreamer had to see the metaphorical significance of the dream to discover the solution to the problem.

How do our dreams solve problems for us? Some psychologists suggest that while dreaming our mind has easier access to our memories and emotions (Cartwright, 1977). Furthermore, these psychologists posit that during dreams our minds are less constrained by the realities of waking life, thus allowing our mental processes to work unhindered with these materials, to experiment, and to create until we arrive at answers. But problem solving in dreams is not limited to mechanical, scientific, or artistic subjects. Perhaps even more common, although less frequently recognized, are dreams that help with emotional dilemmas. Some psychologists believe that we do much of our dreaming in response to emotional concerns in our waking lives (Cartwright, 1977). Research has shown that the very process of dreaming about such difficulties seems to relieve the emotional pressure even if the dream is not understood or remembered (Moorcroft, 1989). Jung (1974) called this process *compensation:* Dreams function to bring emotional balance to our lives. When we awaken we not only feel better, but we are also better able to deal with the traumas of our lives.

REFERENCES

Cartwright RD. 1977. *Night life: Explorations in dreaming.* Englewood Cliffs, N.J.: Prentice-Hall.
Garfield PL. 1974. *Creative dreaming.* New York: Ballantine.
Jung CB. 1974. *Dreams.* Princeton, N.J.: Princeton University Press.
Moorcroft WH. 1989. *Sleep, dreaming, and sleep disorders: An introduction.* Lanham, Md.: University Press of America.

William H. Moorcroft

PROLACTIN

Prolactin is a polypeptide hormone produced by the anterior pituitary gland and released in a pulsatile fashion. Although prolactin is critically important in maintaining electrolyte balance for certain forms of fish as they migrate from saltwater to freshwater, its chief role in humans is limited to reproductive functions and breastfeeding. Prolactin is the most important hormone for production of casein, the essential protein in human breast milk. Prolactin may have other important roles in humans, such as immune regulation, although further research needs to be done in this field.

During pregnancy, prolactin levels increase steadily, and they are maintained at a high level for several months after delivery if breastfeeding is continued. Although this elevated level of prolactin can inhibit return of the normal MENSTRUAL CYCLE in some nursing mothers, it is not a reliable form of contraception as ovulation often resumes during the hyperprolactinemic state. If breastfeeding is not initiated, prolactin levels fall in the first weeks after delivery.

In nonpregnant women and in men, the role of prolactin is still unclear. Although there are receptors for prolactin in both male and female gonadal cells, it is unclear whether this implies that prolactin is indeed necessary for normal function. It is clear that sustained elevations of serum prolactin lead to adverse effects on the reproductive axes of both men and women. In men, hyperprolactinemia causes decreased libido, impotence, and hypogonadism (i.e., complete loss of sexual hormonal function). In women, it can cause irregular, abnormal, or absent menstrual cycles. In either sex hyperprolactinemia may give rise to galactorrhea, an unwanted breast discharge.

Prolactin is probably under both inhibitory and stimulatory hypothalamic control (see HYPOTHALAMUS). Certain common stimulators, such as stress, exercise, eating, breastfeeding, and psychotropic drugs can stimulate prolactin release. Sleep, however, is one of the strongest and best studied stimulators of prolactin secretion. Sassin et al. (1972) studied prolactin levels drawn at 20-minute intervals from three men and three women over 24 hours. Prolactin rose approximately 60 to 90 minutes after sleep onset and peaked at about 5 to 7 A.M. After awakening, prolactin levels fell and reached their minimum between noon and 5 P.M. Further evidence of this sleep-related secretion of prolactin was obtained by Parker, Rossman, and Vanderlaan (1973), who showed that prolactin levels clearly increase during daytime napping, and by Sassin et al. (1973) in sleep reversal studies that demonstrated a rise in prolactin during daytime sleep.

The sleep-related rise in prolactin secretion has been demonstrated in children and in adult men and women (Finkelstein et al., 1978). Some studies have shown a disappearance of this nocturnal rhythm in the elderly (Marrama et al., 1982), whereas others have demonstrated its preservation (Zakria et al., 1988). The nocturnal pattern of secretion is maintained initially in pregnancy, but may become blunted as pregnancy progresses (Schweizer, Kim, and Malarkey, 1984). Studies in both lactating and nonlactating postpartum women reveal that the nocturnal rhythm is again restored (Stern and Reichlin, 1990; Liu and Park, 1988). (See also PREGNANCY, SLEEP IN.)

There is also evidence of an inherent circadian, sleep-independent rhythm of prolactin secretion. Several studies have demonstrated that in the late afternoon or early evening, prolactin levels begin to rise (Sassin et al., 1972; Van Cauter et al., 1981; Tennekoon and Lenton, 1985). In addition, Desir et al. (1982) showed that after westward flight and sleep delay, a brief elevation in prolactin levels occurred at the subjects' normal sleep time, with an additional increase in prolactin when the subject finally did sleep. This "anamnestic peak" provides strong evidence that there may be an inherent circadian rhythm of prolactin that is usually synchronized with sleep. (See also JET LAG; INTERNAL DESYNCHRONIZATION.)

Absence or blunting of the nocturnal sleep-associated rise in prolactin has been demonstrated in a variety of diseases, including labile diabetes mellitus, renal failure, Cushing's disease, cirrhosis, and NARCOLEPSY, in apallic patients, and in some patients with prolactin-producing pituitary tumors. In obese women, the nocturnal prolactin rhythm was observed; however, it was delayed in comparison both to normal-weight controls and to these same obese women after they underwent a 12-day fast (Copinschi et al., 1978). Studies in women with anorexia nervosa have revealed a nocturnal increase in prolactin, but at lower levels than in normal controls (Kalucy et al., 1976). In studies of men with unipolar DEPRESSION, the nocturnal elevation occurred before sleep onset, approximately 2 hours earlier than in normal controls. In both unipolar and bipolar depression, the mid-sleep concentrations of prolactin secretion were blunted and associated with increased fragmentation of sleep (Linkowski et al., 1989).

Although sustained elevations in prolactin can clearly be associated with major reproductive abnormalities, controversy exists as to the role of isolated nocturnal hypersecretion of prolactin. Both endometriosis and luteal phase defects have been associated with elevated nocturnal levels of prolactin (Radwanska, Henig, and Dmowski, 1987; Board, Storlazzi, and Schneider, 1981); however, recent studies using frequent sampling found normal levels of nocturnal prolactin in women with luteal phase deficiency (Soules et al., 1991). Further studies need to be done to define the possible role of prolactin in these disease processes.

In summary, the sleep-related rise in prolactin secretion is a well-described rhythm in humans of most ages and both sexes. Abnormalities of this rhythm are characteristic of several pathophysiological states. Although most studies appear to link this rhythm entirely with sleep, some evidence exists that there may be a circadian, sleep-independent rhythm of prolactin secretion in humans. Further studies are needed to define prolactin's role in both normal human physiology and pathophysiological states.

REFERENCES

Board JA, Storlazzi E, Schneider V. 1981. Nocturnal prolactin levels in infertility. *Fertil Steril* 36: 720–724.

Copinschi G, De Laet MH, Brion JP, Leclercq BR, L'Hermite M, Robyn C, Virasoro E, Van Cauter E. 1978. Simultaneous study of cortisol, growth hormone and prolactin nyctohemeral variations in normal and obese subjects. Influence of prolonged fasting in obesity. *Clin Endocrinol* 9:15–26.

Desir D, Van Cauter E, L'Hermite M, Refetoff S, Jadot C, Caufriez A, Copinschi G, Robyn C. 1982. Effects of "jet lag" on hormonal patterns. III. Demonstration of an intrinsic circadian rhythmicity in plasma prolactin. *J Clin Endocrinol Metab* 55:849–857.

Finkelstein JW, Kapen S, Weitzman ED, Hellman L, Boyar RM. 1978. Twenty-four-hour plasma prolactin patterns in prepubertal and adolescent boys. *J Clin Endocrinol Metab* 47:1123–1128.

Kalucy RS, Crisp AH, McNeilly A, Chen CN, Lacey JH. 1976. Nocturnal hormonal profiles in massive obesity, anorexia nervosa and normal females. *J Psychosomat Res* 20:594–604.

Linkowski P, Van Cauter E, L'Hermite-Baleriaux M, Kerkhofs M, Hubain P, L'Hermite M, Mendelewicz J. 1989. The 24-hour profile of plasma prolactin in men with endogenous depressive illness. *Arch Gen Psychiatry* 46:813–819.

Liu JH, Park KH. 1988. Gonadotropin and prolactin secretion increases during sleep during the puerperium in nonlactating women. *J Clin Endocrinol Metab* 66:839–845.

Marrama P, Carani C, Baraghini GF, Volpe A, Zini D, Celani MF, Montanini V. 1982. Circadian rhythm of testosterone and prolactin in the ageing. *Maturitas* 4:131–138.

Parker DC, Rossman LG, Vanderlaan EF. 1973. Sleep-related, nyctohemeral and briefly episodic variation in human plasma prolactin concentrations. *J Clin Endocrinol Metab* 36:1119–1124.

Radwanska E, Henig I, Dmowski WP. 1987. Nocturnal prolactin levels in infertile women with endometriosis. *J Reprod Med* 32:605–608.

Sassin JF, Frantz AG, Weitzman ED, Kapen S. 1972. Human prolactin: 24 hour pattern with increased release during sleep. *Science* 177:1205–1207.

Sassin JF, Frantz AG, Kapen S, Weitzman ED. 1973. The nocturnal rise of human prolactin is dependent on sleep. *J Clin Endocrinol Metab* 37:436–440.

Schweizer FW, Kim KH, Malarkey WB. 1984. The diurnal variations of serum prolactin levels before and during pregnancy in normal and hyperprolactinemic patients. *Am J Obstet Gynecol* 149:367–371.

Soules MR, Bremner WJ, Steiner RA, Clifton DK. 1991. Prolactin secretion and corpus luteum function in women with luteal phase deficiency. *J Clin Endocrinol Metab* 72:986–992.

Stern JM, Reichlin S. 1990. Prolactin circadian rhythm persists throughout lactation in women. *Neuroendocrinology* 51:31–37.

Tennekoon KH, Lenton EA. 1985. Early evening prolactin rise in women with regular cycles. *J Reprod Fertil* 73:523–527.

Van Cauter E, L'Hermite M, Copinschi G, Refetoff S,

Desir D, Robyn C. 1981. Quantitative analysis of spontaneous variations of plasma prolactin in normal man. *Am J Physiol* 241:E355–E363.

Zakria F, Stern N, McGinty D, Beahm E, Littner M, Sowers JR. 1988. Effect of age on circadian rhythm of prolactin in normal men. *Chronobiologia* 15:219–222.

Joanne Waldstreicher

PROSTAGLANDINS

See Aspirin

PSYCHIC DREAMS

A controversial topic in dreaming concerns so-called psychic or telepathic dreams. Telepathic dreams involve receiving thoughts—while asleep—from another person. The term *telepathic* is also used interchangeably with *psychic* to designate clairvoyant dreams, precognitive dreams, or even out-of-body experiences. In all such psychic dreams, awareness is thought to bypass the normal sensory channels of vision, hearing, smell, touch, and taste, using instead unexplained and unmeasurable energy and unknown mental sensors of such energy. The types of psychic dreams differ in the nature and timing of the content of the dreams (Zusne and Jones, 1989).

Precognitive dreams are dreams in which events seem to be accurately perceived before they occur in waking life. Events seem to occur just as they were dreamed about earlier. The similarities may involve entire dreams or just a single image or event in a dream. For example (Moorcroft, 1989), a young woman reported being in her backyard on a bright, sunny day applying white polish to her nails. Upon looking up, she saw a puppy running toward her down a hill covered with flowers. The puppy approached her and playfully kissed her. At that point she recalled dreaming just a week before of being at her grandfather's farm on a beautiful spring day walking toward a hill. She had new white nail polish on. Suddenly her grandfather's new white puppy ran over the hill toward her and wanted to play. In other instances of precognitive dreams, the similarity between the dream and the subsequent event may be even more precise.

A clairvoyant dream contains events that are actually occurring elsewhere out of sight at the time the dreamer is asleep. A typical example is someone dreaming of a family member being harmed, then finding out that the person actually did suffer some kind of harm around the time the dream was occurring.

During out-of-body experiences dreamers perceive themselves to leave their sleeping body behind as they travel somewhere else. Many times, they report hovering above their sleeping body. The experience, with few exceptions, is described as very realistic.

The experience of psychic dreams can be very vivid and striking. As a result, they tend to be remembered and shared with others more than nonpsychic dreams. Thus psychic dreams may seem to be more common than they really are. Some people view such dreams as authoritative and accurate. To these people, such phenomena point to powers of the mind beyond those of normal sensing, perceiving, and control of movement. However, most accounts of psychic phenomena in dreams are anecdotal and thus impossible to verify.

Scientific investigation of psychic dreams has been infrequent, very difficult, and highly controversial. Most research on psychic dreams has focused on telepathic dreaming because it is easiest to attempt in the laboratory. Such research requires only a sleeper to receive thoughts and a *sender* who remains awake, concentrating thoughts on a specific object otherwise kept secret from the sleeping *receiver*. Dream reports are collected from the receiver and their content reviewed for anything resembling the object. Later the receiver may be given several chances to select the object from a small number of objects.

In one reportedly successful experiment (Ullman, Krippner, and Vaughan, 1989) the sender concentrated on a reproduction of Vermeer's painting *The Wine Taster,* which shows a man wearing a large black hat and holding a wine bottle, with a woman nearby drinking wine from a glass. The dream, as reported by the receiver when awakened during the night, contained references to a nightclub and taking a pill. The next morning the receiver mentioned a man with a black derby hat, a cabaret scene, taking a glass of water to wash down a pill a woman had

offered, and socializing with a drink. Finally, as standard procedure for these experiments, the receiver was given six tries to select *The Wine Taster* from a group of twelve pictures. He was able to do so.

Reported results of research on telepathic dreaming have often shown somewhat greater than expected resemblance of dream content to the object, and selection of the object slightly more frequent than would be predicted on the basis of chance (Ullman, Krippner, and Vaughan, 1989). Such results have been held up as scientific proof of the existence of psychic dreams. However, critics of the research are not convinced (Hansel, 1980). The resemblance of the content of the dream to the object is not always directly obvious but depends on subtle similarities. Furthermore, allowing five errors when picking the object from among twelve does not strongly demonstrate that the receiver was well aware of the identity of the object. Also, other research has been reported that has failed to replicate these results.

On occasion, research on clairvoyant dreams has been attempted. One famous study (Murray and Wheeler, 1937) was done when the baby of the world-famous flier Charles Lindbergh had been kidnapped. In response to newspaper appeals, 1,300 dream reports were submitted concerning the fate of the baby before it was actually known what had happened. Of these, only 7 had content somewhat resembling the characteristics of the burial scene. Most dream reports incorrectly described the baby as still alive. These incorrect reports also contained elements of false speculations widely reported in newspapers.

Research on out-of-body experiences has mostly been limited to collecting anecdotal accounts, with one notable exception (Murray and Wheeler, 1937). A woman who described herself as having frequent out-of-body experiences spent several nights being monitored in a sleep laboratory. One night she awakened from sleep and correctly reported a five-digit number that had been placed out of sight on a high shelf above her bed. She reported that she saw the number while floating above her body.

Research on precognitive dreams has, with rare exceptions, been limited to the collection of anecdotal accounts because of the practical limitations of doing scientifically controlled experiments. Such experiments would entail collecting dreams during or at the end of sleep, then independently, accurately, and objectively documenting subsequent events and comparing them to the dreams. The volume of information involved in this attempt would be overwhelming and unmanageable.

Another problem in validating the existence of psychic dreams lies in the fact that there is no adequate explanation of how such dream phenomena occur. There is no known physical or physiological mechanism for their production nor any known energy by which these kinds of information are transmitted. Furthermore, alternative explanations of such dreams are available, based on well-known and documented abilities of the mind to create illusions and hallucinations (Moorcroft, 1989). The mind is constantly attempting to make sense out of the sensory information fed to it from sources outside of the body as well as from sources within. When awake, the mind is bombarded by information about our environment from our eyes, ears, nose, skin, and other organs. These sensory inputs evoke emotional reactions and may trigger memories. Meanwhile, our brain is using commands to move our muscles. Our mind is constantly synthesizing these various bits of information into our perceptions of reality and our world. In this process, misperceptions, illusions, and hallucinations may sometimes occur.

In sleep, especially in REM sleep, an identical process of synthesis takes place, but now the sensory, emotion, memory, and movement inputs are primarily generated by the brain (McCarley, 1978) (see ACTIVATION–SYNTHESIS HYPOTHESIS). Thus the mind is creating perceptions when asleep just as it does when awake. The difference is the source of the information being synthesized: In sleep, the information is randomly generated from inside the brain.

Since the typical young adult spends an average of 2 hours per night in REM sleep, many perceptions are created. The enormous numbers of dreams produced by vast numbers of people each night mean that some coincidences with current or future events or other peoples' thoughts are inevitable. Furthermore, the anecdotal accounts of psychic dreams are very dependent on memory, and memory of dream content is notoriously poor (Moorcroft, 1989). Everyone has had difficulty recalling the content of dreams—especially the details. Laboratory research has not only verified this but has also shown that people think their memories are more accurate than they actually

are, not only for dream experiences but for waking experiences as well (Alcock, 1981). We forget more than we remember. In addition, our memories are easily changed by later events, thoughts, and interpretations. Therefore, events that appear to resemble our remembered dreams strikingly may not bear great resemblance to the actual dream, and thus the apparent psychic content of dreams is only an illusion.

Another factor may also help account for psychic dreams. Our subconscious mind is capable of doing what has been termed "detective work" (Faraday, 1972). It activates memories of things we have observed but to which we have not paid much attention. Such memories can be combined with other facts in such a way that the dream seems to predict the future or to resemble strikingly what another person has been thinking.

So while it is possible that psychic dreams do exist (since science cannot prove that a given entity does not exist), alternative explanations of such dreams using nonpsychic phenomena of the mind that have been scientifically verified provide strong, compelling alternatives to speculative and unproven psychic explanations.

(See also TELEPATHY AND DREAMING.)

REFERENCES

Alcock JE. 1981. *Parapsychology: Science or magic.* New York: Pergamon.

Faraday A. 1972. *Dream power.* New York: Coward, McCann & Geoghegan.

Hansel CEM. 1980. *ESP and parapsychology: A critical reevaluation.* Buffalo: Prometheus Books.

McCarley RW. 1978. Where dreams come from: A new theory. *Psychology Today* 12:55–65, 141.

Moorcroft WH. 1989. *Sleep, dreaming, and sleep disorders: An introduction.* Lanham, Md.: University Press of America.

Murray HA, Wheeler DR. 1937. A note on the possible clairvoyance of dreams. *J Psychology* 3:309–313.

Ullman M, Krippner S, Vaughan A. 1989. *Dream telepathy: Experiments in nocturnal ESP.* Jefferson, N.C.: McFarland.

Zusne L, Jones WH. 1989. *Anomalistic psychology: A study of magical thinking.* Hillsdale, N.J.: Erlbaum.

William H. Moorcroft

PSYCHOANALYSIS AND DREAMING

See Adler's Dream Theory; Freud's Dream Theory; Jung's Dream Theory

PSYCHOPATHOLOGY, NONDEPRESSION

Schizophrenia, which is far and away the most prominent and important psychotic disorder, is characterized by loss of contact with reality (the patient has loosening of associations and a lack of goal-directed thinking); affects that are inappropriate to the thought content or the situation of the patient; and marked ambivalence—an inability to initiate the activities of daily living, including such things as preparing meals, going to school, and so forth. Furthermore, the patient frequently shows deterioration with repeated relapses and may have bizarre delusions and hallucinations and ideas of self-reference. Delusions such as the belief that the patient's thoughts are broadcast over radio or television, that thoughts are inserted by other people, and elaborate psychotic paranoid delusions of persecution and grandiosity may also characterize the illness. The lifetime prevalence is about 1 percent of the population; the disease is in almost all cases at least partially controlled by use of dopamine receptor blockers, which quiet the patient in general and therefore ameliorate the psychotic hallucinations and agitation.

Sleep disturbances can be quite prominent and important as risk factors in the precipitation of the initial psychotic episode and of subsequent relapses. Sleep disordering of schizophrenia in the prodromal period can be either hypersomnolence or hyposomnolence. The patient most characteristically is agitated and wakeful and may show a polyphasic sleep pattern or a day/night reversal pattern.

Schizophrenia was the first psychiatric syndrome studied at the beginning of the modern era of sleep research in 1955 (see REM SLEEP, DISCOVERY OF). It quickly became apparent that the initial simple hypothesis that psychosis equaled an intrusion of REM sleep into the waking state was not substantiated. The sleep structure of the schizophrenic patient is characteristically marked by prolonged sleep latency, decreased or absent stage 3 and 4 sleep (especially stage 4; in about 40 percent, stage 4 may be nonresponsive to total sleep DEPRIVATION), and short REM LATENCY. These findings are not specific to schizophrenia; they are also seen in major depressive disorder (see DEPRESSION), borderline personality disorder, and obsessive compulsive personality. A serotonin disregulation in schizophrenia has recently become a subject of renewed interest because of the effects of the atypical antipsychotic medications on serotonin systems in the brain.

An early study of the sleep of schizophrenic patients in remission showed that some patients had markedly elevated amounts of REM sleep as though they were responding to REM sleep deprivation. Subsequent studies revealed that this was not true of acutely disturbed patients (see Zarcone and Bennett, 1992, for review). They did not respond to REM sleep deprivation (see DEPRIVATION, SELECTIVE: REM SLEEP) with a compensatory increase in REM sleep on recovery nights; that is, they had REM REBOUND failure. This observation, along with the almost simultaneous demonstration of a behavioral syndrome in serotonin-depleted cats, led to the REM sleep phasic event intrusion hypothesis: The symptoms of schizophrenia are caused by an intrusion of PGO spikelike activity into the waking life of the patient causing hallucinations and disruptions in goal-directed thinking (see PGO WAVES; PHASIC ACTIVITY IN REM SLEEP). Also, these observations were the basis for an animal model of schizophrenia, the cat given *para*-chlorophenylalanine (PCPA), a serotonin-depleting agent. The PCPA cats had a marked depletion of brain serotonin, profound INSOMNIA, a very abnormal distribution of PGO spikes in NREM and waking, a failure to show REM sleep rebound after sleep deprivation, and abnormal sexual and aggressive behavior, and oriented frequently (i.e., exhibited movements and physical changes ordinarily evoked by an unexpected stimulus) with bursts of waking PGO spikes, despite the fact that there were no novel stimuli in the environment (suggesting that they had the equivalent of hallucinations). The "syndrome" of insomnia, abnormal PGO spike distribution, REM sleep rebound failure, and abnormal behavior in these cats responds to neuroleptic drugs, the class of drugs that most benefits schizophrenic patients.

All of the observations on which the REM-sleep-phasic-event intrusion hypothesis was based were questioned in subsequent studies. The REM sleep rebound failure of acute schizophrenia may be caused by dopamine and norepinephrine activation. The PCPA cat's behavior may be the result of a decreased pain threshold produced by serotonin depletion; and the quest for a human scalp recorded analog of the PGO spike failed. Therefore, a possible correlation between REM sleep phasic events and the behaviors of schizophrenia proved impossible to study.

The correlation between stage 4 deficits and brain atrophy seems to be prominent in a subgroup of schizophrenic patients and may indicate trauma before or shortly after birth. In developed countries such as Denmark, perinatal trauma has been reduced by adequate prenatal, obstetric, and pediatric care, and the prevalence of schizophrenia in these countries is decreasing (Weeke and Stromgren, 1978). This finding suggests that longitudinal studies of children at risk for schizophrenia, that is, with a history of perinatal trauma, a strong genetic load for schizophrenia, or both, might reveal abnormalities of sleep structure in the second decade of life, prior to the onset of the first psychotic episode. Sleep structure studies in schizophrenia do seem to indicate that studies of first-degree relatives and the familial/genetic approach using sleep variables as markers to guide psychiatric genetic studies may be important, as they are in major depressive disorder.

REFERENCES

American Sleep Disorders Association. 1990. *The international classification of sleep disorders: Diagnostic and coding manual.* Lawrence, Kans.: Allen.

Weeke A, Stromgren E. 1978. Fifteen years later: A comparison of patients in Danish psychiatric institutions in 1957, 62, 67, and 72. *Acta Psychiatr Scand* 57:129–144.

Zarcone VP, Benson KL. 1992. *Principles and practice of sleep disorders medicine,* 2nd ed. Philadelphia: Saunders.

Vincent P. Zarcone

PSYCHOPHYSIOLOGICAL INSOMNIA

See Insomnia

PSYCHOPHYSIOLOGY OF DREAMING

The psychophysiology of dreaming comprises the relationships between psychological and physiological features of dreams or dream processes. As indicated by Cohen (1979), the psychophysiology of dreaming was "the heart (and soul) of classic sleep research" (p. 183). The hope in the 1950s and 1960s was that clear-cut relationships would be found between physiologic variables and dream characteristics. One major reason for the great interest in the psychophysiology of dreaming was the belief that determining the electrophysiologic correlates of dreaming would provide an exceptional avenue for studying the mind–body problem—an avenue wherein the relationships between physiologic and psychologic events could be studied unencumbered by the confusing impact of uncontrolled environmental input present during the waking state.

Very practical reasons also contributed to the high interest in dream psychophysiology. For example, by knowing the physiological indicators of dreaming, one could identify when dreaming occurs. Thereby, an efficient method of dream collection would be available that would yield detailed and representative dream reports. Further, a method of measuring amount of dreaming would be present; one could then relate other variables of interest (e.g., personality characteristics) to the amount of dreaming. Also, if the physiological correlates of dreaming were known, it was also thought that a better understanding of dreams would eventuate; such an enhanced understanding could be of help in working with individuals and their problems. Some sleep researchers even thought it might become possible to obtain information about specific dream content without awakening the sleeping person.

REM Sleep Versus NREM Sleep as Related to Dreaming

Modern dream research received its impetus from reports published in the mid-1950s by Aserinsky and Kleitman (1953) and by Dement and Kleitman (1957). These two reports indicated that dreaming occurred during REM sleep and that dreaming did not occur during NREM sleep. The primary evidence cited was the dream recall percentages when awakenings were made during these two types of sleep. In the Aserinsky and Kleitman report, 74 percent of awakenings from REM sleep yielded dream recall, whereas only 9 percent of NREM awakenings yielded recall; the comparable percentages reported by Dement and Kleitman were 80 percent and 7 percent, respectively. The most common initial interpretation of these results was that dreaming occurs all of the time during REM sleep and none of the time during NREM sleep. It was assumed that the subjects sometimes forgot their dreams when awakened from REM sleep. As for the dream reports occurring upon NREM awakenings, it was assumed that these reports represented the recall of dreams that occurred during REM periods earlier in the night, or that they were hypnopompic experiences (i.e., experiences that occurred in the process of awakening), or that they were confabulated (i.e., made up to please the experimenter).

There was other evidence supporting the belief that dreaming occurs during REM sleep. First, subjects' estimates of how long they had been dreaming corresponded to some extent with the duration of the REM periods from which they were awakened. Second, external stimuli, accidentally or experimentally introduced to sleeping subjects, sometimes were incorporated into the reported dreams in a timely manner, suggesting an ongoing dream process. Third, the direction of the eye movements during REM sleep seemed to correspond to the reported dream content as if the person were watching dream action. For example, a dream of watching a tennis match would correspond to horizontal eye movements. This point of view was called *the scanning hypothesis.*

Within a few years, evidence was presented that suggested that the simple REM–NREM model of dreaming was not entirely accurate. In particular, several studies indicated that considerable dreaming occurs during NREM sleep. Foulkes (1967) lists nine studies with NREM dream recall percentages ranging from 23 percent to 74 percent. Furthermore, the arguments put forth to explain NREM recall seemed to have little merit (Rechtschaffen, 1973). Some possible factors relevant to why the early reports erred in concluding that NREM sleep is void of

dreaming include subject selection, definition of dreaming, the manner in which the subject was questioned, rating scale and procedure used, influence of awakening schedule (especially regarding time of night), and experimenter expectancy (Herman, Ellman, and Roffwarg, 1978).

Apart from the relative frequency of dream recall percentages, REM and NREM dream reports can be compared with respect to typical qualities or characteristics. On the average, as compared with NREM dreams, REM dreams are reported as more visual, more vivid, more emotional, more implausible (or bizarre), more oriented to the past, more likely to be a distorted representation of something from real life, and less pleasant. Terms such as *dream intensity, dream salience,* and *dreaminess* have been used to summarize the characteristics of REM dreams. An example of a REM dream report would be the following:

Most of it took place in Germany, when I was a child—at this one house where we lived for about 10 years. And supposedly my older brother, who died at the age of 6, was still alive during the dream; and he took a bicycle and rode it on a highway, and I followed after him. I was telling him the bicycle was no good, it made too much noise, but he kept riding. I came back then and told my family, sitting underneath a lilac—no, it was not a lilac—it was, I don't know the name of it, some kind of tree—they were at a table eating, and my mother was looking at me—I came in and she said, "What are you doing, where have you been"? I said, "I just came in from outside—must I always be doing something; I just came in from outside." I was angry. I said, "That everything I did had to be questioned or accounted for." And then she showed me a little—a notebook in which I had done some drawings and some poems and she wanted me to sit down and read them aloud, and I being in a noncommunicative mood said, "No, I don't feel like it at this time." So, she took them, and she was going to pass them around, and I was angry—I didn't feel like having my things passed around. That's when the bell rang—that's the end of the report.

The same subject gave this NREM report:

Somebody, some friend whom I didn't recognize, was learning how to ride a bicycle and I said, "It's just a question of whether you have the endurance to stick with it, whether you will learn it or not." That's the end of the report as far as I now remember.

The REM report was obtained on night 9 in the sleep lab; the NREM report came from night 2; both reports occurred on the fifth awakening of the night.

Even though, on the average, there are some qualitative differences between REM and NREM reports, it should be emphasized that there is considerable variability in both REM and NREM reports and, hence, much overlap between them. For example, it is common to refer to NREM dreams as more like thinking than are REM dreams; however, NREM dreams may be heavily visual. Likewise, REM dreams are referred to as more bizarre than NREM dreams; however, most REM dreams are not bizarre. The following NREM dream report illustrates how a NREM dream may have some of the qualities of a REM dream and illustrates (during the questioning) that experienced subjects seem able to differentiate whether a dream was going on at the moment or some time earlier in the night.

You and I had gone to California, and it was the first time that you were there, and we were just going around seeing different people; and I was introducing you. We went to see Mr. and Mrs. C., that's this little old artist man and his wife, and we were just talking with them—and that's at their house in Campbell—and that's all. I saw them just a year ago before I left. (X: We were talking to them; did you see them in your dream?) Yeah. (X: What was going on just as I awoke you?) We were talking to them, and they said something about the neighbors', the neighbors' cat-and-dog fight. (X: Do you feel anything else was going on?) Well, have you woke me up sometimes and then I went back to sleep? (X: What do you mean?) You know, did you wake me up once or twice and I went right back to sleep? Because I've been waking up. (X: No, I haven't signaled you except the times you've given reports.) Well, I've been waking every once in a while, and I didn't know if I was suppose to talk or what was happening, and I had another whole dream that I haven't told you about. (X: Briefly, what was that? Do you remember now?) (The subject then gave two additional reports, equally or more detailed as the one above. These reports did not seem related to each other nor did either seem related to the above report. The subject emphasized that the action reported above was occurring when she was awakened this time, whereas the two additional reports seemed to have occurred about one-and-a-half hours earlier. She suggested that they may have corresponded with earlier awakenings when she failed to have recall at the time).

A further complication in pinpointing dreaming is the recognition that dreaming may occur at sleep onset, while the subject is in an hypnagogic state (Fiss, 1979; Foulkes, 1985; Vogel, 1978). In one study, the typical subject reported dreaming (i.e., dramatic, hallucinatory imagery that was experienced by the subject as reality) in 75 percent of awakenings (Foulkes, 1985). In addition, Foulkes (1985) reports that upon being signaled when fully awake according to electrophysiological criteria, subjects have given dreamlike reports at a rate of approximately 20 percent recall!

So far nothing has been said of differences among stages 2, 3, and 4 of NREM sleep with respect to dream recall. Dream recall from stage 2 and stage 3 awakenings seems similar in amount and quality (Rechtschaffen, 1973). It is more difficult to make statements regarding stage 4 awakenings, because stage 4 rarely appears during the second half of the night, and it is known that dream recall and dream intensity for other sleep stages are greater the second half of the night. In short, it is difficult to obtain data for stage 4 awakenings independent of time of night.

Another variable that has been studied is the duration of the REM period (REMP) as related to dream characteristics. In one study, comparisons were made between reports from the beginning of REMPs and those made 9 or more minutes into the REMPs (Foulkes, 1966). A second study compared 5-minute REMP awakenings, 12-minute REMP awakenings, controlling for time of night (Verdone, 1965). Both studies found that the longer REMPs produced more dreamlike reports (e.g., more emotional, dramatic, or vivid).

Physiologic Correlates of Dreaming Other Than Sleep Stage

A basic strategy for many years has been to study physiologic variation across REMPs in relation to dreaming. Diverse autonomic (involuntary physiological) variables have been studied fairly extensively with relatively inconclusive, if not disappointing results (Cohen, 1979; Pivik, 1978; Rechtschaffen, 1973). For example, several studies have attempted to relate heart rate to dream characteristics (e.g., emotionality). The results have been almost entirely negative. Much the same can be said of respiratory rate, although some degree of relationship between respiratory rate and qualitative aspects of dreams has been reported. Heart rate variability and respiratory irregularity have been found related to dream emotionality in two studies, but to little else. ELECTRODERMAL ACTIVITY, both basal skin resistance and spontaneous electrodermal changes, seem even less promising than cardiac or respiratory measures. Core BODY TEMPERATURE, measured rectally, has been found to be inversely related to dream recall, vividness, and emotionality (Verdone, 1965); that is, the lower the temperature, the better recalled, more vivid, and more emotional the dream. In the same study, body temperature was related to the overall time setting of the dream, with more recent manifest content corresponding to higher body temperature, whereas less recent dream content corresponded to lower body temperature; this relationship was independent of time of night. Penile ERECTIONS occur during most REMPs, but only a small percentage of dream reports contain sexual content. Hence, it does not seem plausible that most erections correspond to sexual dreams.

A distinction has been made for many years between tonic activity and PHASIC ACTIVITY IN REM sleep. Tonic activity refers to sustained long-lasting physiological activity (e.g., low-voltage electroencephalographic activity), whereas phasic refers to brief intermittent activity (e.g., muscle TWITCHES). Attempts have been made to relate both tonic and phasic muscle activity to dream characteristics and content. The limited research performed with respect to tonic muscle activity recorded from the facial and neck region has been negative; NREM awakenings with low tonic muscle activity are not more apt to produce dreamlike material than NREM awakenings with high tonic muscle activity. During REM sleep, tonic muscle activity from these areas is uniformly low (except during body movements); thus, there is no possibility of finding any relationships with dreams. Phasic muscle activity (i.e., twitches) are frequent during REM sleep, and attempts have been made to relate these muscle twitches to specific dream content. A few studies have reported positive results, but there have been studies with negative results as well.

Another type of discrete motor activity is, of course, the rapid eye movements (REMs) of REM sleep. Some studies have been conducted to study a specific correspondence between REMs and dream content, and other studies have focused on a general nonspecific association between the two types of variables. The first approach pertains to the scanning hypothesis that the eyes are following the dream action. The scanning hypothesis was supported by initial research, but replications have been largely negative. As discussed by Rechtschaffen (1973), however, even if the scanning hypothesis is true, it will be nearly impossible to obtain conclusive evidence to support it because of practical complexities. The second approach (i.e., a nonspecific association between REMs and dreaming) has produced some positive findings. The amount of REM activity has been found related to vividness and emotionality, to activity within the dream, and to the time setting of the dream (Foulkes, 1966; Verdone, 1965). Schwartz, Weinstein, and Arkin (1978), however, point out that REM density is confounded with (i.e., not separable from) time of night in virtually all the studies that have been done. One exception is the study by Hauri and Van de Castle (1973), who controlled for time of night and found a weak association between REM density and involvement of the sleeper in his or her dream (pp. 189–192). (See EYE MOVEMENTS AND DREAMING.)

The discovery of pons-geniculate body-occipital PGO cortex spike waves accompanying REMs in cats led to still another direction in dream psychophysiology research. (See PGO WAVES.) Because of the theoretical importance of PGO spikes (which cannot be recorded from human subjects through surface recording), the search began for alternatives that might be regarded as equivalent. One variable proposed was the K-COMPLEX, characteristic of stage 2 (Pivik, 1978). However, neither K-complexes nor sleep spindles have been found to be related to dream activity (Pivik, 1978; Webb and Cartwright, 1978). Another proposal came from Rechtschaffen (1973), who suggested the use of periorbital PHASIC INTEGRATED POTENTIALS (PIPs), which reflect extraocular muscle activity. MIDDLE EAR MUSCLE ACTIVITY (MEMA) is another phasic event that has been studied. PIPs and MEMA, which occur in both REM sleep and NREM sleep, have been found to be related to dream variables (e.g., bizarreness) in several studies; however, the relationships have been modest and not entirely convincing. Some authors seem to conclude that the research findings using phasic indicators support the tonic-phasic model (Anch et al., 1988; Webb and Cartwright, 1978). On the other hand, Pivik (1978) believes the "phasic-tonic discriminators" yield results that are "meager and sometimes conflicting" (p. 268).

Conclusions

Within the past 10 to 15 years, disillusion with the psychophysiology of dreaming has become widespread. As summarized by Pivik (1978), the early REM–NREM model of dream psychophysiology was oversimplified and the tonic-phasic model "has reached a point of diminishing returns" (p. 271). Foulkes (1985), another leading dream psychophysiology researcher, would seem to be in agreement. The ACTIVATION-SYNTHESIS HYPOTHESIS ("dreaming is the subjective awareness of brain activation in sleep"; Hobson, 1989, p. 147) has gained prominence.

An alternative position to the foregoing is that of Moffitt and Hoffman (1987). Although critical of past progress in dream psychophysiology (which they view as representing simplistic and reductionistic thinking), they believe that dream psychophysiology is still viable. Furthermore, they make some suggestions as to new directions to be taken.

Part of the current widespread disillusion is probably an inevitable outcome of the earlier excessive expectations. Actually, in view of the great complexity involved in dream psychophysiology (Cohen, 1979, pp. 184–187), perhaps the progress to date is not as meager as it seems. If future progress is to be made, it would be advisable to avoid categorical thinking (e.g., REM–NREM, tonic–phasic, awake–asleep, dreaming–not dreaming). Is a lucid dreamer awake or asleep? Do 10 minutes of thoroughly mixed REMs and spindles indicate a period of REM sleep or not? Although appealing, convenient, and of heuristic value, simple dichotomies can be very misleading.

REFERENCES

Anch AM, Browman CP, Mitler MM, Walsh JK. 1988. *Sleep: A scientific perspective.* Englewood Cliffs, N.J.: Prentice-Hall.

Aserinsky E, Kleitman N. 1953. Regularly occurring periods of eye motility and concomitant phenomena during sleep. *Science* 118:273–274.

Cohen DB. 1979. *Sleep and dreaming: Origins, nature and functions.* New York: Pergamon.

Dement WC, Kleitman N. 1957. The relation of eye movements during sleep to dream activity: An objective method for the study of dreaming. *J Exp Psychol* 53:339–346.

Fiss H. 1979. Current dream research: A psychological perspective. In Wolman BB, ed. *Handbook of dreams: Research, theories and applications,* pp 20–75. New York: Van Nostrand.

Foulkes D. 1966. *The psychology of sleep.* New York: Scribner's.

———. 1967. Nonrapid eye movement mentation. *Exp Neurol Suppl* 4:28–38.

———. 1985. *Dreaming: A cognitive-psychological analysis.* Hillsdale, N.J.: Erlbaum.

Hauri P, Van de Castle RL. 1973. Psychophysiological parallelism in dreams. *Psychosom Med* 35: 297–308.

Herman JH, Ellman SJ, Roffwarg HP. 1978. The problem of NREM dream recall re-examined. In Arkin AM, Antrobus JS, Ellman SJ, eds. *The mind in sleep: Psychology and psychophysiology,* pp 59–92. Hillsdale, N.J.: Erlbaum.

Hobson JA. 1989. *Sleep.* New York: Scientific American.

Moffitt A, Hoffman R. 1987. On the single-mindedness and isolation of dream psychophysiology. In Gackenbach J, ed. *Sleep and dreams: A source book,* pp 145–186. New York: Garland.

Pivik RT. 1978. Tonic states and phasic events in relation to sleep mentation. In Arkin AM, Antrobus JS, Ellman SJ, eds. *The mind in sleep: Psychology and psychophysiology,* pp 245–271. Hillsdale, N.J.: Erlbaum.

Rechtschaffen A. 1973. The psychophysiology of mental activity during sleep. In McGuigan FJ, Schoonover RS, eds. *The psychophysiology of thinking,* pp 153–205. New York: Academic.

Schwartz DG, Weinstein LN, Arkin AM. 1978. Qualitative aspects of sleep mentation. In Arkin AM, Antrobus JS, Ellman SJ, eds. *The mind in sleep: psychology and psychophysiology,* pp 143–244. Hillsdale, N.J.: Erlbaum.

Verdone P. 1965. Temporal reference of manifest dream content. *Percept Mot Skills* 20:1253–1268.

Vogel GW. 1978. Sleep-onset mentation. In Arkin AM, Antrobus JS, Ellman SJ, eds. *The mind in sleep: Psychology and psychophysiology,* pp 97–108. Hillsdale, N.J.: Erlbaum.

Webb WB, Cartwright RD. 1978. Sleep and dreams. *Ann Rev Psychol* 29:223–252.

Paul Verdone

PSYCHOTHERAPY

See Adler's Dream Theory; Freud's Dream Theory; Jung's Dream Theory

PTOSIS

See Narcolepsy; Sleepiness

PUBERTY

[*The path between childhood and adulthood crosses through a transitional phase of physiological changes collectively known as puberty. Puberty typically occurs at the age of 10–12 years in girls and slightly later in boys. As might be expected, the host of physical changes accompanying this pivotal stage of life are affected by, and have an effect on, sleep and wakefulness. For example, there is a preferential sleep-related secretion of the* GONADOTROPIC HORMONES, *follicle-stimulating hormone and luteinizing hormone, that is one of the first signs of puberty—even before the more noticeable physical changes occur. Puberty is also accompanied by an increase in daytime* SLEEPINESS, *even though sleep at night remains unchanged. An increased tendency to go to sleep and wake up at later hours occurs in* ADOLESCENCE, *and this may be caused by a pubertal change in underlying* CIRCADIAN RHYTHMS.]

PUBLIC SAFETY IN TRANSPORTATION

Transportation accidents are a major threat to public health. According to Lewis (1990), accidental death, mostly from highway accidents, is the leading cause of death for U.S. citizens aged 10 to 38 years.

Human performance is known to be a factor in a large majority of all transportation accidents. In civil transport aviation, for example, Boeing records indicate that 66 percent of worldwide commercial jet transportation accidents involve the flight crew as a primary cause factor. For general aviation, the rate is significantly higher; approximately 75 percent of such accidents are pilot-caused according to a recent Aircraft Owners and Pilots Association Air Safety Foundation study (1991). For other modes of transportation, the rate of human-error involvement is similar to that found in general aviation; most transportation accidents occur because of some form of human performance failure. It is clear that seeking a means of reducing human error–caused accidents and incidents should be given great priority in transportation research and safety programs.

Many factors affect human performance and lead to human error. Some of these are external to the individual (exogenous), such as poor equipment design, noisy communication channels, and inadequate training. Others are internal to the individual (endogenous) and include stress, drugs and alcohol, and other physiological and psychological factors such as FATIGUE, sleep loss (see DEPRIVATION), SLEEPINESS, and the state of one's internal body clocks, or CIRCADIAN RHYTHMS. Although much is known about how some of these factors—ALCOHOL, for example—affect human performance, and therefore, transportation system safety, others are less well understood. Their role in the causation of incidents and accidents is less defined. Fatigue, sleep, sleepiness, and circadian factors fit into the latter category.

The Role of Fatigue, Sleep Loss, and Circadian Factors in Transportation Accidents

The National Transportation Safety Board (NTSB) is an independent federal agency charged with the responsibility for investigating accidents and serious incidents in all modes of transportation, to determine their probable causes and to make recommendations to any organization or agency for actions that might prevent the reoccurrence of such accidents and incidents. Increasingly, human performance has come under close scrutiny in NTSB investigations. As a result, the role of sleepiness and other related factors in the causation of accidents has received much more attention than before. This has led to several key recommendations for improvements, most notably in the area of better regulations governing duty and rest times, and in the support of additional research. Some illustrative accidents, findings, and recommendations are reviewed here.

Aviation Accidents

Fatigue or sleepiness has rarely been cited as a cause or factor in commercial jet transport accidents investigated by the NTSB. However, this may reflect more about the state of the art of accident investigation techniques than it does about the role of fatigue in aircraft accidents. Metal fatigue leaves telltale signs; mental fatigue does not, and its presence must often be inferred from purely circumstantial evidence. Nevertheless, in an era of increasingly long-haul flight operations (up to 16 hours of scheduled flight time) that cross as many as eight time zones in aircraft designed to be operated by two pilots, circadian variations in human performance, sleep quantity and quality, sleepiness, and fatigue are matters of great concern. At the other end of the spectrum, short-haul flight operations such as those flown by pilots for commuter airlines may not involve any time zone changes, but can involve long duty days (up to 14 hours) and up to 10 hours of flight time before a rest period is required. There is no limitation on the number of take-offs and landings that can be accomplished within these limits.

Despite the low incidence with which sleepiness is cited in NTSB aviation accident reports, there is sufficient concern about these factors in determining aviation system safety that the National Aeronautics and Space Administration (NASA) is conducting a long-term study of such factors in commercial aviation operations (see Graeber, 1988). Underway since 1983, this research has greatly increased our understanding of these issues and has been instrumental in the development of certain countermeasures that can be applied by individual pilots and by airline operators to counteract the adverse effects of these factors in aviation operations. Ultimately, the NASA studies will provide a sound scientific basis for updated flight, duty, and rest time regulations.

Although the NASA work focuses on flight crew members, fatigue and sleepiness can affect many others in the aviation system as well—air traffic controllers and aircraft maintenance and inspection technicians being two examples where the adverse effects of sleepiness, sleep loss, and circadian factors could have a direct impact on

system safety. To address these and many other human performance issues the Federal Aviation Administration has developed the *National Plan For Human Factors,* which provides a bold blueprint for a concerted national effort; fatigue and related human performance issues are major elements of this national plan.

(See also PILOTS.)

Railroad Accidents

Chronic sleep deprivation caused by unpredictable, irregular work shifts and off-duty periods was determined by the NTSB to be causal in a January 1988 head-on collision between two freight trains at Thompsontown, Pennsylvania. The crew of one locomotive was believed to have fallen asleep, despite the presence of a crew "alertness and acknowledging device" that simply required the engineer to depress and release a foot pedal to prevent an automatic application of brakes; as a result, the train proceeded into the path of an oncoming train, resulting in the deaths of all four crew members and more than $6 million of property damage.

Based on its investigations of this and many other railroad accidents, the Safety Board believes that such unpredictable and erratic work schedules are found widely throughout the industry and that both railroad management and unions representing railroad operating crew members have failed to consider adequately the adverse effects of such schedules on human performance and railroad system safety.

Marine Accidents

The infamous EXXON *Valdez* accident in 1989 was determined by the NTSB to have occurred because of the alcohol-impaired decision by the master to leave the vessel in charge of a relatively inexperienced, improperly qualified third mate. Importantly, this third mate was determined to be fatigued because of his extensive duties during the loading and departure of the vessel from Valdez, Alaska. Three months later, on June 23, 1989, the Greek tankship *World Prodigy* ran aground off the coast of Rhode Island, resulting in the release of 7,000 barrels of oil into the waters of Rhode Island Sound and Narragansett Bay. This accident was attributed to the "master's impaired judgment, from acute fatigue, which led to his decisions to decrease the bridge watch and to attend to nonessential tasks during a crucial period in the ship's navigation." It is clear from these and many other marine accidents that sleepiness and fatigue factors play a major role in the safety of ship operations.

Highway Accidents

Major highway accidents involving commercial heavy trucks and buses perhaps provide the most frequent and flagrant examples of adverse human performance effects of fatigue, sleep loss, sleepiness, and circadian factors in transportation operations. For example, the NTSB determined that a cattle truck plowed into the back of a standing school bus in Tuba City, Arizona, because of the truck driver's chronic sleepiness, brought about by a combination of excessive duty time and a prolonged irregular duty pattern. He had been on duty for 88 hours and had driven more than 4,200 miles in the previous 8 days. Two children died and four were seriously injured in the April 1985 collision.

In a 1990 study of fatal-to-driver heavy truck accidents, the NTSB determined that fatigue was the most frequent accident cause, being cited in 31 percent of the sample studied. An additional finding of interest is that 33 percent of fatigued and sleepy drivers were also impaired by alcohol and/or other drugs.

Other studies of highway safety have shown a very prominent circadian variation in highway accident rates. For example, Langolis et al. (1985) demonstrated a very clear 24-hour pattern, with the peak rate occurring at around 3:00 A.M.; driver sleepiness is strongly implicated by these findings.

Public Policy Issues

All commercial transportation operations are governed by some form of federal hours-of-service regulations. Aviation, arguably the most demanding mode of transportation from a human performance point of view, has probably the most well-established and restrictive regulations, but even these have some notable gaps. For example, U.S. regulations governing flight and duty time for pilots do not consider circadian factors in determining maximal duty times or minimal rest periods. The crews of aircraft operating from New

York to Rio de Janeiro, approximately a 9-hour flight, are treated the same as crews operating between New York and Europe, even though only two time zones are traversed in the former and a minimum of five in the latter (see JET LAG). Furthermore, all crew flight, duty, and rest time requirements are the same, regardless of whether the flight departs at 9:00 A.M. or 9:00 P.M.

Hours-of-service regulations in other modes of transportation are equally devoid of consideration of circadian variations in human performance and in quality and quantity of sleep obtained as a function of time of day. Furthermore, most of these regulations have evolved over a period of many years, often being determined by economic factors as reflected in the outcome of labor–management negotiations instead of established criteria for human performance and system safety. In view of significant advances in the scientific understanding of sleepiness, fatigue, and circadian factors as they affect human performance, the NTSB has urged the Department of Transportation (DOT) and its modal agencies to review and upgrade hours-of-service regulations for all transportation modes. In addition, it has asked the DOT to develop and disseminate educational material for all transportation industry personnel and management regarding shift work, work and rest schedules, and rest.

According to the National Safety Council, nearly half of the approximately 100,000 accidental deaths occurring each year in the United States are due to motor vehicle accidents. Furthermore, they estimate that such accidents cost more than $72 billion annually. Although difficult to determine quantitatively, it seems clear from the results of accident investigations such as those conducted by the NTSB, and from scientific studies of human performance, that successful intervention in the prevention of sleepiness-related transportation accidents could have enormous social and economic consequences. Significant progress will be made before the 1990s are over.

REFERENCES

Aircraft Owners and Pilots Association Air Safety Foundation. 1991. *1990 Accident Trends & Factors. Joseph T. Nall general aviation safety report.* Frederick, Md.: AOPA.

Boeing Commercial Airplanes. 1989. *Statistical summary of commercial jet aircraft accidents: World-wide operations 1959–1989*. Seattle: Boeing.

Federal Aviation Administration. 1990. *The national plan for aviation human factors*. December.

Graeber RC. 1988. Aircrew fatigue and circadian rhythmicity. In Wiener EL, Nagel DC, eds. *Human factors in aviation,* pp 305–344. San Diego: Academic.

Langolis PH, Smolensky MH, Hsi BP, Weir FW. 1985. Temporal patterns of reported single-vehicle car and truck accidents in Texas, U.S.A. during 1980–1983. *Chronobiology international* 2:131–140.

Lewis HW. 1990. *Technological risk*. New York: Norton.

National Transportation Safety Board Highway Accident Report NTSB/HAR-85/06. Collision of Tuba City School District schoolbus and Bell Creek, Inc., tractor-semitrailer, US 160 near Tuba City, AZ April 29, 1985.

National Transportation Safety Board Railroad Accident Report, NTSB/RAR-89/02. Head-end collision of Consolidated Rail Corporation freight trains UBT-506 and TV-61 near Thompsontown, PA January 14, 1988.

National Transportation Safety Board Marine Accident Report NTSB/MAR-91/01. Grounding of the U.S. tankship Exxon Valdez on Bligh Reef, Prince William Sound near Valdez, AK March 24, 1989.

———. Grounding of the Greek tankship World Prodigy off the Coast of Rhode Island June 23, 1989.

National Transportation Safety Board Safety Study NTSB/SS-90/01. Fatigue, alcohol, other drugs, and medical factors in fatal-to-the-driver heavy truck crashes, vol 1.

Weiner EL, Nagel DC. 1988. *Human factors in aviation*. San Diego: Academic.

John K. Lauber

PUBLIC SAFETY IN THE WORKPLACE

Sleep is perhaps both the savior and nemesis of today's highly technical world. With the advent of the 24-hour day necessity for the flow of information, cargo, and energy, scheduling time for a basic physiological need like sleep is a problem. Sleep's restorative qualities are necessary for the vigilance required of a modern work force, and the consequences of substandard sleep are enormous given the extended impact of technically advanced industries. Natural selection may have been gentle on prehistoric people who slept poorly; the major killers—war, natural enemies, and pestilence—were much more influential in deciding who lived to conceive and care for children than was sleep deprivation that might lead to falling asleep on the job or sleep disorders, such as sleep APNEA. Today's principal causes of death are very different than in prehistoric times, and what is worrisome today is that so many more people can be hurt by a sleepy or inattentive worker than even a hundred years ago. Historically, societies have been able to ignore the consequences of sleep-related errors in the work environment because, like the stagecoach driver of a hundred years ago, workers rarely controlled more power than that mustered by a few horses. An individual worker in present times may control enough atomic energy to run a city the size of New York. Although this worker's sleep requirements and tendency to fall asleep on the job are the same as those of our prehistoric ancestors, the consequences of this worker's errors are so vast that the well-being of whole countries may be threatened.

Alertness during the day that results from healthful rest during the night can thus be a major life-or-death matter, not only for individual people, but also for whole populations. For example, studies indicate that the near-cataclysmic nuclear accident at Chernobyl on April 26, 1986, was easily avoidable and began when nightshift workers missed or were confused by warning signals on their control panels. Other studies show that nightshift workers have very irregular and poor sleep and, accordingly, have the most difficulty staying alert for long periods. (See also SHIFTWORK.) In our present society, it is clear that poor and unhealthful sleep can lead to catastrophes.

The list of sleep-related, catastrophic human error accidents continues to grow: Chernobyl, Three Mile Island, *Exxon Valdez*, as well as numerous airplane crashes, train crashes, and highway accidents. In each work environment where sustained attention is necessary for safety, research has shown that the probability of an accident rises and falls along with the biological tendency to fall asleep. Thus, catastrophic accidents do not happen at random throughout the day. Rather, they are more likely at times when humans are most prone to sleep.

The U.S. Congress's Office of Technology Assessment (OTA) concluded that the biological cycles (see CIRCADIAN RHYTHMS) underlying fatigue and human error in the workplace have been underestimated. Studies of industrial and transportation accidents report that fully 90 percent are due to human error. The remainder are due to mechanical failure. All available scientific data indicate that people are most likely to make errors between midnight and 6:00 A.M., even when they have slept during the day. People are especially likely to make mistakes if they have not slept at least 7 to 8 hours within the last 24 hours. Fatigue-related errors are linked to our biological need for sleep. The OTA has noted the need for increased public awareness and for legislative action to limit the risks we all face when workers are too tired to do their jobs safely.

Figure 1 shows the rises and falls in the probability that individuals will fall asleep when trying to stay awake for 24 hours. There are two peaks in sleep tendency, one in the early-morning hours and one in the midafternoon. Figure 2 shows the probability of sleep-related auto accidents throughout the 24-hour day, which dovetails with sleep tendency over the same period. Scientists believe that the probability of having an accident while driving a car or, more generally, while doing anything that requires sustained attention for safety is fundamentally affected by the biological tendency to fall asleep. (See also PUBLIC SAFETY IN TRANSPORTATION.)

Increasingly and across all industries, the costs in terms of human life, equipment damage, environmental damage, and litigation are forcing fundamental changes in the way work–rest schedules are determined. Issues of costs and international competitiveness are weighed against the costs of human error accidents. Risk managers scrutinize all aspects of worker alertness, including drug use, the presence of sleep disorders, and the amount of sleep time available to workers when they are not on duty.

Rethinking the needs of workers to sleep has proven to be a difficult task, because there are few well-established guidelines. New concepts are gradually emerging to deal with the need for alertness on the job. Imagine someone arguing against public sanitation because governments should not worry about things that only doctors can see with microscopes. About 100 years ago, this argument often won out because the radical idea that unseen microbes could cause disease was difficult for people to accept. Now, public standards of cleanliness are considered fundamental to society's well-being.

The need to ensure that workers get enough sleep may be another radical idea that people must accept if we are to continue as an advanced society. For the first time in evolution, humans are able to control huge power sources and travel at great speeds any time, day or night. Just as massive epidemics in crowded cities of the 1800s thrust the notion of disease-carrying microbes into the public consciousness, industrial and transportation catastrophes of the present day are forcing worker fatigue into the public consciousness. Modern doctors would never dissect corpses for anatomy class and then, minutes later, deliver babies without even washing their hands; yet this practice was common a hundred years

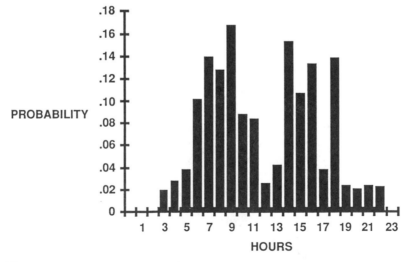

Figure 1. Daily probability of unintended sleep. The hours indicate time of day, with 1 = 1:00 A.M. and 13 = 1:00 P.M.

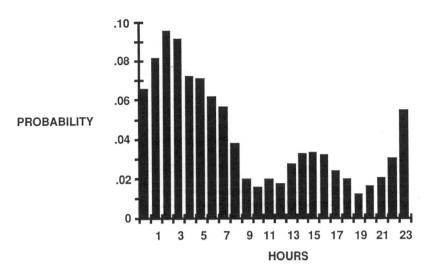

Figure 2. Daily probability of sleep-related auto accidents.

ago. Modern pilots fly transcontinental flights after sleeping only 2 hours; perhaps, in the future, this practice will also seem barbaric.

REFERENCES

Anch AM, Browman CP, Mitler MM, Walsh JK. 1988. *Sleep: A scientific perspective.* Englewood Cliffs, N.J.: Prentice-Hall.

Dinges DF, Broughton RJ, eds. 1989. *Sleep and alertness: Chronobiological, behavioral and medical aspects of napping.* New York: Raven.

Mitler MM, Carskadon MA, Czeisler CA, Dement WC, Dinges DF, Graeber RC. 1988. Catastrophes, sleep and public policy: Consensus report. *Sleep* 11: 100–109.

Merrill M. Mitler

PUPILLOMETRY

Pupillometry is the study of the pupil of the eye—the dark round area bordered by the muscles of the iris. Two muscles, the pupillary sphincter and pupillary constrictor, control the size and behavior of the pupil. These muscles are in turn controlled by different parts of the AUTONOMIC NERVOUS SYSTEM (ANS). The ANS is responsible for many of the involuntary or automatic functions of the body. The sympathetic division of the ANS is responsible for activating or arousing the body when necessary (see SYMPATHETIC NERVOUS SYSTEM). It controls the sphincter muscle of the pupil and causes pupillary mydriasis (large pupil). The parasympathetic division of the ANS has an opposite effect, usually causing relaxation of automatic processes (see PARASYMPATHETIC NERVOUS SYSTEM). It controls the constrictor muscles and causes pupillary miosis (small pupil). Generally, the sympathetic and parasympathetic divisions of the ANS balance each other, resulting in a particular tone and pupil size. The ANS tone varies from moment to moment and across the 24-hour period, resulting in different pupil sizes and behaviors. Because the pupil size and behavior are a direct result of ANS activity, the pupil has been called "the only visible part of the brain" (Janisse, 1977, p. 1)—a place where brain activity can be observed without any special equipment.

It has long been known that sleep and different states of ALERTNESS have a significant effect on the pupil. In the 1700s it was observed that during sleep the pupil becomes miotic (Fontana, 1765). Initially, it was thought that sleep-related miosis occurred because light was blocked by eyelid closure. More recently, however, it was reported that sleep miosis occurs in the blind, suggesting that light stimulation is not the cause of sleep miosis (Berlucchi et al., 1964).

Neurophysiological research has shown that the pupil becomes miotic during sleep because of changes in the ANS. The midbrain area of the brainstem contains a group of parasympathetic neurons whose only function is to make the pupil smaller. During wakefulness, these cells are usually inhibited or suppressed by sympathetic neurons at higher levels of the brain. Because sleep is a state of relatively low sympathetic activity, sympathetic neurons do not suppress the activity of these specialized parasympathetic neurons during sleep. As a result, the pupil gets very small, sometimes as small as a pinpoint, and generally stays small during most of NREM and REM sleep. During certain portions of REM sleep containing bursts of rapid eye movements, however, sympathetic activity is briefly very high and the pupils may dilate. When the eye movements stop, the pupils constrict again and remain very small until the next burst of eye movements. Pupillary dilation during these bursts of eye movements is important evidence that REM sleep is a state of high arousal with significant, sudden changes in ANS activity (see REM SLEEP MECHANISMS AND NEUROANATOMY).

The pupil is also thought to be a useful indicator of alertness or SLEEPINESS. In general, alertness is associated with a large and stable pupil, while sleepiness and fatigue are associated with a small and unstable pupil. Changes in pupil size and alertness are thought to reflect changes in the balance of the two parts of the ANS. During periods of alertness, sympathetic activity is high, parasympathetic activity is low, and the pupil is large; by contrast, during sleepiness or fatigue, sympathetic activity is low, parasympathetic activity is high, and the pupil is small.

Even when alertness is high, the pupil is never completely stable. The changing balance of the two parts of the ANS causes frequent small variations in the pupillary diameter. Pupil size alternates from bigger to smaller and then back again. These changes are called *hippus*. As an individual becomes sleepier, hippus becomes bigger and bigger.

Pupil size and behavior have been studied extensively in patients with NARCOLEPSY, a disorder of the brain in which patients are very sleepy during the day. In untreated patients, pupils are very small and unstable with frequent hippus. When the patients receive treatment with methylphenidate to make them more alert, pupillary diameter increases and becomes more stable with less hippus.

Pupillometry can be performed in many ways. When the doctor shines a light in your eye and watches to see how rapidly the pupil size changes, this is a type of pupillometry. Formal pupillometric studies, however, now use special cameras that can see the pupil in the dark and computers to determine the pupillary diameter automatically (Figure 1). New types of pupillometers may provide better capability to study the ANS and its relationship to sleep and alertness. The pupil remains a place where activity of the ANS can be most easily assessed.

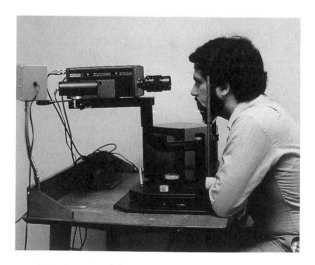

Figure 1.   Testing a patient with a pupillometer.

REFERENCES

Berlucchi G, Moruzzi G, Salvi G, Strata P. 1964. Pupil behavior and ocular movements during synchronized and desynchronized sleep. *Arch Ital Biol* 102:230–244.

Fontana F. 1765. *Dei moti dell'iride.* Lucca, Italy: Giusti.

Janisse MP. 1977. *Pupillometry: The psychology of pupillary response.* New York: Wiley.

Lowenstein O, Feinberg R, Loewenfeld I. 1963. Pupillary movements during acute and chronic fatigue: A new test for objective evaluation of tiredness. *Invest Ophthalmol Vis Sci* 2:138–157.

Schmidt H, Fortin L. 1982. Electronic pupillometry in disorders of arousal. In Guilleminault C, ed. *Sleep and waking disorders: Implications and techniques,* pp 127–143. New York: Addison-Wesley.

Mark R. Pressman

R

REBOUND

[*In the context of sleep,* rebound *refers to an excess of total sleep or of a specific sleep stage, usually occurring after some kind of sleep* DEPRIVATION. *For example, an individual who has gone without sleep for one or more nights will experience a sleep rebound—that is, more total sleep on the subsequent recovery night. In humans, this rebound is notable for an increase of* SLOW-WAVE SLEEP, *NREM sleep stages 3 and 4, which tends to occur in greater quantities than* REM SLEEP *during a recovery episode from total sleep deprivation. In other species, REM sleep may be the favored stage during total sleep deprivation recovery rebound, as found in studies of long-term sleep deprivation in rats. Selective deprivation of a specific stage, as when an individual is prevented specifically from going into REM sleep (though permitted to have all other sleep stages), is followed by a rebound of REM sleep when uninterrupted sleep is allowed. A rebound may be considered a homeostatic mechanism for controlling* SLEEP LENGTH *and the* TIMING OF SLEEP AND WAKEFULNESS. *As such, however, sleep rebound may also interact with the timing mechanisms controlled by* CIRCADIAN RHYTHMS, *which may lessen or enhance the rebound.*

A rebound of various sleep stages also occurs following the withdrawal of drugs or medications that have suppressed a particular type of sleep. Thus, for example, alcoholics may experience a REM sleep rebound when they are abstinent, and the phenomenon of DELIRIUM TREMENS *may be related to this REM sleep rebound. Patients who use* BENZODIAZEPINES *as hypnotics for several nights and then stop using them may experience a rebound of slow-wave sleep, since these compounds tend to suppress the deeper NREM sleep stages. By contrast, many of the* ANTIDEPRESSANT *compounds, such as tricyclic antidepressants and* MONOAMINE OXIDASE INHIBITORS, *suppress REM sleep; thus, their discontinuation is associated with marked REM sleep rebound.*

Because certain sleep disorders are associated with significant sleep FRAGMENTATION, *which may result in suppression of particular sleep states or outright sleep deprivation, effective treatment of these disorders can result in a sleep rebound. The most remarkable example occurs in cases of sleep* APNEA, *particularly with the implementation of treatment with nasal* CONTINUOUS POSITIVE AIRWAY PRESSURE. *For example, the sleep pattern of a patient with sleep apnea syndrome changes after successful treatment with nasal CPAP; the patient may show a marked exaggeration in amount of REM sleep or slow-wave sleep on the first night of treatment, which is the equivalent of a sleep deprivation recovery night since sleep can now occur without interruption.*]

RECALL OF DREAMS

To measure accurately the recall of any event—a word, picture, or dream—an experimenter must have independent control of the stimulus perceived by the individual. Because the dream "stimulus" cannot be observed directly by the experimenter, the measurement of dream recall is necessarily confounded with (cannot be separated from) the process of dream production.

The magnitude of the confound, however, has been considerably reduced by the discovery that dreaming is much more frequent in REM than NREM sleep (Aserinsky and Kleitman, 1953). These findings make it possible to be quite confident if and when dreaming is occurring. Note, however, that scientists speak of the number of minutes of dreaming rather than the number of dreams dreamt because the boundaries between successive dreams are not well defined.

As all healthy people spend approximately 20 percent of their sleep time in REM sleep, scientists are certain that they all dream more than one hour per night. The traditional approach to the study of dream recall has assumed that because everyone dreams every night, variability in dream reporting the next day must result from differences in the ability, or the failure, to recall one's dreams. Such differences may be reliable individual (personality) differences, or they may be day-to-day (state) fluctuations within the same individual. Although no reliable experimental evidence supports Freud's (1900/1955) assumption that failure to recall one's dream is an indicator of repression, the prominence of this assumption in his theories provided incentive for early research interest in failure to recall dreams.

Because dream recall varies greatly with the manner in which it is measured, there is no absolute index of recall. Recall varies with incentive and motivation. People who say they never recall their dreams will generally recall them if a therapist says they are important, or will typically report two dreams a month if they are asked to fill out a dream log every morning. Antrobus, Dement, and Fisher (1964) found that people who say they recall one dream a week may report a dream every morning on the log; 42 percent of subjects reported two or more dreams per week on the log. Note that "dream recall" means simply that some image or information from a dream is reported. The waking verbal "report" may be the first time that the subject actually makes a verbal translation of the characters and events of the dream; prior to that point, parts of the dream may exist only in a visual, imaginal form.

Dream recall is an implicit measure of one's memory of a dream. Recent memory research on brain-damaged patients, who have very poor recall of stimuli when awake, demonstrates that the more cues they are given, the more likely they will eventually recall the stimuli. Thus, one major reason for the failure to recall dreams appears to be the absence of cues in the waking environment that effectively help an individual recall the dreams of the previous night. Consequently, if relevant stimuli are encountered throughout the day, they will often cue the recall of a dream from the previous night. This implies that much more dream information is stored in memory than is identified by measures of dream recall.

Since 1953 when dreaming began to be studied in the sleep laboratory, much of the dream recall research has focused on processes that occur near the point of awakening. Many of these processes are, not surprisingly, similar to the processes of attention and interference identified in waking memory research. Following the work of Peterson and Peterson (1959), who showed that counting backward by threes from, say 78, effectively interferes with memory for the digits or words at the end of a list, many experiments have shown that any distraction at the point of awakening from a dream will interfere with its subsequent recall (Goodenough, 1991). The absence of a distractor seems to permit a brief interval of memory consolidation, that is, the stamping of mental events into memory.

The consolidation process requires either a brief interval of arousal within the sleep interval (dreams fade from memory during ensuing dreamless sleep) or a quiet period immediately on awakening from a dream. Goodenough (1991) and his colleagues have shown that dream recall in the laboratory is greatly enhanced if preceded by a brief interval of electroencephalographic alpha waves, indicating arousal or *cortical activation* (excitement of higher brain centers) within the REM period. Further, most home dreams are recalled from weekend mornings when people sleep late and their REM sleep is frequently punctuated with brief intervals of alpha. Greater activation is also associated with increased dream production within sleep (Antrobus, 1991), so that dreaming and the ability to recall the dream on awakening are jointly tied to cortical activation, which is higher in REM than NREM sleep and higher in the late morning than earlier in the night (Antrobus, 1991).

Finally, as might be expected, interesting dreams are more likely to be recalled than boring ones, and frequent dream recallers produce more interesting and longer dreams than nonrecallers.

REFERENCES

Antrobus J. 1991. Dreaming: Cognitive processes during cortical activation and high afferent thresholds. *Psychol Rev* 98:96–121.

Antrobus S, Dement W, Fisher C. 1964. Patterns of dreaming and dream recall: An EEG study. *J Abnorm Social Psychol* 68:341–344.

Aserinsky E, Kleitman N. 1953. Regularly occurring periods of ocular motility and concomitant phenomena during sleep. *Science* 118:361–375.

Freud S. 1900/1955. *The interpretation of dreams.* New York: Basic Books.

Goodenough D. 1991. Dream recall: History and current status of the field. In Ellman S, Antrobus JS, eds. *The mind in sleep,* 2nd ed., pp. 143–171. New York: Wiley Interscience.

Peterson LR, Peterson MJ. 1959. Short-term retention of individual verbal items. *J Exp Psychol* 58:193–198.

John S. Antrobus

RECIPROCAL INTERACTION THEORY

Natural phenomena are said to be understood by science when they can be described mathematically and when the occurrence of the natural phenomena can be predicted with some degree of accuracy. When this approach is successful in science, it also provides what is commonly referred to as a "model" of complex phenomena. For example, most of us could draw a model of the earth's rotation around the sun and use this model to explain periodic oscillations in light and darkness and seasonal changes based on the earth's tilt along its axis. A corresponding mathematical description of planetary movement provided the predictive power that made it possible to have the lunar landing vehicle and the moon meet at the same point in space. Biologic models similarly help provide simplifying descriptions and predictions concerning complex phenomena. The reciprocal interaction model provided the first and, to date, the only cellularly based, mathematical model of how neurons in the brainstem might generate the regular oscillation between sleep and wakefulness.

A complete history of the reciprocal interaction model has not yet been written, but it draws from many branches of neuroscience and biophysics. Through the work of Cajal, Sherrington,

and Eccles, it became clear that all motor acts and all behaviors occurred as a result of the electrical discharge of cells in the brain. In the late 1950s, it became possible to record the electrical activity of single cells in the brains of sleeping animals. This approach, pioneered by Evarts and Hubel, formed the methodology on which the reciprocal interaction model was based. Hobson's seminal 1972 paper entitled "Cellular Neurophysiology and Sleep Research" made it clear that states of consciousness, like motor acts, could be understood in quantitative cellular terms. Sleep neurobiology continues to clarify which neurons and which neurotransmitters cause the regular oscillation between sleep and wakefulness. Before the reciprocal interaction model, other scientists (notably Michel Jouvet and A. Karczmar et al.) suggested that cholinergic and monoaminergic neurons played a key role in REM sleep generation. (See also CHEMISTRY OF SLEEP.)

McCarley and Hobson's original 1975 reciprocal interaction model extended the cholinergic/monoaminergic concept in important ways. First, the model hypothesized that it was the reciprocal discharge of cholinergic and monoaminergic neurons that causes REM sleep. By reciprocal discharge, the model referred to the then new discovery that certain cells in the brain began to fire more intensely during REM sleep (REM-on cells), while other neurons ceased discharging during REM sleep (REM-off cells). Second, the REM-on population was hypothesized to be cholinergic and the REM-off cell population was hypothesized to be monoaminergic. Furthermore, the model postulated a synaptic interaction between the REM-on and REM-off cell populations. Thus, the observed reciprocal discharge profiles (i.e., REM-on and REM-off) and the postulated synaptic interaction between REM-on and REM-off neurons gave rise to the name reciprocal interaction model. Although these concepts have been revised in light of new evidence (Hobson, Lydic, and Baghdoyan, 1986; McCarley and Massaquoi, 1986), the name has been retained.

The original cellular model was described by differential equations first developed by Lotka and Volterra. The Lotka-Volterra equations were originally used to model, and hence predict, the relationship between prey (rabbit) and predator (lynx) populations in North America. During the colonization of North America, the French fur industry used the Lotka-Volterra equations to model the observation that as the population of lynxes declined, the number of rabbits increased. Reciprocally, as the population of lynxes increased, the number of rabbits declined. Because the REM-on and REM-off cell discharge frequency during REM sleep appeared to follow similar patterns of growth and decline, the reciprocal model applied the Lotka-Volterra equations to the neuronal firing rate data. The published evidence demonstrates that the mathematical model worked so well that the theoretical discharge profiles were able to predict neuronal discharge profiles, which were subsequently recorded. Thus, the model was able to predict when, in time, REM sleep would occur as a function of the discharge of single cells in the pontine brainstem. This was the first time that a behavioral state (i.e., REM sleep) was described and predicted in cellular and formal mathematical terms. McCarley and Massaquoi continue to refine and develop the mathematical model of the neurophysiologic data.

The reciprocal interaction model has greatly promoted the advancement of sleep neurobiology. The 1975 reciprocal interaction model provided a unique interpretive framework. Some hypotheses of the 1975 model have been shown to be incorrect and other hypotheses still offer a cellular-level explanation for how cells in the brain might regulate sleep. Perhaps the most important contribution of the reciprocal interaction model has been its ability to help formalize testable hypotheses.

REFERENCES

Hobson JA. 1972. Cellular neurophysiology and sleep research. In Chase M, ed. *The sleeping brain,* pp 59–82. Los Angeles: UCLA Brain Information Service.

Hobson JA, Lydic R, Baghdoyan HA. 1986. Evolving concepts of sleep cycle generation: From brain centers to neuronal populations. *Behav Brain Sci* 9:371–448.

McCarley RW, Hobson JA. 1975. Neuronal excitability modulation over the sleep cycle: A structural and mathematical model. *Science* 189:58–60.

McCarley RW, Massaquoi SG. 1986. A limit cycle mathematical model of the REM sleep oscillator system. *Am J Physiol* 251:R1011–R1029.

Steriade M, McCarley RW. 1990. *Brain stem control of wakefulness and sleep.* New York: Plenum Press.

Ralph Lydic

RECURRING DREAMS

The phenomenon of the recurrent dream, defined as the very same dream repeated over and over, has long intrigued investigators of human dreaming. Most notably, Freud was perplexed by the role that recurrent, anxiety-laden dreams might play in the mental processes of certain individuals who had been traumatized psychologically. He wondered: "What wishful impulse could be satisfied by harking back in this way to this exceedingly traumatic experience?" Freud (1933/1965) evidently concluded that repetitive dreams in the aftermath of a trauma represent a failure of the dream mechanism itself: Dreaming, which otherwise represents an adaptive outlet for the disguised fulfillment of a repressed wish, here continually fails to achieve its purpose (see FREUD'S DREAM THEORY; FUNCTIONS OF DREAMS).

In fact, a wealth of clinical lore and research data accumulated during the past few decades have established that people enduring a traumatic experience outside the realm of expectable life events can have recurrent, stereotypical dreams of that experience. This form of response to a traumatic stressor can be observed at different stages of the life cycle, for example, in a child who witnessed an act of violence directed toward a parent or other family member (Pynoos and Eth, 1985), as well as in a combat veteran who survived an enemy assault in which a close buddy was killed. The repetitive dreams of people with so-called posttraumatic stress disorder (PTSD) are remarkable in the degree to which they actually replicate the precipitating traumatic scene (Ross et al., 1989). The symptoms of PTSD, including this characteristic sleep mentation, can continue for years following the occurrence of the trauma. Depending on the severity of PTSD in a particular person, the posttraumatic dream may recur once every few months or several times a week (see POSTTRAUMATIC NIGHTMARES).

Aside from PTSD, essentially no other mental disorder recognized in the standard classification of psychiatric diagnoses is characterized by recurrent anxiety-laden dreams. Depressed people seem to have a heightened tendency to enter REM sleep, the stage of sleep when most dreaming occurs, and to have at least some REM sleep periods with particularly abundant eye movements, which perhaps are a correlate of vivid sleep mentation; yet depressed individuals have not been shown to suffer recurrent dreams. A specific condition known as nightmare disorder, seen most commonly in open, trusting, and artistic people, is characterized by repeated awakenings from sleep, with detailed recall of frightening dreams. There may be an underlying theme to many of the dreams of a person with nightmare disorder, but the content usually is not identical from dream to dream (Hartmann, 1984).

Two survey studies (Cartwright, 1979; Robbins and Houshi, 1983) have provided evidence that a history of recurrent dreams may be reported by a significant percentage (60 percent to 65 percent) of adults not otherwise known to have emotional problems. Women are more likely than men to identify such dreams some time in the past. There is also a consensus that these recurrent dreams usually are unpleasant, perhaps even having the qualities of a nightmare (see NIGHTMARES). People who offer a history of recurrent dreams often report that the dreams began in childhood, but retrospective data of this nature may be subject to considerable bias. Although some have suggested that recurrent dreams reflect attempts to cope with psychological stressors—perhaps even the age-specific hurdles encountered in normal human development—substantiation of this conclusion awaits longitudinal studies, including investigations in children.

REFERENCES

Cartwright RD. 1979. The nature and function of repetitive dreams: A survey and speculation. *Psychiatry* 42:131–137.

Freud S. 1933/1965. *New introductory lectures on psycho-analysis.* New York: Norton.

Hartmann E. 1984. *The nightmare.* New York: Basic Books.

Pynoos RS, Eth S. 1985. Children traumatized by witnessing acts of personal violence: Homicide, rape, or suicide behavior. In Eth S, Pynoos RS, eds. *Posttraumatic stress disorder in children.* Washington, DC: Am Psychiatric Press. Pp. 19–43.

Robbins PR, Houshi F. 1983. Some observations on recurrent dreams. *Bull Menninger Clin* 47: 262–265.

Ross RJ, Ball WA, Sullivan KA, Caroff SN. 1989. Sleep disturbance as the hallmark of posttraumatic stress disorder. *Am J Psychiatry* 146:697–707.

Richard J. Ross

RELAXATION THERAPY

"Can't get to sleep? Just relax, empty your mind, let go of the tension, don't worry, and you will sleep like a baby." Unfortunately, it is not always that easy just to relax and fall asleep, especially if worries are running through your mind or you are physically tense or emotionally distressed. For centuries, relaxation techniques have been used to produce an inner state of calm through the reduction of physical, mental, and emotional arousal. Over the years, relaxation techniques have been refined and are now commonly used to treat difficulties falling and staying asleep.

Perhaps the first evidence of a formal relaxation technique comes from India and the Hindu practice of *meditation* between 3000 and 4000 B.C. *Yoga* emerged from these practices and involves specific actions: sitting in a comfortable position, focusing attention on a single object or word (a *mantra*), and breathing slowly (see MEDITATION AND SLEEP). In the 1930s, Edmund Jacobson (considered the father of modern relaxation methods), developed *progressive relaxation*, the basis for many of the current muscular tension-release approaches (Bernstein and Borkovec, 1973; Jacobson, 1929, 1934; Lichstein, 1988). Progressive relaxation involves the sequential tensing and release of the major muscle groups in the body. Attention is focused on the difference between the feelings of muscular tension and the relaxation associated with release. Jacobson (1938) used progressive relaxation to treat many complaints and physical problems, including insomnia. About the same time, another widely used approach, *autogenic training*, was developed by Johannes Schultz (Schultz and Luthe, 1959). Autogenic training is a self-induction technique that combines a focus on physical sensations with pleasant mental imagery. While maintaining passive concentration, a person imagines being in a comfortable and peaceful environment, then rhythmically repeats mental phrases associated with pleasant physical sensations (such as warmth and heaviness). Other relaxation techniques used to promote sleep include hypnosis, biofeedback, and positive guided imagery (see HYPNOSIS AND DREAMING; BIOFEEDBACK; COUNTING SHEEP).

Relaxation therapy is used to reduce the physical, mental, or emotional arousal that may interfere with falling or staying asleep. Scientific research with POLYSOMNOGRAPHY has shown that these techniques can reduce the time it takes to fall asleep by 70 percent (Borkovec, 1982). Relaxation therapy can improve the subjective complaint of poor sleep and also be associated with better physiological sleep as measured objectively. The application of relaxation techniques to a wide variety of sleep and other health complaints has shown clearly that these are skills; they can be learned, practiced, and mastered. Mastery of relaxation skills that can be used at any time and in any environment can provide a critical sense of self-control. Although not always eliminating a sleep problem completely, relaxation therapy can play an important role in the overall improvement and management of difficulties falling or staying asleep (see also BEHAVIORAL MODIFICATION; INSOMNIA).

REFERENCES

Bernstein DA, Borkovec TD. 1973. *Progressive relaxation training: A manual for the helping professionals.* Urbana, Ill.: Research Press. A classic training manual for progressive relaxation.

Borkovec TD. 1982. Insomnia. *J Consulting Clin Psychol* 50(6):880–895.

Jacobson E. 1929. *Progressive relaxation.* Chicago: University of Chicago Press.

———. 1934. *You must relax.* New York: Whittlesey House.

———. 1938. *You can sleep well: The abc's of restful sleep for the average person.* New York: Whittlesey House.

Lichstein KL. 1988. *Clinical relaxation strategies.* New York: Wiley. Good source for specific techniques.

Schultz JH, Luthe W. 1959. *Autogenic training: A psychophysiologic approach in psychotherapy.* New York: Grune & Stratton.

Mark R. Rosekind

RELIGION AND DREAMING

Throughout history people have been very much occupied with their dreams. Primitive people reacted to their dreams as if they were part of real life (see CULTURAL ASPECTS OF DREAMING). For example, Native Americans believed that a snake bite received in dreams had to be treated when the dreamer awakened. In these tribes, dreams were interpreted by the elders or special diviners who advised the dreamer as to what action he or she should take. In other primitive tribes dreams were considered as the actions of the soul that left the body during sleep. Waking up from sleep was a sign that the soul had returned. Thus, they believed that it was very dangerous to be waked abruptly from sleep, because the soul might have no time to be reunited with the body.

In many ancient religions gods were consulted through dreams. From the Sumerian–Babylonian culture in the third millennium B.C. through ancient Egypt and classical Greece, people distinguished between "divine" dreams that had to be interpreted and obeyed, and "ordinary" dreams. The divine dreams were interpreted by priests and magicians, who also made the distinction between "good" and "bad" dreams. "Good" dreams were sent by the gods, "bad" dreams by demons. The ancient Egyptians left behind them catalogues of thousands of dream symbols, to which they turned to find the meaning of their dreams: they believed that dreams either were sent by the gods or were messages sent by spirits of the dead. In dreams, the gods usually demanded that the dreamer perform certain acts, gave the dreamer a warning, or predicted future events. Throughout Mediterranean countries, dreams were also used as a therapeutic means. To this intent, dreams were invoked, or *incubated,* by special rituals in sacred places. The most important temple in Egypt was the temple of Imhotep, the god of healing, at Memphis, where sick persons were brought to sleep in order to induce beneficial dreams. In Greece, during the classical period, there were more than 300 incubation centers. The Greeks, and under their influence the Romans, also believed that dreams were sent by either the dead or the gods, and that most dreams were symbolic, requiring interpretation.

Dreams in the Judeo-Christian tradition were also a means by which God communicated with mortals. "God is departed from me," said Saul, "and answereth me no more, neither by prophets nor by dreams" (Samuel I, 28:5). The word *dream* as a noun occurs sixty-four times in the Old Testament; only six of these were "ordinary" dreams. The verb *to dream* appears twenty-eight times, of which only three occurrences concern "ordinary" dreams. Interestingly, forty-two occurrences of *dream* as a noun or a verb are found in the story of Joseph. Dreams in the Old and New Testaments did not convey any information about the dreamer's internal or psychological problems. The Hebrews had no magical practices to induce therapeutic dreams; the source of their dreams was entirely external to the dreamer. Generally, two types of dreams were reported: the auditory message and the symbolic dream. Dreams conveying messages came to patriarchs, prophets, and kings. Such dreams can be found in Isaiah 6:1–13, Jeremiah 1:11–15, or Amos 7:1–9. Symbolic dreams such as those of Joseph, Pharaoh, and Daniel could appear to ordinary people or to foreigners. Most of the messages were clear and easily understood by the recipients and, therefore, required no intermediary interpreter. Only in a few cases was there a need for dream interpretation, as in the dreams of Pharaoh and Daniel.

Later, the Talmud, the Jewish exhaustive codex of laws, mentioned different classes of dreams: prophetic, oracular, and therapeutic. A dream, the Talmud states, cannot be effective unless it is interpreted, but elsewhere in the Talmud dreams are refuted as nonsense.

The belief that dreams were a means of communication between God and people was fully adopted by emerging Christianity, although later Christian writers paid little attention to dreams. Some attempt was made, however, to distinguish between regular dreams, which were the product of such factors as memories, health, and posture, and incorporeal dreams, which must be ascribed to the agency of the angels, devils, or God himself.

The Arabs also took great account of their dreams. The first part of the Koran, the Islamic sacred book, was first revealed to the prophet Mohammed in a dream. This book categorically states that dreams reveal the secrets of Allah (God).

Dreams also played a role in Far Eastern religions. In the Hindu and Buddhist religions the cause of dreams was believed to be a temporary separation of the earthly body from the spiritual soul, an idea that prevails in many different parts of the world. Once free, the spirit may wander in different places and may communicate with other spirits or with gods.

In conclusion, dreams have had a profound influence in the history of religions, and thus play a decisive part in the religious experience of humankind. Important religious dreams are found at the first appearance of the Judeo-Christian, Islamic, and Buddhist traditions.

REFERENCES

de Becker R. 1964. *The understanding of dreams and their influence on the history of man*. Heron M, trans. New York: Bell.

Gaster TH. 1972. Dreams: In the Bible. In *Encyclopedia Judaica,* vol 6, pp 209–210. Jerusalem: Keter.

Lewin I. 1983. The psychological theory of dreams in the Bible. *J Psychology Judaism* 7:73–88.

MacKenzie N. 1965. *Dreams and dreaming*. London: Aldous Books.

Peretz Lavie

REM LATENCY

[*One of the characteristic features used to describe sleep, particularly in humans, is REM latency—that is, the speed with which an individual achieves* REM SLEEP *after* SLEEP ONSET. *Latency to REM sleep in normal adult humans is usually 100 minutes or longer: this interval is occupied by NREM sleep. A number of factors, however, can alter the length of REM latency; thus, changes in this measurement can serve as a marker for stages of* DEVELOPMENT, *pathological processes, drug effects, circadian influences, or disruptions of the sleep–wake schedule.*

REM latency has an age-dependent component. Newborn human infants fall asleep directly into REM sleep, as do virtually all mammalian newborns (see INFANCY, NORMAL SLEEP PATTERNS IN*). This pattern gradually changes across the first year of life until NREM sleep onset becomes the norm and the interval before REM sleep occurs lengthens to the adult level (see* ONTOGENY; NORMAL SLEEP*). In older, middle-aged and elderly individuals, REM latency then begins to decline in an age-related fashion; while normal REM latency in a young adult may be 100 minutes, normal REM latency in a 65-year-old individual may be 60 minutes (see* AGING AND SLEEP*).*

Decreased latency to REM sleep may also signal a pathological condition. Sleep-onset REM periods, or the occurrence of REM sleep immediately upon falling asleep (as seen normally in newborn infants), are seen in NARCOLEPSY *and* CANINE NARCOLEPSY. *A reduction of REM sleep latency with occasional sleep-onset REM episodes occurring has also been reported in individuals suffering from major* DEPRESSION. *It is interesting to note that many of the drugs used to treat patients who are depressed are also used to treat patients with narcolepsy: A commonality among these drugs is their tendency to reduce the total amount of REM sleep and to increase REM latency. Compounds with this effect include* ANTIDEPRESSANTS *and* MONOAMINE OXIDASE INHIBITORS. *Other drugs known to lengthen REM latency are* ALCOHOL *and many of the* BENZODIAZEPINES *(hypnotics).*

REM latency can also be lengthened or shortened depending upon the time an individual falls asleep with respect to his or her internal body clock. The likelihood of having REM sleep varies on a daily basis because of a strong link with the oscillator for CIRCADIAN RHYTHMS. *In someone who keeps a regular nighttime sleep schedule, the highest likelihood of REM sleep occurring is during the early hours of the morning between 4:00 and 7:00 A.M., whereas the least likely time for REM sleep to occur in such an individual is during the late afternoon and evening; thus, a shiftworker with an inverted sleep–wake pattern will be more likely to experience a short REM latency after going to bed at 9:00 or 10:00 in the morning rather than 9:00 or 10:00 at night. Even the time chosen for* NAPPING *will influence latency to REM sleep: Morning naps are more likely to contain an episode of REM sleep than afternoon or evening naps because the latency to REM sleep is shorter at that time of day.*

REM sleep latency becomes very short following selective REM sleep DEPRIVATION. *Under such circumstances, the tendency to have REM sleep builds as the stage is deprived; as this pressure gets greater and greater, the likelihood of REM sleep occurring earlier than usual, or even at the onset of sleep, increases. A similar finding results when individuals undergo chronic restriction of sleep. Thus, measurable changes in REM sleep latency in adult humans can be used as a signal to help identify psychiatric problems, sleep disorders, and other sleep disturbances.]*

REM SLEEP

[*Sleep can be subdivided into* rapid-eye-movement (REM) *and* non-rapid-eye-movement (NREM) *sleep. NREM sleep is characterized by reduced levels of muscle tone, slow regular breathing, no eye movements or slow eye movements, reduced levels of neuronal activity in most brain regions, and high-voltage spindles and slow-wave brain activity (see* ELECTROENCEPHALOGRAM; SLEEP SPINDLES*).*

REM sleep is characterized by a complete absence of muscle tone in the muscles that support the body against gravity, although this atonia may be interrupted by twitches (see ATONIA; MOTOR CONTROL; PHASIC ACTIVITY IN REM SLEEP*). In humans and cats, the suppression of muscle tone is complete, but in rabbits, opossums, and several other animals, REM sleep atonia is not complete. Animals that move their eyes when awake show rapid eye movements during REM sleep. Respiration tends to be irregular in REM sleep, the most marked irregularity coinciding with rapid eye movement and twitching. Most brain regions show a relatively high level of neuronal activity in REM sleep, exceeding NREM levels and often exceeding levels seen in active waking. Activity in the* AUTONOMIC NERVOUS SYSTEM *is altered, with a marked reduction in sympathetic nerve activity. Brain wave activity tends to look like the waking, low-voltage pattern; the young of many mammalian species, however, have REM sleep while spindles and slow waves are present in the electroencephalogram. REM sleep is the state in which the most vivid dreams occur.*

REM sleep has also been called PARADOXICAL SLEEP, *active sleep, desynchronized sleep, and dream sleep. Entries on dreaming are listed in the guidepost on* DREAMS AND DREAMING. *REM sleep is discussed in greater detail in the following entries:*

CHEMISTRY OF SLEEP
DEPRIVATION, SELECTIVE: REM SLEEP
ERECTILE DYSFUNCTION
ERECTIONS
FEMALE SEXUAL RESPONSE
METABOLIC CONTROL OF REM SLEEP
MIDDLE EAR MUSCLE ACTIVITY
NARCOLEPSY
NOCTURNAL PENILE TUMESCENCE
PGO WAVES

REM SLEEP BEHAVIOR DISORDER

The REM sleep behavior disorder (RBD) is a newly discovered and described parasomnia (i.e., sleep behavior disorder) featuring complex and violent behaviors that emerge during REM sleep, which ordinarily exhibits a generalized muscle paralysis known as "REM ATONIA." REM sleep behavior disorder presents a bold array of findings that interlink the clinical and basic neurosciences.

REM sleep behavior disorder typically affects older men and is characterized by attempts to carry out "violent, moving nightmares" while asleep and by an unawareness of actual surroundings, which results in injury. Although various brain disorders can induce RBD, there is no identified cause in most cases. Fortunately, RBD can be controlled with bedtime medication.

REM sleep behavior disorder was originally discovered by Jouvet and Delorme in 1965 in cats that had received experimental lesions to the PONS region of the brainstem. These French scientists were attempting to locate the part of the brain that generates REM sleep, but instead they identified the group of nerve cells (i.e., neurons) responsible for generating one of the defining features of REM sleep—specifically REM ATONIA. Their laboratory cats exhibited categories of behaviors during REM sleep that are also found in humans with RBD, thus establishing an animal model for clinical RBD.

Although various aspects of human RBD were identified as early as 1966, the full syndrome was not formally identified and named until 1986 (Schenck et al.). RBD has now been included within the international classification of sleep–wake disorders.

RBD commands attention insofar as (1) it is a fascinating syndrome; (2) it is a hazardous sleep disorder requiring treatment; (3) it epitomizes the vital link between basic science and clinical medicine; (4) it offers additional perspectives on human behavior, brain function during sleep, and dreaming; and (5) it provides a scientific explanation for peculiar and bizarre, recurrent nocturnal experiences that can be misunderstood as representing mental illness or epilepsy.

Clinical Features of RBD

Overview and Clinical Course

Complaints of dream disturbance associated with abnormal sleep behaviors require a comprehensive evaluation to determine the proper diagnosis and distinguish the symptoms from other conditions. The protocol employed at the Minnesota Regional Sleep Disorders Center—involving patient and family interviews, extensive polysomnographic monitoring (see POLYSOMNOGRAPHY), and psychiatric-neurological examinations—has yielded the data in Table 1 from seventy consecutive cases of RBD gathered over 6.5 years, the largest such series reported to date (Schenck and Mahowald, 1990). As seen in Table 1, RBD primarily affects older males. Although nearly 25 percent of the patients had a lengthy prodrome eventually culminating in frank RBD, only very few had histories of childhood SLEEP-WALKING or sleep terrors. REM sleep behavior disorder is usually progressive, with both the frequency and severity worsening over time. Most patients have at least one major episode of attempted dream enactment every 2 or 3 weeks; some have had at least one nightly episode for 10 to 20 years. No case of spontaneous remission has yet to be identified. The prevalence of RBD is currently unknown.

Behavioral Abnormalities

The behavioral repertoire during REM sleep in RBD clusters into four categories: (1) a minimal syndrome of twitching and jerking of the limbs and body; (2) orienting and exploratory behaviors, such as staring, head raising, reaching, grasping, searching; (3) attack behaviors; and (4) locomotion, particularly running. These behaviors generally appear more than 60 to 90 minutes after sleep onset, coinciding with the customary latency for REM sleep. Animal-like behaviors reported by the patients' spouses were those resembling large jungle cats, gorillas,

Table 1. Major Findings in Seventy Consecutive Patients With the REM Sleep Behavior Disorder (RBD) Documented by Polysomnography

Categories	% of patients	Comments
Gender		Average age at onset (N=70): 52.6 years (range, 9 to 73 years). Average age at presentation for polysomnography: 59.3 years (range, 10 to 77 years).
Male	90.0	
Female	10.0	
Prodrome	24.3	Sleeptalking, yelling, limb twitching and jerking began an average 22.3 years before RBD onset (range, 2 to 48 years).
Chief complaint		
Sleep injury	77.1	Bruises (N=54), lacerations (N=24), fractures (N=5)
Sleep disruption		
Altered dream process and content	22.9	More vivid, unpleasant, action filled, violent (reported as severe nightmares).
Dream-enacting behaviors	91.4	Talking, laughing, chanting, singing, yelling, swearing, gesturing, reaching, grabbing, arm flailing, punching, kicking, sitting up, jumping out of bed, crawling, running. Animalistic behaviors.
Central nervous system disorders causally linked with RBD	37.5	Degenerative disorders (N=11): 5 dementia, 4 parkinsonism, 2 other; narcolepsy (N=7), stroke (N=3), brainstem tumor (N=1), multiple sclerosis (N=1), Guillain-Barré syndrome (N=1).
Psychiatric disorders causally linked with RBD	8.9	Chronic abstinence states (N=3): 2 from ethanol abuse, 1 from ethanol/amphetamine abuse; adjustment (acute life stress response) disorder (N=2), major depression and rapid withdrawal from tricyclic antidepressant medication (N=1).
Endocrinological disorder	1.4	64-year-old woman developed RBD abruptly after a total surgical removal of her parathyroid glands.
Treatment		
Clonazepam efficacy		
Complete	77.2	Rapid control of problematic sleep behaviors and altered dreams sustained for up to 7 years.
Partial	12.3	
Total	89.5	

Courtesy of the Cleveland Clinic Journal of Medicine, *volume 57 supplement, page S15, Table 1 (modified),* 1990.

bears, and seals. Appetitive behaviors (e.g., feeding, sexual) have not been associated with RBD.

Over 75 percent of RBD patients have sustained repeated injuries, such as bruises, lacerations requiring up to forty sutures to repair, and fractures to the digits, ribs, sternum and vertebrae—including the odontoid process of the second cervical vertebra known colloquially as the "hangman's fracture." Other injuries have involved joint dislocations, sprains, cartilage tears, torn nails, rug burns, pulled hair, nose bleeds, and traumatic headaches. Spouses are also frequently injured. For example, a wife once incurred three broken ribs from a single punch delivered by her sleeping husband.

Self-protection measures chosen by these patients have included restraint devices (sleeping bags and belts, ropes, or dog leashes attaching patients to their beds), padded waterbeds, pillow barricades, and sleeping on a floor mattress in an empty room. Figure 1 on page 501 shows one such device in a man with stroke-induced RBD.

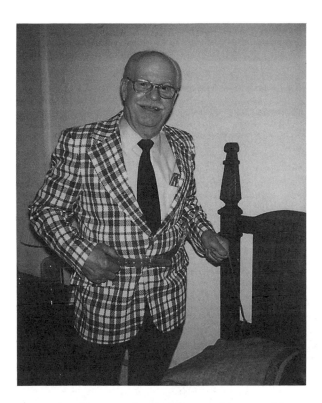

Figure 1. Photograph of a 70-year-old man with RBD who for 6 years had tethered himself to bed with a rope and belt in an effort to prevent injury from leaping out of bed during attempted dream enactments.

Dream Disturbances

There is a very close correspondence between the action in the altered dreams and the observed dream-enacting behaviors. Patients do not enact their usual dreams, but instead carry out distinctly abnormal dreams, which are now known to be stereotypical for RBD. The patients almost never are the primary aggressor in their dreams; rather, they fight to defend themselves or their loved ones from an attacker, who usually is an unfamiliar person or animal. An ironic situation commonly occurs in which a husband dreaming that he was fighting to defend his wife would awaken while actually beating on her in bed.

Neurologic Findings

A substantial minority of RBD patients have neurological disorders that emerged in tandem with RBD. The diversity in the type and location of the brain disorders is great, indicating that human RBD is more complex than its animal model. Pa-

tients with neurodegenerative disorders have been observed by family members to display behaviors during sleep that were not volitionally possible while they were awake and debilitated. Extraordinary feats of strength have included flipping over in bed, jumping out of bed, and running. Such examples indicate how diseases of the brain can paradoxically result in both severe physical debilitation during wakefulness and extreme energization during sleep.

Marital Relations

Of the sixty-seven adults included in Table 1, 91 percent have been married for an average length of 36.5 years, and all but four had been married only once. The wives usually attest to the calm nature of their husbands during wakefulness and do not view RBD as a threat to their marriage. In fact, most wives continue to sleep in the same beds with their husbands despite the risk of injury, in order to protect their husbands from self-injury.

Psychiatric Findings

Of the patients from Table 1, psychiatric disorders were causally linked with RBD in only six cases, or 8.9 percent. In three cases, RBD emerged with chronic abstinence from substances of abuse (ethanol, amphetamine) that are known to suppress REM sleep, suggesting that RBD in these cases may have resulted from a pathologic "REM rebound." In two cases, RBD emerged during acute, severe life-stress reactions (divorce, automobile accident without injury). Of note is that no patient had a history of schizophrenia, manic-depression, or other psychosis.

Polysomnographic (PSG) Findings

PSG studies are essential for establishing the diagnosis of RBD, because there are specific PSG abnormalities distinguishing RBD from other parasomnias and from nocturnal seizures. Figure 2 provides the PSG correlates of dream-enacting behaviors. Figures 3 and 4 are examples of how the arms or legs can be selectively activated in REM sleep. Figure 5 shows a man in the act of repeatedly punching a bed twelve times during REM sleep (see POLYSOMNOGRAPHY).

All PSG findings and behavioral features of RBD are indistinguishable across subgroups, irrespec-

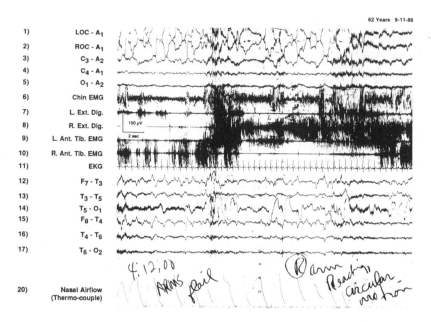

Figure 2. Polysomnographic correlates of dream-enacting behaviors. REM sleep contains dense, high-voltage REM activity (1–2), and there is a fast-frequency, low-voltage, desynchronized electroencephalogram (EEG: 3–5, 12–17) characteristic of REM sleep. The chin electromyographic (EMG) muscle tone is increased (6), as is seen with RBD but not with normal REM sleep. The arms (7–8) and legs (9–10) show bursts of intense twitching, which accompany observable behaviors noted by the technician. The electrocardiogram (EKG: 11) shows a constant rate of 64 beats/minute, despite the vigorous movements, which is consistent with maintenance of REM sleep and inconsistent with an abrupt awakening (which would be accompanied by tachycardia, or increased heart rate). This sequence culminates in a spontaneous awakening, when the man reports a dream of running down a hill in Duluth, Minnesota, and taking shortcuts through backyards, when he suddenly finds himself on a barge that is rocking back and forth. He feels haunted and desperately holds onto anything to prevent falling into the cargo hold, where there are skeletons awaiting him. *Courtesy of Mahowald MW, Schenck CH. 1989. REM sleep behavior disorder. In Kryger M, Dement W, Roth T, eds.* Principles and practice of sleep medicine, *p. 394, figure 42–3 (modified). Philadelphia: W.B. Saunders.*

tive of gender, age, and presence or absence of neurological, psychiatric, or medical disorders. This suggests that a "final common pathway" for RBD exists and can be accessed by a variety of mechanisms.

Treatment

Successful treatment with clonazepam, a BEN-ZODIAZEPINE anticonvulsant, was originally identified through empirical "trial and error." Clonazepam administered at bedtime is very effective in controlling both the behavioral and the dream disturbances of RBD at doses usually well below the anticonvulsant range, which is consistent with the lack of any epileptic abnormalities detected during the PSG studies. Side effects are infrequent and minimal.

Pathophysiology

The pathophysiology of human RBD is hypothesized to involve anatomical and/or functional compromise of the neuronal pathways respon-

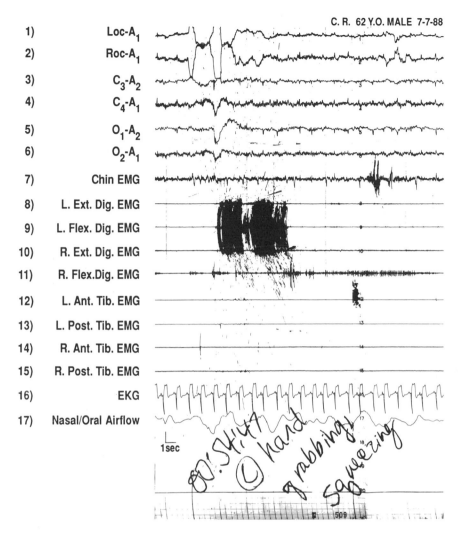

Figure 3. REM sleep polysomnogram revealing selective, dense, high-voltage left arm electromyographic (EMG) muscle twitching (9), which occurs in conjunction with observed grabbing and squeezing behaviors of the left hand. A burst of rapid eye movements (1–2) immediately precedes these behaviors. *Reprinted with permission from Mahowald MW, Schenck CH. 1990. REM-sleep behavior disorder. In Thorpy MJ, ed. Handbook of sleep disorders, p. 579, figure 4. New York: Marcel Dekker.*

sible for the paralysis of REM sleep (see REM SLEEP: MECHANISMS AND NEUROANATOMY). These pathways originate in the brainstem (PONS and MEDULLA) and project to the anterior horn (i.e., motor) cells distributed throughout the spinal cord, which in turn, have neuronal connections with the voluntary (i.e., skeletal) muscles. Another necessary condition for RBD appears to be increased activity of the brainstem motor pattern generators, which are the neuronal source of the observed behaviors. Therefore, RBD apparently emerges in the context of both loss of paralysis and increased drive for behavioral expression in REM sleep.

The male predominance in human RBD raises the possibility of a hormonal effect, perhaps mediated by testosterone. Another possibility is that older men may be at particular risk for developing subtle, age-related changes in their brains that may then promote the appearance of RBD.

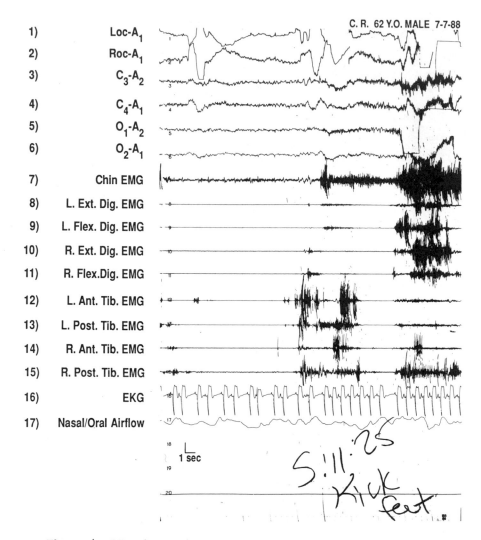

Figure 4. REM sleep polysomnogram demonstrating selective electromyographic (EMG) extensor and flexor twitching of both legs (12–15), which corresponds to the technician's simultaneous observation that the patient is kicking his feet shortly before an awakening (which occurs at the far right side of the figure). *Reprinted with permission from Mahowald MW, Schenck CH. 1990. REM-sleep behavior disorder. In Thorpy MJ, ed.* Handbook of sleep disorders, *page 578, figure 3. New York: Marcel Dekker.*

The close association between the dream and the sleep behavioral disturbances in RBD, along with their shared responsivity to clonazepam treatment, suggests a mutual pathological origin.

The identification of RBD strongly suggests that an important function of REM ATONIA is to protect people, and other mammals, from injury during dreams.

RBD in Veterinary Clinics

RBD has been documented in cats and dogs brought to a veterinary clinic because of abnormal sleep behaviors; clonazepam was documented to be an effective treatment. Thus, the history of RBD demonstrates how an experimen-

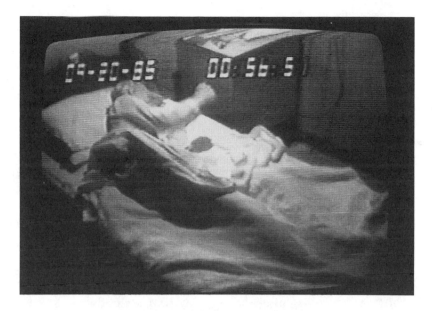

Figure 5. Photograph from sleep lab video footage of a man with RBD throwing a punch during a REM sleep dream. The dark spot on the bed below his raised arm is a shadow cast by the overhead light on his clenched fist.

tal animal model anticipated the discovery of a human clinical syndrome, which then facilitated the recognition and treatment of the corresponding clinical disorder in animals.

REFERENCES

Hendricks JC, Lager A, O'Brien D, Morrison AR. 1989. Movement disorders during sleep in cats and dogs. *J Am Vet Med Assoc* 194:686–689.

Hendricks JC, Morrison AR, Mann GL. 1982. Different behaviors during paradoxical sleep without atonia depend on pontine lesion site. *Brain Res* 239: 81–105.

ICSD—International classification of sleep disorders: Diagnostic and coding manual. 1990. Diagnostic Classification Steering Committee, Thorpy MJ, Chairman. Rochester, Minn.: American Sleep Disorders Association.

Jouvet M, Delorme F. 1965. Locus coeruleus et sommeil paradoxal. *C R Soc Biol (Paris)* 159: 895–899.

Jouvet M, Sastre J-P, Sakai K. 1981. Toward an etho-ethnology of dreaming. In Karacan I, ed. *Psychophysiological aspects of sleep,* pp 204–214. Park Ridge, N.J.: Noyes Medical. Discussion in English of the discovery of the RBD animal model.

Mahowald MW, Schenck CH. 1989. REM sleep behavior disorder. In Kryger MH, Roth T, Dement WC, eds. *Principles and practice of sleep medicine,* pp 389–401. Philadelphia: Saunders. Contains the most comprehensive bibliography available on all aspects of RBD.

Schenck CH, Bundlie SR, Ettinger MG, Mahowald MW. 1986. Chronic behavioral disorders of human REM sleep: A new category of parasomnia. *Sleep* 9: 293–308.

Schenck CH, Mahowald MW. 1990. Polysomnographic, neurologic, psychiatric, and clinical outcome report on 70 consecutive cases with REM sleep behavior disorder (RBD): Sustained clonazepam efficacy in 89.5% of 57 treated patients. *Cleve Clin J Med* 57(suppl):S9–S23.

Carlos H. Schenck

REM SLEEP, DISCOVERY OF

The discovery or identification of the discrete organismic state known as REM sleep should be distinguished from the discovery that rapid eye movements occur during sleep. The historical threads of the discovery of rapid eye movements are identifiable. Nathaniel Kleitman, a professor of physiology at the University of Chicago, had long been interested in the cycle of motor activity and inactivity in infants, and in the possibility that this cycle would ensure a periodic opportunity to awaken and nurse. He postulated that the times infants awakened to nurse on a self-demand schedule would be integral multiples of a basic rest–activity cycle. The second thread was an interest in eye motility as a possible measure of "depth" of sleep. The reasoning for this was that eye movements had a much greater neocortical representation in the brain than almost any other observable motor activity, and that slow, rolling or pendular eye movements had been described at the onset of sleep with a gradual slowing and disappearance as sleep "deepened."

In 1951, Kleitman gave the assignment of observing eye motility to a graduate student in physiology named Eugene Aserinsky. Watching the eyes with the eyelids closed in infants was very tedious and they soon found that it was easier to establish periods of motility if they observed any movement at all, usually a writhing or twitching of the eyelids, versus periods of "no motility." After describing an apparent rhythm in eye motility, they decided they should look for a similar phenomenon in adults. Again, watching a sleeper's closed eyes was very tedious and watching the eyes at night was even worse. Casting about, they came on the method of electrooculography (EOG) and decided this would be a good way to observe eye motility and would relieve the human observer of the tedium of direct observations. Sometime in the course of doing this, bursts of electrical potential changes were seen in the EOG of a sleeping subject that were quite different from the slow movements at sleep onset.

When they were observing infants, Aserinsky and Kleitman had not differentiated slow and rapid movements; however, with the EOG, the different nature of the slow eye movements at sleep onset and the newly discovered "rapid" motility were very obvious. Initially, there was a great deal of concern that these potentials were electrical artifacts. But with their presence in the EOG as a signal, it was possible simultaneously to watch the subject's eyes, and when this was done the movement of the eyes beneath the closed lids was easily identified.

At this point, Aserinsky and Kleitman made two assumptions: (1) These eye movements represented a lightening of sleep, and (2) because

they were associated with irregular respiration and accelerated heart rate, they might represent dreaming. The basic sleep cycle was not identified at this time, primarily because the EOG and other physiological measures, notably the electroencephalogram (EEG), were not recorded continuously, but rather by sampling a few minutes out of each hour or half-hour. The sampling strategy was done to conserve paper (there was no research grant), because there was not a clear reason to record continuously, and because it was possible for the observer to take a nap between sampling episodes.

Kleitman and Aserinsky initiated a series of awakenings to elicit dream recall either when rapid eye movements were present or when rapid eye movements were not present. They did not apply sophisticated methods of content analysis, but the descriptions of dream content were sufficiently different that it was possible to conclude that rapid eye movements were associated with dreaming and this was, indeed, a breakthrough (Aserinsky and Kleitman, 1953, 1955).

In the late 1950s, sleep was widely regarded as a single state. The notion of REM sleep as a separate biological state did not yet exist. The occurrence of the eye movements was quite compatible with the contemporary dream theories that the dream occurred when sleep lightened to prevent or delay awakening; that is, dreaming was regarded as the "guardian of sleep." Furthermore, a leading neurophysiological theory of the time postulated that brain wave patterns, sleep and wakefulness, and levels of consciousness were ineluctably associated in a vertical dimension of brain activity under the mediation of a hypothetical, ascending reticular activating system. Low-amplitude, high-frequency brain wave patterns were thought to indicate high levels of brain activity, wakefulness, and consciousness. High-amplitude, slow brain wave patterns were thought to indicate sleep, low levels of brain activity, and lack of consciousness.

The developing knowledge of the nature of sleep with rapid eye movements was in direct opposition to these notions and constituted a paradigmatic crisis. The following observations were crucial:

1. Arousal thresholds in humans were much higher during periods of rapid eye movement with a low-amplitude, relatively slow (stage 1) EEG pattern than during similar

stage 1 patterns ("light sleep") at the onset of sleep (Dement and Wolpert, 1958).

2. Rapid eye movements during sleep were discovered in cats in which the concomitant brain wave patterns were indistinguishable from active wakefulness; that is, they did not resemble sleep at all (Dement, 1958).

3. By discarding the sampling approach and recording continuously all night, a basic 90-minute cycle of sleep without rapid eye movements, alternating with sleep with rapid eye movements, was discovered. The all-night sleep patterns had a very regular, lawful, predictable pattern of occurrence. Continuous recording revealed a consistent EEG pattern during long periods of sleep within which bursts of rapid eye movement occurred. Additionally, further investigation established these entire periods as periods of vivid dreaming (Dement and Kleitman, 1957).

4. Observations of motor activity during sleep in both humans and animals revealed the unique occurrence of an active suppression of spinal reflex activity, and tonic, nuchal electromyographic potentials present at all other times (Jouvet, 1962).

It was, thus, no longer possible to think of sleep as one state. Sleep had to be conceived as two distinct organismic states, as different from one another as both were from wakefulness. REM sleep was one state, NREM sleep the other. It also had to be conceded that sleep could no longer be thought of as a time of brain inactivity and EEG slowing. By 1960, this fundamental change in our thinking about the nature of the sleep was well established and exists as fact that has not changed in any way since that time.

REFERENCES

Aserinsky E, Kleitman N. 1953. Regularly occurring periods of eye motility and concomitant phenomena during sleep. *Science* 118:273–274.

———. 1955. Two types of ocular motility occurring in sleep. *J Appl Physiol* 8:11–18.

Dement W. 1958. The occurrence of low voltage, fast electroencephalogram patterns during behavioral sleep in the cat. *Electroenceph Clin Neurophysiol* 10:291–296.

Dement W, Kleitman N. 1957. The relation of eye movements during sleep to dream activity: An objective method for the study of dreaming. *J Exp Psychol* 53:339–346.

Dement W, Wolpert E. The relation of eye movements, body motility, and external stimuli to dream content. *J Exp Psychol* 53:543–553.

Jouvet M. 1962. Recherches sur les structures nerveuses et les mécanismes responsables des différentes phases du sommeil physiologique. *Arch Ital Biol* 100:125–206.

William C. Dement

REM SLEEP, FUNCTION OF

Perhaps the greatest mystery in the field of sleep and wakefulness is the function of REM sleep. It seems obvious that REM sleep must have some vital function. Virtually all mammals have REM sleep. In human adults it occupies approximately 90 to 120 minutes of sleep time each night. The intense brain activity during this state is mirrored by intense mental activity experienced as dreams. It is difficult to believe that this physiological state does not have some vital survival role. There is no general agreement among sleep researchers about the function of REM sleep.

Theories of REM sleep function stem from several kinds of evidence. These include data from REM sleep deprivation (*see also* DEPRIVATION, SELECTIVE REM SLEEP), developmental studies, the distribution of REM sleep amounts in different species, the correlation (or lack of correlation) between REM sleep and intelligence, and the role of REM sleep inferred from physiologic studies of the brain.

The most direct approach to answering the question of REM sleep function is to deprive organisms of REM sleep and determine the nature of the ensuing deficit. Early studies in humans and animals found that such deprivation produces a selective increase in the amount of REM sleep when sleep is allowed after deprivation is terminated. This REM rebound indicates that a need for REM sleep exists and accumulates in its absence, analogous to our need for food or water. Early studies also suggested that psychiatric problems occurred during REM sleep deprivation, suggesting that perhaps processes accompanying the dreams of REM sleep facilitated the maintenance of sanity in waking. Further studies have shown that this initial report was not correct. While REM sleep–deprived individuals certainly become irritable, and the frequency of certain behaviors changes in REM sleep–deprived animals, grossly pathologic behavior does not occur after deprivation of normal individuals.

A number of studies have examined the possibility that REM sleep is essential for forming permanent memories, and several studies have reported that REM sleep deprivation produced greater effects on memory retention than deprivation of NREM sleep stages. There is also some evidence suggesting that the amount of REM sleep increases after intense learning experiences. On the other hand, many investigators have failed to find relations between REM sleep and learning. Thus, the effect appears to be a small one, if it exists at all. Others have hypothesized that REM sleep is required for "forgetting" certain types of information, but evidence for this hypothesis is lacking (see also MEMORY; LEARNING).

It is clear, at least in rats, that complete deprivation of REM sleep for periods of weeks results in death. This effect, however, is less marked than that of total sleep deprivation, and it is not clear that the effect of long-term REM sleep–deprivation procedures produce qualitatively different effects than does the deprivation of NREM sleep (see also DEPRIVATION, TOTAL PHYSIOLOGICAL). The cause of death after either kind of deprivation is not yet established, although this is an active area of study (Rechtschaffen et al., 1989).

A second kind of evidence bearing on REM sleep function is the distribution of REM sleep amounts across different species of animals (see PHYLOGENY). In this approach researchers try to correlate other characteristics of animals with the nature of their REM sleep and, in particular, with the amount of REM sleep. Because REM sleep is associated with the dreaming state in humans, it is often assumed that humans and other "intelligent" animals have more REM sleep than "lower" animals. This is clearly not the case. Human REM sleep percentages are neither uniquely high nor low. For example, opossums and ferrets are the current "REM sleep champions," having more than 6 hours of REM sleep each day and devoting more than 30 percent of their sleep time to REM sleep. Adult humans have about 1.9 hours of REM sleep each night, 24 percent of their sleep time. Animals with very low amounts of REM sleep include larger animals such as elephants and hippopotami. Elephants have 1.8 hours of REM sleep each day, indicating that the elephant's legendary memory does not require large amounts of REM sleep. As a group, birds have less REM sleep than mammals. It is unclear whether reptiles and other nonmammalian vertebrates have REM sleep. Only two mammals have been found to lack REM sleep. One is the ECHIDNA, or spiny anteater, a primitive egg-laying mammal found in Australia. The other is the bottle-nosed dolphin. Other aquatic mammals have REM sleep (see PHYLOGENY).

Phylogenetic evidence is at variance with the often expressed belief that REM sleep is related to higher intellectual function. Nevertheless, the variation in REM sleep amounts has been shown to relate to the security of the animals' sleep arrangements. Animals that are subject to predation and have unsafe sleeping places tend to have little REM sleep, whereas predator animals or animals with safe sleeping places have more REM sleep. Since REM sleep is in some sense a deeper stage of sleep, an abundance of REM sleep might be maladaptive for prey animals. This theory explains variations in REM sleep amounts in terms of the danger of the state, but does not really explain what function the state performs.

The issue of an intellectual role of REM sleep has also been addressed by comparisons among humans. While there is some evidence that REM sleep amount may be positively correlated with a person's weight, there is no good evidence that it is correlated with intelligence.

Another variable correlated with the variation in REM sleep percentage among groups of mammals is the maturity of animals at birth. Thus, the opossum with its large REM sleep quota is born in a very immature state, whereas grazing animals such as horses, which have relatively little REM sleep (0.6 hours per day), are born mature enough to begin functioning independently soon after birth. One theory to explain a correlation between REM sleep and level of maturity at birth is that REM sleep aids in the development of the nervous system.

This theory is further supported by the fact that the amount of REM sleep in all animals examined so far is maximum at birth and decreases to a lower "plateau in adulthood." In humans, for example, newborn infants spend more than 6 hours a day in REM sleep—more than 3 times the adult amount (see INFANCY, NORMAL SLEEP PATTERNS IN). For this reason, it has been hypothesized that REM sleep may stimulate the brain and thereby aid in its development. This theory does not, however, explain the function of REM sleep in the adult. Nevertheless, although direct evidence for or against this theory is not available, the developmental decrease in amount of REM sleep is so consistent across species that it seems likely that REM sleep does fulfill some as yet unspecified developmental role.

Investigations of neuronal activity during REM sleep have revealed intense activity within the brainstem. The behavioral expression of this activity is normally blocked by a system that prevents activity in motoneurons and thereby blocks movement. Scientists have hypothesized that this intense neuronal activity is a way in which connections are formed within the central nervous system. Such connections might allow animals to express genetically determined behavior patterns. For example, the complex motor patterns required for stalking prey, getting and storing food, or mating may be imprinted on the central nervous system by the motor sequences commanded during REM sleep. This theory is also difficult to test experimentally, because it would require extended periods of REM sleep deprivation, and again, it does not explain the need for extended periods of REM sleep in the adult.

REM and NREM periods normally alternate within the sleep period. Because brain neuronal activity is greatly reduced during NREM sleep, some have hypothesized that REM sleep's function is to stimulate the brain to allow it to recover from NREM sleep. This theory is consistent with the finding that we are much more alert when we awaken from REM sleep than when we awaken from NREM sleep, and the fact that some animals, such as cats, almost always wake up right after REM sleep. Nevertheless, this theory does not adequately explain the long duration of REM sleep (see ATONIA; CYCLES OF SLEEP ACROSS THE NIGHT).

Although much of the brain is intensely active during REM sleep, several populations of neurons greatly *decrease* their activity at this time. Neurons releasing the neurotransmitters serotonin, histamine, and norepinephrine are continuously active during waking, decrease their level of activity during NREM sleep, but are completely inactive during REM sleep (see CHEMISTRY OF SLEEP; REM SLEEP PHYSIOLOGY). Of these transmitters, the functional role of norepinephrine is best understood. This transmitter appears to increase the efficiency of signal processing throughout the nervous system by increasing the response of neurons to signals produced by other neurotransmitters, while reducing the level of background "noise." There is evidence that uninterrupted release of norepinephrine would cause a gradual degradation of this system by reducing the sensitivity of receptor systems for norepinephrine. It may be this loss of sensitivity that we experience as sleepiness. The interruption of norepinephrine release that occurs in REM sleep would prevent this degradation of receptor sensitivity. This pattern of state-related neuronal activity and inactivity, led Siegel and Rogawski (1988) to hypothesize that the maintenance of receptors for these systems of REM-off neurons is a principal function of REM sleep. There is some limited evidence to support this theory, based on recordings of neuronal activity during sleep deprivation. Related theories have hypothesized other neural recovery functions for REM sleep, including synthesis of various neurotransmitters. Further work needs to be done to monitor neuronal metabolism and structure and to establish the time course of any REM sleep effects.

In conclusion, we do not yet know the function of REM sleep. Several possibilities have been suggested and are under active investigation. One or more of these may prove to be correct. However, it may well be that the most critical functions of REM sleep have yet to be suggested.

REFERENCES

Adam K. 1987. Total and percentage REM sleep correlate with body weight in 36 middle-aged people. *Sleep* 10:69–77.

Allison T, Cicchetti DV. 1976. Sleep in mammals: Ecological and constitutional correlates. *Science* 194:732–734.

Jouvet, M. 1978. Does a genetic programming of the brain occur during paradoxical sleep? In Buser P, Rougeul-Buser A, eds. *Cerebral correlates of conscious experience,* pp 245–261. INSERM symposium. Amsterdam: Elsevier/North-Holland.

Rechtschaffen A, Bergmann BM, Everson CA, Kushida CA, Gilliland MA. 1989. Sleep deprivation in the rat: X. Integration and discussion of the findings. *Sleep* 12:68–87.

Roffwarg HP, Muzio JN, Dement WC. 1966. Ontogenetic development of the human sleep-dream cycle. *Science* 152:604–619.

Siegel JM, Rogawski MA. 1988. A function for REM sleep: Regulation of noradrenergic receptor sensitivity. *Brain Res Rev* 13:213–233.

Zepelin H. Mammalian sleep. In Kryger MH, Roth T, Dement WC, eds. *Principles and practice of sleep medicine,* pp 30–49. Philadelphia: WB Saunders.

Jerome Siegel

REM SLEEP MECHANISMS AND NEUROANATOMY

REM sleep is the state in which our most vivid dreams occur. REM sleep in humans and animals can be recognized by the presence of rapid eye movements during sleep. These rapid eye movements are accompanied by "PGO waves," electrical currents resulting from bursts of neuronal activity (see REM SLEEP PHYSIOLOGY). The ponto-geniculo-occipital (PGO) waves originate in the brainstem region called the pons, and then ascend through a nucleus in the thalamus called the lateral geniculate, to the occipital cortex (see PGO WAVES). Another sign of REM sleep is low-voltage brain waves, resembling those seen during waking. The brain waves of waking and REM sleep contrast with the slower and higher-voltage brain waves seen in NREM sleep. The high-voltage waves of NREM sleep are a result of synchronized "idling" activity in adjacent cortical neurons that produces a bigger signal even though less information processing is going on. During waking, adjacent neurons tend to be active at different times so that the currents produced by the neurons cancel each other out. Therefore, the electrical signals that can be recorded from large groups of neurons in waking are smaller (see AROUSAL).

Whereas muscle tone is low in NREM sleep, it is completely absent in many muscles during REM sleep. This loss of muscle tone is thought to prevent the "acting out" of dreams. The loss of muscle tone results from the action of an inhibitory system that blocks activity in the motor neurons in the spinal cord, even while the higher motor systems within the brain are intensely active (see ATONIA).

Since its discovery, sleep researchers have attempted to localize the areas in the brain that generate the REM sleep state. Some evidence has come from brain-damaged humans; however, most has been derived from experiments on rats and cats. Two profound conclusions emerge from this work. One is that the REM sleep is substantially similar in animals and humans. The second is that the generation mechanisms for REM sleep are in the brainstem and not in the cerebral cortex. Both of these conclusions seem to be at variance with the complex symbolic representations and highly imaginative nature of dreams. One might expect that this state would be generated by higher nervous system structures and perhaps be unique to humans.

The localization of REM sleep mechanisms within the brain derives from three kinds of evidence. The first kind can be termed "lesion" evidence. The experimenter studies animals with certain brain regions removed or disconnected. If REM sleep is present after this removal, it can be concluded that the removed region is not required for generating this state.

A second kind of evidence comes from "stimulation" studies. Electrical and chemical stimulation is administered to see if REM sleep can be induced or blocked. If the critical brain area is identified and the right chemical chosen, it should be possible to control REM sleep.

A third type of evidence comes from recording. Microscopically fine electrodes can be placed near or even within neurons in the brain regions that are believed to have an important role in REM sleep control. The presence of recording electrodes does not disturb the normal pattern of sleep–wake states. The experimenter can not only observe whether the electrical activity of the recorded neurons changes in REM sleep, but also determine the neurotransmitters the cells respond to and what the connections of the cells are.

As explained below, all of these kinds of evidence indicate that a portion of the brainstem called the PONS (Figure 1) is the brain area most critical for REM sleep. It had been known since the work of the English physiologist Charles SHERRINGTON that animals could survive removal of the entire forebrain in front of the midbrain (Figure 1). After the discovery of REM sleep, Michel JOUVET analyzed the sleep and waking states in these "decerebrate" (without cerebrum) animals. He found that they had periods of muscle tone suppression with rapid eye movements. PGO spikes, similar to those seen in REM sleep,

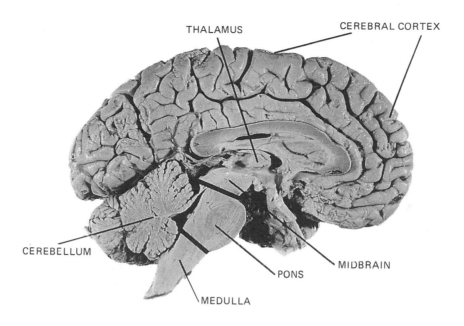

THALAMUS

CEREBRAL CORTEX

CEREBELLUM

MIDBRAIN

PONS

MEDULLA

Figure 1. Midline, or "sagittal," section of the human brain, showing the medial part of the left half. The major subdivisions of the brain have been labeled.

occurred along with the eye movements. The REM sleep state (or PARADOXICAL SLEEP, as Jouvet named it) had a duration similar to that seen in the intact animal. It also recurred cyclically, as it does in the intact animal. This experiment proved that the forebrain was not essential to REM sleep.

Further work showed that REM sleep would occur in animals in which a transection was made just in front of the pons, demonstrating that most of the midbrain was not required for REM sleep. The REM sleep phenomena that can be recorded after such a transection include rapid eye movements, PGO spikes, and suppression of muscle tone. It was also shown that the spinal cord is not required for REM sleep control. Therefore, the pons and MEDULLA alone are sufficient to generate REM sleep.

It is possible to localize the brain regions responsible for REM sleep further by separating the brainstem at the junction of the pons and medulla (Figure 1). We can then look on both sides of the transection to determine which portion of the brain has REM sleep. The medulla of such an animal does not have REM sleep: periods of rapid eye

movement and neuronal activity resembling that seen in REM sleep do not occur, and muscle tone is never completely suppressed. Therefore, unlike the midbrain decerebrate brain, the medullary decerebrate brain is not capable of generating REM sleep.

Whereas the disconnected medulla is not capable of generating REM sleep, the forebrain and pons, when disconnected from the medulla, produce several of the signs of REM sleep. PGO spikes can be observed in the thalamus in association with low-voltage brain waves, as in REM sleep. At these times, the activity of single neurons in the forebrain resembles that seen during REM sleep. These transection studies, therefore, led to the conclusion that the pons contains neurons critical for generating REM sleep. When the pons is connected to the medulla, REM sleep signs occur in the pontine and medullary regions. When the pons is connected to the forebrain, several REM sleep signs are seen in the pons and forebrain.

If the pons is critical for REM sleep control, then damage to it should prevent REM sleep. A number of studies have shown that damage to the pons reduces or eliminates REM sleep. The critical areas are in the reticular formation of the pons. The reticular formation is a region of neuronal cell bodies and axons (the output connections of neurons). The critical portion of the reticular formation is in the lateral regions of a nucleus called the "reticularis pontis oralis" and is just below a group of cells containing norepinephrine called the "locus coeruleus" (see PONS).

Stimulation evidence confirms and extends this conclusion. Injections of chemicals mimicking the actions of the neurotransmitter acetylcholine (see CHEMISTRY OF SLEEP; ACETYLCHOLINE) into the nucleus reticularis pontis oralis can trigger very long periods of REM sleep. This suggests that this chemical is normally released in this area to initiate REM sleep.

Recordings from neurons within the area defined by lesion and stimulation studies have identified several distinct cell types. One type has been called a "REM sleep-on cell." These cells are inactive (i.e., they do not release their neurotransmitter) during waking and NREM sleep, but they are extremely active during REM sleep. Some of these cells may be the ones releasing acetylcholine to trigger REM sleep. It has been shown that most of the REM sleep-on cells do not contain acetylcholine, however, indicating that other neurotransmitters are also important in REM sleep control.

A second major cell type in the critical regions of the pons is the REM sleep-off cell. These cells are continuously active in waking but become inactive in REM sleep. Some of these REM sleep-off cells contain the neurotransmitter serotonin (see PONS). These cells are located on the midline of the brainstem in an area called the "raphe" nucleus. Their activity blocks the expression of PGO waves. The inactivity of these raphe cells in REM sleep allows the PGO waves to appear. Other REM sleep-off cells located in the locus coeruleus nucleus contain the neurotransmitter norepinephrine. While these cells are not essential for generating REM sleep, they may have some role in inhibiting REM sleep. The cessation of activity in REM sleep-off cells may also "rest" the neurons with which REM sleep-off cells connect. This "rest" may be one of the functions of REM sleep (see FUNCTION OF REM SLEEP).

Certain neurons located in the pontine region important in REM sleep control project forward to affect the forebrain. One of these forward-projecting systems contains the transmitter acetylcholine. (Some acetylcholine-containing neurons in the pons project to the forebrain, whereas others project within the brainstem to regions in the pons and medulla.) Certain acetylcholine-containing cells in the pons may be active only during REM sleep, but most are active during both REM sleep and waking. The release of acetylcholine in the forebrain improves the speed and efficiency of information processing (particularly in the THALAMUS, one of the main relays for sensory activity on its way to the cerebral cortex). The release of acetylcholine is thought to be one of the main reasons that brain wave activity is similar in REM sleep and in waking. It may also underlie the similarities between thought processes in these two states. Some acetylcholine systems are particularly active during the PGO waves and associated eye movements of REM sleep. The sudden increases in acetylcholine release during PGO waves may produce the shifting images of dreams.

By activating or inactivating particular cell groups, it is possible to impair or elicit parts of the REM sleep state. For example, damage to a small portion of the nucleus reticularis pontis oralis can disrupt the muscle tone suppression of REM sleep without preventing the rest of the state from occurring. The result is an animal that appears to act out its dreams, a syndrome called REM sleep without atonia (see ANIMALS' DREAMS; ATONIA). A cat with REM sleep without atonia will appear to chase imaginary mice, confront imaginary foes, and explore its environment, while other aspects of its brain activity demonstrate that it is in REM sleep. Humans with damage to this system will in the same way make violent movements during REM sleep as they act out their dreams (see REM SLEEP-BEHAVIOR DISORDER).

Small injections of acetylcholine or of glutamate, another neurotransmitter implicated in REM sleep control, into these same pontine regions can produce a complete suppression of muscle tone without the other aspects of REM sleep. Such animals appear to be fully awake, but cannot move until the chemicals wear off.

This state induced by injections of acetylcholine resembles a state seen in human patients with NARCOLEPSY. Humans with this sleep disorder will collapse when suddenly excited, a condition called CATAPLEXY. During these cataplectic attacks, the patients are awake but are unable to move, just like the animals in which acetylcholine or glutamate has been injected into the pons. It appears that the system normally producing muscle tone suppression in REM sleep becomes active during waking in patients with narcolepsy, although the precise cause of this triggering is not yet known. These patients also experience loss of muscle tone just before going to sleep and when waking up. (This is called SLEEP PARALYSIS.)

The circuit producing muscle tone suppression passes through the pons to the medial medulla on its way to produce suppression of muscle tone in the spinal cord. The critical relay in the medulla is within two cell groups near the midline (the nucleus magnocellularis and paramedianus; see MEDULLA). Damage to the medial medulla can produce the same syndrome of REM sleep without the atonia seen after damage to the pons. Stimulation of these nuclei with acetylcholine and glutamate produces suppression of muscle tone, as in the pons.

The combination of muscle tone suppression with the muscle twitching seen in REM sleep is what makes this state so "paradoxical." Recent work sheds light on how this combination of excitation and inhibition might be generated. Glutamate activates two kinds of receptors in the pons and medulla. One type of receptor ("non-NMDA receptors") produces suppression of muscle tone, while the other type ("NMDA receptors") produces increased motor activity. The simultaneous release of glutamate during REM sleep onto neurons with each of these receptor types may be responsible for this combination of motor excitation, producing rapid eye movements and twitches, with the simultaneous inhibition of motoneurons. The inhibition allows us to have the motor excitation accompanying our dreams, while at the same time protecting us from the injuries that would occur if we actually made these movements while we slept.

If REM sleep is generated in the brainstem, how can it produce dreams with all of their complexity? While REM sleep is present after damage to the forebrain, it is not completely normal. The patterns of eye movements in REM sleep are changed to simpler, more stereotyped sequences after forebrain damage. Studies in humans show that eye movement patterns and intensity are highly correlated with dream content. Therefore, forebrain lesions that change eye movement are likely to have altered dream content. An analogy between forebrain control of breathing and forebrain control of REM sleep can be made. Breath-

ing is known to be controlled by the brainstem. Removal of the forebrain does not prevent normal breathing and regulation of oxygen and carbon dioxide levels in the blood. In the intact individual, however, variations in respiration and related brainstem physiologic variables are sensitive indicators of thought processes, fear, surprise, and other emotions, and can even be used to detect lying, as in polygraph tests. Although respiration is organized in the brainstem, it can clearly be controlled by the forebrain. In the same way, our highest intellectual processes can affect the physiology and dream imagery of REM sleep, even while the generator mechanism resides in the brainstem. Descending connections to the pons from forebrain regions governing complex thought processes (e.g., frontal cortex) and from regions important in emotional control (e.g., the amygdala) have been identified. These descending connections can alter REM sleep generation just as ascending projections from the pons alter forebrain processes during REM sleep. In this way our most subtle thoughts, our most intense fears and desires can interact with brainstem mechanisms to generate our dreams.

REFERENCES

Morrison AR. 1983. A window on the sleeping brain. *Scientific American* 248:94–102.

Siegel JM. 1989. Brainstem mechanisms generating REM sleep. In Kryger MH, Roth T, Dement WC, eds. *Principles and practice of sleep medicine,* pp 104–121. Philadelphia: WB Saunders.

Siegel JM, Rogawski MA. 1988. A function for REM sleep: Regulation of noradrenergic receptor sensitivity. *Brain Res Rev* 13:213–233.

Jerome Siegel

REM SLEEP, PHYSIOLOGY OF

It is widely known that during REM sleep we experience many of the vivid and bizarre hallucinatory episodes known as dreams. However, the striking array of physiologic changes and phenomena that occur during REM sleep are perhaps less familiar to the general public. The following discussion describes the major physiologic occurrences of REM sleep; the possible neuro-physiologic mechanisms underlying the generation of this state; and finally, the possible physiologic functions of REM sleep.

Physiologic Characteristics of REM Sleep

By recording the electrical activity of the brain, eyes, and muscles from mammals while they are asleep, scientists can observe a fascinating phenomenon (see ELECTROENCEPHALOGRAM; REM SLEEP, DISCOVERY OF). Interspersed with slow wave sleep (SWS) episodes are regularly occurring periods of REM sleep. The exact timing of its periodic appearance varies from species to species but REM sleep is usually preceded by SWS and then alternates with periods of SWS throughout the sleep episode (see CYCLES OF SLEEP ACROSS THE NIGHT). This cyclic alternation between REM and SWS is known as the sleep cycle. The cycle is not a circadian rhythm (a rhythm with a period of 24 hours), but rather an ultradian rhythm because its period is less than 24 hours (see CIRCADIAN RHYTHMS; ULTRADIAN RHYTHMS). In humans, REM sleep occurs approximately every 90 minutes during sleep (i.e., four to five times a night) and generally lasts for 5 to 30 minutes—plenty of time for a good dream to play!

During REM periods, a striking paradox occurs. Intense levels of brain activity (representing increased neuronal firing of action potentials throughout the central nervous system)—even greater than that seen in waking—and bursts of rapid eye movements are observed at the same time as a complete loss of muscle tone (Figure 1). Thus, during REM sleep, while we have vivid and fantastic mental experiences, the nervous system is at its highest level of activity and the body's motor system is essentially paralyzed!

REM sleep episodes are also accompanied by ponto-geniculo-occipital (PGO) waves (signs of intense short-lasting bursts of neural activity originating in the brainstem and traveling to the cortex; see PGO WAVES), characteristic "theta" waves originating in an area of the brain called the hippocampus, penile erections, middle ear muscle activity (MEMA), and periodic muscle twitches. Another physiologic phenomenon of REM sleep is a change in the way that the autonomic nervous system functions (see SYMPATHETIC NERVOUS SYSTEM; THERMOREGULATION; RESPIRATION

CONTROL IN SLEEP). The autonomic nervous system is responsible for the modulation of such basic life functions as blood pressure, heart and respiratory rates, and body temperature. During REM sleep, blood pressure and heart rate show increased variability, and the normal regulation of body temperature is lost. Of particular clinical significance is the change in the control of respiratory function. The respiratory response to carbon dioxide levels in the blood, required to keep them in a range compatible with life, is dramatically altered during REM sleep. This may have a critical role in sleep APNEA (cessation of breathing).

It is now known that together all of these physiologic activities comprise the hallmark signs of the enigmatic behavioral state called REM sleep. The unprecedented dissociation of a high level of brain activity from muscle activity (and associated active behavior) has led to another name for this state, "paradoxical sleep." Other researchers have called this state "desynchronized sleep" because of the low-amplitude, high-frequency (i.e., desynchronized) nature of the brain activity. Still another name, signifying the increased neuronal activity, is "active sleep" (as compared with the less "active" brain activity seen in SWS).

Physiologic Mechanisms of REM Sleep Regulation

REM sleep is a state characterized by numerous interesting physiologic activities; the question now posed by many sleep researchers is how these diverse activities are generated and regulated (see REM SLEEP MECHANISMS AND NEUROANATOMY). One of the first questions that must be addressed regarding REM sleep–regulating mechanisms is what parts of the central nervous system are or are not necessary for its generation. A useful way to approach this problem is with experimental lesion studies in which an area of the brain is lesioned (i.e., cut or removed) and the consequent effects on REM sleep determined. One study of fundamental importance demonstrated that in cats a transection of the brainstem at the border between the pons and the midbrain (severing all connections of higher brain centers with those below the midbrain) does not eliminate the periodic appearance of a REM sleep–like

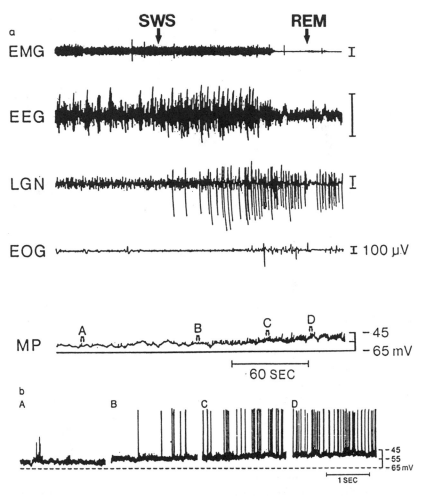

Figure 1. Physiologic characteristics of REM sleep. Top four lines (a): Electrical recordings from muscle (EMG = electromyogram), cortex (EEG = electroencephalogram), thalamus (LGN = lateral geniculate nucleus), and eyes (EOG = electrooculogram). Note that when REM begins (arrow), muscle activity ceases, the EEG becomes desynchronized (low-amplitude waves at high frequencies [speed of recording is too slow to show the frequency]), PGO waves (large deflections) are seen in the thalamus, and periodic rapid eye movements are recorded with the EOG. Bottom two lines (b): Traces showing the transitions from the hyperpolarized (more negative) membrane potential (MP) of SWS to the excited (depolarized, with more action potentials) membrane potential during the REM state of a "REM on" neuron located in the pontine reticular formation. μV, microvolts; mV, millivolts. *Reprinted in modified form from Ito K and McCarley RW. 1984.* Brain research *292:169–175.*

state. This state is like REM sleep in that there is muscle atonia periodically appearing together with pontine (the lower brainstem component "P" of the PGO wave) waves and rapid eye movements. Because there is no connection with the higher brain centers, this experimental state differs in that a highly activated brain and geniculo-occipital (the "GO" component of the PGO wave) waves are no longer present. The conclusion drawn from these studies is that the neural tissue sufficient to generate the periodic appearance of REM sleep is located caudally to the pons–midbrain junction (i.e., in the pons and medulla).

How can the neural tissue of the pons and medulla generate REM sleep? To begin to answer this question it is necessary to realize that this neural tissue is composed of thousands upon thousands of simple neurons interacting in an organized and specific fashion to bring about the complex physiologic changes that define the behavioral state of REM sleep.

Interaction between neurons occurs at the synapse, a specialized structure where two cells communicate, one to another, by an electrochemical mechanism (Figure 2). The presynaptic neuron sends an electrical signal (called an action potential) down its long threadlike process (called an axon) somewhat like a telegraph message traveling down a telegraph wire. When the action potential reaches the presynaptic ending, it causes the release from this ending of a small amount of chemical called the neurotransmitter. The neurotransmitter molecules diffuse across the very narrow region between the pre- and postsynaptic membranes, called the synaptic cleft. On the postsynaptic membrane are specialized molecules that will bind only to the neurotransmitter molecules or to molecules of a shape that mimics the neurotransmitter molecule's shape. These molecules are called receptors. The binding of the neurotransmitter to the receptor activates an effector mechanism within the postsynaptic cell that causes a change in the electrical properties (and sometimes other biochemical properties as well) of this neuron. These changes can either be excitatory or inhibi-

tory in nature depending on the particular receptor–effector complex activated.

A molecule that mimics a neurotransmitter's action by binding to its receptor and activating the effector is called an "agonist" of that neurotransmitter. An important series of studies using neurotransmitter agonists in cats has yielded key information on the neural mechanism of REM sleep generation. These experiments involved the injection of carbachol, an agonist of the neurotransmitter acetylcholine (ACh), into a part of the PONS called the medial pontine reticular formation (mPRF) (see CHEMISTRY OF SLEEP, ACETYLCHOLINE). Surprisingly, the application of this ACh agonist to the mPRF elicits a behavioral state indistinguishable from natural or "physiologic" REM sleep. Under physiologic conditions, specific ACh receptor–effector complexes in the mPRF are activated only when an action potential traveling down the presynaptic ACh-containing neuron's axon has caused the release of ACh into the synaptic cleft. In contrast, under experimental conditions, when the ACh agonist is injected into the mPRF, most of the ACh receptor–effector complexes surrounding the injection site are simultaneously activated. In general terms then, the experiment mimics what would physiologically be a very nonspecific activation of ACh-releasing neurons. It is a very rare occurrence in neurobiology that a highly complex association of physiologic changes (like those seen in REM

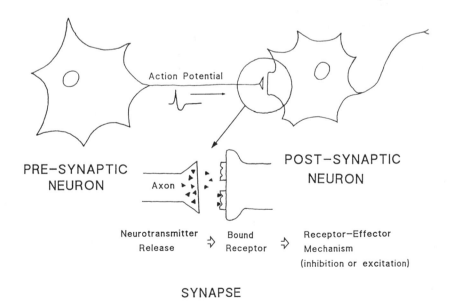

Figure 2. Schematic diagram of a chemical synapse.

sleep) can be evoked by the application of a single neurotransmitter agonist to a very localized area of the brain. One is left with the supposition that the orchestration of the REM sleep phenomena is likely to be derived from the organization of the postsynaptic, ACh receptor–effector complexes located in or near the mPRF.

Although studies like those already described do not exclude the possibility of other mechanisms (e.g., the involvement of other neurotransmitters and/or brain centers), they indicate the likelihood of a very significant involvement of ACh in the generation of REM sleep. To date, ACh agonists are the only chemical substances that have been shown to induce a REM sleep–like state that closely mimics the physiologic REM state. Furthermore, other studies have lent support to the validity of the ACh model of REM sleep generation. These include the demonstration of the necessary anatomic connections between ACh-containing neurons and neurons in the mPRF, and the demonstration of the mimicry of REM effects at the cellular level (i.e., membrane depolarization and excitation) by ACh agonists (Figure 1).

An aspect of REM sleep that is intimately related to its generation is its striking periodicity (SEE CYCLES OF SLEEP ACROSS THE NIGHT; ULTRADIAN RHYTHMS). In fact, any explanation of REM sleep generation should be able to account for the oscillation between SWS and REM sleep during a sleep episode. A most appealing source of this oscillation might be at the cellular level with a pacemaker neuron (i.e., a neuron that fires in periodic bursts, such as those observed in invertebrate nervous systems). Unfortunately, no pacemaker neurons have been observed in the mammalian brainstem, and thus some other kind of oscillator is required. A model of REM sleep cycle oscillation has been proposed that does not require a cellular pacemaker (see RECIPROCAL INTERACTION THEORY). Instead, oscillatory activity may be generated by the reciprocal interaction of two populations of neurons. One population is proposed to be comprised of "REM on" neurons, which excite themselves and the other population, called the "REM off" neurons, which in turn inhibit themselves and the "REM on" neurons. The activity of "REM on" cells peaks when the activity of "REM off" cells is at its lowest, and then the situation reverses itself to complete one period of the oscillatory cycle.

Physiologic Functions of REM Sleep

Closely related to the question of the mechanism of REM sleep generation is the question of REM sleep function (SEE REM SLEEP, FUNCTION OF). Whereas the gross physiologic phenomena of REM sleep are fairly well characterized and the mechanisms underlying REM sleep generation are beginning to be better understood, the physiologic function of REM sleep remains one of the great enigmas of biology. A useful technique researchers have employed to determine the function of physiologic processes has been to eliminate that process and observe the results. For example, to determine the function of eating, the process can be curtailed with the result that the subject becomes malnourished. Thus the function of eating may be deduced to be a means to nourishment. When laboratory rats are prevented from entering REM, their health deteriorates and they eventually die (see DEPRIVATION, SELECTIVE, REM SLEEP). A series of clever experiments have addressed the question of REM sleep function by examining the difference between REM sleep–deprived (experimental) and nondeprived (control) rats. While the control animals appeared absolutely no worse for wear, the experimental animals died after about 30 days of REM sleep deprivation. Preliminary observations of the experimental animals after several weeks of REM deprivation indicate a severe dysfunction of metabolic homeostasis (see METABOLIC CONTROL OF PARADOXICAL SLEEP; METABOLISM). In particular, the REM-deprived rats ate more food but lost weight and lost the normal control of their body temperatures. A similar deficit occurred after deprivation of the "deeper" phases of NREM sleep and after total sleep deprivation. Therefore, it is unclear whether REM sleep has a metabolic function distinct from that of NREM sleep. Clearly, at least in rats, REM sleep is crucial to metabolic well-being and the prolonged loss of REM sleep can be incompatible with life.

Another function proposed for REM sleep is a cognitive one, namely, MEMORY consolidation and the related function of LEARNING (see COGNITION). Studies have demonstrated a correlation between REM deprivation and decreased learning abilities. As with metabolic dysfunction after REM deprivation, it is unclear whether REM sleep itself is directly necessary for normal cognitive function. An analogous situation to the relationship of REM sleep and metabolic homeostasis, or learning, might be the relationship between eating and breathing. Namely, after prolonged food deprivation, respiration will become weaker and eventually cease, yet under normal circumstances, eating is not directly required for breathing. While they do not provide all the answers, REM sleep deprivation studies provide important clues that may lead to a more definitive understanding of the function of REM sleep.

In conclusion, the physiology of REM sleep remains in large part an enigma and thus an exciting challenge to sleep researchers. Currently, REM sleep can be defined only in phenomenologic terms because neither its mechanism of generation nor its function is understood. It is all the more intriguing because we all have first-hand experience of the REM sleep state (in the form of vivid dreams), and perhaps even more important, REM sleep appears to be essential for good health and even life. The elucidation of the physiologic regulation and function of REM sleep is made difficult because of the very nature of the central nervous system itself. Unlike other organ systems, the brain is comprised of a large heterogeneous group of cells that rarely act in a homogeneous fashion to accomplish a given function. The heterogeneity of the central nervous system may demand a detailed understanding at the cellular level to gain insight into the more systemic manifestations, such as REM sleep. Currently, research at both the cellular and molecular level is beginning to yield some very exciting data needed for an understanding of the fascinating behavioral state of REM sleep.

REFERENCES

Kryger MH, Roth T, Dement WC, eds. 1989. *Principles and practice of sleep medicine.* Philadelphia: WB Saunders.

Steriade M, McCarley RW. 1990. *Brainstem control of wakefulness and sleep.* New York: Plenum Press.

Robert W. Greene
Jennifer I. Luebke

REPTILES, SLEEP IN

Nonmammalian vertebrates, such as fish, amphibians, and reptiles, with a longer evolutionary history than mammals may provide clues about the origins of sleep. The living reptiles whose major representatives include the turtles and tortoises, crocodiles and alligators, and lizards and snakes have changed little from their ancient fossil ancestors. Thus, reptiles may provide a living window to the past in better understanding the function of sleep.

Controversy exists as to whether, in fact, reptiles sleep. Like mammals, reptiles meet the behavioral criteria for sleep. These criteria include (1) behavioral inactivity, (2) a characteristic sleep posture, (3) decreased responsiveness to stimulation, and (4) a rapid return to waking with moderate stimulation. Although reptiles show behavior that looks like the behavior of mammalian sleep, this does not guarantee that the underlying physiology is the same. Resting with the eyes closed can look like sleep, but the brain activity during rest and during sleep are very different. Reptiles, in fact, do not show the same electroencephalographic (EEG) patterns during their behavioral sleep that appear on the brain surface of sleeping mammals. Instead of the cyclic alternation between slow wave sleep (SWS) and REM sleep, the most distinctive feature of reptilian brain activity during behavioral sleep is an high-amplitude (300 microvolts), fast (50 to 150 milliseconds) spike potential that occurs throughout the forebrain. This difference between reptilian and mammalian brain activity during behavioral sleep might suggest that reptiles do not exhibit true sleep. However, the reptile brain surface lacks a thick neocortex where the slow waves of mammalian SWS are generated. Recordings from the reptilian brain surface reveal spike activity in brain areas most similar to the limbic system—the "old brain"—of mammals. Recordings from the mammalian limbic system, particularly the ventral hippocampus (VH), reveal a high-amplitude, fast spike potential similar to the reptilian spike. This VH spike is most frequently present in SWS and least frequently present in waking and REM sleep (Hartse et al., 1979). In other words, during behavioral sleep, reptiles show a brain activity that resembles the activity of certain subcortical brain regions of mammals in SWS.

There are striking similarities between the mammalian VH spike and the reptilian spike. Both spikes (1) are high-amplitude, fast waveforms recorded from a similar noncortical brain area; (2) are most frequent during behavioral sleep and least frequent during behavioral wakefulness; (3) increase in number after deprivation of behavioral sleep; and (4) respond similarly to administration of pharmacologic agents. Although reptiles do not display mammalian slow waves, the reptilian spike is similar to the mammalian VH spike, which strongly supports an analogy between mammalian SWS and reptilian sleep. The most detailed studies (Hartse, 1989) do not support the presence of REM sleep in reptiles.

Crocodiles and Alligators

Four distinct postures correspond to progressive behavioral inactivity and an increasing frequency of spikes in crocodiles and alligators (Flanigan, Wilcox, and Rechtschaffen, 1973). The reversibility of behavioral sleep and a decrease in spikes, elevated arousal thresholds during behavioral sleep, and a rebound in both behavioral sleep and spikes after enforced wakefulness show that behavioral sleep is present and that the spikes are a correlate of sleep. Several studies have suggested that behavioral sleep and spikes in the alligator are temperature dependent, because both increase at high ambient temperatures. Because of this relationship to temperature, it has been suggested by some researchers that reptiles do not have true sleep. Although extremes of temperature may affect reptilian behavior and brain activity, this does not eliminate the reptilian spike as a valid indicator of sleep. Mammalian sleep can also be affected by temperature extremes.

Lizards and Snakes

Behavioral sleep, defined by distinctive postures and an increase in spike activity with the most relaxed postures, is present in the iguana. Elevated arousal thresholds to electrical stimulation dur-

ing behavioral sleep and rebounds in behavioral sleep and spikes after enforced wakefulness are present. Disagreement exists as to whether lizards have REM sleep because apparent eye movements have been recorded during behavioral sleep. However, detailed analysis suggests that they are movements of the nictitating membranes that cover the eyeball or retractions of the eyeball that occur during brief arousals from behavioral sleep rather than true eye movements of REM sleep. The loss of muscle tone seen with mammalian REM sleep has not been recorded in conjunction with these apparent eye movements, further suggesting that REM sleep is not present in lizards.

Only one study of sleep has been carried out in a snake. High-amplitude brain waves and elevated arousal thresholds during behavioral sleep were observed.

Turtles and Tortoises

Turtles and tortoises also exhibit behavioral sleep and associated spike activity, elevated arousal thresholds to electrical stimulation and a decrease in spike activity following stimulation, and a rebound in behavioral inactivity and spikes after prolonged wakefulness. The sea turtle, however, has been reported not to exhibit an association between behavioral sleep and spike potentials. In contrast, SWS and REM sleep as well as spike activity during behavioral quiescence has been reported in the European pond turtle. One study of the tortoise failed to show a difference in arousal thresholds during spiking and nonspiking states. Under extremes of temperature, the correlation between behavioral sleep and spikes was no longer present; one research group concluded that spikes are temperature dependent and are not true indicators of sleep. There is clearly disagreement about the presence of behavioral sleep in turtles and tortoises and whether the spikes are indicators of their sleep. Nevertheless, the most carefully controlled studies provide convincing evidence that these reptiles meet the criteria for sleep and that the spikes are correlated with sleep. The administration of pharmacologic agents that act on the brain to cats and tortoises reveals a similar response of the reptilian spike and mammalian VH spike, thus further strengthening the position that the spike is an indicator of sleep in reptiles.

In summary, evidence is strong for behavioral sleep in reptiles and for the reptilian spike as an indicator of sleep, despite some disagreement. Additionally, the best evidence indicates that the reptilian spike is similar to the mammalian VH spike, thus suggesting that sleep in reptiles is most like mammalian SWS. Although we still do not know the exact function of sleep, the presence of sleep in living reptiles suggests that it has ancient origins and that certain sleep states fulfill similar functions in reptilian and mammalian existence.

REFERENCES

Flanigan WF, Wilcox RH, Rechtschaffen A. 1973. The EEG and behavioral continuum of the crocodilian, *Caiman sclerops. Electroencephalogr Clin Neurophysiol* 34:521–538.

Hartse KM, Eisenhart SF, Bergmann BM, Rechtschaffen A. 1979. Ventral hippocampus spikes during sleep, wakefulness, and arousal in the cat. *Sleep* 3: 231–246.

Hartse KM. 1989. Sleep in insects and nonmammalian vertebrates. In Kryger MH, Roth T, Dement WC, eds. *Principles and Practice of Sleep Medicine*, pp 64–73. Philadelphia: WB Saunders.

Kristyna M. Hartse

RESPIRATION CONTROL IN SLEEP

Breathing is controlled by a closed-loop system comprising several elements. Respiratory centers in the nervous system excite muscles whose actions cause ventilation of the lungs where oxygen is taken up by the blood and carbon dioxide is removed from it. The concentrations of oxygen and carbon dioxide in the blood are monitored by sensors that send information back to the respiratory centers (Figure 1). This information signals the adequacy or inadequacy of breathing to the respiratory centers that then adjust their output as needed. This closed-loop system is controlled also by systems outside of the loop: in particular, breathing is influenced greatly by states of consciousness (sleep and wakefulness).

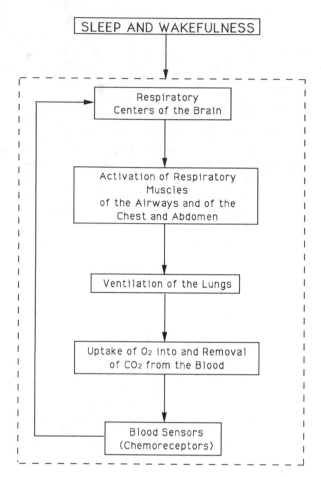

Figure 1. Closed-loop, automatic system for breathing is shown within the box delimited by dashes. As indicated, sleep and wakefulness influence the closed-loop, automatic system. O_2, oxygen; CO_2, carbon dioxide.

The Closed-Loop, Automatic Respiratory System.

The purpose of breathing is to bring oxygen from the atmosphere into the lungs and, on exhalation, to expel carbon dioxide. Without oxygen, consciousness is lost within 10 to 20 seconds, and the brain is damaged irreversibly within 3 to 5 minutes. Levels of oxygen and carbon dioxide in the blood are continuously monitored by chemoreceptors. Low oxygen levels are sensed by chemoreceptors located in the aortic and carotid arteries. These chemoreceptors communicate oxygen debt to the respiratory centers of the brain and cause these centers to increase breathing. High levels of carbon dioxide lead to an increase in hydrogen ion concentration, which is detected by chemoreceptors that are located on the lower surface of the brainstem.

The respiratory centers are located in the PONS and MEDULLA of the brainstem. These centers coordinate breathing: they cause dilation (widening) of laryngeal, pharyngeal, and nasal airways while activating inspiratory muscles (principally the diaphragm muscle and the external intercostal muscles) to create the negative pressures that "suck" air into the lungs. They also control exhalation, either by stopping inspiration and allowing expiration to occur passively (the usual case in quiet breathing) or by activating expiratory muscles such as the abdominal and internal intercostal muscles. Within these centers, the respiratory commands to inspire and expire are produced either by interactions between neurons, by pacemaker neurons, or by combinations of the two.

Control of Breathing in Wakefulness and in NREM Sleep

In mythology, there is the story of Ondine who took automatic breathing from her unfaithful lover. Thus, he was unable to breathe in sleep and died when he could resist sleep no longer (see ONDINE'S CURSE). Fortunately, most of us are not faced with the choice between breathing and sleeping. For us, breathing can occur automatically as we sleep; however, just as with Ondine's lover, patients having lesions in brainstem respiratory areas, or in whom the chemoreceptors are not functioning, can breathe adequately in wakefulness but not in sleep. This finding indicates that, in NREM sleep, breathing depends entirely on the automatic system and that, in wakefulness, breathing is controlled by something more than the automatic system (Figure 2). These differences in the control of breathing in wakefulness and NREM sleep are evident from the different patterns of breathing in the two states: In NREM sleep, the pattern is slow and regular (Figure 3, Table 1); changes in oxygen and carbon dioxide concentrations lead to appropriate changes in breathing. In contrast, the pattern in wakefulness is more rapid and irregular, reflecting state effects on the closed-loop, automatic system. Breathing responses to changes in oxygen and carbon dioxide concentrations are also variable

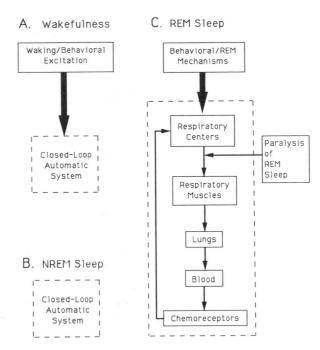

Figure 2. Models of breathing in wakefulness (*A*), NREM sleep (*B*), and REM sleep (*C*). In wakefulness, breathing is stimulated by behavioral or waking neural systems. In NREM sleep, the closed-loop, automatic system functions without influences from outside of it. In REM sleep, behavioral or REM-specific mechanisms, including the paralysis characteristic of that state, influence the closed-loop, automatic system.

in wakefulness and indicate that behavioral or waking influences can override the closed-loop system.

There are two interpretations of the control of breathing in wakefulness. One proposes that multiple behavioral influences in wakefulness excite the respiratory centers. For example, speaking, coughing, crying, and playing a wind instrument are behavioral acts that use respiratory muscles for purposes other than ventilation of the lungs. For these behaviors to occur, the respiratory centers must be controlled by behavioral systems in the brain, and the mere readiness to perform these acts may cause some tonic excitation of these centers. With the onset of sleep, these behavioral waking influences are lost, and the respiratory centers receive less excitatory input. The other interpretation is based on results showing that neural systems that cause wakefulness also excite the respiratory centers. The reticular formation of the midbrain and pons is necessary for waking consciousness. Destruction of this reticu-

522 Respiration Control in Sleep

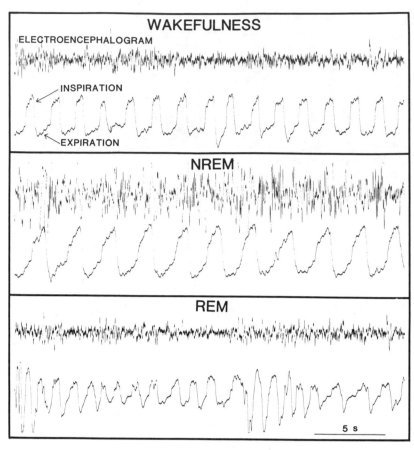

Figure 3. Examples of breathing in the cat in wakefulness, NREM sleep, and REM sleep. Breathing in this case was measured by recording pressures within the airway. Upward deflections (negative pressures) signal inspiration. In wakefulness, breathing was rapid, vigorous, and variable. In NREM sleep, breathing was slow and regular. In REM sleep, it was extremely variable.

lar formation causes coma, and stimulation of it causes not only a cortical and behavioral arousal but also an excitation of breathing. These stimulated effects on breathing are similar to the effects of wakefulness on breathing (see also AROUSAL; COMA).

Control of Breathing in REM Sleep

Breathing depends entirely on the automatic system in NREM sleep, but breathing in REM sleep, as in wakefulness, may depend in part on behavioral systems. The salient feature of breathing in REM sleep is its variability: at one moment it is rapid and irregular, the next slow and regular, or it may even be stopped briefly (Figure 3). One interpretation of this varying respiratory pattern

is that it is related to the content of the dream. Just as the rapid eye movements of REM sleep may arise from the dreamer scanning the dream, the varying respiratory patterns in REM sleep may result from various dreamed activities, such as speech. Another interpretation is that the variable breathing pattern is a manifestation of basic REM sleep processes or phasic events. Other manifestations of these processes are rapid eye movement bursts and muscle twitches; these and the irregular breathing may result from pulsatile activity originating in the pons (see PGO WAVES). This interpretation is attractive because newborns, who have not developed the higher nervous structures necessary for dreaming mentation, have irregular breathing, muscle twitches, and rapid eye movements during REM sleep (see EYE MOVEMENTS AND DREAMING).

Table 1.   Characteristics of Breathing in Sleep and Wakefulness

State	Pattern of Breathing	Respiratory Centers	Respiratory Muscles	Ventilation[a]	Arterial O_2 and CO_2[b]	Responses to O_2 and CO_2
Wakefulness	Vigorous/ variable	High tonic and respiratory activity	Tone/vigorous contractions	12–15 breaths/ min, 0.5 L/breath	$P_{O_2} \approx 100$ mm Hg $P_{CO_2} \approx 40$ mm Hg	Intact; can be overridden behaviorally
NREM sleep	Slow/ regular	Decreased tonic and respiratory activity	Some reduction in tone and vigor	<12–15 breaths/ min, >0.5 L/breath	$P_{O_2} \leq 100$ mm Hg $P_{CO_2} \geq 40$ mm HG	Intact
REM sleep	Variable	Variable; some centers are more active, others are less active	Some muscles lose tone; diaphragm remains active	Variable; difficult to determine because there is no steady state	Variable; difficult to determine because there is no steady state	Variable; difficult to determine because there is no steady state

[a]Values are for a normal 70-kg adult.
[b]P_{O_2} is the partial pressure of oxygen in the blood. P_{CO_2} is the partial pressure of carbon dioxide in the blood.

Certain muscles of breathing are paralyzed or minimally active in REM sleep. Paralysis is a characteristic of REM sleep, and without it, we would act out our dreams. On the other hand, if this paralysis were complete, we would die because of respiratory arrest. The diaphragm, the major inspiratory muscle, is spared the paralysis of REM sleep, but some of the other respiratory muscles are not. The paralysis or lesser activity of these muscles may compromise breathing if the diaphragm is ineffective or if the upper airways are too narrow or collapsible. There is much information on the neural mechanisms responsible for paralysis in REM sleep, but it is not known how the diaphragm is spared this paralysis (see MOTOR CONTROL; REM SLEEP BEHAVIOR DISORDER).

REFERENCE

Phillipson EA, Bowes G. 1986. Control of breathing during sleep. In Cherniack, Widdicombe, eds. *Handbook of physiology.* Sect. 3: *The respiratory system,* Vol. II: *Control of breathing,* Part 2, pp 649–689. Bethesda, MD: American Physiological Society. This is the single best review of the subject, but it is not for the fainthearted.

John Orem

REST

In everyday speech and even in dictionary definitions, the words "rest" and "sleep" are often used interchangeably. People often say that they "need a good night's rest" when, in actuality, they really mean that they "need a good night's sleep." Sleep research studies have determined that just resting—that is, just lying awake in bed—is not the same as being truly asleep. It has been shown that sleep is a unique state of consciousness with special restorative functions that only take place when one is sleeping.

This distinction addresses the issue of the "forced rest" theory of sleep function. While this theory has had many proponents, an early version attributed by Wilse B. Webb to Claparede (1905) suggested that the FUNCTION OF SLEEP is to ensure that the organism regularly enters a period of unresponsiveness to the environment. The period of nonresponding was postulated to be important because it kept the organism safely in its bed during the night away from predators and helped the organism to conserve energy by lowering metabolic rate.

The most simple and direct test of the forced rest theory is to determine whether sleep itself becomes unnecessary when a person just lies in bed quietly. Nathaniel Kleitman first examined the difference between sleep and rest in studies begun in 1922. His sleep research subjects undressed and went to bed at their usual bedtimes but were required to remain awake throughout the night. Dr. Kleitman noted that it was possible for these subjects to stay awake during the first night of the study but that, on the second night, they kept falling asleep and had to be awakened repeatedly. Bed rest did not take the place of sleep in these subjects, and despite lying down, they still became sleepy and showed a need to go to sleep.

Sleep deprivation research studies have also shown that resting does not prevent the performance changes that occur when people are deprived of sleep (Lubin et al., 1976). These studies showed that subjects who are permitted to rest in bed but are not allowed to sleep show the same types of psychomotor and cognitive performance decrements as do sleep loss subjects who are not confined to the bed during the vigil (see DEPRIVATION, TOTAL, BEHAVIORAL EFFECTS).

Many other common experiences and research data converge to underscore the concept that rest and sleep are distinct activities. Bedridden patients sleep and humans in prolonged social and temporal isolation also need to go to sleep. In research on the effects of weightlessness in space, long-term bed rest has been used as a research model in studying the effects of weightlessness on physiological functions; it is noteworthy that subjects who participate in these extended bed rest studies also show true sleep.

More recently, it has been learned that too much rest may cause sleep problems. Chronic bed rest interferes with the circadian sleep–wake rhythm and leads to sleep fragmentation. In the elderly, who often spend a great deal of time lying down, sleep is often highly fragmented. Going to bed too early and just lying awake until the natural bedtime occurs may cause insomnia. Conversely, sleep restriction is a procedure for treating patients who complain that their sleep is broken and fragmented. In this procedure, the patient is allowed to lie down to sleep for only limited periods of time, in an effort to consolidate sleep and make sleep more efficient (see also SLEEP RESTRUCTION: THERAPEUTIC).

Based on current knowledge, the old adage that if one cannot fall asleep one should just rest awake in bed is poor advice.

REFERENCES

Kleitman N. 1963. *Sleep and wakefulness*. Chicago: University of Chicago Press.

Lubin A, Hord DJ, Tracy ML, Johnson LC. 1976. Effects of exercise, bedrest, and napping on performance decrement during 40 hours. *Psychophysiology* 13:334–339.

Webb WB. 1974. Sleep as an adaptive response. *Percept Mot Skills* 38:1023–1027.

Webb, WB, Agnew HW. 1973. Effects on performance of high and low energy-expenditure during sleep deprivation. *Percept Mot Skills* 37:511–514.

Cheryl L. Spinweber

RESTLESS LEGS SYNDROME

See Insomnia; Periodic Leg Movements

RESTORATION

See Fatigue—Recovery Model; Functions of Sleep; Slow-Wave Sleep

RHYTHMIC MOVEMENT DISORDER

Rhythmic movement disorder refers to the various patterns of stereotyped and repetitive large body movements that occur during drowsiness, often continue into light sleep, and sometimes appear within deep sleep. These behaviors are common and usually normal in early childhood but occasionally persist or occur in older children or adults. The cause of these behaviors is not always clear, and treatment (if necessary) may be difficult.

This pattern was described as far back as 1727. Terms used previously, *jactatio capitus nocturna* and *rhythmie du sommeil*, have been largely replaced by *rhythmic movement disorder* because the newer term is easier to understand and it includes all of the various motor patterns that may been seen in this condition.

Three main forms predominate: headbanging, bodyrocking, and headrolling.

- *Headbanging:* The child may rock on his hands and knees and bang the front of his head into the headboard or wall, he may lie on his stomach and bang his face into the pillow or mattress, or he may sit upright and bang his head backward against the headboard or wall.
- *Bodyrocking:* Bodyrocking is similar to headbanging, except the child rocks either on her hands and knees or while sitting upright but does not bang her head.
- *Headrolling:* The child lies on her back and rolls her head from side to side. Older children and adults may simply roll their legs back and forth.

Most of these movements seem to help the child fall asleep and disappear soon after sleep is established. They may recur after middle-of-the-night awakenings, and some children will rock or bang in the morning before they are fully awake. Most often events stop within 15 minutes but some children are able to continue for up to 1 hour or longer. Although similar patterns are seen in some individuals within well-established and deep sleep (REM and all stages of NREM), this is less common.

Rocking at some point in the day is common in young children. Most infants and toddlers do this occasionally, and about 20 percent of them do this frequently. Perhaps 10 percent have well-established rocking patterns linked to the night and sleep, and another 5 percent have nighttime headbanging or headrolling.

Although there is considerable variation, these rhythmic behaviors typically start at 6 to 9 months of age. It is uncommon for the onset to occur after 18 months. Regardless of when they start, these behaviors are usually gone within 18 months and generally are not present after a child reaches age 4. Headbanging is more common in boys but the other forms occur with equal frequency in both sexes. Occasionally this tendency seems to run in families.

It is easy to imagine how rocking may be pleasurable to children and help them fall asleep (parents frequently rock their children to sleep). It is harder to understand how a child might find headbanging soothing and how this might help him or her fall asleep. Perhaps it is similar to being patted on the back. There is no good explanation yet available to explain the occasional persistence of these behaviors into deep sleep.

Bodyrocking and headbanging (day and night) as well as other self-stimulatory behaviors are also common among children with certain major disorders, especially mental RETARDATION, blindness, and autism (see BLINDNESS). The physical and psychological problems are usually readily apparent, and some of these children may bang hard enough to injure themselves and need special protection such as a helmet. But serious injury in an otherwise normal child is not common. Nighttime rocking or banging is almost never a symptom of epilepsy.

Rhythmic movements can reflect anxiety, emotional needs, and anger, especially in older children. Perhaps a child's concentration on these movements helps "take his mind off" his worrisome thoughts. Or by banging, she may "force" her parents to come into the room: she gets more attention and sees that her parents are all right, but she may also make them very angry.

The usual form of rhythmic movement disorder seen in early childhood is considered a developmental problem because it is outgrown with age. Usually no treatment other than reassurance is necessary. The main problems come from the noise associated with prolonged vigorous headbanging or sometimes from the loud rhythmical humming that may accompany rocking. These may keep other family members awake. Sometimes environmental changes help, such as letting the child sleep on a mattress away from the wall or placing a metronome near the child's bed. If the child is old enough and aware of these behaviors, various behavior modification programs are possible, including contracts, rewards, and star charts, as well as rocking or humming practice sessions ("overpractice") when wide awake. Limiting a child's time in bed to the actual number of hours he or she sleeps may eliminate the extra wake time that is only spent rocking or banging. Anxiety or emotional needs must be met directly and appropriately during the day, not through a pattern of angry interventions at night. Medication, particularly a class of tranquilizers called BENZODIAZEPINES, is sometimes helpful. Finally, children with major physical or psychological disturbances need special therapy for their particular problems.

Rhythmic movement disorder is a common developmental behavior seen in normal young children as an aid to sleep and usually is outgrown by age 4. Sometimes the behaviors are unusually violent, long-lasting, and disruptive. They may occur in much older individuals and within deep sleep. And they may occur in children with neurological, sensory, and psychological abnormalities. In such cases, treatment may be warranted.

REFERENCES

American Sleep Disorders Association. 1990. *International classification of sleep disorders,* pp 151–154. Lawrence, Kans.: Allen Press.

DeLissovoy V. 1962. Head banging in early childhood. *Child Dev* 33:43–56.

Ferber R. 1985. Headbanging, body rocking, and head rolling. In Ferber R, ed. *Solve your child's sleep problems,* pp 191–200. New York: Simon & Schuster.

Klackenburg G. 1971. Rhythmic movements in infancy and early childhood. *Acta Paediatr Scand [Suppl]* 224:74–83.

Sallustro F, Atwell CW. 1978. Body rocking, head banging and head rolling in normal children. *J Pediatr* 93:704–708.

Thorpy M. 1990. Rhythmic movement disorders. In Thorpy MJ, ed. *Handbook of sleep disorders,* pp 609–629. New York: Marcel Dekker.

Thorpy MJ, Glovinsky P. 1989. Jactatio capitis nocturna. In Kryger M, Roth T, Dement WC, eds. *Principles and practice of sleep medicine,* pp 648–654. Philadelphia: Saunders.

Richard Ferber

S

SANDMAN

The Sandman has been delivering dreams for many centuries, but his origins are as elusive as the character himself. References to the Sandman can be traced back to the Middle Ages (1100 to 1300 A.D.) and are believed to originate in German or Scandinavian folklore. Throughout the twentieth century, the Sandman has been a popular subject of children's stories, songs, and poetry in many different languages.

Described as either an elf or a bearded old man wearing a nightcap, the Sandman carries a large sack of magic dust that he sprinkles in the eyes of children to induce sleep and pleasant dreams. In the past, he has also been referred to as the "Dustman," but this name may have faded because of its more modern association with garbage collection. The Sandman travels on moonbeams when darkness falls; thus, the phrase *Sandman time* has been used to describe the time when parents gather their children together for an evening of storytelling and lullabies. In some stories, the Sandman sings or plays a magic pipe to make children sleepy. Legend says that the small grains found in the eyes after sleeping are proof of the Sandman's nocturnal visits.

Although the Sandman is usually associated with children's literature, several novels titled *Sandman* have been published in recent years (Martins, 1990; Crockett, 1990). A British murder story mentions the Sandman in a darker context (Gibson, 1984).

In 1954, the Sandman made his musical claim to fame in a number-one hit song written by Pat Ballard and performed by the Chordettes called *Mr. Sandman*. This tune can still be heard on the radio from time to time, often inspiring people to sing along with the familiar first words, "Mr. Sandman, bring me a dream." Also included in the Sandman's musical repertoire is a children's operetta in which a goblin steals the Sandman's bag of sand, and none of the children can sleep until at last it is returned (Maler, 1901).

It is said that children who lie awake hoping to catch a glimpse of the Sandman as he goes about his work will be sadly disappointed, for he stays out of sight and disappears with the first rays of the sun; however, those who close their eyes and let him cast his spell will find their slumber filled with plenty of sweet dreams. (See also BEDTIME STORIES; LULLABY; LITERATURE, SLEEP AND DREAMS IN; POPULAR MUSIC, SLEEP AND DREAMS IN.)

REFERENCES

Bonte W. 1904. *The Sandman rhymes.* New York and Boston: HM Caldwell Co.

Crockett L. 1990. *Sandman.* New York: Tor.

Gibson M. 1984. *Sandman.* London: Heinemann.

Maler A. 1901. *The Sandman: A fairy operetta for the grades.* San Diego, Calif.: Silver, Burdett, & Co.

Martins R. 1990. *Sandman.* New York: Macmillan.

Mayhew R, Johnson B. 1924. The Sandman. In *The chimney corner bubble book that sings.* Camden, N.J.: Victor Talking Machine Co.

Semra A. Aytur

SAWTOOTH WAVES

The sawtooth wave is the only electroencephalographic feature characteristic of REM sleep.

527

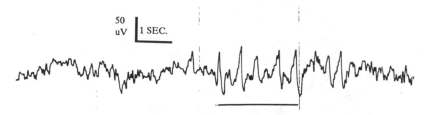

Figure 1. Electroencephalogram recording during REM sleep from the left central scalp (C$_3$ electrode) using the right ear as a reference electrode. Five consecutive sawtooth waves are underlined. SEC., second; uV, microvolts.

With the onset of REM sleep, the ELECTROENCEPH-ALOGRAM (EEG) changes its appearance from a pattern dominated by K-COMPLEXES, SLEEP SPIN-DLES, and slow waves, to a faster, lower-amplitude irregular pattern similar to that seen in stage 1 sleep. Sawtooth waves are 2 to 6 cycles per second and occur intermittently throughout the REM period, usually in runs lasting 1 to 5 seconds (Figure 1). They frequently accompany bursts of rapid eye movements, although they can also appear just before the onset of the REM period. The waves are most apparent over the frontal and central scalp. In a typical recording, with negativity of the active electrode producing an upward deflection, the waves have a triangular shape: A slow initial upward phase is followed by a sharp downward deflection, so that the wave resembles a sawtooth. Sawtooth waves help to distinguish the EEG of REM sleep from the EEG of stage 1 NREM sleep, which is also a low-amplitude irregular pattern of mixed frequencies. (See also ELECTROENCEPHALOG-RAPHY; STAGES OF SLEEP.)

REFERENCE

Erwin CW, Somerville ER, Radtke RA. 1984. A review of electroencephalographic features of normal sleep. *J Clin Neurophysiol* 1:253–274.

Michael Aldrich

SCANNING HYPOTHESIS

See Eye Movements and Dreaming; Psychophysiology of Dreaming

SCHIZOPHRENIA

See Hallucinations; Psychopathology (nondepression)

SEASONAL AFFECTIVE DISORDER (SAD)

Seasonal affective disorder (SAD) is a form of clinical DEPRESSION in which a person regularly (virtually every year) becomes depressed in certain months and then, without treatment, becomes well again during other months. In the 1980s, researchers in the United States at the National Institute of Mental Health began working with patients who became depressed in the fall and winter months. They found that fall/winter SAD could be treated by exposing the patients to bright light (Rosenthal et al., 1984) (see LIGHT THERAPY). In addition, some medications have been reported effective (Teicher and Glod, 1990). Subsequently, patients with the opposite annual pattern of affective disorder have been described (Wehr et al., 1989, 1991). Among the few patients with spring/summer SAD who have participated in studies so far, most did not respond to light therapy. However, it seems that exposure to heat makes depression worse for many summer SAD patients and exposure to cooler temperatures may bring improvement.

SAD has been found throughout the world. Survey studies along the east coast of the United States have shown that the proportion of people affected by SAD varies with changes in latitude (Rosen et al., 1990). In addition, many individual cases have been described in which moving to a more northern (polar) latitude has brought on fall/winter SAD or made it more severe, whereas moving nearer to the equator has led to improvement. Overall, approximately 5 percent of the U.S. population surveyed have described SAD in which the annual depression becomes severe enough to be categorized as a major depressive episode. Up to another 15 percent to 20 percent of the population report seasonal changes that are similar in kind, but less severe. This has been called "subsyndromal" SAD (Kasper et al., 1989). Among the total 20 percent to 25 percent of the population estimated to experience problematic seasonal changes, at northern (polar) latitudes the vast majority have the fall/winter type. However, closer to the equator, a greater proportion have the spring/summer type.

The term "depression" has many different uses. In mental health, depression is diagnosed when a person has a number of symptoms that last for at least several days (but can last for months) and that include feeling sad, "down," or unable to get interested in things that used to be enjoyable. In addition, a negative thought pattern and a tendency to withdraw from others are common. The diagnosis of depression is also based on signs of physical change, such as in energy level, sleep, and appetite. In the case of fall/winter SAD, the most common complaint is lack of energy. These patients tend to oversleep in the fall and winter, both going to bed earlier and arising later. Many report NAPPING; however, they do not report irresistible needs to sleep during the day. Although survey studies suggest that similar seasonal changes in sleep length are commonly found even in people without depression (Wirz-Justice, Kräuchi, and Wirz, 1991), electroencephalographic recordings (see EEG) during sleep in a small number of fall/winter SAD patients have suggested that in the winter, before light treatment, they have decreased sleep efficiency, decreased delta sleep percentage, and increased REM density (but normal REM LATENCY) compared with the summer months and compared with nondepressed individuals in winter (see SEASONAL EFFECTS ON SLEEP). Light therapy seems to reverse these electroencephalographic changes. It is not clear at the present time how they relate to other symptoms of SAD.

Patients with spring/summer SAD more frequently experience INSOMNIA when depressed, and also tend to eat less and lose weight. Fall/winter SAD patients usually report having an increased appetite, particularly for carbohydrates, and they seem to eat more starchy foods in the late afternoon and evening (Kräuchi, Wirz-Justice, and Graw, 1990). The carbohydrate craving typical of fall/winter SAD has led to a hypothesis that these patients have a disturbance of the neurotransmitter serotonin, and that carbohydrate consumption restores their brain serotonin (Wurtman and Wurtman, 1989). This theory led to therapeutic tests of an experimental serotonin-enhancing drug, d-fenfluramine, which was reportedly successful in treating fall/winter SAD. However, the serotonin hypothesis requires further evaluation (Anderson et al., 1991).

Initially, it was reported that fall/winter SAD patients also tended to become extremely overactive and overly optimistic (hypomanic) in the spring. This has led people to think of SAD as a form of bipolar affective disorder (a disorder that includes not only episodes of depression, but also episodes of mania or hypomania). However, since that time many research centers have failed to find a high proportion of fall/winter SAD patients with hypomania (National Institute of Mental Health, 1990). Hypomania also has not been reported by a high proportion of spring/summer SAD patients.

At the present time it is not known what causes seasonal affective disorders. In addition to the hypotheses regarding serotonin, researchers have suggested that disturbances of 24-hour body rhythms (see CIRCADIAN RHYTHMS) are involved (National Institute of Mental Health, 1990). Mental health professionals had long recognized that some people tend to have relapses at the same time of year; but before the 1980s this had been thought about mainly from a psychosocial standpoint. The relapses were attributed to seasonal situational factors, such as job availability or stresses, or to psychological factors (sometimes called "anniversary reactions").

More recently, the definition of SAD and interest in light exposure as a treatment (see LIGHT THERAPY) grew out of speculation that depressions might be regulated within the body in a similar way as hibernation is in animals (see HIBERNATION). Annual cycles such as hibernation are known to be regulated primarily by seasonal changes in the length of the day (photoperiod). Day length influences the times at which the hormone MELATONIN is released within the body, and in many species it is the pattern of melatonin availability that regulates seasonal changes in physiology and behavior. When it was demonstrated in the early 1980s that bright light could affect melatonin in humans, researchers tested to see whether bright light could also influence depressions that developed as the days grew shorter in the fall. Although the bright light exposures have been successful in treating the fall/winter depressions of SAD patients, the role of melatonin in this process is not clear. In addition, there are many important differences between hibernation behavior and SAD. The most influential hypothesis regarding fall/winter SAD has been that patients undergo a shift in the timing of certain circadian rhythms that can be shifted back by exposure to bright light (Lewy, Sack, and Singer, 1990; National Institute of Mental Health, 1990). This and other hypotheses continue to be tested.

In the United States, an interest group formed in the 1980s comprised of members of the general population as well as mental health professionals. The National Organization for Seasonal Affective Disorders (NOSAD; P.O. Box 40133, Washington, D.C. 20016) helps to foster research and education regarding SAD.

REFERENCES

Anderson JL, Wirz-Justice A, Graw P, Kräuchi K. 1991. Light therapy and fall/winter depression: Links to serotonin, melatonin, and headache. In G Nappi et al., eds., *Headache and depression: Serotonin pathways as a common clue,* pp 109–132. New York: Raven.

Kasper S, Wehr TA, Bartko JJ, Gaist PA, Rosenthal NE. 1989. Epidemiological findings of seasonal changes in mood and behavior: A telephone survey of Montgomery County, Maryland. *Arch Gen Psychiatry* 46:823–883.

Kräuchi K, Wirz-Justice A, Graw P. 1990. The relationship of affective state to dietary preference: Winter depression and light therapy as a model. *J Affective Disord* 20:43–53.

Lewy AJ, Sack RL, Singer CM. 1990. Bright light, melatonin and winter depression: The phase-shift hypothesis. In Shafi MA, ed. *Biological rhythms, mood disorders, light therapy, and the pineal gland,* pp 143–173. Washington D.C.: American Psychiatric Press.

National Institute of Mental Health. 1990. Seasonal mood disorders: Consensus and controversy. *Psychopharmacol Bull* 26:465–530.

Rosen LN, Targum SD, Terman M, Bryant MJ, Hoffman H, Kasper SF, Hamovit, JR, Docherty JP, Welch B, Rosenthal NE. 1990. Prevalence of seasonal affective disorder at four latitudes. *Psychiatry Res* 31: 131–144.

Rosenthal NE. 1989. *Seasons of the mind.* New York: Bantam.

Rosenthal NE, Sack DA, Gillin J, Lewy AJ, Goodwin FK, Davenport Y, Mueller PS, Newsome DA, Wehr TA. 1984. Seasonal affective disorder: A description of the syndrome and preliminary findings with light therapy. *Arch Gen Psychiatry* 41:72–80.

Smyth A. 1990. *SAD: Winter depression—Who gets it, what causes it and how to cure it.* London: Unwin.

Teicher MH, Glod CA. 1990. Seasonal affective disorder: Rapid resolution by low-dose alprazolam. *Psychopharmacol Bull* 26:197–202.

Wehr TA. 1989. Seasonal affective disorders: A historical overview. In Rosenthal NE, Blehar MC, eds. *Seasonal affective disorders and phototherapy,* pp 11–32. New York: Guilford.

Wehr TA, Giesen H, Schulz PM, Joseph-Vanderpool JR, Kasper S, Kelly KA, Rosenthal NE. 1989. Summer depression: Description of the syndrome and comparison with winter depression. In Rosenthal NE, Blehar MC, eds. *Seasonal affective disorders and phototherapy,* pp 55–63. New York: Guilford.

Wehr TA, Giesen HA, Schulz PM, Anderson JL, Joseph-Vanderpool JR, Kelly K, Kasper S, Rosenthal NE. 1991. Contrasts between symptoms of summer depression and winter depression. *J Affective Disord* 23:173–183.

Wirtz-Justice A, Kräuchi K, Wirz H. 1991. Season, gender and age: Interaction with sleep and nap timing and duration in an epidemiological survey in Switzerland. World Federation of Sleep Research Societies Congress; Cannes, France; Abstract submitted.

Wurtman RJ, Wurtman JJ. 1989. Carbohydrates and depression. *Sci Am* 260:68–75.

Janis Anderson

SEASONAL EFFECTS ON SLEEP

Seasonal effects on sleep have been of interest to researchers at least since the early 1920s. The major variables that have been studied in this regard are changes in total sleep duration and, to a lesser extent, alterations in sleep quality. In one of the earliest empirical studies to focus on this question, Haas (1923), a German scientist, reported that sleep was deeper in winter than in summer. Later studies seemed to confirm this finding, as it was found that movements during sleep were reduced in winter compared with summer. It was also reported that the ability to recall dreams followed a seasonal pattern, with poorest recall coinciding with the highest motility levels in summer. Neither of these measures, however, was found to be associated with how well rested people felt on awakening in the morning.

Several (though not all) studies have also found that people generally sleep longer in fall and winter than in spring and summer. For example, after studying the sleep habits of several hundred children, one investigator found sleep to be longer in winter than in summer (Erwin, 1934). Yet, a similar study in a different group of children found no such seasonal variations in sleep length (Garvey, 1929). Kleitman and Kleitman (1953) interviewed a group of citizens of Tromsö, a Norwegian town situated north of the Arctic Circle, and found that their reported sleep lengths were about an hour less in summer (7.5 hours) than in winter (8.5 hours). Later studies of the same population, however, and of people from other towns in northern Norway found less dramatic seasonal effects on sleep duration, with sleep lengths differing only by about 15 minutes between summer and winter, again with winter sleep being longer (Weitzman et al., 1975). Differences between these studies are likely to be the result of using more refined data collection techniques in the more recent investigations.

Researchers investigating usual sleep lengths of people living at much lower latitudes (i.e., closer to the equator) have also reported similar seasonal differences. A questionnaire survey of 249 Australian medical students found that they slept about a half-hour less in summer than in winter (7.8 hours compared with 7.3 hours) (Johns et al., 1971). This difference was the result not of seasonal changes in the time of going to bed, but rather of earlier rising times during the summer months; by contrast, in Kleitman's earlier study the shorter sleep in summer was attributed not to earlier rising times, but to later bed times. A similar reduction in average nighttime sleep duration from winter to summer was also reported for a large group of American college students (White, 1975). In this sample, however, NAPPING was also considered separately. When total sleep per 24 hours was examined, no differences were found between winter and summer months. In other words, the college students made up for their shorter nighttime sleep in summer by more frequently taking daytime naps.

Though it must be kept in mind that most studies of seasonal effects on sleep have relied on self-reports rather than actual sleep laboratory measures, there is general agreement that small differences in usual nighttime sleep length and sleep quality do exist between winter and summer. What factors are most likely to account for these apparent seasonal effects? A number of possibilities have been put forth, including seasonal variations in ambient temperature, humidity, and precipitation, as well as changes in body temperature, urinary metabolites, and other internal circadian rhythms. For example, one investigator reported that people slept best in the late fall, when calcium metabolism was at its highest (Laird, 1934). Another study (Kleitman, Cooperman, and Mullin, 1933) concluded that motility was less in winter, primarily because the bed sheets were colder!

Probably the most evident factor, however, and the one believed by most researchers to be instrumental in bringing about seasonal changes in sleep is the change in the ratio between day and night that characterizes the different seasons. This notion is supported by the general finding that seasonal differences in sleep tend to be greater as one moves further from the equator, that is, as seasonal differences in day/night ratios become larger. North of the Arctic Circle, for example, summertime is characterized by constant daylight, whereas winter days have no real daylight and only a few hours of twilight (see LIGHT). The longer nighttime hours of winter may make going to bed earlier and/or waking up later more likely. Moreover, and perhaps more important, the natural alteration in day length associated with the change in seasons can strongly influence our social and work schedules. In turn, these alterations in our daily regimens are likely to have an impact on our sleep–wake patterns.

REFERENCES

Erwin D. 1934. An analytical study of children's sleep. *J Genet Psychol* 45:199–226.

Garvey C. 1929. An experimental study of the sleep of preschool children. In *Proceedings of the 9th International Congress on Psychology*, pp 176–177.

Haas A. 1923. Ueber Schlaftiefenmessungen. *Psychol Arb* 8:228–264.

Johns M, Gay T, Goodyear M, Masterton J. 1971. Sleep habits of healthy young adults: Use of a sleep questionnaire. *Br J Prev Soc Med* 25:236–241.

Kleitman N. 1963. *Sleep and wakefulness*. Chicago: University of Chicago Press. Contains exhaustive bibliography, including the early studies referred to in this article.

Kleitman N, Cooperman N, Mullin J. 1933. Motility and body temperature during sleep. *Am J Physiol* 105:574–584.

Kleitman N, Kleitman H. 1953. The sleep–wakefulness pattern in the Arctic. *Sci Mon* 76:349–356.

Laird D. 1934. Seasonal changes in calcium metabolism and quality of sleep. *NY Med J Med Rec* 139:65–67.

Weitzman E, deGraaf A, Sassin J, Hansen T, Godtlibsen O, Perlow M, Hellman L. 1975. Seasonal patterns of sleep stages and secretion of cortisol and growth hormone during 24-hour periods in northern Norway. *Acta Endocrinol* 78:65–76.

White R. 1975. *Sleep length and variability: Measurement and interrelationships*. Unpublished Ph.D. dissertation, University of Florida.

Scott S. Campbell

SEIZURES

See Epilepsy

SENOI DREAM THEORY

The Senoi of Malaysia were a peaceful society, described as a highly civilized people who were protected by their isolation until they were largely destroyed by modern, mechanized warfare by both the Allied and Japanese troops during World War II. Studies of these people found that they were nonviolent and that there were no obvious cases of mental illness in this culture, possibly as a result of their theory of dream control and utilization. Knowledge of the Senoi dream control technique is based mostly on this particular culture of the past, but today, dream researchers continue to study the people that they call the Senoi, who are actually two groups that are closely related culturally, the Temiar and the Semai (Domhoff, 1985).

The Senoi hold a unique cultural perspective on dreaming, viewing dreams as a "co-reality" with waking life. Co-reality in this sense is the existence of the dream world along with the waking world, so that if something occurs in one, it occurs in the other. The Senoi rely on dreams as an important guiding force throughout their lives, believing that dreams are a reflection of ongoing life events and a result of accumulated tensions. Senoi children are encouraged from an early age to use their dreams to manipulate reality. Children tell their dreams to their fathers every morning and then receive advice about how to correct the situation in the waking world. Parents teach their children not to fear dreaming, as the unpleasant or threatening aspects of dreams merely represent parts of themselves with which they must come to terms. Instead of ignoring their fear or allowing it to continue, they must either fight and conquer it, make friends with it, or allow it to conquer them (Cartwright, 1977).

In adulthood, the Senoi view sleep as an opportunity for the soul to leave the body during dreaming and to interact with people and objects from distant lands. In the morning, Senoi adults gather in groups to analyze and discuss the experiences from their dreams the night before. They often attempt to bring something back from their dream to share, such as a song, considering dreams to be a source of artistic inspiration. Overall, the Senoi believe there is much to be gained from the close correspondence between dreaming and waking life; for example, it is said that when a dreamer wins a dream battle with an enemy spirit, that enemy becomes a friend who, in waking life, will help the dreamer (Moorcroft, 1989).

(See also CULTURAL ASPECTS OF DREAMING.)

REFERENCES

Cartwright R. 1977. *Night life: Explorations in dreaming*. Englewood Cliffs, N.J.: Prentice-Hall.

Domhoff, G. W. 1985. *The mystique of dreams: A search for Utopia through Senoi dream theory*. Berkeley: University of California Press.

Gackenbach J, Bosveld J. 1989. *Control your dreams*. New York: Harper & Row.

Moorcroft WM. 1989. *Sleep, dreaming, and sleep disorders: An introduction*. Lanham, Md.: University Press of America.

Wolman BB, ed. 1979. *Handbook of dreams: Research, theories, and applications*. New York: Van Nostrand Reinhold.

Krista Hennager

SENSORY PROCESSING AND SENSATION DURING SLEEP

In humans and animals, sleep usually occurs in a quiet and dark environment. We try to minimize sensory stimulation while we sleep. Our ability to perceive and to respond to external sensory information is also greatly reduced during sleep. Yet, sleep is not a state of total unresponsiveness. Sensory transmission in the periphery (the regions in which nerves terminate) is mostly preserved in sleep, basic processing of sensory information is actually not affected or only slightly suppressed at many levels of the central nervous system, and humans can perform certain simple tasks during sleep. Brain processing of sensory information is determined by many factors other than sleep stages. These may include intensity, meaningfulness, and prior experience with the stimulus; accumulated sleep time; the amount of prior sleep deprivation; and individual differences in reaction to sensory stimulation.

Auditory

Auditory processing in the periphery does not appear to change greatly across sleep–wake states. The evoked response in the round window of the cochlea, an indication that sounds have been transformed to neural impulses, is not affected by state changes. The primary evoked responses in auditory relay nuclei (e.g., cochlear nucleus, inferior colliculus, and medial geniculate nucleus of the thalamus) are also either unchanged or only slightly reduced during sleep. Some sleep-related modulation may come from phasic contractions of the middle ear muscles (i.e., tensor tympani and stapedius), as sound transmission is reduced during these middle ear muscle activities (MEMA). MEMA are normally elicited by loud sounds, presumably to protect the ear from damage by the sound, and are activated during movements of the body, head, jaw, and face in waking. They also occur spontaneously during REM sleep in association with PGO spikes, when information transmission in higher auditory centers may be altered (see PGO WAVES). Spontaneous PGO-like spiking activities can be recorded in the cochlear nucleus during REM sleep, and PGO-like waves can be evoked by novel stimuli of several sensory modalities. These phasic events may facilitate information transmission within the brain. (See also MIDDLE EAR MUSCLE ACTIVITY.)

Sleep states affect how the cerebral cortex processes auditory information. In general, the amplitude of the electrical response evoked by auditory stimuli is augmented during slow-wave sleep (SWS), and reduced during REM sleep, as compared with waking.

Humans show a variety of responses to auditory stimulation during sleep. They are seen in the electroencephalogram (as a K-complex or desynchronization), in the autonomic nervous system (e.g., heart rate, finger plethysmograph, and galvanic skin response), or in the motor system (e.g., reflexes, finger movement, and button push). These responses also differ in different stages of sleep. For example, the ability to make differential responses to meaningful versus non-meaningful stimuli (e.g., one's own name versus other people's names) is greater during stage 2 and REM sleep than in stages 3 and 4. Auditory awakening threshold in humans follows a similar trend, as they are more easily awakened from stage 2 and REM sleep than from SWS. The significance of the stimulus also determines how easily a person can be awakened. For example, a recorded baby's cry awakens mothers more easily after they deliver than before they deliver.

Most reflexes are reduced during SWS and diminished or greatly reduced during REM sleep, except for the auditory-evoked eye blink reflex. This orbicularis oculi reflex is either not changed or only slightly reduced during REM sleep as compared with waking, but is greatly reduced during SWS as compared with waking.

Visual

Visual processing is affected by sleep in much the same way as auditory processing. Visual stimulus response in the periphery (e.g., retina) is not changed by sleep. However, as the information is transmitted through higher brain centers and to the visual cortex, its processing is increasingly diminished by sleep stages. In animal studies, light stimulation produces a reduced response in the LATERAL GENICULATE NUCLEUS (LGN) and cortex during sleep. As in auditory transmission, the visual signal is also modified, even facilitated, during the occurrence of PGO waves. It has been suggested that these phasic changes in sensory processing during REM sleep may function to preserve the stability of the visual image, much like the "corollary discharge" of the visual system that stabilizes the image during eye movements in waking. (See also VISUAL SYSTEM.)

Humans can respond to visual stimulation during sleep. This capability is higher during stage 2 and REM sleep than during stage 3 and 4 sleep.

Somatosensory

Tactile transmission in the periphery (i.e., through the dorsal column of the spinal cord) does not change across sleep stages, except during bursts of rapid eye movements. Somatic transmission is greatly suppressed during the phasic eye movements of REM sleep. In contrast to the situation in the spinal cord, somatic transmission in the central relay station, the THALAMUS, is generally suppressed during sleep. Cortical response to somatic afferent stimulation is also depressed during sleep. Transmission through these higher centers, however, may be enhanced during bursts of rapid eye movements in REM sleep.

The subjective pain threshold in humans is increased in sleep, as is the itching threshold, determined by the frequency of spontaneous scratching in patients with skin disease. People are less likely to scratch in stages 3 and 4 than in REM sleep or stages 1 and 2. Our bodily response to environmental temperature change is diminished in SWS and greatly suppressed in REM sleep. Eye movements in response to head acceleration (vestibular nystagmus response) is greatly suppressed during SWS, but is preserved to some degree during REM sleep.

The eye blink reflex can also be evoked by somesthetic stimulation during sleep. This reflex is affected by state changes, as is its elicitation by auditory stimulation: the amplitude is not changed or only slightly reduced during REM sleep, but is greatly reduced in SWS.

Olfactory

There are only a handful of studies on olfaction during sleep (see SMELL DURING SLEEP). The available evidence suggests that olfactory processing occurs during sleep, though greatly suppressed. Humans react to odors behaviorally, autonomically, and centrally during SWS and REM sleep about 15 percent of the time.

Other

Behavioral responses to internal stimulation are also affected by sleep stages. Both humans and animals can be awakened by an increase in blood pressure. In humans, arousal threshold to blood pressure elevation induced by intravenous infusion of the vasoconstrictor angiotensin II is lower in stage 2 and REM sleep periods than in stages 3 and 4.

Summary

State-dependent modulation of sensory processing has been found at several levels in all modalities. Our brain, on the one hand, tries to preserve basic sensory information during sleep, yet on the other hand suppresses our ability to perceive and to respond to sensory inputs. In this way the brain assures prompt processing of important or life-threatening information, but also assures sleep continuity if the signal is insignificant. Much of our knowledge about sensory processing during sleep derives from experiments measuring electrical potentials and neuronal activities evoked by sensory stimulation. The sleep-related changes in these parameters do not provide an obvious explanation of the diminished perception and behavioral responses to sensory stimulation during sleep. The complete explanation may await a true understanding of the functional connection of those objective physiologic measures to the subjective perception of sensory signals.

REFERENCES

Bonnet MH. 1982. Performance during sleep. In Webb, WB, ed. Biological rhythms, sleep, and performance, pp 205–237. New York: John Wiley.

Jones GM, Sugie N. 1972. Vestibulo-ocular responses in man during sleep. *Electroenceph Clin Neurophysiol* 32:43–53.

Livingston MS, Hubel D. 1981. Effects of sleep and arousal on the processing of visual information in the cat. *Nature*, 291:554–561.

McGinty DJ, Seigel JM. 1983. Sleep states. In Satinoff E, Teitelbaum P, eds. *Handbook of behavioral neurobiology: 6. Motivation*, pp 105–181. New York: Plenum Press.

Oswald I, Taylor AM, Treisman M. 1960. Discriminative responses to stimulation during human sleep. *Brain* 73:440–453.

Poitras R, Thorkildsen A, Gagnon MA, Naiman J. 1973. Auditory discrimination during REM and non-REM sleep in women before and after delivery. *Canadian Psychiat Assoc J* 18:519–526.

Price LJ, Kremen I. 1980. Variations in behavioral response threshold within the REM period of human sleep. *Psychophysiology* 17:133–140.

Reding GR, Fernandez C. 1968. Effects of vestibular stimulation during sleep. *Electroenceph Clin Neurophysiol* 24:75–79.

Savin JA, Paterson WD, Oswald I. 1973. Scratching during sleep. *Lancet* 2:296–297.

Schneider-Helmert D. 1983. Experimental elevations of blood pressure induced as an internal stimulus during sleep in man: effects on cortical vigilance and response thresholds in different sleep stages. *Sleep* 6:339–346.

M. F. Wu

SENTINEL HYPOTHESIS

In the 1960s, there was intense speculation on the function of the newly discovered state of REM sleep, shown to be present in essentially all mammals and birds. Dr. Fredrick Snyder of the National Institutes of Health proposed that REM sleep served a "sentinel" function for survival. It had already been noted that, after arousals from REM sleep, mental activity is quite clear and performance levels generally high, whereas slow-wave sleep is followed by mental confusion, poor memory, and much poorer performance. It was also known that REM periods are often terminated by a brief arousal. Snyder (1966) proposed that in REM sleep the brain is prepared for optimal waking function and that the arousals after and in REM sleep were nature's way of permitting recurrent "sentinel" scanning of the environment for predators. This would serve survival better than would long periods of continuous sleep. However, when predatory cats were placed near rats, the sleep of the latter did not show any changes that the theory would predict, such as more frequent or longer arousals from REM sleep. This intuitively appealing evolutionary hypothesis therefore remains unconfirmed.

REFERENCE

Snyder F. 1966. Towards an evolutionary theory of dreaming. *Am J Psychiatry* 123:121–136.

Roger J. Broughton

SEROTONIN

See Chemistry of Sleep: Amines and Other Transmitters; L-tryptophan

SEX AND SLEEP

The bed constitutes the physical point of intersection between sleep and sexual activity. Although both sleep and sexual activity can and do occur elsewhere, sexual intercourse is traditionally a presleep, bedtime activity in Western society. Normally, sexual activity concludes with orgasm. For most individuals, orgasm is associated with a deep feeling of relaxation and well-being; therefore, the notion that presleep sexual activity should augment or in some manner improve sleep has great intuitive appeal. It is on this basis that many clinicians believe sexual activity before sleep may be therapeutic for some patients with sleep onset insomnia. If sexual performance anxiety and/or failure to reach orgasm occur, however, the resulting tension and frustration are likely to prolong the latency to sleep and possibly create additional sleep problems. Indeed, a case series exists describing several patients with sleep disruption after coitus (Wise, 1981).

In some individuals, however, even successfully consummated sexual activity produces an overall increase in general arousal that may interfere with sleep. This reaction, which reputedly occurs more often in women, may be related to adrenocorticoid release. Orgasm in women is accompanied by uterine contractions, which in turn are associated with oxytocin release. This can stimulate adrenocorticoid release. Obviously, this chain of effects does not occur in men. Studies demonstrating sex differences (elevation in females) in plasma adrenocorticoid levels 30 minutes after sexual activity are reported for humans.

Several prospective, systematic investigations of the effects of presleep sexual activity on subsequent sleep have been done. Overall, no consistent differences in sleep were found between nights preceded by sexual activity and those in which participants abstained from sexual behavior. Polygraphic indices of sleep integrity and architecture were neither improved nor adversely affected by sexual activation in humans. Even in young adult heterosexual men who abstained from sex for an average of 10 days and then had presleep intercourse, the only finding was a slight increase in sleep stage 3 during the post-intercourse night. Moreover, no change in the duration of sleep-related erections was found between sexual deprivation and sexual satiety nights in these individuals. The number of erections, however, was slightly lower on sexual deprivation nights.

The effect of viewing an erotic movie just before going to sleep at night has also been studied. Symbolic sexual dream content (see CONTENT OF DREAMS; SEXUAL SYMBOLISM) under these circumstances increases; however, dramatic increases in sexual themes are not observed. One must realize that if one's "dream day" ends with erotic visual stimulation under laboratory conditions in which sexual arousal is under observation, these events can make a significant contribution to the "daytime residue" directing dream content. Surprisingly, presleep visual erotica, with or without masturbation, has no effect on the frequency, magnitude, or duration of nocturnal penile tumescence. The relationship between sexual dream content and erectile or genital activation during sleep is a complex one (for more detail, see SEXUAL ACTIVATION). In general, manifest sex-

ual dream content is rare; however, when dreams are about sex we may be more likely to remember them.

NIGHTMARES are a different story. In some cases, dreams about being raped or sexually assaulted can be an expression of a specific fear or a more general metaphor for the violation of self and personal boundaries. By contrast, victims of sexual assault with posttraumatic stress disorder often have "flashback" nightmares that are detailed re-enactments of the incident (see POSTRAUMATIC NIGHTMARES; RECURRING DREAMS). In some patients, the memory of a sexual assault during childhood can be repressed; however, the trauma may become manifest in the form of a recurrent, frightening dream. The recurrent nightmare and its associated disruption of sleep usually remit with successful treatment of the condition.

Genital and reproductive organs activate periodically during sleep. Penile erections, clitoral erections, increased vaginal blood flow, and uterine contractions all occur in close association with REM sleep (see NOCTURNAL PENILE TUMESCENCE and SEXUAL ACTIVATION for more detail).

The discovery of REM sleep quickly led to intense investigation of selective sleep stage deprivation. In the hope of uncovering the differential functions of REM and NREM sleep, experimenters deprived laboratory animals and volunteer subjects of REM sleep. They then observed and recorded changes in a wide variety of physiological and behavioral activities. Perhaps one of the most dramatic and unexpected findings was a substantial increase in sexual activity in many laboratory animals deprived of REM sleep. Increased sexual pursuit and mounting occurred in both normal and hyposexual animals. Cats and rats would sometimes have frenzied sexual activity and mount virtually anything, including blocks of wood. An analogous sleep-related increase in sexual interest in humans was demonstrated in a rather ingenious study by Zarcone, De La Pena, and Dement (1974). Reproductions of several famous paintings containing sexual features were viewed by volunteers after sleep deprivation. The duration of gaze at specific sections of the paintings with high sexual content increased after sleep deprivation and was highest after REM sleep deprivation. (See DEPRIVATION: SELECTIVE NREM SLEEP; DEPRIVATION: SELECTIVE REM SLEEP; FEMALE SEXUAL RESPONSE)

Sexual activation produced by experimentally

induced sleep deprivation stands in stark contrast to self-reports from individuals with sleep disorders. Patients with INSOMNIA often report feelings of "sexlessness" and decreased sexual desire (libido). Loss of libido also characterizes DEPRESSION (also a leading cause of insomnia). Furthermore, many ANTIDEPRESSANTS cause impotence. Laboratory sleep studies have shown diminished nocturnal penile tumescence among men suffering from major depressive disorders. This indicates that erectile failure in men with depression reflects more than decreased sexual desire.

Sleep–wake disorders that cause excessive daytime sleepiness are also frequently associated with sexual problems. Erectile failure afflicts 30 percent to 48 percent of men with clinically significant sleep APNEA. Moreover, in some cases, successful treatment leads to the return of sexual potency. The mechanisms linking sleep apnea and impotence are not known; furthermore, they may differ from one patient to the next. Loss of libido secondary to excessive sleepiness or apnea-related depression may be the cause. However, decreased testosterone levels in men with sleep apnea have been reported. Libido and erectile function vary directly with testosterone. Finally, autonomic nervous system changes produced by chronic periodic hypoxia can undermine normal sexual functioning.

Prevalence estimates for impotence among patients with NARCOLEPSY vary widely, from 17 percent to 67 percent. In some, the problem develops as a side effect of the medications used to treat the disorder (especially tricyclic antidepressants and MONOAMINE OXIDASE INHIBITORS). In others, the comorbid presence of diabetes mellitus (a powerful cause of organic impotence) is responsible. CATAPLEXY, an ancillary symptom of narcolepsy, is a sudden muscle weakness usually evoked by strong emotion. Cataplexy induced by sexual arousal can wreak havoc with some patients' sexual pursuits. Impaired libido secondary to excessive daytime sleepiness, such as is thought to occur in sleep apnea, may play a role. Finally, the theorized underrelease of the neurotransmitter dopamine may contribute to sexual problems in patients with narcolepsy. In men with Parkinson's disease, treatment with *l*-dopa sometimes restores erectile function.

Sleep and sex interrelate in a variety of ways. Sexual and reproductive organs activate during REM sleep, and experimental sleep deprivation can stimulate sexual activity. In contrast, patients suffering from sleep-wake disorders are often sexually dysfunctional. In general, sexual activity before sleep has little effect on sleep integrity, sleep architecture, or the sleep-related erection cycle.

REFERENCES

Karacan I, Howell JW. 1988. Use of nocturnal penile tumescence in diagnosis of male erectile dysfunction. In Tanagho EA, Lue TF, McClure RD, eds. *Contemporary management of impotence and infertility*, pp 95–103. Baltimore: Williams & Wilkins.
Ware JC. 1989. Monitoring erections during sleep. In Kryger MH, Roth T, Dement WC, eds. *Principles and practice of sleep medicine*, pp 689–695. Philadelphia: WB Saunders.
Wise TN. 1981. Difficulty falling asleep after coitus. *Med Aspects Human Sexuality* 15:144ff.
Zarcone V, De La Pena A, Dement WC. 1974. Heightened sexual interest and sleep disturbance. *Percept Motor Skills* 39:1135–1141.

Max Hirshkowitz

SEX DIFFERENCES

See Content of Dreams; Depression; Individual Differences; Normal Sleep

SEXUAL ACTIVATION

During sleep, especially during REM sleep, activation occurs in the sexual and reproductive organs in both men and women. In boys and men, penile ERECTIONS accompany REM sleep episodes. These sleep-related erections have also been called NOCTURNAL PENILE TUMESCENCE (NPT) and periodic penile erections. Under normal circumstances these episodes of tumescence closely follow the pattern of REM sleep; however, this synchrony can uncouple in extraordinary situations. For example, a "REM sleep–like" cycle of erectile activity, recurring every 90 to 120 minutes, will persist even in the presence of drug- or HEAD INJURY–induced REM sleep suppression.

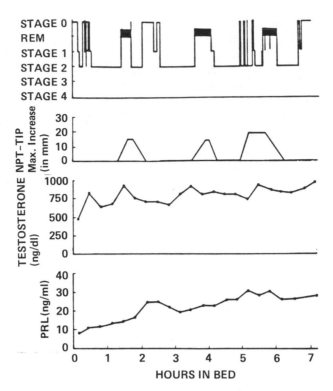

Figure 1. Sleep stages, penile circumference increase recorded from the coronal sulcus (NPT-TIP), and hormonal levels. This figure illustrates a normal pattern of coordination between sleep-related erections and REM sleep. It also shows the normal nocturnal pattern for testosterone level—peaking near each NREM–REM sleep transition. The continual sleep-related increase in prolactin (PRL), peaking near the end of the sleep period, is typical.

Neither presleep sexual activity nor sexual abstinence alters the nocturnal erectile duration (see SEX AND SLEEP). Ontogenetic studies reveal that nocturnal penile tumescence reaches its peak at approximately the time of puberty in young boys. Although some age-related decline occurs in sleep-related tumescence, the quantity, quality, and general pattern persists with only modest changes after 25 to 30 years of age in healthy, sexually potent men. Furthermore, high anxiety does not produce diminished nocturnal erections unless it interferes with REM sleep. Dream anxiety may produce perturbations in nocturnal erections; however, overall erectile activity is not impaired. In the early 1970s, these and other considerations led Ismet Karacan to speculate that polysomnographic assessment of sleep erections could be useful for differentiating between psychogenic and organic impotence. Stated simply, the operating principle

regards the presence of normal erections during sleep as evidence of functional erectile capacity. In such cases, therefore, the impotence is thought to be related to psychological, situational, or relationship factors. There are several known exceptions to this formulation, including pelvic steal syndrome, Peyronie's disease, neurologically decreased penile sensation, and acute androgen deficiency. Additional diagnostic procedures should be used in conjunction with nocturnal penile tumescence testing to rule out these conditions.

In contrast to the regular and persistent cycle of sleep erections in sexually potent men, tumescence is markedly reduced or absent in many men with complaints of erectile impotence. This is especially true when diseases are present that are known to adversely affect vascular or neural processes. If sleep-related erections fail to occur or are substantially diminished in men who sleep well and have reasonably intact REM sleep, then an organic cause of impotence is strongly suspected. When interpreting sleep erection patterns, one must consider the contribution of concurrent drug therapies. A wide variety of medications adversely affect erectile function and can suppress sleep-related penile tumescence. Such drugs include antihypertensives, antipsychotics, and ANTIDEPRESSANTS. Additionally, recent investigations have revealed sleep erection decrements in patients with major depression. Controversy exists as to whether this indicates that psychological factors can alter nocturnal tumescence or, alternatively, that major depression is principally an organic condition. (See DEPRESSION; ERECTILE DYSFUNCTION.)

Several research groups have attempted to find a sexual activation in women that is analogous to nocturnal penile tumescence. A study of two women with congenital clitoral enlargement sufficient to permit recording with strain gauges revealed an erectile pattern similar to that observed in men. Other studies indicate the presence of REM sleep–related increases in vaginal blood flow and uterine contractility. However, measurement and quantification of these activities are more difficult than with strain gauge monitoring of erections in men. Parameter variability and technical difficulties have impeded the use of these female sexual and reproductive organ activity recordings for differentiating the causes of female sexual dysfunction. (See FEMALE SEXUAL RESPONSE.)

The discovery of a close relationship between sexual organ activation and REM sleep generated renewed interest in sleep among psychiatrists and psychologists. REM sleep, as the neurophysiological state underlying dreams, seemed an appropriate time for psychosexual release (see REM SLEEP PHYSIOLOGY). High hopes of finding a key to the "royal road to the unconscious" and the dream-related "release of instinctual drives" led to dream studies in which REM sleep, nocturnal erections, and vaginal blood flow were scrutinized. Disappointingly, erotic dream content does not characteristically accompany the occurrence of sleep-related erections in man. In fact, notwithstanding the nightly occurrence of nocturnal erections in men and REM sleep–related increased vaginal blood flow in women, laboratory and nonlaboratory sleep studies reveal a low general incidence in overtly sexual dream content. Very stimulating dreams with exceptional

sexual content, however, are more likely to be remembered. Even nocturnal emissions—the so-called "wet dreams"—need not be accompanied by overtly sexual dream content. Nocturnal emission occurs during sleep-related erections, most commonly in adolescent boys.

Presleep exercise and laboratory conditions in which sex organ measurement devices are used may increase the occurrence of sexually symbolic or erotic dream content. This likely reflects the "daytime residue" phenomenon, in which dreams will include features related to significant events of the past day or two ("the dream day"). Under such laboratory conditions that may stimulate sexual dreams, overtly erotic dream content reportedly follows sudden changes in sleep-related erections and vaginal blood flow. In a fascinating but largely anecdotal report, sexual dream content was found when men were awakened after sharp increases in penile circumference. In a more systematic investigation, a similar pattern was found for women. Manifest erotic dream content was highest when awakenings were made during sustained high levels of vaginal blood flow. Sudden increases in vaginal blood flow and sexual dreams were also related.

The overall picture of REM sleep and its features are sometimes framed in terms of the accompanying "autonomic storm" (see AUTONOMIC NERVOUS SYSTEM). The development and maintenance of erectile activity requires parasympathetic nervous system innervation. In contrast, changes in the skin's conductance (i.e., electrodermal activity) usually ceases during REM sleep–related erections. This and the body's reduced thermoregulatory capacity during REM sleep suggest decreased sympathetic involvement. Sympathetic discharge is thought to control detumescence.

Another underlying mechanism relating penile tumescence to sleep involves hormonal changes (see GONADOTROPHIC HORMONES). Specifically, hypogonadism in men can produce impaired libido and potency that can be restored by testosterone replacement therapy. Diminished erectile activity during sleep accompanies acute cessation of testosterone replacement in androgen-deficient men. Sleep-related erections are most frequent in boys around the age of puberty, suggesting that increasing serum testosterone levels may facilitate nocturnal erections. Mean testosterone levels calculated for each stage of sleep do not show a REM sleep elevation. However, studies investigating the pattern of testosterone release throughout the night reveal a relationship. Testosterone levels vacillate throughout the night. However, within each NREM–REM sleep cycle, testosterone levels usually peak during the 30-minute segment surrounding the transition from NREM to REM sleep. By contrast, PROLACTIN increases 60 to 90 minutes after sleep onset and usually is greatest during the last 1 to 2 hours of sleep. Figure 1 illustrates the interrelationships among sleep stage, nocturnal penile tumescence, testosterone levels, and prolactin levels. Prolactin release is sleep dependent; a sleep–wake schedule reversal promptly shifts prolactin secretion so that it remains coordinated with sleep. Diminished libido and impotence commonly occur in patients with hyperprolactinemia (especially when caused by prolactin secreting tumors). Normalization of prolactin with surgery or the use of dopamine agonists restores potency. Nocturnal penile tumescence reportedly diminishes with hyperprolactinemia and recovers after treatment; however, testosterone is also usually subnormal before treatment and normal afterwards.

Finally, one must exercise caution when characterizing REM sleep phenomena as "sexual activity." Although the organs relating to sexual or reproductive function increase in physiological activity, the behavior is not sexual. It is not known whether the mechanisms underlying these sleep-related activities are the same as those involved during daytime sexual arousal. The use of nocturnal indicators for psychogenic and organic impotence in men has proven useful; however, the function of these REM sleep–related events still eludes our understanding.

REFERENCES

Karacan I. 1982. Evaluation of nocturnal penile tumescence and impotence. In Guilleminault C, ed. *Sleeping and waking dsorders: Indications and techniques,* pp 343–371. Menlo Park, Calif.: Addison-Wesley.
Ware JC. 1989. Monitoring erections during sleep. In Kryger MH, Roth T, Dement WC, eds. *Principles and practice of sleep medicine,* pp 689–695. Philadelphia: Saunders.

Max Hirshkowitz

SEXUAL SYMBOLISM

The concept of sexual symbolism in dreams derives primarily from the work and theories of Sigmund Freud. He suggested that male and female sexual organs are often depicted symbolically in dreams; thus, in the interpretation of a dream one can take a dream image (for instance, a cigar) and "interpret" it as referring to the penis. In his discussion of symbolic interpretations of "typical dreams," Freud states, "All elongated objects, such as sticks, tree-trunks and umbrellas, may stand for the male organ; also all long sharp weapons such as knives, daggers and pikes." Rooms, boxes, interior spaces, and doorways will sometimes represent the vagina or the female genitals. He also suggested that riding horses or playing exciting games can sometimes be considered symbols for sexual intercourse.

Sexual symbolism also includes the idea that shapes such as hills can represent the breast or that emerging from water can represent birth. Large numbers of insects, mice, or small creatures of any kind may represent sperm, and so on.

It is difficult to prove the existence of sexual symbolism or of any kind of symbolism in dreams, although case examples can be quite convincing. And in fact, looking for sexual symbols in dreams is not generally considered a major part of dream interpretation, and it was not a major part of dream interpretation for Freud (see FREUD'S DREAM THEORY; INTERPRETATION OF DREAMS). The principal technique introduced by Freud was the method of free association. He emphasized above all that one can understand a dream only by obtaining the dreamer's associations to it and that the same dream image can have very different meanings for different dreamers. When attempting to examine or interpret the dream, one uses the dreamer's associations insofar as possible. It is only when for some reason the dreamer does not provide any associations that Freud suggests one can fall back, with caution, on standard symbols, prominent among which are the sexual symbols mentioned above.

Thus, even Freud emphasizes the minor role that should be assigned to sexual symbolism in interpreting dreams. Others, such as Carl Gustave Jung, or French and Fromm, also pay attention to sexual symbolism but assign it a relatively minor role (see JUNG'S DREAM THEORY).

It is obvious that the dream does not always

treat sexual organs or sexual acts symbolically; in fact, sexual organs and the act of sexual intercourse frequently appear directly in the manifest content of the dream. Possibly, sexual symbolism plays a more prominent role in dreams—and for that matter in jokes, stories, etc.—in settings such as late nineteenth-century Vienna when sex could not be discussed openly and straightforwardly.

REFERENCES

French TM, Fromm E. 1964. *Dream interpretation.* New York: Basic.
Freud S. 1965. *The interpretation of dreams.* Standard Edition, Vols. 4–5. Strachey J ed. London: Hogarth.
Jung CG. 1974. *Dreams.* Princeton, N.J.: Princeton University Press.

Ernest Hartmann

SHIFTWORK

Humans are diurnal, endowed with a biological clock specifically tailored to prepare the body and mind for sleep at night and active wakefulness during the day. Human society is also inherently diurnal in its temporal orientation—expecting work during the day, recreation during the evening, and sleep at night. Thus, the 20 percent or so of the population who are shiftworkers, required to be at work at "unusual" hours, are fighting against both biological and social pressures. These pressures, coupled with the inherent "inertia" of the human circadian system, will inevitably lead to disrupted sleep and impaired waking performance.

Surveys of shift workers (e.g., by Knauth et al., 1980) reveal that they get an average of 7 fewer hours of sleep per week compared with their day-working colleagues. Sleep is often rated as the shiftworker's number one problem, with 20 percent reporting significant sleep disruption. Not surprisingly, shiftworkers also report significant sleepiness at work. Åkerstedt's study of 1,000 train drivers (1982) reports that 11 percent of them admit to "dozing off" at the wheel on most night shifts, and 70 percent "dozing off" at least once.

There are two reasons why a night worker's day sleep is impaired. First, the daylight hours are inherently noisy, with more traffic, children playing, and other outside distractions. Second (and probably more important), is the sleep disruption that comes from within the individual. As mentioned before, the function of the human circadian system (biological clock) is to prepare the body and mind for sleep at some times of the day and wakefulness at others (see CIRCADIAN RHYTHMS). Without this preparation, sleep will be impaired by lack of sleepiness, hunger, and the need to use the bathroom. Waking performance will be impaired by the "shutting down" of processes as the body prepares itself (mistakenly) for a nocturnal sleep episode. Åkerstedt and Gillberg (1982) nicely showed that even in an acoustically shielded laboratory, sleep duration depends on the timing of sleep onset. Even after a missed night of sleep, healthy young volunteers sleep 50 percent less at 7 A.M. than at 11 P.M. Unfortunately, under normal conditions, the human circadian system takes well over a week to adjust to a night work routine (if it ever completely adjusts), and the sleep disruption is therefore chronic.

Sleep is not the only part of the shiftworker's life that is affected, however. While the circadian system is in the process of realigning to a new routine, the individual may suffer from the malaise, irritability, and gastrointestinal distress equivalent to a chronic version of "jet lag." Such effects are a natural consequence of the breakdown in the normal harmony of the circadian system and, as well as affecting the individual himself or herself, can cause significant disruption to the family or household. As Walker (1985) has discussed, shiftwork is a major domestic stressor because of its interference with social interaction and family roles. Parenting roles and the spousal roles of social companion, caregiver, and sexual partner are all compromised by shiftwork, even for evening shift workers, for whom the biological disruptions are minimal.

Health consequences of shiftwork are hard to determine accurately, because the group is inherently a self-selected one, transferring to daywork if they are unable to cope. However, Gordon et al. (1985) have found evidence of increased alcohol and sleeping pill use in rotating shift workers, Rutenfranz, Knauth, and Colquhoun (1976) report increased incidence of gastrointestinal problems, including peptic ulcers; and Knutsson, Åkerstedt, and Orth-Gomer (1986) discovered an increased incidence of cardiovascular disease and the risk factors associated with it. At this stage it is not possible, though, to ascribe a shortening of life expectancy to shiftwork.

Not all shiftworkers are affected equally. A small proportion actively prefer shiftwork, contrasting with an equal-sized group who find it almost intolerable. As Monk and Folkard (1985) report in their review of interindividual differences, people who seem particularly at risk are those over 50 years of age, those who require more than 9 hours' sleep per "night," and those whose natural tendency is to be "morning types"—waking up and retiring to bed early (see MORNINGNESS/EVENINGNESS). Gadbois (1981) reported that women often find shiftwork particularly difficult to cope with because of the additional domestic and child-rearing responsibilities that are expected of them.

Clearly, with all these problems and negative consequences, it is desirable that countermeasures be mounted to improve the shiftworker's lot. Because the problem is a multifaceted one, solutions should be multifaceted too, involving a general education of the shiftworker to chronobiological and SLEEP HYGIENE principles, as well as to the specific mechanics of speeding up the circadian realignment process. Certainly more benign shift schedules can be recommended, and a move away from counterclockwise weekly shift rotation has been shown to reap significant benefits. Also, Czeisler and colleagues (1990) have shown that the use of daylight levels of artificial illumination at work on the night shift and precise specification of 8 hours of total darkness at home from 9 A.M. to 5 P.M. will dramatically speed up the circadian realignment process (see LIGHT). Although sleeping pills may improve daytime sleep, they do not affect the speed of circadian realignment and their long-term use is not recommended. Much more research needs to be done on shiftwork so that the many millions of people affected can be usefully helped.

Conclusions

Shiftwork is a multifaceted problem involving disruptions in sleep, circadian rhythms, and social/domestic harmony. Health can be nega-

tively affected, particularly when the shift schedule is a rotating one. Promising lines of research are concerned with the improvement of shift schedules and the manipulation of time cues that might speed up the phase-alignment process. Education of the shiftworker and his or her family is also a vital component of any shiftwork countermeasure.

REFERENCES

Åkerstedt T, Gillberg M. 1982. Displacement of the sleep period and sleep deprivation: Implications for shift work. *Hum Neurobiol* 1:163–171.

Åkerstedt T, Torsvall L, Froberg JE. 1983. A questionnaire study of sleep/wake disturbances and irregular work hours. *Sleep Res* 12.

Czeisler CA, Johnson MP, Duffy JF, Brown EN, Ronda JM, Kronauer RE. 1990. Exposure to bright light and darkness to treat physiologic maladaptation to night work. *N Engl J Med* 322:1253–1259.

Folkard S, Monk TH, eds. 1985. *Hours of work: Temporal factors in work scheduling*. New York: John Wiley. Brings together such leading international experts as Åkerstedt, Knauth, Kogi, Rutenfranz, and Walker, among others.

Gadbois C. 1981. Women on night shift: Interdependence of sleep and off-the-job activities. In Reinberg A, Vieux N, Andlauer P, eds. *Night and shift work: Biological and social aspects*, pp 223–227. Oxford: Pergamon Press.

Gordon NP, Cleary PD, Parker CE, Czeisler CA. 1985. Sleeping pill use, heavy drinking and other unhealthful practices and consequences associated with shift work: A national probability sample study. *Sleep Res* 14:94.

Knauth P, Landau K, Droge C, Schwitteck M, Widynski M, Rutenfranz J. 1980. Duration of sleep depending on the type of shift work. *Int Arch Occup Environ Health* 46:167–177.

Knutsson A, Åkerstedt T, Orth-Gomer K. 1986. Increased risk of ischaemic heart disease in shift workers. *Lancet* 89–92.

Monk TH, Folkard S. 1985. Individual differences in shiftwork adjustment. In Folkard S, Monk TH, eds. *Hours of work—Temporal factors in work scheduling*, pp 227–237. New York: John Wiley.

Scott AJ, ed. 1990. *Shiftwork*. Occupational Medicine: State of the Art Reviews, vol 5, no 2. Philadelphia: Hanley & Belfus. Offers a contemporary approach and a North American–oriented perspective; chapters give key insights into the problems of shiftwork and ways to ameliorate them.

Rutenfranz J, Knauth P, Colquhoun WP. 1976. Hours of work and shiftwork. *Ergonomics* 19:331–340.

Walker JM. 1985. Social problems of shift work. In *Hours of work—Temporal factors in work scheduling,* pp 211–225. Folkard S, Monk TH, eds. New York: John Wiley.

Timothy H. Monk

SHORT SLEEPERS IN HISTORY AND LEGEND

Psychological investigations of PERSONALITY and sleep have suggested that people who sleep for short periods of time (6 hours or less per night) and function well with this amount of sleep are more calm and efficient than people who require a great deal of sleep (more than 9 hours per night). One research team found that short sleepers typically handled stress by keeping busy, and employed denial as a primary coping strategy when confronted with problems; in addition, short sleepers had negative or neutral attitudes towards sleep in comparison to long sleepers, and also reported fewer dreams (Hartmann, Baekeland, and Zwillig, 1972). It cannot yet be concluded, however, that differences in sleep length or physiological need for sleep are either the cause or the consequence of observed personality differences (see INDIVIDUAL DIFFERENCES).

Many famous historical figures reportedly functioned well with very little sleep each night. For instance, it is said that former British Prime Minister Winston Churchill had remarkable endurance, slept very little, and believed that there was no excuse for fatigue. One biographer recounts the tale of a middle-aged Churchill chiding a younger colleague about sleepiness; when the newly elected official complained of exhaustion in the smoking room of the House of Lords, Churchill reportedly replied, "You have no business to be tired, a young man like you. I have never been tired in my life" (Broad, 1963). Coincidentally, another former British Prime Minister, Margaret Thatcher, is reputed to need only 3 to 4 hours of sleep each night (Holt, 1991).

United States President John F. Kennedy is also said to have been a short sleeper. Accounts of his presidency indicate that Kennedy usually worked in the Oval Office until 2 or 3 A.M. and arose each morning at 7:30, often napping for an hour during the day. Biographers state that JFK showed incredible stamina and worked at a very fast pace. Perhaps in acknowledgment of his own vitality, he frequently recited the famous lines "but I have promises to keep, and miles to go before I sleep, and miles to go before I sleep," from the Robert Frost poem "Stopping by Woods on a Snowy Evening."

As a young man, Napoleon Bonaparte claimed to need only 4 hours of rest in order to feel alert and satisfied. Reports state that as he grew older, however, Napoleon sometimes underestimated his need for sleep and performed badly as a result of fatigue (Hall, 1911).

Thomas Alva Edison was another short sleeper, requiring less than 4 hours' rest per day. It is said that the American inventor kept a couch in his workroom and slept only when he felt fatigued, rather than adhering to a regimented sleep schedule. Edison also investigated the sleep habits of 200 of his factory workers and not only concluded that they were getting "too much" sleep but also succeeded in convincing many of them of this opinion (Hall, 1911).

Nikola Tesla, the Yugoslavian electrical engineer whose inventions include alternating electric current systems, wireless radios, and mechanical oscillators, was reputed to be a short sleeper. According to those who knew him, he worked almost continuously and claimed that the only sleep he got each day consisted of 2 hours during the early morning. During the middle of the night, Tesla conducted experiments with various electrical devices. It is said that local law-enforcement officials grew accustomed to complaints regarding the strange noises and eerie lights emanating from his laboratory at all hours.

Tesla was both a colleague and competitor of Thomas Alva Edison and scoffed at Edison's claim of sleeping only 4 hours per night, insisting that Edison also dozed off for at least two 3-hour naps each day without even realizing it. Ironically, some of Tesla's employees report that Tesla had similar habits. For instance, hotel staff revealed that they frequently saw Tesla standing motionless in his room, as though he was in a trance. During these episodes he became so oblivious to his surroundings that the workers were able to clean his room around him. Perhaps both inventors shared such a strong work ethic and such disdain for sleep that they not only curtailed their nighttime sleep but also repressed their daytime naps.

Certain short sleepers display a different sleep pattern, scattering their few hours of sleep throughout the day in the form of short naps. For instance, Spanish Surrealist painter Salvador Dali seemed to rejoice in sleep but reportedly needed only a quick nap in order to feel refreshed (Parinaud, 1976). One legend holds that Dali would doze in a chair with a tin plate placed on the floor beside it. At the beginning of his nap, he would hold a spoon above the plate and shut his eyes. When the spoon fell from his hands and crashed onto the plate at the onset of sleep, the artist would awaken, feeling completely rejuvenated (Dement, 1972).

Leonardo Da Vinci also spread out his sleep by taking short naps during the day (Stampi, Moffat, and Hoffman, 1990). Da Vinci was reputed to work almost continuously by engaging in a 15-minute nap every 4 hours—a total of 1.5 hours of sleep per day. Centuries later, research is being conducted to examine the advantages and pitfalls of this method of sustained performance in the hopes that it may prove useful to people who work around the clock, such as medical workers, emergency crisis teams, military personnel, and long-distance sailors (see NAPPING). Although the idea of such increased stamina is appealing, experts are quick to caution that true short sleepers are rare, whereas disasters resulting from insufficient sleep are not uncommon (Mitler et al., 1988).

REFERENCES

Broad L. 1963. *Winston Churchill—The years of achievement.* New York: Hawthorn.

Dement WC. 1972. *Some must watch while some must sleep.* New York: Norton.

Hall B. 1911. *The gift of sleep.* New York: Moffat, Yard.

Hartmann E, Baekeland F, Zwillig G. 1972. Psychological differences between long and short sleepers. *Arch Gen Psychiatry* 62:463–468.

Holt J. 1991. Zzzzzzzz: The case for sleep. *The New Republic,* 7 Oct, 25–27.

Mitler MM, Carskadon MA, Czeisler CA, Dinges D, Graeber RC, Dement WC. 1988. Catastrophes, sleep and public policy: Consensus report. *Sleep* 11:100–109.

O'Neill, J.J. 1944. *Prodigal genius: The life of Nikola Tesla.* New York: Ives Washburn.

Parinaud A. 1976. *The unspeakable confessions of Salvador Dali.* Salemson HJ, trans. New York: William Morrow.

Sorenson TC. 1965. *Kennedy.* New York: Harper & Row.

Stampi C. 1989. Ultrashort sleep/wake patterns and sustained performance. In Dinges DF, Broughton RJ, eds. *Sleep and alertness: chronobiological, behavioral and medical aspects of napping,* pp 139–169. New York: Raven.

Stampi C, Moffat A, Hoffman R. 1990. Leonardo DaVinci's polyphasic ultrashort sleep: A strategy for sleep reduction? *Sleep Res* 19:408.

Katherine M. Sharkey

SIESTA

The siesta is a midday nap or rest that is primarily culturally determined. The word *siesta* is Spanish in origin, taken from the Latin *sexta hora,* literally meaning "the sixth hour," counted from the time of awakening in the morning (Ulrich, 1983). Approximately 1 to 2 hours in length, the siesta is usually taken during the afternoon following the noon meal. This allows people in tropical climates to avoid the hottest and most unpleasant part of the day, returning to work in the cooler evening hours. It also takes advantage of the body's normal postlunch "dip" in alertness (see NAPPING; POSTPRANDIAL; CIRCADIAN RHYTHMS). Among siesta cultures the length of nighttime sleep is typically reduced to an average of 4 to 6 hours. Therefore, the total amount of sleep within the 24-hour period still averages about 8 hours (Thorpy and Yager, 1991). Siestas are, therefore, an example of replacement napping.

Tropical regions, between latitudes 45 degrees north and 45 degrees south of the equator, contain most siesta cultures (Webb and Dinges, 1989). The siesta is common in Mediterranean countries such as Spain and Italy and in many parts of Central and South America. In Greece all businesses close in the afternoon for the *messi medianos ipnos* or "sleep in the middle of the day" (Ulrich, 1983). The siesta is also practiced in China, where it is called *xiu-xi (hsiuhsi).* Such napping is sanctioned by the Chinese constitution which states "the working population has a right to rest" (Borbély, 1986). Both peasant farmers and Chinese heads of state take these naps, and sleeping bodies are observed along streets and alleys during the afternoon (Ulrich, 1983). The cultural practice of daytime napping is not common in northern and central Europe or in North America. As Noël Coward wrote, mad dogs and Englishmen go out in the midday sun! It does appear that climate is the greatest determining factor in whether a country has a siesta culture, but not all tropical or equatorial countries indulge in the practice. Another factor that might influence siesta in tropical climates is that excessive heat tends to disrupt nocturnal sleep, which could require a daytime nap to replace lost sleep.

In some countries the practice of siesta has given way to increasing industrialization, leading to the view that "time is money." Studies have shown that fewer daytime naps are taken by people in countries that previously had a siesta culture. For example, as Spain has become more modern and industrialized, the practice of siesta has declined (Rezsohazy, 1972). The siesta, a pleasant and practical means of regaining midday alertness, is one of the first casualties of the pressure of modern society to fit more and more work into the day, cutting into our leisure time and nighttime sleep as well.

REFERENCES

Borbély A. 1986. *Secrets of sleep*. New York: Basic Books.

Rezsohazy R. 1972. The methodological aspects of a study about the social notion of time in relation to economic development. In Szalai A, ed. *The use of time*, pp 449–465. The Hague/Paris: Mouton.

Thorpy MJ, Yager J, eds. 1991. *The encyclopedia of sleep and sleep disorders*. New York: Facts on File.

Ulrich E. 1983. Napping. *Health* 15:50–52.

Webb WB, Dinges DF. 1989. Cultural perspectives on napping and the siesta. In Dinges DF, Broughton RJ, eds. *Sleep and alertness: Chronobiological, behavioral, and medical aspects of napping*, pp 247–265. New York: Raven Press.

Nancy Barone Kribbs

SLEEP ATTACKS

The term *sleep attacks* refers to episodes of irresistible sleep. The first reference to sleep attacks in the medical literature dates to 1877, when Westphal described a patient afflicted with sudden sleep attacks; however, descriptions of inappropriate and abnormal sleep episodes can be found earlier in the medical literature. Today, sleep attacks are believed to be the culmination of a variety of manifestations that are an expression of excessive daytime sleepiness. These manifestations may include feelings of overwhelming sleepiness, pressure or irritation of the eyes, heaviness in the extremities, and occasionally dry mouth. There may also be lapses of memory and automatic behaviors, blurring of vision, diplopia, or vertigo. The objective behavioral signs may include inactivity, closure of the eyes, relaxation of facial musculature, and a need to rest the head. These episodes occur mostly during times of boredom; however, they may occur while one is talking, eating, driving, cycling, swimming, skiing, and even during sexual intercourse. Some people recognize the sleep attacks as imminent, whereas others describe them as occurring without warning. The electroencephalographic features of these episodes would reveal NREM or REM sleep. The attacks often last 15 minutes or less and may occur once or several times during the day. The first descriptions of sleep attacks were in individuals in whom other associated features were also described. These included CATAPLEXY, HYPNAGOGIC HALLUCINATIONS, and SLEEP PARALYSIS, all symptoms associated with NARCOLEPSY. More recently, sleep attacks have also been recognized in other medical conditions such as sleep APNEA syndrome, idiopathic central nervous system HYPERSOMNIA, and insufficient sleep syndrome. It is now recognized that people suffering from sleep attacks always have some degree of excessive daytime sleepiness between attacks. Thus, these episodes are likely to be a manifestation of pathological sleepiness. (See Figure 1 on page 546.)

REFERENCES

Westphal C. 1877. Eigenthümlich mit Einschlafen verbundene Anfälle. *Arch Psychiatr Nervenkr* 7:631–635.

Leon D. Rosenthal

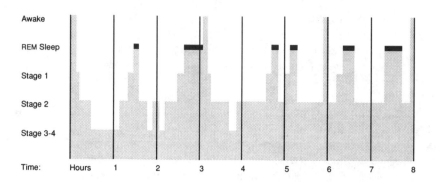

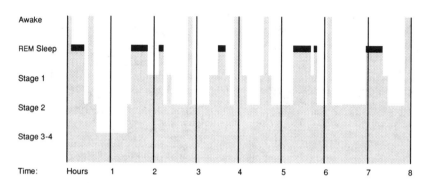

Figure 1. Sleep histogram of a normal adult (on top) and of a patient with narcolepsy (bottom).

SLEEP CYCLE

See Cycles of Sleep Across the Night

SLEEP DISORDERS CENTERS

The disorders covered by sleep medicine extend beyond the boundaries of any single medical specialty (Lemmi, 1990). As a result, sleep disorders centers are the principal medical setting in which sleep-related conditions are diagnosed and treated. In response to a long-standing demand from the public for help with inability to sleep and unexplained daytime sleepiness, the first sleep disorders centers evolved in the early 1970s for the purpose of carrying out inclusive explorations of these difficulties. By 1992, approximately 200 centers will be accredited in the United States. This number only surpassed 50 in

1986 (Figure 1). Sleep disorders centers are now also emerging in Europe.

The Sleep Disorders Center: Opportunity for a Comprehensive Diagnostic Approach

Some sleep disorders centers are "free-standing" but most are part of general hospitals. A significant number are connected with hospitals that are affiliated with medical school and specialty training programs. Though a sleep disorders center is medically staffed usually by one or several sleep medicine specialists, and may also be directed by a psychologist sleep-specialist, all centers are operationally committed to an active, multidisciplinary team approach in diagnosing and caring for patients. With rare exception, patients with sleep difficulties present chief complaints of either INSOMNIA, excessive daytime SLEEPINESS, or abnormal behaviors during sleep

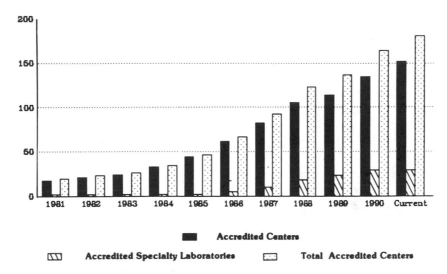

Figure 1.   The steady expansion of sleep disorders centers in the United States accredited by the American Sleep Disorders Association between 1981 and 1991. *Adapted from The APSS Newsletter 6:30,* June 1991.

(see also PARASOMNIAS; HYPERSOMNIA; CIRCADIAN RHYTHM DISORDERS). It has been found that each of these symptoms can have its source in one or a combination of psychological, physical, circadian, or medical disturbances. For this reason, the data gathered in a sleep disorders center by the sleep disorders specialist from the patient's initial, comprehensive interview are used to formulate a *differential diagnosis,* that is, a group of diagnostic possibilities that are the most likely ones to explain the clinical picture. The specialized nature of these candidate conditions may require that either a neurologist, psychiatrist, pulmonary physician, or cardiologist help in confirming the final diagnosis. Such specialists either are on the full- or part-time staff of the center or are available to consult on the center's patients. Sleep disorders centers also frequently provide psychological testing services.

A sleep disorders center optimally brings together under one roof the capacity, just described, for a multispecialty, clinical assessment of patients with the opportunity for round-the-clock, comprehensive, laboratory assessment of their behavioral and physiological sleep–wake functioning (Thorpy and Yager, 1991). Every sleep center performs, when indicated, sleep medicine's primary laboratory test, a polysomnogram—the simultaneous recording of a number of important physiological systems during sleep—and also the MULTIPLE SLEEP LATENCY TEST

(MSLT), which delivers objective quantification of the patient's severity of sleepiness during waking hours. Ultimately, the sleep specialist of a center, when evaluating a patient, must decide whether the ability to make a definitive diagnosis requires either of these polysomnographic studies. If sufficiently confident of his or her clinical, working diagnosis, the specialist may decide to omit sleep recordings. (See POLYSOMNOGRAPHY.)

Physical Facilities of Sleep Disorders Centers

In addition to waiting room, reception, secretarial, transcription, and record-holding areas, most centers have offices for patient intake and follow-up appointments. Generally, a small conference room accommodates case review sessions, teaching, and staff meetings. Virtually all accredited sleep disorders centers have at least two comfortable, temperature-controlled and quiet, individual patient sleep rooms. Privacy is maintained for undressing and changing clothes. Many centers have a special area for patient "set up," the application of electrodes and transducers.

A central "control room" houses the recording polygraphs (Figure 2). All centers have at least one computer for entry, analysis, and storage of epoch-by-epoch sleep recording data. Audio

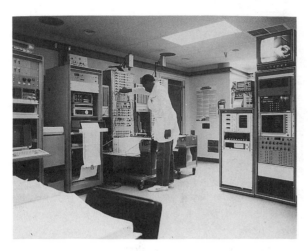

Figure 2. Central control room of the Presbyterian Hospital Sleep Disorders Center, Dallas, Texas. The technician is adjusting the settings during a sleep recording on one of the several polygraph machines, chart recorders, and computers. Three patients are being polysomnographically studied on this night. Note the split-screen video recording that permits a simultaneous picture of the electrophysiological recordings in apposition to the patient's body positions and sleep behaviors.

communication and facilities for video monitoring of motoric activity, body position, vocalization, and facial expression during sleep are standard. Small workshop and supply areas typically support the recording instruments and other apparatus.

All sleep recordings are no longer carried out within the physical confines of sleep centers. Increasingly, sleep disorders centers also exploit portable, "ambulatory," recording instruments. These devices permit survey recordings in the patient's home sleep environment that are stored on optical disk or tape or electronically transmitted on-line back to the center. The recording transducers for such monitoring are usually applied at the center. The tracings are interpreted at the center. Additional recordings may be carried out in the center to check on the survey recordings. (See ACTIVITY-BASED MEASURES OF SLEEP; AMBULATORY MONITORING.)

Accreditation of Sleep Disorders Centers: Why Is It Necessary?

In accordance with state-of-the-art sleep medicine standards, the American Sleep Disorders As-

sociation (ASDA) maintains rigorous criteria that must be met before sleep disorders centers can be accredited or reaccredited. The ASDA Accreditation Committee conducts "site visits" to check on the critical areas of center functioning: the physical facility; emergency cardiopulmonary-resuscitation capability; quality of the clinical diagnostic evaluation procedure; testing and recording techniques; record keeping; report writing; and treatment recommendations (American Sleep Disorders Association, 1988).

A small group of diagnostic facilities, which may be accredited, restrict their sphere of interest to breathing disorders during sleep. They are called specialty laboratories. Recently, several centers of a different type have also been accredited that concentrate on the distinctive disturbances of sleep behavior seen in infants and children. Accurate information does not exist concerning the number of nonaccredited facilities carrying out sleep recordings, but a complete listing of ASDA-accredited sleep disorders centers may be obtained from

The American Sleep Disorders Association
1610 14th Street NW
Rochester, MN 55901–2200
(507) 287–6006

Meeting the standards established for sleep disorders center accreditation depends, in reality, on quality of staffing. The concept of an accredited center presupposes that diagnostic interviewing is conducted or closely supervised by board-certified sleep disorders experts. Such specialists are carefully trained to listen for diagnostically relevant subtleties in the patient's symptom presentation and 24-hour sleep/alertness description. Further, sleep disorders specialists are superior at using patient feedback to alter the course or sequence of available treatments. Experience has shown that, as with diagnostic evaluation, treatment, when left to noncertified sleep specialists, has a lower success rate. Analysis and interpretation of the polysomnogram are the final responsibility of a board-certified sleep disorders specialist. Carefully trained technologists perform the polysomnographic recordings. In sum, accredited sleep disorders centers bring specialized expertise to bear in the three critical encounters with patients: diagnostic interviewing, laboratory assessment (if needed), and treatment delivery.

Case reviews by the entire professional staff of

sleep disorders centers take place at least weekly to establish the diagnosis(es) and treatment plan for every evaluated patient. Most comprehensive sleep disorders centers not only offer treatment recommendations but, in collaboration with the referring doctor, typically begin and may fully carry through the treatment course. Increasingly, centers are developing insomnia treatment programs encompassing psychological, "sleep hygiene," stress reduction, and medication therapies. Specialists in a sleep disorders center are also called on to consult outside the center with practitioners in regard to whether patients require a sleep disorders evaluation.

Research In Sleep Disorders Medicine

Medical schools in the United States have not yet created specific departments and postgraduate training programs in sleep medicine. Consequently, sleep disorders centers constitute the physical as well as academic setting of sleep disorders research and training. The major portion of all sleep disorders research has unquestionably been performed in sleep disorders centers. For this reason, these centers have been vital to the progress in understanding the primary disorders of sleep and also the medical conditions that frequently manifest themselves during sleep.

An additional function of sleep disorders centers is their educational role. They put on a variety of didactic programs concerning the types and treatments of sleep disorders. These programs are geared to the interests of patients, members of patients' families, general physicians, and the public. Centers also offer seminars on public health and transportation and workplace safety risks that result from abnormalities of sleep and sleepiness (see PUBLIC SAFETY IN THE WORKPLACE; PUBLIC SAFETY IN TRANSPORTATION).

REFERENCES

American Sleep Disorders Association. 1988. *Standards for accreditation of sleep disorders centers.* Rochester, Minn.: American Sleep Disorders Association.
Lemmi H. 1990. Sleep disorders centers and polysomnographic evaluation. In Thorpy MJ, ed. *Handbook of sleep disorders,* pp 179–193. New York: Marcel Dekker.
Thorpy MJ, Yager J, eds. 1991. *The encyclopedia of sleep and sleep disorders,* p 203. New York: Facts on File.

Howard P. Roffwarg

SLEEP DRUNKENNESS

See Violence

SLEEP EXTENSION

Sleep extension refers to individuals sleeping longer than their habitual sleep times. Two important questions arise about this phenomenon: (1) Does it exist, and if so, what types of individuals exhibit it and under what circumstances do they do it? (2) What is the significance of sleep extension? Does sleep extension reflect compensatory sleep—that is, do people extend their sleep to make up for an accumulated sleep debt—or are they simply OVERSLEEPING (i.e., consuming sleep beyond their biological sleep need)?

Studies using self-report measures as well as POLYSOMNOGRAPHY show that when people have the opportunity to extend their sleep, they do. According to questionnaire and sleep diary studies, in which individuals report their sleep patterns in their normal environments, sleep extension typically occurs on weekends, and individuals typically report sleeping 1 to 2 hours longer on weekend nights than on weekday nights. In one sleep diary study, subjects who reported they were sleepy extended their sleep on weekends more than those who rated themselves as alert (Rosenthal et al., 1991). In a polysomnographic study evaluating sleep extension, subjects slept in a sleep laboratory in the absence of any time cues and were allowed to sleep as long as they desired (Webb and Agnew, 1975). In this situation, subjects slept longer than their habitual times.

Such data show that people sleep more if given the opportunity; before concluding that people have an accumulated sleep debt resulting from chronically insufficient sleep relative to their sleep need, one must examine the daytime consequences of sleep extension. Several studies have addressed this issue by allowing subjects to sleep 2–3 hours longer than their habitual bed times for 1 to 6 days. In early studies evaluating the effects of sleep extension for 1 or 2 nights, impaired psychomotor PERFORMANCE was found when subjects arose (e.g., Taub, 1980). More recently, studies involving sleep extension for longer periods of time and evaluating daytime functioning across the entire day have shown that sleep extension is in fact associated with improved levels of daytime alertness, as measured by the MULTIPLE SLEEP LATENCY TEST and improved performance on psychomotor tasks (Carskadon et al., 1986; Roehrs et al., 1989). Interestingly, subjects shown to be sleepy before sleep extension showed greater improvements in alertness with sleep extension than did alert subjects.

Taken as a whole, these studies show that many people get less sleep than they require relative to their biological sleep need. This insufficient sleep results in a chronic sleep debt. The sleep debt leads individuals to extend their sleep when given the opportunity. Finally, extended sleep alleviates the chronic sleep debt and provides an accompanying increase in alertness.

(See also FATIGUE-RECOVERY MODEL; FUNCTIONS OF SLEEP; NEED FOR SLEEP; SLEEP LENGTH; THEORIES OF SLEEP FUNCTION.)

REFERENCES

Carskadon MA, Mancuso J, Keenan S, Littell W, Dement WC. 1986. Sleepiness following oversleeping. *Sleep Res* 15:70.

Roehrs T, Timms V, Zwyghuizen-Doorenbos A, Roth T. 1989. Sleep extension in sleepy and alert normals. *Sleep* 12(5):449–457.

Rosenthal L, Kozler C, Roehrs TA, Roth T. 1991. Nap behaviors and subjective daytime sleepiness among college students. *Sleep Res* 20a:241.

Taub JM. 1980. Effects of ad lib extended-delayed sleep on sensorimotor performance, memory and sleepiness in the young adult. *Physiol Behav* 25:77–87.

Webb WB, Agnew HW. 1975. Are we chronically sleep-deprived? *Bull Psychon Soc* 6:47–48.

Thomas Roth

SLEEP FACTORS

See Chemistry of Sleep: Sleep Factors

SLEEP HYGIENE

Sleep hygiene refers to those practices of daily living that promote good sleep and daytime functioning. It does not rely on specialized knowledge, extensive training, high technology, or medical intervention. Sleep hygiene practices are in accord with commonsense as well as with the principles of sleep regulation. For example, a quiet room, winding down after a stressful work day, and restricted caffeine consumption are indeed all conducive to sleeping well.

While nearly everyone has had first-hand experience with the daytime consequences of sleeping poorly, it is less appreciated that our actions during waking hours influence how well we sleep. Sleep hygiene practices represent a distillation of the most important ways in which we are capable of enhancing sleep. Most people will abide by these guidelines intuitively, thereby maintaining the quality of their sleep. However, under the stress of a few sleepless nights, it is not uncommon for panic to set in—and sleep hygiene practices are among the first casualties. Those who can cling to these principles will weather the storm, while those who begin to improvise risk developing a chronic sleep disturbance.

Sleep hygiene comes into play throughout the day, from the moment one chooses to arise with the buzz of the alarm clock until one finally decides to turn off the light. In between, there are all kinds of opportunities to influence sleep for good or ill. The following list is not meant to be exhaustive, but it may yet help you to sleep well.

Regular Bedtimes Foster a Reliable Sleep–Wake Cycle. Retiring and arising at roughly the same time every day synchronizes sleep and other biological rhythms, much as the steady beat of a drummer keeps the rest of the band in step. Repeatedly going to bed at the same time of night also establishes and strengthens associations between factors in the bedtime environment and the process of falling asleep. For example, a sizable number of American adults developed the habit of falling asleep "after the monologue," by which they meant after Johnny Carson's opening monologue on the "Tonight" show. Not only did this cue establish regular bedtimes, it also served to "condition" a relaxed readiness for sleep. Viewers learned to associate the specific cue of the monologue with the drowsiness typically present around 11 P.M. After repeated pairings, the monologue itself could elicit sleep.

Limiting Napping Promotes Nocturnal Sleep and Helps Sustain Alertness During the Day. NAPPING is an effective short-term solution for fatigue and sleepiness. In some SIESTA cultures, a regular nap has been incorporated into the daily routine, resulting in later nocturnal bedtime and shorter nocturnal sleep. Napping in such a regulated fashion may make sense for some individuals in other cultures as well. However, irregular napping appears to be detrimental for most individuals. It reduces nocturnal sleep time; results in light and fragmented sleep; and leads to a vicious cycle of poor sleep, daytime sleepiness, and compensatory napping (see CIRCADIAN RHYTHMS).

The Sleeping Environment Should Be Both Physically Comfortable and Psychologically Conducive to Sleep. Excessive noise and light as well as temperature extremes are some environmental factors that commonly disturb sleep. More subtle disturbers of the peace include the pet that insists on sharing the bed or the human bed partner who begins to snore in the middle of the night.

The bedroom may be a hub of activity rather than a place of repose. It may become the preferred location for television viewing, dining in bed, talking on the phone, or finishing work from the office. In the process, the bedroom loses its association with sleeping. Precluding inappropriate activities from the bedroom will help reclaim the bed as the province of sleep.

The Bed Is No Place to Wait for Sleep. If lying in bed fails to bring on sleep within a short while, then get out of bed. Tossing and turning will only increase agitation and transform what should be a refuge into a battlefield. Spend the time out of bed engaged in quiet activity and return to bed when drowsiness occurs.

Sleep Comes More Readily When the Mind is Tranquil. Thoughts and moods, whether troubling or elating, have the potential to disrupt sleep. Many of these cognitions and emotions are appropriate responses to events occuring during the day; nonetheless, they are incompatible with sleep and should be addressed or set aside at bedtime. The hours before sleep should be a time for gradually "winding down," with less attention paid to the pressing issues of the day. The last hour before retiring might be reserved as a "buffer period" between activity and sleep, when telephone calls are routed to an answering machine, gory newscasts are avoided, and unfinished work is returned to the briefcase.

Sleep Comes More Readily When the Body Is Relaxed. Agitated worry, anger, and strenuous exercise can all lead to physiological arousal that interferes with sleep. Such arousal may be manifest by muscle tension, sweaty palms, and elevated heart rate and body temperature. When somatic tension is present, relaxation exercises have proven effective in reducing the sleep disturbance. EXERCISE can either interfere or enhance sleep, depending on its timing. Although it is prudent to avoid exercising late at night, sustained exercise as well as hot baths taken in the late afternoon may promote sleep at night.

Restricting Time Spent in Bed Consolidates Sleep. Just as the confining banks of a river maintain the water's depth, so restricting time in bed leads to deep, consolidated sleep. There is no set amount of sleep that an individual must accumulate each night; rather, there is a range of sleep times yielding more or less adequate functioning. An individual may consistently opt for the high end of this range in order to minimize the discomfort of fatigue or sleepiness. When this is done, sleep is spread thin and arousals may proliferate. If a shorter bedtime is selected, then nocturnal arousals and light sleep are diminished and the continuity of sleep is preserved. (See SLEEP RESTRICTION, THERAPEUTIC.)

Outdoor Light at the Beginning and the End of the Day Tends to Reset the Biological Clock. To maintain a stable sleep–wake cycle, exposure to outdoor light must be appropriately timed. While this timing will vary among individuals, the following guidelines should prove useful. Exposure to outdoor light in the early morning will "advance" the clock, resulting in earlier evening sleepiness, earlier sleep onset, and morning awakenings. Trouble falling asleep or awakening in the morning can be addressed by exposure to outdoor light in the morning and by avoiding it at dusk. Conversely, exposure to outdoor light at dusk and avoiding outdoor light in the morning will "delay" the clock, leading to prolonged alertness, a later sleep onset, and well-maintained sleep through the early morning hours. These effects are particularly useful for elderly individuals whose biological clocks have become too "advanced"—that is, those who tend to go to sleep and get up too early. (See ADVANCED SLEEP PHASE SYNDROME; LIGHT THERAPY.)

Restricting Moderate Caffeine and Nicotine Consumption to the Early Part of the Day Promotes Good Sleep. The effects of CAFFEINE are stronger and last longer than people realize. In young adults two cups of COFFEE consumed at a midafternoon break will maintain an arousal level at bedtime equivalent to that produced by half a cup taken just before retiring. In older individuals the arousal produced by the same two cups equals the effect of a full cup of coffee taken just before bedtime. The sleep-disturbing effects of caffeine may occur without any subjective sense of arousal. Caffeine is also present in TEA, COLA BEVERAGES, CHOCOLATE, headache remedies, diet pills, and other over-the-counter preparations. As with the effects of napping, habitual use of caffeine leads to a vicious cycle because satisfactory daytime performance comes to depend on continued usage.

NICOTINE is another widely consumed stimulant that disrupts sleep. Smokers think nothing of lighting up after dinner, even as they conscientiously switch to decaffeinated coffee. Cigarettes do exert a calming influence on the habitual smoker, so much so that they are often consumed before bedtime and during nocturnal awakenings. However, the immediate subjective calm produced by smoking belies its subsequent arousing effects.

When Sleep Becomes a Problem, Resist the Temptation of Alcohol and Sleeping Pills, Think Sleep Hygiene. An important goal of good sleep hygiene is learning how to achieve a good night's sleep regularly without relying on sedating drugs and ALCOHOL. It is just at the onset of a sleep problem that some self-regulation is most helpful. Beware of the quick fix, whether it be getting into bed early or staying in bed late to catch up on sleep, napping, or resorting to SLEEPING PILLS or alcohol. Sleep hygiene is an effective long-term strategy for re-establishing a good sleep pattern, but it may require tolerating a period of less-than-optimal sleep and daytime functioning.

Sleep hygiene is of little comfort in the face of calamity. When a short-term solution is essential, the use of pills or alcohol for sleep may be effective. However, there are risks associated with their use, including daytime drowsiness, impaired performance, dysphoric mood, psychological dependence, drug interactions, and drug overdose. In addition, long-term use of these substances diminishes their effectiveness.

Conclusions

Sleep hygiene may be intuitively appealing, but it is not necessarily simple. Often an individual must choose between competing demands—the pull to join the gang for a night out versus the need to be alert for a presentation the next afternoon. We all have our priorities and act accordingly, but the issue does not end with our decision. If it is for a night out, then one still has to decide whether simply to lose sleep or try to compensate by sleeping late into the morning. This latter strategy will not be found in the guidelines listed above, but it is not without benefit. Sleep loss is avoided, as is sleepiness during the presentation. However, sleeping in will affect the timing of the next night's sleep. It may take longer to fall asleep at one's usual bedtime and be more difficult to wake in the morning. So after straggling home at 2 A.M. our party-goer must decide whether to give priority to the short-term objective of maintaining alertness the next day or to the long-term goal of maintaining a stable sleep–wake cycle.

Sleep hygiene puts the findings of sleep research, clinical experience, and popular wisdom into practice. It clears the way for the endogenous rhythm of sleep and wakefulness. When sleep is disturbed, sleep hygiene provides the foundation on which effective treatment is built.

(See also STIMULUS CONTROL FOR INSOMNIA.)

REFERENCES

Hauri PJ, ed. 1991. *Case studies in insomnia.* New York: Plenum.

Hauri PJ, Linde S. 1990. *No more sleepless nights.* New York: Wiley.

Spielman AJ, Caruso L, Glovinsky PB. 1987. A behavioral perspective on insomnia treatment. In Ermin M, ed. *Psychiatric clinics of North America,* pp. 541–553. Philadelphia: Saunders.

Arthur J. Spielman
Paul B. Glovinsky

SLEEP INERTIA

The ability to think and perform is reduced on awakening from sleep. Awakening typically requires a few minutes before it is possible to orient to and interact with the environment. Sometimes this period of transition from sleep to wakefulness can be especially difficult. Confusion, grogginess, and cognitive performance impairment can accompany the effort to awaken. This phenomenon is sleep inertia—the sleeping brain is indisposed to change.

Hypnopompic Period

Sleep inertia includes the hypnopompic period of semiconsciousness preceding waking (in contrast to the hypnagogic period of drowsiness preceding sleep). During sleep inertia one can experience hypnopompic reverie, which refers to dreamlike thoughts. The reverie can be so intense that it intrudes into waking conversation (e.g., during a phone call after being awakened from a deep sleep). The dramatic nature of hypnopompic disorientation and performance impairment has also been described by other names, including sleep drunkenness and postdormital sleepiness, which are now used to describe sleep pathology. Sleep inertia refers to awakenings in healthy persons.

Sleepiness and Performance

During sleep inertia alertness is low and the tendency to return to sleep is high, suggesting that sleepiness underlies the phenomenon. Several aspects of sleep inertia, however, make it difficult to explain as merely heightened sleepiness. For example, when performance impairment from sleep inertia is very severe, the person experiencing it often denies feeling sleepy. At the same time, the ELECTROENCEPHALOGRAM shows a pattern that is not distinguishable from that seen in a sleep-deprived subject, despite the fact that the cognitive performance impairment during sleep inertia is many times worse than that seen when the same person is sleep deprived.

More than anything else, sleep inertia is defined by poor performance on awakening. The poorer the performance, the more severe the sleep inertia. There have been many scientific studies in which sleepers were abruptly awakened from different stages of sleep to determine their cognitive processes (see DEPRIVATION, TOTAL: BEHAVIORAL EFFECTS). Often these studies compare awakenings from REM sleep with awakenings from NREM sleep. A consistent finding is that performance on most cognitive tasks, such as mental arithmetic, is impaired for 1 to 15 minutes after awakening from NREM sleep. The magnitude of the impairment is smaller for psychomotor and perceptual tasks, suggesting that sleep inertia affects information processing (thinking) more so than sensory input or response output. Memory appears to be especially affected by sleep inertia. Following a severe sleep inertia, the person often fails to remember what transpired during the performance task or interaction. This failure of memory makes sleep inertia similar to PARASOMNIAS such as SLEEPWALKING and SLEEP TERRORS, which involve partial arousals out of NREM sleep and subsequent amnesia for the event.

Sleep Depth

The physiological basis of sleep inertia remains unknown. It can occur on awakening from nocturnal sleep as well as from daytime naps. It is usually not very severe on awakening in the morning after a night of normal sleep, because the awakening is gradual and tends to occur naturally out of REM sleep. There are circumstances, however, in which sleep inertia can be very dramatic and difficult to overcome. Sleep inertia is almost always worse when the sleeper is awakened abruptly. Although it is commonly assumed that sleep inertia is primarily the result of the stage of sleep from which the sleeper is awakened, many other factors influence it. Most of the factors that affect the severity of sleep inertia are associated with the DEPTH OF SLEEP from which the sleeper was awakened. Abrupt awakenings from slow-wave sleep produce the greatest sleep inertia, especially if the person has been in slow-wave sleep for 30 to 60 minutes. Sleep inertia becomes more dramatic when the awakening occurs from SLOW-WAVE SLEEP following a period of sleep deprivation. Thus, the most severe sleep inertia can be seen in healthy sleepers who are abruptly awakened late in the first slow-wave sleep period following 2 full days without sleep. Fortunately, even in the most severe cases, sleep inertia is typically dissipated in a matter of minutes, giving way to a normal level of waking performance and alertness.

REFERENCE

Dinges DF. 1990. Are you awake? Cognitive performance and reverie during the hypnopompic state. In Bootzin D, Kihlstrom J, Schacter D, eds. *Sleep and cognition,* pp 159–175. Washington, D.C.: American Psychological Association.

David F. Dinges

SLEEPINESS

The simplest definition of sleepiness is that it is an awake condition that is associated with an increased tendency for an animal or a person to fall asleep. Sleepiness is manifested both as an elemental feeling labeled *sleepy* or *drowsy* and as a physiological drive. It is helpful to compare sleepiness with another biological drive in which the feeling or conscious part is experienced as being thirsty and the behavior motivated by the biological drive is seeking or drinking water or other suitable fluid to relieve dehydration. Dehydration would correspond to the state of sleep deprivation.

The Psychological Side of the Coin: Feeling Sleepy

Subjective sleepiness is an elemental feeling. It should, as such, be readily identified or introspected. If people are asked how they feel after having no sleep at all for one whole night most say, "I feel sleepy," but many would say, "I feel tired," "I feel fatigued," or "I feel irritable." In American society, the association between the psychological feeling state of sleepiness and the words used to describe it is inconsistent. Another important word that is the reciprocal of sleepiness is ALERTNESS. It has other connotations, such as being more intelligent, more interested in things, and quicker. These qualities, however, are impaired by increasing sleepiness and enhanced by decreasing sleepiness or increasing alertness.

Quantifying the level of subjective sleepiness as precisely as possible is desirable because the level of sleepiness has strong performance and/or diagnostic implications. Measuring psychological sleepiness or subjective sleepiness requires introspection, assessment of how one feels over some brief period, and then use of a scale on which to rank the intensity or level of sleepiness. Two types of scales are usually used. One is a numerical scale, the most popular of which is the STANFORD SLEEPINESS SCALE, a 7-point Likert self-rating scale with statements that are used to aid the introspection. Because no matter how many words are provided they will never mean the same thing to everyone, investigators also like to use an analog scale in which individuals mark their level of sleepiness on a line from most sleepy to most alert or most sleepy to least sleepy. In this case, the level of subjective sleepiness is measured as the distance (in millimeters) of the mark from one of the anchor points.

Objective Sleepiness: The Physiological Side of the Coin

Physiological sleepiness, in the absence of knowledge about a biochemical substrate, is defined as an increased tendency to fall asleep, implying an underlying physiological drive state. This tendency can be assessed directly by measuring the number of minutes it takes a human being to fall asleep in a standardized test situation. This value is called the *sleep latency.* In ordinary circumstances it is possible to keep anyone awake by stimulating them. Therefore, the measurement of sleep latency must be performed in the absence of stimulation. For all practical purposes, lying quietly in a darkened, sound-attenuated room on a comfortable bed with an empty bladder, no hunger pangs or pain, and comfortable loose clothing removes enough disturbing stimuli that the speed of falling asleep can be assumed to represent the underlying physiological sleep tendency.

In a standardized approach known as the MULTIPLE SLEEP LATENCY TEST (MSLT), the speed of falling asleep is measured by detecting the onset of sleep in continuous brain wave recordings five times a day at 2-hour intervals—10:00 A.M., noon, 2:00 P.M., 4:00 P.M., 6:00 P.M. Occasionally the last test is dropped. The test itself is allowed to continue for 20 minutes, at which time, if the person being tested has not fallen asleep, the test is terminated. If the individual falls asleep earlier, the test is terminated as soon as 1 minute of sleep is detected. The reason for abruptly ending the test is that allowing sizable amounts of sleep to accumulate across the day would actually change the level of sleepiness and confound the measurement. (See also MULTIPLE SLEEP LATENCY TEST.)

The five measurements, displayed as a figure or graph, are called the *sleep latency profile,* and test results for the day are usually expressed as the mean of the five individual tests (Figure 1). When the mean is zero to 5 minutes, the level of physiological sleepiness is clinically significant; 5 to 10 minutes is considered a borderline to troublesome level; 10 to 15 minutes is considered within normal limits; and 15 to 20 minutes is considered to be a high level of alertness.

Determinants of Physiological Sleepiness

Just as the drive to seek fluids is a homeostatic response to deprivation, so the increased tendency to sleep is a homeostatic response to prior sleep deprivation or amount of wakefulness. In other words, a homeostatic mechanism in the brain

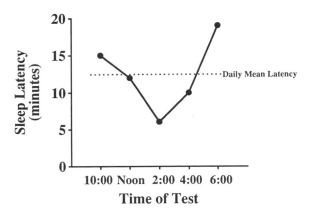

Figure 1. Sleep latency profile in a "typical" young adult sleeping 8 to 9 hours a night. The standard Multiple Sleep Latency Test (MSLT) is performed at 2-hour intervals beginning at 10:00 A.M. No appreciable amount of sleep accrues, because the subject is awakened from each test as soon as the technician can unequivocally identify the onset of sleep (i.e., within about 1 minute). The midday trough is characteristic in all adults. To make comparisons across days or from subject to subject, the mean latency from the five tests can be used. In this example, the mean is about 12 minutes.

responds to sleep reduction by increasing the tendency to fall asleep and, presumably, decreases the tendency to fall asleep by neurochemical and neurophysiological means in response to an increase in the amount of sleep.

Prior Amount of Sleep

Although not the only determinant of physiological sleepiness level, the length of sleep on one or several nights is the most important. Studies measuring MSLT scores during a variety of sleep schedules in human beings have found a very lawful, almost linear, relationship between the mean daytime sleep tendency or sleep latency profile and nocturnal amounts of sleep (Figure 2). Varying sleep allotments, from 10 hours to zero, on the night before are associated with a nearly linear decrease in the mean MSLT the next day (Carskadon and Dement, 1987). In addition, sleep loss accumulates from night to night (Figure 2). It is the accumulation of lost sleep over time that is probably the most important feature of this physiological regulatory system (Carskadon and Dement, 1981). Because individuals often do not feel sleepy even when they have accumulated a large amount of sleep depri-

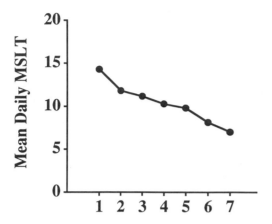

Consecutive Days of Sleep Reduction

Figure 2. Accrual of a cumulative sleep debt. Mean daily MSLT scores across nine young adults are shown for 7 consecutive days when sleep was held at 5 hours a night. The MSLT shows that the subjects accumulated a greater level of physiological sleepiness (faster sleep onset on MSLT) across the 7 days. Subjects in this study did not perceive that they were getting progressively sleepier.

vation, they do not realize they have a strong underlying tendency to fall asleep at any moment and are, therefore, at risk for a sleep-related error or accident. (See also PUBLIC SAFETY IN TRANSPORTATION; PUBLIC SAFETY IN THE WORKPLACE).

Although many more experiments need to be done, today we may assume that every hour of his or her needed amount of sleep that an individual fails to obtain is carefully registered by the brain as a debt and this debt is precisely tabulated over time. It is quite possible that the debt includes an hour lost a month ago or a week ago as well as last night. Obviously this assumes that there is an amount of nightly sleep that over time will maintain the same degree of daytime physiological alertness. It is also assumed with relatively sparse data that this amount varies from individual to individual. Assuming that the amount is 9 hours in a young adult, it is clear that sleeping 6 hours per night for a week can accumulate a severe level of sleepiness. Sometimes called the *sleep debt,* this debt would equal 21 hours for a whole week.

Continuity of Nocturnal Sleep

Sleep must be relatively continuous to reduce the tendency to fall asleep in the daytime. Experimental volunteers who are awakened briefly all night long every time several minutes of sleep have taken place are very sleepy in the daytime, even when nearly normal amounts of sleep have accumulated. (See also FRAGMENTATION.)

Maturation and Aging

It is widely believed that the need for sleep decreases with age. Thus, very young children, below 2 years of age, get very sleepy if they do not have around 10 to 12 hours of sleep at night plus a nap or two in the daytime. As the absence of a measurable tendency to fall asleep in the daytime can be used as an indicator that the amount of sleep the night before has fulfilled the daily need for sleep, the general assumption that sleep need continuously decreases with age can be tested.

As mentioned earlier, round-the-clock measurements of nocturnal sleep and daytime sleepiness are very sparse; however, human beings have been fairly well studied across the second decade of their lives. If it is possible, such studies should be longitudinal, that is, the same individual should be studied over time. One such study was carried out from 1976 to 1985 by Mary Carskadon, though not all the subjects were observed for the same number of years. The research protocol required children to go to bed at 10:00 P.M. and get out of bed at 8:00 A.M.; sleep latency was then measured at 2-hour intervals across the day. Prepubertal adolescents were fully alert, MSLT near 20, all day long with between 9.5 and 9.75 hours a night. With the same time in bed and the same amount of sleep, daytime sleepiness increased as puberty developed (Carskadon et al., 1980) (Figure 3).

If adolescent maturation has an impact on waking alertness, is this maturational change limited to the second decade or does it persist into later life? The data on this are not clear because it is difficult for adults in their twenties or thirties to sleep the same amount as adolescents; however, on an 8-hour schedule, many young adults show fairly severe levels of daytime sleepiness. Thus, in larger samples, the sleep latency profiles of young adults reveal that approximately one quarter show severe sleepiness (0 to 5 minutes); and only 10 percent are in the range from 15 to 20 minutes; 25 percent in the range from 5 to 10 minutes; and 25 percent in the range from 10 to 15 minutes. Overall, older individuals tend to be more sleepy in the daytime than prepubertal

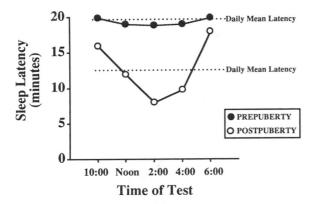

Figure 3. Effects of puberty on physiological sleepiness. Children were evaluated at age 10, 11, or 12, before they showed physical signs of puberty, and then again after they showed clear signs of puberty (ages 14, 15, 16). All children slept about 9 hours and 30 minutes each night. This schematic drawing of sleep latency profiles shows that prepubertal children are not at all sleepy, but postpubertal adolescents have a midday alertness trough even though they get as much sleep at night.

adolescents, but again, obtaining the same amount of sleep is difficult for young adults. Nonetheless, the notion that adults need less sleep as they grow older is not supported by clear evidence. Many elderly people are very sleepy, but their sleep at night is very fragmented, and this also contributes to the daytime sleep tendency. (See also AGING AND SLEEP.)

Circadian Determinants

Another physiological determinant of sleepiness is the influence of the circadian timing system (see CIRCADIAN RHYTHMS). This influence is reflected in the occurrence of a major sleep period once every circadian cycle in time-isolation environments. A secondary sleep episode is also seen when napping is permitted (Zulley and Campbell, 1985). Multiple measurements of sleep latency across the day show a U-shaped curve, with sleep latency measures tending to decrease until a midafternoon trough is reached and then tending to increase again. The midday maximum of sleep tendency is independent of the midday meal and occurs in the absence of food and drink. When the MSLT is repeated throughout the 24 hours, a nocturnal trough is also seen (Richardson et al., 1982) (Figure 4).

Sleep Extension

If measurable sleepiness occurs, increasing the amount of sleep the next night is associated with improved alertness. This improvement may be very slow. For example, it may take four or more consecutive nights of an extra hour of sleep to achieve an unambiguous decrease in physiological sleepiness on the following day. A single night of extended sleep is not always associated with a feeling of rejuvenation. Often, the opposite feeling occurs. This has given rise to the widespread belief that one can obtain "too much" sleep; this effect, however, appears to be transitory. Individuals who have a chronically increased sleep tendency in the daytime and then are able to habitually obtain more sleep uniformly show a clear improvement of physiological sleepiness and, generally, attest to feeling more alert, having more initiative, and so on (Carskadon et al., 1986). (See also SLEEP EXTENSION).

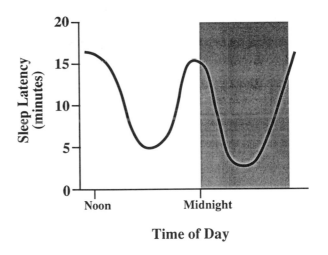

Time of Day

Figure 4. Sleep latency across 24 hours depicts the effects of circadian rhythms on physiological sleepiness. The MSLT was performed every 2 hours across the day in eighteen subjects, and a the averaged results are schematically represented by the curve. The white background represents the usual waking hours; the gray background is the usual nighttime. MSLTs performed during the usual nighttime were performed by allowing subjects to sleep, waking them every 2 hours, and then measuring the time it took to return to sleep. Two distinct times of sleepiness are apparent: one in the middle of the night, the other in the middle of the day.

Other Determinants

Nonphysiological factors that increase the tendency to fall asleep are sedating drugs and ALCOHOL; conversely, drugs that decrease the tendency to fall asleep include CAFFEINE and other STIMULANTS. Sleep disorders are commonly associated with daytime sleepiness. The most common clinical disorder in which patients appear to be very sleepy is called sleep APNEA syndrome. When the MSLT is measured in these patients, it usually shows a very severe level of sleepiness, in the range 0 to 5 minutes. Another sleep disorder associated with a severe (sometimes called "pathological") level of sleepiness is NARCOLEPSY.

The Need for Sleep

It should be clear from the foregoing that an individual's need for sleep at night (or the daily quota) may be defined in terms of a standard level of physiological sleepiness or alertness in the daytime in the same manner as we might define the need for fluid. A human being of a certain age must drink a certain amount of water each day to avoid either dehydration or diuresis. By the same token, a human being must sleep a certain amount each day to maintain a nominal level of alertness. From a practical point of view, there is usually a maximal amount of sleep that fits into an individual's daily schedule beyond which more sleep is difficult to obtain. In individuals who are sufficiently sleepy in the daytime that they can fall asleep and take a nap, the nap has an ameliorating effect on daytime sleepiness. Viewed in this manner, it is clear that every individual needs a certain amount of sleep, and that this need varies in a lawful manner.

Keeping in mind that stimulation can offset the momentary tendency to fall asleep and the associated feeling of sleepiness or drowsiness, it is clear that subjective sleepiness is determined in large part by the intensity of ongoing stimulation. Furthermore, stimulation can arise from both external and internal sources. At an exciting event, for example a championship football game, one would not feel sleepy even with fairly substantial degrees of physiological sleepiness. Endogenous stimulation is less clear, but certainly includes pain, competing behavioral drives, such as thirst and hunger, and, almost certainly, some kind of internal circadian fostering of AROUSAL. An internal circadian or clock-dependent alerting is currently the best explanation of the evening decrease in physiological sleepiness without intervening sleep. Thus, adolescents and young adults who can barely struggle out of bed in the morning are often vivaciously wide awake in the late evening.

It is clearly possible to have a very severe sleep tendency without feeling sleepy, but it is not possible to feel sleepy when one has no physiological sleep tendency at all. Removing stimulation will allow subjective sleepiness to become manifest. Because this is such a commonplace experience, human beings construe the stimulation-reducing factors, such as monotony, eating and drinking, quietness, and warmth, as the *causes* of sleepiness; it must, however, be clearly understood that these factors cannot cause a feeling of sleepiness in an individual who is physiologically fully alert.

Conclusion

Sleepiness is a positive feeling when it occurs at bedtime and one intends to go to sleep. It is a negative feeling when it pervades the waking hours and has to be resisted. Sleepiness is dangerous when it is intense and an individual is not aware of it, or worse, does not understand how it works. Perhaps the most dangerous misattribution is that strong waves of drowsiness are caused by something other than the amount of prior sleep and that they will permanently dissipate once the "cause" is removed (e.g., being sedentary, a warm bed, a monotonous committee meeting). Although, as is obvious, a great deal is known about sleepiness, none of this knowledge is communicated at any educational level—not in elementary school, or high school, or college, or medical school, or any graduate program, or in the medical profession at any continuing medical educational level. As a result, both the American public and health professionals have a pervasive ignorance about the determinants and consequences of sleep deprivation and its associated cognitive impairment. To lead a healthy and productive life, individuals should cultivate a level of alertness that fosters their life objectives on a day-to-day basis, as well as a long-term basis.

REFERENCES

Carskadon MA, Dement WC. 1981. Cumulative effects of sleep restriction on daytime sleepiness. *Psychophysiology* 18:107–113.

———. 1987. Daytime sleepiness: Quantification of a behavioral state. *Neurosci Biobehav Rev* 11:307–317.

Carskadon MA, Harvey K, Duke P, Anders T, Litt I, Dement WC. 1980. Pubertal changes in daytime sleepiness. *Sleep* 2:453–460.

Carskadon MA, Mancuso J, Keenan S, Littell W, Dement WC. 1986. Sleepiness following oversleeping. *Sleep Res* 15:70.

Dinges DF, Broughton RJ, eds. 1989. *Sleep and alertness: Chronological, behavioral, and medical aspects of napping.* New York: Raven.

Richardson GS, Carskadon MA, Orav EJ, Dement WC. 1982. Circadian variation of sleep tendency in elderly and young adult subjects. *Sleep* 5:S82–S94.

Roth T, Roehrs T, Carskadon M, Dement W. 1989. Daytime sleepiness and alertness. In Kryger MH, Roth T, Dement WC, eds, *Principles and practice of sleep medicine,* pp 14–23. Philadelphia: Saunders.

Zulley J, Campbell SS. 1985. Napping behavior during "spontaneous internal desynchronization": Sleep remains in synchrony with body temperature. *Human Neurobiol* 4:123–126.

William C. Dement

SLEEPING PILLS

The modern history of sleeping pills began in the mid-nineteenth century, and largely grew out of the development of anesthetics used in obstetrics and gynecology (see ANESTHESIA). Potassium bromide was developed in the 1850s by Charles Locock, a London gynecologist who, while using it for dysmenorrhea, noted that it had sedative properties. It rapidly came to be used for INSOMNIA and SLEEPWALKING, as well as a variety of Victorian complaints including "frightful imaginings" in pregnancy and "undue indulgence in bed." In his book *Home Remedies for Man and Beast* ... (1893), Dr. B. G. Jeffries recommended what we would now call SLEEP HYGIENE: ("Sleepless persons should avoid exciting conversation ... or any kind of mental excitement during the evening") as well as 5 to 10 grains of bromide. The bromides are very toxic, as they replace chlorine atoms in the body with bromine, and result in irritability, depression, and confusion. For that reason, they are rarely used although they occasionally appear in over-the-counter medicines. Nonetheless, to this day, doctors are trained to look for a skin rash on the faces of a confused and toxic patient, as a characteristic sign of bromide poisoning.

Although when James Young Simpson, a Scottish physician, introduced chloroform for anesthesia during childbirth he was met with a variety of criticisms (it was argued by some that birth should be a painful process), the discovery led a number of scientists to look for new kinds of anesthetics and hypnotics. In the 1850s, Oscar Liebreich created chloral hydrate by combining chlorine atoms with acetaldehyde. He predicted it would induce sleep because, he thought, it would be chemically broken down (metabolized) into chloroform. Although his chemistry was mistaken, chloral hydrate did indeed turn out to be a potent hypnotic. Unfortunately it, too, had a number of drawbacks including gastrointestinal irritation and a liability for developing dependence. Indeed, it was a popular drug of abuse during the late nineteenth century, claiming among its victims a number of artists such as Dante Gabriel Rosetti. It has had limited use for the last few decades. Ironically, because of recent restrictions on prescribing benzodiazepine hypnotics, both chloral hydrate and barbiturates are once again beginning to be prescribed more frequently.

In 1882, another derivative of acetaldehyde, paraldehyde, was introduced by Vincenzo Cervello. It rapidly gained a role as an anticonvulsant and sedative for agitated psychotic patients, as well as for sleep. It, too, had many qualities that ultimately limited its use, including stomach irritation, damage to muscle tissue when injected, and an unpleasant odor that was very noticeable on the patient's breath. While still in the bottle it decomposes into acetaldehyde and acetic acid, and a number of deaths have been attributed to injections of medicine that was stored for too long.

Another family of potent anesthetics, the urethanes, were known in the nineteenth century, and prompted studies of other derivatives of urea that might induce sleep. Among these were the barbiturates, formed by combining malonic acid and urea (see BARBITURATES). Veronal, or diethylbarbituric acid, became widely used as an anticonvulsant and hypnotic after the turn of the century, followed by phenobarbital in 1912. During World War I, the Allied blockade of German shipping cut off the supply of a number of drugs that were patented and manufactured exclusively in Germany, including Veronal, Novacaine, and Salvarsan. By an act of Congress, the patent laws were changed so that Veronal began to be manufactured in the United States as Barbital. During the 1920s and 1930s, the intermediate-acting barbiturates—pentobarbital, secobarbital, and amobarbital—became available and rapidly became the most widely used hypnotics. This remained the case until the introduction of benzodiazepines in the 1960s (see BENZODIAZEPINES). Because of a number of perceived advantages, including decreased toxicity, they rapidly became the most popular hypnotics. Although the particular benzodiazepines used have changed over the years, they remain the most widely prescribed hypnotics. The last few years have also seen the introduction of new nonbenzodiazepine hypnotics and tranquilizers which may enter the American market in the near future.

General Description

In one sense, a "sleeping pill" is any medication a doctor gives a patient to aid sleep. On the other hand, it is useful to understand that all prescription medications are assigned official "indications" as part of the approval process when a pharmaceutical manufacturer applies to the Food and Drug Administration for permission to market a medicine. Those medicines that carry an official indication to aid sleep are known as *hypnotics* or, more casually, as sleeping pills. Hypnotics, however, represent only about three fourths of the prescriptions doctors write to help sleep. The remaining compounds are medicines that are indicated for other purposes, but may have sedating properties. These include drugs used as ANTIDEPRESSANTS and ANTIHISTAMINES and the "major TRANQUILIZERS," which are indicated for psychotic patients. The former two groups may have some usefulness in a treatment regimen for insomnia; the latter medications may have significant side effects and are probably better reserved for their psychiatric indications.

It is also important to distinguish between hypnotics, which can be obtained only by pre-scription, and medicines that can be purchased "over-the-counter" at drug stores (see OVER-THE-COUNTER SLEEPING PILLS). The over-the-counter medicines are usually antihistamines, including doxylamine and pyrilamine. These have mild sleep-promoting effects, but are not entirely benign: Many antihistamines have significant anticholinergic properties (i.e., they inhibit the normal functioning of the chemical acetylcholine in the nervous system) and can cause elderly patients to become confused and forgetful. Some naturally occurring substances that may aid sleep can be purchased at health food stores (see FOLK AND OTHER NATURAL REMEDIES FOR SLEEPLESSNESS). Probably the best known of these is L-tryptophan. It has generally been considered a benign substance, but in recent years there has been concern that taking it in large amounts may cause liver damage, and that some people may develop very severe blood disorders (it is not yet known if the latter problem is due to tryptophan itself or to a material that comes along with it in the capsule). Thus, all of these medicines and substances should be taken seriously and used in a manner that maximizes their many beneficial effects while minimizing possible difficulties. We focus primarily on the use of prescription hypnotics. To learn about their pharmacological properties, please see BENZODIAZEPINES and BARBITURATES.

Therapeutic Uses

To see if hypnotics are helpful, it is necessary to understand a little about insomnia. INSOMNIA is primarily a complaint on the part of a patient that he or she is not getting enough sleep or that the sleep is of poor quality. Many different causes can result in the complaint of sleeping poorly. A person with PERIODIC LEG MOVEMENTS, for instance, may have very disturbed sleep, as can an elderly person who is kept awake by pain from ARTHRITIS or a person suffering from depression. When insomnia results from such specific causes, it is best to treat it with medicines specific to the problem. Thus if a person suffers from poor sleep as a result of depression, an antidepressant medication is the best approach. Similarly, if pain is keeping a person awake, an analgesic may be a more appropriate medicine. (Hypnotics, incidentally, do not have pain-reducing qualities except in extremely high doses that result in unconsciousness.) Many persons, however, suffer from long-term difficulty sleeping but do not seem to have any of these known disorders that lead to insomnia. At this time, the causes of their poor sleep are best described in psychological terms, which include "sleep state misperception" and "conditioned insomnia" (Thorpy, 1990). These are the persons for whom hypnotics are often used and to whom we refer as *insomniacs.*

One of the hardest parts about understanding the effectiveness of hypnotics is determining what measures to use. Many insomniacs, particularly those with sleep state misperception, have minimal alterations in sleep as measured by POLYSOMNOGRAPHY, although their subjective experience is that they sleep very poorly. As the polygraphic measures of sleep are minimally disturbed, it is not surprising that drug-induced improvement in polygraphic sleep may be relatively small and (even if it were bigger) might not fully reflect the benefits of the medication to the subjective experience of sleeping (Mendelson, 1990). The strength of polygraphic measures of sleep, however, is that they are very quantitative and hence amenable to modern scientific methods of analysis. On the other hand, relying only on the patient's subjective report of effectiveness may not be optimal either. A patient may prefer a drug for the wrong reasons; for instance, he or she may describe a hypnotic in very positive terms if it produces a euphoric effect, when in fact the goal was to enhance sleep. Because each method has certain benefits and drawbacks, it seems best to use information from both the polygraphic and patient report techniques in determining the benefits of a hypnotic (efficacy) for insomniacs.

Most prescription hypnotics improve standard polygraphic measures of sleep during the first few weeks of administration. Sleep latency (the time from administration of the medicine or from when the lights are turned out until sleep onset) is shortened, and the total duration of sleep is increased. The amount of waking time after initial sleep onset is reduced. The speed with which these changes take place differs with various drugs. Short-acting hypnotics may show these beneficial alterations on the first night medication is taken (Kripke et al., 1990). Longer-acting agents may not reach full effectiveness until the second or third night. Individ-

ual sleep stages may also be altered. Most of the older hypnotics including the barbiturates and chloral hydrate potently decrease REM sleep. The BENZODIAZEPINES do this to a much smaller degree. Although common sense suggests that this might be a marked advantage, it is not really clear that this is true. In the 1960s, the popular belief was that decreased REM sleep might lead to psychological harm or even psychotic behavior, but more recent experiments indicate that this is probably not the case. Indeed, in certain circumstances REM deprivation may even be beneficial, and has been used as a treatment for depression (see DEPRIVATION, SELECTIVE: NREM SLEEP; DEPRIVATION, SELECTIVE: REM SLEEP). Moreover, the benzodiazepines potently suppress SLOW-WAVE SLEEP (stages 3 and 4) and at this point in our understanding it is not clear whether this is any better or worse than suppressing REM sleep. Some newer hypnotics that are available in Europe, but not the United States, actually increase slow-wave sleep. Until we achieve a better understanding of the functions of the sleep stages, the best we can say is that it makes sense that a pill that does not alter sleep stages at all might be best, but we truly do not know the implications of altering one stage or another. For these reasons, polygraphic measures of efficacy usually focus on sleep latency, total sleep time, and reduction in wake time after sleep onset. (Later when we talk about daytime sleepiness caused by hypnotics, we will also consider polygraphic measures of alertness.)

Patient reports of sleep tend to focus on the subjective counterparts of sleep latency, total sleep time, and awakenings during the night, as well as qualities such as the depth and restfulness of sleep. Again, as with the polygraphic measures, most prescription sleeping pills are reported to be very beneficial. This happy prospect is dimmed, however, by the realization that after several weeks of nightly use of medicine, the effectiveness seems to decrease, a phenomenon known as *tolerance.* Because of the possibility of tolerance, a number of alternative strategies have been developed. Among these have been the use of sleeping pills in conjunction with nonmedicine (behavioral) techniques to improve sleep, and the use of sleeping pills on an occasional (rather than nightly) basis (see BEHAVIORAL MODIFICATION). This leads us to the broader question of factors that limit the usefulness of sleeping pills.

Limitations on the Use of Sleeping Pills

Issues that need to be considered when a patient is given a sleeping pill prescription include the following.

Possibility of Overdose and Interaction with Alcohol

Older hypnotics including the barbiturates are extremely toxic in overdose, and ten therapeutic doses are often lethal. Perhaps the most lethal of all is methaqualone, which is excreted into the gastrointestinal system and then cyclically reabsorbed into the bloodstream to repeat the process. Chloral hydrate is very toxic in overdose but, because of the large size of the capsules and the frequent vomiting resulting from stomach irritation, is somewhat less likely to result in death. The benzodiazepines are substantially less dangerous in overdose when a medically healthy person takes them alone (Mendelson, 1980). It is important to remember, however, that overdoses are often taken in combination with alcohol, and in this setting benzodiazepines can be lethal. The concern about overdose emphasizes the importance of considering the possibility of clinical depression in patients who complain of insomnia; if the poor sleep in a particular patient is indeed associated with depression, then specific drugs such as the tricyclic antidepressants are much more appropriate. (It should be noted that they, too, can be very toxic in overdose and should be used with care.)

Withdrawal Sleep Disturbance

Sleep may be transiently disturbed after cessation of any hypnotic. The timing and duration of this difficulty vary with the duration of action of the drug. In general, the longer-acting hypnotics result in milder withdrawal sleep disturbance, which starts a few nights after stopping medication. With the shorter-acting hypnotics, sleep disturbance may be manifest on the first night after stopping the drug (National Institute of Mental Health, 1984). This phenomenon has been reported after a single night of medication. In general, however, sleep disturbance on withdrawal from short-acting benzodiazepines is most evident at high doses which have minimally more benefits than lower doses (Roehrs et al., 1986).

There is also some evidence that there may be a wide range in individual susceptibility to withdrawal sleep disturbance. At least one factor involved is degree of initial sleep improvement with medication, such that patients with the greatest initial increase in sleep may have the most withdrawal sleep disturbance. These types of concerns point to the importance of discussing withdrawal insomnia with the patient at the time medication is started.

Effects on Daytime Functioning

Although the usual therapeutic goal for taking hypnotics is to improve nighttime sleep, these compounds may have profound effects on a patient's daytime life. Much of the original concern was focused on the longer-acting benzodiazepines. Because of their long half-lives, these drugs linger in the body and can accumulate substantially with nightly use. After 2 weeks of taking one popular agent, for instance, blood levels during the daytime may be seven times greater than the peak level after the first dose. Although there may be some tolerance to these continued high blood levels, there is ample evidence that patients taking long-acting benzodiazepines may be impaired in various ways during the daytime (Mendelson, 1980, 1987). This has been manifested in studies of motor activity (as measured by wrist actigraphs), simulated driving tests (and in one case in actual measures of driving cars), and various psychomotor batteries. Daytime multiple sleep latency tests (MSLTs) also demonstrate increased propensity to fall asleep (see MULTIPLE SLEEP LATENCY TEST). For these reasons, the shorter-acting benzodiazepines, which do not accumulate in the bloodstream, became very popular. In more recent years, however, concern has been voiced about the possibility that the short-acting agents may themselves be associated with some unique difficulties. Among these have been the possibility of enhanced daytime anxiety and memory disturbances. Although some studies have reported enhanced anxiety, many others have not observed it. One possible resolution of this apparent disagreement is that rare patients may have this response, but that it is so uncommon that it is usually not manifest in studies of groups of patients. When a patient does have increased anxiety, the appropriate therapeutic action would be to lower the dose or try a longer-acting agent.

Alterations in Memory

All benzodiazepine hypnotics affect cognition, particularly episodic MEMORY, the ability to learn new material. The study of the practical significance of this observation is difficult because the act of falling asleep by itself produces a form of amnesia for events immediately prior to sleep onset. Thus, in principle, a hypnotic might alter memory either by "direct" effects on the nervous system or indirectly by inducing sleep. Studies of memory function are also complicated by the high frequency with which unmedicated insomniacs complain of trouble remembering events around bedtime. There have also been claims that short-acting benzodiazepines induce a global amnesia in which patients have no remembrance at all of their behavior for extended periods (Morris and Estes, 1987). Careful analysis of these allegations usually reveals that there was a combination of factors involved, including concomitant use of ALCOHOL, sleep deprivation, and external circadian desynchronization ("jet lag").

Respiratory Suppression

One clear advantage of the benzodiazepines is that the degree of respiratory suppression is much less than that produced by older hypnotics. On the other hand, they do have this property to some degree, which may be significant in patients with compromised respiration (Dolly and Block, 1982). Clinical settings in which this problem may become evident would include situations in which benzodiazepines are given to patients with chronic obstructive pulmonary disease or sleep APNEA. These effects can of course be compounded by the use of alcohol.

Special Needs of the Elderly

Persons over 65 have a higher frequency of side effects from all medications, and hypnotics are no exception. Several factors contribute to this, including increased nervous system sensitivity and decreased serum albumin (which binds the drug). Many hypnotics have longer half-lives in the elderly, especially in men (Greenblatt et al., 1981). Depending on the particular agent, this may result either from altered hepatic clearance or from increased absorption of drug into fatty tissue. Clinically, then, it is best to use minimal doses and short-acting agents in older patients, as well as to emphasize nondrug treatments. (See AGING AND SLEEP.)

Appropriate Use of Hypnotics

In general, most sleep researchers agree that the brief use of hypnotics is appropriate in patients with short-term insomnias that result from emotional trauma, illness, or sleeping in new settings (National Institute of Mental Health, 1984). Using hypnotics to aid sleep in SHIFTWORK or jet travel situations is still being evaluated. In general, most data have suggested that short-acting hypnotics can improve sleep at the new sleeping time, but that they do not actually increase the rate at which a person adjusts to the new schedule. In chronic insomnia that has gone on for at least 6 months, the first thing to consider is whether the sleep disturbance results from other drugs, a physiological disorder such as sleep apnea, or a psychiatric illness such as depression. When these are not found, and there is some evidence that the patient has conditioned insomnia or sleep state misperception, hypnotics may have a useful therapeutic role. Because of the development of tolerance, nightly use for more than a short period is usually only minimally helpful. Many clinicians prefer to prescribe hypnotics as adjunctive therapy, perhaps twice a week, while treating the patient with nondrug techniques. Addressing sleep habits and attitudes about sleep, decreasing caffeine, and lowering anxiety about not sleeping can help many insomniacs considerably.

REFERENCES

Dolly FR, Block AJ. 1982. Effect of flurazepam on sleep-disordered breathing and nocturnal oxygen desaturation in asymptomatic patients. *Am J Med* 73:239–243.

Greenblatt DJ, Divoll M, Harmatz JS, MacLaughlin DS, Shader RI. 1981. Kinetics and clinical effects of flurazepam in young and elderly non-insomniacs. *Clin Pharmacol Res* 30:475–486.

Jeffreis BG. 1893. *Home remedies for man and beast; the household guide; or practical helps for every home.* Naperville, IL: JL Nichols.

Kripke DF, Hauri P, Ancoli-Israel S, Roth T. 1990. Sleep evaluation in chronic insomniacs during 14 day use of flurazepam and midazolam. *J Clin Psychopharmacol* 10:32S–43S.

Mendelson WB. 1980. *The use and misuse of sleeping pills.* New York: Plenum Press.

————. 1987. *Human sleep: Research and clinical care.* New York: Plenum Press.

————. 1990. Do studies of sedative/hypnotics suggest the nature of chronic insomnia? In Montplaisir J, Godbout R, eds. *Sleep and biological rhythms,* pp 209–218. New York: Oxford University Press.

Morris HH, Estes ML. 1987. Traveler's amnesia: Transient global amnesia secondary to triazolam. *JAMA* 258:945–946.

National Institute of Mental Health. 1984. Consensus conference report: Drugs and insomnia—The use of medication to promote sleep. *JAMA* 251: 2410–2424.

Roehrs TA, Zorick R, Wittig M, Roth R. 1986. Dose determinants of rebound insomnia. *Br J Clin Pharmacol* 22:143–147.

Thorpy MJ. 1990. Classification and nomenclature of the sleep disorders. In Thorpy MJ, ed. *Handbook of sleep disorders,* pp 155–178. New York: Marcel Dekker.

Wallace B. Mendelson

SLEEPING SICKNESS

Sleeping sickness is the term originally applied to the disease *African trypanosomiasis* because of the apparent sleepiness suffered by its victims. It is caused by infection with the parasite *Trypanosoma* (species *brucei, gambiense,* or *rhodesiense*), which is transmitted by the tsetse fly. The "sleeping sickness" corresponds to the stage of the disease when the parasite penetrates into the brain and causes an inflammatory process therein. The resultant meningoencephalitis lasts several months to several years before progressing to a terminal stage, when massive lymphoplasmocytic infiltration is associated with profound gliosis and diffuse demyelinization in the brain.

In the early stages of neurological involvement, patients suffer from headache and feel tired and listless. This state progresses to one of somnolence in which the patient apparently falls asleep unless actively stimulated; however, as in the case of other forms of ENCEPHALITIS, the apparent sleep does not correspond to normal sleep. The electroencephalographic activity during waking is characterized by predominant alpha and theta rhythms of low amplitude often interrupted by bursts of high-amplitude delta waves. The cycle of sleep is disrupted. Stages 1 and 4 are often absent. REM sleep persists though may partly invade other stages of sleep and also occur with sudden onset from waking. The CIRCADIAN RHYTHM is often disturbed, with daytime SLEEPINESS being reciprocated by nighttime INSOMNIA. With progression of the disease motor signs also appear as a loss of initiative and akinesia (immobility). Somnolence progresses to stupor, and electroencephalographic activity shows increasing slow waves accompanied by spike and wave complexes. Eventually, the patient dies in a coma.

Neuropathological examination of the brain reveals a diffuse inflammatory process that involves maximally the rostral midbrain, HYPOTHALAMUS, and BASAL FOREBRAIN. The somnolence may thus be caused by lesions and progressive dysfunction of the brainstem reticular activating system and its forebrain continuation in the posterior hypothalamus and basal forebrain (see BRAIN MECHANISMS).

REFERENCES

Gallais P, Badier M. 1952. Recherches sur l'encéphalite de la trypanosomiase humaine africaine. Correlations cliniques, anatomiques, électro-encéphalographiques, biologiques. *Med Trop* 12:633–675.

Schwartz BA, Escande C. 1970. Sleeping sickness: Sleep study of a case. *Electroencephalogr Clin Neurophysiol* 29:83–87.

Van Bogaert L. 1956. De quelques aspects neurologiques de la trypanosomiase africaine. *Ann Soc Belg Med Trop* 36:645–654.

Barbara E. Jones

SLEEP LEARNING

See Amnesia; Cognition; Learning; Memory; Problem Solving and Dreaming

SLEEP LENGTH

[*A wide variety of factors are involved in determining sleep length, including species, age, disease, drugs, and others. Within the class of* MAMMALS, *for example, daily sleep needs range from about 3.5 hours in the cow to more than 12 hours of sleep per day in the opossum. Age also has a major effect on sleep length. In human infants, the length of a sleep episode is generally limited by the need for frequent feeding; over the first year of life, the infant gradually consolidates sleep into one long nocturnal sleep episode and two or three daytime naps (see* INFANCY, NORMAL SLEEP PATTERNS IN*). Across* CHILDHOOD, *the nocturnal sleep episode decreases and* NAPPING *eventually drops out (see* CHILDHOOD SLEEP DURING*). Sleep length continues to decline across adolescence (see* ADOLESCENCE AND SLEEP*) and into old age. To a large extent, sleep length can also be reduced by volitional intervention—that is, the adolescent or adult may reduce the amount of sleep obtained at night in order to fulfill waking obligations; in many Western countries, this is often achieved through the use of* ALARM CLOCKS.

When environmental constraints, whether social, academic, or otherwise, are not an issue—for example, during an experiment when a person is placed under constant conditions without external time cues—the regulation of sleep length by CIRCADIAN RHYTHMS *becomes quite apparent. Under such conditions, the length of sleep appears to be determined by a strong circadian influence on the time of* WAKING UP. *At a particular phase of its circadian cycle, the brain shows a greater tendency to arouse. Therefore, if one has fallen asleep shortly before this circadian phase, then the sleep episode will be short-lived; if one has fallen asleep long before this circadian phase, then the sleep episode will last considerably longer. In constant conditions, the length of sleep episodes can be quite variable but is always influenced markedly by the subject's internal circadian rhythm. (See also* TIMING OF SLEEP AND WAKEFULNESS.)

Environmental or related factors can influence length of sleep, sometimes as a result of a mismatch with circadian rhythms. For example, shiftworkers may experience short sleep episodes because they are attempting to sleep out of phase with their normal circadian rhythms, going to bed only a short while before the internal phase of waking up begins (see SHIFTWORK*). Adolescent and college-age students influence their length of sleep by "pulling* ALL-NIGHTERS," *often in response to academic demands; thus, nocturnal sleep on one night may be nonexistent but recovery sleep the next night may be greatly extended. Even after conditions of significant sleep* DEPRIVATION, *there may exist a finite limitation to such* SLEEP EXTENSION. *Randy Gardner, a high school student whose science fair project was to stay up longer than any other person had been known to previously, deprived himself of sleep for more than 11 consecutive days. When he had his recovery sleep, however, he was only able to sleep 14 hours and 40 minutes (see* GARDNER, RANDY*).

For many animals, the season of the year influences sleep length. In certain species, winter sleep or sleep under conditions of low environmental sustenance may not terminate in arousal but may instead progress into a dormant, nonsleep state such as ESTIVATION, TORPOR *or* HIBERNATION. *In humans,* SEASONAL EFFECTS ON SLEEP *appear to be particularly acute for people living above the Arctic Circle and for those with* SEASONAL AFFECTIVE DISORDER. *Other mood disorders such as* DEPRESSION *are associated with alterations in the length of the sleep period. For example, adolescents diagnosed with major depression often report very long episodes of sleep; these depressed young people may be described as hypersomnolent. Many adults with major depression, by contrast, have short nocturnal sleep. A very consistent complaint among adults with major depression is known as* EARLY MORNING AWAKENING, *or waking up long before the desired rising time.

Hypnotic medications such as BENZODIAZAPINES, BARBITURATES, *and* OVER-THE-COUNTER SLEEPING PILLS *typically lengthen sleep;* ALCOHOL, *on the other hand, may act in the early part of the night to induce sleep but in the latter part of the night acts to shorten the sleep episode. Withdrawal of hypnotic medications may result in a rebound effect, in which sleep is shortened. Individuals who routinely take* STIMULANTS *may also have reduced sleep, whereas withdrawal from stimulant medications may have the opposite impact, leading to prolonged sleep episodes.

The length of sleep an individual obtains

under normal circumstances appears to be determined largely by GENETICS. *Therefore, there are many* INDIVIDUAL DIFFERENCES *in sleep length. Various* PERSONALITY *characteristics have been linked with either long or short sleep, although whether sleep length results in the personality differences or vice versa is debated. One study looked at the usual amount of sleep at night in more than 1 million adults, and determined how many of those people died over the course of the next 6 years; results indicated that* LONGEVITY *may be influenced by sleep length. Of course, many stories (if not tall tales) concern characters who were very short sleepers or very long sleepers (see* SHORT *and* LONG SLEEPERS IN HISTORY AND LEGEND).*

Finally, many specific sleep disorders are associated with consistent variations of sleep length. People who have INSOMNIA *generally have short sleep; people with* HYPERSOMNIA *often have long sleep. Interestingly, people with* NARCOLEPSY *usually do not have excessive sleep lengths but often fall asleep at the wrong time—that is, during the daytime. In fact, nighttime sleep in narcoleptics is often quite disrupted. Other medical disorders may also influence sleep length, such as* MONONUCLEOSIS *and* CHRONIC FATIGUE SYNDROME, *which are often associated with long sleep.*]

SLEEP ONSET

Although falling asleep is normally experienced as a simple, even effortless process, sleep onset actually involves a complex series of adjustments in central nervous system functioning. During the sleep onset period (SOP), changes are evident in behavioral responsiveness, level of consciousness, brain wave or electroencephalographic (EEG) activity, the firing patterns of many neural systems, and most physiological measures. The process of moving from a state of relaxed drowsiness to the first signs of unmistakable sleep is characterized by moment-to-moment oscillations in these systems as the person—or animal—slides erratically down the arousal continuum from wakefulness into sleep (Kleitman, 1957). The time course of this descent into sleep may range from several seconds to many minutes or even hours, depending on factors such as

length of prior wakefulness, sleep habits, familiarity with the sleep setting, and personality. Typically, the SOP processes can be reversed voluntarily by the potential sleeper or by external stimulation; in certain sleep disorders, such as narcolepsy, voluntary maintenance of wakefulness is not possible and the sleep onset process itself is atypical (see NARCOLEPSY; SLEEP ATTACKS; MULTIPLE SLEEP LATENCY TEST). In other disorders, such as certain forms of insomnia, voluntary initiation of the SOP process is difficult and latency to sleep onset is increased (see INSOMNIA).

Physiological Changes During Sleep Onset

The human SOP has been studied carefully recently, and it is now possible to describe a series of orderly changes in a wide variety of indices of arousal level. EEG changes have been the most common means of assessing sleep onset and sleep–wake stages, because EEG activity varies with level of arousal and can be measured continuously and relatively unobtrusively (see ELECTROENCEPHALOGRAPHY). During wakefulness, the dominant EEG patterns contain a mixture of relatively high-frequency, low-amplitude activity, primarily in the beta (17 to 25+ cycles per second) frequencies. As relaxed drowsiness approaches and particularly when people close their eyes, alpha activity (8 to 13 cycles per second) appears as the dominant frequency. Alpha levels drop again, just before sleep (see ALPHA RHYTHM). As sleep approaches, slower theta (3.5 to 7.5 cycles per second) frequencies take over, and around the moment of behavioral sleep (the cessation of responses to faint auditory stimuli), there is a pronounced rise in delta activity (0.3 to 3.5 cycles per second). In fact, computer quantification of EEG power shows that there is a significant increase in power across all frequencies at the beginning of sleep (Ogilvie et al., 1991).

People looking for distinctive EEG signs of sleep have relied on the appearance of two EEG waveforms not observed during wakefulness. SLEEP SPINDLES are bursts of regular 12- to 14-cycle-per-second activity that are clearly visible early on in NREM sleep. Spindles are produced by the activity of neurons in a midbrain structure called the thalamus (see THALAMUS). Johnson (1973) found that these waves are often accompanied by K-COMPLEXES, which appear very early in sleep as sharp, biphasic waves of high amplitude. K-complexes occur spontaneously in sleep, seemingly in response to internal central nervous system stimulation, but they may also be triggered by external stimuli (noises or light flashes). Together, spindles and K-complexes provide good indicators that their producer is asleep (see SLEEP SPINDLES; K-COMPLEX; STAGES OF SLEEP).

Ogilvie and Wilkinson (1984) have shown that reaction time lengthens as the EEG-defined stages of wakefulness and early sleep are entered. Corresponding changes in respiratory patterns are seen then, too. At the point of behaviorally defined sleep, abdominal respiratory amplitude drops, signaling a change in respiratory control processes at sleep onset (see RESPIRATION CONTROL IN SLEEP).

Hypnagogic Reverie

Hypnagogic reverie refers to the mental activity occurring during the transition into sleep. Foulkes (1966) aroused people from different points within the SOP and asked them to describe their mental activity. Almost all arousals resulted in reports, many of which were dreamlike, containing hallucinated and dramatic material. As

people moved further toward definite sleep, the proportion of arousal reports containing dreamlike content increased from 31 to 76 percent but then dropped off as stage 2 sleep developed. Foulkes' work shows that there is a mixture of wake and dreamlike mentation near sleep onset and that the dreamlike reports differ in several ways from typical REM sleep dreams, with hypnagogic experiences being generally briefer, more present oriented, and less personally meaningful, perhaps to assist the dreamer to maintain the developing sleep process (see HYPNAGOGIC REVERIE; HYPNAGOGIC HALLUCINATIONS).

Falling Asleep in a Sleep Onset Study

Let us look at a sleep researcher's view of the sleep onset process. Figure 1 is a 1-minute recording from a very sleepy person as she moves from relaxed wakefulness (left side) to definite sleep (right side). The S/W line shows that her arousal level, determined by standard criteria (Rechtschaffen and Kales, 1968), initially indicated wakefulness (W) and later stages 1 and 2 of NREM sleep. The thick line immediately below recorded large body movements and shows that none was evident. The Cz-A1 and Pz-A1 lines show EEG activity during this transition period.

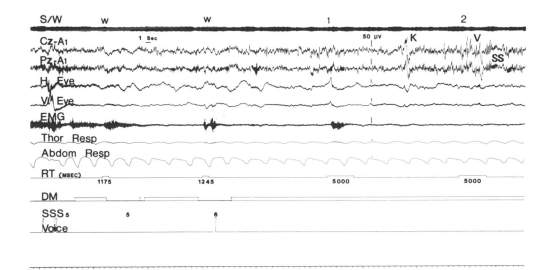

Figure 1. See text above for a complete description of sleep onset as defined by the pattern of brain activity, eye movements, muscle tone, respiration, and behavioral responses shown in this polysomnogram tracing.

Alpha activity typical of wakefulness occupies the first one third of the record (seen as the darker segments of Pz-A1). Diminished alpha consistent with stage 1 sleep is seen next, and the first distinctive EEG sign of sleep is the K-complex (K) found approximately 5 seconds after the calibration marks. Note that after the K-complex, the amplitude [height or voltage in microvolts (μV)] increases due to the presence of vertex sharp waves (V), which are seen clearly only during the transition into sleep (see VERTEX SHARP WAVES). Two sleep spindles (SS) confirm stage 2 sleep at the end of the figure.

Horizontal and vertical eye movements were recorded on the next two lines (see ELECTRO-OCULOGRAPHY). On the horizontal eye movement recording, the slow oscillations (each lasting about 5 seconds) demonstrate the slow rolling eye movements normally seen just prior to sleep. Note that these have ceased by the end of the record. Below them, the EMG tracing indicated chin muscle tension (see ELECTROMY-OGRAPHY). As expected, there is more activity in this system during wakefulness, with periodic activity when verbalizations were made. Thoracic and abdominal respiratory amplitudes were also recorded. You can see that abdominal respiratory amplitude is reduced as sleep begins.

The RT line shows the subject's response time to faint tones presented by a computer. Upward deflection of the line indicates the beginning of the tone; the reaction time is indicated in milliseconds—the time taken to acknowledge having heard the tone by pressing a switch to turn it off. The response time gives a good measure of how "wide awake" the person is at the moment the tone is generated, and failure to respond indicates behaviorally defined sleep (shown here when the computer turns the tones off after 5 seconds).

On the next line, a Deadman's switch (DM) provides a continuous behavioral measure of state. The subject was asked to keep this button switch depressed while awake. As sleep sets in, finger muscles relax and the release of the switch (double line) provides another indicator of sleep onset.

The final task required of this sleepy volunteer was to provide a verbal estimate of her subjective sleepiness by saying a number from 1 to 7 describing how sleepy she felt as she responded to each tone. On this Stanford Sleepiness Scale (SSS), a "6" means the person is "fighting sleep" (see STANFORD SLEEPINESS SCALE). That value was given after the last tone to which the person responded; sleep won the battle shortly after that, for all responses ceased by the middle of the figure, and by the end of the figure, all indices show that sleep has begun.

Mechanisms of Sleep Onset

As researchers continue to study sleep–wake control, there is growing realization that no single brain area turns sleep on or off. Damage to many cortical, forebrain, and/or brainstem structures seriously disrupts sleep–wake regulation. McGinty (1985) argues that sleep is controlled by structures widely distributed throughout the brain and states that other physiological control systems cannot be distinguished from sleep control systems. The interaction of sleep–wake and respiratory control in the brainstem is an important example of McGinty's point: we have seen respiratory changes at sleep onset but have difficulty deciding whether respiratory changes or sleep–wake changes are primary. (See also NREM SLEEP MECHANISMS.)

Conclusions

As Figure 1 shows, there is good agreement on what constitutes definite wakefulness and clearly developed sleep. An exact transition point is probably impossible to discern because the changes being examined are continuous ones. Many researchers view stage 1 activity not as sleep, but as part of the transition period leading to sleep (see STAGES OF SLEEP). People are still quite responsive to external events during stage 1, which has as much in common with wakefulness as with sleep. Hypnagogic mental activity from stage 1 arousals shows features of both waking thoughts and sleeping dreams. The beginning of stage 2 sleep, with its K-complexes and spindles which are unique to sleep, is also the time when people become much less responsive to things around them; that is, they have attained sleep onset—the sleep state has truly been entered.

REFERENCES

Foulkes D. 1966. *The psychology of sleep.* New York: Scribner's.

Johnson LC. 1973. Are stages of sleep related to waking behavior? *Am Sci* 61:326–338.

Kleitman N. 1957. Sleep, wakefulness and consciousness. *Psychol Bull* 54:354–359.

McGinty DJ. 1985. Physiological equilibrium and the control of sleep states. In McGinty DJ, Drucker-Colin R, Morrison A, Parmeggiani PL, eds. *Brain mechanisms of sleep.* New York: Raven Press.

Ogilvie RD, Simons IA, Kuderian RH, MacDonald T, Rustenburg J. 1991. Behavioral, event-related potential, and EEG/FFT changes at sleep onset. *Psychophysiology* 28:54–64.

Ogilvie RD, Wilkinson RT. 1984. The detection of sleep onset: Behavioral and physiological convergence. *Psychophysiology* 21:510–520.

Rechtschaffen A, Kales A, eds. 1968. *A manual of standardized terminology, techniques and scoring system for sleep stages of human subjects.* Los Angeles: UCLA, Brain Information Service/Brain Research Institute.

Robert D. Ogilvie

SLEEP PARALYSIS

Sleep paralysis, a brief episode of partial or total paralysis occurring at the beginning or end of a sleep period, has been recognized by physicians at least since 1876. It has been called *night palsy, sleep numbness, cataplexy of awakening,* and *hypnagogic cataplexy.*

Sleep paralysis is an unforgettable experience. The paralysis, which prevents limb movement and eye opening, is frequently accompanied by a sensation of struggling to move or speak or of fighting to wake up. The subject may believe that he or she is dying or unable to breathe. Frightening illusions or hallucinations, such as visions of animals or monsters in the room or a sense that persons are about to enter the room, often accompany the paralysis. The subject often feels awake or half-awake and is usually aware of being in bed. The sensations accompanying the first episode of sleep paralysis are often so vivid and terrifying that the person recalls them clearly for years afterward. With repeated episodes, the experience becomes more familiar and there is less associated anxiety and fear.

Despite the intense psychic experience of sleep paralysis, the subject appears to be asleep with eyes closed. There may be occasional twitches, slight moans, or irregular respirations. The episodes usually last a few seconds or minutes and may end abruptly during an intense effort to move, or may terminate after brief stimulation such as the touch of another person. Less commonly, the paralysis continues despite vigorous attempts by observers to arouse the subject. After an attack, the subject usually feels entirely normal although there may be some residual anxiety.

Relationship to Narcolepsy

In medical practice, sleep paralysis is encountered most often in persons with NARCOLEPSY. Sleep paralysis occurs in about 60 percent of narcoleptic patients and is one of the classical tetrad of narcoleptic symptoms along with SLEEPINESS, CATAPLEXY, and HYPNAGOGIC HALLUCINATIONS. It usually develops between ages 15 and 30 years and may occur just a few times per year or as often as every night. With advancing age, attacks of sleep paralysis often become less frequent.

Pathophysiology

Electrophysiological studies during attacks of sleep paralysis in patients with narcolepsy have demonstrated muscle ATONIA that appears to be identical to the loss of tone that accompanies REM sleep. These studies have also shown that sleep paralysis at the onset of sleep occurs in association with SLEEP-ONSET REM periods and almost never when the initial sleep is NREM. The facial twitches and irregular respirations are also similar to events of REM sleep and suggest that sleep paralysis is caused by an overlap of REM SLEEP PHYSIOLOGY with wakefulness. The hallucinations accompanying the paralysis are identical to hypnagogic hallucinations and are probably a consequence of dream imagery occurring during wakefulness.

Isolated Sleep Paralysis

Sleep paralysis without other symptoms of narcolepsy is called isolated sleep paralysis. It usually occurs at the end of a period of sleep, often following a nap, whereas sleep paralysis in NARCOLEPSY can occur at the beginning or at the end of a sleep period. Isolated sleep paralysis is most common during adolescence, when up to 5 percent of persons may experience it. In rare instances, isolated sleep paralysis occurs in several members of a family. Isolated sleep paralysis is most likely to occur after a period of sleep disruption or a change in sleep schedule, situations that increase the likelihood that naps will include REM sleep.

Treatment

Although sleep paralysis can be a frightening experience, it is not harmful and usually does not require treatment. Some patients with narcolepsy, however, experience sleep paralysis with such regularity when they lie down to sleep that they resort to sleeping in chairs or in a semi-upright position in which sleep paralysis is less likely to occur. Tricyclic antidepressant medications, which suppress REM sleep and are effective treatment for cataplexy and sleep paralysis, are sometimes prescribed for these individuals.

REFERENCES

Goode GB. 1962. Sleep paralysis. *Arch Neurol* 6: 228–234.
Hishikawa Y. 1975. Sleep paralysis. In Guilleminault C, Dement WC, Passouant P, eds. *Narcolepsy,* pp 97–124. New York: Spectrum.

Michael Aldrich

SLEEP POSITIONS

Sleep is the only time when the body is allowed to relax completely. Thus, without muscular tonus, the body assumes a lateral position as a result of the force of gravity. It remains in this recumbent position for the duration of the sleeping period. However, sleepers exhibit postural variations. One may go to bed in a certain position and awaken in yet another contorted state. Some people maintain that these nocturnal body shifts do not occur in their sleep. However, research has dispelled this belief.

In 1930, for a study sponsored by a mattress company, Johnson, Swan, and Weigand photographed 112 subjects asleep with use of a 16-millimeter camera. This pioneering work discovered that each subject exhibits his/her own repertoire of preferred positions and confirmed the occurrence of postural shifts during sleep. The periods of immobility present during sleep varied in length, and position changes occurred between twenty and forty-five times per night. Although the experiment was limited to the technology of the time, the study has been replicated with similar results, providing reliable evidence to support previous anecdotal observations and clinical speculations about changes in sleep positions. Further techniques were later developed that utilized various measurement devices such as the "sensitive bed," which measures movement displacements; time-lapse photography (Hobson, Spagna, and Malenka, 1978); videotaping; direct observations; and electroencephalographic/electromyographic recordings. It has been found that the most accurate recordings of sleep positions combine at least two of these various measures.

Most individuals have a preferred position for sleep, whether it be on one's back, stomach, side, or a variation of one of these. A question often asked is whether there exists a proper sleeping position. Although this query remains not fully explored, there is some research that may provide insight. In terms of sleep satisfaction, sleep positions appear to be related to the quality of sleep one receives. Poor sleepers spend more time in the dorsal position (on the back with head straight), whereas good sleepers occupy more periods of immobility in a contorted position, similar to the healthy position reported by Johnson, Swan, and Weigand over 50 years earlier. The sleep position of these poor sleepers also appears to correspond with the normal position of sleepers who complain of respiratory problems (see APNEA). Sound sleepers spend more sleep time immobile than poor sleepers. The poor sleepers tend to have more movement patterns, which seem to disrupt their sleep. Sound sleep is also characterized by eight to twelve shifts per night, which corresponds with the dozen gross postural changes during 8 hours of sleep observed by Johnson, Swan, and Weigand (1930).

These studies do suggest the "proper" sleep position to be a curved, "fetal," side position with longer periods of immobility generally accompanying sound sleep. There exists large variations among individuals, and the same sleepers often vary from night to night, but this pattern of postures and postural changes remains consistent.

> All of them [sleeping subject's positions] that are maintained for fairly long periods are contorted; in particular, the spinal column is always curved laterally, and usually bowed backward, and also twisted (Johnson, Swan, and Weigand 1930, p. 2062).

Although research tends to agree with this observation, there remains a lack of evidence in complete support of one "proper" sleeping position. At best, it seems that a combination of postures is recommended.

Abnormal Sleep Positions

The relationship between sleep positions and quality of sleep may be compounded by an uncomfortable bed or sleeping surface, which may also result in poor sleep. For instance, a soft mattress may place excessive stress on certain parts of the body, especially the spine. Such pressure on nerves and blood vessels can cause numbness or more severe pain; however, these discomforts are usually transient. In response to this discomfort, sleeping positions may change more frequently. Snoring can also be reduced by a change in sleep positions. Sleeping on the side position as opposed to flat on one's back reduces heavy snoring. Postural changes may also be an indicator of a more severe problem (see APNEA), in which case a sleep disorders professional should be consulted.

In addition, alcohol may affect sleep position changes and movement. It is known that alcohol disrupts sleep, which may result in more brief awakenings and consequent movement. Alcohol's inhibitory effect on movement may also cause temporary immobility ("Saturday night paralysis") if there is excessive alcoholic con-

sumption (see ALCOHOLISM). Heavy sedative medication also tends to create this "loglike" slumber. These forms of immobility, although from different exogenous sources, are quite similar.

Relation to Sleep Stages

Major postural changes during sleep are associated with changes in sleep stages. This correlation between the change of position and electroencephalographic stage generally occurs at the cyclic end of NREM (stage 4 sleep) and REM sleep. Two shifts per sleep cycle are typical. "Tossing and turning" sleep is usually more than two shifts per cycle, which typifies the sleep of an insomniac. Postural shifts do not always mark sleep stages. A shift may be merely preceding or following a brief arousal, whereas sleep stage changes from stage 4 or REM sleep are often marked by major body shifts.

In addition to major postural shifts, there is an increase in the frequency of general body movement as the night progresses. This is known as the "crescendo effect," which also corresponds with the distribution of sleep stages. In the early night, when "deep" or slow-wave sleep is abundant during sleep cycles, there is a longer duration of body immobility. The latter half of sleep, which is dominated by REM sleep, is characterized by more frequent body movements (see CYCLES OF SLEEP ACROSS THE NIGHT).

Sleep positions are characterized by the relaxation or paralysis of muscular activity. In the latter case, which occurs during REM sleep, atonia is caused by the brain suppressing muscular movements. The period of body immobility, when the sleep position remains stable, is thought to be associated with the regenerative aspects of sleep, corresponding to the lack of mobility during slow-wave sleep. Insufficient evidence is available to draw any final conclusions concerning this possible correlation.

Sleep Positions in Animals

In the first century B.C., Lucretius observed small movements in horses and dogs and related them to dreaming. Since that time, numerous animal studies have been done examining sleep postures in horses, cats, hyenas, foxes, kangaroos, mice, etc. Foxes curl up with their tails touching their head. Cats prefer their sides, either stretched or rolled up. Whereas most animals exhibit atonia, birds that sleep in a perched position require the use of certain muscles to maintain balance. And similarly, bats sleep hanging upside down. Lions, bears, and rabbits are some of the few animals that favor sleeping on their backs. Thus, animals have their own characteristic sleep positions just as humans do. Horses exhibit four resting and sleeping positions: standing with head held free, standing with head resting on a structure, lying on its belly, or lying on its side. In addition, the deeper the sleep, the more likely that the horse will sleep on its side. In relation to sleep stages, it has been found that as in humans, REM sleep in mice can be identified by measuring body movements. These observations in animals support the findings that sleep positions are distinctive characteristics that correlate with various other aspects of sleep, for example, sleep stages. (See also ANIMALS IN SLEEP RESEARCH.)

REFERENCES

Borbély A. 1986. *Secrets of sleep,* pp 106–108. New York: Basic Books.

De Koninck J, Gagnon P, Lallier S. 1983. Sleep positions in the young adult and their relationship with the subjective quality of sleep. *Sleep* 6(1):52–59.

Hobson JA, Spagna T, Malenka R. 1978. Ethology of sleep studied with time-lapse photography: Postural immobility and sleep-cycle phase in humans. *Science* 201(29):1251–1253.

Johnson HM, Swan TH, Weigand GE. 1930. In what positions do healthy people sleep? *JAMA,* June 28, pp. 2058–2062.

Richard Lee

SLEEP RESTRICTION, THERAPEUTIC

Sleep restriction is a treatment for INSOMNIA in which reducing time spent in bed is the chief intervention. The treatment grew out of the observation that many individuals with sleep disturbance spent extra time in bed in an attempt to redress their sleep loss. On most occasions, however, the extra time in bed did not yield more sleep but rather more tossing and turning. It was hypothesized that a significant reduction in time in bed would not only cut out the extra wakefulness but also consolidate sleep and render it less susceptible to interruption.

The first step in sleep restriction is to assess how much sleep the patient thinks he or she obtains. The restricted bedtime is set initially equal to this subjective estimate. Thus, a patient who spends 7.5 hours in bed and reports sleeping 5.5 hours would be prescribed 5.5 hours in bed. The timing of arising is set at the habitual wakeup time. Retiring time is therefore later than usual to accomplish the restriction. Total time in bed is not reduced below 4.5 hours for anyone, even for those patients who claim not to sleep at all. This minimum is designed to limit the extent of daytime drowsiness.

This restricted regimen is then repeatedly modified according to one of two decision rules. One rule is based on sleep efficiency, defined as the percentage of time in bed spent asleep over the past 5 to 7 days. Sleep efficiency will almost certainly improve on the restricted regime. When it reaches 85 percent or 90 percent, the individual is given more time in bed. The rationale for this increment is that the patient is using nearly all of the allotted time in bed for sleep and may be able to consistently sleep for a longer period. If, on the other hand, a substantial time in bed is still spent awake, then time in bed may be further reduced. Typically, the retiring time is altered by 15 minutes.

Another decision rule used to alter time in bed involves preprogrammed increases from the initial restricted level on a weekly basis. This approach has the benefit of bolstering patient morale in that only increases in time in bed are scheduled. It also addresses the problem posed by that subgroup of patients who invariably report little or no change in their amount of sleep. A typical schedule might entail an initial 2.5-hour reduction of time in bed followed by a 30-minute increase after 1 week and 15-minute increases for the next 2 or 3 weeks.

Prospects for successful treatment are improved when the patient is prepared for the challenges inherent in sleep restriction. It is likely that the patient will sleep less than usual for the first few weeks of treatment. Significant daytime sleepiness must be anticipated. Patients are cautioned against driving or operating dangerous machinery if they are feeling drowsy. Patients are also told that the process of sleep consolidation triggered by sleep restriction typically takes 2 or 3 weeks and that, overall, they may feel that their functioning gets worse before it gets better. In addition, the first few weeks of treatment require the patient to stay up hours later than usual. The patient should plan specific activities to help stay awake. Tasks such as light housekeeping, organizing a shelf, and cleaning out a desk drawer are not too mentally or physically demanding and will help preclude inadvertent sleep episodes.

Another feature of sleep restriction that patients may find daunting is that it effectively precludes the possibility of their obtaining a "great night's sleep." Many patients have come to rely on such sleep occurring intermittently, and they may argue that it is only the prospect of such a night that keeps them functioning at all. Sleep restriction replaces the variability that is one of the hallmarks of insomnia with a predictable string of barely adequate nights of sleep. In doing so, it addresses the anticipatory anxiety that most insomniacs feel regarding the upcoming night's sleep: Will tonight be a disaster and ruin my plans for tomorrow? The heightened need for sleep at the beginning of treatment helps protect against disastrous nights of little sleep.

Sleep hygiene approaches to sleep problems often incorporate some features of sleep restriction, and the reverse is also true (see SLEEP HYGIENE). A course of sleep restriction therapy will benefit from a prohibition of daytime NAPPING; reduction of CAFFEINE, cigarette, and ALCOHOL consumption; and other commonsense guidelines.

REFERENCES

Glovinsky PB, Spielman AJ. 1991. Sleep restriction therapy. In Hauri P, ed. *Case studies in insomnia,* pp 49–63. New York: Plenum Press.

Spielman AJ, Saskin P, Thorpy MJ. 1987. Treatment of chronic insomnia by restriction of time spent in bed. *Sleep* 10(1):45–56.

Arthur J. Spielman
Paul B. Glovinsky

SLEEP SPINDLES

Spindle waves are one of the major components of the electroencephalogram (EEG). They appear during the early part of sleep in humans as well as in cats, the animal of choice for cellular studies of the sleep cycle. As such, spindles are a landmark of the transition from drowsiness to full-blown sleep. The study of the origin and cellular mechanisms of spindles allows a better understanding of brain processes involved in shifting the adaptive state of waking to the sleep state, when we are disconnected from the external reality. (See also SLEEP ONSET.)

Description

Spindles are so termed because of their waxing and waning envelope. They are defined as 7- to 14-cycle-per-second waves, clustered within sequences lasting 1 to 2 seconds and recurring periodically every 3 to 10 seconds (see bottom panel in Figure 1). Thus, there are two spindle-related rhythms: an *intra*spindle oscillation (7 to 14 cycles per second) and a slower *inter*spindle rhythm (0.1 to 0.3 cycles per second). Both rhythms should be taken into consideration, because other EEG activities (such as alpha waves occurring during wakefulness) have a frequency similar to that of the intraspindle oscillation.

Origin

Spindles originate in the thalamus, a neuronal mass consisting of about 40 cellular aggregates (nuclei) and located deep within the brain, between the cerebral cortex and the brainstem. During the mid-1940s, it was demonstrated that spindles can still be recorded in the THALAMUS after complete removal of the cerebral cortex and disconnection from the brainstem. It is now established that spindles survive in the thalamus even after more radical procedures involving the removal of other brain structures.

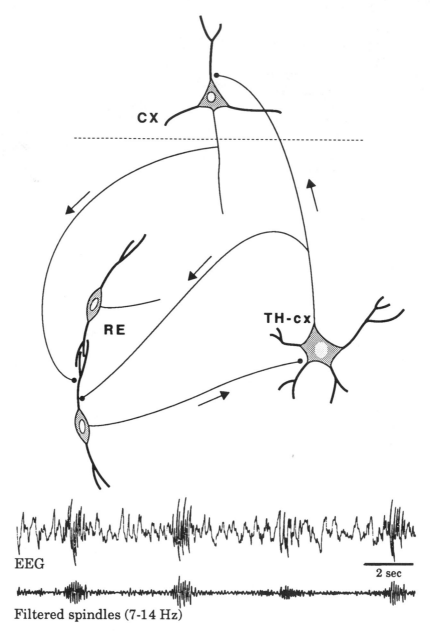

EEG

2 sec

Filtered spindles (7-14 Hz)

Figure 1. Neuronal circuit producing electroencephalographic spindle waves. The upper diagram shows a thalamic cell with axon projecting to the cerebral cortex (TH-cx) and an axonal collateral to the reticular (RE) thalamic nucleus; two thalamic RE inhibitory cells (one of them projecting back to a TH-cx cell); and a cortical pyramid-shaped cell with a collateral to the RE cell (cx). Arrows indicate the direction of axons. Below, EEG waves are shown during an epoch of quiet sleep in cat. In the upper trace, spindle sequences are shown to occur between slow (delta) waves. The lower trace, from the same epoch, depicts only spindles, as the EEG trace was filtered to illustrate 7- to 14-cycle-per-second waves in isolation.

Cellular Mechanisms: The Spindle Pacemaker

The cellular events associated with spindle rhythms have been revealed by recording the electrical activity of two thalamic cell types: (1) thalamocortical (TH-cx) neurons, which have axons projecting to the cerebral cortex, and (2) thalamic reticular (RE) neurons, which receive information from TH-cx neurons as well as from cortical neurons, but do not project to the cortex; instead, RE cells project back to TH-cx cells (Figure 1). TH-cx cells use excitatory amino acids as neuronal transmitters, whereas RE cells use a potent inhibitory transmitter, γ-aminobutyric acid (GABA) (see CHEMISTRY OF SLEEP: AMINES AND OTHER TRANSMITTERS). The thalamic circuit involved in the genesis of spindles is a feedback inhibitory loop, consisting of TH-cx neurons exciting RE neurons, which in turn inhibit TH-cx neurons (Figure 1).

The activities of RE and TH-cx neurons, recorded intracellularly with a fine pipette, are shown in Figure 2 depicting a single sequence of spindle waves. In RE neurons, a spindle sequence appears as a continuous excitation, with successive spike bursts at 7 to 14 cycles per second. A mirror (inverse) image is seen in target Th-cx cells where a spindle sequence consists of cyclic inhibitory potentials lasting about 70 to 150 milliseconds (thus recurring with a frequency of 7 to 14 cycles per second). As with some other types of central neurons, long-lasting periods of inhibition uncover in TH-cx cells a special conductance for calcium ions, which gives rise to bursts of high-frequency action potentials. These bursts are transferred along TH-cx axons and they excite, within the frequency range of spindles, cortical neurons (see neuron Cx in Figure 2). These are the cellular bases of spindles recorded on the EEG.

It was proposed that the inhibitory potentials in TH-cx cells are produced by GABAergic (i.e., cells using GABA as a transmitter) RE neurons, which would function as spindle generators in TH-cx systems. Experimental evidence has confirmed this hypothesis. Indeed, selective destruction of RE cells is followed by loss of spindling in the remaining thalamus as well as in the cerebral cortex. On the other hand, RE neurons isolated

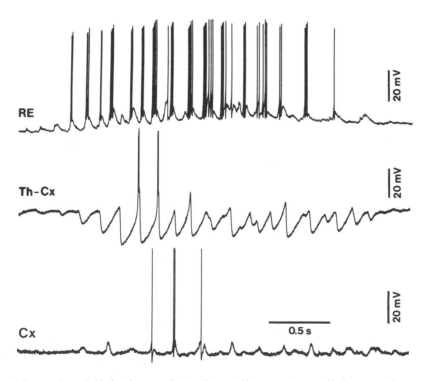

Figure 2. Cellular bases of spindle oscillations. Intracellular recordings of reticular thalamic (RE), thalamocortical (TH-cx), and cortical (cx) cells of cat. The recordings are taken from one spindle sequence. For details, see text.

from any input still display spindle oscillations. These results point to the RE thalamic nucleus as the spindle pacemaker.

Functions of Spindles

The primary role of spindles is thought to be the inhibition of the very special function of the thalamus in wakefulness; that is, the thalamus is a primary sensory way station for transmitting information from the environment to the cortex. TH-cx cells spend about 80 percent of the time during sleep in long-lasting inhibitory periods, consisting of either spindling oscillations that prevail in stage 2 sleep or delta oscillations that prevail in stages 3 and 4. When these TH-cx neurons are inhibited, signals from different sense organs are not allowed to pass the thalamic gates en route to the cerebral cortex. Thus, the thalamus is the first central station where incoming messages are blocked at sleep onset. This is a prerequisite for a well-deserved rest in the cerebral cortex during NREM sleep. (See THALAMUS; AROUSAL; STAGES OF SLEEP; NREM SLEEP.)

REFERENCES

Steriade M, Jones EG, Llinás RR. 1990. *Thalamic oscillations and signaling.* New York: Wiley–Interscience.

Steriade M, Llinás RR. 1988. The functional states of the thalamus and their associated neuronal interplay. *Physiol Rev* 68:649–742.

M. Steriade

SLEEPTALKING

Sleeptalking (somniloquy) is an ubiquitous phenomenon characterized by verbal vocalizations during sleep. These vocalizations are usually difficult to understand and are often nonsensical. There may be a familial tendency, and episodes may be triggered by incomplete arousals. Despite its frequency, surprisingly little research has been conducted on sleeptalking. Sleeptalking can occur during any or all stages (both REM and NREM) of sleep. Those episodes occurring during REM sleep may more often be associated with recall of sleep mentation. Sleeptalking probably carries no psychological or psychiatric significance, and the content should be taken very lightly (Mahowald and Ettinger, 1990). It rarely causes problems to the talker, except when very frequent or loud, or under circumstances involving multiple roommates or dormitory-style sleeping facilities. There have been no scientific reports of treatment attempts.

REFERENCE

Mahowald MW, Ettinger MG. 1990. Things that go bump in the night: The parasomnias revisited. *J Clin Neurophysiol* 7:119–143.

Mark W. Mahowald

SLEEP TERRORS

Sleep terrors, or night terrors (pavor nocturnus), exemplify the extreme form of "disorders of arousal," which include SLEEPWALKING and sleep drunkenness. Night terrors are common in children (up to 6 percent prevalence), with a peak prevalence between 5 and 7 years of age (Thorpy, 1990). Contrary to popular opinion, they also occur in adults, and there is little evidence that the majority of either children or adults experiencing sleep terrors have any significant underlying psychiatric disease or psychological problems. The most important underlying factor is a genetic predisposition (Mahowald and Rosen, 1990). As in the case of sleep drunkenness and sleepwalking, they may be triggered by sleep deprivation, fever, stress, and medications or drugs (i.e., alcohol).

Sleep terrors represent the simultaneous occurrence of incompletely declared wakefulness and NREM sleep. Polygraphic monitoring during an episode reveals elements of both wakefulness and NREM sleep. Their tendency to occur during the deepest stages of NREM sleep (slow-wave sleep, stage 4) explains their usual appearance within the first 2 hours of the sleep period and their infrequent appearance during daytime naps.

Like sleepwalking, sleep terrors can occasionally be triggered by sensory (usually auditory) stimulation. This suggests that they are not the culmination of ongoing, complex, emotionally laden thought processes occurring during sleep. They are typically heralded by a "blood-curdling" shriek accompanied by signs of intense fear and cataclysmic panic, such as sweating and dilated pupils, with significant increases in heart rate, respiratory rate, and blood pressure. Frantic yelling and frenzied movements, including arm-flailing and running as though attempting to escape a perceived dreadful threat, are common. Such violent behaviors may result in inadvertent injury to the victim or the protector. Inconsolability during an attack is almost universal, and attempts at consolation are not only futile, but may serve to prolong the episode. These phenomena demonstrate a curious paradox: profound internal arousal immune to external arousal.

Although often confused with "bad dreams," "nightmares," or "dream anxiety attacks," sleep terrors represent a completely different phenomenon. Conventional dream anxiety attacks arise from REM (dream) sleep, whereas sleep terrors arise from NREM sleep. During REM sleep there is paralysis of all muscles (except for the diaphragm and eye-movement muscles) (see ATONIA), which would preclude such vigorous behaviors. The anxiety accompanying sleep terrors is much more severe, and unlike dream anxiety attacks, there is usually no remembered complex mentation or theme that led to the arousal. There may be recall of simple, fragmentary frightening imagery such as the apparition of a wild animal, fire, or other perceived danger. Also, unlike the dream anxiety attack, there is usually complete AMNESIA of the event. They are clearly more frightening to the observer than to the victim.

Inasmuch as sleep terrors are usually infrequent and do not result in violent or potentially injurious behavior, reassurance of their benign nature is often effective treatment. It is understandably difficult to convince parents that their "panic-stricken" child is, in fact, unaware of the event. The episodes typically decrease in frequency with increasing age. It should be stressed that these are usually not the manifestation of psychiatric disease. If they are associated with potentially violent or injurious behavior, or ex-

tremely disruptive to family members, formal evaluation may be indicated. It may be impossible on clinical grounds to differentiate sleep terrors from other parasomnias such as unusual nocturnal seizures, REM SLEEP BEHAVIOR DISORDER, or psychogenic dissociative conditions such as fugue states or multiple-personality disorders (Mahowald and Schenck, 1992). Precipitating factors such as sleep deprivation, medication, or drug ingestion should be avoided. Treatment with a variety of medications (BENZODIAZEPINES) or simple hypnosis is often effective. (See EPILEPSY.)

Erroneously applied synonyms include *incubus* and *succubus*.

REFERENCES

Mahowald MW, Ettinger MG. 1990. Things that go bump in the night: The parasomnias revisited. *J Clin Neurophysiol* 7:119–143.

Mahowald MW, Rosen GM. 1990. Parasomnias in children. *Pediatrician* 17:21–31.

Mahowald MW, Schenck CH. 1992. Parasomnia purgatory—the epileptic/non-epileptic parasomnia interface. In Rowan AJ, Gates JR, eds. *The dilemma of non-epileptic (pseudoepileptic) seizures.* Springfield, Md.: Butterworths.

Thorpy MJ. 1990. Disorders of arousal. In Thorpy MJ, ed. *Handbook of sleep disorders,* pp 531–549. New York: Marcel Dekker.

Mark W. Mahowald

SLEEP THERAPY

Sleep therapy, or *electrosleep therapy,* is an unconventional technique developed in Russia to treat many medical disorders. Treatments are given several times weekly for several weeks: Patients lie in a darkened room, and a small electric current (approximately 0.5 volts, 0.2 amps) is applied to the brain using small surface electrodes attached to each side of the head. This stimulus produces sufficient drowsiness, especially when combined with hypnotics, for patients to fall asleep for 1 to 2 hours. Although there is no conclusive documentation of electrosleep's effectiveness, the procedure is used to treat many medical conditions, including nervous system disorders, high blood pressure, ulcers, and heart disease. Electrosleep may alleviate these and other symptoms as a result of the relaxation it produces.

REFERENCE

Fenichel M. 1958. Electro-sleep in a chronic disturbed service. *Dis Nerv Syst* 19 (Monogr. Suppl.):84–86.

Martin A. Cohn

SLEEPWALKING

Sleepwalking (somnambulism) is a mild form of the "disorders of arousal." Other forms include SLEEP TERRORS and sleep drunkenness. Sleepwalking is extremely common, occurring in up to 40 percent of children, with a peak incidence at 11 to 12 years of age. The reported incidence in adults (2.5 percent) is likely understated. It may even begin in adulthood. Sleepwalking can be induced in normal children by arousing them during NREM sleep. This fact indicates that there is often no antecedent emotionally laden thought process (Mahowald and Ettinger, 1990; Kavey et al., 1990; Mahowald and Rosen, 1990).

Mild forms consist of simply sitting up in bed and mumbling (often incoherently). More complex forms involve leaving the bed, walking around in or outside the house, or even driving an automobile. The eyes are usually open, but appear not to be focusing. Some degree of awareness of the environment is apparent, as often objects of furniture are bypassed or stairs negotiated safely. Although the individual appears to be awake, he or she is unable to perceive the environment properly or to exercise proper judgment. Sleepwalking undoubtedly represents a mild form of the night terror. Sleepwalking episodes are usually associated with complete amnesia. If the victims do not awaken during the spell, or do not awaken later in the sleep cycle to find themselves in a place different from where they went to sleep, they are often none the wiser. Although there is no truth to the old wives' tale that

one "should never awaken a sleepwalker," it is usually difficult to awaken a sleepwalker during an episode (see MYTHS ABOUT SLEEP). Gently guiding the sleepwalker back to an appropriate sleeping place is the best management.

Most sleepwalking episodes are benign; however, more extreme cases may involve potentially injurious or violent behavior: loading shotguns, turning on the stove, or misperceiving a bed partner as a source of danger.

Physiologically, there is the simultaneous occurrence of incompletely declared wakefulness and NREM sleep. Polygraphic monitoring during an episode of sleepwalking reveals electroencephalographic elements of both wakefulness and NREM sleep. All of the disorders of arousal occur during NREM sleep, particularly during the deepest stages (SLOW-WAVE SLEEP). Because the majority of slow-wave sleep occurs during the early portion of the sleep period, sleepwalking episodes most often take place within 2 hours of falling asleep. Slow-wave sleep (and therefore sleepwalking) rarely occurs during daytime naps. Complex motor behaviors during sleep are rarely the manifestation of "acting out of dreams," because during REM, or dream, sleep there is paralysis of all muscles except for the diaphragm and those controlling eye movements, which prevents acting upon dream mentation (see ATONIA).

One interesting variant of conventional sleepwalking is the "sleep-related eating disorder." Some individuals without eating disorders while awake will manifest eating behaviors during sleepwalking episodes. This sleep-related behavior may result in difficult to explain weight gain, fear of choking on food while eating asleep, or concern about starting fires or sustaining burns while cooking asleep (Schenck et al., 1991).

Contrary to popular opinion, there is little evidence that conventional sleepwalking is indicative of significant underlying psychiatric disease in either children or adults. The tendency to sleepwalk is genetically determined, and may be precipitated by sleep deprivation, fever, stress, or drugs and medications (i.e., alcohol). Most cases are best managed by reassurance of its benign nature, with emphasis upon lack of psychiatric significance. In most cases, the sleepwalking episodes gradually resolve spontaneously, becoming less frequent with increasing age. Instances resulting in potentially injurious or violent behavior, or causing severe disruption to other family members, may require formal sleep laboratory evaluation. Such evaluation is necessary because other conditions such as unusual nocturnal seizures, the REM SLEEP BEHAVIOR DISORDER, and psychogenic dissociative states (fugues or multiple personality disorders) may be impossible to differentiate from sleepwalking by clinical history alone. Effective treatment includes medications, such as BENZODIAZEPINES, or simple hypnosis (Hurwitz et al., 1991). Long-term treatment with medications is to be discouraged, unless the behaviors are frequent, violent, and unresponsive to behavioral therapy. Precipitating factors such as sleep deprivation or medications and drugs should be avoided. (See EPILEPSY.)

REFERENCES

Hurwitz TD, Mahowald MW, Schenck CH, Schluter JL, Bundlie SR. 1991. A retrospective outcome study and review of hypnosis as treatment of adults with sleepwalking and sleep terror. *J Nerv Ment Dis* 179:228–233.

Kavey NB, Whyte J, Resor SR Jr, Gidro-Frank S. 1990. Somnambulism in adults. *Neurology* 40:749–752.

Mahowald MW, Ettinger MG. 1990. Things that go bump in the night: The parasomnias revisited. *J Clin Neurophysiol* 7:119–143.

Mahowald MW, Rosen GM. 1990. Parasomnias in children. *Pediatrician* 17:21–31.

Schenck CH, Hurwitz TD, Bundlie SR, Mahowald MW. Sleep-related eating disorders: Polysomnographic correlates of a heterogeneous syndrome distinct from daytime eating disorders. *Sleep* 14:419–431.

Mark W. Mahowald

SLOW-WAVE SLEEP

Slow-wave sleep (SWS) is usually defined as that part of NREM sleep characterized by a high proportion of electroencephalographic (EEG) slow waves, termed *delta waves*. In humans, SWS traditionally has been considered to be confined to stage 3 and 4 sleep in the visual scoring system (see STAGES OF SLEEP). However, the development in recent years of computer analysis techniques has made it clear that SWS may occur within any portion of NREM sleep. Slow-wave sleep constitutes about 20 percent of a normal night's sleep for young adults, and it is in this state that SLEEP-WALKING (somnambulism) and sleep terrors (pavor nocturnus; see SLEEP TERRORS) usually occur (Guilleminault, 1989). Young children tend to show relatively more SWS, and older people generally exhibit less than healthy young adults. Most SWS occurs during the first 3 hours of a normal night's sleep, but a second, less robust period of SWS has also been observed in people napping in the middle of the day (Campbell and Zulley, 1989) or in people who extend their night's sleep beyond about 12 hours (Broughton, 1975; Gagnon and DeKoninck, 1984; Webb, 1986). For any individual, the absolute amount (i.e., minutes) of SWS per 24 hours remains quite constant from one day to the next.

Slow-wave sleep is often considered to be the "deepest" state of sleep, and is also considered by certain researchers to be the most "important" part of sleep. That it is very deep sleep is reflected in the finding that a much greater stimulus, for example, a louder noise, is required to awaken a person from SWS than from other sleep states (see DEPTH OF SLEEP). The depth of SWS is particularly impressive in young children. One study, for example, found that a group of 10-year-olds could not be awakened from SWS, even with a 123-decibel tone, a sound approaching the intensity of artillery fire or a jet airplane taking off (Busby and Pivik, 1983)! Moreover, a large number of waking functions, such as short- and long-term MEMORY and cognitive and psychomotor performance, are impaired on awakening from SWS when compared with awakenings from other sleep states.

The "importance" of SWS is underscored by several characteristics of its occurrence. For example, when people are deprived of all sleep for, say, 48 hours, they tend to make up the lost SWS preferentially, before making up other types of sleep (such as REM sleep). They also make up *more* of the lost SWS during recovery sleep than any other sleep state. In addition, when a night's sleep is restricted from the typical 7 to 8 hours down to 4 or 5 hours, the usual amount of SWS persists (see COGNITION; REBOUND). That is, the 3 to 4 hours of lost sleep is at the expense of other sleep states, but not SWS. Because of these characteristics, the occurrence of SWS is generally considered to be a reflection of the degree of one's sleep need (see DEPRIVATION).

Although most researchers agree on the importance of SWS, there is less consensus regarding exactly *why* SWS is so important. There are three general theories as to the function of SWS. It has long been hypothesized that sleep in general, and SWS in particular, serves to restore or reverse some process(es) that degrades during wakefulness. Many researchers believe that if SWS does serve a *restorative function,* it may be more closely tied to the restoration of brain processes rather than to bodily restitution. The exact nature of such brain restoration remains unclear (see FATIGUE-RECOVERY MODEL).

It has also been proposed that SWS may serve an *energy conservation* function. According to this theory, SWS serves to counterbalance, during periods when activity is not required, the high energy costs that are associated with the regulation of body temperature during waking hours (see ENERGY CONSERVATION). Evidence to support this notion includes the finding that METABOLISM and body temperature are substantially reduced during SWS. A third, *ecological theory* of SWS function maintains that we enter this state as a behavioral means of guaranteeing the avoidance of predator danger, during times when activity is not necessary. That is, sleep forces us to remain still and quiet when it is advantageous to do so. Why sleep is required for this function, rather than simply quiet wakefulness, remains unclear. None of these theories of SWS function is necessarily at odds with another, and it is unlikely that a process as complex and as widely observed across the animal kingdom as SWS has any single function. Rather, SWS may serve a number of functions simultaneously (see FUNCTIONS OF SLEEP).

REFERENCES

Broughton R. 1975. Biorhythmic variations in consciousness and psychological functions. *Can Psychol Rev* 16:217–239.

Busby K, Pivik RT. 1983. Failure of high intensity auditory stimuli to affect behavioral arousal in children during the first sleep cycle. *Pediatr Res* 17(10):802–805.

Campbell S, Zulley J. 1989. Evidence for circadian influence on human slow wave sleep during daytime sleep episodes. *Psychophysiology* 26:580–585.

Chase M, Roth T, eds. 1990. *Slow wave sleep: Its measurement and functional significance.* Los Angeles: Brain Information Service/Brain Research Institute. Contains an annotated bibliography of studies on slow-wave sleep from 1986 to 1989.

Gagnon P, De Koninck M. 1984. Reappearance of EEG slow waves in extended sleep. *Electroencephalogr Clin Neurophysiol* 58:155–157.

Guilleminault C. 1989. Sleepwalking and night terrors. In Kryger M, Roth T, Dement W, eds. *Principles and practice of sleep medicine,* pp 379–384. Philadelphia: WB Saunders.

Scott S. Campbell

SMELL DURING SLEEP

To what extent do we remain sensitive to environmental changes during sleep? Specifically, does our sense of smell function while we sleep? Can we detect the odor of smoke? Burning fabric? Perfumes? Coffee? Do odors judged alerting or relaxing during waking affect our nighttime sleep? These are interesting questions and researchers are beginning to address them.

Investigating the sense of smell, in waking or in sleep, poses special problems. The main difficulty is determining whether an odor relates only to smell or provides other stimulus qualities such as touch, pain, and temperature. The human nasal cavity is innervated by branches of both the olfactory and trigeminal nerves. The trigeminal nerve provides the face (nose) with cutaneous sensitivity giving rise to sensations of pungency, irritation, warmth, and cold. Some odors are relatively free of trigeminal stimulation (e.g., vanillin, coffee); others (e.g., menthol, ammonia) produce considerable trigeminal stimulation. If an individual responds to an odor in sleep (or at any time), is the individual reacting to the odor purely on the basis of the sense of smell or is the individual reacting to the odor because of the other, trigeminal sensations?

The procedure for determining whether an odor has trigeminal cues is straightforward. An odor that excites only the olfactory nerve does not permit the subject to localize (identify) the nostril (left/right) to which the odor was delivered. In contrast, odors with a high trigeminal component permit the subject to identify the nostril.

Obviously, if a researcher is interested in

purely olfactory stimuli, then great care must be taken to choose odors without trigeminal cues. Often, however, researchers are interested in a particular odor and are not concerned with analyzing its properties. They are simply interested in whether the odor can be detected in sleep and what effect it has on sleep quality.

One of the earliest studies of olfaction during sleep recorded the electrical activity of the brain in cats following presentation of an odor (Hernandez-Peon et al., 1960). It was found that olfactory stimuli presented during sleep changed the rhythm of the brain waves as recorded on the electroencephalogram. This finding indicates that odors do in fact stimulate the sleeping brain. Others testing newborn human infants showed that odors presented during behavioral sleep increased activity level (Murray and Campbell, 1970).

Several systematic studies with adults tested olfaction during sleep using a method similar to the following. Either an odor or room air was randomly presented to subjects for a 3-minute period during stage 2 sleep. Before going to sleep, subjects were instructed that an odor would be presented to them while they slept. They were also instructed to press a switch and to awaken when they detected it. Measures of brain wave changes, heart rate changes, awakenings, and switch closures were all higher when a fragrance was presented than when only room air was presented. Various odors have yielded similar effects with this procedure, showing that subjects are responsive during sleep but far less so than during waking (Badia et al., 1989, 1990; Carskadon et al., 1990)

Others have investigated whether odors judged to be alerting or relaxing during waking would have an effect on nighttime sleep (see INCORPORATION). It was expected that odors judged as relaxing during waking might enhance sleep and odors judged alerting might degrade sleep. Although this research is only beginning, to date odors presented to sleeping subjects, whether judged alerting or relaxing during waking, tend to be disruptive to sleep.

A different approach concerning reactions to odors presented during sleep was used by Trotter, Dallas, and Verdone (1988). They were interested in whether olfactory stimuli presented to a person while dreaming (i.e., in REM sleep) would be incorporated into dreams (become part of the dream). Odors were presented to subjects

in REM sleep each night across four nights. Subjects were awakened after 1 minute of odor presentation and asked to report their dreams. Seventy-nine dreams were recalled on awakening; 15 were judged to involve incorporation. Others have reported similar low incorporation results using auditory, tactile, and visual stimuli.

The research described indicates that our sense of smell continues to function during sleep, although at a greatly diminished level. These findings are similar to those reported with other sensory modalities. (See also PERCEPTION DURING SLEEP; SENSORY PROCESSING AND SENSATION DURING SLEEP.)

REFERENCES

Badia P, Wesensten N, Lammers W, Culpepper J, Marsh J. 1990. Responsiveness to olfactory stimuli presented in sleep. *Physiol Behav* 48:87–90.

Badia P, Wesensten N, Lammers W, Hughes R, Boecker M. 1989. Olfactory sensitivity in sleep. *Sleep Res* 18:151.

Carskadon MA, Bigler PJ, Carr J, Gelin J, Etgen G, Davis SS, Herman KB. 1990. Olfactory arousal thresholds during sleep. *Sleep Res* 19:147.

Hernandez-Peon R, Lavin A, Alcocer-Cuaron C, Marcelin JP. 1960. Electrical activity of the olfactory bulb during wakefulness and sleep. *Electroencephalogr Clin Neurophysiol* 12:41–58.

Murray B, Campbell D. 1970. Difference between olfactory thresholds in two sleep states in the newborn infant. *Psychon Sci* 18:313–314.

Trotter K, Dallas K, Verdone P. 1988. Olfactory stimuli and their effects on REM dreams. *Psychiatry J Univ Ottawa* 13:94–96.

Pietro Badia

SMOKING AND SLEEP

Numerous studies have demonstrated that the physiological effects of NICOTINE, a major component of cigarette smoke, include effects on sleep and AROUSAL. In addition, many reports have documented the risks of smoking in terms of a wide range of health measures. Physical complaints related to chronic smoking include INSOMNIA, shortness of breath, loss of appetite, and fatigue. Smoking in bed is a particularly hazardous practice, especially for people who are hypersomnolent. The U.S. Fire Administration (1992) has estimated that in 1990 alone, smoking in bed caused 7,700 fires, which resulted in 1,300 injuries and 190 deaths. The specific effect of smoking on sleep has been less well studied, in part because of the difficulty of designing a study with appropriate controls (e.g., the difficulty of having subjects inhale smoke without their knowledge), and in part because of the fact that individuals who smoke often use other substances that affect sleep, such as CAFFEINE and ALCOHOL. Furthermore, cigarette smoke contains substances other than nicotine, such as carbon monoxide, and individuals who smoke may be different from nonsmokers in other subtle ways.

Survey studies have indicated that smokers report more difficulty with sleep than do nonsmokers (Wheatley, 1985; MacGregor and Balding, 1988), and one laboratory study used data from three nights of POLYSOMNOGRAPHY to investigate the sleep of smokers and nonsmokers. The smokers had greater difficulty falling asleep than the nonsmokers, although there were no differences between the two groups on other sleep measures. These researchers also found no differences between smokers and nonsmokers in terms of several psychological measures, and caffeine use was not related to the sleep differences between the two groups (Soldatos et al., 1980). An interesting study from Japan reported that university students who rated themselves as being more "evening" types ("owls") were more likely to smoke than those who rated themselves as being more "morning" types ("larks") (see MORNINGNESS/EVENINGNESS; CIRCADIAN RHYTHMS). The "owls" were also more likely to drink more caffeinated beverages and alcohol than the "larks" and reported less regular sleep–wake habits than the "larks" (Ishihara, Miyasita, and Inugami, 1985). In the United States, Carskadon (1990) has shown that high school students who work 20 hours or more each week were likely to sleep less and have more difficulty staying awake in school, and were more likely to smoke and to drink caffeine, than those students working less than 20 hours per week. Much more research is needed to tease apart the relationships between the effects of smoking, other substance use, and psychological variables with respect to sleep and AROUSAL.

A second laboratory study by Soldatos and colleagues (1980) investigated the effects of abrupt smoking withdrawal on the sleep of eight male smokers. Sleep was monitored in the laboratory for four nights while subjects continued to smoke and then for at least five nights after the subjects had stopped smoking. During the first two withdrawal nights, there was a significant decrease in sleep latency (time until subjects fell asleep) compared with the nights the subjects smoked. On the following nights, subjects showed a decreased sleep latency as well as decreased time spent awake after sleep onset, as compared with smoking nights. Thus, withdrawal from smoking appears objectively to improve sleep, although one of the primary subjective complaints of people trying to quit smoking is that of insomnia.

REFERENCES

Carskadon MA. 1990. Adolescent sleepiness: Increased risk in a high-risk population. *Alcohol Drugs Driving* 5/6:317–328.

Ishihara K, Miyasita A, Inugami M. 1985. Differences in the time or frequency of meals, alcohol and caffeine ingestion, and smoking found between "morning" and "evening" types. *Psychol Rep* 57: 391–396.

MacGregor ID, Balding JW. 1988. Bedtimes and sleep duration in relation to smoking behavior in 14-year-old English schoolchildren. *J Biosocial Sci* 20: 371–376.

Soldatos CR, Kales JD, Scharf MB, Bixler EO, Kales A. 1980. Cigarette smoking associated with sleep difficulty. *Science* 207:551–553.

U.S. Fire Administration. 1992. *Fire in the United States.* Washington, D.C.

Wheatley D. 1985. Insomnia in general practice. *Acta Psychiatr Scand* 74:142–146.

Christine Acebo

SNORING

The word *snore* is derived from eleventh-to fifteenth-century low German (*snorren*), Dutch (*snarren*), and English (*snoren*). The words meant "to drone" or "to hum." The word today is used in a much more vigorous context to refer to the noise made by people when they sleep, but it also refers to the noise a ship makes when it cuts the waves with a roar.

Snoring noises arise in the throat and are

caused by vibration of soft pliable tissues. Figure 1 shows the soft structures that play a role in snoring. This part of the upper airway is vulnerable because it is not supported by any skeletal structures and so can collapse just as a straw collapses when the suction pressure inside the straw is very negative.

People do not snore when they are awake. On falling asleep there occurs a reduction in the tone of the muscles that surround and prevent the throat from collapsing. All people have a loss in the tone of these muscles during sleep, but only some people snore. Several factors contribute to snoring: An airway is at risk if it is already smaller than normal because of increased bulk of the tissues in the throat. Such increase in bulk can be caused by obesity, large tonsils and adenoids, a larger-than-normal tongue, or a smaller-than-normal jaw. Second, people who snore almost always breathe through their mouths during sleep. In many people who snore there is as yet no adequate explanation for why they breathe through their mouths, because their airways are often entirely normal. Medications (sleeping pills, alcohol, and even some cold medications) can make snoring worse because they may relax the muscles in this region. Smoking cigarettes irritates the throat region, which may also make snoring more common. Blocked nostrils, by forcing the person to breathe through the mouth, also can result in snoring.

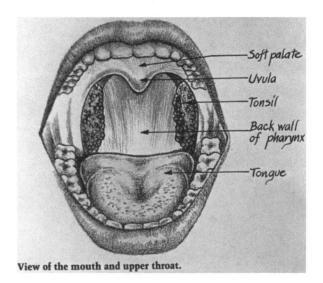

View of the mouth and upper throat.

Figure 1. Structures of the mouth and upper throat involved in snoring. *Reproduced with permission from Lipman, 1990.*

Thus some people snore only when they have nasal obstruction with a cold or during an allergic episode such as hay fever.

Snoring can be extremely loud. Normal speech is usually approximately 40 decibels of loudness. A baby crying or a radio will often register about 60 decibels. Loud snorers may generate a noise equivalent to about 80 decibels, which is about the same loudness as the barking of some dogs or some jackhammers. The loudest snoring ever recorded is almost as loud as the continuous ringing of a telephone or the revving up of a motorcycle. Thus, it is not surprising that some bed partners of snorers and some snorers themselves may suffer from hearing loss. In fact the noise from snoring in some persons is severe enough that it exceeds the government standards for noise in a workplace.

Snoring is extremely common. About 25 percent of all men snore every night. Snoring is unusual among young people, and the prevalence of snoring increases beyond age 35. There is a progressive increase in the prevalence so that in the age group between 41 and 64 years of age, 60 percent of men snore almost every night. For the entire population snoring is found almost twice more frequently in men than women. In women who are between 41 and 64 years of age the prevalence of snoring is about two-thirds the male prevalence. Figure 2 shows the frequency of snoring for men and women at different ages.

The differences related to age are thought to be explainable by the fact that with age there is a loss of tone of the muscles of the throat. Soft tissue distribution including distribution of fat is different in men and women; however, after menopause women lose the protective effect of the hormone progesterone, a respiratory stimulant that may stabilize the muscles of the upper airway.

Although for many years snoring was thought of as more a noisy nuisance than a medical problem, it now appears as though snoring may in fact be a risk factor for the development of cardiovascular disease. Research suggests that arterial hypertension, heart disease, and stroke may be much more common in people who snore than in those who do not snore. Some research suggests that snorers are three times more likely to have a stroke than nonsnorers! If research confirms these findings, then physicians will have to take snoring very seriously.

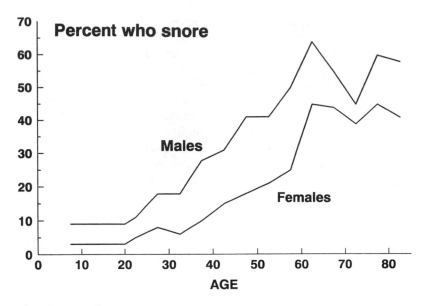

Figure 2.   Snoring in men and women. These data were obtained from 5,713 people living in San Marino. *Data from Lugaresi E, Cirignotta F, Coccagna G, Piana C. 1980. Some epidemiological data on snoring and cardiocirculatory disturbances.* Sleep *3:222.*

Relationship with Sleep Apnea

Patients with sleep APNEA snore. The snoring in sleep apnea patients is not constant. These persons will have regularly repeating periods when they make snoring noises which are then followed by relative quiet followed again by the snoring noises. It is during the quiet snoring intervals that the patients are not breathing (apneic) and when their major abnormalities occur. To start breathing effectively again, sleep apnea patients have a brief awakening which just precedes the resumption of the snoring or snorting. Many awakenings lead to daytime sleepiness. People who snore who do not have sleep apnea (the vast majority of the snoring population) do not have this pattern—the intensity of the snoring is relatively constant. People who have snoring with sleep apnea almost always have severe sleepiness during the daytime, whereas people who simply snore do not.

Because snoring is so disruptive to other people, many cures have been proposed over the years, many having been designed by the bed partner of a loud snorer! The U.S. patent office has hundreds of patents for devices claiming to stop snoring. Figure 3 shows a device designed to stop snoring. Most of the treatments assume that the open mouth plays an important role in the genesis of the snoring, and many devices have been designed to keep the mouth closed. Other suggested cures include devices to keep the snorer off his or her back, because it is known that change in posture from lying flat on the back to the side will reduce snoring. Some people sew tennis balls into the backs of pajamas to keep persons off their backs. The angry spouse sometimes inflicts pain on the snoring bed partner to get him or her to stop snoring. There have been patients who have been evaluated for a mysterious injury suffered during the night that was later proven to be caused by a angry spouse inflicting pain to get her or him to change position. Sometimes snoring is such a serious problem that surgical treatment is used in an operation called UVULOPALATOPHARYNGOPLASTY. Some of the tissues (uvula, tonsils, parts of the soft palate, see Figure 1) that cause the snoring are removed with the operation. If the patient also has sleep apnea, other treatments to treat the apnea are then initiated.

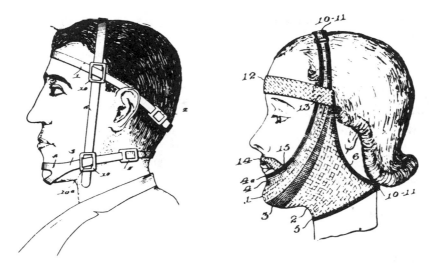

Figure 3. One of many devices invented to stop snoring.

REFERENCES

Lipman D. 1990. *Stop your husband from snoring: A medically proven program to cure the night's worst nuisance.* Emmaus, PA: Rodale Press.

Lugaresi E, Cirignotta F, Montagna P. 1989. Snoring: Pathogenic, clinical, and therapeutic aspects. In Kryger M, Roth T, Dement WC, eds. *Principles and practice of sleep medicine.* chap 53, pp 494–500. Philadelphia: WB Saunders.

M. Kryger

SOMNAMBULISM

See Sleepwalking

SOMNILOQUY

See Sleeptalking

SOMNOLENCE

See Hypersomnia; Sleepiness

SPACE SHUTTLE SLEEPING ARRANGEMENTS

Just as on earth, it is necessary for astronauts to sleep from time to time during spaceflight. However, the time chosen to sleep and the duration of that sleep is something that is precisely regimented. This regimentation is necessary because the most precious commodity during a Space Shuttle flight is the crewmembers' time. To make the best use of the available crew time, therefore, the people in the Mission Control Center on earth carefully choreograph the crew's day in a document known as a *timeline.* Generally, the crew is given an 8-hour block of time in each 24-hour period for sleep.

Having an 8-hour allotment for sleep is one thing; using it for that purpose is quite another. Because the normal work day is completely filled on most flights, the crew's only opportunity to look out at the earth tends to occur during the allotted sleep period. For this reason, many crewmembers choose to sacrifice some of their sleep time to "look out the window" or engage in other desired activities.

Once they get around to it, there are several factors that influence the manner in which the crewmembers try to get their sleep. The first major factor involves whether the crew is on a one- or two-shift mission. On a one-shift mission, the crew are all scheduled to sleep at the same time, whereas on a two-shift mission, half the crew is awake while the other half sleeps. On single-shift missions, the crew is supplied with a piece of equipment called a *sleep restraint,* which resembles a cross between a sleeping bag and a hammock (Figure 1). Its name is descriptive of its function, which is not to keep the crewmember warm but to keep him or her from floating around. When the body is unrestrained and relaxed, as in sleep, an individual tends to assume a position in which the elbows, knees, and hips are all slightly flexed, similar to the position seen in a person who is practicing "drownproofing." Restraint is necessary because the crew is weightless and could possibly, if left unrestrained while asleep, bump into equipment or jostle other sleeping crewmembers causing them to awaken. So as much out of courtesy to other crewmembers as to maintaining a safe working environment, the crewmembers are encouraged to remain restrained while asleep. On single-shift missions, this is sometimes accomplished in rather unorthodox ways, which can include the use of duct tape or elastic "bungee" cords.

Besides restraint, the crew frequently takes

measures to insulate themselves from the ambient light and noise present in the cabin environment. The ambient noise level in the Shuttle typically ranges between 70 and 95 decibels during the work day and remains around 70 to 75 decibels during the sleep period. On single-shift missions the crew uses foam ear plugs to limit problems with sleep stemming from this noisy environment. Another problem stems from the fact that an orbit of the earth takes only approximately 90 minutes, which means that 45 minutes of every 90 minutes are spent in sunlight, which is annoying to some individuals. This is remedied by most crewmembers through the use of eyeshades or Shuttle window shades.

On two-shift missions, the noise and light problem are addressed in a different manner, although the modalities mentioned above are still available for use. On these two-shift missions, bunks that are light-tight, noise-proof, and hardly larger than a full-length gym locker enclose each crew member (Figure 2). In this way, the environmental nuisances are eliminated and at the same time the crewmembers who are at work can perform their jobs without concern for disturbing the crew-

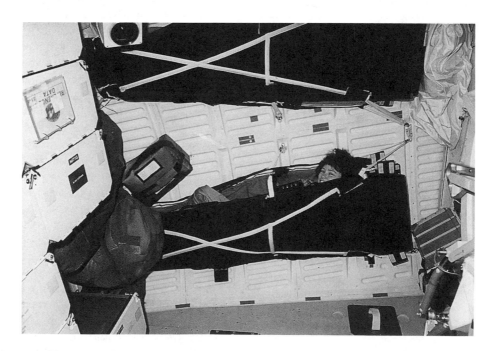

Figure 1.   Astronaut Anna L. Fisher demonstrates the versatility of Shuttle sleep restraints to accommodate the preference of crewmembers as she appears to have configured hers in a horizontal hammock mode. Stowage lockers, one of the mid-deck walls, another sleep restraint, a jury-rigged foot-and-hand restraint are among other items in this 35-millimeter frame.

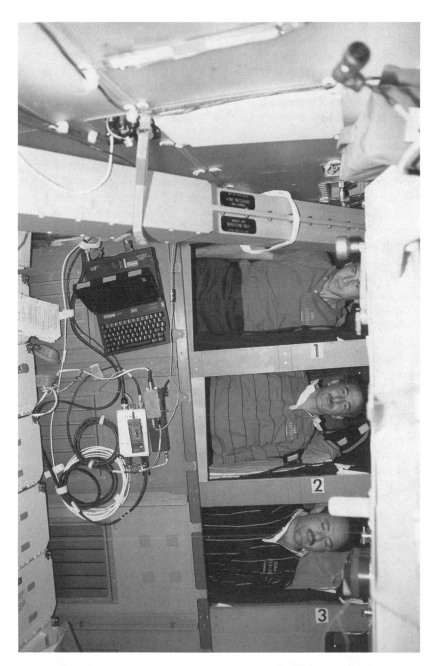

Figure 2.   Although they're not actually asleep, three crewmembers demonstrate the bunk-style sleep quarters onboard *Columbia*. From top to bottom are Payload Specialist Samuel T. Durrance and Astronauts Jeffrey A. Hoffman and John M. (Mike) Lounge, mission specialists. At left is the Shuttle amateur radio experiment (SAREX). The frame was exposed with a 35-millimeter camera.

members who are asleep. Were it not for the considerable space that these bunks occupy, they would be used on single-shift missions as well, because they perform their intended function superbly.

From a subjective standpoint the majority of Shuttle crewmembers report sleep of good quality. This is probably the result of the long work hours that they put in. For crewmembers who experience difficulty sleeping or are concerned that they may encounter difficulty, various sleep medications are made available.

While dreaming is reported, it is not identified as being different from what is experienced on earth. Sleep studies done aboard Skylab in the early 1970s showed that sleep latency was not significantly different in flight from either pre-or postflight. In flight, there did not appear to be significant disturbances in REM sleep as compared with preflight, but an increase in REM sleep was observed postflight. The Skylab investigators' conclusions were that, if anything, the readaptation to 1-g (i.e., back on earth) was more disruptive than the flight itself. They also felt that there was no degradation of performance resulting from sleep disturbances while in orbit.

Except for the absence of gravity and the particular tasks and constraints related to this absence, sleeping in space is not unlike sleeping on earth. The major obstacle to sleep, if there is one, tends to be self-imposed and relates to the voluntary sacrifice of sleep in favor of time to "look out the window" or pursue other activities in the limited time available while in orbit.

James P. Bagian

SPORTS AND SLEEP

Because of known relationships between sleep and daytime PERFORMANCE, one may predict that sleep quality and quantity should affect athletic performance. Moreover, because the demands of different athletic pursuits differ, some ought to be more influenced than others by sleep management. Actual data to demonstrate any of this are sparse, however. As sleep loss adversely affects reaction time, sleep loss prior to contests in events that depend heavily on rapid, correct reactions—baseball or boxing, for example—should affect

outcomes. Similarly, because sleep loss adversely affects motivation, and because high levels of motivation are required to sustain high levels of practice and performance, sleep management should be part of any athlete's training regimen.

Sleep management within contests is important in events that continue across days or weeks. The Tour de France, the Iditarod, the cycling Race Across America (RAAM), or long-distance yachting events whether single-handed or crewed are examples. Issues more basic even than ultimate performance, for example, safety and survival, are likely to be affected if sleep loss leads to failures of vigilance or judgment in critical situations.

Claudio Stampi has studied single-handed long-distance sailing races and has found that the winners are those who maintain their performance taking only catnaps. That is, the sailors best able to go days or weeks taking only short (less than 2-hour) naps were best able to attend to the constant task of making their boats go fast (see NAPPING). Conversely, those who maintained more "normal" sleep schedules (i.e., at least one longer primary sleep period) finished significantly lower in the standings, presumably because of the longer periods in which optimum sail trim was perforce neglected.

Other long-distance competitions place a premium not so much on managing sleep but on the ability to deprive oneself of sleep systematically. The Race Across America is a nonstop event, a bicycle race that has taken the top contenders 8 to 11 days to cover about 3,100 miles. Reward accrues to those able to ride the longest without taking time to sleep. Competitors typically ride the first 2 to 3 days before once dismounting to nap; thereafter they subsist on less than 4 hours of sleep per day.

The Iditarod dog sled race from Anchorage to Nome, Alaska, is a continuous, typically 2-to 3-week event save for one compulsory 24-hour stopover. Obviously, taking time to sleep costs competitors time and distance. Mushers in 1978 reported an average of 6 hours of sleep per night prior to the race. In the first 72 hours, they slept as little as 2 hours total, routinely augmenting alertness with caffeinated beverages such as coffee, tea, and colas (see COFFEE; COLA; TEA). At midrace the competitors reported an average of 3.6 hours of sleep in the preceding 24 hours. The leaders reported shorter sleep times than did slower mushers. Clearly this, too, is competition that rewards the ability to deprive oneself of sleep. Management strategy for such events should maximize a competitor's ability to perform as long as possible (i.e., as many days as possible) with the absolute minimum amount of sleep. There has been little research directly pertaining to how this might best be done, though one thought is to sleep as much as possible for several days before the event starts. The Iditarod is even more complicated when one considers that not one but two species are involved.

In those sports in which the entire event lasts only seconds (e.g., sprints, throwing events), minutes (e.g., longer races, swimming events), or hours (e.g., professional team sports, marathons), circadian factors become important (see CIRCADIAN RHYTHMS). Physiological parameters (e.g., aerobic capacity, muscular endurance) as well as cognitive functions (e.g., memory, reaction times, vigilance and alertness) vary across the day, and the optimum performance of one type of task may well occur at a different time than another. The highest pain thresholds, for example, are reported in the morning hours, whereas the greatest aerobic capacity develops in late afternoon or evening. An athlete's performance at his or her specialty will vary across the day and will be suboptimum if competitions occur outside of peak hours. The range of this variation may be 10 to 30 percent of the mean, depending on the task's complexity. A 10-percent decrease in performance can occur in more than one way and is about what would result from achieving a legal-limit (0.09-percent) blood alcohol level or from restricting the prior day's sleep to 3 hours.

Fatigue certainly affects professional sports, especially those with demanding schedules involving travel across several time zones and more than 80 games per season. The outcomes of these sports are closely watched by gamblers who would like to find patterns predicting small changes in the probability that one team will defeat another. In baseball, with 162 games per season per team, more games are won at home than on the road, 54 percent versus 46 percent for 1984 to 1986. In the National Basketball Association the figures skew even more, 64.5 percent versus 35.5 percent in the same time period. Of course many factors contribute, but the fatigue of travel, JET LAG, and attendant sleep loss and disruption must be among them.

Athletes rely on the advice of champions or trainers and use any approach, scientific or otherwise, they think might yield the slightest edge over competitors. The demands of different contests differ so much that the simple strategy of regular, adequate sleep and careful preparation prior to events that occur outside the optimum circadian period cannot help everyone and is not possible much of the time. Good advice on how to optimize sleep schedules and relevant circadian functions can come only from someone with intimate knowledge of both the event and the athlete.

REFERENCES

Silberstang E. 1988. *The winner's guide to sports betting,* Appendices II and III, pp 371–420. New York/Scarborough, Ontario: New American Library.

Stampi C. 1989. Ultrashort sleep/wake patterns and sustained performance. In Dinges DF, Broughton R, eds. *Sleep and alertness: Chronobiological, behavioral, and medical aspects of napping,* pp 139–171. New York: Raven Press.

Stillner V, Popkin MK, Pierce C. 1982. Biobehavioral changes in prolonged competitive stress: Observations of Iditarod Trail sled dog mushers. *Alaska Med,* January/February 1982: pp 1–6.

Robert M. Wittig

STAGES OF SLEEP

[Sleep in birds and mammals is generally considered to consist of two distinct states: non-rapid-eye-movement or NREM sleep, and rapid-eye-movement or REM SLEEP. *In humans, NREM sleep is subdivided into four stages defined primarily on the basis of the* ELECTROENCEPHALOGRAM (EEG), *which is one of the measures obtained in* POLYSOMNOGRAPHY. *A number of specific brain wave patterns are used to identify different sleep states. For example, four types of EEG wave forms help to distinguish the various NREM sleep stages:* K-COMPLEX, SLEEP SPINDLES, VERTEX SHARP WAVES, *and high-voltage slow waves. Vertex sharp waves are seen at the onset of sleep; sleep spindles and K-complexes characterize stage 2 sleep; and high voltage slow waves are predominant in stages 3 and 4 of*

NREM sleep, leading to the combined description of these two stages as SLOW-WAVE SLEEP. The ALPHA RHYTHM seen in the EEG of the awake brain may also appear occasionally during slow-wave sleep, and the resulting EEG pattern is called ALPHA–DELTA SLEEP. The EEG of REM sleep (also known as PARADOXICAL SLEEP) is characterized by SAWTOOTH WAVES in humans and by PGO WAVES in nonhuman mammals. PGO waves are named for their occurrence in the PONS, the LATERAL GENICULATE NUCLEUS of the THALAMUS, and the occipital cortex.

Sleep stages are also closely related to DEPTH OF SLEEP—in humans, one considers stage 1 sleep to be the lightest and stage 4 sleep the deepest. The partition of a night's sleep into different stages can be affected by many factors, perhaps most by the individual's age or stage of DEVELOPMENT. For example, the slow-wave stages of NREM sleep are predominant in childhood and then decline across adolescence and adulthood to very low levels in the elderly. Another example is REM sleep, which peaks in infancy (taking up approximately 50 percent of sleep time in newborns) and declines over the first few years of life to approximately 20 to 25 percent of sleep time, a level maintained through most of adolescence and adulthood. This interesting developmental progression of sleep stages has led to an ontogenetic theory for REM sleep need (see REM SLEEP, FUNCTION OF; see also ONTOGENY).

Other factors that exert consistent effects on the composition of sleep stages within a night of sleep include drugs, ALCOHOL, EXERCISE, and specific sleep disorders. One of the most impressive influences, however, is prior sleep history. Someone who has undergone DEPRIVATION of all sleep or selective deprivation of a certain stage of sleep will subsequently show altered sleep patterns; thus, a person recovering from total sleep deprivation will have an increase in slow-wave sleep, while a person recovering from selective REM sleep deprivation will have an increase in REM sleep. This sleep stage REBOUND is a very characteristic feature of the sleep process. Rebounds also occur following selective sleep stage deprivation induced by such drugs as ALCOHOL, BENZODIAZEPINES, MONOAMINE OXIDASE INHIBITORS, tricyclic ANTIDEPRESSANTS, STIMULANTS, and certain SLEEPING PILLS.

Although several conditions mimic various sleep stages, they are now known not to be true sleep as they do not share the necessary defining characteristics—such states resembling sleep include ANESTHESIA, COMA, and PASSING OUT (see also ALTERED STATES OF CONSCIOUSNESS). Thus, the stages of sleep are very well-defined and well-characterized aspects of the normal sleep process. Alterations in sleep stages are clear responses to many situations; the precise function of these stages, however, is not yet known (see FUNCTIONS OF SLEEP).

The article that follows discusses the stages of NREM sleep in additional detail.]

STAGES OF SLEEP

Stage 1 Sleep

Stage 1 NREM sleep is often described as a "transitional" stage of sleep in humans. Using the accepted polysomnographic measurements, stage 1 sleep is identified chiefly by its electroencephalographic (brain wave) pattern, although the electrooculographic (eye movement) and electromyographic (muscle tone) patterns may also contribute to identification of this stage (see POLYSOMNOGRAPHY). Stage 1 sleep is usually the first stage of sleep to occur in the transition from wakefulness to sleep.

In the awake, relaxed state that normally precedes sleep onset, the brain wave pattern often shows a very rhythmic and characteristic frequency called alpha rhythm (8 to 13 cycles per second) (see ALPHA RHYTHM). During the transition to sleep, this rhythmic alpha activity begins to break up and a more mixed frequency pattern of waves appears (Figure 1). As defined by standard criteria, the ELECTROENCEPHALOGRAM (EEG) pattern of stage 1 sleep is "relatively low voltage, mixed frequency" (Rechtschaffen and Kales, 1968). Activity in the theta frequency band (3 to 7 cycles per second) may occur, but it is not regular or rhythmic. One specific EEG waveform may be seen in stage 1 sleep: the vertex sharp wave. Vertex sharp waves usually appear as fairly distinct, fast, monophasic, negative waves (upward deflections) and show greatest amplitude when recorded over the vertex of the scalp (top of the head).

Another feature of stage 1 NREM sleep is the

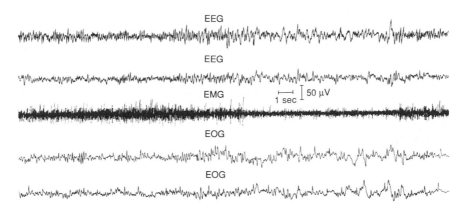

Figure 1. Polysomnographic recording showing transition from wakefulness to stage 1 sleep. Alpha rhythm can be seen to drop out of the two electroencephalogram tracings approximately halfway across the chart.

presence of slow, rolling eye movements. At the transition from wakefulness to sleep, these slow eye movements often precede the EEG change from alpha rhythm to the stage 1 sleep pattern. After sleep onset, stage 1 sleep generally persists only a few moments before the next NREM sleep stage ensues (see Stage 2 Sleep). Stage 1 often reappears as a transitional state following arousals during the night, at which time the stage may last a half-minute or less but will still show the characteristic EEG waveforms and often slow eye movements as well (Figure 2).

An important characteristic of stage 1 sleep is that it is the "lightest" phase of NREM sleep. An individual in stage 1 sleep is generally quite sensitive to sensory input: a soft whisper of the person's name or a gentle touch will often wake someone from stage 1 sleep (Rechtschaffen, Hauri, and Zeitlin, 1966). Another characteristic of stage 1 sleep, particularly on falling asleep, is the accompaniment of visual imagery and wandering, somewhat dreamlike thoughts. Hypnic starts or hypnic jerks that occur while falling asleep are thought to arise in this NREM sleep stage (Carskadon and Dement, 1989; see HYPNIC JERKS; HYPNAGOGIC REVERIE).

Although stage 1 sleep is usually a fleeting, transitional stage, it is quite prominent in several

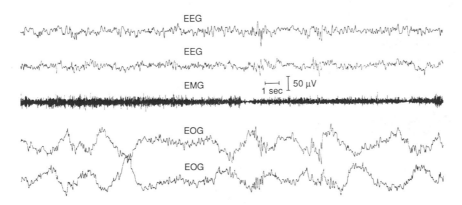

Figure 2. Polysomnographic recording showing characteristic waveforms of stage 1 sleep. Electroencephalogram tracings display relatively low-voltage, mixed-frequency activity, including a vertex sharp wave visible over the 1-second calibration mark. Electrooculogram tracings display the slow, rolling eye movements that often accompany stage 1 sleep.

sleep disorders: those disorders in which sleep is most disrupted. For example, in a patient with sleep apnea, who must wake up to breathe, stage 1 sleep becomes quite pronounced and follows virtually every arousal, if only for a brief period (see APNEA). Although a normal young adult may spend as few as 10 or 15 minutes per night in stage 1 sleep, a patient with sleep apnea may show the stage 1 sleep pattern for a total of several hours a night. Thus, an increased amount of stage 1 sleep can be an important marker of sleep disturbances (see FRAGMENTATION).

Stage 2 Sleep

Stage 2 sleep is one of the four phases of NREM sleep in humans. The distinguishing feature of stage 2 sleep is its EEG pattern; the other standard polysomnographic measures—ELECTROOCULOGRAPHY and ELECTROMYOGRAPHY—contribute little to its identification. The EEG of stage 2 sleep is distinguished by episodic waveforms that occur in the context of a background of relatively low-voltage, mixed-frequency EEG activity. As the background activity of stage 2 sleep is very similar to the EEG pattern of stage 1 sleep, the transition from stage 1 to stage 2 is marked by the appearance of two distinct EEG waveforms: the sleep spindle and the K-complex (Rechtschaffen and Kales, 1968).

Figure 3 illustrates the classical appearance of sleep spindles as a waxing and waning, rhythmic pattern with a frequency range of 12 to 14 cycles per second. The name *spindle* refers to their shape, which resembles the spindle on a spinning machine. In normal young adults, sleep spindles occur in stage 2 sleep with an average frequency of three to eight per minute, although there is marked variation in this pattern from individual to individual. Sleep spindles are not present in newborn infants, but usually develop by age 3 months. The lack of sleep spindles at birth in humans is thought to indicate the relative immaturity of the central nervous system. A certain level of neurological development is required to produce these complex brain wave patterns. Sleep spindles also occur during sleep in other mammals (see SLEEP SPINDLES).

The second brain wave pattern that distinguishes stage 2 sleep is the K-COMPLEX first described in the 1930s by Loomis, Harvey, and Hobart (1937). K-complexes stand out very clearly from the background EEG, as illustrated in Figure 4. This form consists of a sharp negative (upward) spike followed by a somewhat slower positive component. Often, a sleep spindle may "ride" over a K-complex. K-complexes arise spontaneously during stage 2 sleep and can also be produced by external sensory stimulation. Thus, if one were to make a sharp noise near a person who was in stage 2 sleep, one would either wake the person or induce a K-complex, which would be visible on the chart if the EEG were recorded. Such K-complexes may be thought of as cortical evoked potentials caused by sensory stimulation (see EVOKED POTENTIALS). In normal young adults, K-complexes occur spontaneously during stage 2 sleep with a frequency of about three per minute, though as with sleep spindles, there is marked variability from person to person.

Occasionally, the electrooculogram (EOG) of stage 2 sleep may show the persistence of the

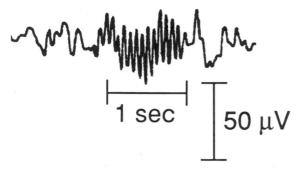

Figure 3. A distinct sleep spindle in the background electroencephalogram of stage 2 sleep.

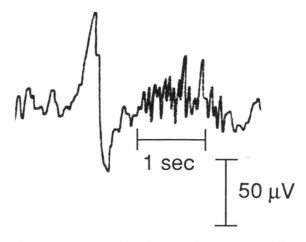

Figure 4. A K-complex followed by a sleep spindle.

same slow eye movements that characterized stage 1 sleep. In general, however, the EOG of stage 2 sleep is free of any eye movements. Another feature of stage 2 sleep is that the AROUSAL threshold in most individuals is somewhat higher than the stage 1 arousal threshold; that is, a more intense stimulus is required to awaken someone from stage 2 sleep than from stage 1 sleep (see DEPTH OF SLEEP). A stimulus that woke a person from stage 1 sleep might only induce a K-complex in the same person during stage 2 sleep. Nevertheless, as with all normal sleep stages, stage 2 sleep is reversible: people can be awakened by a sufficiently intense stimulus. This is an important difference between sleep and the comatose state (see COMA; HEAD INJURY).

Stage 3 Sleep

Stage 3 sleep is a phase of NREM sleep in humans that is often, along with stage 4 sleep, called slow-wave sleep. The distinguishing feature of stage 3 sleep is the EEG pattern, which is characterized by waveforms having higher amplitude (voltage) and slower frequency than in stage 1 or stage 2 sleep. In stage 3 sleep, these high-amplitude slow waves make up between 20 and 50 percent of specific portions of the EEG record (Figure 5). The transition from stage 2 sleep to stage 3 sleep occurs with a gradual increase in the EEG amplitude and a corresponding decrease in frequency. When the amount of high-amplitude (greater than 75 microvolts) and slow-frequency (2 cycles per second or slower) EEG activity reaches *at least* 20 percent but *less than* 50 percent of the EEG segment, the pattern is called stage 3 sleep (Rechtschaffen and Kales, 1968).

Electrooculographic and electromyographic patterns do not contribute substantially to the identification of stage 3 sleep. In general, no eye movements are visible in this stage. In most people, stage 3 sleep is deeper than stage 1 or stage 2 sleep; that is, it takes a more intense stimulus (e.g., louder noise) to wake someone from stage 3 sleep (see DEPTH OF SLEEP). Sleep spindles and K-complexes may be seen in stage 3 sleep, although the stage determination is made by the high-voltage, slow EEG activity (see also SLOW-WAVE SLEEP).

Stage 4 Sleep

Stage 4 sleep is a phase of NREM sleep in humans, often considered together with stage 3 sleep as slow-wave sleep. Stage 4 sleep is defined by a predominance (more than 50 percent) of high-voltage (greater than 75 microvolts), slow-frequency (2 cycles per second or slower) EEG waves (Rechtschaffen and Kales, 1968). Figure 6 illustrates this pattern. In a normal young adult, stages 3 and 4 generally occur in the early sleep cycles of the night (see CYCLES OF SLEEP ACROSS THE NIGHT; NORMAL SLEEP).

The arousal threshold during stage 4 sleep is generally the highest of all the NREM sleep stages. Thus, a more intense stimulus (i.e., louder noise) is needed to wake someone from stage 4 sleep than any other stage of NREM sleep (see DEPTH OF SLEEP). The arousal threshold in slow-wave sleep is typically much higher in young children than in young adults and older people (Zepelin, McDonald, and Zammit, 1984) (see CHILDHOOD, SLEEP DURING; AGING AND SLEEP). This developmental change in arousal threshold is accompanied by a developmental change in the amplitude of the EEG waves in slow-wave sleep. For example, the stage 4 sleep EEG pattern in a 15-year-old may have an amplitude of several hundred microvolts, whereas the stage 4 EEG in a

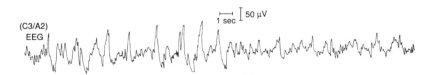

Figure 5. A typical segment of electroencephalogram recorded during stage 3 sleep, showing large slow waves occupying between 20 percent and 50 percent of the record.

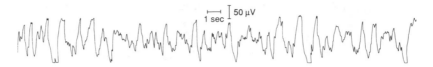

Figure 6. A typical segment of electroencephalogram recorded during stage 4 sleep, dominated by high-voltage slow waves.

65-year-old may barely achieve the 75-microvolt amplitude criterion level (Figure 7). For this reason, certain sleep researchers choose to evaluate stage 3 and 4 sleep in elderly individuals by examining the EEG frequency alone and not taking amplitude into account (Webb and Dreblow, 1982). It is interesting to note that both stages 3 and 4 decline with age and that many older people report that their sleep is "lighter" than it was when they were young (Carskadon and Dement, 1989). (See also SLOW-WAVE SLEEP.)

REFERENCES

Carskadon MA, Dement WC. 1989. Normal human sleep: An overview. In: Kryger MH, Roth T, Dement WC, eds. *Principles and practice of sleep medicine,* pp 3–13. Philadelphia: Saunders.

Loomis AL, Harvey EN, Hobart GA. 1937. Cerebral states during sleep as studied by human brain potentials. *J Exp Psychol* 21:127–144.

Rechtschaffen A, Hauri P, Zeitlin M. 1966. Auditory awakening thresholds in REM and NREM sleep stages. *Percept Mot Skills* 22:927–942.

Rechtschaffen A, Kales A, eds. 1968. *A manual of standardized terminology, techniques and scoring system for sleep stages of human subjects.* Los Angeles: UCLA Brain Information Service/Brain Research Institute.

Webb WB, Dreblow L. 1982. A modified method for scoring slow wave sleep of older subjects. *Sleep* 5:195–199.

Zepelin H, McDonald CS, Zammit GK. 1984. Effects of age on auditory awakening thresholds. *J Gerontol* 39:294–300.

Sharon Keenan
Kate B. Herman
Mary A. Carskadon

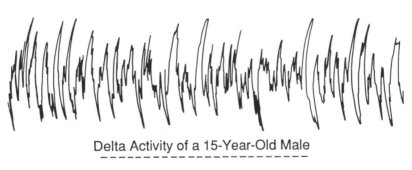

Delta Activity of a 15-Year-Old Male

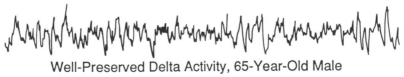

Well-Preserved Delta Activity, 65-Year-Old Male

Figure 7. Stage 4 sleep electroencephalogram amplitude changes with age.

STANFORD SLEEPINESS SCALE

The Stanford Sleepiness Scale (SSS) is a self-rating scale developed to quantify sleepiness for any period of the day or night. The scale consists of seven statements. In using the scale, individuals select the statement that best indicates their state of sleepiness. The statements and their scale values are as follows:

1. Feeling active and vital; alert; wide awake
2. Functioning at a high level, but not at peak; able to concentrate
3. Relaxed; awake; not at full alertness; responsive
4. A little foggy; not at peak; let down
5. Fogginess; beginning to lose interest in remaining awake; slowed down
6. Sleepiness; prefer to be lying down; fighting sleep; woozy
7. Almost in reverie; sleep onset soon; lost struggle to remain awake

The scale was developed by using a scaling technique known as the method of equal-appearing intervals (Thurstone and Chave, 1929), and it was found to be reliable using an "alternative-forms" reliability check. The scale was found to cross-validate with performance on long, monotonous mental tasks and to be sensitive to changes in sleepiness that occurred with sleep deprivation and subsequent recovery (Hoddes, Zarcone, and Dement, 1972).

The SSS appeared to work best when sleepiness ratings were averaged over an hour-long period rather than 15-minute periods.

In research settings, using normal, college-aged participants, the scale appears to be accurate in documenting subjective SLEEPINESS; however, in sleep disorder clinical populations, the scale has less accuracy. Consequently, the SSS has typically been used in sleep disorder centers in conjunction with objective measurements of sleepiness such as the MULTIPLE SLEEP LATENCY TEST.

REFERENCES

Hoddes E, Zarcone V, Dement W. 1972. Cross-validation of the Stanford Sleepiness Scale. *Sleep Res* 1:91.

Thurstone LL, Chave EJ. 1929. *The measurement of attitudes.* Chicago: University of Chicago Press.

Eric Hoddes

STIMULANTS

There are a great number of drugs whose actions stimulate the central nervous system (CNS). Three general classes of stimulant drugs may be identified: (1) amines that mimic the action of norepinephrine, such as AMPHETAMINE; (2) toxic agents that cause abnormal neuronal activity and seizures, such as strychnine; and (3) xanthines that block adenosine receptors and stimulate respiration, such as CAFFEINE.

Amines

Stimulants like AMPHETAMINE are called CNS sympathomimetics because they affect the sympathetic nervous system by mimicking the effect of norepinephrine, the primary neurotransmitter of the SYMPATHETIC NERVOUS SYSTEM and one of the important stimulating neurotransmitters in the brain (see CHEMISTRY OF SLEEP: AMINES AND OTHER TRANSMITTERS). Drugs in this class can produce pleasurable alerting effects on the CNS that may lead to abuse and dependency. Amphetamine and COCAINE are the best known stimulant DRUGS OF ABUSE. With low doses, fatigue and sleepiness are reduced, movement is increased, and a sense of effectiveness and strength is produced. With very high doses, complex movements are replaced by stereotyped, simple movements, and a sense of anxiety and danger is engendered.

Stimulants also have important medical uses. Amphetamines are most commonly prescribed to control appetite in obese patients and to increase attention in children with hyperactivity/attention deficit disorder. Cocaine is used medically as an intranasal anesthetic and vasoconstrictor. Stimulants, in addition to causing CNS arousal, constrict blood vessels, open breathing passages, increase heart rate, and increase blood pressure. To avoid the addictive potential of amphetamines and retain medically useful effects outside the CNS, drugs such as phenylpropanolamine and pseudoephedrine were developed.

Phenylpropanolamine and pseudoephedrine are chemically related to amphetamines, but are safe enough to be sold without a physician's prescription. These drugs do not greatly affect the CNS and yet retain vasoconstricting and bronchodilating effects.

These compounds exert their effects on the sympathetic nervous system by releasing norepinephrine from storage sites in the sympathetic nerves. This, in turn, activates alpha and beta-adrenergic receptors. It is believed that these compounds work in the CNS by increasing the release from nerve terminals of the biogenic amines, dopamine, norepinephrine, and serotonin. The increase in movement associated with the use of these drugs depends on dopamine release. The alerting effect, the appetite-suppressing effect, and some of the increased locomotor effects probably depend on the release of norepinephrine. The disturbances in perception and overt psychotic behavior seen after high doses of an amphetamine may result from the release of serotonin.

Prevention and reduction of fatigue are well-known effects of centrally acting sympathomimetic drugs. These agents increase the duration of adequate performance on tasks, reduce unfavorable attitudes toward certain types of work, and improve performance on tasks requiring sustained attention. Such stimulants alter normal sleep architecture by delaying the onset of sleep, disturbing sleep in general, reducing stage 3 and 4 NREM sleep, and reducing REM sleep to about half of normal levels. After use of amphetamine-like drugs, there is an increase in total sleep time and a large increase in REM sleep relative to normal levels (REM REBOUND).

Under physician supervision, stimulant drugs are used to treat abnormal sleepiness resulting from certain sleep disorders. Table 1 summarizes the most common stimulant drugs prescribed to treat the sleepiness of sleep disorders such as NARCOLEPSY and idiopathic CNS HYPERSOMNIA.

Studies in narcoleptic patients treated with some stimulant drugs have employed objective measurements of sleepiness (MULTIPLE SLEEP LATENCY TEST) or of the ability to stay awake (Maintenance of Wakefulness Test). In these studies, none of the stimulant drugs produced long-term normalization of alertness in narcoleptic patients, but several drugs improved alertness to a significant degree. In this respect, methamphetamine appears to be the most effective. The drugs most often used for treating excessive sleepiness in patients with narcolepsy, in order of efficacy, are methamphetamine, methylphenidate, d-amphetamine, modafinil (an experimental alpha-adrenergic receptor agonist available in Europe), and pemoline. With all stimulant drugs, it is necessary to balance the desirable alerting effects against the undesirable side effects such as agitation, gastrointestinal upset, and insomnia by adjusting daily dose or otherwise limiting the quantity ingested over time.

A perplexing question concerning CNS stimulants is why they seem to calm children with ATTENTION DEFICIT HYPERACTIVITY DISORDER (ADHD) and yet energize people who are fatigued. One idea that has been studied is that the excessive movements and attentional problems of children with ADHD are manifestations of underlying excessive sleepiness. According to this hypothesis, when an alerting drug is given, the behavioral and attentional problems diminish. Another important idea is that children with ADHD may actually suffer from continual overstimulation of the

Table 1

Chemical Name	Brand Name	Usual Daily Dose (milligrams)
Amphetamine	Benzedrine	5–60
d-Amphetamine	Dexedrine	5–60
Methamphetamine	Desoxyn	2.5–40
Methylphenidate	Ritalin	5–60
Modafinil	None available	200–300
Pemoline	Cylert	18.75–150
Mazindol	Sanorex	1–8
Diethylpropion	Tenuate	75–150

dopamine system. When this system is even more stimulated by CNS stimulants, a decrease in activity is brought about by the same mechanisms that cause reduced gross locomotor activity when very high doses of amphetamine are given.

Toxic Agents

Drugs such as strychnine produce their activating CNS effects by blocking neuronal inhibition. Most drugs in this class do not produce pleasurable CNS arousal and are not used in the treatment of disease. These agents are, however, helpful as research tools in developing anticonvulsant medications and in understanding the connections between different parts of the brain.

Xanthines

The xanthines form a group of closely related plant alkaloids that have a number of properties in common with the CNS sympathomimetics. Their activating effects are most pronounced on CNS control of breathing. The xanthines are used predominantly in the treatment of certain respiratory diseases. The most likely mechanism for CNS action is through blockade of receptors for adenosine; however, the xanthines also affect the translocation of calcium ions within neurons and cause neurons to accumulate energy-rich cyclic nucleotides. (See CHEMISTRY OF SLEEP: ADENOSINE.)

Patients with narcolepsy and idiopathic CNS hypersomnia are not commonly treated with xanthines; however, sleep-deprived people and some sleep disorder patients with excessive sleepiness report improvement of sleepiness after taking caffeine in the form of a caffeinated beverage or in the tablet form available in drug stores and markets. Furthermore, studies have shown that sleep-deprived people can perform work more efficiently and accurately after taking caffeine or a caffeinated beverage. It is these effects of caffeine that make it virtually ubiquitous among cultures of the world. Often caffeine-containing drinks or foods become fundamental features of a society. For example, consider the roles of tea in the United Kingdom and China, coffee in North America and the Middle East, and chocolate in Mexico and many other tropical societies.

(See also AMPHETAMINE; CAFFEINE; CHEMISTRY OF SLEEP: ADENOSINE; NARCOLEPSY.)

REFERENCES

Gilman AG, Goodman LS, Gilman A. 1980. *Goodman and Gilman's the pharmacological basis of therapeutics.* New York: Macmillan.

Lyon M, Robbins TW. 1975. The action of central nervous system stimulant drugs: A general theory concerning amphetamine effects. In Essman WB, Valzelli L, eds. *Current developments in psychopharmacology,* vol 2, pp 79–163. New York: Spectrum.

Mitler MM. 1987. Alerting drugs: Do they really work? *Psychopharmacol Bull* 23:435–439.

Merrill M. Mitler

STIMULUS CONTROL FOR INSOMNIA

The goals of stimulus control instructions are to help the insomniac learn to fall asleep quickly and to maintain sleep. They do that by strengthening the bed as a cue for sleep, weakening it as a cue for activities that might interfere with sleep, and helping the insomniac acquire a consistent sleep rhythm. Although there are many causes of INSOMNIA, poor sleep habits are often an important contributor.

Insomniacs often engage in activities at bedtime that are incompatible with falling asleep. They may, for example, use their bedrooms for reading, talking on the telephone, watching television, snacking, listening to music, or worrying. Many insomniacs seem to organize their entire existence around the bedroom, with television, telephone, books, and food within easy reach. For others, bedtime is the first quiet time during the day available to rehash the day's events and to worry and plan for the next day. Under these conditions, bed and bedtime become cues for AROUSAL rather than cues for sleep.

Another source of arousal for the insomniac is that the bedroom can become a cue for the ANXIETY and frustration associated with trying to fall asleep. Insomniacs often can sleep any place other than their own bed. They might fall asleep in an easy chair or on a couch, and they often have less difficulty sleeping when away from home. In contrast, people who have no difficulty falling asleep in their own bed often have difficulty in strange surroundings. For them, there are strong cues for sleep associated with their bed, and it is only when these cues are not available that they have difficulty.

The following rules constitute the stimulus control instructions (Bootzin, 1972; Bootzin, Epstein, and Wood, 1991). They form the foundation for the development of new permanent sleeping habits and are to be followed even after the insomniac is falling asleep more quickly and sleeping better.

1. Lie down intending to go to sleep *only* when you are sleepy.
2. Do not use your bed for anything except sleep; that is, do not read, watch television, eat, or worry in bed. Sexual activity is the only exception to this rule. On such occasions, the instructions are to be followed afterward when you intend to go to sleep.
3. If you find yourself unable to fall asleep, get up and go into another room. Stay up as long as you wish and then return to the bedroom to sleep. Although we do not want you to watch the clock, we want you to get out of bed if you do not fall asleep immediately. Remember the goal is to associate your bed with falling asleep *quickly!* If you are in bed more than about 10 minutes without falling asleep and have not gotten up, you are not following this instruction.
4. If you still cannot fall asleep, repeat step 3. Do this as often as is necessary throughout the night.
5. Set your alarm and get up at the same time every morning irrespective of how much sleep you got during the night. This will help your body acquire a consistent sleep rhythm.
6. Do not nap during the day.

Stimulus control instructions have been found to be a highly effective intervention in controlled studies in which the instructions are explained and progress is monitored in individual or group sessions. Although the focus of most evaluations has been on sleep-onset insomnia (Espie et al., 1989; Lacks et al., 1983), improvement in sleep-maintenance insomnia in older adult pa-

tients has also been demonstrated (Morin and Azrin, 1987, 1988).

REFERENCES

Bootzin RR. 1972. A stimulus control treatment for insomnia. *Proceed Am Psychol Assoc,* 395–396.

Bootzin RR, Epstein D, Wood JM. 1991. Stimulus control instructions. In Hauri P, ed. *Case studies in insomnia.* New York: Plenum Press.

Espie CA, Lindsay WR, Brooks DN, Hood EM, Turvey T. 1989. A controlled comparative investigation of psychological treatments for chronic sleep-onset insomnia. *Behav Res Ther* 27:79–88.

Lacks P, Bertelson AD, Gans L, Kunkel J. 1983. The effectiveness of three behavioural treatments for different degrees of sleep-onset insomnia. *Behav Ther* 14:593–605.

Morin CM, Azrin NH. 1987. Stimulus control and imagery training in treating sleep-maintenance insomnia. *J Consult Clin Psychol* 55:260–262.

Morin CM, Azrin NH. 1988. Behavioral and cognitive treatments of geriatric insomnia. *J Consult Clin Psychol* 56:748–753.

Richard R. Bootzin

STRESS

See Anxiety; Content of Dreams; Insomnia; Personality and Sleep Deprivation; Posttraumatic Nightmares; Psychopathology

STROKE

A stroke is defined as an injury to the brain resulting from disease of the cerebrovascular system. A synonym for *stroke* is *cerebrovascular accident* (CVA). The two most common causes of stroke are ischemia, in which a lesion results from decreased or complete loss of the blood flow to a part of the brain, and hemorrhage from a ruptured blood vessel. The focus of this article is on ischemic strokes. These may be caused by thrombosis, narrowing of a vessel, usually due to atherosclerosis ("hardening of the artery"); embolus, defined as a clot, originating in the heart or another site that lodges in a cerebral blood vessel; or a drastic decrease in blood pressure. Whatever the cause, the clinical effects depend on the size and location of the lesion and will vary from no symptoms at all to complete coma, as in the case of a stroke in the brainstem, in which there are vital structures within a relatively small space. Between these clinical extremes, a wide variety of disabilities may be seen, including hemiplegia (partial paralysis), blindness in a visual field, and loss of sensation. In addition, a left-cerebral-hemisphere stroke may lead to language dysfunction, known as *aphasia*, whereas damage to the right hemisphere is often associated with lack of directed attention to the opposite side.

Effects of Stroke on Sleep and Dreaming

Most patients have disrupted sleep during the acute phase of a stroke. The degree of disruption may have predictive value in that an early appearance of normal stage 2 sleep means better recovery. Some patients may show a loss of the 24-hour organization of the sleep–wake cycle, leading them to more wakefulness at night and abnormal sleepiness during the day. However, it is difficult to separate the effects of disability and inactivity from an actual dysfunction of biological rhythms. Another factor is the high incidence of obstructive sleep APNEA (OSA) (see below), which also leads to excessive daytime SLEEPINESS. Whatever the cause, the sleepy or lethargic stroke patient has an additional impediment in the path of his or her successful rehabilitation.

Brainstem strokes are especially likely to cause somnolence because of the relatively small size of this structure and the presence of a collection of neurons called the *reticular formation*, which is responsible for AROUSAL and tonic wakefulness. The larger the lesion, the more likely that COMA will occur. After smaller destructive lesions and also in certain degenerative diseases affecting the brainstem, REM sleep is specifically inhibited and/or rapid eye movements during REM sleep are sparse or absent. This is no doubt secondary to impairment of structures within the PONS (the part of the brainstem between the MEDULLA and MIDBRAIN) that normally trigger the onset of recurrent REM periods (see REM SLEEP MECHANISMS

AND NEUROANATOMY). In contrast, strokes of the THALAMUS (located just above the midbrain) may impair NREM sleep because messages from the thalamus to the overlying cerebral cortex are responsible for the slow waves and spindles of this sleep stage (see NREM SLEEP MECHANISMS).

A paucity or absence of dreams after cerebral hemisphere strokes has been reported. Some have hypothesized that right cerebral hemisphere activation plays a key role in the phenomena of REM sleep (dreaming sleep). This theory is consistent with the notion that the right hemisphere has a dominant role in visuospatial, as opposed to verbal, brain activity; dreams are particularly visual, bizarre experiences. However, posterior lesions in either hemisphere are likely to suppress dreaming. It may be that dreams originate in the right hemisphere and acquire their distinctive features there but communication between the two hemispheres is necessary for dreaming to propagate and to be experienced.

Circadian Rhythms of Stroke

Numerous epidemiological studies have demonstrated a significant peak of ischemic stroke onset between 6:00 A.M. and 10:00 A.M. These data are similar to those reported for myocardial ischemia, myocardial infarct, and sudden cardiac death. The explanation for this phenomenon is unknown, but the following possibilities can be considered:

1. The morning peak of incidence could be the immediate result of obstructive sleep apnea (OSA), which tends to be worse in the hours just before awakening. Obstructive sleep apnea is accompanied by hypoxia, increased blood pressure, and cardiac arrhythmias; all these complications are risk factors for stroke.

2. Blood pressure and heart rate increase in all individuals around the time of awakening.

3. In the early morning hours, adrenocortical hormones and norepinephrine increase as part of a circadian rhythm (see CIRCADIAN RHYTHMS). These biochemical changes might lead to deleterious effects such as constriction of blood vessels, resulting in changes in blood flow.

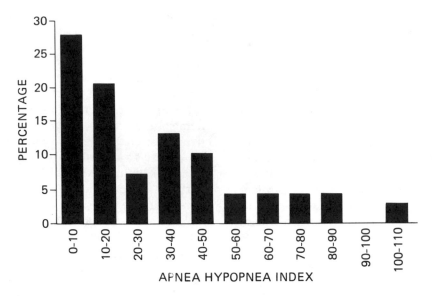

Figure 1. The height of the bars represents the percentage of stroke patients with numbers of stop-breathing events as noted below each bar. The number of stop-breathing events per hour is known as the apnea–hypopnea index.

4. Blood platelets have a greater tendency to aggregate in the early morning, thus increasing the clotting tendency.

Stroke and Sleep Disorders

SNORING is more common in stroke patients than in nonstroke control subjects. Because a history of snoring is an index of OSA, apnea can be considered to be a risk factor for stroke, which means that stroke is more likely in patients who snore. Furthermore, snoring is significantly more common in patients having onset of stroke between 6:00 and 10:00 A.M.

Sleep laboratory evaluation of male stroke victims have confirmed the above epidemiological data. Seventy-five percent of these patients have significantly increased apneic (stop-breathing) events during sleep (Figure 1). Over 50 percent have twenty events or more per hour of sleep, a level which has been shown to be associated with increased morbidity and mortality. In addition to OSA being a risk factor for stroke, it is conceivable that the stroke itself might provoke or exacerbate a preexisting case of OSA.

Poststroke Depression and Sleep

Depression is not uncommon after an ischemic stroke. The frequency of DEPRESSION seems to be greater after lesions in the anterior left cerebral hemisphere (the dominant hemisphere). An important finding in spontaneous depression is short REM LATENCY (time from sleep onset to the first REM period). It is therefore significant that left hemisphere stroke patients have abnormally short REM latencies compared with right hemisphere subjects. The similarity of left-hemisphere stroke patients' sleep to that of individuals with spontaneous depression is consistent with the idea that poststroke depression is caused by a specific disruption of brain function rather than a simple reaction to illness.

REFERENCES

Partinen M, Palowaki H. 1985. Snoring and cerebral infarction. *Lancet* 2:1325–1326.
Zamula E. 1986. Stroke; fighting back against America's No. 3 killer. *FDA Consumer* 20:6.

Sheldon Kapen

SUDDEN DEATH

See Apnea; Death; Sudden Death Syndrome in Asian Populations; Sudden Infant Death Syndrome

SUDDEN DEATH SYNDROME IN ASIAN POPULATIONS

Sudden death syndrome in Asian populations is a mysterious and terrifying disorder. Its victims are young, previously healthy males of Southeast Asian descent who die mysteriously at night during sleep. The official Centers for Disease Control definition requires the presence of the following findings: The deceased person must have been older than two years; the deceased person must have been born in or have had at least one parent born in a Southeast Asian country or the Philippines; no other obvious cause of death is found on the postmortem examination. The disease, known as *pok-kuri* in Japan and as *bangungut* in the Philippines, has been recognized for years in Southeast Asia, but has been reported in the United States only since 1977. This coincides with the influx of Southeast Asian refugees during the 1970s. Ninety-nine percent of its victims have been male, with a mean age of thirty-two years. Almost three quarters of the U.S. victims were of Laotian descent.

Episodes of this syndrome invariably occur during sleep. Typically, others in the room or in the house are awakened by sounds of gurgling, gasping, or labored breathing. Often the victim is described as being stiff or rigid, and occasionally generalized seizure activity is noted. In patients with acute heart monitoring, ventricular fibrillation (disorganized fatal heart rhythm) is usually found, if any electrical activity of the heart is noted at all. No specific or consistent findings have been reported at postmortem examinations.

No single theory completely explains all aspects of sudden death syndrome in Asian populations. The following theories have been proposed:

1. *Cardiac disease.* In the largest series of autopsy examinations in sudden death syn-

drome victims, all hearts studied showed evidence of left ventricular hypertrophy (enlargement), and all but one showed abnormalities in the heart's electrical conduction system. Three known survivors of this syndrome all presented with ventricular fibrillation; two of these three continued to have dangerous heart rhythms, and one later died suddenly. These cases suggest that underlying structural heart abnormalities may lead to electrical instability in these patients. This theory does not, however, explain the exclusive nocturnal occurrence of sudden death syndrome or the male predominance.

2. *Sleep apnea.* The occurrence of breathing pauses (apneas) during sleep with associated arterial oxygen desaturation could precipitate abnormal heart rhythms. Such an explanation would certainly address the nocturnal occurrence of the syndrome and the male predominance, as both of these factors are also characteristics of obstructive sleep apnea. Furthermore, obstructive sleep apnea has been associated with systemic hypertension, which could explain the ventricular enlargement often seen at postmortem assessment. Yet, there is little other supporting evidence for this theory. For example, all victims have been relatively young and of normal height and weight, which are not typical of sleep apnea. In addition, retrospective interview with family members has shown no consistent history of snoring, stridor (harsh, high-pitched respiratory sound), previous sleep disturbance, daytime sleepiness, or systemic hypertension in most victims. Pathologists have been unable to find consistent upper airway pathology or evidence of systemic and/or pulmonary hypertension at autopsy. Unfortunately, the three known survivors had no formal sleep evaluation; therefore, this theory remains unproven.

3. *Sleep terrors.* Resembling intense anxiety attacks, sleep terrors are nocturnal episodes of extreme levels of autonomic nervous system output, as well as thrashing, screaming, grunting, and groaning. Such sounds have been noted in many cases of sudden death

syndrome. Furthermore, the agitated movements sometimes seen prior to true seizure activity in certain cases have been compared with the frenzied movements seen with night terrors. Researchers suggest that in certain patients who have an abnormal heart to begin with, the intense autonomic discharge of a sleep terror may precipitate or lower the threshold for ventricular fibrillation and, thus, lead to death. (See SLEEP TERRORS.)

Certain aspects of sudden death syndrome in Asian populations, however, suggest that sleep terrors alone are also an inadequate explanation. Sleep terrors usually begin in individuals younger than these victims, but there has been no prior history of such parasomnias in any of the reported cases. Death rarely, if ever, complicates sleep terrors, and it would be exceedingly unlikely that death would be the initial presentation of this parasomnia.

4. *Environmental factors.* Many of these victims had emigrated from their native Southeast Asian country or had parents who had emigrated. It has been speculated that the resulting change in their environment may have led to these nocturnal deaths. Dietary changes or deficiencies, disruption of social and/or religious foundations, and airborne or ingested toxic substances have all been implicated as possible contributing factors. Nevertheless, it is unlikely that environmental changes can account for either the syndrome's nocturnal occurrence or its predilection for males. Furthermore, this theory certainly becomes irrelevant with regard to the long history of this disease in the victims' native Southeast Asian countries.

The etiology of this bizarre and frightening sleep disorder therefore remains unclear, and probably involves a structural or anatomical cardiac abnormality, possibly hereditary, that predisposes development of malignant arrhythmias. These arrhythmias are then unmasked by a poorly characterized nocturnal event, resulting in sudden death during sleep. More information is needed to formulate measures to reduce or prevent the occurrence of sudden death in Southeast Asia, as well as in the growing Southeast Asian population in the United States.

BIBLIOGRAPHY

Baron RC, Thacker SB, Gorelkin L, Vernon AA, Taylor WR, Choi K. 1983. Sudden death among Southeast Asian refugees. *JAMA* 250:2947–2951.

Kirschner RH, Eckner AO, Biron RC. 1986. The cardiac pathology of sudden, unexplained nocturnal death in Southeast Asian refugees. *JAMA* 256:2700–2705.

Melles RB. 1987. Sudden, unexplained nocturnal death syndrome and night terrors. *JAMA* 257:2918–2919.

Otto CM, Touxe RV, Cobb LA, Greene HL, Gross BW, Werner JR, Burroughs RW, Samson WE, Weaver WD, Trobaugh GD. 1984. Ventricular fibrillation causes sudden death in Southeast Asian immigrants. *Ann Intern Med* 100:45–47.

Parrish RG, Tucker M, Ing R, Encarnacion L, Eberhardt M. 1987. Sudden unexplained death syndrome in Southeast Asian refugees: A review of CDC surveillance. *MMWR* 36:43SS–53SS.

Scott E. Eveloff
Richard P. Millman

SUDDEN INFANT DEATH SYNDROME

Sudden infant death syndrome (SIDS), also known as *crib death* or *cot death*, has been recognized since biblical times. Sudden infant death syndrome is the leading cause of death in infants between the first month and the first year of life. The number of babies who die of SIDS has varied geographically and from year to year, but it has not decreased in parallel with other causes of infant mortality over the past 2 decades. In the United States, SIDS is responsible for 5,000 to 10,000 deaths per year, or about 1 to 2 per 1,000 live births. Worldwide, the range is from 0.4 to 8 SIDS deaths per 1,000 births. A panel organized by the National Institutes of Health (NIH, 1987) defined SIDS as "the sudden death of an infant under 1 year of age which remains unexplained after a complete postmortem examination, including an investigation of the death scene and a review of the case history."

Who Is at Risk for SIDS?

Although the majority of SIDS victims do not have identifiable risk factors (Figure 1), epidemiological studies have linked the occurrence of SIDS with a consistent pattern of mother and infant risk factors: low socioeconomic status, young mothers, many pregnancies, short intervals between births, multiple birth, male gender, race, and low birth weight. The peak age for SIDS is 2 to 4 months; deaths occur throughout the year, but there are more cases during the winter months; and SIDS most often occurs when the infant is thought to be asleep. No medical tests can identify an individual infant at higher risk. Certain groups of infants are at a somewhat higher risk, including siblings of SIDS victims (especially where there are two or more SIDS victims in a family) and infants born to substance-abusing mothers.

Some SIDS victims have a history of an *apparent life-threatening event* (ALTE). In an ALTE, someone has been frightened because the baby has some combination of: (1) APNEA (cessation of breathing), (2) color change (usually pale or blue/grey), (3) choking, or (4) gagging. The observer often fears that the infant has died. It is important to note that most infants with an ALTE do not subsequently die of SIDS.

Causes of SIDS

Most SIDS victims are born at full term, appear to be well developed and nourished, and have been considered to be in good health prior to death, although a large body of evidence suggests that SIDS victims may differ from normal infants very early in development. Studies of brainstem pathology (Kinney, Filiano, and Harper, 1992) are particularly interesting because the brainstem is important for integrating many body functions. Respiration, cardiovascular and thermal stability, sleep, and AROUSAL are all regulated in part by the brainstem, and all these factors are likely to play important roles in SIDS. Because some SIDS victims are found with high body temperatures or covered with sweat, it is important to study the complex interactions between temperature regulation, sleep, arousal, and control of breathing (Glotzbach and Heller, 1989). Many SIDS cases

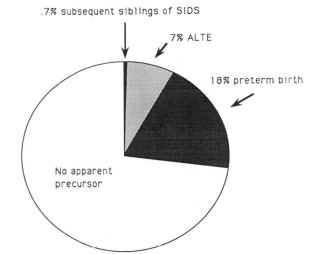

Figure 1. Distribution of SIDS deaths by risk group.

show tiny hemorrhages within the chest cavity that suggest increased breathing efforts and airway obstruction at the time of death. For this reason, the influence of sleep state and temperature on airway muscle tone, and maintenance of an open airway, is an important area for future investigation.

One very active area of research has been the "apnea hypothesis," the theory that apnea is the main cause of death in SIDS. Although many research groups have extensively evaluated the role of apnea, no conclusions have resulted because of the differences in infants studied and methods used. Some of these factors include variations in the time of day and duration of the recording, laboratory conditions (e.g., warm environment versus normal room temperature), the age and development of the infants, and the clinical conditions of the infants examined. The enthusiasm for the apnea hypothesis has diminished because less than 10 percent of SIDS victims were seen to have apnea before death.

Tests purported to be predictive of SIDS, including electrocardiography (ECG; see ELECTROCARDIOGRAM), pneumocardiography (breathing patterns), POLYSOMNOGRAPHY (sleep patterns), and high carbon dioxide and/or low oxygen challenges (provoking respiratory or arousal responses) have been reviewed by Bentele and Albani (1988). Although many of these evaluations in infants considered to be at higher risk have shown some differences from control groups, these studies have not had sufficient specificity (i.e., few false-positive results) or sensitivity (few false-negatives) to identify individuals at risk. Moreover, the majority of SIDS victims do not belong to these "at-risk" groups.

Newborn infants spend approximately two-thirds of the 24-hour period asleep, and at 6 months they still spend half of their day asleep (see INFANCY: NORMAL SLEEP PATTERNS IN). Major alterations in sleep organization (with changes in the amount and characteristics of active sleep and quiet sleep) occur during the peak incidence of SIDS, at 2 to 4 months. Yet, no data exist that show consistent abnormalities in sleep patterns in individual infants presumed to be at risk for SIDS. Many questions remain, and any model or proposed mechanism for SIDS must incorporate a multifactoral cause that explains the particular vulnerability in the young infant 2 to 4 months of age during sleep. New research approaches are needed to explore the interaction between sleep and other physiologic control systems in the developing infant.

SIDS Prevention and Home Apnea Monitoring Status

The results of the 1987 NIH Consensus Development Conference on Infantile Apnea and Home Monitoring now serves as a guide for pediatricians. This report gives recommendations for further research in the controversial area of the efficacy of home monitoring in preventing SIDS. At least four groups of infants were identified by the consensus committee to be considered as candidates for a home monitor that alerts parents in the event of problems with breathing and heart rate: (1) infants with one or more severe ALTE's requiring mouth-to-mouth resuscitation or vigorous stimulation; (2) premature infants with apnea; (3) subsequent siblings of SIDS victims in families with a history of two or more SIDS, or the twin of a SIDS victim; and (4) infants with certain diseases affecting breathing (e.g., congenital or acquired alveolar hypoventilation). Home monitoring is not indicated for normal infants or healthy preterm infants. When home monitoring is done, it is most effective with the combined efforts of physicians, parents, health care providers, monitor vendors, and community resources such as parent support groups. Monitoring can be very helpful in the management of apnea, but it is

no guarantee that SIDS can be totally averted: SIDS has occurred in infants during monitoring. (See ONDINE'S CURSE; RESPIRATION CONTROL IN SLEEP.)

Management of the SIDS Death

If an infant is found lifeless and not breathing, the immediate response should be cardiopulmonary resuscitation (CPR) and a call to emergency services. If the child does not revive, many resources are needed to support the family. It is common for parents of a SIDS baby to feel guilty and confused as well as grief-stricken. All these feelings must be addressed by the physician and health care providers. Furthermore, the community police, fire department, and other emergency personnel must be knowledgeable about SIDS: SIDS is unexpected, it cannot be prevented, and the cause is not known. Parents should be assured that they are not at fault. Local chapters of the National SIDS Foundation or the Guild for Infant Survival provide support and information to SIDS families, health professionals, and the general public. Other important resources are the National SIDS Clearinghouse (8201 Greensboro Drive, Suite 600, McLean, VA 82102; 703-821-8955) and the SIDS Alliance (10500 Little Patuxent Parkway, Suite 420, Columbia, MD 21044; 800-638-7437).

Summary

Advances in understanding the causes and possible prevention of SIDS will be achieved by (1) rigorous application of the NIH definition of SIDS; (2) carefully designed, prospective studies on the efficacy of home cardiorespiratory monitoring; and (3) interdisciplinary research designed to investigate the development and interaction of the central nervous system elements of cardiorespiratory control, sleep, and arousal. The continuing search for the causes and prevention of SIDS must involve a detailed understanding of the normal development of the central nervous system as well as examination of infants in "high-risk" categories.

REFERENCES

Bentele KHP, Albani M. 1988. Are there tests predictive for prolonged apnoea and SIDS? A review of epidemiological and functional studies. *Acta Paediatr Scand Suppl* 342:3–21.

Glotzbach SF, Heller HC. 1989. Thermoregulation. In Kryger MH, Roth T, Dement WC, eds. *Principles and practice of sleep medicine.* Philadelphia: Saunders.

Kinney HC, Filiano JJ, Harper RM. 1992. The neuropathology of the Sudden Infant Death Syndrome: A review. *J Neuropathol Exper Neurol* 51:115–126.

National Institutes of Health Consensus Development Conference on Infantile Apnea and Home Monitoring. 1987. Consensus statement. *Pediatrics* 79: 292–299.

Steven F. Glotzbach
Ronald L. Ariagno

SUNDOWN SYNDROME

Sundown syndrome is the recurrent appearance or exacerbation of behavioral disturbances such as agitation, pacing, restlessness, aggression, and inappropriate verbalization in the afternoon or evening. It derives its name from the characteristic daily timing of its onset and from the belief that its cause is a reduction in ambient light. More recent research has confirmed the aptness of the term only partially. Sundowning is most prevalent among elderly persons with cognitive impairment, especially those residing in institutions. Its disruptiveness to staff and other residents in such settings and the apparent discomfort attributed to the sundowning patient often result in treatment attempts that include physical restraint or chemical sedation. These interventions tend to have mixed efficacy, with some patients actually becoming worse. Sundowning is therefore an important public health problem and one in need of additional research.

Evans's (1987) study supports the clinical impression that sundowning is a definable syndrome and that the risk in elderly subjects increases with greater mental impairment. Other clinical factors that may predispose to sundowning include recent changes in environment, such as admission to a new facility or a room change, and sensory deficits. An association between sundowning and declines in ambient light is suggested by the finding that confusion and agitation may be induced in demented patients (see DEMENTIA) by placing them in a dark room during the day, and by a report of an apparent increase in sundowning behavior in nursing home patients during the winter months.

Sundowning behavior is often associated with acute increases in confusion, decreased attention and alertness, hyperactivity of the autonomic nervous system, and psychotic (usually paranoid) ideas. These features, as well as the association with dementia, suggest that sundowning may be a form of delirium; however, delirium typically has an identifiable organic or medical cause and, unlike sundowning, is usually of brief duration and either resolves or progresses to death. To date there are no data strongly connecting sundowning with acute medical illness or with metabolic, electrolyte, endocrine, or other acute physiological imbalances.

Sundowning may develop as part of the syndrome of fragmented sleep–wake rhythms in the elderly and in demented patients in particular. Prinz et al. (1982) have found that patients with ALZHEIMER'S DISEASE have a sleep–wake pattern characterized by increased awakenings from sleep, increased time awake at night, and numerous daytime naps. Sleep APNEA, which is markedly increased in elderly demented individuals, may further fragment nighttime sleep and increase daytime napping (see AGING AND CIRCADIAN RHYTHMS; AGING AND SLEEP; FRAGMENTATION; NAPPING). Feinberg, Koresko, and Heller (1967) reported that some demented patients awaken repeatedly from REM sleep and, on awakening, exhibit a delirious activated state with delusional ideas. The combination of an increased tendency to daytime sleep and decreased ability to maintain a sleeping state with the effects of awakening from REM sleep may result in the sundowning syndrome.

Sundowning's possible relationship to the sleep disturbances of dementia suggests that it may reflect a more generalized dysfunction of CIRCADIAN RHYTHMS. The hypothesis of a disordered circadian pacemaker in some demented patients is supported by chronobiological studies of the rest–activity cycle and endocrine measures, and by neuropathological studies reporting cell loss in the SUPRACHIASMATIC NUCLEUS OF THE HYPOTHALAMUS, the putative endogenous pacemaker.

These findings may have important implications for our understanding of sundowning and other behavioral disorders and for devising more effective treatments.

REFERENCES

Bliwise DL, Carroll JS, Dement WC. 1989. Apparent seasonal variation in sundowning behavior in a skilled nursing facility. *Sleep Res* 18:408.

Cameron DE. 1941. Studies in senile nocturnal delirium. *Psychiatr Q* 15:47–53.

Evans LK. 1987. Sundown syndrome in institutionalized elderly. *J Am Geriatr Soc* 35:101–108.

Feinberg I, Koresko RL, Heller N. 1967. EEG sleep patterns as a function of normal and pathological aging in man. *J Psychiatr Res* 5:107–144.

Prinz PN, Peskind ER, Vitaliano PP, Raskind MA, Eisdorfer C, Zemcuznikov N, Gerber CJ. 1982. Changes in the sleep and waking EEGs of nondemented and demented elderly subjects. *J Am Geriatr Soc* 30:86–93.

Satlin A, Teicher MH, Lieberman HR, Baldessarini RJ, Volicer L, Rheaume Y. 1991. Circadian locomotor activity rhythms in Alzheimer's disease. *Neuropsychopharmacology* 5:115–126.

Andrew Satlin

SUPRACHIASMATIC NUCLEUS OF THE HYPOTHALAMUS

The suprachiasmatic nucleus (SCN) in the anterior HYPOTHALAMUS is a paired nucleus straddling the midline, bordering the third ventricle, and bounded anteroventrally by the optic chiasm (Figure 1). This nucleus is the site of a circadian pacemaker in mammals. No other discrete area of mammalian brain has yet been found with the circadian pacemaking properties of the SCN. The homolog of the nucleus also appears to play a crucial timekeeping role in a few species of lizards and birds that have been examined.

The architecture of the SCN has been studied most extensively in rodents, especially in the albino rat. Suprachiasmatic nucleus cells are among the smallest in the brain and are very densely packed. A combination of various anatomic techniques suggests that the nucleus is composed of distinct dorsomedial and ventro-lateral subdivisions. Cell bodies in the dorsomedial SCN are smaller, contain fewer organelles, and are more closely apposed than those located ventrolaterally. A number of neural peptides have been identified in these neurons. Vasopressin is synthesized within some of the dorsomedial SCN neurons, and smaller amounts of somatostatin, enkephalin, atrial naturietic peptide, and angiotensin are also found. By contrast, cell bodies in the ventrolateral SCN are usually larger and give rise to extensive dendritic arbors (branching of dendrites). Some of these neurons synthesize vasoactive intestinal polypeptide or gastrin-releasing peptide. Cells from both SCN subdivisions interact extensively with one another in a dense and complex neuropil. Most SCN axons terminate locally within the nucleus amidst a myriad of synaptic interactions, including dendrodentritic contacts (contacts between dendrites). Immunoreactive gamma-aminobutyric acid (GABA) is the most plentiful substance identified in SCN axons and dendritic boutons. (See CHEMISTRY OF SLEEP: PEPTIDES.)

Many of the neural afferents to the SCN preferentially innervate its ventrolateral portion. Visual inputs are conveyed directly to the dendrites of neurons in this subdivision from retinal ganglion cells via a "retino-hypothalamic" tract (RHT), which appears to be both necessary and sufficient for entrainment of overt CIRCADIAN RHYTHMS to the environmental day–night cycle. The neurotransmitter of the RHT is unknown but may be an excitatory amino acid. Additional photic information is channeled indirectly to the ventrolateral SCN via fibers from the intergeniculate leaflet, and lesions of the leaflet suggest that it may mediate some of the effects of light *intensity* on overt circadian rhythmicity. Some of the fibers of this "geniculo-hypothalamic" tract (GHT) indicate immunoreactive neuropeptide Y when stained. Finally, serotonergic fibers from the raphe nuclei of the MIDBRAIN ramify within the ventral portion of the SCN. Interestingly, some of the RHT, GHT, and serotonergic fibers appear to terminate onto cells containing vasoactive intestinal polypeptide. Besides neural afferents, the SCN also receives hormonal input; for example, the nucleus contains high-affinity receptors for the pineal hormone MELATONIN. Suprachiasmatic nucleus efferents emanate from the dorsocaudal aspects of the nuclei, mainly innervating neighboring parts of the hypothalamus. (See NEUROENDOCRINE HORMONES.)

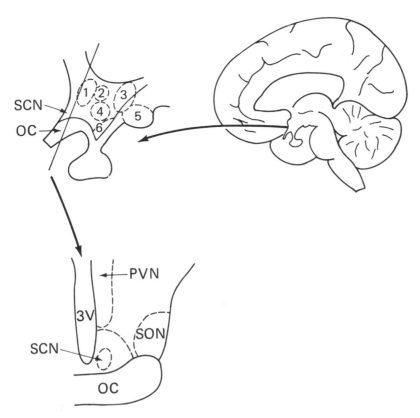

Figure 1. Diagrams of the human brain showing the location of the SCN. Right top, a sagittal view. Left top, the hypothalamus expanded. OC, optic chiasm; SCN, suprachiasmatic nucleus; 1, paraventricular nucleus, PVN; 2, dorsomedial nucleus; 3, posterior nucleus; 4, ventromedial nucleus; 5, mammillary body; 6, arcuate nucleus. Left bottom, a coronal section taken at the level of the line, above. SON, supraoptic nucleus; 3V, third ventricle.

Extracellular recordings of the SCN's electrical activity show a low frequency of spontaneous discharges. About one-third of the recorded units respond to light, usually by increasing their firing rates. These responses are sustained, proportional to light intensity, and elicited from large receptive fields lacking a retinotopic organization such as is found in visual system neuron populations. These SCN neurons appear to code for luminance (especially in the range of illumination intensities corresponding to dawn and dusk). These data, as well as the anatomy of the RHT and GHT, suggest that the system for photic entrainment of circadian rhythms is distinct from the other visual systems for eye movements and pattern vision.

There is strong evidence (mostly in rodents) that the SCN contains a functioning circadian pacemaker. Electrical or pharmacologic stimulation of the nucleus causes predictable phase shifts of overt circadian rhythms, whereas destruction of the SCN results in a breakdown of the entrainment or generation of a wide array of such rhythms. More than 75 percent of the nucleus must be ablated to eliminate expressed rhythmicity, and no recovery of function is found even after prolonged postoperative survival. Three intrinsic properties of the SCN (energy metabolism, neuronal spike activity, and vasopressin secretion) exhibit circadian rhythmicity both *in vivo* and *in vitro*; all of these rhythms peak during the subjective day in both diurnal and nocturnal mammals. Finally, neural grafts of fetal SCN tissue re-establish overt rhythmicity in arrhythmic SCN-lesioned recipients, and the rhythms restored by the transplants display properties that are characteristic of the circadian pacemakers of the donors rather than those of the hosts. Of course, these kinds of experiments have not been done in humans. Nevertheless, the human SCN and its retinal input have been identified, and disturbed rhythmicity may follow damage to this region of the human hypothalamus.

The cellular and molecular processes that constitute the SCN's actual timekeeping mechanism are unknown. Nicotinic or glutamatergic antagonists block light-induced phase shifts of overt circadian rhythms in rodents and inhibit SCN neuronal responses to optic nerve stimulation in hypothalamic slices, although administration of the agonists (carbachol or glutamate) to the animals does not exactly reproduce light's phase-shifting action. Manipulation of brain GABAergic and serotonergic systems also alters the circadian pacemaker's responsivity to light and entrainment to the light–dark cycle, but the observed effects are quite complex (see CIRCADIAN RHYTHM DISORDERS). Of note, the SCN's endogenous oscillatory mechanism seems to persist even when neuronal action potentials are blocked pharmacologically (with the drug tetrodotoxin), and the oscillation begins in fetal animals in the uterus even when the nucleus is morphologically immature (the SCN is nearly devoid of conventional synapses at this time). Factors such as membrane potential, calcium metabolism, cyclic nucleotides, protein synthesis, and transcriptional regulatory proteins are suspected to play roles in SCN clock function, but it is unclear how these elements might work in an oscillatory mechanism.

REFERENCES

Klein DC, Reppert SM, Moore RY, eds. 1991. *Suprachiasmatic nucleus: The mind's clock.* New York: Oxford University Press.

Meijer JH, Rietveld WJ. 1989. Neurophysiology of the suprachiasmatic circadian pacemaker in rodents. *Physiol Rev* 69:671–707.

William J. Schwartz

SYMBOLISM IN DREAMS

Symbolism has been defined as "the art or practice of using a symbol, which is something that stands for or suggests something else by reason of relationship, association, convention, or accidental resemblance" (*Webster's,* 1986). It is widely thought that the mind employs symbolism in dreaming to convey meaningful messages to the dreamer through images (see PICTORIAL REPRESENTATION.) Several theorists consider dreams to be a symbolic language expressing the most intimate and individual aspects of our lives; thus, these dream symbols often have unique and special significance to the dreamer.

Researchers and clinicians have also identified many common symbols that appear frequently in dream reports; these symbols are found as well in artistic and literary depictions of dreams throughout history. Such symbols are often derived from basic human experiences, suggesting similar meanings for dreams of people from very different cultures or time periods. One example is symbolism representing the dreamer's relationship with members of the immediate family, a fundamental life experience for most people. Instances of universal dream symbolism abound, from the obscure to the ordinary. The snake has been interpreted as temptation since Biblical times; in the ancient Greco-Roman world, snakes were also symbols of the medical arts, and people often dreamed of snakes when seeking or undergoing treatment for an illness (Faraday, 1974).

Houses, another common symbol in dreams, are often considered in a general sense as an extension of oneself or one's life style, or seen as the symbol of a marriage or a family relationship. Dreaming of a childhood home may indicate that something in the present is reminiscent of events that happened earlier in the dreamer's life. Similarly, dreaming of the destruction of a home may symbolize the dissolution of a marriage by divorce, separation, remarriage, or the death of a spouse. Symbolic interpretation can be still more specific: a dream of being in someone else's house may express a wish to be married to someone else, or dreaming of a Victorian-style house may be indicative of "Victorian" attitudes that are causing problems for the dreamer. (See also INTERPRETATION OF DREAMS.)

Perhaps the most common dream symbols are people. Although some characters may simply represent themselves, strangers or anonymous figures may stand for actual people, situations, or even psychological aspects of oneself (see SENOI DREAM THEORY). Theorists have suggested that children in dreams represent undeveloped sides of our personalities or parts of ourselves that are stuck in the conflicts of childhood; alternatively, they may symbolize a new phase of life or a period of personal growth. The symbolic language of dreams, then, can be seen at least as an efficient way to convey a wide array of attitudes and emotions. Interpretation of these symbols may provide a rich source of psychological insights to the dreamer.

(See also ADLER'S DREAM THEORY; CHARACTERISTICS OF DREAMS; FLYING IN DREAMS; FREUD'S DREAM THEORY; JUNG'S DREAM THEORY.)

REFERENCES

Delaney G. 1981. Living your dreams. San Francisco: Harper & Row.

Faraday A. 1974. *The dream game.* New York: Perennial Library.

Von Grunebaum GE, Caillois R. 1966. *The dream and human societies.* Berkeley: University of California Press.

Krista Hennager

SYMPATHETIC NERVOUS SYSTEM

The sympathetic nervous system is one of the two major subdivisons of the autonomic nervous system (see also PARASYMPATHETIC NERVOUS SYSTEM). The autonomic, or visceral, nervous system is responsible for the control of the heart, blood vessels, intestine, smooth muscles, and glands. Activation of sympathetic function expends energy by increasing heart rate, blood pressure, and respiratory rate; blood flow to the skin and gastrointestinal tract is diverted to the skeletal muscles, heart, lungs, and brain; dilation of the pupil of the eye is stimulated as is increased secretion from sweat glands; the rectal and urinary sphincters contract. Thus, strong sympathetic activation occurring during emotional crises quickly mobilizes the body's reserves for intense muscular action needed in offense and defense (the fight-or-flight reaction). Although during these times of stress, the actions of the sympathetic system

may be thought of as antagonistic to parasympathetic actions, routine sympathetic activity balances and closely integrates with parasympathetic activity to regulate bodily functions.

The sympathetic output pathway involves two types of neuron. The first, or preganglionic, neuron is situated in the spinal cord and sends its axon out of the CENTRAL NERVOUS SYSTEM with the motor output (ventral roots) of the spinal cord. The fibers travel a short distance where they terminate in groups of cells called ganglia. Most preganglionic fibers terminate in ganglia that lie beside the spinal column from the base of the skull to the coccyx (bottom of the spine). Other preganglionic fibers end in ganglia that are found around a major blood vessel, the abdominal aorta. In the ganglia, the preganglionic cells make synaptic connections with postganglionic neurons. The postganglionic neuron sends its axon out of the ganglia to innervate the visceral organs, such as heart, gut, and pupillary muscles. The neurotransmitter released by preganglionic neurons is acetylcholine. Postganglionic neurons release norepinephrine, except for those innervating the sweat glands, which release acetylcholine. (See CHEMISTRY OF SLEEP.)

General sympathetic activity is reduced in NREM sleep. In REM sleep tonic sympathetic outflow is suppressed further, but is also characterized by phasic increases (see AUTONOMIC NERVOUS SYSTEM).

REFERENCES

Carpenter MB, Sutin J, eds. 1983. *Human neuroanatomy,* pp. 209–231. Baltimore, MD: Williams and Wilkins.

Diamond MC, Scheibel AB, Elson LM. 1985. *The human brain coloring book.* New York: Harper and Row.

McGinty DJ, Drucker-Colin R, Morrison A, Parmeggiani PL, eds. 1985. *Brain mechanisms of sleep.* New York: Raven Press.

Orem J, Barnes CB, eds. 1980. *Physiology in sleep.* New York: Academic Press.

Stephen Morairty

T

TEA

Chinese legend holds that aboriginal tribesmen of Asia first prepared tea nearly 4,700 years ago by boiling raw, green leaves of wild tea trees in kettles over outdoor fires. By about A.D. 590, tea was in common use as a social beverage in China and thereafter throughout Asia. Tea was first introduced in Europe in the 1500s by Jesuit missionaries throughout Asia. Tea truly came into vogue in England in the middle of the seventeenth century when Catherine of Braganza, wife of King Charles II, brought chests of tea leaves from Portugal as part of her dowry. The beverage came to America with the colonists in the 1700s, and was dumped into Boston Harbor on December 16, 1773, as part of the Boston Tea Party, a protest by American revolutionaries who opposed tea taxes levied by King George III.

Tea comes from the leaves and buds of the *Camellia sinensis* plant, native to China and India. After picking, tea leaves are withered and crushed to release a sap containing the enzyme *tea polyphenol oxidase*. This organic catalyst causes fermentation, a process that affects the flavor-producing chemicals in tea and also turns the leaves dark brown. The tea is then dried and crumbled in preparation for blending. Depending on its level of fermentation, tea is said to be of the black (fully fermented), oolong (partially fermented), or green (unfermented) variety.

Regardless of the level of fermentation, dry tea leaves from the *C. sinensis* plant contain approximately 3.5 percent caffeine by weight, or about 40 milligrams per one 8-ounce cup of tea. Tea can be decaffeinated by rinsing moistened tea leaves with methylene chloride, a solvent that extracts caffeine from the leaves. Herbal teas blended without any leaves from the *C. sinensis* plant usually have no caffeine. To be called "caffeine-free," tea may contain no more than 5 milligrams of caffeine per one 8-ounce cup. Some people use caffeinated tea's stimulating effect to promote alertness (see CAFFEINE); others use caffeine-free or herbal tea to soothe, calm, and promote sleep (see FOLK AND OTHER NATURAL REMEDIES FOR SLEEPLESSNESS). Studies have shown that the level of caffeine in tea can affect sleep; the results of caffeine consumption include an increase in the time a person takes to fall asleep, increased movement during sleep, decreased total sleep time, and a decrease in quality of sleep.

REFERENCES

Florio D. 1991. A toast to tea. *Health* 22:74–78.
Gilbert RJ. 1986. Caffeine—The most popular stimulant. In *The Encyclopedia of Psychoactive Drugs 18*. New York: Chelsea House.
Isles J. 1987. *A proper tea.* New York: St. Martin's Press.
Ryan R. 1988. The gentleman's guide to perfect tea. *Gentleman's Q* 12:95–98.
Ukers WH. 1935. *All about tea.* New York: The Tea and Coffee Trade Journal.

Katherine M. Sharkey

TEDDY BEARS

Since 1903, when Teddy bears first appeared, they have been cherished companions for children of all ages. The Teddy bear generally appears at about the same time the newborn child arrives home. Parents, grandparents, and friends compete to be the first one to give that special Teddy bear; each wants to be a part of the lifelong friendship that develops. By six months, many infants make a strong attachment to a stuffed animal. It becomes a reminder of the mother and of the child's lasting connection with her. It also provides a harmless and safe means of relieving anxiety. The stuffed animal is the infant's first tool for comforting himself or herself.

As the child grows older, the Teddy bear becomes a magical protector and friend who helps the child to overcome fear of the unknown, especially in the loneliness of nighttime. At bedtime, the Teddy bear's presence is essential, and if it has been misplaced, there will be upset and tension for both the parents and the child until the bear is back in its proper place in the child's arms. All of these quali-

ties make the Teddy bear into what the English psychoanalyst Winnicott has described as a *transitional object,* the importance of which is well recognized, particularly in assisting the child to fall asleep (see TRANSITIONAL OBJECTS).

Historical research indicates that a cartoon in the *Washington Star* by Clifford Berryman, in 1902, unleashed Teddy fever in this country. He had drawn a caricature of President Theodore Roosevelt refusing to shoot a baby bear while on a hunting trip. People who saw the drawing began to associate the bear cub with President Roosevelt. A New York City shopkeeper was inspired to sew up a stuffed brown plush bear, complete with movable limbs and button eyes. He placed it in his shop window along with a copy of the Berryman cartoon and the sign "Teddy's bear." The bear was an immediate success, and in reply to a request, the President authorized the use of his name for the Teddy bear. This inspiration gave birth to an industry that continues to supply millions of bears and other stuffed animals to the children who love them.

Ivan Herman

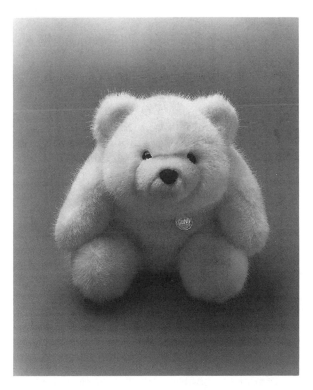

Figure 1. Typical modern teddy bear. Photo courtesy of Gund Manufacturing Company, New York.

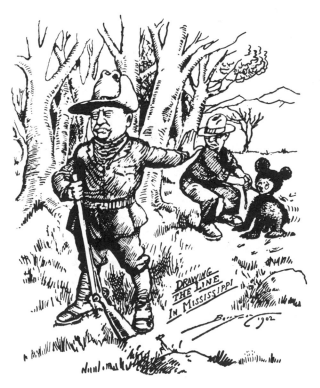

Figure 2. Later version of Clifford Berryman cartoon originally published in the *Washington Post* on November 16, 1902. Courtesy of the Theodore Roosevelt Collection, Harvard College Library.

TELEPATHY AND DREAMING

Telepathy is a word used to describe purported information obtained by one individual from another, supposedly through "mind-to-mind" contact. It is one manifestation of the events that parapsychologists refer to as potential *psi phenomena*—anomalous (or unexplained) interchanges of information or influence that appear to exist apart from currently identified physical mechanisms. Other manifestations of psi include clairvoyance (reported anomalous perception of information), precognition (reported anomalous perception of future events), and psychokinesis (reported anomalous influence on objects or organisms). Considerable overlap exists, especially between telepathy and clairvoyance. For example, Carlos claimed to dream of a gift that Maria, who lived overseas, had decided to buy him for his birthday. Was this a possible instance of telepathy? Or could Carlos have had clairvoyant knowledge of Maria's thought processes? Or was it merely a coincidence?

A survey of more than 7,000 self-reported anecdotal telepathic experiences was tabulated by Rhine (1961); nearly two thirds of these experiences were said to have occurred in dreams. These data supported Freud's conjecture that sleep and dreams create favorable conditions for telepathy. Jung incorporated the concept of telepathic dreams into psychotherapy, using the term *crisis telepathy* to refer to instances in which a dream contains anomalous information about a loved one whose death is imminent or who has suffered an accident, an assault, or other life-threatening situation.

Anecdotal reports of telepathy in dreams are unreliable because one cannot guard against coincidence, dishonesty, self-delusion, or logical or sensory clues of which the dreamer was unaware. The Parapsychological Association insists that the term *psi phenomenon* be used only to describe events obtained under conditions in which all known sensorimotor channels for anomalous interactions have been eliminated. The first attempt to study telepathic dreams experimentally was reported in 1895 by Ermacora, who worked with an Italian medium who attempted to influence the dreams of a child telepathically. Although amateurish by contemporary standards (e.g., the child in question was

the medium's cousin), Ermacora's design was the first serious investigation of telepathic dreams.

It was not until 1966 that telepathic dream studies using the monitoring of REM sleep were reported. Designed by Ullman and his colleagues at Maimonides Medical Center in Brooklyn, these studies paired a volunteer subject with a "telepathic transmitter"; the pair interacted briefly, then separated and spent the night in distant rooms. An experimenter randomly selected an art print (from a collection or "pool") and gave the print to the transmitter in an opaque sealed envelope, to be opened only when the transmitter was in the distant room. The experimenter awakened the subject near the end of each REM period and requested a dream report. These reports were transcribed and sent to outside judges who, working independently, matched them against the pool of potential art prints from which the actual print had been randomly selected. Statistical evaluation was based on the average of these matchings, as well as by self-judgings of the subjects following the conclusion of the experiment. Ullman and his collaborators claimed that there was no way in which sensory cues or fraudulent subject/transmitter collaboration could have influenced the dream reports and statistical results. The results showed an overall pattern of statistical significance supporting the telepathy hypothesis.

One example of a finding in an experiment that obtained statistical significant results occurred on a night when the randomly selected art print was "School of the Dance" by Degas, depicting a dance class of several young women. The subject's dream reports included such phrases as "I was in a class made up of maybe half a dozen people; it felt like a school." "There was one little girl that was trying to dance with me." An examination of the dream reports and the matched art prints indicates a similarity in this process to the way in which day residue, psychodynamic processes, and subliminally perceived stimuli find their way into dream content. Sometimes the material corresponding to the art prints was intrusive (for example, "There was one little girl that was trying to dance with me"), and sometimes it blended easily with the narrative (for example, "It felt like a school"). At times it was direct, at other times symbolic. Although these dream reports had presumptively telepathic characteristics, their construction and description did not appear to differ in significant ways from other dreams collected in laboratory studies.

A statistical reanalysis of the Maimonides experiments was reported by Child in 1985. He found that six of the fifteen studies attained statistically significant results and that data from one other study were nearly significant. Including the latter study, statistical significance varied from the 0.06 level of probability (only 6 possibilities in 100 that chance was responsible for the results) to the 0.000002 level (less than one chance in several thousand that the matches between dream report and art print were sheer coincidence). On the other hand, several critics (for example, Zusne and Jones, 1982) would not go this far, and claimed that there were serious flaws in the procedure; in response, Child declared that some of these criticisms were irrelevant and that others reflected actual misrepresentation and distortion of the original experiments. A lack of reliable replication by other researchers is the most important criticism that can be made of these dream telepathy studies.

Another analysis of the Maimonides data provided provocative results. Persinger and Krippner (1989) examined the first night that each of sixty-two subjects in telepathic or clairvoyant dream experiments spent at the Maimonides laboratory. A significant difference was observed between "high psi" nights and "low psi" nights: the former were more likely in the absence of electrical storms and sunspots. These data may indicate that the telepathic and clairvoyant capacities of the human brain are sensitive to geomagnetic activity.

In summary, the evidence supporting telepathic dreams is modest, consisting of a variety of interesting but unproven anecdotal reports and a small number of controversial experimental studies whose replication record is unimpressive. Nevertheless, Ullman, Krippner, and Vaughan (1988), Wilson and Barber (1982), and others have made the point that enough is already known to prevent psychotherapists from automatically labeling a report of a telepathic dream as psychopathology, or assuming that people reporting them are necessarily lying, hallucinating, or deluding themselves or others. Future research studies may provide naturalistic, conventional explanations for some or all of these cases, but it is not improbable that the telepathic dream contains unresolved lessons for students of human behavior and experience.

REFERENCES

Child IL. 1985. Psychology and anomalous observations: The question of ESP in dreams. *Am Psychol* 40:1219–1230.

Ermacora GB. 1895. Telepathic dreams experimentally induced. *Proc SPR* 11:235–308.

Persinger MA, Krippner S. 1989. Dream ESP experiments and geomagnetic activity. *J Am Soc Psychical Res* 83:101–106.

Rhine LE. 1961. *Hidden channels of the mind.* New York: William Sloane.

Ullman M, Krippner S, Vaughan A. 1988. *Dream telepathy,* 2nd ed. Jefferson, NC: McFarland.

Wilson S. Barber TX. 1982. "The fantasy-prone personality": Implications for understanding imagery, hypnosis, and parapsychological phenomena. *Psi Res* 1:94–116.

Zusne L, Jones WH. 1982. *Anomalous psychology.* Hillsdale, N.J.: Erlbaum.

Stanley Krippner

TEMPERATURE EFFECTS ON SLEEP

Humans and other warm-blooded animals sleep best when they are in their thermal comfort zone, the range of ambient (air) temperatures within which they do not have to spend energy on shivering or increasing metabolic rate in the cold or sweating or panting in the heat. Under conditions of cold or heat stress both the quality and quantity of sleep are disturbed. Figure 1 shows that as the ambient temperature gets very low or very high, both REM sleep and SLOW-WAVE SLEEP (SWS) become poorer, but REM sleep is more affected.

Even short-lasting peripheral temperature

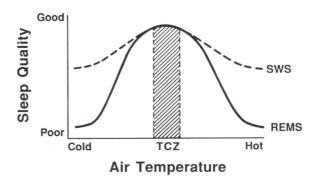

Figure 1. Diagram showing the relationship between the thermal comfort zone (TCZ) and the quality of SWS and REM sleep.

changes toward or away from the thermal comfort zone can affect REM sleep. Rats enter REM sleep only after SWS. In one experiment, when the rats had entered SWS, warm air was blown over them when they were sleeping in cool temperatures or cool air was blown when they were sleeping in hot temperatures (Szymusiak et al., 1980). Within only a few minutes, the sleep state changed to REM sleep in 70 to 80 percent of the trials. During control SWS bouts, when the air that was blown over them was the same as their sleeping temperature, the rats entered REM sleep on only about 23 percent of the trials, and woke up the rest of the time. When the rats were sleeping within their thermal comfort zone, at about 25°C, 46 percent of the control SWS bouts ended in REM sleep. Skin warming decreased this to 22 percent and skin cooling to 9 percent. Rats showed the most REM sleep when they were near the upper end of their thermal comfort zone.

In humans, as air temperature decreases lower than the preferred temperature of about 30°C (the same temperature rats prefer!), there is an increase in the number and length of waking periods. This occurs partly because body temperature influences sleep duration: the higher your body temperature when you go to sleep (within normal limits, of course), the longer you will sleep. In the heat, people move around in bed much more, often causing them to wake up and thus fragmenting their sleep. In animals, thermoregulatory responses to thermal stress are lower during SWS than in waking, but not as low as in REM sleep. At one level this explains why REM sleep is more sensitive to thermal stress: because thermoregulatory mechanisms are absent in REM sleep, it is more dangerous to have REM sleep in an environment where the animal's body temperature may deviate too far from normal. At another level, of course, such an explanation is not satisfactory. We would have to know *why* thermoregulatory mechanisms are lowered or suspended during REM sleep. (See THERMOREGULATION.)

Why do people (and rats, too) feel sleepier when they are comfortably warm? One possibility is that we need more sleep when we are warm; we may be metabolizing some needed substance faster or using up something that keeps us awake, and only sleep can restore it. Another more likely possibility depends on a distinction between *core* sleep and *optional* sleep, made by the British psychologist James Horne. Core sleep is essential, although no one knows why. Optional sleep is thought to fill time, and is under a behavioral drive to sleep. It is the same distinction as between hunger and appetite. Hunger requires us to eat a certain amount of food that is essential to maintaining energy balance; appetite causes us to eat the chocolate cake after a full meal, although we certainly do not need it. A warm environment may be to optional sleep what a piece of chocolate cake is to appetite: it stimulates sleep even though we do not need it. No one knows what the required amount of sleep is at different ambient temperatures. Rats have almost three times as much REM sleep at 30°C as they do at 23°C. Does this mean that they are REM sleep deprived at 23°C? Or are they laying down "REM sleep fat" at 30°C?

Because sleep is so much affected by body temperature, which in turn is affected by environmental temperature, it is experimentally complicated to study basic neurophysiological and neuropharmacological mechanisms of sleep. This is because many drugs and many parts of the brain also influence thermoregulation. Thus, if a treatment were found to alter sleep, it would not necessarily mean that the treatment was directly affecting brain areas or brain chemicals that control sleep. Rather, the treatment might be interfering with an important requirement for normal sleep—thermal comfort. A level of thermal comfort before the treatment might be uncomfortable afterward, and this might reverse the effects of a drug or a brain lesion on sleep. This important relationship means that experiments studying sleep should be conducted within the zone of thermal comfort for the species under study, and this thermal comfort zone itself might change with the treatment.

REFERENCES

Horne J. 1988. Why we sleep. New York: Oxford University Press.

Satinoff E. 1988. Thermal influences on REM sleep. In Lydic R, Biebuyck J, eds. *Clinical physiology of sleep,* pp 135–144. New York: Oxford University Press.

Szymusiak R, Satinoff E, Schallert T, Whishaw IQ. 1980. Brief skin temperature changes towards thermoneutrality trigger REM sleep in rats. *Physiol Behav* 25:305–311.

Evelyn Satinoff

TEMPERATURE REGULATION

See Body Temperature; Temperature Effects on Sleep; Thermoregulation.

TEMPORAL ISOLATION

External time cues, such as light and air temperature, can both entrain the circadian clock (see ENTRAINMENT) and also affect observed behavior directly (as when someone wakes up during the night because the temperature is too warm; see TEMPERATURE EFFECTS ON SLEEP). These time cues can thus greatly complicate the interpretation of circadian experiments. In order to study the circadian timekeeping system directly, one must separate the organism from all external environmental influences that can affect either the circadian clock or the behaviors controlled by it. Such a condition is called *time isolation* or *temporal isolation*.

Although temporal isolation is relatively easy to achieve with laboratory animals, it is difficult to separate humans completely from the ubiquitous timing cues of the environment and society. Even such subtle cues as the sounds of traffic outside or the noise of air conditioners turning off and on with night and day must be removed from the subject's environment. In order to achieve temporal isolation, researchers have recorded the sleep, behavior, and physiology of human subjects living for months at a time in caves, underground bunkers, and specially designed apartments. These experiments are difficult for both experimenter and subject (who, sometimes, are the same person). Michel Siffre spent 6 months alone in an underground cave to study his own rhythms. He wrote:

> Overcome with lethargy and bitterness, I sit on a rock and stare at my campsite in the bowels of Midnight Cave, near Del Rio, Texas. Behind me lie a hundred days of solitude; ahead loom two and a half more lonely months. But I—a wildly displaced Frenchman—know none of this, for I am living "beyond time," divorced from calendars and clocks, and from sun and moon, to help determine, among other things, the natural rhythms of human life.

While most laboratory animals in temporal isolation continue indefinitely to free-run with a constant period (see FREE RUNNING), a large fraction of humans show a more complicated organization under these conditions. Although the daily cycling of the BODY TEMPERATURE rhythm shows a free-running period of about 25 hours, after a few days to a few weeks the sleep–wakefulness rhythm begins to free-run with a 30-to 36-hour period. These people stay awake for about 20 hours at a time and then sleep for about 12 hours. Since they are in temporal isolation, they do not know how long they have been sleeping and think that their sleep is normal. This phenomenon of decoupling between the body temperature and sleep–wakefulness rhythms is called spontaneous *internal desynchronization*. The mechanisms underlying INTERNAL DESYNCHRONIZATION are not known.

The expense and difficulty of running temporal isolation experiments with human volunteers has reduced their use in recent years. Several other techniques, most notably an abbreviated version of temporal isolation called CONSTANT ROUTINE, have supplanted temporal isolation as a means for studying the human circadian clock.

(See also CIRCADIAN RHYTHMS.)

REFERENCES

Siffre M. 1975. Six months alone in a cave. *National Geographic* 147:426–435.
Strogatz SH. 1986. *The mathematical structure of the human sleep-wake cycle.* New York: Springer-Verlag.

Russell N. Van Gelder

THALAMUS

The thalamus is a collection of nerve cells clustered into distinct cell populations, or nuclei, interposed between the brainstem and higher cortical structures. One major function of the thalamus is to relay sensory and movement information to the neocortex. The thalamus is there-

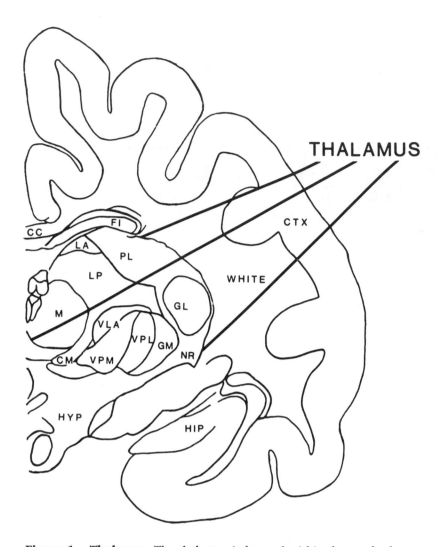

Figure 1.   Thalamus: The thalamus is located within the cerebral cortex adjacent to the midline of the brain. This cross section shows the right side of the brain, indicating the major subdivisions of the thalamus, and adjacent regions of the brain.

CC – corpus callosum (white matter pathway interconnecting the left and right sides of the cerebral cortex)

CM – centro median nucleus

CTX – cerebral cortex

FI – fimbria of the hippocampus (a pathway originating in the hippocampus)

GL – lateral geniculate of the thalamus

GM – medial geniculate nucleus of the thalamus

HIP – hippocampus

HYP – hypothalamus

LA – anterior lateral nucleus of the thalamus

LP – posterior lateral nucleus of the thalamus

M – medial dorsal nucleus of the thalamus

NR – reticular nucleus of the thalamus

PL – pulvinar nucleus of the thalamus

VLA – ventro-lateral nucleus of the thalamus

VPL – ventral posterolateral nucleus of the thalamus

VPM – posteromedial nucleus of the thalamus

White – white matter connecting regions of the cerebral cortex fore in a position to process and control much of the information received by the cortex. The major thalamic nuclei can be classified into three functional classes. Most lateral thalamic nuclei are the specific relay nuclei that project to well-defined cortical areas related to specific functions, such as vision and hearing. These would include the lateral (vision) and medial (hearing) geniculate nuclei of the thalamus. The second group of thalamic relays, lying closer to the midline of the brain, are called associational nuclei. They receive input from the specific thalamic nuclei and project output to association areas of cortex that deal with higher-order integrative functions. Third are the most centrally located intrinsic thalamic nuclei that have diffuse projections to cerebral cortex and receive their major input from the brainstem reticular formation. The intrinsic thalamic nuclei are in an ideal position to relay the influences of the reticular activating system to the entire cerebral cortex and are at least partially responsible for the cortical activation observed during wakefulness and REM sleep.

During waking, thalamic neurons are highly excitable and accurately relay incoming messages to the cortex. On entrance into NREM sleep, thalamic neurons are actively inhibited by a mechanism that at present is poorly understood. Relay neurons under inhibition exhibit a bursting pattern of discharge and are less responsive to incoming messages. This mechanism is largely responsible for the attenuation of sensory input, which is necessary for the maintenance of uninterrupted sleep. A group of neurons located at the lateral margin of the thalamus and called the *thalamic reticular nucleus* (not part of the reticular formation) express a pronounced rhythmic pattern of activity in NREM sleep. These neurons do not project to the cortex, but through extensive connections within the thalamus, synchronize bursts of activity in thalamic relay neurons to produce rhythmic activity and spindle waves, brain waves recorded in the cortex, which are characteristic of NREM sleep. During REM sleep, thalamic relay neurons are as excitable as during waking. Increased excitability is due to the renewal of reticular activation and the unique phasic excitations, of brainstem origin, associated with PGO waves. (See also AROUSAL; LATERAL GENICULATE NUCLEUS; NREM SLEEP MECHANISMS; PGO WAVES; SENSORY PROCESSING AND SENSATION DURING SLEEP; SLEEP SPINDLES.)

REFERENCE

Steriade M. 1990. Thalamocortical systems: Inhibition at sleep onset and activation during dreaming sleep. In Mancia M, Marini G, eds. *The diencephalon and sleep,* pp 231–247. New York: Raven Press.

Gerald A. Marks

THEORIES OF SLEEP FUNCTION

[*One of the most persistent questions asked of sleep researchers is "Why do we sleep?" This question, which has driven much of the research in the field, is also one of the most resistant to straightforward answers. At present, there exist innumerable theories of sleep's purpose, and the wide variety of these theories points to the likelihood that sleep has multiple functions rather than a single one. For example, a number of scientists have proposed that* REM SLEEP *and NREM sleep subserve entirely different sets of functions; furthermore, the cyclic alternation of these two states within the architecture of sleep itself may have functional utility for the organism.*

EARLY SLEEP THEORIES *and* DREAM THEORIES OF THE ANCIENT WORLD *survive from the prescientific era. In addition, anthropologists have documented the* ABORIGINAL DREAMING *lore of Australia and the* SENOI DREAM THEORY *of Malaysia (see also* RELIGION AND DREAMING*). Numerous anecdotes suggest that one of the functions of REM sleep may be to promote* CREATIVITY IN DREAMS *or* PROBLEM SOLVING IN DREAMING*. Different schools of psychology have proposed functions for dreams in psychoanalysis and daily life (see* ADLER'S DREAM THEORY; COGNITIVE DREAM THEORY; FREUD'S DREAM THEORY; JUNG'S DREAM THEORY*).*

Observational and experimental studies suggest functional roles for sleep in the areas of LEARNING *and* MEMORY, *as well as general* COGNITION *(see also* AMNESIA*). The REM sleep state may serve specific physiological functions (see* REM SLEEP, FUNCTION OF*). A number of functional theories have been posited regarding the cyclic organization of sleep and wakefulness and the stages within sleep. For example, the* BASIC REST–ACTIVITY CYCLE *was proposed by Nathaniel*

Kleitman (the father of U.S. sleep research) as a fundamental means of behavioral organization that is evidenced most clearly by the CYCLES OF SLEEP ACROSS THE NIGHT. CIRCADIAN RHYTHMS *related to sleep and wakefulness may also have some functional underpinnings; in addition, these rhythms have an impact on the duration and* TIMING OF SLEEP AND WAKEFULNESS.

Wilse Webb's overview of the FUNCTIONS OF SLEEP *encompasses many present-day theoretical positions. Much of current thinking on the topic is based upon sleep* DEPRIVATION *studies that examined the consequences of denying all sleep or a single type of sleep—that is, REM sleep or NREM sleep—to the organism. An early theory arising from such studies and from naturalist observation was the* FATIGUE–RECOVERY MODEL. *Additional theories of sleep function are touched upon in the entries concerning the* EVOLUTION OF SLEEP, ONTOGENY, LONGEVITY, SLOW-WAVE SLEEP, *and the* SENTINEL HYPOTHESIS. *Finally, sleep's unique thermoregulatory physiology, accompanying changes in metabolic rate, and the known thermal consequences of long-term sleep deprivation have led to theories invoking* ENERGY CONSERVATION *as a major function of sleep.*]

THERMOREGULATION

Scientists have known since the nineteenth century that body temperature decreases during sleep (see Kleitman, 1963); this observation has been confirmed in many mammals and birds. Later it was found that brain temperature rises during REM sleep in most species, almost to levels found in waking (Kawamura and Sawyer, 1965). The possible significance of these changes has been studied extensively, first to discover how the changes in body temperature during sleep are brought about, but also because theories about sleep control place much importance on temperature regulation.

In order to maintain a relatively constant temperature, homeotherms (mammals and birds) compensate for changes in environmental temperature by increases or decreases in heat production and heat loss. The mechanisms controlling heat loss and heat production are often tested and quantified by raising or lowering envi-

ronmental temperature and measuring the animal's responses, including processes such as increased or decreased metabolism, shivering, sweating, panting, or the extent of vasodilation of blood vessels in the skin. In the latter case, for example, the skin is warmed by increased blood flow during vasodilation and more heat can be "lost" to the environment through convection. Behavioral processes, such as increasing motor activity, putting on more clothes, fluffing the fur for insulation, or seeking a warm nest may be thermoregulatory processes. Thermoregulation is also studied by warming or cooling certain parts of the brain, particularly the preoptic-anterior HYPOTHALAMUS (POAH), because such brain sites are found to be directly thermosensitive and to control thermoeffector responses, that is, responses that alter temperature. For example, warming the POAH is like warming the whole animal in that this treatment elicits cooling responses such as vasodilation, panting, and reduced motor activity.

Tests such as these have shown that the onset of sleep actively induces a reduction in metabolic rate and heat-loss responses. Evidence for these conclusions includes the findings that the threshold and rate of change of the metabolic response to hypothalamic cooling are lowered in NREM sleep in kangaroo rats (Glotzbach and Heller, 1976) and that sweating is increased in humans (Satoh, Ogawa, and Takaji, 1965). These experiments support the hypothesis that there is a lowering of the regulated temperature during sleep, a change analogous to lowering the setting on the thermostat of a building heating system during the night. The decrease in temperature during sleep is brought about by both reduced heat production and increased heat loss. Several studies have shown that overall and cerebral metabolic rate are reduced during NREM sleep (see ENERGY CONSERVATION; METABOLISM). The temperature decrease during sleep is independent of changes in temperature mediated by CIRCADIAN RHYTHMS (Gillberg and Akerstedt, 1982), although when sleep occurs at its usual circadian time, sleep-related and circadian rhythmic temperature drops are superimposed, so cooling is maximized.

Changes in thermoregulation during REM sleep are different from those in NREM sleep, and seem to constitute a loss of the homeostatic control that normally characterizes many aspects of mammalian physiology. Parmeggiani (1980) has shown by several techniques that thermoregulation seems to cease in REM sleep. For example, panting in a warm environment and shivering and vasoconstriction in a cold environment are suppressed in cats during REM sleep (Parmeggiani and Rabini, 1967); metabolic responses to POAH cooling are absent in kangaroo rats, and thermoregulatory sweating is suppressed in humans (Henane et al., 1977). Thus, a variety of tests suggest loss of thermoregulatory homeostasis in REM sleep. In humans, however, some thermoregulatory responses to heat and cold are preserved in REM sleep (Libert et al., 1982; Haskell et al., 1981).

As already noted, brain temperature rises during REM sleep in many species, although monkeys may be an exception (Reite and Pegram, 1968). Factors such as local heat production resulting from increased cerebral metabolic activity may contribute to the REM sleep–related brain temperature elevation. A theory that the brain temperature elevation in REM sleep is controlled primarily by increases in arterial blood temperature resulting from vasoconstriction and reduced peripheral heat loss (Baker and Hayward, 1967) remains controversial. Another finding is that REM sleep is sensitive to ambient temperature and is more easily suppressed in either warm or cool environments than is NREM sleep (Szymusiak and Satinoff, 1984). The amount of REM sleep within a sleep period is maximized in warm "thermoneutral" environmental temperatures, in which the animal's metabolism is at a minimal level (Szymusiak and Satinoff, 1981). These diverse and fascinating aspects of REM sleep thermoregulation have not yet engendered a unifying hypothetical explanation. (See TEMPERATURE EFFECTS ON SLEEP.)

Thermoregulatory aspects of NREM sleep fit a more coherent framework. The POAH region that controls temperature also participates in the regulation of NREM sleep, and these two functions of the POAH seem to be closely integrated (see BASAL FOREBRAIN). For example, POAH lesions both suppress sleep and disturb heat loss responses (McGinty and Szymusiak, 1990). Warming of the POAH induces heat loss responses such as vasodilation, as well as increased NREM sleep (Sakaguchi, Glotzbach, and Heller, 1979). In humans, deep NREM sleep (stage 3 and 4 sleep) is increased after daytime temperature elevations produced by hot bath immersion or intense aerobic exercise (Horne and Moore, 1985; Horne and Reid, 1985). Increases in stage 3 and 4 sleep are interpreted as increases in the DEPTH OF SLEEP. Because NREM sleep induces brain and body cooling, increased NREM sleep could produce thermoregulatory compensation for heating while awake.

These findings have nourished hypotheses that NREM sleep is, at least in part, a thermoregulatory process under control by the POAH and that cooling is the functional end point (Obal, 1984). This idea is consistent with other facts about sleep. For example, sleep functions can be explored by assessing effects of sleep deprivation (see DEPRIVATION, TOTAL: PHYSIOLOGICAL EFFECTS). Among the most critical changes produced by sleep deprivation is dysregulation of body temperature and metabolism (Rechtschaffen et al., 1989). Such a result is consistent with the hypothesis that sleep has important thermoregulatory functions, although further studies are needed to discover the exact nature of these functions.

That sleep may have a thermoregulatory function is also consistent with our knowledge concerning the evolution of sleep (see EVOLUTION OF SLEEP). Sleep in homeotherms (mammals and birds) is different from that in poikilothermic animal groups such as reptiles, amphibians, and fish. Unlike homeotherms, poikilotherms show large changes in body temperature accompanying changes in environmental temperature. It is reasonable to hypothesize that the unique qualities of sleep in homeotherms are related to the unique characteristics of their temperature regulation. Mammals and birds are thought to have evolved separately from ancestral poikilotherms. Thus, we can ask why mammals and birds may have independently evolved similar sleep processes. Independent evolution of functional mechanisms is not unusual. For example, vision is thought to have evolved separately many times, with obvious adaptive advantages. But independent evolution supports a hypothesis that adaptive pressures related to homeothermy itself underlie the evolution of the special features of sleep in homeotherms. For example, sleep-related cooling could provide energy conservation (see ENERGY CONSERVATION) or other adaptive benefits in homeothermic animal species that must maintain a high waking temperature (Allison and Van Twyver, 1970; Zepelin and Rechtschaffen, 1974; Berger, 1975). Lowering of temperature in NREM sleep would fit this model, but it is not yet clear how events in REM sleep can be understood. Alternatively, the evolution of sleep could be required for some as yet not understood support of mechanisms of homeothermic thermoregulation, or to interrupt the sustained exposure of certain heat-sensitive cells to the high body temperatures associated with waking.

REFERENCES

Allison T, Van Twyver H. 1970. The evolution of sleep. *Nat Hist* 79:56–65.

Baker MA, Hayward JN. 1967. Autonomic basis for the rise in brain temperature during paradoxical sleep. *Science* 157:1586–1588.

Berger RJ. 1975. Bioenergetic functions of sleep and activity rhythms and their possible relevance to aging. *Fed Proc* 34:97–102.

Gillberg M, Akerstedt T. 1982. Body temperature and sleep at different times of day. *Sleep* 5:378–388.

Glotzbach SF, Heller HC. 1976. Central nervous regulation of body temperature during sleep. *Science* 194:537–539.

Haskell EH, Palca JW, Walker JM, Berger RJ, Heller HC. 1981. Metabolism and thermoregulation during stages of sleep in humans exposed to heat and cold. *J Appl Physiol* 51:948–954.

Henane RA, Buguet A, Roussel B, Bittel J. 1977. Variations in evaporation and body temperatures during sleep in man. *J Appl Physiol* 42:50–55.

Horne JA, Moore VJ. 1985. Sleep EEG effects of exercise with and without additional body cooling. *Electroencephalogr Clin Neurophysiol* 60:33–38.

Horne JA, Reid AJ. 1985. Night-time sleep EEG changes following body heating in a warm bath. *Electroencephalogr Clin Neurophysiol* 60: 154–157.

Kawamura H, Sawyer CH. 1965. Temperature elevation in the rabbit brain during paradoxical sleep. *Science* 150:912–913.

Kleitman N. 1963. *Sleep and wakefulness.* Chicago: University of Chicago Press.

Libert JP, Candas V, Muzet A, Ehrhart J. 1982. Thermoregulatory adjustments to thermal transients during slow wave sleep and REM sleep in man. *J Physiol (Paris)* 78:251–257.

McGinty D, Szymusiak R. 1990. Keeping cool: a hypothesis about the mechanisms and functions of slow wave sleep. *Trends Neurosci* 12:480–487.

Obal F, Jr. 1984. Thermoregulation during sleep. *Exp Brain Res Suppl* 8:157–172.

Parmeggiani PL. 1980. Temperature regulation during sleep: A study in homeostasis. In Orem J, Barnes CD, eds. *Physiology in sleep,* pp 97–143. New York: Academic Press.

Parmeggiani PL, Rabini. 1967. Shivering and panting during sleep. *Brain Res* 6:789–791.

Rechtschaffen A, Bergmann BM, Everson CA, Kushida CA, Gilliland MA. 1989. Sleep deprivation in the rat: Integration and discussion of finding. *Sleep* 12(1):68–87.

Reite ML, Pegram GV. 1968. Cortical temperature during paradoxical sleep in the monkey. *Electroencephalogr Clin Neurophysiol* 25:36–41.

Roberts WW, Bergquist EH, Robinson TCL. 1969. Thermoregulatory grooming and sleep-like relaxation induced by local warming of the preoptic area in opossum. *J Comp Psychol* 67:182–188.

Sakaguchi S, Glotzbach SF, Heller HC. 1979. Influence of hypothalamic and ambient temperatures on sleep in kangaroo rats. *Am J Physiol* 237:R80–R88.

Satoh T, Ogawa T, Takaji K. 1965. Sweating during daytime sleep. *Jpn J Physiol* 15:523–529.

Szymusiak R, Danowski J, McGinty D. 1991. Exposure to heat restores sleep in cats with preoptic/anterior hypothalamic cell loss. *Brain Res* 541:134–138.

Szymusiak R, Satinoff E. 1984. Ambient temperature-dependence of sleep disturbances produced by basal forebrain damage in rats. *Brain Res Bull* 12:295–305.

Szymusiak R, Satinoff W. 1981. Maximal REM sleep time defines a narrower thermoneutral zone than minimal metabolic rate. *Physiol Behav* 26: 687–690.

Zepelin H, Rechtschaffen A. 1974. Mammalian sleep, longevity and energy conservation. *Brain Behav Evol* 10:425–470.

Dennis McGinty

THUMBSUCKING

Thumbsucking is a self-generated rhythmical behavior that can be observed in infants as early as birth and even in the womb before birth. A recent study conducted in Cleveland indicated that more than 20 percent of children between 6 months and 4 years old suck their thumbs (Wolf and Lozoff, 1989). The prevalence of thumbsucking may vary greatly among cultures, since the phenomenon is closely linked to child-rearing practices and other cultural differences. In an Israeli infant sleep survey, for example, only 8.4 percent of the infants reportedly fell asleep while sucking their thumbs. However, more than 80 percent of the sample used other sucking behaviors (pacifier or bottle) during the transition to sleep (Scher et al., 1987).

Thumbsucking, like other nonnutritive sucking and rhythmical behaviors (e.g., using a pacifier, rocking), serves a self-soothing function. Woodson, Drinkwin, and Hamilton (1985) demonstrated the soothing qualities of nonnutritive sucking for full-term and preterm babies, showing decreased restlessness in infants following periods of sucking behavior. Thumbsucking is related to another self-soothing phenomenon: Infants who suck their thumbs are also more likely to be attached to a transitional object such as a piece of cloth, blanket, or TEDDY BEAR (see TRANSITIONAL OBJECTS). Breast-fed infants are also more likely to suck their thumbs than bottle-fed babies (Wolf and Lozoff, 1989).

In addition to the general soothing effects of sucking behaviors, these studies have also shown that thumbsucking in infants is closely linked to the particular process of falling asleep. Wolf and Lozoff (1989) as well as Ozturk and Ozturk (1977) have demonstrated that infants who suck their thumbs are more likely to be left by their parents to fall asleep alone than are infants who do not use thumbsucking as a self-soothing behavior. Because these correlative studies simply associate one phenomenon with another, their findings can be interpreted using two alternative explanations: (1) that infants who are born with or acquire this self-soothing technique very early in life do not need the help of a care-giver to fall asleep; or (2) that infants who are left alone to fall asleep tend to develop self-soothing behaviors such as thumbsucking out of necessity. It appears, from developmental and clinical perspectives, that both explanations are relevant, and that longitudinal research is still needed to clarify the complex relationship of thumbsucking to sleep during infancy and childhood. (See also INFANCY, NORMAL SLEEP PATTERNS IN; CHILDHOOD, SLEEP DURING.)

REFERENCES

Ozturk M, Ozturk OM. 1977. Thumbsucking and falling asleep. *Br J Med Psychology* 50:95–103.
Scher A, Tirosh E, Jaffe M, Rubin E. 1987. Survey of sleep patterns of Israeli infants and young children. *Sleep Res* 16:209.
Wolf AW, Lozoff B. 1989. Object attachment, thumbsucking, and the passage to sleep. *J Am Acad Child Adolescent Psychiatry* 28(2):287–292.
Woodson R, Drinkwin J, Hamilton C. 1985. Effects of nonnutritive sucking on state and activity: Term-preterm comparisons. *Infant Behav Development* 8:435–441.

Avi Sadeh

THYROID DISEASE AND SLEEP

Abnormalities of thyroid function collectively represent the most common type of endocrine disease. In countries such as the United States where iodine deficiency is rare, the principal cause of both hypothyroidism (an underactive thyroid gland) and hyperthyroidism (an overactive gland) is autoimmune dysfunction. In the United States, both hypo- and hyperthyroidism are much more common in women than in men, and as many as 5 percent of adult women have or have had one or the other disorder. Thyroid hormone has important effects on virtually every part of the body and brain, so even small deviations of thyroid hormone concentration from normal levels can have complex and important effects on general health. The normal expression of sleep and wakefulness also depends on thyroid hormone, and sleep complaints are among the most consistently reported symptoms of thyroid hormone excess or deficit. While the mechanism linking abnormalities of thyroid hormone concentration to specific sleep problems is not always clear, enough is known about the two physiological functions to allow a productive exploration of their relationship.

The Normal Thyroid Gland

The thyroid is the two-lobed, butterfly-shaped endocrine gland in the anterior neck just below the larynx (the "Adam's apple"). The normal thyroid gland weights just 20 grams and can barely be felt on palpation. Prominent enlargement, termed a *goiter,* is inevitably a sign of thyroid disease. The thyroid gland secretes thyroid hormones that act at specific receptors on peripheral tissues to exert their effect (see ENDOCRINOL-OGY). The diverse actions of the thyroid hormones are difficult to characterize collectively, but they are typically described as acting to increase metabolic activity and protein synthesis. Thyroid hormones are essential for normal growth and development, and appear to provide important signals for the selective differentiation of tissues throughout the body. In concert with the catecholamines (epinephrine and norepinephrine), thyroid hormones act to facilitate many of the actions of the SYMPATHETIC NERVOUS SYSTEM. They increase the output of the heart, raise blood pressure, and increase heat production. Exactly how thyroid hormone is involved in normal sleep–wake expression is not known; thyroid hormone has diverse actions throughout the brain, but no specific role in the control of sleep and wakefulness has been documented.

Thyroid Dysfunction

As mentioned above, the two broad categories of thyroid disease are hypothyroidism and hyperthyroidism. In much of the world, dietary iodine deficiency is the most common cause of thyroid disease. Iodine is essential for the synthesis of thyroid hormone by the thyroid gland. In developed countries, where iodine deficiency is rare, thyroid dysfunctions occur for other reasons. While the specific diseases that lead to both hyper- and hypothyroidism are many and varied, two diseases exemplify the effects of these abnormalities on sleep.

Hashimoto's disease is a common disorder in which the body's own immune cells (see IMMUNE FUNCTION) attack the thyroid gland and, over a variable period of time, destroy the functional tissue. When inadequate thyroid tissue remains, thyroid hormone levels fall below normal and hypothyroidism results. Infiltration of the thyroid gland by the immune cells and the resultant inflammation result in growth of a goiter. On the opposite end of the spectrum, *Graves's disease* results from stimulation of the thyroid gland by an "autoantibody" that abnormally recognizes the thyroid-stimulating hormone receptor (see THYROID-STIMULATING HORMONE). The thyroid gland responds to this incessant stimulation with excessive growth (*hypertrophy*) and ever-increasing levels of the thyroid hormones. The

hypertrophy of the thyroid gland from this cause also results in a goiter.

Sleep Disruption in Thyroid Disease

Few objective studies of sleep have been done in patients with hyperthyroidism of any kind, but clinical observations of patients with Graves's disease suggest that these patients commonly complain of difficulty falling asleep, frequent awakenings, and light and restless sleep. Daytime sleepiness is not a common complaint, being presumably overwhelmed by the direct stimulating effects of excess thyroid hormone.

More data have been collected to describe the relationship of hypothyroidism in general, and Hashimoto's disease specifically, to sleep and sleep disorders. Patients with severe untreated hypothyroidism have diminished consciousness that presages *myxedema coma,* a life-threatening condition. In less severe hypothyroidism, patients complain of daytime fatigue and daytime sleepiness. The basis for the former complaint is complex, but the daytime sleepiness seems to be related to nocturnal sleep disruption that may be due to a number of causes. For example, certain patients with hypothyroidism have PERIODIC LEG MOVEMENTS of sleep, although the causal link between the two problems is not well established.

More typically, patients with hypothyroidism due to Hashimoto's disease have obstructive sleep APNEA syndrome (OSAS). The relationship appears to be due to a number of factors. First, hypothyroidism is associated with obesity and an increase in soft tissue mass. This increased weight and tissue presumably contributes to OSAS just as it does in obese people with normal thyroid function. Second, patients with Hashimoto's disease appear to have selective enlargement of the soft tissue of the pharynx, contributing to upper airway obstruction. In extreme cases, the goiter itself may play a role in airway obstruction. Third, hypothyroidism is associated with muscle weakness, presumably including the muscles of respiration in the upper airway. Finally, thyroid hormone is important to normal respiratory drive, and hypothyroid states are associated with centrally mediated hypoventilation states. This latter problem may result in a component of central or mixed apnea superimposed on OSAS.

Summary

In summary, abnormalities of thyroid function, both hyperthyroidism and hypothyroidism, are associated with disrupted sleep. The best-studied relationship is between hypothyroidism and obstructive sleep apnea syndrome, but clinical observations suggest that a broader relationship exists.

REFERENCES

Grunstein RR, Sullivan CE. 1988. Sleep apnea and hypothyroidism: Mechanisms and management. *Am J Med* 85(6):775–779.

Ingber SH, Braverman LE, eds. 1986. *Werner's The thyroid: A fundamental and clinical text.* Philadelphia: Lippincott.

Passouant P, Passouant FT, Cadilhac J. 1967. Influence on sleep of hyperthyroidism. *Electroencephalogr Clin Neurophysiol* 23(3):283–284.

Gary S. Richardson

THYROID-STIMULATING HORMONE

Thyroid-stimulating hormone (TSH; also known as *thyrotropin*) is secreted from the anterior PITUITARY GLAND and consists of an alpha and a beta subunit. The alpha subunit is almost identical to the alpha subunits of the other glycoproteins secreted from the anterior pituitary. Secretion of TSH is regulated by thyrotropin-regulating hormone (TRH), by feedback inhibition by the thyroid hormones it promotes, and by the body's biological clock. It stimulates the secretion of the thyroid hormones thyroxine (T4) and triiodothyronine (T3) from the thyroid gland. T4 is often converted to T3 after secretion from the thyroid gland. Thyroid hormones affect almost every cell in the human body. An excess concentration of thyroid hormone in plasma results in more rapid glucose metabolism, increased oxygen uptake, and alteration of skin/nail growth. If there is a limited level of thyroid hormone in blood circulation, metabolism and cholesterol turnover are decreased; in children, bone maturation and the onset of puberty are delayed if the thyroid hormone level is subpar. (See also ENDOCRINOLOGY.)

Thyroid-stimulating hormone is secreted in pulses throughout the day and night with 1 to 3 hours between episodes. The distinct pattern of the frequency and amplitude of these pulses is evidence of circadian rhythmicity (see CIRCADIAN RHYTHMS). No significant sex-dependent differences in TSH secretion or in the response of TSH to TRH have been found in humans. TSH serum concentration remains relatively constant throughout the day and then reaches a peak just before sleep onset, between 8:00 P.M. and 4:00 A.M. depending on the usual time sleep occurs. From there, TSH decreases through the night and reaches a nadir around noon the next day. Pulse analysis of the nocturnal rise of TSH demonstrates that this peak is caused by an increase in both pulse frequency and pulse amplitude. Animal studies indicate that TSH also has a circannual (yearly) rhythm, but this does not appear to be the case for humans.

Secretion of TSH is modulated by sleep, but the exact mechanism is unclear. Parker and colleagues (1976) demonstrated that TSH levels begin to fall immediately upon sleep onset, indicating that the nocturnal rise in TSH is dampened by sleep. Thus, subjects put to bed 3 hours earlier than normal show a smaller rise and shorter duration of TSH concentration across the following normal day. Conversely, when sleep onset is delayed 3 hours, TSH concentration reaches a higher than normal level, again with a drop beginning at sleep onset. If sleep is entirely prevented, TSH concentration levels off at an above-normal concentration level for the first part of the following day. Studies have also reported indirect evidence of correlation between TSH and SLOW-WAVE SLEEP. Furthermore, TSH response to TRH is decreased in REM sleep as compared with slow-wave sleep. Brabant and colleagues (1990) confirmed Parker's findings, but found no significant correlation between TSH and any sleep stage.

In hyperthyroidism, where there is an overabundance of TSH, patients have increased slow-wave sleep times and increased REM sleep times. Similarly, in central hypothyroidism, a decrease in the sleep-related TSH peak is accompanied by a decrease in slow-wave sleep. Kales and colleagues (1967) showed that when the hypothyroid patients were treated for their hypothyroid condition, the slow-wave sleep time returned to normal, indicating that slow-wave sleep and TSH secretion may be controlled by a single mechanism.

The TSH circadian fluctuation is generally agreed to be reduced in depressed patients; whether the circadian pattern returns to normal after recovery or remains altered is unknown. Sleep DEPRIVATION transiently improves DEPRESSION, and a significant rise in maximum TSH secretion due to TRH may be predictive of a successful sleep deprivation treatment (Kvist and Kirkegaard, 1980).

REFERENCES

Brabant G, Prank K, Ranft U, Schuermeyer Th, Wagner TOF, Hauser H, Kummer B, Feistner H, Hesch RD, Muhlen A. 1990. Physiological regulation of circadian and pulsatile thyrotropin secretion in normal man and woman. *J Clin Endocrinol Metabolism* 70:403–409.

Kales A, Heuser G, Jacobsen A, Kales JD, Hemley J, Zwaizig JR, Paulson MJ. 1967. All night sleep studies in hypothyroid patients, before and after treatment. *J Clin Endocrinol Metabolism* 27:1593–1599.

Kvist J, Kirkegaard C. 1980. Effect of repeated sleep deprivation on clinical symptoms and the TRH test in endogenous depression. *Acta Psychiatr Scand* 62:494–502.

Mendelson WB. 1987. Neuroendocrinology and sleep. In *Human sleep,* pp 129–179. New York: Plenum.

Parker DC, Pekary AE, Hershman JM. 1976. Effect of normal and reversed sleep-wake cycles upon nyctohemeral rhythmicity of plasma thyrotropin: Evidence suggestive of an inhibitory influence of sleep. *J Clin Endocrinol Metabolism* 46:318–329.

Laura Walbof

TIME ZONES

Before the creation of time zones, standard time was determined by each country. Geographically, this meant that time changed at irregular intervals of distance along the east–west axis, since different parts of the globe are in different positions relative to the sun at the same moment in time. The need for a uniform system of time became apparent with the onset of the industrial era and increased travel by sea and then by air. In 1884, the International Date Line and twenty-four time zones were established. The date line lies in the mid-Pacific Ocean near Western Samoa. Each day "begins" at this line, so that when traveling westward across the line, one moves into the next calendar day, and, likewise, when traveling eastward across the line one moves into the previous calendar day. Time zone boundaries were drawn at intervals of 15 degrees of latitude, starting at the date line, with the poles as endpoints. Thus, the conterminous United States has four time zones (Pacific, Mountain, Central, and Eastern), each separated by 1 hour from those on either side. In addition, various countries adopted DAYLIGHT SAVINGS TIME during World War I in order to reduce the need for artificial light at night, thereby conserving fuel: Clocks were advanced 1 hour during part of the year to create longer days. Since then, further variations on the time zones have been adopted by some countries, but they do not greatly affect the whole system. "Spring forward, fall back" is a popular phrase used as a reminder for Daylight Savings Time, meaning to turn the clock forward in spring and then back in the fall.

REFERENCE

Winfree A. 1987. *The timing of biological clocks,* pp 1–19. New York: Scientific American.

Richard Lee

TIMING OF SLEEP AND WAKEFULNESS

Impressive regularities are evident in the timing of sleep episodes. These regularities are reflections of how different physiological processes interact with each other and with an animal's environment and behavior to determine when an animal will fall asleep and when it will awaken. A clear understanding of the biological factors that determine sleep timing is particularly valuable because it provides some insight into the possible FUNCTIONS OF SLEEP.

General Features

Sleep patterns vary considerably with species. Humans typically sleep 7 to 9 hours each night in a single block with few interruptions. Rats, on the other hand, sleep in short episodes of just a few minutes each, mostly during the daytime, that add up to 12 hours or more per day. Sleep also varies with age. Human infants may sleep 16 hours per day, in short episodes scattered around the clock. Sleep is not consolidated to the night-time hours until at least 3 to 6 months after birth. Even among individuals of the same species and AGE there can be substantial differences in sleep timing characteristics, some of which are genetically determined.

Within a sleep episode, mammals alternate between REM sleep and NREM sleep. REM sleep makes up 20 percent to 25 percent of total sleep time in humans. It is typically divided into four to six REM periods during the night, with NREM sleep in between. The period of this ultradian REM–NREM cycle varies from 50 to 60 minutes in newborns to about 90 minutes in adults, but it also varies significantly from one cycle to the next. Across species, the period generally varies inversely with body size. The proportion of REM sleep increases toward the end of the daily sleep period, because of the influence of the circadian clock. (See also CYCLES OF SLEEP ACROSS THE NIGHT; CIRCADIAN RHYTHMS; BIOLOGICAL RHYTHMS.)

Physiological influences on the timing of sleep episodes include both circadian and homeostatic processes. The circadian clock tends to confine sleep to a particular phase of the daily cycle. Humans tend to sleep at night, whereas many rodents are active at night and sleep mostly during the day. This suggests that sleep is a device for conserving energy and ensuring inactivity at times of day when activity would not be adaptive. There is also a homeostatic tendency to preserve a balance between amounts of sleep and wakefulness. People who are kept awake for long periods are likely to sleep for a long time when given the opportunity to do so (see DEPRIVIATION, TOTAL). Sleep–wake homeostasis is an expression of the commonsense notion that sleep serves a restorative purpose. Current experimental findings show how the phase of an animal's circadian clock, its recent sleep–wake experience, its environment, and its behavior all interact to determine when sleep will occur.

Circadian Phase

"Circadian" (approximately daily) influences on sleep timing have been demonstrated in experiments in which environmental conditions are held constant. Much of what is known about the timing of human sleep comes from long-term studies of subjects in a special environment without information about time of day. These are known as TEMPORAL ISOLATION or FREE RUNNING studies. Many experiments of this type were conducted at the Max Planck Institute in Germany and elsewhere during the 1960s, 1970s, and early 1980s. Other mammals have been studied under equivalent conditions.

It has been known for some time that daily rest–activity rhythms in mammals persist under constant conditions with periods close to (but not exactly) 24 hours. Corresponding rhythms of sleep–wake have been documented by continuous electroencephalographic recordings—first in humans, then in mice, rats, and squirrel monkeys. Similar rhythms exist in a host of other physiological and behavioral variables, all of them mutually synchronized. Free-running circadian rhythms have a period of approximately 25 hours in humans. The entire system is normally synchronized to, or "entrained" by, a 24-hour light–dark cycle. The phase of the system can be delayed or advanced predictably by LIGHT pulses given at appropriate times. Nonphotic cues such as social events, meals, and episodes of physical activity may also contribute to ENTRAINMENT (see ZEITGEBERS). Thus, not only is sleep expressed under constant conditions in a regularly recurring circadian pattern, but it is also part of a complex biological system that regulates daily timing of many other variables.

In humans, sleep is ordinarily coupled tightly to the circadian clock, such that it always occurs at a definite phase of the circadian cycle. After several weeks in time isolation, this coupling often breaks down, so that sleep episodes are distributed more widely across circadian phase. This is known as spontaneous INTERNAL DESYNCHRONIZATION (Figure 1). Unusually long (noncircadian) cycles of sleep and wakefulness are often seen in desynchronized subjects, and such cycles have been interpreted as manifestations of a second (noncircadian) oscillator. The long (30- to 50-hour) cycles do not appear, however, if subjects are encouraged to take naps. Under these

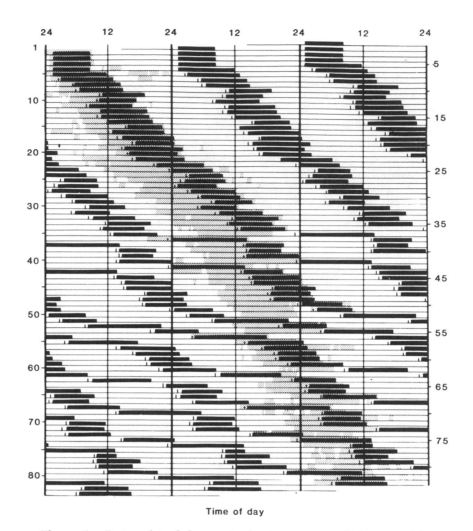

Time of day

Figure 1. Raster plot of sleep episodes in a young male human subject living on a normal daily schedule (days 1–5), and thereafter in time isolation, with instructions to avoid napping. Spontaneous internal desynchronization occurs at day 36. Thin vertical lines before thick bars represent times when the subject started preparing for bed. Dark bars represent time in bed. Phase of the circadian clock is indicated by stippled areas, which represent time when core body temperature was below a normal daily mean value. Data are triple-plotted to improve appreciation of long-term patterns that cross midnight; that is, each day's raster line is extended horizontally to 72 hours, duplicating data on the following two lines. (Reproduced, with permission, from Czeisler CA, Weitzman ED, Moore-Ede MC, Zimmerman JC, Knauer RS. 1980. *Science* 210:1265. American Association for the Advancement of Science.)

conditions of more fragmented sleep, the only long-term rhythm observed is a circadian modulation of the duration and timing of sleep episodes. The same result applies in rodents, which always have a highly fragmented sleep–wake pattern. In such cases, the alternation between sleep and wake is much faster than the circadian cycle and does not appear as a long-term oscillation.

Thus, the hypothesized second oscillator can be seen as a homeostatic tendency to alternate between episodes of sleep and wake, superimposed on the cyclic modulatory influence of the circadian clock (Figure 2). On the other hand, the long sleep–wake cycles of desynchronized subjects are usually perceived as subjective days, complete with proportionally longer meal spac-

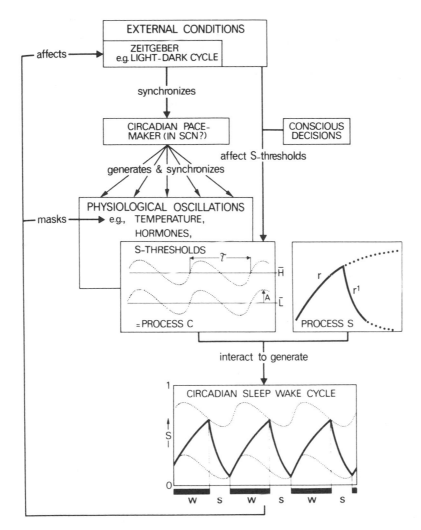

Figure 2.   Model of sleep timing by Daan, Beersma, and Borbély. Process *S*, indexed by the spectral power of sleep electroencephalogram, rises exponentially during wakefulness and declines exponentially during sleep, reflecting the homeostatic contribution to sleep timing. Sleep begins when *S* rises to an upper threshold and ends when *S* falls to a lower threshold. Process *C*, which oscillates with a circadian period determined by the SCN, sets the threshold values of *S* at which sleep–wake transitions occur. The fragmented sleep patterns characteristic of rodents may be achieved by setting the upper and lower thresholds closer together. Environmental and behavioral factors may influence sleep timing by adding to or subtracting from the upper or lower threshold levels determined by *C*. Human sleep patterns similar to those seen in time isolation can be produced by lengthening the period of the threshold oscillations. Spontaneous internal desynchronization can be reproduced by reducing the amplitude of the threshold oscillations, so that sleep episodes occasionally skip a circadian cycle. The model does not consider phase shifts of *C*. (Reproduced, with permission, from Daan S, Beersma DGM, Borbély AA. 1984. *Am J Physiol* 246:R163. American Physiological Society.)

ing and subjective estimates of elapsed time. This implicates a noncircadian timing mechanism that controls more than just sleep and wake times. Whatever its biological basis may be, spontaneous internal desynchronization has provided an opportunity to study sleep episodes initiated over a broad range of circadian phase.

In desynchronized human subjects, sleep duration varies systematically with circadian phase, as indexed by the circadian rhythm of core body temperature. Sleeps initiated near the temperature minimum tend to be short, whereas sleeps initiated near the temperature maximum are often 12 to 16 hours long (Czeisler et al., 1980). For a typical young adult on a normal daily schedule arising at 8 A.M., these two phases of short and long sleeps correspond roughly to 6 A.M. and 6 P.M., respectively. The dependence of sleep duration on circadian phase is summarized by the equivalent result that wake onsets tend to occur on the rising phase of the circadian temperature rhythm. Similar results have been obtained from experiments using an imposed 90- or 180-minute sleep–wake cycle, or scheduled NAPPING. (See SLEEP LENGTH.)

In desynchronized human subjects, sleep onsets are more frequent at two distinct circadian phases: one phase near the temperature minimum and the other approximately 40 percent of the circadian cycle later. Similar results have been obtained under entrained conditions by encouraging napping. For a typical young adult arising at 8 A.M., these two phases correspond roughly to 6 A.M. and 3:30 P.M. Subjective feelings of sleepiness tend to be maximal at these times. There are also two circadian phases, "forbidden zones," where sleep onsets are highly improbable; these correspond roughly to 11:30 A.M. and 9:30 P.M. Though evidence is limited, this biphasic pattern may have a counterpart in other mammals. Chimpanzees and gorillas living in natural conditions nap habitually at around noon, a phase consistent with their early-morning rising time. In squirrel monkeys, midday naps have been documented by laboratory electroencephalographic recordings. Even in rodents, activity patterns often show prominent early and late components with less activity in between. Thus, there seems to be a biphasic circadian rhythm of sleep propensity in several primates and in humans.

Occurrence of REM sleep also varies with circadian phase, whereas slow-wave sleep shows no such correlation. Near the circadian temperature minimum, REM sleep latency is reduced (see REM LATENCY), and there are increases in duration of REM sleep, number of rapid eye movements, and length of the REM–NREM cycle. This accounts for the increasing proportion of REM sleep normally observed during the early-morning hours.

The circadian clock is located in the suprachiasmatic nuclei (SCN) of the hypothalamus. Destruction of the SCN abolishes circadian rhythmicity of sleep and wakefulness in rats and in squirrel monkeys. Little is known about how the SCN generates circadian oscillations of sleep–wake, but it seems to promote both sleep and wakefulness at appropriate circadian phases: SCN-lesioned rats and squirrel monkeys express a constant level of sleep that is intermediate between active-phase and rest-phase levels in intact animals. (See SUPRACHIASMATIC NUCLEUS OF THE HYPOTHALAMUS.)

Homeostasis

Sleep is an appetitive behavior. Just as an animal deprived of food becomes increasingly hungry, an animal deprived of sleep becomes increasingly sleepy. Just as an animal prefers feeding to other behaviors when it is hungry, an animal prefers to sleep when it is sleepy. And just as feeding relieves the desire for food, sleeping relieves the desire for sleep. Thus, there is a tendency to preserve a balance between amounts of sleep and wakefulness, and this is referred to as sleep–wake homeostasis.

One difference between sleep and other appetitive behaviors is that the nature of the physiological need satisfied by sleep is not immediately obvious. People kept awake for long periods become irritable, express a growing desire for sleep, and tend to perform poorly on various physical and mental tasks (see DEPRIVATION, TOTAL). Rats that are continuously deprived of sleep for several weeks become ferociously aggressive and eventually die. Because sleep is a phenomenon of the brain, it seems likely that sleep is important for reversing or complementing some brain process that occurs during wakefulness. For instance, there is limited evidence that REM sleep plays a role in MEMORY consolidation. Beyond this, the restorative purpose of sleep is a mystery.

Homeostatic influences on sleep timing have been demonstrated by keeping people awake. After prolonged wakefulness, there is increased sleepiness, reduced sleep latency, and longer sleep on recovery. Furthermore, restricting sleep modestly over several nights can have a cumulative effect on daytime sleepiness (see DEPRIVATION, PARTIAL), and extending sleep by providing more time in bed can reduce daytime sleepiness in normal young adults. Sleep interruptions can also increase daytime sleepiness.

Recovery sleep after sleep deprivation is not lengthened by the same amount as wakefulness is lengthened. Even after extremely long sleep deprivations, sleep is lengthened by only a few hours. But recovery sleep is also characterized by an increase in large-amplitude slow-wave activity in the ELECTROENCEPHALOGRAM compared with baseline, and is deeper in the sense that more intense auditory stimuli are required to produce arousal. Several investigators have explained these results by proposing that sleep has an intensity dimension reflected in electroencephalographic spectral power and arousal threshold, and that restorative capacity is a function of a sleep episode's intensity as well as its duration. When rats are deprived of sleep, the results are similar to those obtained in human studies. Sleep propensity, sleep duration, and sleep intensity are all enhanced by prolonging wakefulness (see DEPTH OF SLEEP).

In contrast to the considerable recent progress in circadian physiology, little is known about the physiological basis of homeostatic influences on sleep timing, except that these influences are not eliminated by destruction of the SCN in rats.

Circadian Phase Versus Homeostasis

Normally, circadian and homeostatic processes are mutually reinforcing. For instance, the occurrence of nocturnal sleep in humans may result from the homeostatic sleep drive from the preceding day's wakefulness as well as circadian phase-specific potentiation of sleep by the SCN. Circadian and homeostatic influences will conflict only in situations where there is opportunity for sleep to occur at unusual circadian phases, as in desynchronized subjects in time isolation, or

after extended sleep deprivations. In these situations, effects of prior wakefulness are often surprisingly small, or even absent. Homeostatic effects tend to be apparent only after very long intervals without sleep, and even then are modulated by circadian phase. For example, in an analysis of data from human subjects in time isolation, Strogatz (1986) found (1) no effect of prior wakefulness on sleep duration when controlling statistically for circadian phase and (2) a modest effect of prior wakefulness on sleep onset frequency, but only at the circadian phase of maximal sleepiness (near the temperature minimum). Thus, under most conditions circadian influences on sleep timing predominate over homeostatic effects.

Environment

Environmental stimuli are perhaps the most obvious influences on sleep timing. Cyclic changes in light intensity can synchronize circadian rhythms of sleep through effects on the SCN, an effect known as entrainment. Light can also directly suppress sleep in day-active animals or enhance sleep in nocturnal animals, a phenomenon referred to as *masking*. Loud noises or extremes of ambient temperature can also reduce the probability of falling asleep or increase the probability of awakening. The arousing effects of environmental stimuli depend on such variables as sleep stage and age. Young children, for example, are very deep sleepers. Susceptibility of sleep timing to environmental influences is adaptive because it allows an animal to respond to unpredictably timed environmental challenges. (See AGE; SLEEP STAGES; TEMPERATURE EFFECTS ON SLEEP.)

Behavior

Behavioral factors are important determinants of sleep onset timing. In the extreme case, sleep onset is unlikely during vigorous motor ACTIVITY, regardless of circadian phase. In mice, voluntary wheel-running activity significantly prolongs wake episodes and reduces the frequency of sleep onsets. Similarly, human subjects can resist sleep onset for many days if permitted to be active and motivated to do so. On the other hand, short daytime sleeps are remarkably frequent during continuous bedrest, even if subjects are explicitly instructed to remain awake. This effect is greatly pronounced if social contact and intellectual stimulation are restricted. Thus, even low levels of motor activity or cognitive activity may reduce sleep propensity. The influence of waking behavior on sleep timing can be particularly complex in humans, because the timing of waking behaviors themselves may involve conscious decisions.

Environment and behavior can also influence sleep timing through more subtle interactions with the circadian clock. For example, environment or behavior may influence phase setting of the circadian clock by keeping an animal awake, thereby prolonging its exposure to light. When environmental variables oscillate with a 24-hour period, they may reinforce circadian sleep–wake rhythms by either (1) helping to synchronize the endogenous oscillations of the SCN (entrainment), or (2) exerting a direct, periodic influence on sleep (masking). Similarly, behaviors that keep an animal awake may themselves be expressed in a circadian pattern determined by the SCN, so that they reinforce circadian patterns of sleep and wakefulness.

Models

Several quantitative models of sleep–wake timing have been advanced in recent years. These models have had varying success in capturing the subtle interplay of circadian, homeostatic, environmental, and behavioral influences on timing of sleep and wakefulness. The most widely known is the model devised by Daan, Beersma, and Borbély (1984) (see Figure 2).

REFERENCES

Czeisler CA, Weitzman ED, Moore-Ede MC, Zimmerman JC, Knauer RS. 1980. Human sleep: Its duration and organization depend on its circadian phase. *Science* 210:1264–1267.

Daan S, Beersma DGM, Borbély AA. 1984. Timing of human sleep: Recovery process gated by a circadian pacemaker. *Am J Physiol* 246:R161–R178.

Dinges DF. 1989. The influence of the human circadian timekeeping system on sleep. In Kryger MH, Roth T, Dement WC, eds. *Principles and practice of sleep medicine.* Philadelphia: Saunders.

Moore-Ede MC, Czeisler CA, eds. 1984. *Mathematical models of the circadian sleep–wake cycle.* New York: Raven.

Strogatz SH. 1986. *The mathematical structure of the human sleep–wake cycle.* Berlin: Springer-Verlag.

David K. Welsh

TOBACCO

See Nicotine; Smoking and Sleep

TONSILLITIS

The tonsils and adenoids are lymph glands located in the pharynx (throat). Tonsils sit on either side of the oropharynx, the part of the throat at the level of the mouth just behind the tongue (Figure 1). Adenoids are located in the nasopharynx just behind the nasal canals. These glands can become inflamed and infected and swell in size. If the tonsils are involved it is called *tonsillitis*; if both are involved it is called adeno-*tonsillitis*. The accompanying figure demonstrates enlarged tonsils that touch the uvula and obstruct the throat. Most people are aware of common symptoms associated with adenotonsillitis, specifically a sore throat, difficulty swallowing, a blocked nose, and a feeling of fullness in the ears as a result of blockage of the eustachian tubes.

Acute adenotonsillitis may cause a child or an adult to awaken choking from a sound sleep, especially if the tonsils are as enlarged as those shown in Figure 1. Acute and chronic swelling of the tonsils and adenoids from recurrent infections can also lead to the development of obstructive sleep apnea. Often adenotonsillar hypertrophy (enlargement) is the sole cause of sleep APNEA in a child, and surgical removal of these glands will frequently correct the problem. Removal of tonsils and adenoids in an adult, how-

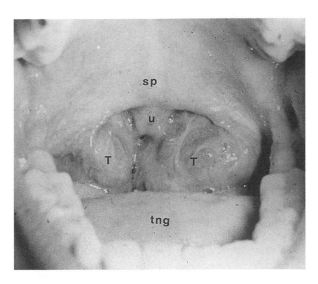

Figure 1. Acute tonsillitis in a child. This photograph was taken with the child's mouth wide open. The tonsils (T) are so large that they meet in the midline and touch the uvula (U). The soft palate (sp) and tongue (tng) are also shown.

ever, often does not cure the sleep apnea, as most adults with sleep apnea are obese as well, which contributes to upper airway obstruction.

When children with enlarged tonsils and adenoids have sleep apnea, they snore (see SNORING) and can be observed to stop breathing frequently while sleeping. Prior to puberty, they frequently do not exhibit the excessive sleepiness seen in adults with sleep apnea. Instead, they demonstrate hyperactivity, aggressive behavior, and learning difficulties in the daytime. BEDWETTING (enuresis) has been associated with sleep APNEA caused by enlarged tonsils and adenoids in children. In severe cases, children may demonstrate a failure to thrive because of a paucity of SLOW-WAVE SLEEP and occasionally signs of right-sided heart failure.

It is now well accepted that obstructive sleep apnea is a reasonable indication for removal of the tonsils and adenoids, especially in children. This actually represents a change in thinking about the need for this type of surgery. Since about 1970, the role of adenotonsillectomy has been quite controversial, with as many physicians against removal of the tonsils and adenoids as advocating it. Part of the controversy stems from a misconception that these lymphoid glands are a necessary immune system barrier to fight infection. The potential severe consequences of

obstructive sleep apnea have overshadowed these concerns.

REFERENCES

Ahlqvist-Rastad J, Hultcrantz E, Svanholm H. 1988. Children with tonsillar obstruction: Indications for and efficacy of tonsillectomy. *Acta Paediatr Scand* 77:831–835.
Moser RJ, Rajagopal KR. 1987. Obstructive sleep apnea in adults with tonsillar hypertrophy. *Arch Intern Med* 147:1265–1267.
Singer LP, Saenger P. 1990. Complications of pediatric obstructive sleep apnea. *Otolaryngol Clin North Am* 23:665–676.
Stradling JR, Thomas G, Warley ARH, Williams P, Freeland A. 1990. Effect of adenotonsillectomy on nocturnal hypoxaemia, sleep disturbance, and symptoms in snoring children. *Lancet* 335:249–253.

Richard P. Millman

TOOTHGRINDING

Toothgrinding, or *bruxism*, occurs during sleep at some time in about 70 percent of all people. For most of these individuals toothgrinding will not have other noticeable effects. However, 5 percent of those with nocturnal bruxism develop symptoms such as excessive tooth wear, jaw pain, or muscle contraction headaches. In severe instances, the range of motion of the jaw is restricted because of damage to the temporomandibular joint.

The precise cause of toothgrinding is unknown, but the episodes of grinding are more severe after emotionally or physically stressful days. Hormones secreted in response to stress may act to initiate episodes of grinding. Use of ALCOHOL or STIMULANT medications can also exacerbate grinding. Because of the nature of these triggering events, experts presume that grinding is mediated by the CENTRAL NERVOUS SYSTEM (CNS). However, the exact CNS mechanism underlying grinding is unknown.

The diagnosis of toothgrinding is made most easily when it is observed by a bed partner. Only about 22 percent of grinding episodes produce the characteristic "grinding" sound, so tape recordings or bed partner interviews are not foolproof. Examination of the pattern of tooth wear is more likely to confirm the presence of pathological grinding. Grinding is measured directly on a sleep recording by obtaining an ELECTROMYOGRAM (EMG) with electrodes on the masseter muscle. Even without this special EMG, all standard sleep recordings use a chin EMG, which should also reveal any tooth-grinding activity that occurs. Grinding occurs in all stages of sleep, although it is most often reported in stage 2 sleep. Some evidence suggests that grinding that occurs in REM sleep is more likely to cause pain and other pathological symptoms. This may occur because certain reflexes that mitigate against the destructive effects of grinding are absent or suppressed during REM sleep.

Many treatment approaches can be helpful in reducing the effects of toothgrinding. For individuals experiencing chronic stress or anxiety, coping skills to aid in stress management should be at least a part of the overall treatment plan. This approach may include relaxation training, time management, or psychotherapy, and it is time-consuming and may require dramatic lifestyle changes. Therefore, only very highly motivated patients will be successful.

Another approach is to use a plastic bite splint during the night. The amount of grinding is not reduced, but the pressure is more evenly distributed, and 80 percent to 90 percent of patients report a remission of their symptoms with use of this device. Pharmacological treatments, such as hypnotics or muscle relaxants taken at bedtime, are also helpful. However, long-term use of any of these medications may produce tolerance to them.

REFERENCES

Rugh JD, Harlan J. 1988. Nocturnal bruxism and temporomandibular disorders. In *Advances in neurology, vol. 49: Facial dyskinesias,* Jankovic J, Tolosa E, eds. New York: Raven.

Ware JC, Rugh JD. 1988. Destructive bruxism: Sleep stage relationship. *Sleep* 11(2):172–181.

Wruble MK, Lumley MA, McGlynn FD. 1989. Sleep-related bruxism and sleep variables: A critical review. *Journal of Craniomandibular Disorders: Facial and Oral Pain* 3:152–158.

Edward J. Stepanski

TORPOR

The term torpor is derived from the Latin *torpere,* which means to become numb or stiff. Torpor is a physiological state in which animals are inactive and relatively unresponsive to environmental stimuli. The metabolic rate of animals in torpor is extremely low, and their body temperature may approach environmental temperature. Animals assume a stereotypical posture during torpor in which certain muscles are contracted, resulting in an animal that appears to be stiff.

Although torpor is found among many vertebrates and even invertebrates, the term *torpor* has at least two different scientific meanings, depending on the animal being discussed. The body temperature of all animals except birds and mammals is dependent on ambient or environmental temperature. Thus, as environmental temperature decreases, the body temperature of these animals will decrease and all biochemical reactions within these organisms will slow or even cease. Thus, animals such as insects, amphibians, and reptiles will become torpid passively as a result of decreased environmental temperature. In harsh environments, animals may exist in this state of torpor for several months until warmer temperatures occur. The term diapause describes the "overwintering" of eggs or juvenile stages of many species of insects whose development is slowed or stopped by cold environmental conditions. Most species must find an environment in which ambient temperature remains above 0°C while they are in torpor. Some species, however, experience subfreezing temperatures while torpid. A question of great interest to physiologists is how such animals can survive below-freezing temperatures for long periods of time.

Torpor has a different meaning when applied to birds and mammals. These animals can use metabolic heat production to regulate their body temperatures above environmental temperatures. At some times of the year, however, these animals allow their body temperatures to approach those of the environment. In these species, torpor is an adaptation used to conserve energy during periods of harsh environmental conditions and/or restricted food availability. Because body temperature is decreased, less energy will be required, as all biochemical reactions that occur within the body are slowed. The absence of vigorous activity contributes to decreased energy consumption during torpor.

This need for energy conservation is particularly acute in small birds and mammals. Because of their small size, such animals lose heat to the environment at a higher rate than larger animals and thus have a high demand for energy. Also due to their small size, these animals have a limited ability to store energy in the form of fat. Consequently, some birds and mammals enter torpor on a daily basis at specific times of the year. This phenomenon has been extensively studied in hummingbirds, which have an extremely high rate of metabolism and have a preferred food source, nectar, that is not available at all times of year. Torpor in hummingbirds was not described in the scientific literature until 1948, yet the Hopi used the word "Holchko," meaning "the sleeping one," to describe torpid hummingbirds.

Torpor can either be seasonal or nonseasonal in its occurrence. The daily torpor of hummingbirds and small mammals already described can either be seasonal or occur throughout the year. Daily torpor is sometimes also called "nocturnal hypothermia" if the body temperature decrease occurs at night. Seasonal torpor is of two types depending on the time of year during which it occurs: HIBERNATION (winter) or ESTIVATION (summer). Although the terms are sometimes used interchangeably, in warm-blooded animals torpor is distinguished from hibernation on the basis of the length of time the animal remains inactive, the time of year at which it occurs, and the degree to which body temperature is lowered. Whereas a bout of daily torpor lasts less than 24 hours (usually less than 12 hours), a bout of hibernation can last for a week or more. Daily torpor can occur at any time of year in many small birds and mammals, but hibernation occurs only during winter (a similar adaptation during the warmer time of the year is called estivation).

Birds and mammals generally do not lower their body temperature below 15°C during daily torpor, whereas body temperature may approach 0°C in small mammals during hibernation. Although bears are commonly described to hibernate in the winter, their body temperatures do not decrease much below 32°C because they are so large and well-insulated. Thus, some scientists describe the sleeplike state of bears in winter as either torpor or "seasonal lethargy," rather than hibernation. Physiological evidence suggests that these distinctions may simply be a matter of degree rather than indicating unique physiological adaptations. For example, both daily torpor and hibernation are entered through NREM sleep with an apparent suppression of REM sleep. The electrophysiological patterns recorded during torpor and shallow hibernation are very similar to those observed during slow-wave sleep at higher body temperatures. Furthermore, the time of day at which the entrance to hibernation and torpor occurs appears to be related to the normal body temperature rhythm. To blur the distinction further, hibernating animals are often referred to as being "torpid," and, as indicated above, daily torpor can occur on a seasonal basis in animals that inhabit environments where access to food is limited to certain times of year.

REFERENCES

French AR. 1988. The patterns of mammalian hibernation. *Am Sci* 76:569–575.

Lyman CP, Willis JS, Malan A, Wang LCH. 1982. *Hibernation and torpor in mammals and birds*. New York: Academic Press.

Thomas S. Kilduff

TRACHEOSTOMY

Tracheostomy is a surgical procedure that involves the creation of an opening in the trachea, the part of the airway that connects the bronchial tubes to the lower part of the pharynx. A small curved tube is placed into the opening to allow the unobstructed flow of air into the lungs. This procedure is performed in patients who have chronic or acute obstruction of the upper airway, or in patients who need assisted ventilation. Because patients with obstructive sleep APNEA characteristically have numerous episodes of complete airway occlusion (closure) during sleep, this procedure is one of several available treatments for patients with this syndrome. By allowing the flow of air to be initiated below the level of the upper airway obstruction, the afflicted patient can breathe quite normally during sleep. This procedure generally produces a dramatic and, in most cases, complete resolution of the patient's symptoms (usually, excessive daytime sleepiness, morning fatigue, and on some occasions heart failure).

Shortly after the discovery of upper-airway obstruction in sleep, and for several years after that, the treatment of choice in most instances was the tracheostomy. The only other option known to improve upper-airway obstruction during sleep in many patients was weight loss. Although the tracheostomy is a definitive cure in the vast majority of cases, it presents many obvious drawbacks to the patient. It results in a rather restricted lifestyle (no swimming or showers) and creates an increased risk for infection in the lungs.

Many patients have great difficulty adjusting psychologically to having a tube placed in their throat, and not uncommonly it is a source of chronic inflammation and irritation. The vast majority of patients, however, adjusted well to these problems in exchange for what amounted to a new life. Any individual involved in the treatment of patients with sleep apnea syndrome can recall extraordinary changes in patients who underwent tracheostomies for the treatment of sleep apnea. In many instances, these were individuals who were severely ill with congestive heart failure, could barely keep awake even at stop lights, and whose lives had become almost completely meaningless. Tracheostomy restored daytime alertness and intellectual functioning, as well as leading to resolution of personality changes such as depression and irritability. These changes are indeed dramatic, but the inherent drawbacks and complications have made acceptance of the tracheostomy as a cure for sleep apnea syndrome very difficult to accept as routine therapy. Newer therapies for sleep apnea syndrome include CONTINUOUS POSITIVE AIRWAY PRESSURE (CPAP) and MAXILLOFACIAL SURGERY.

REFERENCES

George C, Kryger MH. 1988. Management of sleep apnea. *Semin Respir Med* 9(6):569–576.

He J, Kryger MH, Zorick FJ, Conway W, Roth T. 1988. Mortality and apnea index in obstructive sleep apnea: Experience in 385 male patients. *Chest* 94(1):9–14.

William C. Orr

TRANQUILIZERS

Tranquilizers are used to help control a variety of unwanted behaviors and feelings. The term *tranquilizers* is confusing because of the diversity of drugs it encompasses. Generally, tranquilizers include antianxiety drugs (anxiolytics), major tranquilizers (antipsychotic drugs such as the phenothiazines), and SLEEPING PILLS (hypnotics). Most commonly tranquilizers are used to treat ANXIETY and anxiety-related disorders. Anxiolytics are perceived as drugs that can improve well-being by slowing down an overactive nervous system, a nervous system that is spinning its wheels and not progressing toward a desired goal. Antipsychotic drugs can often be helpful in managing extreme levels of anxiety as well as such behavior as agitation and delirium. Major tranquilizers also can be used in the treatment of psychotic symptoms such as delusional thinking and HALLUCINATIONS.

Tranquilizers may be used to overcome anxiety that specifically disturbs sleep. The difference between a hypnotic and an anxiolytic is primarily a matter of the degree of sedation created by the drug. Sedation is largely determined by the dose and drug half-life (a measure of the amount of time the drug stays in the body) rather than by unique pharmacological properties. At least theoretically, an anxiolytic allows the patient to function more effectively, whereas hypnotics and sedating medications are typically used to turn off functioning for a certain period. An example of a drug with the opposite effects, an anxiogenic drug, is CAFFEINE.

Tranquilizers are among the drugs most frequently prescribed. Librium (chlordiazepoxide), Valium (diazepam), and Miltown (meprobamate) all have prominent places in the tranquilizer hall of fame. A contender is Xanax (alprazolam), which currently is one of the more commonly used medications. An impressive diversity of drugs can be used for their tranquilizer-like properties although they are not specifically tranquilizers. These include ALCOHOL, NICOTINE (in certain doses), some ANTIDEPRESSANT medications, and even the cardiovascular medication propranolol. Propranolol, normally used to treat high blood pressure and certain heart arrhythmias, has been used to treat fear of public speaking.

One reason for the prevalent use of tranquilizers is that stress and anxiety are thought to cause a number of physical and behavioral disorders. Another reason is that unlike an antibiotic that makes one feel better only if there is an infection that responds to the drug, tranquilizers are not disease specific and may affect mood and behavior even in the absence of a pathological state. This creates the potential for abuse. Fortunately, the most commonly used type of tranquilizers, a class of drugs referred to as the BENZODIAZEPINES, are endowed with an extraordinary margin of safety. Even a relatively large dose is unlikely to produce death. More than 2000 benzodiazepines have been synthesized and more than a dozen are on the market today. (See DRUGS FOR MEDICAL DISORDERS.)

No drug is entirely benign. Even the benzodiazepines can produce reduced alertness, loss of coordination, slurred speech, loss of memory, unintentional and inappropriate sleep episodes, and dependence. The elderly, who are commonly prescribed tranquilizers, are especially susceptible to side effects because of (1) their reduced ability to eliminate the drug from their body, (2) the prolonged periods for which the drug is prescribed, and (3) the presence of concomitant illnesses and medications. The chronic use of tranquilizers also can lead to tolerance in which the same dose no longer produces the desired effect. Increasing the dose increases the risk of side effects, and stopping the drug may result in a temporary rebound of the initial symptoms.

Do tranquilizers normalize behavior, moderate the extremes, or slow down the entire range of nervous system activity? Tranquilizers have been assumed to be nonspecific; however, this view may be changing. For example, a relatively new class of medication, currently represented by the anxiolytic buspirone, appears to function as an antianxiety medication without producing sedation.

In conclusion, tranquilizers, although dominated by the benzodiazepines, are still a heterogenous and somewhat loosely defined group of drugs. They are used to treat a variety of real and perhaps imagined disorders. With the tranquilizers that are available, as much consideration needs to be given to potential side effects, tolerance, and dependence as given to the potential beneficial effects; however, as an understanding of anxiety evolves, as knowledge of the action of drugs improves, and as ability to tailor drugs for exact effects develops, treatment of specific behaviors can be more successfully targeted with specific drugs.

REFERENCES

Gilman AG, Goodman LS, Rall TW, Murad F. 1990. *The pharmacological basis of therapeutics*. New York: Macmillan.

Schatzberg A, Cole J. 1986. *Manual of clinical psychopharmacology*. Washington, D.C.: American Psychiatric Press.

J. Catesby Ware

TRANSITIONAL OBJECTS

Transitional object is a term coined by Winnicott (1953) to describe the inanimate objects that infants use in their self-soothing activities. Winnicott, a pediatrician and psychoanalyst, was particularly interested in infants' development from a period of total dependence on caregivers for external regulation of their needs to a state of relatively independent self-soothing capacities. One phenomenon that Winnicott noted was infants' apparent interest in inanimate objects such as a piece of cloth or diaper, a blanket, a teddy bear, or even a bottle or pacifier (see TEDDY BEARS).

Winnicott described a number of features common to transitional objects: (1) They seem to be chosen by the infant; a mother may offer an object and facilitate attachment, but she cannot impose a specific object. (2) The objects have special characteristics that must be maintained, for example, the blanket that is not washed to preserve the smell or texture recognized by the child. (3) Such objects provide comfort during times of distress; the child intentionally seeks them out in self-soothing efforts. (4) Loss of the object causes distress and disrupts self-soothing skills. Winnicott (1953) also suggested that the acquisition of a transitional object is determined by nonverbal two-way infant–mother communication, by which the partners negotiate the transfer of maternal soothing skills to the infant. Physical or emotional unavailability of the mother was therefore considered to be a facilitating factor in this process.

Other clinicians have challenged Winnicott's formulation that transitional objects are necessary for normal, healthy development. Bowlby (1969) considered transitional objects to be a simple redirection of attachment behavior when the mother or other caregivers become unavailable. Similarly, Brody (1980) questioned the universality and developmental necessity of transitional object use. Brody suggested that although this phenomenon is related to physical and emotional distance between the child and the mother, it bears no necessary adverse or positive implications for child development.

As an easily observed and prevalent phenomenon, the use of transitional objects has elicited significant research efforts. Klackenberg (1987) found that only 7 percent in a sample of 212 Swedish children never used a transitional object between the ages of 4 and 14 years. A progressive decrease was found in habitual use of transitional objects when going to sleep, from 45 percent at the age of 4 years to 7 percent at the age of 14 years. No significant relationships between sleep problems and the use of transitional objects were shown in this study. Wolf and Lozoff (1989) examined relationships between transitional objects and other child-rearing practices. In their sample of 126 American children under 4 years of age, 44.4 percent habitually used transitional objects at bedtime. The use of transitional objects was also more common in children who fell asleep alone (57 percent) compared with children who fell asleep in the presence of a caregiver (30%), and older children were more likely to use transitional objects than younger children (see CHILDHOOD, SLEEP DURING).

Child-rearing practices vary significantly with families' socioeconomic status, race, and other cultural differences. Similarly, cross-cultural studies indicate that the prevalence of transitional object use is dramatically different among populations (Gaddini and Gaddini; 1970; Hong and Townes, 1976; Litt, 1981). For example, compared with American children in the middle class, rural Italian children and Korean children used transitional objects considerably less, as did black children at a lower socioeconomic level. The three latter groups of children were also much more likely to sleep with their parents during the night and to be breastfed for prolonged periods; this finding supports an inverse association between transitional object use and parent–child proximity during bedtime (see CO-SLEEPING; CULTURAL ASPECTS OF SLEEP).

Thus, several studies support Winnicott's no-tion regarding the role that transitional objects play in substituting for parental presence in the developing child. There is no clear evidence, however, linking the use of transitional objects with better adjustment or other developmental benefits. In the specific domain of infant sleep, research has associated parental presence at bedtime with higher prevalence of sleep problems (Adair et al., 1991), but transitional object use was not found to be directly related to infant sleep patterns (Johnson, 1991) (see INFANCY, SLEEP DISORDERS IN; INFANCY, NORMAL SLEEP PATTERNS IN; NIGHT WAKING IN INFANCY; THUMBSUCKING).

REFERENCES

Adair R, Bauchner H, Phillip B, Levenson S, Zuckerman B. 1991. Night waking during infancy: Role of parental presence at bedtime. *Pediatrics* 87(4):500–504.

Bowlby J. 1969. *Attachment and loss.* Vol 1, *Attachment.* London: Hogarth Press.

Brody D. 1980. Transitional objects: Idealization of a phenomena. *Psychoanal Q* 49:561–605.

Gaddini R, Gaddini E. 1970. Transitional objects and the process of individuation. *J Am Acad Child Psychiatry* 9:347–365.

Hong K, Townes B. 1976. Infants' attachment to inanimate objects. *J Am Acad Child Psychiatry* 15:49–61.

Johnson CM. 1991. Infant and toddler sleep: A telephone survey of parents in one community. *J Dev Behav Pediatrics* 12:108–114.

Klackenberg G. 1987. Incidence of parasomnias in children in a general population. In Guilleminault C, *Sleep and its disorders in children.* New York: Raven Press.

Litt C. 1981. Children's attachment to transitional objects. *Am J Orthopsychiatry* 51:131–139.

Winnicott DW. 1953. Transitional objects and transitional phenomena. *Int J Psychoanal* 34:89–97.

Wolf AW, Lozoff B. 1989. Object attachment, thumbsucking and the passage to sleep. *J Am Acad Child Adolescent Psychiatry* 28(2):287–292.

Avi Sadeb

TRICYCLIC ANTIDEPRESSANTS

See Antidepressants; Depression

TRUCKERS

Because of diurnal patterns of wholesale production and of retail sales, truck deliveries are quite often required during the nighttime hours or shortly after dawn. Thus, truck drivers quite often drive at night. Twenty percent of interstate drivers may be on duty at noon, whereas 30 percent may be on duty at midnight. Interstate drivers usually spend at least one night sleeping away from home on each trip. While traveling, they sleep most often in motels. Some sleep in truck sleeper berths while the truck is parked. Thus, interstate drivers, just as night- and shiftworkers, deal with the problems associated with sleeping during the day and sleeping in strange environments (see SHIFTWORK).

In the United States, interstate truck operations must contend with federal hours-of-service regulations (Title 49 of the Code of Federal Regulations, Subchapter B, Part 395.3), established by the Motor Carrier Act of 1935. Following 8 consecutive hours off duty, drivers may not be scheduled to drive more than 10 hours nor to be on duty more than 15 hours. An exemption to the consecutive 8 hours of off-duty time allows two separate off-duty periods to be spent in a truck sleeper berth. The periods must total at least 8 hours, with neither period being shorter than 2 hours. In addition, drivers are limited to 60 hours of duty in 7 days (for carriers operating fewer than 7 days per week) or to 70 hours of duty in 8 days (for carriers operating 7 days per week). In Canada, 13 hours of driving are allowed after 8 hours off duty.

Intrastate hours-of-service regulations vary. Many allow more hours of driving per duty day than for interstate operations. For local, around-the-clock operations, such as gasoline deliveries, however, this often translates into 12-hour shift lengths with two shifts per day (day shift and night shift) and about four teams of drivers who seldom rotate from one shift to the other. Each driver works four or five shifts per week.

Driver Fatigue, Drowsiness, and Sleep

Irregular schedules associated with interstate truck operations may induce sleep disorders in the drivers.

Drivers' perceptions and demonstrations of fatigue may be divided, in theory, into acute fatigue, which accumulates during a single duty period; cumulative fatigue and sleepiness, which accumulate across duty periods separated by inadequate recovery, usually including sleep disruption; and CIRCADIAN RHYTHM fatigue, which is greatest during the predawn hours. Work by Mackie and Miller (1978) and by Jovanis, Kaneko, and Lin (1991) showed that interstate drivers appear to face the greatest risk of accidents when all three types of fatigue are combined, for example, a long trip ending just before dawn after a week of night work.

Single-vehicle, run-off-the-road accidents represent situations in which the driver presumably fell asleep at the wheel. Harris's (1977) analysis of 493 such accidents used the proportion of trucks on the highway across the hours of the day and night as a covariate in estimating accident risk as a function of the time of day. He showed proportional accident ratios of 31 percent at 1300 hours and 460 percent at 0400 hours, a 15-fold increase from midday to the predawn hours. This strong circadian pattern supports the hypothesis that driver vigilance is lowest during the predawn hours. Similarly, Prokop and Prokop (1955) found bimodal peaks in the tendency to fall asleep at the wheel, one peak stretching from midnight to 0400 hours and the other at 1400 hours.

Substance Abuse

Stimulant abuse occurs to some degree among interstate drivers. The National Transportation Safety Board (1990) investigation of factors associated with fatal-to-the-driver accidents found stimulants in the blood of 33 of 182 fatally injured truck drivers. These included cocaine (14) and over-the-counter (OTC) and/or prescription stimulants (20, five with both OTC and prescription stimulants). The OTC stimulants were ephedrine, pseudoephedrine, and phenylpropanolamine (see STIMULANTS).

CAFFEINE was detected in 56 drivers, with five samples in excess of 5,000 nanograms per milliliter and a maximum of 16,000 nanograms per milliliter. (This driver was also positive for AMPHETAMINES and for ephedrine.) Another of the five was positive for high levels of AMPHETAMINES and MARIJUANA; two others were fatigued and two more used other stimulants. FATIGUE was listed as a causal factor in 57 (31%) of the 182 fatal accidents included in the study.

The fact that truckers have run-off-the-road accidents indicates inadequate work/rest cycle management in the industry. The interactions of very old hours-of-service regulations with newer economic pressures force truckers to operate with inadequate sleep and to sleep inadequately. Sleep disruption-induced and circadian rhythm-induced accident rates peak during the predawn hours. A few drivers deal with their fatigue and sleepiness by taking stimulant drugs. New research using modern, clinical sleep analysis may reveal some ways to revamp hours-of-service regulations.

REFERENCES

Harris WA. 1977. Fatigue, circadian rhythm, and truck accidents. In Mackie RR, ed. *Vigilance: Theory, operational performance, and physiological correlates,* pp 133–146. New York: Plenum Press.

Jovanis PP, Kaneko T, Lin, T-D. 1991. Exploratory analysis of motor carrier accident risk and daily driving patterns. *Transport Res Rec,* 1322.

Mackie RR, Miller JC. 1978. *Effects of hours of service, regularity of schedules, and cargo loading on truck and bus driver fatigue.* Goleta, Calif.: Human Factors Research, Inc. HFR Report No. 1765-F. NHTSA Report No. DOT-HS-803-799. NTIS Accession No. PB-290-957.

National Transportation Safety Board. 1990. *Fatigue, alcohol, other drugs, and medical factors in fatal-to-the driver heavy truck crashes.* Washington, D.C.: NTSB. NTSB Report No. SS-90. NTIS Accession No. PB 90-917003.

Prokop O, Prokop L. 1955. Ermüdung und Einschlafen am Steuer. *Z Gerichtliche Med* 44: 343–355.

James C. Miller
Merrill M. Mitler

TRYPTOPHAN

See Chemistry of Sleep: Amines and Other Transmitters; L–tryptophan

TWITCHES

Twitches are one of our best clues to detect REM SLEEP. Twitching in REM sleep usually consists of brief contractions of hand, feet, and face muscles. They are noticeable in REM sleep because the body is otherwise paralyzed except for breathing and heart beats (see ATONIA). In normal REM sleep, such paralysis prevents movement. Failure to develop such paralysis results in a disorder where patients act out their dreams (see REM SLEEP BEHAVIOR DISORDER). In normal sleepers, this paralysis is briefly overridden but not removed during the twitch. Studies of cells in the brain stem (MEDULLA) have shown that some are active only during movements that occur in REM sleep or wakefulness. These medullary reticular cells discharge specifically in relation to movements of facial muscles, to which they are connected (Vertes, 1984).

Twitches are often closely correlated with bursts of rapid eye movement. They usually occur at irregular intervals after the REM episode has been present for several minutes. They result in grimaces, finger movements, or wrist flexing. Dogs make running motions, babies smile, and some twitches may move the entire body. They are easily noted in the cat, whose whiskers quiver as the face muscles contract. Twitches are part of a broader class of activity during REM sleep called *phasic* events (see PHASIC ACTIVITY IN REM SLEEP). These include rapid eye movements, contraction of middle ear muscles, irregularities in heart and respiratory rate, and whimpers or other vocal attempts. Their association with dreams has been documented only in recent times. Wolpert, based upon his study of dream content and limb movements in humans, has suggested that some of these movements can be related to specific activity in our dreams (Kleitman, 1963, p. 96).

REFERENCES

Kleitman N. *Sleep and wakefulness.* 1963. Chicago: University of Chicago Press.

Vertes RP. 1984. Brainstem control of the events of REM sleep. *Prog Neurobiol* 22:241–288.

Edgar Lucas

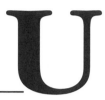

ULTRADIAN RHYTHMS

Ultradian rhythms are biological rhythms that exhibit a period shorter than 24 hours (i.e., a frequency greater than once every 24 hours); hence the name, which is derived from the Latin words *ultra,* "beyond," and *dies,* "day" (24 hours).

The most prominent ultradian rhythm is the REM/NREM rhythm of sleep, with a period of about 90 to 100 minutes. Sleep is characterized by the regular recurrence of REM sleep and the four stages of NREM sleep. The NREM sleep stages are also called *quiet sleep,* whereas REM sleep represents a form of active sleep with a high level of brain activity, increased variability of vegetative functions, activation of the sexual organs, and blockade of skeletal muscle tone. (See also CYCLES OF SLEEP ACROSS THE NIGHT; STAGES OF SLEEP; REM SLEEP PHYSIOLOGY.)

The ultradian REM/NREM sleep cycle with its deeply rooted alternations of physiological and mental experiences is so prominent that Nathaniel Kleitman, one of the founders of modern sleep research, proposed that this cycle is only the sleep-dependent expression of a BASIC REST–ACTIVITY CYCLE (BRAC), which persists during sleeping and waking. The Danish researcher Niels Engelsted elaborated this idea further and hypothesized that the recurrence of REM episodes during sleep represents the periodic reactivation of motivational structures during sleep, while the inhibition of muscle tone prevents the release of motor patterns during sleep.

On the basis of this hypothesis, many scientists have searched for the postulated waking counterpart of the sleep-dependent REM/NREM rhythm. In addition to typical laboratory studies, observational studies on ultradian rhythms were performed in infants and children and in adults under conditions of everyday social interaction in different cultural settings. In general, ultradian rhythmicity during wakefulness is far less prominent and less regular than during sleep. Nevertheless, numerous studies provide evidence that a variety of overt behaviors and internal experiences are neither continuous in time nor unpredictable, but instead are organized in a rhythmic fashion. These phenomena in human adults predominantly involve intervals of about 1 to 2 hours, a period length similar to that of the REM/NREM sleep cycle. This rhythmicity holds for physiological processes such as gastric motility or urine production as well as for sensory functions (e.g., pain perception) and performance on certain psychological tests (see Table 1). In addition to these positive findings of physiological and behavioral waking ultradian rhythms, however, a number of studies have had negative results, including a failure to reproduce certain earlier findings. Thus, the topic of ultradian rhythms during wakefulness and the BRAC hypothesis are still under debate.

The identification of ultradian rhythms during wakefulness may also be hampered by the fact that these rhythms are flexible and can be modified by situational demands. This view is in line with the observation that ultradian rhythms can be detected more easily at an early developmental age, or in some pathological conditions (e.g., mental retardation, narcolepsy) in which internal factors may be more prominent than external ones.

During ontogeny, ultradian rhythms appear before CIRCADIAN RHYTHMS. A number of weeks are

Table 1. Examples of Ultradian Rhythms in Different Functions during Wakefulness in Human Adults

Variable	Mean ultradian cycle duration (minutes)	Duration of observation (hours)	Measurement intervals (minutes)	Number of subjects
Physiology				
Urine volume	100	10	10	20
Gastric activity	90–100	8	Continuous	11
Heart rate variations	90	23	Continuous	12
Oxygen consumption	60–120	2–6	25	10
Vigilance				
EEG frequency parameters	60–100	11	20	9
Sleep propensity (shift to sleep stage 1)	100	12	15	9
Motor and oral activity				
Gross motor activity	72–144	12	5	14
Oral intake under free choice conditions	90	6	5	10
Psychometry				
Continuous performance test	100	6	10	19
Simple psychomotor task	100	10	10	16
Tracking task	100	12	10	9
Daydreaming	72–120	10	5	11

Most of these studies are cited in Kleitman, 1982.

required before a progressive coalescence of shorter episodes of sleep and wakefulness leads to the establishment of a basically monophasic sleep–wake cycle. Later in life, ultradian and circadian rhythms coexist (see Figure 1). The Canadian neurophysiologist Roger Broughton has proposed a hierarchy of biological rhythms, whereby 1.5-hour, 3-hour, and semicircadian (12-hour) rhythms are understood as submultiples of circadian rhythms. This concept assumes a system of mutually coupled oscillators that drive ultradian and circadian rhythms.

The biological significance of ultradian rhythms is suggested by the observation that many hormones are released in a pulsatile manner. One such hormone—renin, which is involved in the regulation of body fluids—has been shown to be closely coupled with the REM/NREM sleep cycle. Others, such as the sexual hormones luteinizing hormone (LH) and follicle-stimulating hormone (FSH), show a pulsatile secretion pattern with a period of about 1 hour in mammals, including the human. Knobil (1980) has clearly demonstrated that the ultradian pulsatile discharge of gonadotropin-releasing hormone (GnRH), which activates LH and FSH, is required for a normal menstrual cycle; continuous (experimental) release of GnRH does not have the same physiological effect (Knobil, 1980). These investigations strikingly illustrate the importance of the temporal organization of physiological functions. (See also ENDOCRINOLOGY.)

Ultradian and circadian rhythms represent a basic schedule for the temporal organization of rest and activity and a wide range of bodily functions across the 24 hours of the day.

REFERENCES

Kleitman N. 1963. *Sleep and wakefulness*. Chicago: University of Chicago Press.

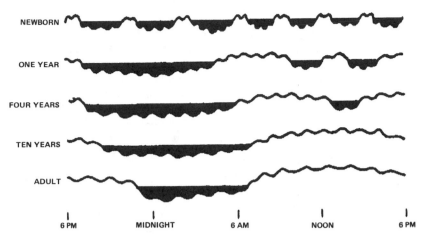

Figure 1.   A schematic representation of the ontogenetic transition from the primitive polyphasic (ultradian) alternation of sleep and wakefulness in the newborn infant to the monocyclic (circadian) sleep–wakefulness rhythm in the adult. The 50- to 60-minute basic rest-activity periodicity in the infant, shown in the secondary undulations, is gradually lengthened to 80–90 minutes in the adult. Black areas represent sleep. *Reproduced with permission from Kleitman, 1963.*

———. 1982. Basic rest-activity cycle 22 years later. *Sleep* 5:311–317.

Knobil E. 1980. The neuroendocrine control of the menstrual cycle. *Rec Prog Horm Res* 36:53–88.

Lloyd D, Rossi EL, eds. 1992. *Ultradian rhythms in life processes: An inquiry into fundamental principles of chronobiology and psychobiology.* London: Springer.

Schulz H, Lavie P, eds. 1985. *Ultradian rhythms in physiology and behavior. Exp Brain Res* 12, suppl.

Stampi C, ed. 1992. *Why we nap: Evolution, chronobiology, and functions of polyphasic and ultrashort sleep.* Boston: Birkhäuser.

Hartmut Schulz

UNCONSCIOUS

In many modern theories of dreaming the source, elements, and construction of dreams are unconscious. The *unconscious* designates all of the content and processes of the mind that exist below the level of awareness and that are not directly accessible to the conscious mind. Sigmund Freud (1901/1980) was the first to make major use of this concept and to introduce it into Western culture, although others before had noted its existence. Thereafter the concept of the unconscious or variations of it became an important element of most dream theories, especially the theory of Jung. Today it is almost impossible to think about or to discuss dreams and dreaming without considering unconscious processes.

For Freud, most of the motivation for all human behavior, including dreaming, resides in the unconscious (see FREUD'S DREAM THEORY; JUNG'S DREAM THEORY). What he called *Trieb* (often translated "instinct" but more properly meaning "drive") resides in the unconscious together with memories and associations. *Trieb* is very powerful but is too threatening to manifest itself directly in consciousness and thus must be transformed into more acceptable forms by various processes residing in the unconscious. Freud named the *Trieb* that underlies a dream the *latent content* of the dream; he termed the transformed version of the *Trieb* the *manifest content.* Included among the unconscious processes of dream transformation are displacement, condensation, and overdetermination, which serve to convert the latent content into the highly symbolic manifest content. He called this entire transformation process *dream work.* Thus a single object or action in a dream may serve to represent an entirely different object or event (*displacement*) and several unconscious objects or events (CONDENSATION), any one of which could have been sufficient by itself to produce the object or action in the dream (*overdetermination*). For example, a fast ride in a red sports car might represent the desire for a more exciting girlfriend (displacement), the desire to own something enviable, and the desire to not always be in control (not being the driver; condensation), all at the same time (overdetermination).

Freud viewed the analysis of dreams as an avenue to the unconscious. His main interest was not in the dream itself but in the dream as a means to get at the underlying psychological processes of the dreamer. Carl Jung, who early in his career worked with Freud, also adopted the concept of the unconscious and its importance for the determination of dreams from Freud. However, Jung made several significant changes. The unconscious, Jung maintained, reveals, not conceals, itself through images in our dreams. This serves to put emotional energy back into our otherwise bland conscious mind, especially calling attention to things we have been ignoring, suppressing, or not using.

Jung also expanded the notion of the unconscious. He agreed with Freud that many uniquely individual thoughts, memories, and drives exist in what Jung called the *personal* unconscious. But, in addition, he stated that we all have a *collective* unconscious. The collective unconscious contains more primitive, more colorful, and more imaginative forms of expression. In the collective unconscious reside predispositions or instincts we have inherited from our primitive human ancestors in the form of *archetypes* (common symbols that transcend time and space and thus have a universal, mystical aspect). Some of the more important archetypes include the shadow (the dark, repressed aspect of our personality) and the animus and anima (the male and female elements). For example, a religious person may dream of robbery and murder (shadow) and a very macho male may dream of mothering a baby (anima).

Freud also described the *subconscious,* another nonconscious process distinct from the unconscious and also affecting dreams. The subconscious, Freud maintained, contains information readily available to the conscious mind but to which it is not presently attending. The subconscious may also have its own mechanisms for influencing the content of dreams. For example, things being ignored or not being paid sufficient attention may become a part of a dream in the form of a warning or revelation (Faraday, 1972).

REFERENCES

Faraday A. 1972. *Dream power.* New York: Coward, McCann & Geoghegan.

Freud S. 1901/1980. *On dreams.* New York: Norton.

Jung CG. 1974. *Dreams.* Princeton, NJ: Princeton University Press.

Moorcroft WH. 1989. *Sleep, dreaming, and sleep disorders: An introduction.* Lanham, MD: University Press of America.

William H. Moorcroft

UVULOPALATOPHARYNGOPLASTY

Uvulopalatopharyngoplasty (UPPP) is the most commonly performed surgical procedure currently available to eliminate loud snoring and treat obstructive sleep APNEA. SNORING is a breathing noise generated while asleep by a vibration of the soft palate and uvula (the soft tissue hanging in the back of the throat). It usually occurs when a partial airway obstruction is present during sleep, for example, enlarged adenoids and tonsils, nasal congestion frequently associated with upper respiratory infection, allergy, and obesity. Snoring improves when these underlying conditions are eliminated.

Individuals with habitual snoring sometimes have structural abnormalities, such as an enlarged uvula or low-position soft palate. Snoring is also not uncommon for those with a receding jaw (retrognathia) or small chin (micrognathia), which forms a relatively small passageway for air to flow behind the tongue base.

The upper airway opening is protected from collapsing during sleep by maintaining the tension of the throat and tongue muscles (muscle tone) through reflex mechanism. The tension of these muscles keeps the airway open in order for breathing to continue throughout the night. This muscle tension may diminish as a result of several factors, including ALCOHOL, sedative drugs, constant airway obstruction, muscular disorders, and the aging process.

When upper airway narrowing and the loss of muscle tone are combined, the airway becomes more compromised and tends to collapse. Therefore, normal exchange of oxygen in the lungs is impaired. This is the basic mechanism seen in obstructive sleep apnea syndrome. UPPP was

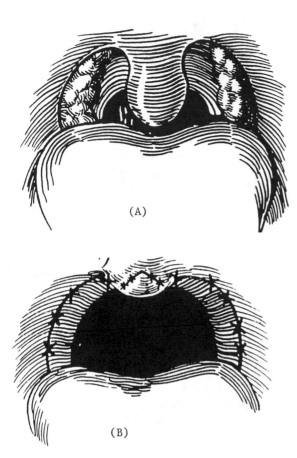

(A)

(B)

Figure 1.   Front view of the throat before (top) and after (bottom) uvulopalatopharyngoplasty.

designed to enlarge the airspace by surgically trimming excessive tissue of the soft palate (including uvula and tonsils) and reconstructing the airspace (see Figure 1).

Complications of this procedure (bleeding, infection, temporary nasal regurgitation, nasal speech, breathing and swallowing difficulty) are rare when the appropriate surgical technique is implemented. If patient evaluation, selection, and surgical technique for this procedure are appropriate, UPPP is quite effective in eliminating loud snoring, physical fatigue, and excessive daytime SLEEPINESS associated with obstructive sleep apnea syndrome.

REFERENCES

Fairbanks D, Fujita S, Ikematsu T, Simmons FB. 1987. Snoring and obstructive sleep apnea. New York: Raven.

Guilleminault C, Partinen M. 1990. Obstructive sleep apnea syndrome, Clinical research and treatment. New York: Raven.

Shiro Fujita

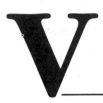

V

VAGINAL BLOOD FLOW

See Female Sexual Response

VERTEX SHARP WAVES

One of the characteristic waves seen during normal sleep on the ELECTROENCEPHALOGRAM (EEG) is the vertex sharp wave, a sharply contoured wave that is most apparent over the center, or vertex, of the scalp and that is usually the most distinctive EEG feature of light sleep (Figure 1). It has a prominent negative phase that may exceed 200 microvolts in amplitude and that is sometimes followed by a smaller positive phase. Vertex sharp waves, which may appear singly or in repetitive salvos every 1 to 2 seconds for 10 seconds or longer, can occur spontaneously or as an evoked response to auditory or other stimulation.

The vertex sharp wave first appears at about 5 months of age, is most prominent at 2 to 4 years of age, and remains a feature of light sleep throughout life, although the amplitude may decline in aged individuals. It is seen most commonly in stage 1 sleep, less so as sleep deepens into stage 2, and not at all in the deeper stages (see STAGES OF SLEEP). Synonyms for vertex sharp waves include vertex waves, V-waves, vertex sharp transients, and biparietal humps.

REFERENCES

Erwin CW, Somerville ER, Radtke RA. 1984. A review of electroencephalographic features of normal sleep. *J Clin Neurophysiol* 1:253–274.

Niedermeyer E. 1987. Sleep and EEG. In Niedermeyer E, Lopes da Silva F, eds. *Electroencephalography. Basic principles, clinical applications and related fields,* 2nd ed, pp 119–133. Baltimore: Urban & Schwarzenberg.

Michael Aldrich

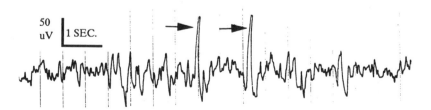

Figure 1. Electroencephalogram recording during stage 1 sleep from the left central scalp (C$_3$ electrode) with the right ear signal used as a reference. Two vertex sharp waves are shown at the arrows. SEC., second; uV, microvolts.

VIOLENCE

Cases of purported bizarre sleep-related escapades, including murder, have received sensational coverage in the popular press, inciting vigorous debate as to whether such behavior is possible—much less defensible in court. It has been well established that violent or injurious behavior may arise during the sleeping state—resulting in bruises, lacerations, fractures, automobile accidents, and even murder. Some "suicides" may actually be the result of these conditions (e.g., the fatal "leap" [fall] from a second-story window during an episode of frenzied sleepwalking).

The underlying physiological phenomenon involved in all cases is a dissociation between motor activity and consciousness. This disengagement permits the execution of complex, apparently goal-directed behaviors of which the performer is unaware. A wide variety of unrelated conditions may result in such actions (Mahowald et al., 1990).

The majority of sleep-related violent or injurious acts are attributable to the "disorders of arousal," which include SLEEP TERRORS, SLEEPWALKING, and sleep drunkenness. Sleep drunkenness is a variation on the theme of sleep terrors and sleepwalking, and is characterized by delirium occurring during the transition between sleep and wakefulness. Such confusional arousals have been experienced by most normal individuals, usually with harmless outcomes. Common minor forms include getting out of bed, walking across the room, and turning off the alarm, or carrying on complex phone conversations without memory of them in the morning.

These "arousal disorders" appear to represent the simultaneous occurrence of incompletely declared states of both wakefulness and NREM sleep, permitting the appearance of complex motor behavior in the absence of conscious awareness (see PARASOMNIAS). Motor activity during such periods of incomplete wakefulness is permitted by the activation of locomotor centers in the brain. These centers are usually not active during sleep. The lack of conscious awareness is most likely a result of an inactivation of memory and attentional systems of the brain that occurs during the sleeping state. An extreme form of cognition/motor activity dissociation may be seen in the case of the headless barnyard chicken.

Common precipitants of sleep drunkenness are sleep DEPRIVATION and medications or drugs (e.g., ALCOHOL). Sleep deprivation–induced sleep drunkenness explains the complex nocturnal behaviors exhibited by some patients with primary sleep disorders, such as obstructive sleep APNEA. Alcohol and other sedative/hypnotic drugs have been a factor in many of the more dramatic cases of violent behaviors arising from sleep.

Complex arousals can be triggered by auditory or tactile stimulation during sleep, so the victim may be an unwitting innocent bystander, becoming the target of violent behavior by a confused, frightened, incompletely awakened person. The fact that such arousals can be suddenly induced suggests that the ensuing behaviors are not the culmination of ongoing, complex, psychologically important sleep mentation.

Other causes include the following:

1. The REM SLEEP BEHAVIOR DISORDER (RBD). This condition is characterized by the absence of somatic muscle paralysis normally present during REM sleep, permitting the "acting out" of dream mentation. It usually occurs in older men, and has resulted in injury to the dreamer or bed partner when the victim attempts to escape or disable a dreamed threat. Unlike the behavior associated with disorders of arousal, these behaviors are appropriate to remembered complex dreamlike mentation (Schenck et al., 1986).

2. Nocturnal seizures. Seizures originating from the frontal lobe region of the brain may result in frantic and elaborate behaviors as their sole manifestation. Other types of seizures may result in "episodic nocturnal wanderings" that may perfectly mimic disorders of arousal (Schenck et al., 1989a).

3. Psychogenic dissociative states. Such states as fugues or multiple personality disorders may manifest themselves predominately or exclusively during the sleep period. These behaviors may be bizarre, dangerous, and very elaborate (Schenck et al., 1989b).

With the uncommon exception of the RBD, injurious or violent sleep-related behaviors are never the result of "acting out of dreams," because normally during dream sleep there is total body muscle paralysis (except the diaphragm and eye muscles), which would preclude the appearance of complex motor activity (see ATONIA). Most of these conditions are readily diagnosable by sleep laboratory techniques, and the majority are treatable.

Sleep-related violence may result in accidental injury or death and occasionally has legal and forensic science implications (i.e., "somnambulistic homicide"). After-the-fact proof of such behaviors as having occurred during sleep, and therefore without conscious (legally responsible) awareness, may be very difficult. In general, to entertain the possibility of violent or injurious acts as being the manifestation of sleep-related behavior, there should be a history of prior, similar, but less violent events. The behaviors usually should have been brief, out of (waking) character for the perpetrator, and followed by shock or horror—without attempts at "covering up" the act. There is typically only fragmentary recall of the act.

REFERENCES

Mahowald MW, Bundlie SR, Hurwitz TD, Schenck CH. 1990. Sleep violence—forensic science implications: Polygraphic and video documentation. *J Forensic Sci* 35:413–432.

Schenck CH, Bundlie SR, Ettinger MG, Mahowald MW. 1986. Chronic behavioral disorders of human REM sleep: A new category of parasomnia. *Sleep* 9:293–308.

Schenck CH, Milner DM, Hurwitz TD, Bundlie SR, Mahowald MW. 1989a. A polysomnographic and clinical report on sleep-related injury in 100 adult patients. *Am J Psychiatry* 146:1166–1173.

———. 1989b. Dissociative disorders presenting as somnambulism: Polysomnographic, video and clinical documentation (8 cases). *Dissociation* 11:194–204.

Mark W. Mahowald

VISUAL SYSTEM

Visual sensation is the hallmark feature of human dreams. As visually intense dreams are most typically found in REM SLEEP, a natural question about this sleep phase is whether the brain visual system is equally active. Our rather extensive knowledge of this subject is based on studies on nonhuman animals, and we are fortunate in that the basic physiology of animal REM sleep appears quite similar to that of humans. Knowledge of brain visual system activity in animals will thus shed light on the possible neural counterparts of the subjective state of dreaming in humans. A related question is whether animals "dream" during their REM sleep episodes. We cannot definitively answer this question but we can come to a more informed opinion by determining if visual system activity during REM sleep in animals resembles that normally associated with visual processing or "seeing" when the animal is awake. (See also ANIMALS' DREAMS.)

Eye Movements

The term *rapid eye movement (REM) sleep* highlights eye movements as one of the defining features of the physiology of this sleep phase. The eye movements are termed *rapid* because of their speed; this resembles that of waking eye movements and contrasts with either no eye movements or the occasional very slow, rolling eye movements of NREM sleep. We know that the movements of each eye in REM sleep are coordinated, like those in waking, rather than independent. Despite these similarities, there are some characteristics of eye movement that are distinctive for REM sleep as compared with waking. During REM sleep, most eye movements are in the horizontal plane, and there are fewer up and down movements than in waking. Also during REM sleep, eye movements tend to occur more in clusters and with a slower velocity than the rapid eye movements of waking. These characteristics of REM sleep eye movements are relatively stereotyped and are about the same in all individuals and in all REM periods. This constancy likely reflects the stereotyped nature of brain activation during REM sleep.

What causes the eye movements of REM sleep? We have to admit that the answers are incomplete. Eye movements are controlled by a complex brain system that has a hierarchical organization. Lower centers, especially those in the brainstem, may be the ones that are primarily activated during REM sleep. (The brainstem is a primitive structure at the base of the brain; it is stemlike in appearance, and the higher brain regions, collectively called the forebrain, emerge from its top. See REM SLEEP MECHANISMS AND NEUROANATOMY for diagram.) REM sleep eye movements persist in the absence of higher forebrain centers, and we know that neural activity in the pons, a particular region of the brainstem, is especially intense in REM sleep. The pons is the site of the neural center controlling horizontal eye movements, which may account for the preponderance of horizontal eye movements during REM sleep.

Activity in the Brain Centers for Vision

The brain visual system is organized in a series of steps of progressive complexity of processing, each managed by different brain areas. During waking, the visual image falling on the retina is transformed by nerve cells into nervous impulses that code aspects of form and color. Retinal nerve cells transmit these impulses via projections to the next visual system waystation, the LATERAL GENICULATE NUCLEUS (LGN). During waking, the level of excitation of LGN nerve cells acts to control and regulate the flow of information from the retina. The LGN neurons, in turn, communicate via projections to the visual cortex, the highest visual center of the brain. Nervous impulses arrive at the visual cortex primary receiving area and then begin a complex cascade throughout other brain regions as the information is processed.

During the NREM phase of sleep, transmission in the visual system is shut down. Whereas during waking, specialized areas of the brainstem provide the excitatory tone necessary for efficient information processing in LGN and in visual cortex, this ascending activation system indeed "falls asleep" during NREM sleep. There is a marked reduction in its activity. The consequences of a reduction in excitatory input for cell activity in the LGN are dramatic. During NREM sleep, LGN cells cannot transfer information at a rapid rate. This means that even if the eyes were opened, LGN neurons could not transfer retinal input to the visual cortex, and thus no visual images could be produced.

In contrast to the "shutdown" in the visual system during NREM sleep, some parts of the visual system are activated during REM sleep without any external visual stimuli. In waking, the chain of visual system activation runs thus: retina →

LGN → visual cortex. This is dramatically altered in REM sleep. Nerve cells in the LGN and visual cortex are activated *in the absence of retinal input,* that is, in the absence of input from the "external world." During REM sleep nerve cells in the LGN and visual cortex receive excitation from sources entirely within the brain, a situation we refer to as *internal activation.*

What are the sources of this internal activation? We know that nerve impulses from the brainstem are especially important. During REM sleep there are distinctive waves of excitation termed PGO WAVES, because they are recorded in the pons (where they originate), in the LGN, and in the occipital cortex (visual cortex).

Of course, a central question is whether this internal visual system activation might provide the substrate for the experience of "seeing" in REM sleep. We must acknowledge that a definitive answer is not currently possible; however, we do know that in humans, almost any form of visual system stimulation, even very crude electrical stimulation, will give rise to some kind of visual sensation. It would thus seem plausible that the internal visual system stimulation that occurs during REM sleep would also evoke a visual sensation. In fact, one theory of dream formation, the ACTIVATION–SYNTHESIS HYPOTHESIS, has as its foundation the notion that this internal brain stimulation forms the initial impetus for dreams, with additional elaboration dependent on the individual's experiences and current state.

We should also note that careful study of the animal visual system has shown that these intense waves of internal visual system stimulation, PGO waves, not only occur during REM sleep episodes, but start even before a REM sleep episode. Thus, somewhat surprisingly, these waves of excitation that herald the onset of a REM period can occur when the cortex of the animal shows the EEG signs of NREM sleep. It has been suggested that the human equivalent of NREM PGO waves might be linked to dreams that occur in the NREM phase of sleep.

The heightened duration of intense REM sleep visual system activation in the brain of very young animals (even before birth) suggests that this activation may promote growth and development of the nervous system (see ONTOGENY). A related speculation on the function of REM sleep in the adult is that this activity may represent "exercise" of neural machinery that is necessary for circuit maintenance.

REFERENCE

Steriade M, McCarley RW. 1990. *Brainstem control of wakefulness and sleep*. New York: Plenum.

Robert W. McCarley

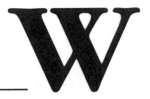

WAKING UP

Waking up is a difficult process for many people. Some people spring out of bed to face the day but a majority of adults in Western society rely upon ALARM CLOCKS to awaken them at the appropriate time. Factors such as quality of sleep and sleep schedule can influence the ability to get up in the morning. Furthermore, the transition from sleep to wakefulness is not instantaneous. Responding to a morning questionnaire immediately after waking, many people do not feel refreshed. However, this feeling does not usually extend into the day.

The length of sleep and consequently the termination of sleep are closely linked to the circadian rhythm of BODY TEMPERATURE. A sleep "terminator" appears to coincide with the rise in body temperature in the morning. Czeisler and others as well as Zulley and others reported independently that irrespective of bedtime, sleep typically ends on the upturn of the circadian rhythm of body temperature. Waking up appears so reliably associated with this circadian rhythm marker in humans that sleep length is actually more dependent on the phase of the circadian cycle than it is on the length of prior wakefulness. (See also CIRCADIAN RHYTHMS.) Patients with severe DEPRESSION often have EARLY MORNING AWAKENINGS, which may be due to abnormal circadian rhythm phase.

Awakenings and brief arousals occur as a normal part of a night's sleep. Waking up due to external stimuli exposes an interesting differentiation between SLOW-WAVE SLEEP and REM SLEEP. The ability of a stimulus to wake a sleeper depends not only on the magnitude of the stimulus but also on its meaning. Horne (1988, p. 167) summarizes: "In the case of sounds, the factors are loudness and meaning." If a stimulus carries no personal significance to the sleeper, then it will take louder levels of that noise to cause an arousal. This auditory threshold varies with sleep stage; it is easier to awaken out of stage 1 than stage 2, and so on through stage 4 (see STAGES OF SLEEP). REM sleep depth is generally equivalent to that of stage 4. However, if the sound is meaningful (e.g., saying the sleeper's name), then REM sleep will appear as light as stage 1 or 2. (See also DEPTH OF SLEEP.)

Despite the demonstrable importance of minute physiological factors in the timing of awakening, some people claim to have the ability to wake up when they want to without the aid of external stimuli. This ability was studied long before the advent of the modern sleep laboratory. In 1892, Child and colleagues reported that 59 percent of 200 respondents to a questionnaire were able to wake when they desired. Since that time, a small number of studies have been designed to determine whether the aptitude for "programmed awakening" really exists. (See INTERNAL ALARM CLOCK.)

In summary, waking up from sleep depends upon a number of factors. The phase of the circadian rhythm is a principal factor. If circadian phase is held constant, then one's tendency to wake up to an internal or external stimulus is related to stage of sleep, with stage 1 the "lightest" NREM sleep stage and stage 4 the "deepest." REM sleep can be either "light" or "deep" depending upon the meaningfulness of the stimulus. Finally, depth of sleep is generally increased with prior wake extension or sleep *deprivation*, though circadian phase remains a major determinant of waking up even after sleep loss.

REFERENCES

Child CM, et al. 1892. Statistic of "unconscious cerebration." *Amer J Psychol* 5:249–259.

Czeisler CA, Weitzman ED, Moore-Ede MC, Zimmerman JC, Knauer RS. 1980. Human sleep: Its duration and organization depend on its circadian phase. *Science* 210:1264–1267.

Horne J. 1988. *Why we sleep.* New York: Oxford University Press.

Lavie P, Oksenberg A, Zomer J. 1979. "It's time, you must wake up now." *Percept Motor Skills* 49: 447–450.

Parkes JD. 1985. *Sleep and its disorders.* Philadelphia: Saunders.

Webb WB. 1978. The spontaneous ending of sleep. *Percept Motor Skills* 46:984–986.

Zulley J, Wever R, Aschoff J. 1981. The dependence of onset and duration of sleep on the circadian rhythm of rectal temperature. *Pflügers Arch* 391:314–318.

Jason Sullivan

WARM MILK

See Folk and other natural remedies for sleeplessness; Nutrition

WATERBEDS

See Beds; Mattress

WEIGHT LOSS

See Apnea; Eating Disorders

Y

YAWNING

Yawns are slow, involuntary, gaping movements of the mouth that begin with a slow inspiration of breath and end with a briefer expiration. The word *yawn* is derived from the Old English *ganien*, meaning to open wide or gape. The association of yawning with SLEEPINESS or boredom is indicated by the popular media's description of boring sporting events or speeches as "yawners." Yawning is a widespread, complex, and vigorous act that is interesting in its own right and a source of valuable insights in the neural, behavioral, medical, and social sciences.

Yawning in Humans and Animals

A glance at a dog or a cat or a trip to the local zoo provides ample evidence of the wide distribution of yawning among vertebrate animals. Behavior resembling human yawning is performed by diverse animals including crocodiles, snakes, fish, birds, and mammals, although contagious yawning may be exclusive to humans.

Humans of all races and cultures yawn. Spontaneous yawning begins in human embryos near the end of the first prenatal trimester and remains prominent throughout life. Contagious yawning does not develop until the second year after birth.

Yawning in humans and other animals is highly regular in form, the reason why yawns are so easily recognized (Figure 1). The typical human yawn lasts about 6 seconds, but some yawns are longer or shorter in duration. Yawns are automatic and under little conscious control. Once a

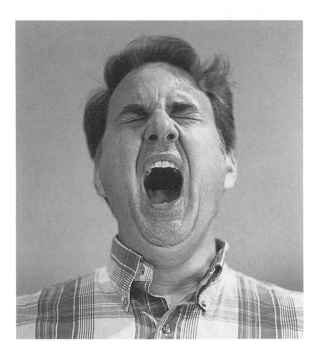

Figure 1. A typical yawn.

yawn begins, it tends to go to completion; everyone is aware of the difficulty of stifling a yawn. Yawns often recur at variable intervals averaging about 1 minute. No one minds yawning: On a 1 (bad) to 10 (good) scale, people rate yawning as about an 8.5.

Folklore about Yawning

There is rich folklore about yawning and its causes, some of which stand the test of scientific scrutiny.

651

1. You yawn when you are sleepy

Sleepy people do yawn a lot. Most yawning occurs during the hours shortly before bedtime and after waking when people are presumably sleepy. This is the basis for simulated yawns as a rude gesture for drowsiness or boredom. You usually yawn when you stretch, but most yawns are not accompanied by stretches.

No one knows if yawning hastens or impedes sleep or has neither or both effects. Although sleepy people yawn, so do paratroopers before their first jump and they are certainly not drowsy or bored. Yawning may have a homeostatic function—it may maintain some optimal level of activity.

2. You yawn when you are bored

Bored people are prolific yawners. However, it is not known whether the yawning of a student in a classroom is a valiant effort to remain alert or a preparation for sleep.

3. You yawn because of a build-up of carbon dioxide or a low level of oxygen in the blood

These widely cited "facts" about yawning are false. Increasing blood carbon dioxide levels by breathing a 5 percent carbon dioxide mixture (over 100 times the naturally occurring amount in air) does not increase yawning, although it increases breathing rate. The complementary procedure of breathing 100 percent oxygen does not inhibit ongoing yawning. Thus, yawning is neither a response to an excess of carbon dioxide nor to a shortage of oxygen. Yawning and breathing are controlled by different physiologic processes.

You can participate in two additional tests challenging the respiratory hypothesis of yawning. When you begin to yawn (reading about yawning stimulates yawns), inhale through clenched teeth. Although you can breath normally through clenched teeth, clenched-teeth yawns are unsatisfying and often give the experience of "being stuck" in mid-yawn. The stretching of the jaws seems to be a central, if not a primary, component of the yawning act. "Nose yawns" are another informative yawn variant. Try yawning through your nose while keeping your lips sealed. Unlike breathing, which can be performed with equal facility through nose or mouth (or through clenched teeth), most people find it impossible to perform a satisfactory nose yawn. Clearly, yawning is more than a deep breath.

4. Yawning is contagious

Yes! People yawn or are tempted to yawn when they observe someone yawning. However, important ramifications of this remarkable and bizarre behavior for the neural and social sciences have not been appreciated.

Contagious yawning is an ancient, neurologically programmed form of social behavior shared by all cultures and races. Observed yawns produce a chain reaction of yawning that synchronizes the behavioral and physiologic state of a group. For example, synchronized yawning of group members may coordinate bedtime. Yawners influence the physiology of others at a distance. Unfortunately, we know little about the physiologic changes produced by yawning.

Observed yawns trigger a visual recognition process in our brains programmed to detect yawns. When this "yawn detector" is activated, it triggers yawns in observers. Scientists have used the contagion response as a tool for analyzing how the brain analyzes information about yawns, faces, and other complex visual patterns.

Yawn detection is not orientation specific. Video images of a yawning face evoke as many yawns when inverted or rotated 90° clockwise or counterclockwise as they do when erect. If video images of a yawning face are edited so that such features as the gaping mouth are deleted, the contagious response can be used to assay the yawn-evoking potency of the missing or remaining facial features. (You can examine these effects by rotating or masking parts of the yawning face in the figure). Surprisingly, the video image of the gaping mouth, the most obvious feature of the yawning face, stimulates few yawns. The isolated yawning mouth is ambiguous—it could be yelling or singing. A complementary analysis shows a yawning face lacking a mouth to evoke as many yawns as an intact yawning face. Thus, yawn detectors are activated by the overall configuration of the yawning face, not by a single facial feature. This finding bears on a point of etiquette: Shielding your mouth during a yawn does not prevent its contagion.

The discovery of a perceptual process activated by visually observed yawns establishes a precedent for facial-expression detectors in humans. Similar detectors may exist for smiles and frowns, but they would be difficult to detect because of the lack of a contagious response to assay their activity.

Although the primary vector of contagious yawning is visual, virtually any stimulus associated with yawning can trigger yawns. As readers may already suspect, even reading or thinking about yawning triggers yawns. This is a convenient response for those wishing to stimulate yawns for study.

Yawning in the Clinic and Laboratory

Yawning is of medical interest because it is symptomatic of human pathology including brain lesions and tumors, hemorrhage, motion sickness, chorea, ENCEPHALITIS, and opiate withdrawal. Psychotics are reported to yawn rarely, except when suffering from organic brain syndrome. This finding in conjunction with schizophrenics' presumed excess brain dopamine and the production of yawns by antidopaminergic drugs is provocative; yawning may provide a behavioral measure of pathogenesis and drug response in schizophrenia. In regard to neurotransmitters, yawning is associated with cholinergic and peptidergic excitation and dopaminergic inhibition. Because yawning is stimulated by hormones (i.e., testosterone, oxytocin, corticotropin, melanocyte-stimulating hormone) and drugs (i.e., apomorphine, piribedil, pilocarpine) with known mechanisms of action, yawning is a useful behavioral index of chemical events within the brain.

Old clinical folklore (unconfirmed) notes that patients suffering from acute physical illness never yawn when their condition is serious; a return of yawning signals convalescence. Yawning is therapeutic in preventing atelectasis, the collapse of the alveoli, a frequent postoperative respiratory complication. Yawning is also useful for equalizing the pressure between the ambient environment and the middle ear. Because yawning is a vigorous act involving much of the body, it probably has many more such physiological correlates. It may not be possible to identify a single beneficial consequence as the "function" of yawning.

The neurological mechanism for yawning is poorly understood, but because yawning is performed by anencephalics having only the brainstem and rudimentary midbrain structures, the neural circuits necessary for yawning are probably in the brainstem near other respiratory and vasomotor centers. The neural mechanism for yawning probably involves both respiratory and vasomotor components because hemiplegics, people with paralysis of the right or left side of their body, are unable to separate these acts. Much to their amazement, hemiplegics may perform involuntary "associated" stretching movements of their otherwise paralyzed arm during yawns. This strange phenomenon, the fact that drugs inducing yawning often induce stretching, and the normal concurrence of yawning and stretching all suggest a strong relationship between the two acts. The yawn may have evolved as the craniofacial component of a generalized stretch response. The facial stretch of yawning is certain to alter intracranial pressure and blood flow to produce yet unspecified neural and behavior consequences.

Conclusion

Human yawns are stereotyped, involuntary, innate, behavioral signals of sleepiness, boredom, and perhaps other behavioral states, but not of blood levels of carbon dioxide or oxygen. Yawning provides valuable insights into brain chemistry and drug effects. Although yawning produces many physiologic changes in the body, no specific "function" of yawning has been identified. Most vertebrate animals yawn, although contagious yawning may be exclusive to humans. Contagious yawning is an ancient form of neurologically programmed social behavior that is useful in studying how the brain perceives complex visual features such as the yawning face.

REFERENCES

Heusner AP. 1946. Yawning and associated phenomena. *Physiol Rev* 25:156–168. A good review of the early work.
Huyghe P. 1989. The big yawn. *Discover,* June, pp 78–81.
Ingram J. 1989. This chapter is a yawner. In *The science of everyday life,* pp 167–176. New York: Viking.

Provine RR. 1986. Yawning as a stereotyped action pattern and releasing stimulus. *Ethology* 72:109–122. A description of yawning, contagion, and how to study yawning in the laboratory and classroom. A good place to start.

———. 1989. Faces as releasers of contagious yawning: An approach to face detection using normal human subjects. *Bull Psychon Soc* 27:211–214. The use of yawning to study visual perception and brain function.

Provine RR, Hamernik HB, Curchack BC. 1987. Yawning: Relation to sleeping and stretching in humans. *Ethology* 76:152–160. This and the previous article confirm the folklore that sleepy and bored people yawn.

Robert R. Provine

Z

ZEITGEBERS

Most mammals exhibit continuing CIRCADIAN RHYTHMS when isolated from environmental time cues. The animal's activity–rest cycle drifts in relation to clock time and "free-runs" in self-sustaining periods displaced slightly from a 24-hour cycle (see FREE RUNNING). Free-running periods distinct from the environmental period of 24 hours indicate that circadian rhythms are driven by endogenous clocks or pacemakers within the organism. In the natural setting, the non-24-hour circadian clocks are normally entrained or "reset" to a 24-hour period each day by time synchronizers in the environment called *zeitgebers*. Aschoff (1951, 1954) originated the term, derived from the German word meaning "time giver." Other designations to denote the aspect of the environment that provides temporal information include *synchronizer, entraining agent,* and *time cue*.

For most mammals, the mother is often the first effective zeitgeber. Studies suggest that entrainment begins in utero, where the concentrations of placental nutrients and hormones entering the fetal bloodstream reflect maternal circadian rhythmicity and appear to provide a strong enough signal to entrain the circadian pacemaker of the fetus. After birth, the newborn gradually develops an intrinsic circadian rhythmicity, and a free-running rhythm emerges followed by a developing capability to entrain to zeitgebers. Data in human infants are limited, but one study suggests similar development of rest–activity patterns in the first weeks of the infant's life (Kleitman and Engelmann, 1953). The lag time between the free-running period and entrainment ability in infants is attributed to the gradual development of the neural pathways responsible for zeitgeber recognition and entrainment.

In natural environments, multiple potential time cues exist. In order to demonstrate that an oscillating environmental variable acts as a zeitgeber to the circadian system, one must study animals or humans in controlled environments (see TEMPORAL ISOLATION). In such conditions, zeitgebers can be selectively eliminated and reintroduced. To be considered zeitgebers, potential time cues must meet four important criteria. First, they must be able to entrain the circadian clock in the absence of other time cues. The monitored rhythm must be independently free-running before exposure to the synchronizer and must resume a free-running period after the synchronizer is removed. Second, the period of the circadian rhythm—once exposed to the environmental cycle—must adjust to equal the period of the environmental cycle. Third, a stable and reproducible phase relationship between the timing of the observed rhythm and the timing of the zeitgeber must emerge and be maintained. The entrained rhythm must be independent of clock time and dependent only on the imposed time cue. The fourth criterion involves phase control. When the zeitgeber is removed, the rhythm must start to free-run from a phase position determined by the environmental cycle and not by the rhythm as it existed prior to entrainment (see also PHASE RESPONSE CURVE).

Research suggests that several environmental stimuli can entrain circadian rhythms in mammals. An important time cue for both nocturnal and diurnal mammals is the light–dark (LD) cycle. The wavelength of the light, the difference in intensity between light and dark portions, and the inclusion or exclusion of dawn and dusk transitions are important variables determining the efficacy of LD cycle entrainment. Food availability cycles provide another effective zeitgeber. Cycles of eating and fasting (EF) entrain temporal behavior in animals, particularly in natural conditions when food availability varies according to the time of day. Other environmental cycles such as hot–cold temperature cycles, social contact and isolation cycles, noise and quiet sound cycles, electromagnetic field strength cycles, atmospheric cycles, and water availability cycles appear to be effective zeitgebers in entrainment studies. In general, these secondary zeitgebers are not as effective or universal as the LD or EF cycles in entraining most mammalian circadian rhythms. Definitive biochemical or physiological explanations of how zeitgebers entrain the circadian clock remain to be worked out.

(See also ENTRAINMENT.)

REFERENCES

Aschoff J. 1951. Die 24-stunden-Periodik der Maus unter konstanten Umgebungsbedingungen. *Naturwissenschaften* 28:506–507.

———. 1954. Zeitgeber der tierischen Tagesperiodik. *Naturwissenschaften* 41:49–56.

Czeisler CA, Richardson GS, Coleman RM, Zimmerman JC, Moore-Ede MC, Weitzman ED. 1981. Entrainment of human circadian rhythms by light-dark cycles: A reassessment. *Photochem Photobiol* 34:239–247.

Kleitman N, Engelmann TG. 1953. Sleep characteristics of infants. *J Appl Physiol* 6:269–282.

Moore-Ede MC, Sulzman FM, Fuller CA. 1982. *The clocks that time us.* Cambridge: Harvard University Press.

Reppert SM, Chez RA, Anderson A, Klein DC. 1979. Maternal fetal transfer of melatonin in the nonhuman primate. *Pediatr Res* 13:788–791.

Eleanore S. Kim

Appendix: Organizations Involved with Sleep

The **American Sleep Disorders Association** (ASDA) is an outgrowth of the Association of Sleep Disorders Centers (ASDC). Incorporated in New York State in 1979, the ASDC limited its membership to sleep disorders centers. In 1984 the ASDC changed its name to the Association of Sleep Disorders Centers/Clinical Sleep Society (ASDA/CSS). This change reflected the addition of individual members into the organization. In 1987, new articles and by-laws were adopted and the ASDC/CSS was incorporated in the State of Minnesota as the American Sleep Disorders Association. More than 200 sleep disorders centers across the United States and more than 2,000 clinicians and researchers are members.

The ASDA establishes standards for evaluation and treating sleep and sleep-related disorders. It provides a vehicle for exchanging information pertaining to human sleep, and promotes education, training, and research in sleep disorders medicine. The association also represents the sleep disorders discipline before health regulatory agencies and other health organizations.

The ASDA is responsible for the establishment of two other organizations, the Board of Sleep Medicine and the National Sleep Foundation.

For further information: American Sleep Disorders Association, 1610 14th Street Northwest, Suite 300, Rochester, MN 55901-2200, (507) 287-6006.

The **Sleep Research Society** (SRS) was established informally in the early 1960s as the Association for the Psychophysiological Study of Sleep. In the early 1980s the association took on a more hierarchical structure, adopting new bylaws, and changed its name to the Sleep Research Society. The SRS is an association of 520 members whose primary interest is in basic sleep research. Research conducted by members ranges from psychology to biochemistry and brainstem neurophysiology. Breakthroughs in understanding the sleeping brain have led to an increasing clinical interest in sleep disorders. The SRS provides a forum for dialogue and scientific debate among sleep researchers and also actively encourages young professionals to enter the field.

For further information: Sleep Research Society, 1610 14th Street Northwest, Suite 300, Rochester, MN 55901-2200, (507) 287-6006.

The **Association of Polysomnographic Technologists** (APT) was founded in April 1978 at Stanford University in California. The membership of 1,175 reflects a wide geographic distribution, including members from Europe, Canada, and Australia. The Association sets standards for polysomnography (sleep recordings), provides training and education, and helps build a professional identity for its members. The APT has established the Board of Registered Polysomnographic Technologists and publishes its own journal.

For further information: Association of Polysomnographic Technologists, 1610 14th Street Northwest, Suite 300, Rochester, MN 55901-2200, (507) 287-6006.

The **Association of Professional Sleep Societies** (APSS) was founded in 1986 as a federation of three organizations: the Sleep Research Society, the American Sleep Disorders Association, and the Association of Polysomnographic Technologists. Although these organizations retain their own character and individual goals, the APSS was established to facilitate activities that would benefit by the associations' joint participation. The activities include an annual meeting and publication of a quarterly newsletter and a professional journal (*Sleep*).

For further information: Association of Professional Sleep Societies, 1610 14th Street Northwest, Suite 300, Rochester, MN 55901-2200, (507) 287-6006.

The **Board of Sleep Medicine** was incorporated as an independent, nonprofit, self-designated board on January 28, 1991. Its establishment was the result of many years of planning. In 1978 the Association of Sleep Disorders Centers formed a committee to produce an examination for the purpose of establishing and maintaining standards of individual proficiency in clinical polysomnography. This committee, which became the Examination Committee of the American Sleep Disorders Association, certified 432 physicians and Ph.D.s as Accredited Clinical Polysomnographers (A.C.P.s).

The Board of Sleep Medicine directs all aspects of the certifying process, including establishment of criteria to qualify for the examination, review of training and qualifications of applicants, and the development and administration of the two-part examination. The Board has discontinued the term *A.C.P.* and instead refers to its diplomates as Board-certified sleep specialists.

For further information: Board of Sleep Medicine, 1610 14th Street Northwest, Suite 300, Rochester, MN 55901-2200, (507) 287-9819.

The **National Sleep Foundation** was established in 1990 with an unrestricted grant from the American Sleep Disorders Association. The foundation is a nonprofit national medical charity, dedicated to improving the health and quality of life of all people suffering from sleep disorders and to preventing the catastrophic accidents that are related to poor or disordered sleep. Through its programs, the foundation seeks to enhance public and professional awareness of sleep disorders and to foster scientific research, education, and training in their diagnosis and treatment.

Encompassing all sleep-related disorders, the National Sleep Foundation serves medical professionals, news and science writers, government agencies, and the general public as a clearinghouse for information about sleep.

For further information: National Sleep Foundation, 122 South Robertson Boulevard, Suite 201, Los Angeles, CA 90048, (310) 288-0466.

The **American Narcolepsy Association** (ANA) was founded in 1975 by nine people afflicted with narcolepsy. Currently, the ANA is governed by a nine-member board of directors and has 4,000 members nationwide. The primary goal of the ANA is to improve the quality of life for everyone with narcolepsy through funding basic research; providing direct information and services to members and others with narcolepsy; and educating physicians, the media, and the general public about the symptoms and treatment of narcolepsy.

For further information: American Narcolepsy Association, P.O. Box 26230, San Francisco, CA 94126-6230, (415) 788-4793.

The **American Sleep Apnea Association** (ASAA) was founded in 1990 as a national voluntary health agency committed to individuals with sleep apnea and their families. The mission of the ASAA is to reduce disability and death from sleep apnea. Its objectives are to sponsor public and professional education, support groups, and community service programs addressing sleep apnea. The ASAA promotes basic and clinical research into the causes and treatment of breathing abnormalities during sleep.

ASAA patient support groups, referred to as the AWAKE Network, were started in 1989. Associated primarily with sleep disorders centers, there are approximately 90 AWAKE groups throughout the United States.

For further information: American Sleep Apnea Association, P.O. Box 3893, Charlottesville, VA 22903.

The **Narcolepsy Network** was incorporated in May 1986 by a group of people who suffer from narcolepsy. The primary focus of the Narcolepsy Network is the development of chapters to provide information and support for individuals suffering from narcolepsy at the local level.

For further information: The Narcolepsy Network, P.O. Box 1365, FDR Station, New York, NY 10150.

Carol C. Westbrook

Index

Page numbers in **boldface** indicate a major discussion. Page numbers in *italic* indicate illustrations.

monoamine oxidase inhibitors,
379–80
narcolepsy and, 93, 397
neuroendocrine hormones, 401–3
neurologic disorders and, 403
NREM sleep mechanisms, 419
opiate receptors, 400
Parkinson's disease effects, 437
peptides, 107–8, 606
PGO waves, 448
phenylketonuria and, 368
reciprocal interaction theory and,
493
REM sleep physiology, 516–17
sleep factors (biochemical), 108–9
sleep spindles, 575–76
thermoregulation, 614
yawning and, 653
see also Drugs of abuse; Drugs for
medical disorders; specific
names and types of drugs
Chernobyl nuclear accident, 487
Cheyne, John. *See* Cheyne-Stokes
respiration
Cheyne-Stokes respiration, 29, 46,
109–11
Childhood, sleep during, **111–13**
arousal disorder parasomnias, 435–36
bedtime lullaby, 340–42
bedtime stories, 68–69
bedtime transitional objects, 611,
621, 635–36
bedwetting, 69–71
circadian rhythm disorders, 120
co-sleeping with parents, 142–48
cultural aspects, 156
cycles across the night, 425, 157
daytime sleepiness, 556
depression and, 111
dreams, 79, 113–15, 127, 407, 527,
532
high auditory thresholds, 187, 629
individual differences, 300–301
K-complex presence, 324
lullaby, 340–42
mental retardation-related problems,
367–68
napping patterns, 112, 300–301,
302, 303, 392, 393, 556, 565
nightwear, 433, *434*
nocturnal eating/drinking, 202
rhythmic movement disorder, 436,
524–26
sleep duration, 424, 565
sleep needs, 112, 401
sleep terrors, 576, 577
sleepwalking, 578
slow-wave sleep arousal threshold,
593
slow-wave sleep increase, 112, 113,
159, 570, 590
teddy bears, 611, 621, 635
thumbsucking, 620–21

total daily sleep, 302
transitional objects, 611, 621,
635–36
waking up songs, 342
see also Fetal sleep-wake patterns;
Infancy, normal sleep patterns
in; Infancy, sleep disorders in;
Milk allergy and infant sleep;
Night wakening in infancy;
Puberty
Children
aboriginal dreams stories to educate,
1
attention deficit hyperactivity disorder, 34, 59–60, 595, 596–97
Down syndrome, 190–91
head injuries, 273–74
sleep and development. *See* Childhood, sleep during
as symbols in dreams, 608–9
tonsillitis, 630, *631*
Children's dreams, 79, **113–15**
and cognitive dream theory, 127
deaf themes, 163
nightmares, 407
Sandman folklore, 527
Senoi theory, 532
Chili, 388
China
headrests, 455
midday siesta (*xiu-xi*), 544–45
tea, 510
Chirico, Giorgio de, 55
Chloral hydrate, 559, 562
Chlordiazepoxide, 72, 634
Chloride ion channel (ionophore), 72
Chloroform, 559
Chocolate, **115–16**, 248
caffeine in, 88, 116, *116*, 426, 552,
597
Cholecystokinin-8 (CCK-8), 107
Cholesterol, 141
Choline acetyltransferase (ChAT), 102
Cholinergic activity. *See* Acetylcholine;
REM sleep mechanisms and
neuroanatomy
Cholinergic REM induction test, 263
Chopin, Frédéric, 342
Chordettes (musical group), 527
Christianity, 496–97
artists' sleep and dreaming imagery,
53
dream theories, 193, 497
Chromosome 6, 90, 284, *285*
Chromosome 15, 368
Chromosome 21, 30, 190
Chronic fatigue syndrome, **117–18**,
307, 409, 414, 566
Chronic mountain sickness, 29
Chronic obstructive pulmonary dis-
ease, 355
see also Apnea
Chronic paroxysmal hemicrania, 270

Chronobiology, **118**, *see also* Biological rhythms; Circadian rhythms;
Ultradian rhythms
Chronotherapy, 9, 10, **118–19**, 120,
166, 200
Chüang Tzu, 152
Churchill, Winston, 394, 543
Cicero, 193–94
Cigarettes. *See* Nicotine; Smoking and
sleep
Cingulate gyrus, 97
Circadian rhythm disorders, **120**,
122–23
advanced sleep phase syndrome, 10–
11, 120, 122
alertness impairment and, 25
Alzheimer's disease link, 30
ambulatory monitors, 31
blindness and, 81–82, 287, 330, 367
chronotherapy for, 118–19
delayed sleep phase syndrome, 120,
122, 166
depression and, 173
early morning awakening, 199–200
hypernychthemeral syndrome, 120,
286–87
hypersomnia-causing, 120, 288
insomnia-causing, 310–11
internal desynchronization and,
315–16
irregular sleep-wake cycle and, 120,
318–19
jet lag, 80, 81, 120, 320–21, 331
light therapy, 82, 120, 332
melatonin therapy, 360
PMS-linked, 470
SAD and, 529, 530
shiftwork and, 120, 122–23, 541–42
sleep disorders centers, 546–47
sleeping sickness, 564
space flight-related, 372, 373
sundown syndrome link, 168, 605–6
Circadian rhythms, 118, **120–23**
accident relationship, 485, 486,
487–88
activity measurement, 4
aging and, 12–14
all-nighters and, 26
ambulatory monitor studies, 31
basal forebrain and, 64
benzodiazepines and, 73
birds, 77–78
blind people's, 81–82, 330, 359, 360
body temperature variations with,
83–84, 120, 618
change between entrained and free-
running conditions, 251
constant routine studies, 134, *135*,
136
cortisol secretion and, 142, 174
Daylight Saving Time adjustment, 162
and death, 164–65

H